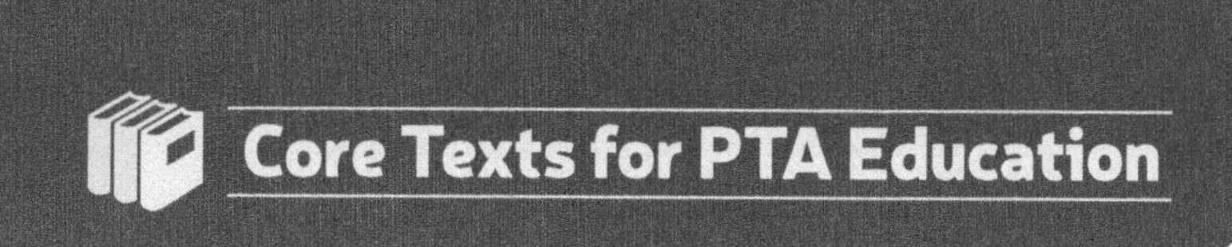



Principles of

# Therapeutic Exercise

for the Physical Therapist Assistant

Series Editor
Mia L. Erickson, PT, EdD, CHT, ATC

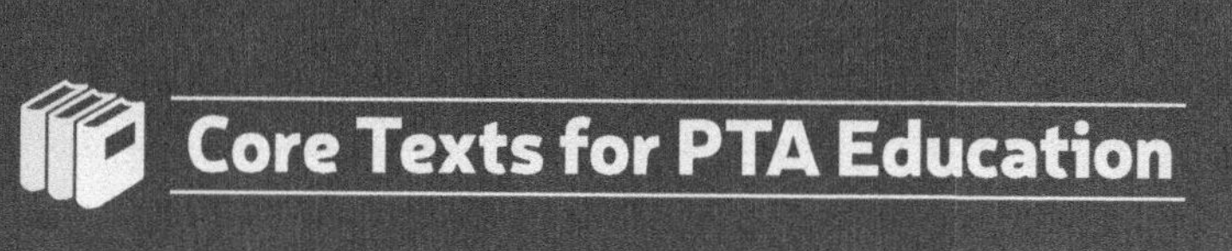


# Principles of Therapeutic Exercise for the Physical Therapist Assistant

Jacki Klaczak Kopack, PT, DPT

Karen A. Cascardi, PhD, MS, ATC, PTA

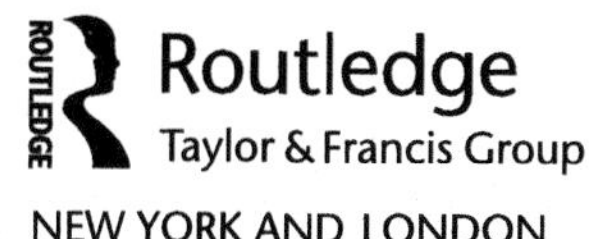


NEW YORK AND LONDON

First published in 2023 by SLACK Incorporated

Published in 2024 by Routledge
605 Third Avenue, New York, NY 10158

and by Routledge
4 Park Square, Milton Park, Abingdon, Oxon, OX14 4RN

*Routledge is an imprint of the Taylor & Francis Group, an informa business.*



*Library of Congress Cataloging-in-Publication Data*

Names: Klaczak Kopack, Jacki, author. | Cascardi, Karen A., author.
Title: Principles of therapeutic exercise for the physical therapist
assistant / Jacki Klaczak Kopack, Karen A. Cascardi.
Description: Thorofare, NJ : SLACK Incorporated, [2023] | Includes
bibliographical references and index.
Identifiers: LCCN 2023001775 (print) | ISBN 9781630913533 (paperback)
Subjects: MESH: Exercise Therapy--methods | Physical Therapist Assistants |
Exercise Movement Techniques | Exercise--physiology | BISAC: MEDICAL /
Allied Health Services / Physical Therapy
Classification: LCC RM705 (print) | NLM WB 541 | DDC
615.8/2023--dc23/eng/20230516
LC record available at https://lccn.loc.gov/2023001775

ISBN 13: 9781630913533 (pbk)
ISBN 13: 9781003525943 (ebk)

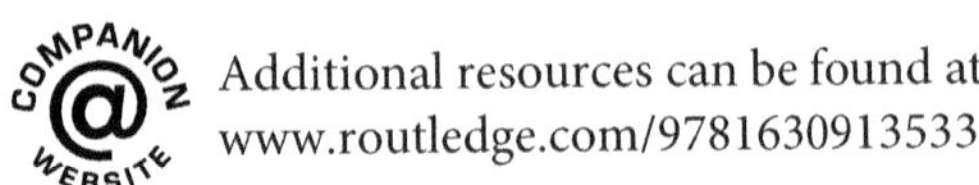


Additional resources can be found at
www.routledge.com/9781630913533

DOI: 10.4324/9781003525943

# Dedication

John, Johnny, and Jimmy, you live in my heart. Your unwavering faith in me supports me in everything I do. I love you all the most. John, I am grateful every day for your love, your support, and your ability to make me laugh.

Mom and Dad, I wish you were here to see this. You provided love and faith in me and emphasized the importance of hard work. I think you would be proud of this project!

I appreciate the support and love from my sisters, Carolyn and Kristen, as well as from the best in-law family ever, each of my "heart" sisters, my friends, and an awesome work family. Karen, you are the absolute best coauthor and friend and your unwavering support motivates me.

*—Jacki Klaczak Kopack, PT, DPT*

Gary, your constant love and support have been paramount during this long, but rewarding, process. You are my soulmate. Dad, thanks for your patience and support with this project. Mom, you always knew I wanted to write a textbook, and I wish you were here to see my long last desire completed. Jacki, your dedication, tenacity, and relentless perseverance made this book happen. I am honored and humbled that you asked me to join you on this journey.

*—Karen A. Cascardi, PhD, MS, ATC, PTA*

# Contents

Instructors: *Principles of Therapeutic Exercise for the Physical Therapist Assistant* includes ancillary materials specifically available for faculty use, including an *Instructor's Manual* and PowerPoint Slides. Please visit www.routledge.com/9781630913533

# Acknowledgments

We express our sincere gratitude to the clinicians (Patricia A. Crane, Kevin Kunkle, and John Morris) who contributed their expert knowledge to this textbook. We also want to thank our students, clinicians, colleagues, and friends (Emily, Maxime, Barbara, Cecilia, Diana, Isabelle, Jennifer, Johnny, Julie, Kelli, Matt, Marcus, Richard, Alexa, Gabby, Pete, Jimmy, Shaun, Danette, and Rosalie); our photographers (Tracy and John); Johnny for his editing assistance; and our artists (John, Jimmy, and Buzzy) who contributed their time and energy to help bring this book to life.

We very gratefully acknowledge and appreciate the wide circle of professional colleagues and friends who were willing to answer "one more question," take "one more call," or who generously read or discussed rough drafts of ideas to ensure we were not missing key content. We especially acknowledge our many friends from our work with the Federation of the State Board of Physical Therapy who supported and encouraged us when the writing process seemed daunting. Our work teams provided support, laughter, and the occasional eye roll, but their consistent faith in our abilities helped to keep this project on track.

A special thank you to Tony Schiavo from SLACK Incorporated for his unwavering confidence in us as we went through this process over the years. We are grateful and appreciative of the expert editing skills that Erin O'Reilly provided. Her matter-of-fact, positive feedback, and calm direction helped to consolidate our thoughts into a more user-friendly and accessible text.

Our students are the future of our profession. To each student we have had the privilege of teaching or working with, know that we have learned as much from you as you did from us. Our hope is that you never stop learning and that you use your knowledge and skills every day to improve the outcomes and quality of life of the patients you work with.

*— Jacki Klaczak Kopack, PT, DPT and Karen A. Cascardi, PhD, MS, ATC, PTA*

# About the Authors

*Jacki Klaczak Kopack, PT, DPT,* has served as a professor and physical therapist assistant program director at Harcum College in Bryn Mawr, Pennsylvania, for 23 years. Her teaching responsibilities have included pathophysiology, kinesiology, functional anatomy, therapeutic exercise, rehabilitation, and evidence-based practice. She completed her bachelor's degree and master's degree in physical therapy from the University of the Sciences in Philadelphia, Pennsylvania (now St. Joseph's University), and her doctorate in physical therapy from Temple University in Philadelphia, Pennsylvania. She is currently working toward a doctorate of education degree (executive leadership) from the University of St. Augustine for Health Sciences in St. Augustine, Florida. She is a 2013 recipient of the Lindback Foundation Award for Distinguished Teaching and a 2005 recipient of the Philip Klein Memorial Award for outstanding service to Harcum College.

Dr. Kopack's clinical practice spans 30 years across the inpatient continuum of care, including intensive care unit, acute care, acute rehabilitation, and subacute rehabilitation settings. Dr. Kopack served as a clinical instructor, a center coordinator of clinical education, and a director of rehabilitation in the clinical setting before transitioning to academia.

Dr. Kopack strives to support the physical therapy profession and has done so in a variety of ways throughout her career. She served as an item writer for the Federation of the State Board of Physical Therapy (FSBPT) and the Practice Exam and Assessment Tool from 2011 to 2018. She was inducted into the FSBPT Academy of Advanced Item Writers in 2015. Dr. Kopack completed an extended term as a board-appointed member of the FSBPT Physical Therapist Assistant Exam Development Committee (2019–2022), and is currently serving as a co-chair for the FSBPT Physical Therapist Assistant Exam Development Committee. Dr. Kopack has served as an American Physical Therapy Association reviewer for physical therapist assistant recognition of advanced proficiency applicants and as a Combined Sections Meeting and Educational Leadership Conference proposal and abstract reviewer. She is a Commission on Accreditation in Physical Therapy Education–appointed physical therapy education on-site reviewer and team leader. Dr. Kopack served as an elected Pennsylvania delegate to the American Physical Therapy Association House of Delegates from 2020 to 2022 and currently serves as an alternate delegate. Dr. Kopack is a frequent reviewer for physical therapist assistant textbook publishers, providing content analysis specific to physical therapist assistant curriculum content. She has presented regionally and nationally on topics related to evidence-based practice, physical therapist assistant education, and the development of the faculty team.

*Karen A. Cascardi, PhD, MS, ATC, PTA,* was the director of clinical education and an assistant professor at South University Physical Therapist Assistant Program in West Palm Beach, Florida, for 20 years. In addition to her clinical education responsibilities, her teaching responsibilities in the physical therapist assistant program included therapeutic exercise, kinesiology, habilitation/rehabilitation, and current issues. She completed her bachelor's degree at Ashland College in Ashland, Ohio; her master's of science degree at Indiana State University in Terre Haute, Indiana; her associate's degree in physical therapist assistant at Lynn University in Boca Raton, Florida; and her PhD in health sciences education and research from Touro University International in Cypress, California. She published her dissertation in 2008 (*The Relationship of Vestibulo-Ocular Reflex [VOR] Function to Falling in the Past Year Among Physically Active Community-Dwelling Adults 75 Years and Older*).

Dr. Cascardi's clinical experience spans more than 40 years as a certified athletic trainer and physical therapist assistant mostly in the outpatient setting with specialties in sports medicine, orthopedics, and vestibular rehabilitation. She continues to lecture on balance and vestibular rehabilitation.

During her career and now in retirement, she continues to give back to the physical therapy profession by volunteering as an advanced item writer and item writer coordinator for the FSBPT. She was inducted into the Academy of Advanced Item Writers and received the Outstanding Service Award twice. Dr. Cascardi served 6 years on both the Item Bank Review Committee and the Exam Development Committee. She also works with the Area Agency on Aging Healthy Living in West Palm Beach, Florida, and is on the Advisory Council and Strategic Planning Committee.

# Contributing Authors

*Kenneth R. Amsler, PT, PhD, CHCQM (Foreword)*
Director of Clinical Education
Keiser University
West Palm Beach, Florida

*Patricia A. Crane, PT, DPT, MBA, OCS, Cert MDT (Chapter 14)*
Assistant Professor
Temple University
Philadelphia, Pennsylvania

*Kevin Kunkel, PT, MSPT, PhD (Chapter 19)*
West Palm Beach, Florida

*John Morris, PT, MBA, OCS, Cert MDT (Chapter 12)*
Clinical Manager
Moss Rehab
Lansdale, Pennsylvania

# FOREWORD

As a physical therapist assistant educator for the past 30 years, I have always been expected to adapt texts focused on physical therapist education for my therapeutic exercise courses. Considering the excellent texts available, this has not been difficult, but experience has convinced me that a text, written and organized for physical therapist assistants by physical therapist assistant educators, would be most desirable.

*Principles of Therapeutic Exercise for the Physical Therapist Assistant* is a welcome addition to the educational materials specific to physical therapist assistant education. I am not aware of another text so focused and relevant to this area of education.

The authors and their 3 contributing authors have years of education, teaching, and research, including the development and accreditation of physical therapist assistant education programs and a high level of involvement in the Federation of the State Board of Physical Therapy's examination writing process. A quick perusal of the About the Authors' section of this text should convince us of the breadth of their expertise and the passion that they bring to education.

The perennial challenge of getting students to utilize the text for class preparation and study is solved with the organization of this text. It is prepared by experienced educators and incorporates a number of features that make it ideal for students and instructors. Every chapter begins with Key Terms and Chapter Objectives clearly listed to guide the student's review. Interspersed throughout the chapters are boxed Questions for Thought, Eye on the Research, and Key Safety Considerations; these are frequent and cleverly icon-highlighted features. Documentation tips are included. Each chapter ends with a list of Review Questions, a Conclusion, and at least one Case Study allowing immediate application of the material.

The text is clear and concise with relevant illustrations and frequent use of tables to highlight and organize principles and to support the emphasis on developing exercise interventions and using critical thinking to produce effective progression of patients through the therapist's plan.

This text maintains careful focus on the knowledge, attitudes, and skills that are specific to the successful practice of a physical therapist assistant and provides those of us committed to their education a useful, comprehensive tool to accomplish this.

*—Kenneth R. Amsler, PT, PhD, CHCQM*

# Introduction

Therapeutic exercise is a highly effective tool in the physical therapist assistant's "toolbox." This textbook provides vital information and practical steps for developing and implementing safe and effective therapeutic exercise programs for persons with different conditions and disorders. The textbook focuses on therapeutic exercise principles that can be applied throughout the continuum of care; it is written by physical therapist assistant educators and physical therapy clinicians who treat patients in their respective areas of expertise.

The first section of the textbook provides an introduction to a variety of therapeutic exercise foundational concepts, knowledge, and skills. These "building blocks" of knowledge and skills are necessary; they enable the physical therapist assistant to provide treatments and exercise progressions that are safe and effective. The second section focuses on common orthopedic diagnoses and treatments for the upper quarter, lower quarter, and spine. Other rehabilitative considerations in the third section include neurologic pathologies, amputations, pulmonary conditions, cancer and lymphedema, sex-related conditions, medically complex patients, and special considerations for the athlete.

There are several highlighted items throughout the textbook that provide the reader with valuable information relevant to physical therapy treatment interventions. Eye on the Research sections provide brief summaries of current evidence-based research. Considerations for the Physical Therapist Assistant sections include important information that a physical therapist assistant needs to perform safe treatment, whereas Key Safety Considerations sections provide guiding principles that are important for the physical therapist assistant to know when monitoring and assessing patients. Clinical Tips boxes provide easy "tricks of the trade" that can assist the clinician to improve treatment interventions. Some chapters include Quick Class Activities, Questions for Thought, or Documentation Tips to enhance student learning. Each chapter has review questions and case studies so the reader can apply the concepts presented and progress patient treatments. An *Instructor's Manual* that includes lab activities, chapter review questions with answers, and quizzes and PowerPoint slides are also accessible electronically.

Physical therapy is a wonderful and rewarding career; clinicians who are effective at creating, modifying, and progressing therapeutic exercise programs play an important role in improving the functional outcomes and quality of life of our patients/clients.

*—Jacki Klaczak Kopack, PT, DPT and Karen A. Cascardi, PhD, MS, ATC, PTA*

Section I

# Theory and Principles of Therapeutic Exercise

Chapter 1

# Introduction to Therapeutic Exercise

*Jacki Klaczak Kopack, PT, DPT and Karen A. Cascardi, PhD, MS, ATC, PTA*

**KEY TERMS** Body functions | Body structures | Impairment | *International Classification Functioning, Disability and Health* model | Red flags | Therapeutic exercise

## Chapter Objectives

1. Define therapeutic exercise.
2. List the types of therapeutic exercise.
3. Explain the role of the physical therapist assistant in the development and implementation of therapeutic exercise programs and wellness/fitness programs.
4. Describe the *International Classification of Functioning, Disability and Health (ICF)* model and the role of this model in the rehabilitation process.
5. Discuss the development and importance of clinical decision-making skills and effective questioning techniques.
6. Describe considerations that guide the selection and progression of exercise interventions in the clinical setting.
7. Identify topics that a physical therapist assistant should provide education about to a patient.
8. Explain why accurate documentation is important when treating patients.

### Questions for Thought

Is there a magic tool that can improve health? What if there was a medicine or intervention that demonstrated the potential to lower blood sugar, promote maintenance of a healthy weight, decrease the risk of cardiovascular disease, increase endurance, and improve overall health?

*Exercise can help achieve all of these outcomes.*

Exercise has been demonstrated to effectively address all of those health issues. So, why isn't everyone exercising?

*Exercise can improve health and restore function.*

How can the physical therapy profession best leverage our knowledge and skills to improve the health and function of our patients and the general population?

*Let's find out.*



Kopack JK, Cascardi KA. *Principles of Therapeutic Exercise for the Physical Therapist Assistant* (pp 3-12).

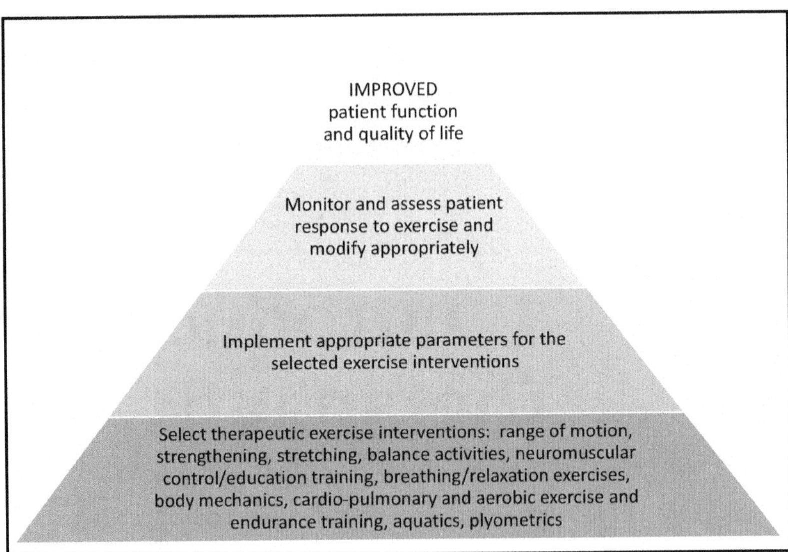


**Figure 1-1.** The therapeutic exercise pyramid.

## Introduction to Therapeutic Exercise

Many patients and clients who seek physical therapy interventions do so for 1 of 2 reasons: They are in pain and/or they are unable to perform those activities or tasks they want or need to perform. Exercise is one of many tools a physical therapist or physical therapist assistant can use to help patients decrease pain and return to their desired activities and prior level of function.

"Therapeutic exercise is the systematic performance or execution of planned physical movements or activities intended to enable the patient or client to remediate or prevent impairments of body functions and structures, enhance activities and participation, reduce risk, optimize overall health, and enhance fitness and well-being."[1] Therapeutic exercises include stretches or strengthening activities that target specific muscles (eg, hamstring stretches or biceps curls) or several groups of muscles at once (eg, squats). Other therapeutic exercise categories that can be used to achieve the patient's goals include aerobic training, coordination exercises, developmental or neuromuscular education, vestibular exercises, balance training, breathing exercises, relaxation techniques, aquatics, and plyometric training.

Physical therapists and physical therapist assistants prescribe, develop, and implement individualized exercise programs for all patients across the continuum of care; they integrate knowledge of the individual's health status and medical conditions when creating a treatment plan. Physical therapists and physical therapist assistants are educated on health, wellness, illness, pathologies, anatomy and physiology, the stages of healing, therapeutic exercise theory and application, and appropriate monitoring of patients with different diagnoses in different clinical settings. The physical therapy team has the skills to select appropriate therapeutic exercises, to administer the exercise interventions using appropriate parameters (ie, frequency, intensity, and duration/repetitions), and to monitor and assess patient performance in order to achieve the patient's goals (Figure 1-1). The physical therapy team is uniquely qualified to create exercise programs that are individualized and targeted to maximize the patient's function, decrease pain, and improve the patient's quality of life.

The general health of the population is declining, and regular exercise can assist with reversing this trend. The physical therapy team can and should play a role in preventative exercise and wellness programs. The health and wellness business is booming, and there is a demand for exercise books, fitness and wellness training programs, training videos, and do-it-yourself exercise programs. However, even with all of these resources available and access to new and affordable tracking tools (ie, Fitbit devices [Google]), the percentage of Americans who participate in regular fitness programs/activities remains low. The American Physical Therapy Association (APTA) states that "Movement is a key to optimal living and quality of life for all people that extends beyond health to every person's ability to participate in and contribute to society."[2] The APTA recognizes the global role that therapists should take in promoting the health of the population.[2] When the APTA's vision for the physical therapy profession is melded with the abilities of the physical therapy team, it is clear that therapists and assistants can guide both patients and the general population in maximizing function and health.

Physical therapists and physical therapist assistants understand why exercise is beneficial and necessary to maintain or improve overall health and well-being. Physical therapy clinicians know how to perform the following:

- Select specific exercises/activities that are most appropriate for individuals to perform (those who are healthy and those with underlying diseases/conditions).
- Monitor for accurate and safe performance.
- Implement fitness/wellness programs effectively.
- Monitor physiologic response to activities.

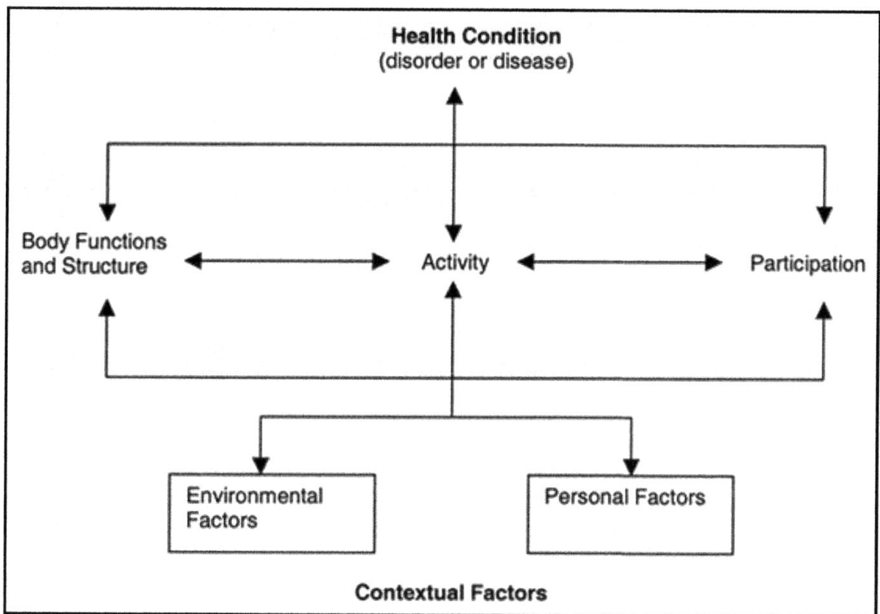


**Figure 1-2.** The *ICF* model. (Reproduced with permission from the World Health Organization.)

- Modify a program for continued progression.
- Motivate and encourage patients to help ensure exercise program compliance.

## International Classification of Functioning, Disability and Health

The APTA endorsed the ***ICF*** model of care to standardize the language used to describe people with a health condition and how they function during their daily lives.[3] The *ICF* model (Figure 1-2) focuses on a person's level of health and functional abilities in society.[4] Conversely, a medical model views disability as the direct result of trauma, injury, disease, or other health conditions (ie, stress or aging) and as a feature of the person. The medical model focuses on medical care and intervention. The *ICF* model is a biopsychosocial model; it considers the biological, social, and individual factors that impact a patient's ability to function in society. "The social model of disability, on the other hand, sees disability as a socially created problem and not at all an attribute of an individual ... brought about by attitudes and other features of the social environment."[4]

According to the *ICF* model, *health condition* is the overarching term for disorders, diseases, or injury that may include congenital or predisposing problems, aging, or stress-related conditions. **Body functions** are the physiologic functions of the various body systems. The anatomical parts, such as organs, limbs, and their components, are **body structures**. An **impairment** is a problem with a body structure or function. The health condition usually results in a significant impairment or loss; it can be mild, moderate, severe, temporary, or permanent. Impairments can improve as the patient progresses through treatment, or they can get progressively worse. The evolution is based on both the typical progression of the underlying disease as well as the individual's response/coping and the impact of other contextual factors. An activity is a task or action, so a person having difficulty executing an activity is considered to have an activity limitation. There is a difference between an activity limitation and a participation restriction. A person who has trouble with societal interactions or daily life situations as a result of the health condition is said to have participation restrictions.[4]

There are external and internal factors that are factored into the model. The environmental factors are external factors that include the physical (ie, home/work environment, terrain, and climate), social (ie, spiritual beliefs and the presence of a support system), and attitudinal (ie, personal attitudes and feelings) environment where people live and conduct their lives. Personal factors are internal factors that are specific to the individual; these include sex, age, past personal experiences, upbringing, level of education, and coping abilities. Personal factors play an important part in how patients experience or view their current level of ability/disability.[4]

The physical therapist considers all of the factors that may affect a patient's potential to make progress toward functional goals. These factors include, but are not limited to, the pathology, the patient's health status and functional abilities, social roles, available support, and the environment. The *ICF* model encourages the rehabilitation team to treat the *whole* person when creating and carrying out a treatment plan. Physical therapists use the *ICF* as a guide when determining the patient's impairments, activity limitations, and participation restrictions; this information is used to create and determine the patient's physical therapy goals and plan of care (POC).[4-6] The physical therapy team focuses on treating and correcting the health condition, and the team addresses the impact that the health diagnosis has on the patient's ability to function in society. The therapist and assistant will educate the patient during treatment. Physical therapy education addresses fear-based behaviors, the benefits of exercise, proper body mechanics, energy conservation, joint protection, and education about the individualized interventions that are being used to maximize the patient's function. Interventions and education that address the patient's fear of pain and avoidance of physical activity are prioritized. The therapy team provides education in a positive manner; education is focused on changing personal attitudes so that the patient can resume daily activities and return to societal interactions.

## The Role of the Physical Therapist and the Physical Therapist Assistant

The role of the physical therapist is to examine, evaluate, and diagnose the patient. The examination includes a review of medical and social history and incorporates testing that helps the therapist to identify impairments, activity limitations, and participation restrictions. The physical therapist evaluates the gathered information/data, establishes a diagnosis and prognosis, and creates an individuated POC for the patient.[7]

The physical therapist assistant and physical therapist share the role of implementing the physical therapist's POC. The assistant collects data so an ongoing assessment of patient performance can be made.[8] The primary focus of therapy interventions is to maintain the patient's safety while promoting progress toward the patient's goals (jointly established by the physical therapist and the patient). To prepare the assistant for this role, students must successfully complete courses in a Commission on Accreditation for Physical Therapy Education–accredited physical therapist assisting curriculum and pass the Federation of State Boards of Physical Therapy National Physical Therapy Examination for physical therapist assistants. This textbook provides vital information on developing and implementing safe and effective therapeutic exercise programs for persons with different conditions and disorders. A licensed physical therapist assistant understands and recognizes the indications, contraindications, and benefits of the various types of exercise that can be prescribed for a patient. Physical therapist assistants must be competent performing therapeutic exercises, including range of motion (ROM), strengthening, stretching, postural, balance activities, neuromuscular control training, cardiopulmonary aerobic and endurance training, and aquatics; they must also be able to appropriately modify and progress the interventions. Foundational knowledge is necessary for the assistant to be able to select and safely implement therapeutic exercise interventions.

### *The Physical Therapist Assistant and Clinical Decision-Making Skills*

Knowledge gained during the education process does not by itself result in the ability to develop and implement programs that optimize patient function and safety. To maximize effectiveness, the physical therapist assistant must be able to pair foundational knowledge and clinical skills with consistent effective clinical decision making/problem solving. Clinical decision making is a skill that evolves with experience; yet, a novice can follow key steps to improve their problem-solving skills. Regular practice helps students develop and strengthen their clinical decision-making abilities. Decision-making skills improve when the student integrates feedback from faculty members, clinical instructors, or clinical mentors. Developing a standardized and organized decision-making "process" is beneficial to students; this promotes the integration of these skills so that they become routine.

Reviewing the initial evaluation and subsequent progress notes provides necessary information about the patient's current status and the treatment POC; this guides in the development of an appropriate treatment plan. There are key questions the assistant can ask to assist when making clinical decisions before and during the treatment session (Table 1-1). The assistant should use open-ended questions (see Table 1-1) and actively listen to the responses. Compiling this information helps guide the assistant in selecting those therapeutic exercises that are most appropriate. Students can use Figure 1-3 as a general problem-solving algorithm. It serves as a guide for progression through therapeutic exercise selection and implementation, providing an example of the decision-making process for a patient with a painful shoulder diagnosis based on what skills/abilities are needed to achieve the patient's goal (eg, reaching in a cabinet for dishes). This algorithm can be modified for any functional skill.

The physical therapist assistant focuses on safety while using clinical decision-making skills to monitor and modify a patient's program. The assistant must learn to implement therapeutic exercise interventions using the appropriate parameters, and the assistant should be aware of typical/expected and unexpected vital sign responses to activities. **Red flags** are observations or events that indicate that a high risk or medically significant event is evolving. Red flags require immediate response and appropriate follow-up by the assistant. Because all **therapeutic exercise** interventions cause changes in a patient's physiologic status (and these changes affect multiple body organ systems), the use of appropriate monitoring techniques helps to ensure patient safety. Vital sign monitoring and patient observation provide the clinician with pertinent information regarding the patient's physiologic status.

**Table 1-1**

Decision-Making Skills: Key Questions to Consider

| Questions for the Physical Therapist Assistant to Consider When Developing a Treatment Plan | Open-Ended Questions to Ask Patients Before and During Treatment |
|---|---|
| • Which goal will be addressed? Review and select a short- or long-term goal from the initial evaluation.<br>• Which interventions can be used to create progress toward the goal?<br>• Which intervention is *most* appropriate given the patient's current status, health history, or orthopedic precautions?<br>• Are any of the interventions selected contraindicated or inappropriate given the patient's current status, health history, or orthopedic precautions?<br>• Is there any equipment needed for the selected intervention?<br>• What treatment parameters are most appropriate given patient presentation (consider standards of practice and evidence-based practice)?<br>Implement the treatment intervention. Then ask yourself the following:<br>• What methods are best to monitor the patient's response to the intervention (patient report, observation, vital sign, and other physiologic data)?<br>• What data are most relevant to collect to show progress toward patient goals (eg, strength, ROM, functional performance, balance)?<br>• Is the patient improving? If so, continue with or make the treatment intervention more challenging. If not, consider reasons why and potential alternate interventions; discuss other options in the POC or with the physical therapist. | • How are you feeling today?<br>If the patient states they have pain, then ask the following questions about pain:<br>• Can you grade your pain right now, 0 to 10?<br>• Can you point to where your pain is located?<br>• Can you describe it (eg, sharp, dull, achy, burning, stabbing)?<br>• What makes your pain better? Or worse?<br>• Did you perform any tasks or activities that may have changed your pain since your last visit?<br>Questions on other important information:<br>• What activities do you have the most difficulty doing?<br>• Have you seen a physician since your last visit?<br>• Have you had any tests performed or medication changes since your last visit?<br>During the selected treatment intervention or therapeutic exercise performance, monitor the patient's response and ask the following questions:<br>• How does this feel (eg, too easy, good, a bit challenging, too hard, or does it alter your pain)?<br>• Would you like to choose another exercise/ intervention to perform next?<br>At the end of the treatment session ask the following:<br>• How do you feel after your session today?<br>• Do you have any questions for me or comments regarding your treatment or home exercises? |

Therapeutic exercise treatment interventions are used across the continuum of care and in different health care settings. Physical therapy is provided to patients who range from being critically ill in the intensive care unit to those who are otherwise healthy but dealing with an orthopedic injury in an outpatient clinic. The level of monitoring depends on the patient's acuity, diagnoses, and comorbidities as well as the type of clinical setting (Figure 1-4).

## Introduction to Patient Education

Patient education was defined by Bartlett in 1985 as "a planned learning experience using a combination of methods such as teaching, counseling and behavior modification techniques which influence patients' knowledge and health behavior."[8] Education should be included as a component of every treatment. In order to successfully educate patients, the physical therapist assistant needs to establish rapport and demonstrate effective communication skills. Patient education can empower patients to self-manage their care and prevent further injury.[9,10] Clinicians should be aware of all aspects of patient communication. Adjustments to education techniques are indicated when treating patients across the life span (consider generational differences); from different cultures (consider cultural differences); and those with visual, auditory, or cognitive impairments. Like patient care, education is individualized to the patient.

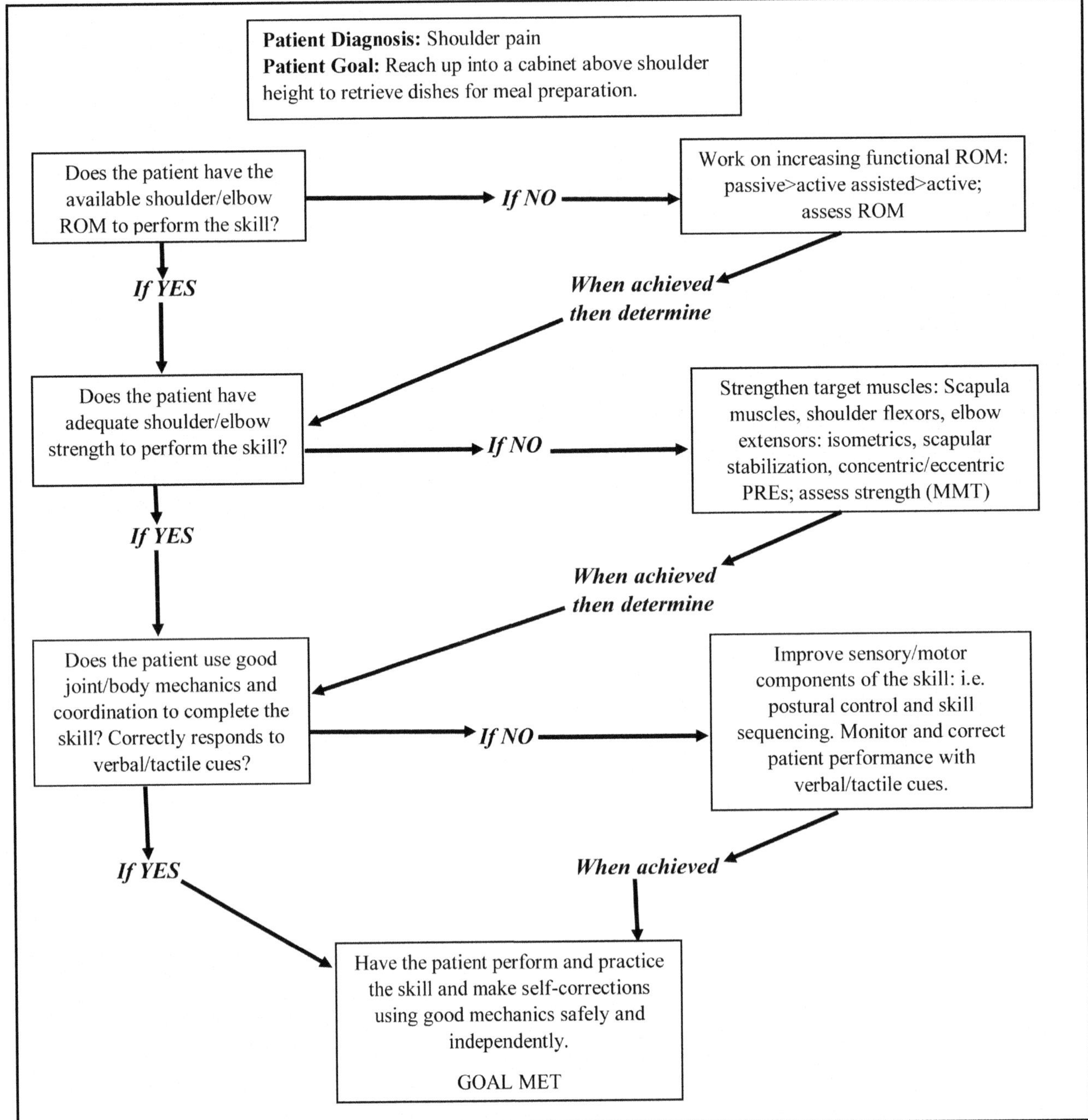


**Figure 1-3.** An algorithm for a therapeutic exercise progression and functional skill performance. (PREs = progressive resistive exercises; MMT = manual muscle tests.)

The physical therapist assistant may provide education related to the patient's health condition/diagnosis, the patient's complaints, a home exercise program (instructions and/or compliance), the goals and benefits of treatment interventions, and/or caregiver education. Keeping the patient motivated and focused on their functional goals can improve understanding and compliance with physical therapy interventions. Patient education and tips to maximize exercise compliance are discussed in depth in Chapter 2, and tips regarding education about specific exercises are provided throughout this textbook.

## Documentation and Reimbursement

There are several types of electronic documentation systems or programs. Regardless of the system, the ability to complete concise, accurate, and thorough documentation

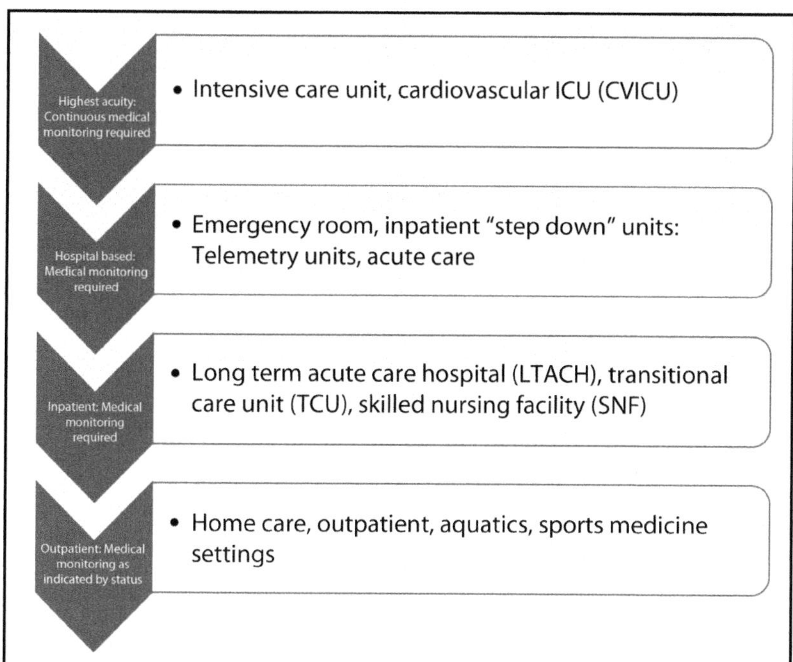


**Figure 1-4.** Monitoring patients across the continuum of care.

is critical for every clinician. Each clinician must complete documentation each time a patient is treated. Thorough documentation paints a picture for the clinician, allowing a clinician to understand what the patient has been doing (and their response to treatment) throughout their therapy program. Accurate and specific documentation for all aspects of treatment include the subjective portion and the plan for the next treatment session; this information is important for continuity of care. Table 1-2 provides a detailed checklist of critical elements that should be included in physical therapy documentation. It is important to document how the physical therapy care provided was skilled and medically necessary. Include copies of any team communication (ie, updates to the physical therapist or physician), exercises, and/or home program instructions issued to the patient in the medical record. Identify and document the reason for any missed or canceled appointments, and document how this information was provided to the prescribing physician. Proper documentation is vital to appropriate reimbursement for care. There are situations when payers will not reimburse for physical therapy services; oftentimes, these situations are related to poor documentation. Two common scenarios in which reimbursement is denied are cases in which the stated therapy goals are not measurable and attainable because of vague descriptions of goals or progress or cases in which there is a lack of evidence that the patient is making progress toward goals.[11] The physical therapist assistant should review the goals and provide documentation that indicates patient performance and progress toward the goals.

## Considerations for the Physical Therapist Assistant

The physical therapist develops the POC based on the patient's needs. If therapy services are declined by a payer, the physical therapy team must consider the ethical obligation of providing appropriate care, and the team may need to appeal the insurance company's denial. The therapy team can consider best practices as it relates to the patient's diagnosis/presentation. For example, rather than treating a patient 2 or 3 times a week for 1 month, it may be more clinically appropriate to treat a patient twice a week for 1 week to establish the patient's independence with a home exercise program and then once a week or every other week for the next month to assess, modify, and progress the patient's home exercise plan. The team can refer to the *Guide to Physical Therapist Practice* for length of stay guidelines; those guidelines may provide support when the therapy team is advocating for additional visits or services. When the physical therapy team focuses on providing appropriate interventions and education that promote effective self-management for the patient, the outcome is that patients are discharged with the tools/education needed to maintain their improved status independently.

**Table 1-2**

## Documentation Checklist

- Include the treatment date and time
- Clinician signature at the end of note (include student physical therapist assistant or physical therapist assistant after your signature)
- Limit the use of abbreviations (use only facility-approved abbreviations)
- Write legibly (if your employer still uses handwritten notes)
- Fill in all required text areas in the electronic medical record
- Whenever possible, document at point of service (do not wait until the end of the day; it is too easy to forget key information or mix up patient data)
- Be specific about patient/caregiver subjective reports and complaints
    - Grade pain with a specific function (eg, 6/10 with sit-to-stand transfers)
    - State the specific location of the patient's pain (eg, medial aspect right knee)
    - List functional limitations or improvements
    - Report response to current and/or previous treatment
- State objective tests and measures results and record interventions in detail including exercise parameters, modality parameters, gait training distance/assistance/device, balance activities, patient education, etc
- The physical therapist assistant should document their clinical judgment (assessment) or impression of the patient's response to the treatment specific to the goals and outlined in the initial evaluation
    - Address functional gains and relate progress to tests/measures or specific interventions performed
    - Document any inconsistencies between subjective reports and objective findings
    - Report any findings or changes in the patient's status (ie, impairments or functional limitations)
    - State how improvements in the patient's impairments will improve function and lead to increased activity performance and participation, not just general well-being
    - Comment on the ineffectiveness of an intervention or complications arising from it
    - Clearly state reasons delaying progress toward goals (eg, medical status, comorbidity, complications)
- Avoid using the term "Tolerated treatment well"; this term is nonspecific and does not verify the presence of skilled observation
- State specific plans for the next treatment session, including new exercises, exercise progression, changes in the POC as discussed with the physical therapist, changes in treatment frequency, any upcoming consultations (ie, physician and medical testing), and physical therapist re-evaluation or discharge for next session
    - Avoid writing "As per PT POC"; this term is nonspecific and does not verify the presence of skilled problem solving

Tips

- Clearly tie each intervention to an impairment and functional goal (many electronic medical record systems prepopulate this for the clinician)
- Maintain APTA membership and regularly review new literature to stay current with new evidence-based practice

Health care reimbursement is a process by which health care providers are paid for health care services. Most physical therapy clinics receive payment after the services are rendered. This is a retrospective method. In a prospective payment system method, reimbursement is determined and paid for before services are provided.[12] Discussion regarding the different insurance companies and reimbursement methods is outside the scope of this textbook. In-depth information specific to various reimbursement methods can be reviewed in the resource located at the end of this chapter. The most current reimbursement issues and changes related to physical therapy practice are located on the APTA website.

Insurance companies review documentation to determine if the care provided was medically justified. Physical therapy documentation is a legal document; it is used to justify reimbursement as well as in situations requiring legal review (ie, a lawsuit). The assistant should accurately document each patient treatment session. Tips on how to document each new intervention/technique are provided in each unit (as appropriate) to assist the student with streamlining the documentation while ensuring all critical information is conveyed; the learner is referred to physical documentation textbooks for more comprehensive direction.

## Conclusion

The physical therapist assistant uses the physical therapy evaluation and POC as a guide when creating a treatment plan. The assistant considers the *IFC* model when selecting which rehabilitation interventions will help the patient meet their long-term goals. Exercise plays an important role in improving overall fitness, functional mobility, and quality of life. Most physical therapy interventions across the continuum of care will include education and therapeutic exercise. The assistant will select, implement, modify, and progress therapeutic exercises. Clinical decision-making and observation skills allow the assistant to appropriately supervise and monitor the patient in order to maintain patient safety.

## Review Questions

1. List 5 types of therapeutic exercise.
2. What are the responsibilities of the physical therapist assistant when incorporating therapeutic exercise into a patient's treatment plan?
3. Describe 3 reasons why physical therapists and physical therapist assistants are logical practitioners to establish and carry out a fitness/wellness program.
4. List and briefly describe each component of the *ICF* model.
5. List at least 3 items that the physical therapist assistant should consider to guide the selection and progression of exercise interventions.
6. What is clinical decision making? How can a student begin to develop/improve their clinical decision-making skills?
7. Outline 4 questions an assistant could use to gather patient data before starting a treatment intervention.
8. List 3 topics that a physical therapist assistant could educate a patient about.
9. Explain why accurate documentation is important when treating patients.
10. What are red flags? What should the assistant do if a patient presents with a significant change in status?

## Case Study

A 61-year-old patient has a diagnosis of a moderate right knee sprain that occurred 4 weeks ago; the patient currently has full ROM. The patient complains of knee pain and difficulty with stair climbing at home and is unable to participate in normal activities, which include walking 2 miles every day and playing golf twice a week. The patient is very motivated and would like to return to their prior level of function and activities.

1. Based on the patient diagnosis and information provided in the scenario, relate the patient's presentation to each *ICF* term.
2. List the questions a physical therapist assistant should consider during the decision-making process to determine which treatment interventions are most appropriate.
3. Write 3 open-ended questions that would provide additional important information about the patient's pain.

## Suggested Resource

Song PH, Reiter KL. *Gapenski's Fundamentals of Healthcare Finance.* 3rd ed. Health Administration Press; 2018. Accessed February 14, 2023. https://search.ebscohost.com/login.aspx?direct=true&db=cat03948a&AN=usa.9004&site=eds-live

## References


1. American Physical Therapy Association. *Guide to Physical Therapy Practice.* Accessed January 23, 2023. http://guidetoptpractice.apta.org/content/1/SEC40.extract
2. American Physical Therapy Association. Vision statement for the physical therapy profession and guiding principles to achieve the vision. APTA website. Accessed January 23, 2023. https://www.apta.org/Vision/
3. Bemis-Dougherty A. Practice matter: what is the ICF? *PT Now.* February 2009. Accessed January 23, 2023. https://www.apta.org/PTinMotion/2009/2/Feature/PracticeMatters/ICF/
4. World Health Organization. *Towards a Common Language for Functioning, Disability and Health ICF.* World Health Organization; 2002.
5. World Health Organization. The ICF: an overview. Accessed January 23, 2023. https://www.cdc.gov/nchs/data/icd/icfoverview_finalforwho10sept.pdf

6. CAPTE standards and required elements for accreditation of physical therapy education programs. 2017. 7D21. Accessed January 23, 2023. http://www.capteonline.org/uploadedFiles/CAPTEorg/About_CAPTE/Resources/Accreditation_Handbook/CAPTE_PTStandardsEvidence.pdf
7. American Physical Therapy Association. *Guide to Physical Therapy Practice 3.0*. American Physical Therapy Association; 2014.
8. Bartlett EE. Eight principles from patient education research. *Preventive Medicine*. 1985;14(6):667-669. doi:10.1016/0091-7435(85)90065-9
9. Sluijs EM. A checklist to assess patient education in physical therapy practice: development and reliability. *Phys Ther*. 1991;71:561-569. doi:10.1093/ptj/71.8.561
10. Purtilo R, Haddad A. Health *Professional and Patient Interaction*. 8th ed. Elsevier; 2014.
11. Bohnett C. 4 common reasons for PT claim denials (and what to do about them). August 21, 2019. Accessed January 23, 2023. https://www.webpt.com/blog/post/4-common-reasons-for-pt-claim-denials-and-what-to-do-about-them/
12. Gapenski R. Chapter 2: healthcare insurance and reimbursement methodologies. In: *Healthcare Finance: An Introduction to Accounting & Financial Management*. 6th ed. Health Administration Press; 2016.

Chapter 2

# Implementing a Therapeutic Exercise Program

*Karen A. Cascardi, PhD, MS, ATC, PTA and Jacki Klaczak Kopack, PT, DPT*

**KEY TERMS** Evidence-based practice | Extrinsic (augmented) feedback | FITT (frequency, intensity, time, and type) principle | Intrinsic feedback | Knowledge of performance | Knowledge of results | Motor learning | Motor performance

## Chapter Objectives

1. Describe the role of the physical therapy team in the initiation and implementation of a therapeutic exercise program.
2. Explain the monitoring procedures a physical therapist assistant should use with patients across the continuum of care.
3. Explain the various elements of an exercise program.
4. Describe the basic principles of motor learning.
5. Summarize the types of practice and list the selection parameters that will yield the best outcomes for a patient.
6. Explain the role of feedback in learning.
7. Identify suggestions to improve patient exercise performance and home exercise compliance.

## Introduction: The Role of the Physical Therapist Assistant

The physical therapist assistant selects, modifies, and progresses treatment interventions in order to address the treatment goals outlined in the initial evaluation and included in the physical therapy plan of care (POC). An effective physical therapist assistant understands the physiology of various structures (ie, bones, joints, ligaments, tendons, and muscles) and has the ability to palpate those structures accurately, apply biomechanical/kinesiology principles, and use good decision-making skills in order to select and apply appropriate interventions (Table 2-1). The clinician selects each intervention based on the stage of healing of the affected tissue and knowledge of the typical healing time for that tissue. In the early stages after injury, therapeutic physical agents may be used to decrease inflammation and pain. As the tissues heal, it is important to introduce controlled/graded stress to the healing tissues to promote appropriate alignment of the healing collagen and connective tissues.[1] The assistant can use the information in Appendix A to guide treatment through the various stages of healing.



Kopack JK, Cascardi KA.
*Principles of Therapeutic Exercise for the Physical Therapist Assistant* (pp 13-29).

**Table 2-1**

**Depth of Knowledge and Physical Therapist Assistant Decision Making**

| Strong Physical Therapist Assistant Knowledge Regarding: | Will Allow the Physical Therapist Assistant To: |
|---|---|
| Anatomy: The structures involved, their location, and physiologic properties | Select appropriate interventions and apply to appropriate structures |
| Tissue healing times, target tissues involved, and the signs/symptoms for the stages of healing | Select appropriate interventions and apply at appropriate time, maintain patient safety, and prevent reinjury |
| General screening processes and patient's vital sign monitoring | Maintain patient safety and modify treatment interventions |
| Selection of exercise interventions and therapeutic physical agent interventions (as per POC) | Improve function, decrease pain, and progress patient toward goals safely and efficiently |
| Appropriate intervention parameters (ie, FITT) | Select appropriate interventions and parameters; apply at the right time to obtain optimal outcomes |
| Appropriate application including motor learning theory, practice, and feedback schedule | Provide effective progressions and achieve optimal outcomes |
| Exercise progression vs maintenance vs return to prior level of function or sport | Prevent reversibility of gains and stress the importance of patient education |

FITT=frequency, intensity, type, time.

The physical therapist examines the patient (Figure 2-1) and creates patient-centered, measurable, and functional goals based on the patient's diagnosis, current medical status, impairments and limitations, and prior level of function. The physical therapist creates a problem list that outlines the patient's current functional impairments and limitations and then creates a POC that addresses the limitations and the patient's goals. The assistant will consider evidence-based or clinical practice guidelines (CPGs) when developing a POC (Figure 2-2) that addresses the problem list. The physical therapist assistant will review key information (ie, contraindications, precautions, weight-bearing status, and level of assistance) from the initial evaluation to ensure patient safety and will include interventions in the POC that address the patient's goals. The physical therapist assistant should (1) prioritize the problem list, (2) select and apply the appropriate interventions to address patient goals, (3) provide patient education, (4) continually reassess the patient's physiologic response to the interventions selected, and (5) communicate patient responses appropriately to the supervising physical therapist. Appendix B is a template that can guide the physical therapist assistant in organizing treatment and providing rationales to justify the selected interventions.

Many patients seek out physical therapy for the treatment of pain. A thorough physical therapy evaluation should correctly determine the cause of the patient's pain. The general information about treating pain in this chapter is just an overview; Chapter 11 discusses pain more in depth. Typically, the clinician will address the patient's pain first. Patient education regarding pain reduction with sitting, standing, and sleeping positions is an important part of the treatment intervention and should be implemented during the first treatment session. Providing information regarding the neurophysiology of pain can promote improved clinical outcomes because it allows the patient to start to better understand their body's response to injury.

Common treatments for pain include physical agents, relaxation exercises, imagery,[2] and correction of the biomechanical or physical issues that were the initial cause of the pain. Patients perceive active interventions to treat pain (ie, exercise, imagery, and stress management) as very helpful.[3] Physical agents may be used as a short-term pain relief option to decrease symptoms so that the patient can better tolerate the interventions needed to address the underlying cause of the pain; however, there is limited benefit to long-term modality use.[4,5]

It is imperative that the physical therapist assistant monitor the patient during treatment for red flags that might indicate that the root cause of pain is not a result of a musculoskeletal or neuromuscular issue. The ability to reproduce symptoms is a strong indicator that the diagnosis is musculoskeletal and treatable by therapeutic interventions. The physical therapist assistant should monitor the patient's progression, presentation, and symptoms. Signs, symptoms, or patient reports that are inconsistent with the diagnosis or are incompatible with the expected timeline for recovery must be discussed with the supervising

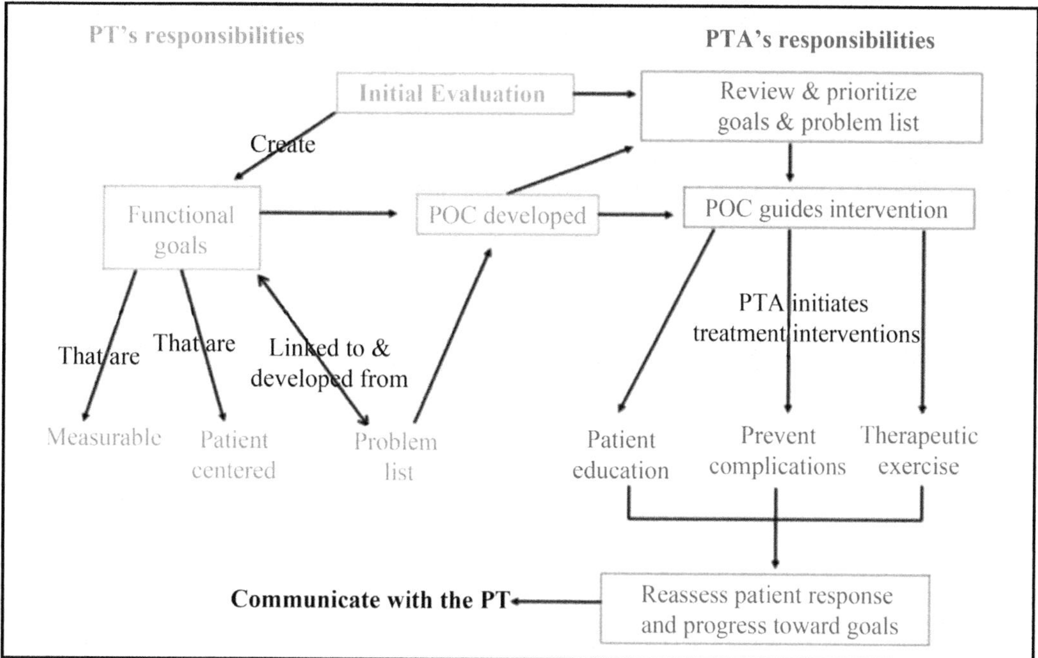


**Figure 2-1.** Physical therapist and physical therapist assistant team roles and responsibilities. (PT = physical therapist; PTA = physical therapist assistant.)

physical therapist. Any of the following signs or symptoms should be reported to the physical therapist immediately:

- Any new medical red flags such as a severe increase in the severity of symptoms or new neurologic, cardiovascular, or pulmonary signs/symptoms
- Any signs/symptoms that are inconsistent with the physical therapy treatment diagnosis
- Any signs/symptoms that are inconsistent with the stage of healing[6]

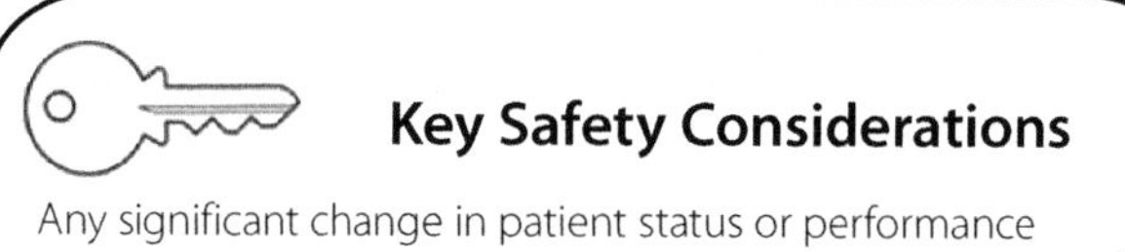

**Key Safety Considerations**

Any significant change in patient status or performance should be brought to the attention of the physical therapist.[7]

## Selecting Treatment Interventions

The physical therapist assistant reviews the patient's physical therapy evaluation, POC, and the problem list and creates a treatment plan that includes specific interventions for the patient. The physical therapist assistant discusses the plan with the patient to gain consent and to determine if any new adverse events, precautions, or contraindications to the selected interventions are present. This allows the assistant to eliminate, revise, or modify any of the interventions that were selected before initiating the treatment to ensure that the treatment plan is safe for the patient. Optimal treatment interventions address the patient's impairments, respect the stage of healing, promote progress to the functional goals, and are aligned with the POC. A list of general treatment goals and interventions are described in Table 2-2.

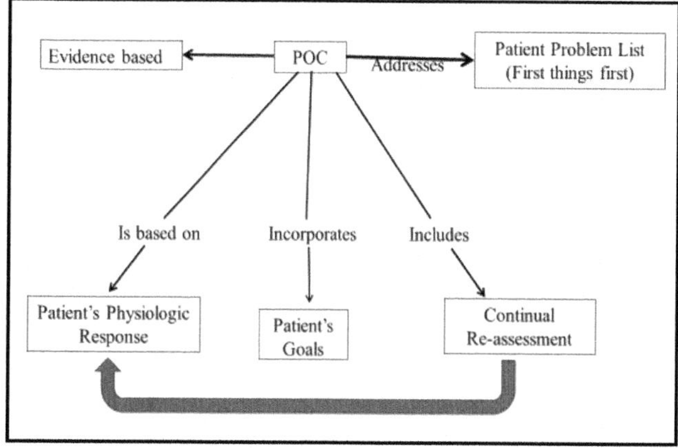


**Figure 2-2.** Elements of the physical therapist's POC.

The physical therapist assistant will determine (1) the best sequence to administer the selected interventions, (2) progression/modification of the exercises (ie, easy to hard, gravity minimized to against gravity, and light vs heavier resistance), and (3) dosage/parameters of the exercise (intensity, repetitions, sets, and/or duration). The frequency of exercise performance and rest periods are considerations when designing a home exercise program (HEP) for the patient.

**Table 2-2**

Treatment Goals and Possible Interventions

| Treatment Goal | Possible Interventions |
|---|---|
| Decrease pain[a] | • Protection, rest, ice, compression, and elevation (PRICE)<br>• Grade I/II joint mobilizations<br>• Pain related to tightness/adhesions:<br>  ○ Therapeutic physical agents/modalities<br>  ○ Stretching<br>  ○ Strengthening<br>• Patient education regarding pain and pain modulation |
| Decrease inflammation | • Therapeutic physical agents/modalities<br>• PRICE<br>• Pain-free passive range of motion (ROM; based on acuity of inflammation) |
| Increase circulation | • Therapeutic physical agents/modalities<br>• Active range of motion (AROM)<br>• Graded ambulation program (for peripheral arterial disease)<br>• General aerobic exercise (ie, as a warm-up activity)<br>• Resistance exercise (increase circulation to muscles) |
| Increase joint stability | • Bracing<br>• Strengthening<br>• Stabilization exercises<br>• Taping |
| Increase ROM/flexibility[b] | • Passive ROM, active assisted range of motion (AAROM), and AROM<br>• Stretching (static and dynamic)<br>• Grade III/IV joint mobilizations<br>• Therapeutic physical agents/modalities, instrument-assisted soft tissue mobilization<br>• Proprioceptive neuromuscular facilitation techniques |
| Increase strength/power | • AROM/AAROM (only increases strength for muscles with strength $< 3/5$)<br>• Neuromuscular electric stimulation<br>• Resistance exercises (ie, isometrics, concentric, and eccentric)<br>• Plyometrics (if indicated) |
| Increase cardiovascular endurance | • Aerobic exercise |
| Increase balance | • Core stability exercises<br>• Static balance activities<br>• Dynamic balance activities |
| Increase pulmonary function | • Breathing exercises<br>• Coughing exercises<br>• Aerobic exercise |

[a]Determine the root cause of pain (ie, is pain related to acute inflammation; referred pain).
[b]Determine the root cause for the limitation (ie, joint restriction, muscle tightness/guarding, or weakness).

## *Frequency, Intensity, Type, and Time: The FITT Principle*

After creating a treatment outline (verifying that the interventions are included in the POC), the assistant will select the most appropriate treatment parameters based on the patient's current status (ie, stage of healing, ROM, and strength). The **FITT (frequency, intensity, time, and type) principle** includes treatment parameters that the clinician modifies to individualize exercise programs (based on the patient's presentation/goals); these variables include frequency, intensity, time, and type.[8,9] Appropriate selection of these parameters is crucial; it allows the clinician to develop a program that provides adequate stimulus/stress to improve strength or aerobic conditioning. Appropriate parameter selection also allows enough rest so that the body can recover between sessions, and it prevents overtraining. See Chapter 6 for the application of these parameters to resistance/strength training and Chapter 9 for aerobic conditioning/cardiorespiratory training programs.

Selecting an appropriate frequency for the exercise allows the body to adapt to the training stresses and to heal between sessions. The recommended frequency for aerobic training is a minimum of 3 sessions per week up to 5 to 6 sessions per week. The frequency may fluctuate between 2 and 6 days per week based on the duration of each session.[10] The frequency for resistance training should allow the patient to rest the body part 1 day between each training session; the American College of Sports Medicine recommends strength training 2 to 3 days per week.[10,11] Elite athletes and other competitive athletes may train outside these guidelines (their training programs are individualized and must still build in adequate time for rest).

Intensity refers to the amount of effort a person puts forth in any training session. This reflects how hard a person is working. Adequate effort to produce a training stimulus must occur to see improvement, but exercise at too high of an intensity must be avoided to prevent injury. The heart rate (HR) response measures the intensity of cardiorespiratory training. The recommended intensity is determined using the Karvonen formula, exercise stress test results, or the rate of perceived exertion (RPE) tool (Chapter 9). Aerobic program intensity is adjusted by increasing or decreasing the speed or elevation (if using a treadmill or elliptical machine) or increasing or decreasing the resistance (if using a stationary bike or NuStep bike [NuStep, Inc]).

A clinician selects resistance training intensity by determining how much weight a person can lift for a set number of repetitions (called a *repetition maximum*). A program can be modified by adjusting the amount of weight, the number of repetitions, or the length of time to complete a set of exercises; the adjustments selected are dependent on the treatment goals. Only one of these parameters should be adjusted at a time. Muscle adaptation to strength training occurs when progressive overloading of a muscle takes place.

The third parameter a therapist will individualize is the type of exercise. Cardiorespiratory or aerobic training incorporates continuous movement and involves motion of the large muscle groups. The purpose of aerobic training is to improve heart and lung efficiency. Resistance training exercises can include concentric and eccentric training using weights, resistance bands, equipment, or body weight resistance. The purpose of resistance training is to progress the difficulty of the exercises in order to increase strength, muscle endurance, and/or power to achieve the patient's task/activity goals.

The final parameter is time, reflecting the duration of time a person exercises in one session. With aerobic conditioning, the overall time depends on the person's current fitness level. Patients who are less fit will benefit from 20 to 30 minutes of aerobic exercise, and as fitness levels increase, the time may increase to 45 to 60 minutes. Exercise time can be cumulative throughout the day; it does not need to be continuous.[9] For individuals who are in better physical condition, cardiorespiratory training is recommended at a moderate intensity (ie, greater than 30 minutes for 5 days per week), or vigorous or high-intensity cardiorespiratory training should occur for greater than 20 minutes at least 3 days per week.[10]

Overtraining can occur if any of these parameters are progressed too quickly or if a patient is not following the suggested nutritional and hydration guidelines. Signs and symptoms of overtraining include excessive fatigue, delayed-onset muscle soreness, loss of strength or endurance, and/or increased recovery times after exercise.[12] Overtraining can be avoided by ensuring adequate rest periods between sessions, adequate diet/hydration, and gradual progression of exercise intensity.

A person who stops exercising will experience a relatively quick decline in the functional gains they experienced from exercise. Typically, the frequency and intensity of exercise required to maintain gains are less than the frequency and intensity it took to make the gains. Even so, regular exercise is required to maintain strength and aerobic capacity. Detraining effects (ie, loss of endurance and muscle strength) begin within the first 2 weeks after terminating exercise.[9,13] To maintain aerobic performance, the American College of Sports Medicine recommends moderate-intensity aerobic exercise 5 days per week. Muscular strength can be maintained by training the muscle groups (at the same intensity) 1 to 2 days per week.[9]

## Evidence-Based Medicine/Practice

Most students and new graduates tend to rely heavily on textbook information when learning and applying basic treatment interventions. Physical therapist assistants develop lifelong learning skills through continuing education courses and personal learning activities. Ongoing professional development enhances critical decision-making skills and treatment techniques while maintaining clinical currency.

All clinicians should strive to develop skills that include research review and critical appraisal of new evidence.[14] Incorporating evidence-based medicine or **evidence-based practice** is a basic expectation in clinical care, and it includes the integration of the best available research, clinical expertise, and patient information in the development of treatment plans. Many of the barriers to the use of evidence-based medicine revolve around finding and applying the recommendations of recent research. There are many online resources available to the physical therapy team to assist them. The American Physical Therapy Association (APTA) website provides APTA members with access to contemporary research, including research articles, clinical summaries, and clinical practice guidelines (CPGs). CPGs are defined by the Institute of Medicine as systematically developed statements that guide practitioner and patient decision making when determining appropriate health care in specific clinical circumstances.[15] There are numerous CPGs that apply to physical therapy interventions. The practitioner must assess the quality of the research and the relevance to the patient, but these guidelines often provide a useful guide to practice decisions.

# Patient Monitoring

The depth of pretreatment patient screening that a clinician completes typically depends on the acuity of the patient. The depth and breadth of patient monitoring often vary based on the treatment setting because the level of medical acuity/stability may be very different for patients in an outpatient physical therapy clinic vs those in acute care. However, vital sign monitoring should be performed in all environments. Vital sign monitoring includes monitoring of, at a minimum, HR, blood pressure (BP), and respiratory rate. The clinician may also monitor the RPE, oxygen saturation level, and pain level. Patients in the acute care or inpatient setting typically require more comprehensive monitoring compared with those in an outpatient setting because of the increased acuity of the patient's medical condition.

## Monitoring Patients in the Acute Care or Inpatient Setting

Before treating any patient, the physical therapist assistant completes a thorough review of the medical record to determine if there are any recent changes in laboratory values, vital signs, cognition, medication, new operative reports, procedures, imaging, consults with specialists, or test results since the last physical therapy treatment session. The physical therapist assistant will also talk to the nurse on duty to see if any adverse events or changes have occurred. If the physical therapist assistant thinks that the information collected indicates that physical therapy needs to be put on hold, the assistant will notify the physical therapist. If physical therapy services are discontinued by the medical team, new physician orders must be obtained, and a new evaluation must be performed by the physical therapist in order for physical therapy to be reinstated.

Reviewing the comprehensive list of laboratory values in the acute care setting is imperative to maintaining patient safety, especially in the intensive care unit where a patient's medical status may change even more frequently. Table 2-3 provides a list of normative values for vital signs, hematology, electrolytes, and other laboratory values that should be reviewed before treatment.[6,16] Laboratory values near or at a critical value should be reviewed with the supervising physical therapist and/or nurse before initiating treatment. As with all reference values included in this text, these laboratory values are a reflection of the current standard of practice. Individual facility protocols and critical values may vary. The clinician should be prepared to integrate any updates to standards of care.

Before the start of each treatment session, the physical therapist assistant should also review the patient's physical therapy evaluation, short-term goals, and the last few therapy treatment notes. The assistant determines if there have been any changes in contraindication/precautions, exercises performed, weight-bearing status, level of supervision, distance walked, type of assistive device, and/or medical equipment (ie, oxygen tank, intravenous pole, or urinary catheter). Once this information is reviewed, the clinician can enter the patient's room/treatment area, introduce themselves, and gain consent for treatment. Vital sign data (HR, BP, respiratory rate, oxygen saturation, and RPE) are collected and recorded in the medical record. Any significant change in resting vital signs from the patient's normal values warrants a follow-up with the physical therapist or the medical team before initiating treatment. Any resting BP greater than 140/90 mm Hg or less than 90/60 mm Hg or the presence of any new symptoms (ie, severe headache or light-headedness) should be discussed with the physical therapist and/or nurse before proceeding with treatment.

**Table 2-3**

Vital Signs and Laboratory Values[6,16]

| Category | Adult | Older Adult | Child | Infant | Abnormal Values/Consideration to Hold Physical Therapy Intervention |
|---|---|---|---|---|---|
| *Vital Signs* | | | | | |
| HR/pulse (beats/minute) | 60 to 100 | 60 to 100 | 80 to 120 | 100 to 130 | Abnormal response to exercise, new arrhythmia, change in amplitude |
| BP (mm Hg) | 110/70 (< 120/< 80) | 90 to 140/60 to 90 | 75 to 120/45 to 84 | 60 to 90/30 to 60 | Abnormal response to exercise, < 10 mm Hg change in diastolic BP, narrowing of pulse pressure |
| Respiratory rate (breaths/minute) | 12 to 18 | 10 to 20 | 20 to 30 | 35 to 55 | Resting value < 10 or > 20 |
| Oxygen saturation (%) | > 95% | | | | < 90% |
| Temperature (°F) | 96.8 to 99.5 | | | | Caution with any patient who is febrile |
| *Hematology* | | | | | |
| Hemoglobin (g/dL) | Men: 13 to 18<br>Women: 12 to 16 | | 14 to 17 | 17 to 19 | < 8 |
| Hematocrit (%) | Men: 37 to 49<br>Women: 36 to 46 | | 30 to 49 | Up to 60 | < 25% |
| Platelets | 100,000 to 450,000 | 150,000 to 400,000 | 150,000 to 400,000 | 150,000 to 300,000 | < 20,000 |
| White blood cell count (K/mm$^3$) | 3.8 to 11.0 | | 4.6 to 4.8 | 5.5 to 6.0 | < 5000 with fever |
| International normalized ratio | 1 to 2<br>Heparin: 2 to 3<br>3.5 to 4.5 | | Atrial fibrillation<br>Prosthetic valve 3 to 4 | | > 5 |
| Prothrombin time | 11 to 13 (with heparin: 16.5 to 32.5 or 1.5 to 2.5 × normal value) | | | | > 32.5 |
| Partial thromboplastin time | 21 to 35 (with heparin: 50 to 88) | | | | > 110 (hold 1 hour after drip stopped) |

*(continued)*

**Table 2-3 (continued)**

Vital Signs and Laboratory Values[6,16]

| Category | Adult | Older Adult | Child | Infant | Abnormal Values/Consideration to Hold Physical Therapy Intervention |
|---|---|---|---|---|---|
| *Electrolytes/pH/Other Values* | | | | | |
| Sodium (Na; mEq/L) | 135 to 145 | 135 to 145 | 135 to 145 | 134 to 150 | < 110, weakness/neurologic surgery<br>> 155, cardiovascular/renal surgery |
| Potassium (K; mEq/L) | 3.5 to 5.3 | 3.5 to 5.3 | 3.5 to 5.5 | 3.6 to 5.8 | < 2.8<br>> 6.2 |
| Calcium (Ca; mEq/L) | 9 to 11 | 9 to 11 | 9 to 11.5 | 10 to 12 | < 7, tetany<br>> 12, coma |
| pH | 7.4 | | | | > 7.45, metabolic alkalosis<br>< 7.35, metabolic acidosis |
| $PCO_2$ (mm Hg) | 40 | | | | < 40, hypocapnia, hyperventilation<br>> 40, hypercapnia, hypoventilation |
| $PO_2$ (mm Hg) | 97 | | | | |
| $HCO_3$ (mEq/L) | 24 | | | | < 22<br>> 26 |
| Erythrocyte sedimentation rate | Men: 0 to 17<br>Women: 1 to 25 | | 1 to 13 | | Any value significantly higher than reference |
| Blood glucose (mg/dL) | 80 to 120 | | | | < 70, give carbohydrate<br>> 300 |

The physical therapist assistant will monitor the patient's vital sign response to activity and should expect to see an appropriate change in vital signs based on the level of exertion. The physical therapist assistant will plan to adjust vital sign and RPE monitoring when a patient is taking a drug from any of the following medication classes: beta blockers and calcium channel blockers (expect a lower HR response to activity and risk for orthostatic hypotension), diuretics (monitor for orthostatic hypotension and electrolyte imbalance), or antiarrhythmics (monitor for irregular HR and dizziness). Orthostatic hypotension causes a drop in BP and an increase in HR as a patient moves from supine to sitting or standing. Additionally, many medication classes (pain medications, antianxiety medications, antiepileptics, and drugs to treat affective disorders) can cause dizziness and/or lethargy, warranting additional monitoring for fall prevention.[17] For a list of medication side effects, refer to Appendix E.

Observing the medically complex patient can provide meaningful information to the assistant. The assistant will observe facial expressions, chest movement, and the use of accessory muscles (assessing for pain or difficulty breathing). A patient who is perspiring excessively, making abnormal noises during breathing, and/or displaying abnormal skin color (ie, red/flush, pale/pallor, or blue-gray/cyanotic) may have cardiac or pulmonary issues. If these signs or symptoms are observed, the assistant will notify the nurse immediately and discuss the situation with the physical therapist before initiating treatment.

The assistant can proceed with treatment with a medically stable patient who has consented to treatment. To maintain a safe treatment environment, the assistant will need to perform the following:

- Manage all tubes and lines when transferring and walking with patients
- Seek assistance when needed
- Transition patients from supine to sitting to standing positions slowly (to avoid orthostatic hypotension)
- Provide the appropriate level of supervision and guarding (using a gait belt) during all activities to prevent patient falls
- Monitor the patient throughout treatment

## *Monitoring Patients in the Outpatient Setting*

Supervising patients in an outpatient physical therapy setting is just as important as when working in an inpatient setting. The physical therapist assistant needs to be able to quickly recognize the signs and symptoms that indicate a change in patient status. An adverse incident or medical emergency, although less likely, can occur at any time and any place. Similar to the inpatient setting, the assistant will review the patient's physical therapy evaluation, previous medical history, list of medications, and previous treatment documentation to understand the patient's current status. Imaging, laboratory values, operative reports, and other information may or may not be available for review; therefore, ongoing discussions with the evaluating physical therapist before initiating treatment are important.

After a greeting and introduction, the assistant will observe several factors as the patient moves to the treatment area. Facial expressions, posture, and compensatory body movements may indicate pain or muscle weakness. The assistant also observes the patient's body mechanics (during transfers), the use of an assistive device (safely/correctly), and the quality of gait.

The physical therapist assistant should collect the following data before initiating treatment at each session:

- The location of pain and any changes in pain levels at rest and with specific activities
- Any unusual incidents or occurrences since the last visit
- Any changes or new development in signs/symptoms
- An improvement or a decline in any functional activities
- Compliance with an HEP (if applicable)
- Any changes in medications since the last visit
- Any upcoming physician consultations or recent or pending tests

Before initiating treatment interventions, the assistant will explain the risks, benefits, indications, contraindications, and precautions of the treatment; obtain consent for treatment; and gather and record baseline vital sign data. Any unusual subjective reports, objective changes, or responses should be brought to the attention of the physical therapist.

During treatment, the physical therapist assistant will monitor, modify, and/or correct the patient's exercise performance (for accuracy and muscle fatigue), posture and body mechanics (ie, transfers, lifting, and static/dynamic activities), and gait patterns. The assistant will monitor for signs and symptoms of pain, inflammation, muscle fatigue, and exercise intolerance. An inappropriate response to activity or exercise may warrant terminating performance of the intervention, discontinuing the treatment, and notifying the physical therapist and/or seeking medical attention.

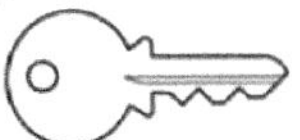

**Key Safety Considerations**

- Pay attention to detail! Is the intervention too hard? Is it causing pain? Is the patient performing the activity correctly? Is the patient completing the activity with compensatory movements because of excessive weakness or fatigue? Improper form can cause injury!
- Use a gait belt to maximize safety for the patient and the clinician and to reduce fall risk for the patient.
- Patients require continual monitoring throughout the physical therapy session for safe and effective treatment (monitor patient subjective reports; clinical observations; and vital signs before, during, and after treatment).

**Table 2-4**

Standard Precautions

| | |
|---|---|
| Handwashing | Wash hands before and after each patient contact. Wash hands before and after donning gloves. Use soap for handwashing for at least 20 to 30 seconds. Wash hands between tasks or procedures on the same patient to prevent cross-contamination; follow facility regulations regarding the use of antimicrobial agents. |
| Gloves | Wear gloves (clean, nonsterile gloves) when touching mucous membranes; nonintact skin; or in the presence of blood, body fluids, secretions, or known contamination. Don a new pair of gloves between procedures on the same patient to prevent cross-contamination. Remove gloves promptly after patient care and wash hands immediately. |
| Patient care equipment | Discard single-use items properly. Disinfect all equipment (assistive devices, BP equipment, weights, etc) before using with another patient. |
| Environment | Follow facility protocol for disinfection of all surfaces. |
| Linen | Handle, transport, and process contaminated linen to avoid contact/contamination to self, others, or environment. |
| Waste | Appropriately discard trash contaminated by blood or potentially contaminated bodily fluid (eg, vaginal secretion, synovial, amniotic, cerebrospinal fluid; red bag waste). |

### *Standard Precautions*

In addition to monitoring patients, the physical therapist assistant will maintain compliance with standard precautions during all patient care in order to prevent the spread of infection from patient to patient (Table 2-4). Proper hand hygiene (especially handwashing between every patient care intervention) and proper cleaning and disinfection of equipment and treatment areas are important for the safety and health of both patients and clinicians.

**Clinical Tips**

- If it is wet and it is not yours, do not touch it.
- Make sure you wash your hands with soap and water for at least 20 seconds (as long as it takes to sing the "happy birthday song" 3 times).

## Motor Learning Theory, Environment, Practice, and Feedback to Enhance Learning

**Motor performance** is the patient's ability to perform a task or skill. **Motor learning** involves both skill or task acquisition and retention through repetitive practice.[18] Retention is the ability to remember how to complete a task over time. By addressing key concepts of motor learning, the therapist can set up a training program geared toward promoting the best outcomes.[19] There is a difference between motor performance and motor learning. One cannot see actual learning because learning occurs using higher levels of central nervous system processes that are not visible. However, through repeated observation of a patient's motor performance, the clinician can infer whether the person has learned the skill/task based on changes that occur over time. Motor learning relative to the treatment of patients with neurologic diagnoses is discussed in Chapter 16.

Before teaching a patient a skill, exercise, or task, the clinician considers the following: the learner (ie, the patient), the task to be performed, and the environment in which the task will be performed. Appropriate selection of the environment, practice schedule, and optimal types of feedback is determined based on the task to be learned and the patient's stage of motor learning.

There are 3 stages of motor learning: cognitive, associative, and autonomous. In the first stage of motor learning, the cognitive stage, the patient is focused on how to complete the task safely, how to move the body, and how the activity/task feels. All of the patient's attention is hyperfocused on task performance, and distractions may make learning the task more difficult. In the associative stage, the patient understands the basics of how to complete the new task, and focus shifts to refining the movement pattern (focusing on how to make the motion most effective/efficient). In the autonomous stage, the patient can perform the task automatically without hesitation and without concentrating on the actual performance. The patient can

**Table 2-5**

Motor Learning and Suggestions to Enhance Learning

| Motor Learning Stage | Typical Presentation of the Learner | Suggestions to Enhance Learning |
|---|---|---|
| Cognitive | Learning what to do<br>Requires increased attention/focus on task<br>Unable to split attention<br>Must focus on each step of task | Complete training in closed environment<br>Demonstrate task first<br>Encourage attention to internal sensory feedback<br>Provide manual guidance (fade use as soon as possible)<br>Offer concurrent, specific, and accurate feedback<br>Provide feedback (knowledge of results) after each trial initially<br>Practice in blocked order<br>Practice subtasks (part practice) as needed initially |
| Associative | Learning how to do it more efficiently/effectively<br>Motions completed with fewer errors<br>Beginning to self-correct errors in task<br>Decreased reliance on extrinsic feedback | Move from closed to more open environment<br>Remove manual guidance<br>Transition to random order practice<br>Decrease use of concurrent feedback and immediate feedback; transition to delayed and summary feedback<br>Begin fading feedback<br>Increase task complexity |
| Autonomous | Able to complete tasks automatically<br>Can focus on other activities while completing task<br>Can complete the task efficiently | Increase task complexity<br>Integrate tasks into activities of daily living (ADLs) and instrumental ADLs<br>Complete tasks in community settings |

also perform the task in varied conditions (changes in task demands or environmental circumstances).[18] Table 2-5 lists the stages of motor learning and provides tips to promote learning.

Motor tasks are described as being discrete, serial, or continuous tasks. Discrete tasks have a specific beginning and end. Most exercises (ie, a biceps curl or long-arc quadriceps) are discrete tasks. Serial tasks are made up of a number of discrete tasks completed in a particular sequence. A transfer board transfer is an example of a serial task. Continuous tasks are made up of repetitive motions with no clear beginning or end. Examples include many aerobic training activities (eg, elliptical, swimming) as well as functional tasks (eg, walking, wheelchair propulsion).

## *Environments and Practice*

Training can occur in a closed or an open environment. Closed environments are predictable environments with minimal distractions. There is limited activity occurring around the patient, and the patient is often in a stable position. Training in a closed environment allows the patient to control the pace of the task and to focus their full attention on the task, which can lead to improved performance and retention. Oftentimes, task training is initiated in a closed environment to facilitate new learning.

Open environments include ones with multiple distractions and where there is activity occurring near/around the patient. The patient must be able to attend to multiple stimuli, adapt to an environment, and pace the activity based on the demands of a changing environment. Open environments are unpredictable. Most training progresses to practicing activities in an open environment to replicate real-life demands.

The therapist can manipulate practice types and schedules to enhance learning and retention. The therapist can have the patient practice the entire task (whole practice), or the patient can complete part practice. Part practice occurs when a task is broken down into discrete tasks; more difficult component tasks can be practiced repetitively. Once the patient has the ability to complete each subtask, the tasks are practiced in sequence, preparing for whole-task practice. The therapist can vary practice order to promote new learning or to promote retention and generalizability. Generalizability is the ability to complete key portions of a task in an altered environment or with a modified configuration of the task. A patient who learns an exercise sequence and can demonstrate the sequence accurately 1 month later is demonstrating retention of the task. A patient who learns how to complete a squat pivot transfer from the wheelchair to a mat and is then able to problem solve to complete a squat pivot transfer from the wheelchair onto a commode demonstrates that they have generalized the task. Clinicians often determine true learning by verifying a patient's ability to generalize the task.

To promote early learning, the therapist may start a program using blocked practice. Blocked practice is repetition of the same task in the same order and under the same conditions. When there is limited variability of the task, it promotes faster improvement in skill performance. However, to obtain better retention and generalizability of the task, practice order should progress to random/block order practice or random order practice. Random order practice occurs when tasks are completed in an unpredictable order, and the task is varied slightly each time. Random/block order practice occurs when variations of the same task are performed in a random order, but each variation is practiced a couple of times in a row before moving to the next variation. Random/block order practice results in better retention than blocked order practice and quicker skill acquisition than random order practice.

Mental practice (visualization/motor imagery practice) is a mental/cognitive review of the steps to complete a task. Research indicates that mental practice, when used with physical practice, can enhance and improve the speed of skill acquisition.[20] Physical practice involves actual performance and practice of the motor task. The best way to learn a new task is by physically practicing the task.

## *Types of Feedback*

After an optimal practice schedule is selected and practice begins, the clinician will provide feedback to help guide the patient's performance. Feedback must be accurate to be useful to the patient. It must also be offered at the best time, without overwhelming the patient with too much information. Feedback that is provided about components of task performance is called **knowledge of performance**. Feedback that is provided about the outcome of a motor task is called **knowledge of results. Intrinsic feedback** is feedback that occurs within the patient/learner; it occurs naturally when a task is being completed. Intrinsic feedback includes the sensory feedback (proprioceptive, kinesthetic, visual, tactile, and auditory information) that is received during task completion.

**Extrinsic (augmented) feedback** is provided by an external source. The external source can be the therapist providing verbal or tactile cues or a mechanical source, such as a limb load monitor or biofeedback. Extrinsic feedback can be used to provide knowledge of performance during or right after task performance, or knowledge of results can be provided after task completion. Research suggests that directing a patient's attention to the outcomes of a task (knowledge of results) is a more effective teaching tool than focusing attention on task performance, indicating that emphasis on the results of task performance is appropriate.[21]

The timing and frequency of extrinsic feedback can impact skill acquisition and retention. Feedback that occurs during task performance is concurrent feedback. The use of concurrent feedback can enhance early skill acquisition, but excessive use may impede retention. Visual cues (the use of a mirror), verbal cues during a task, and manual guidance are types of concurrent feedback. The key to effective use of concurrent feedback is to use it as much as necessary but as little as possible. The use of frequent concurrent feedback may improve early skill acquisition as well as retention in tasks that are new to the learner.[22] Research suggests that varying practice trials by using concurrent and terminal feedback in one trial followed by a practice trial without extrinsic feedback can improve both skill acquisition and retention.[23] Summary feedback is feedback that is given at the end of several task trials. Summary feedback allows the patient some time to self-evaluate before receiving the feedback; this brief delay in offering feedback promotes retention and generalizability. Immediate feedback is given immediately after task completion; this can enhance early skill acquisition. Delayed feedback is offered after each trial but after a brief delay to allow the patient to problem solve what was successful and what did not work. Delayed feedback promotes improved retention.

As the patient moves from the cognitive to the associative stage of learning, the clinician should decrease the type and timing of extrinsic feedback as the patient demonstrates accurate skill performance. The clinician will encourage more intrinsic feedback, where the patient makes the necessary corrections on their own.

# Developing an Appropriate Exercise Program

The factors that should be considered when designing an exercise program for a patient include, but are not limited to, injury/condition/disease pathology, current medical

**Table 2-6**

Suggestions for Modifying Exercises or Activities

| Making an Exercise Less Challenging | Making an Exercise More Challenging |
|---|---|
| • Increase stability: Increase the size of the base of support.<br>• Use a stable surface: Sitting on a chair, standing on the floor.<br>• Gravity: Perform exercises gravity assisted or gravity minimized before performing against gravity. Consider patient positioning, easiest to move when segment moves in the horizontal plane.<br>• Lever arm: A shorter lever arm will make the exercise easier to perform (ie, shoulder motion with the elbow flexed vs extended).<br>• Speed: Dependent on the environment (ie, pool vs on land). Performing shoulder abduction/adduction slowly in the water provides less resistance and is easier. Oftentimes, performance on land is easier with rapid motion (momentum).<br>• Dosage: Decrease repetitions. | • Challenge the patient's stability: Decrease the size of the base of support; normal stance, Romberg tandem standing, single-leg standing.<br>• Transition to a surface that is unstable: Sitting on a therapy ball, standing on a foam or compliant surface, rocker board, balance beam.<br>• Gravity: Perform against gravity. Be aware of patient positioning.<br>• Lever arm: A longer lever arm will make the exercise more difficult to perform (ie, hip motion with the knee extended/leg straight).<br>• Speed: Dependent on the environment. Performing shoulder abduction/adduction in the pool quickly provides more resistance and is harder. Slow, controlled motion on land is often more difficult than quicker motions that include momentum.<br>• Dosage: Increase repetitions. |

status, comorbidities, age, pain level and tolerance, current level of function, impairments, functional limitations, stage of healing, and patient goals. Exercise modification, patient education, and home exercise compliance are also important to consider during the implementation of a therapeutic exercise program. The assistant will strive to select exercises that will address the patient's impairments while helping a patient attain their goals. It may be beneficial to break a task into parts, targeting the muscles that perform various aspects of the task. For example, if a patient's goal is to climb a flight of stairs, the clinician can problem solve the subtasks and determine which subtasks the patient is having difficulty completing. The clinician can determine if the patient struggles to perform adequate hip flexion to clear a 4-inch (in) step, to maintain balance on one leg, or has inadequate hip extension/knee extension strength to complete the activity. The clinician can determine the appropriate FITT dosage and can make the exercises as specific as possible based on these factors. These activity components are practiced before practicing ascending stairs. If the patient has adequate ROM, strength, and balance but is unable to go up a 4-in step, a 1-in step can be used, and the assistant can progress the step height to achieve the goal. The numerous variables may appear daunting, but a systematic approach to exercise program development can guide the learner in effective program development.

## *Exercise Modifications*

When modifying an exercise or activity, the clinician needs to make it challenging but not to the point where it cannot be performed correctly and/or safely. The clinician will select exercises that address the patient's impairments and that will improve function and progress the patient toward their goals as safely and efficiently as possible.

There are a number of ways an exercise can be modified. The clinician can vary each element (ie, weight/resistance, duration, the number of repetitions and/or sets, the number of exercises to be performed in a session, the type of contraction being performed, and the rest period time). Table 2-6 provides suggestions on how to make an activity/exercise more or less challenging. Only alter one of the variables at a time. Consider this example; a patient is unable to complete a short-arc quadriceps (SAQ) exercise in supine due to decreased quadriceps strength. The assistant can cue the patient to move into the side-lying position where the patient is able to complete the motion (SAQ) on a powder board. By changing the patient position, the muscles were able to perform the activity with gravity minimized. The assistant could also have the patient perform muscle setting with the knee in full extension (quad sets), which would strengthen the quadriceps muscles at the end of the ROM. Once the patient can contract the muscles with the knee straight and can complete the motion in the side-lying

Box 2-1

**Questions to Consider Before Teaching a Task/Exercise**

- The learner: What are the underlying abilities of the learner to perform the task? Is the task appropriate for the learner? Has the patient had previous experiences with such tasks? Are there individualized factors (ie, level of cognition or physical abilities) that will influence the ability to perform the task?
- The task: What body movements are required? How complex is the task/does it demand high concentration/attention? Does an object need to be manipulated by the patient? Is the task performed under a variety of conditions or the same way each time?
- The environment: How/when is the task to be performed? Is that context predicable or unpredictable? Does time play a factor in task completion/is there a time limitation to complete the task?

Box 2-2

**Questions Used to Determine the Cause of Pain or Symptoms**

- What activities/positions increase or decrease your symptoms?
- Where is your pain located?
- Can you grade the intensity from 0 to 10?
- Can you describe your pain (ie, sharp, radiating, dull, achy, or muscle soreness)?
- What time of day and/or with what activity is your pain level better or worse?
- How long does the pain last? Does it stop after exercise/activity or with change in position?
- What do you do to make the pain/symptoms better (eg, cold, heat, nonsteroidal anti-inflammatory drugs, rest)?

position, the assistant can increase the repetitions and then increase the intensity (add manual resistance) in this position. Progressions can then be initiated as follows: supine SAQ, seated long-arc quadriceps exercises, working the muscle through a larger ROM, SAQ with resistance, and then standing mini-squats and full squats.

Once an exercise is selected, the patient's performance is monitored for accuracy and safety. The physical therapist assistant can modify the exercise's level of difficulty by increasing the complexity or intensity (necessary to ensure progress toward goals) or decreasing it (to reduce the risk of injury and in response to fatigue or pain). The assistant must continuously monitor and assess patient responses to the exercises and any changes in functional limitations and impairments.

## *Patient Education and Exercise Compliance*

Patient education is an important component of the rehabilitation process. It is important for the patient to understand the mechanism of injury or potential contributing factors that may be responsible for causing their pain and/or condition. Instruction regarding the importance of activity modification and the reasons associated with any restrictions can be useful in increasing patient compliance with their rehabilitation program.

Clinicians instruct their patients on ways to reduce their pain and improve their function and/or prevent injury (or reinjury) as well as how to properly perform exercises, how to use proper lifting techniques, and proper positioning techniques (ie, sleeping, sitting, standing, and workstations). Clinicians can use the questions provided in Box 2-1 as a framework for exercise selection. Patients often ask the following questions: Why am I doing this exercise? What can I do to sleep better? and When can I resume my normal activities? The clinician should address patient questions honestly and directly and justify why and how exercise performance is important. If the clinician can explain how a particular exercise can help the patient achieve their goals, the patient may be more invested in completing the exercise. If a clinician does not know the answer to a patient's question, it is alright to state that, but plan to follow up by researching the answer and sharing it with the patient during the next session.

Effective communication skills are important when providing patient education, and they can facilitate patient compliance during a treatment session with an HEP. Patients tend to respond better when the clinician takes time to listen intently and to respond honestly and succinctly to patient questions or comments. The assistant should clearly communicate instructions, expectations, and recommendations. Provide the patient an opportunity to express their feelings about their pain level and/or to reflect on the current or previous treatment. The physical therapist assistant can use the list of questions in Box 2-2 to gain pertinent information about the patient's pain/symptoms. Answers to these questions will help guide the assistant's decision as to what may be included in an HEP.

There are a number of ways to improve exercise performance and compliance (Table 2-7). It is helpful if the patient understands why the exercise/activity is important for them to perform. The physical therapist assistant will monitor the patient's exercise performance for correct form, appropriate level of intensity, dosage (repetitions/sets/duration), and onset of fatigue. The patient should be able to correctly and safely complete the exercise independently

**Table 2-7**

**Suggestions to Improve Exercise Performance and Compliance**

Suggestions to improve exercise performance:

- Provide patient instructions in a quiet, distraction-free environment.
- Explain the importance of properly performing the exercise selected and the rationale for including the exercise.
- The assistant should demonstrate the activity/exercise first.
- Provide clear and concise verbal directions.
- Provide manual/tactile cues (if needed) while the patient performs the exercise/activity.
- Have the patient demonstrate the exercise correctly without verbal cues before including it in the HEP.
- Include written instructions and pictures (or links to videos) with the HEP.
- Give the patient no more than 3 exercises at 1 time. As the patient improves and can perform an exercise without difficulty, add resistance or discontinue it and add another that is more challenging.
- Clearly tie the exercises to the patient's goals and problem list; the patient must see the value and the benefit of performing the HEP.

Suggestions to improve compliance:

- Identify and resolve barriers; reiterate how the exercises will help achieve their goals, discuss the patient's progress, modify exercises, and use motivational techniques.
- Work within the patient's time constraints; how much time are they willing to devote to the exercise program (keep it short).
- Break up the exercises so they can be performed throughout the day during ADLs vs completing them all at one time.
- Include the exercise program on a daily calendar; schedule it like a meeting.
- Encourage the patient to exercise with a friend.

before including it in the HEP. Appendix C includes an example of an exercise prescription form. A worksheet to guide the physical therapist assistant student in designing and progressing interventions for a patient with a specific diagnosis is found in Appendix D.

When the patient returns to therapy for the next visit, the assistant will observe the patient's HEP performance to ensure accurate completion; the assistant will ask about exercise tolerance and compliance. If the patient reports not having enough time to do the exercises, the clinician can work with the patient to problem solve. For example, if the patient is at work during the day, are they able to interrupt their work schedule and perform one exercise for 2 or 3 minutes? Can they do a few of them during their lunch hour? If the patient watches television in the evening, can one exercise can be performed during each commercial? Identifying the cause of poor compliance is the first step in improving it. If the exercise causes pain, it may need to be modified, changed, or discontinued. Determining the cause of the patient's pain or symptoms is important. The physical therapist assistant can ask specific open-ended questions to help reveal the root cause and intensity of pain and which activities increase patient symptoms. Having the patient describe their pain and when or what reduces it to a tolerable level generates important information. Data should be reported to the supervising physical therapist.

Patient motivation or a lack thereof can be a barrier to exercise compliance. The physical therapist assistant can use specific strategies to help motivate patients. It is useful to develop a good rapport with the patient. Determining what incentivizes the patient is helpful. For example, if a patient wants to dance at a granddaughter's wedding, then the assistant can encourage the patient to perform lower extremity strengthening exercises at home so they can get stronger (more quickly than if they only exercise during the therapy appointments). The assistant may also suggest including dancing practice in the clinic if the patient is compliant with completing the exercises at home. Having family and friends encourage the patient can also have a positive impact. The clinician should strive to maintain a positive attitude about how the patient is progressing (acknowledge all "baby steps"), even if the patient does not feel the progress is fast enough. It can be helpful to reflect on how much progress the patient has achieved in the past 2 or 3 weeks; this can help with putting a longer rehabilitation process into perspective.

To maximize exercise program compliance, it is helpful if the patient understands the benefits and value in performing the exercises and the role of each exercise in improving function. Compliance may also increase once fear of moving the involved segment is reduced. Patient education can emphasize the importance of continuing with the exercises (after being discharged from physical therapy) to maintain the improvements achieved in physical therapy. The goal is for exercise to become a regular part of the patient's routine.

## Conclusion

The physical therapist assistant plays a crucial role in implementing physical therapy treatment interventions. Strong clinical decision making, knowledge, and a willingness to incorporate evidence-based practice into treatment interventions will provide the assistant with the core abilities to select appropriate treatment interventions to address physical therapy goals. Appropriate exercise application can have many positive outcomes, including improving pain, inflammation, ROM, strength, balance, and cardiovascular endurance. The selection of optimal interventions, paired with appropriate and continuous monitoring of the patient, will maximize patient outcomes and safety. The incorporation of motor learning theory with the selection of optimal exercise parameters will allow the assistant to effectively guide the patient in meeting the treatment goals set in the physical therapy POC.

## Review Questions

1. What activities should the physical therapist assistant complete before initiating any therapeutic exercise intervention? What patient monitoring is indicated?
2. What role does the physical therapist assistant have in the development of an exercise program? What data or information should the assistant use in this process?
3. What are the most common exercise interventions a therapist might use?
4. Describe the parameters that are described by the acronym FITT.
5. List and describe 3 ways to improve exercise performance.
6. Compare and contrast the types of practice. Which are most effective for early skill acquisition? For retention?
7. Describe the optimal application of feedback from early task performance through practice and refining of task completion.
8. List 3 suggestions to maximize patient compliance with an HEP.
9. A patient can perform an upper extremity exercise using a resistance band while standing on foam without cues or hesitation. Which stage of motor learning is this completion most consistent with?
10. A patient is practicing going up and down steps at 2, 4, and 6 in in height. With each practice task, the physical therapist assistant instructs the patient to perform 6 repetitions before changing the height of the practice step. What type of practice is this an example of?

## Case Study

A patient presents with left shoulder flexion strength of 3+/5 and full AROM of both upper extremities. The patient reports having difficulty with the left arm when blow drying their hair and reaching into cabinets to take dishes out or put them away.

- Which muscle(s) is most likely weak?
- Select an exercise to target the weak muscles.
- Provide 3 modifications to the selected exercise that make the exercise easier to complete.
- Describe at least 2 reasons a clinician might need to modify an exercise by making it less challenging to complete.
- Provide 3 modifications to the exercise that will make the exercise more challenging.
- When would this type of modification be indicated?
- Would completing the exercise in a gravity-minimized position increase or decrease the challenge? Why?

## Suggested Resources

American Physical Therapy Association. Evidence-based practice & research. 2022. Accessed February 14, 2023. https://www.apta.org/patient-care/evidence-based-practice-resources#:~:text=Evidence%2Dbased%20practice%20includes%20the,and%20health%20policy%20decision%20making

Centers for Disease Control. Standard precautions for all patient care. Reviewed January 26, 2016. Accessed January 24, 2023. https://www.cdc.gov/infectioncontrol/basics/standard-precautions.html

## References


1. Meir EP. Composition and function of connective tissue. In: Manske RC, ed. *Fundamental Orthopedic Management for the Physical Therapist Assistant*. 4th ed. Elsevier; 2006:143-152.
2. Fernandez E, Turk DC. The utility of cognitive coping strategies for altering pain perception: a meta-analysis. *Pain*. 1989;38(2):123-135.
3. O'Gara T, Kemper KJ, Birkedal J, Curl W, Miller N, Abadie B. Survey of conventional and complementary and alternative therapy in patients with low back pain. *J Surg Orthop Adv*. 2016;25(1):27-33.
4. Santiesteban AJ. The role of physical agents in the treatment of spine pain. *Clin Orthop Relat Res*. 1983;179:24-30.
5. Fedorczyk J. The role of physical agents in modulating pain. *J Hand Ther*. 1997;10(2):110-121.
6. Irion G. Laboratory tests and values. In: Goodman CC, Fuller KS, eds. *Pathophysiology Implications for the Physical Therapist*. 5th ed. Elsevier; 2015:1703-1730.
7. Ethics and Judicial Committee, American Physical Therapy Association. APTA guide for conduct of the physical therapist assistant. October 1981. Updated March 2019. Accessed January 24, 2023. http://www.apta.org/uploadedFiles/APTAorg/Practice_and_Patient_Care/Ethics/GuideforConductofthePTA.pdf_
8. Dick F. *Sports Training Principles*. 5th ed. A&C Black Ltd; 2007.
9. Pescatello L, ed. *ACSM Guidelines for EX Testing and Prescription*. 9th ed. Wolters Kluwer; 2014.
10. Garber CE, Blissmer B, Deschenes MR, et al. Quantity and quality of exercise for developing and maintaining cardiorespiratory, musculoskeletal, and neuromotor fitness in apparently healthy adults: guidance for prescribing exercise. *Med Sci Sports Exerc*. 2011;43(7):1334-1359. doi:10.1249/MSS.0b013e318213fefb
11. Ratamess NA, Alvar BA, Evetoch TK, et al. Progression models in resistance training for healthy adult. *Med Sci Sports Exerc*. 2009;41(3):687-708. doi:10.1249/MSS.0b013e318191567
12. Kuipers H. Training and overtraining: an introduction. *Med Sci Sports Exerc*. 1998;30:1137-1139.
13. Mujika I, Padilla S. Muscular characteristics of detraining in humans. *Med Sci Sports Exerc*. 2001;33(8):1297-1303.
14. Masic I, Miokovic M, Muhamedagic B. Evidence based medicine – new approaches and challenges. *Acta Inform Med*. 2008;16(4):219-225. doi:10.5455/aim.2008.16.219-225
15. Field MJ, Lohr KN. *Clinical Practice Guidelines: Directions of a New Program*. National Academy Press; 1990.
16. American Academy of Acute Care Physical Therapy. Laboratory values point-of-care document. 2017. Accessed December 9, 2017. https://www.aptaacutecare.org/store/viewproduct.aspx?id=10758078
17. Ciccone C. *Davis's Drug Guide for Rehabilitation Professionals*. FA Davis; 2013.
18. Humphrey VN, Colby LA. Therapeutic exercise: foundational concepts. In: Kisner C, Colby LA, Borstad J. *Therapeutic Exercise Foundations and Techniques*. 7th ed. FA Davis Company; 2018:27-34.
19. Schmidt R, Lee T. *Motor Control and Learning: A Behavioral Emphasis*. 4th ed. Human Kinetics Publishers; 2005.
20. Malouin F, Richards C. Mental practice for relearning locomotor skills. *Phys Ther*. 2010;90(2):240-251.
21. McNevin NH, Wulf G, Carlson C. Effects of attentional focus, self-control, and dyad training on motor learning: implications for physical rehabilitation. *Phys Ther*. 2000;80(4):373-385.
22. Fujii S, Lulic T, Chen JL. More feedback is better than less: learning a novel upper limb joint coordination pattern with augmented auditory feedback. *Front Neurosci*. 2016;10:251. doi:10.3389/fnins.2016.00251
23. Park JH, Shea CH, Wright DL. Reduced-frequency concurrent and terminal feedback: a test of the guidance hypothesis. *J Mot Behav*. 2000;32(3):287-296.

# Chapter 3

# Injuries, Tissue Healing, and Surgical Interventions

*Jacki Klaczak Kopack, PT, DPT and Karen A. Cascardi, PhD, MS, ATC, PTA*

**KEY TERMS** Allograft | Arthrodesis | Arthroplasty | Autograft | Fracture | Mechanism of injury | Prehabilitation | Sprain | Strain | Tendinopathy

## Chapter Objectives

1. Define various musculoskeletal injuries or lesions.
2. Describe 3 classifications of ligamentous injuries.
3. Explain the cardinal signs/symptoms of inflammation.
4. Differentiate the phases of healing and the indicated treatments based on the phase of healing.
5. Describe the healing times of various tissues.
6. Define and describe the term *prehabilitation.*
7. Differentiate between an allograft and autograft.
8. Identify common surgical procedures.
9. Summarize postoperative complications associated with orthopedic surgical procedures.

## Types of Injuries or Lesions

Musculoskeletal injuries affect a person's ability to function in a normal manner. Injury to the musculoskeletal system can result from disease or pathology, trauma, a fall, or an insidious or seemingly indirect cause. Injuries can affect bony structures or soft tissue. Common orthopedic injuries include sprains, strains, fractures, dislocations, subluxations, tendinopathies, synovitis, bursitis, contusion, hemarthrosis, and overuse injuries (eg, compartment syndrome, carpal tunnel syndrome; Table 3-1).

The **mechanism of injury (MOI)** is the description of how an injury occurs. Knowing the MOI provides the clinician with a good idea of which structures may be involved or injured. If a patient steps down off a curb and their ankle "twists" into plantar flexion and inversion, the ligaments on the lateral aspect of the ankle would be stretched beyond their normal limits. The muscles on the lateral side (peroneal muscles) could abruptly contract to prevent the overstretching of the ligaments and capsule. This MOI could result in an ankle sprain and/or a peroneal musculotendinous strain and potentially an avulsion fracture of the base of the fifth metatarsal (peroneus brevis muscle attachment) depending on the severity of the injury.

Dislocations and subluxations are painful and are often associated with other soft tissue, nerve, and/or vascular damage. The joints most prone to dislocation are the fingers, thumbs, and shoulders. Typical presentations of a dislocation include joint deformity and the inability to move the dislocated joint.



Kopack JK, Cascardi KA.
*Principles of Therapeutic Exercise for the Physical Therapist Assistant* (pp 31-42).

**Table 3-1**

Types of Injuries and Descriptions

| Injury | Description |
|---|---|
| Sprain | Stretching or tearing of a ligament and/or joint capsule beyond its normal limit |
| Strain | Stretching or tearing of muscle and/or tendon (most commonly the musculotendinous unit) |
| Dislocation | Disruption of joint continuity; bones are displaced from their normal positions |
| Subluxation | Incomplete or partial dislocation. |
| Tendinosis | Degeneration of the tendon due to overuse or repetitive microtrauma or advanced age (often without localized inflammatory response) |
| Paratenonitis | Inflammation of the synovial membrane (paratenon) covering a tendon |
| Tendinitis | Acute inflammation of a tendon; possible scarring or calcium deposits that occur during the healing process |
| Bursitis | Inflammation of a bursa |
| Synovitis | Inflammation of synovial membrane producing excessive synovial fluid in a joint or around a tendon |
| Hemarthrosis | Blood in a joint (commonly results after significant trauma to a joint) |
| Contusion | Bleeding within soft tissue, usually due to a direct blow; resulting in pain, localized edema, and loss of motion |
| Overuse syndrome (cumulative trauma disorder) | Injury due to repetitive submaximal overload tasks/activities causing inflammation and pain |
| Compartment syndrome | Acute compartment syndrome is typically a result of a fracture or crush injury; it is caused by excess pressure within an anatomical compartment (usually forearm or lower leg) and presents with severe pain, paresthesia, decreased pulse in the affected area, pallor, and decreased ability to move the affected area |

**Tendinopathy** is a broad term used to describe tendon-associated conditions. The American Academy of Orthopedic Surgeons describes and classifies types of tendinopathies; the current definitions for tendinosis, tendinitis, and paratenonitis are described in Table 3-1. Paratenonitis typically results from excessive friction between the paratenon and a bony prominence. *Paratenonitis* is the preferred term, replacing the terms *tenosynovitis* and *tenovaginitis.*[1] The Achilles tendon is prone to this condition.

Overuse injuries occur when structures are repeatedly stressed or overloaded submaximally, resulting in pain and inflammation. Stress fractures and lower extremity chronic anterior compartment syndrome, carpal tunnel syndrome, and some tendinopathies are examples of overuse or cumulative trauma disorders. These injuries can be prevented with proper training techniques, using proper mechanics, and/or adequate rest; the physical therapy team is qualified to provide the education and training to patients to decrease injury risk.

### *Classifications of Sprains and Strains*

There are 3 grades/degrees or classifications of ligament **sprains** and musculotendinous **strains** (Table 3-2). Grades I/first degree (mild) and II/second degree (moderate) are most common and can be treated with conservative measures. The patient may require a brace/splint; the use of an assistive device to limit weight bearing; and education on joint protection, rest, ice, compression, and elevation of the involved extremity. Grade I and II sprains/strains usually respond well to physical therapy interventions. Grade III sprains result in joint instability because of the severe tearing or total separation of a ligament and require surgical intervention to repair the ligament(s) and often the surrounding tissues.

## Soft Tissue and Bone Healing

Various tissues have different healing times and healing capabilities. The severity of the initial injury will also affect healing times. The physical therapist assistant must be able to select treatment interventions based on the structure (muscle, tendon, ligament, or bone) involved and the phase of healing. The phases of healing for different tissues are described in Table 3-3. Inappropriate interventions or interventions applied too early or too aggressively may jeopardize the healing process.

**Table 3-2**

Classifications of Ligament Sprains and Muscle/Tendon Strains

| Classification | Tissue Involvement | Swelling | Amount of Pain | Weight-Bearing Status |
|---|---|---|---|---|
| Grade I<br>Mild<br>First degree | Microscopic tearing of fibers of ligament or muscle/tendon; no joint laxity | Mild | Sprain: Mild up to 24 hours after injury; pain only when ligament stressed; local point tenderness<br>Strain: Some pain with active contraction but able to complete full ROM | Full; ADLs not usually affected, limited sport participation |
| Grade II<br>Moderate<br>Second degree | Sprain: Partial torn ligament fibers, some joint laxity<br>Strain: Indentation of muscle belly with palpation at the site of the tear | Moderate | Sprain: Moderate with ligament stress and palpation<br>Strain: Significant pain with active contraction, moderate weakness | Partial; all weight-bearing activities are restricted |
| Grade III<br>Severe<br>Third degree | Sprain: Significant or complete rupture; joint instability<br>Strain: Significant or complete rupture, total loss of movement | Severe | Sprain: Minimal pain when joint is stressed, obvious deformity with stress or palpation<br>Strain: Minimal pain; muscle usually retracts proximally with total rupture (ie, biceps) | Non–weight bearing; usually requires surgical intervention or immobilization |

ADLs = activities of daily living; ROM = range of motion.

**Table 3-3**

Phases of Healing and Tissue Repair Times[2,3,a]

| Tissue | Acute Phase Maximal Protection | Subacute Phase Moderate Protection | Chronic Phase Return to Function | Approximate Total Healing Time |
|---|---|---|---|---|
| Muscle | 4 to 6 days | 2 to 3 weeks | > 3 weeks | 6 to 9 weeks |
| Tendon | 4 to 6 days | 2 to 6 weeks | > 6 weeks | 12 weeks to 6 months |
| Ligament | 1 to 3 weeks | 3 to 6 weeks | > 6 weeks | 6 to 12 months |
| Cartilage | | | | 6 to 8 weeks |

| General Fracture Healing Times[b] | | Types of Fracture Healing |
|---|---|---|
| Bone | 4 to 6 weeks children<br>6 to 8 weeks adolescents<br>10 to 18 weeks adults → | Clinical union (normal/initial healing)<br>Radiologic union (normal/optimal outcome)<br>Nonunion or malunion (abnormal) |

[a]These are estimated times; individual healing times will depend on the severity of the injury, thickness/depth of the tear or break, injury location, and vascularity availability.
[b]Fracture healing time is impacted by the following factors: Age, general health, smoker, type/location of fracture, displaced/nondisplaced, and surgical fixation/nonsurgical.

## Soft Tissue Healing

A number of factors affect soft tissue healing. Similar types of tissue (ie, cartilage) may heal at different rates because of blood supply availability. For example, a tear of the medial meniscus (fibrocartilage) in the knee on the outer edge (periphery) of the joint is likely to heal because there is adequate vascular supply located there. Conversely, if the tear occurs deep within the joint, there is an increased likelihood that the meniscus will not heal well because of reduced vascularity (requiring subsequent surgical repair). Superficial damage to articular (hyaline) cartilage that covers the ends of bone will not heal as well as a deeper (full-thickness) injury. The full-thickness tear disrupts the subchondral (bone) blood supply, which increases vascularity and facilitates healing. The healing ability of any structure is related to the presence of adequate vascular supply; cartilage typically has limited capabilities for healing.

Scar tissue that forms as a result of the healing process is not as strong as the original (uninjured) tissue. The assistant should consider the potential implications for the return to function/recreation/sports if a patient has sustained a significant injury. The postinjury training must account for potential diminished tensile strength of the injured structure(s).

Grade I and II sprains are common; they can occur at any joint (most commonly knees and ankles). These injuries can occur during sport participation, ambulation tasks, or stepping off a curb/step; they may occur with any movement that results in a twisting action at the joint. Sprains and/or fractures can also occur when falling on an outstretched arm or with any significant trauma.

For ligament healing to occur, the ends of the ligaments must remain in contact with each other, and there must be adequate blood supply. Low-load activities are used to gently stress the healing tissues while excessive stresses are prevented (ie, bracing). Controlled movement and the resumption of activity aid in stimulating repair and restoration of function, whereas prolonged rest can delay recovery and adversely affect ligament healing.[4] Low-load stresses promote scar tissue formation in the direction of the stresses placed on it, thereby creating a stronger and more organized ligament repair/scar.

Approximately 75% of Achilles tendon ruptures occur in men 30 to 49 years old, and they most commonly occur during sport participation.[5] Rotator cuff full-thickness tears are more commonly observed in older adults, and occurrence tends to be multifactorial. Approximately 25% of adults in their 50s and up to 50% of those in their 80s will experience a full-thickness tear, partially due to age-related degenerative changes and microtrauma(s) to the rotator cuff tendons.[5]

Different tendons have different levels of vascularity. Vascularization (and therefore blood flow) of tendons tends to be better than that of ligaments. For this reason, it is common to use a portion of the patella tendon to replace or reconstruct a torn anterior cruciate ligament (ACL). After repair, revascularization of the surgical tissue occurs up to 16 to 20 weeks, and by week 26 the revascularization response ceases.[6] Over time (when assessed at 52 and 104 weeks after repair), the tendon structure changes, and it appears physiologically more like the ACL ligament, with vascularity only noted at the bony ends.[6] Additionally, the tissue tends to demonstrate increased strength and mechanical properties more closely aligned with typical ACL presentation.[6]

Tendon healing is very complicated and depends on the actual tendon anatomy and shape (ie, the Achilles tendon is round, and rotator cuff tendons are flatter), the type of repair performed, and the function the tissue will perform. The physical therapy program must carefully take into account the fact that the recommended immobilization period (ie, bracing), although important for healing, may increase adhesion formation and joint stiffness. Overloading the tissues too soon can lead to reinjury or tendon repair failure.[5] Most physicians provide postoperative protocols and timelines for therapy interventions. These protocols are based on the type of repair and typical healing times for the repaired tissues and are focused on providing appropriate levels of stress to the healing tissues at the appropriate point in the healing process. Following the protocol should promote optimal healing and optimal integrity of the repaired tissue.

## Bone Healing

A **fracture** is defined as a disruption in bone continuity. Fractures range from a slight disruption as seen in a stress fracture to severe fractures resulting in several bony fragments. Fractures can occur due to experiencing an abrupt trauma, from overuse or repetitive overloading (ie, stress fractures), or they can be pathologic (ie, secondary to osteoporosis or cancer metastasis). Fractures are categorized as nondisplaced, displaced, or comminuted. In a nondisplaced fracture, the bone fragments remain aligned/in position. With displaced fractures, the bone segments are out of alignment. Comminuted fractures have more than 2 bony segments, but often multiple bony fragments can be present. Fractures are closed or open (compound). The bone ends pierce through the skin with compound/open fractures, and the skin remains intact with closed fractures.

Transverse or oblique fractures result from a forceful bending of a long bone (cortical bone) that breaks the shaft in half. Greenstick fractures are more common in children; the break does not fully separate the bone into 2 pieces. This fracture resembles the damage that occurs when a person tries to break a newly cut/fresh tree branch in half. The branch does not completely separate; rather, there is splintering because many fibers remain intact. Spiral fractures occur when a long bone is twisted. Avulsion fractures occur when a tendon or ligament is pulled away from its bony attachment. Compression fractures usually occur with crushing or compressing forces; these are a common cause of vertebral fractures.

Immediately after a fracture, bleeding occurs followed by clotting (hematoma formation); this process is part of the inflammatory phase of healing. The amount of bleeding that occurs depends on the severity of the fracture and the amount of soft tissue involvement and damage. The second phase of bone healing is called the *reparative phase*, and it lasts for several weeks after the initial fracture. During this phase, soft callus forms. This soft callus consists of chondroblasts and osteoblast cells. Chondroblasts create a cartilaginous callus, and osteoblast cells begin to form woven bone near the fracture site. The point in healing when the fracture site is considered stable (the bone ends do not move) is called *clinical union*. The remodeling phase begins once clinical union has occurred, and it continues as the callus becomes bony (hard callus). This hard callus is replaced with lamellar bone as the bone continues to heal. Complete fracture healing is called *radiologic union*. At that point, the callus is fully absorbed, and the bony callus is replaced by mature lamellar bone.

There are instances when fractures do not heal or when they heal abnormally. A nonunion fracture is a fracture that failed to heal. Nonunion may occur due to poor blood supply or because of too much movement between bone ends during the healing process. A nonunion fracture will require surgical intervention to repair the fracture. Delayed union describes fractures that take longer than typical to heal. Malunion fractures have healed in an undesirable position, often resulting in a bony deformity.

## Soft Tissue Phases of Healing

The physical therapist assistant must recognize the cardinal signs/symptoms of inflammation because inflammation can be an indication of the stage of injury/healing. The cardinal signs/symptoms of inflammation include swelling (edema), redness (rubor), heat (calor), loss of function, and pain (dolor) at rest. Inflammation decreases as the tissues move through the stages of healing. Interventions may be applied to reduce inflammation. Understanding the healing process is important because introducing a treatment intervention too early in the healing process or too aggressively can disrupt the healing process, prolong a patient's symptoms, and damage healing tissue.

After a structure sustains an injury or requires a surgical intervention, the tissue(s) progress through 3 phases of healing. Commonly, physical therapy practitioners will refer to these phases as they relate to the level of tissue protection indicated during the rehabilitation process. The acute or inflammatory phase of healing is also referred to as the *maximal protection phase*, the proliferation or subacute phase is referred to as the *moderate protection phase*, and the maturation/remodeling or chronic phase is considered the *minimal protection phase* or *return-to-function phase*.[3]

The general exercises included in this section target improving ROM, flexibility, or strength, with a focus on how implementation should pertain to stages of healing. Appendix A provides a template for problem-solving treatment interventions, with consideration of the stages of healing. Examples of these exercises are discussed in more detail in Chapters 4, 5, and 6 and the corresponding orthopedic chapters in Section II.

### Acute or Maximum Protective Phase

During the acute phase of healing, the body's initial and immediate response to an insult or injury (or surgical intervention) is an inflammatory response. This first step initiates the process to promote healing.[7] The physiologic tissue response during the acute phase includes an increase in blood flow, blood vessel permeability, edema, and white blood cells (leukocytes). The increase in blood cells and platelets sent to the injured area allows clotting to occur so that the bleeding stops. It is typical to observe redness, soft tissue swelling (or joint effusion), and heat. Pain is the fourth cardinal indicator of inflammation, but it cannot be observed, only reported subjectively by the patient. There is a decrease in function and mobility, and the patient typically reports experiencing pain at rest and may try to avoid moving the injured body part. This phase can last up to 4 to 7 days.

The treatment goals during this phase are to limit damage to the surrounding tissues from immobilization, promote healing, decrease inflammation/swelling, and decrease pain. Because this is the maximum protective phase of rehabilitation, the treatment interventions are protective of the healing process. Interventions may include joint protection, rest, ice, compression, and elevation; gentle joint mobilizations (Chapter 4); gentle pain-free passive motion; and patient education. Note that not all interventions will be appropriate; the selection and application must be based on the individual injury/presentation.

During the first 24 to 48 hours, rest, cold application, compression, and elevation are most effective at reducing pain and controlling the inflammatory response. Joint protection (promoting restricted weight bearing by using an assistive device, a splint/brace, or a cast) will also be beneficial immediately after the injury. After the first 24 to 48 hours and depending on the severity of the injury, passive movements to the involved joint in a pain-free range may be initiated to help maintain tissue and joint mobility. Passive motion frequency and rest periods must be gauged carefully because too much movement can exacerbate pain and swelling, but long periods of immobilization may increase muscle spasms/guarding, decrease tissue extensibility, decrease joint mobility, and increase the risk of motion-restricting scar tissue formation. Some patients can tolerate a few degrees of motion, and others may not tolerate any motion at all during this time. The incorporation of passive ROM is dependent on the injury type (ie, passive ROM will not be applied in the region of a new fracture or in the direction that stresses a newly injured tendon or ligament).

It is appropriate to educate the patient on indications, contraindications, and precautions and what to expect during this phase. The patient may be permitted to perform active range of motion (AROM) and/or light, limited resistance training to uninvolved joints. For example, if a patient had a rotator cuff repair and the shoulder is immobilized, active finger and wrist flexion and extension with the forearm supported are permitted. Gentle submaximal isometric (or muscle setting) exercises may be indicated for the surrounding stabilizing muscles to reduce muscle guarding and prevent atrophy. The physical therapist assistant will review the physical therapist's initial evaluation and plan of care (POC) and the physician protocol to verify which activities are indicated and which are contraindicated. The assistant can confirm which activities are indicated with the physical therapist before initiating these exercises.

The patient should be instructed on the proper techniques for cold application (the type and duration of application and contraindications to use), compression (monitor for signs of impaired circulation), body part elevation (above the heart), and donning/doffing/usage of orthoses (including splints/braces). The physical therapist assistant will ensure that the patient understands that if pain is experienced when performing an activity, the body is sending a message to stop; they should discontinue the activity and follow up with the physical therapist.

## Subacute or Moderate Protective Phase

As the swelling and pain decrease and the patient transitions into the subacute phase of healing (fibroblastic repair phase), some activity will be gradually increased. Capillaries and fibroblasts (cells that form collagen) form and replace the initial clotting material. This phase typically lasts less than 3 to 4 weeks. Typical presentation during this phase includes diminishing signs and symptoms of inflammation, minimal to no pain with active motion (except near or at the end of the available ROM), muscle weakness, and decreased function. During this phase, new collagen is produced and deposited, but the initial alignment of the fibers is random. The patient will begin to feel better; it is critical that the patient understand that overdoing it because they feel better can lead to increased injury because the new tissue repair is very fragile early during this phase. Better alignment of scar tissue formation will occur when safely controlled stresses are applied to healing tissues.

Active assisted ROM and/or AROM introduce gentle stresses to the healing tissues. These activities are appropriate to initiate during this phase to help healing tissue lay down collagen and elastin longitudinally in the direction of the stresses and in line with the surrounding healthy tissue fibers. It is often appropriate to initiate exercise in the end range of the patient's available AROM in a gravity-eliminated position. This enables the patient to gain additional ROM before progressing to motion against gravity.

Submaximal isometric contractions may be appropriate to initiate and can be performed at various angles as long as pain is not produced. This strengthening exercise can be progressed by having the patient increase the amount of muscle force (working toward a maximal isometric contraction) when performing the exercise. The likely progression from isometrics and AROM is to incorporate concentric and eccentric exercises based on patient tolerance. These activities are initially performed in one plane at slow speeds to allow the patient to better control the motions. Open kinetic chain exercises allow isolated joint motion and muscle control. Gentle stretching and massage can also introduce stress to the healing tissues, but these must be carefully controlled. All activities mentioned previously can be increased gradually in the later portion of this phase of healing as long as healing is progressing and the patient's symptoms do not increase.

The physical therapist assistant monitors the healing times of the involved tissues and the time that has passed from the injury; this, together with the patient's presentation/symptoms, informs decisions about when it is appropriate to increase the patient's exercise parameters or advance the program. The physical therapist assistant reviews the patient's goals and discusses any changes or additions to the goals and/or POC with the physical therapist before progressing the patient.

## Chronic or Minimal Protection/ Return-to-Function Phase

As healing progresses to the chronic phase (the maturation/remodeling phase), scar tissue begins to remodel, and the collagen becomes stronger and thicker. This phase can last from several months up to more than 1 year. This phase is characterized by no remaining signs of inflammation, and the patient may present with contractures or adhesions. Muscle weakness may be present. At the beginning of this phase, the patient may feel pain but typically only at the end of the ROM or with stretching. The patient may present with poor endurance and decreased neuromuscular control. The primary goal in this phase is to optimize tissue function so that the patient can return to their prior level of function. It is critical to remember that the tissue is not fully healed, but it can tolerate a gradual increase in progressive loading until it achieves normal function and significantly less pain toward the end of this phase.

The patient's pain is typically associated with residual muscle weakness and/or joint limitations, so interventions in this phase often include multiplanar AROM and resistance strengthening to address muscle weakness and endurance issues, gentle progressive stretching to address end-range limitations, and static/dynamic balance and coordination activities to improve neuromuscular control. Patient education in this phase includes education regarding safe and appropriate progressions, the importance of rest between exercise sessions, the use of ice as needed, and activity modification to prevent reinjury.

Progression to dynamic closed kinetic chain exercises and high-speed functional training (ie, plyometrics) are appropriate once the patient has normal strength and ROM, does not experience an increase in symptoms, and has been cleared for progression. Research indicates that the use of eccentric exercises may be significantly more effective at increasing strength and promoting return to function compared with other interventions when treating patients with tendon injuries (tendinopathies).[8] High-intensity exercises are implemented at the very end of this phase if the patient is preparing to return to sport. These exercises will not be appropriate or included for all patients.

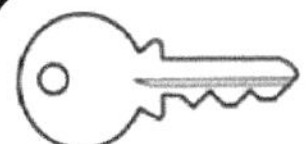

### Key Safety Considerations

- "No pain, no gain" is not an acceptable thought process and can create further injury.
- To prevent reinjury, knowledge of specific tissue healing times is critical when progressing a patient's exercise program.
- The goal of treatment is to challenge the patient's healing tissues (to promote adaptation) without causing further injury.

## Prehabilitation Before Surgery

Many health care practitioners have anecdotal experience that supports the use of preadmission physical therapy, education, and exercise (referred to as **prehabilitation**) to improve patients' health and fitness before an elective surgical procedure. Many patients undergo surgery to correct or reduce disease or orthopedic impairments (ie, hip or knee arthroplasty), but patients are at risk during the postoperative recovery period for a decrease in function, deep vein thrombosis (DVT), and pulmonary issues (atelectasis and pneumonia). Prehabilitation programs include supervised preoperative exercises, a review of the postoperative precautions/restrictions, proper fitting and use of an assistive device, safe bed mobility and transfer training instruction, and postoperative exercises to reduce postoperative complications, decrease the length of hospital stay, and improve patient recovery.

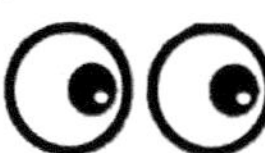

### Eye on the Research

Several studies have examined the benefits of a prehabilitation program for a number of surgical interventions. One study reported that a 6-week presurgical exercise program improved preoperative functional status and muscle strength levels in people scheduled to have total hip arthroplasty.[9] Participation in a preoperative exercise program significantly lowered the percentage of patients requiring inpatient rehabilitation before discharge home.[9]

Researchers are reviewing the potential benefits of prehabilitation for other surgical candidates. Mayo et al[10] determined that patients who had colorectal surgery who demonstrated meaningful changes in functional capacity over several weeks of prehabilitation were more likely to have recovered to their baseline walking capacity postoperatively compared with those who did not improve during the prehabilitation period. For patients undergoing colorectal resection for cancer, a higher proportion of the group who received prehabilitation recovered to (or above) baseline exercise capacity at 8 weeks compared with the group who only received rehabilitation after surgery.[11] The inclusion of a prehabilitation program for persons scheduled for intra-abdominal surgery was successful in decreasing the incidence of postoperative complications.[12]

In a large systematic review, researchers noted that the inclusion of prehabilitation was beneficial in decreasing postoperative pain, length of stay, and physical function but that prehabilitation was not consistently associated with improved health-related quality of life or cardiorespiratory fitness in those studies that examined these outcomes.[13] Some studies did not find significant improvements in patients' functional status but noted improvements measured by decreases in postoperative length of hospital stay or a decreased need for an acute rehabilitation stay.[13-15] These results may indicate that the inclusion of a prehabilitation program can present opportunities to save limited health care resources.

## Types of Surgical Interventions

Surgical procedures are indicated for patients if the injury or condition is so severe that physical therapy intervention is not an option or when physical therapy does not produce the desired results to improve function and reduce pain. There are numerous common orthopedic surgical procedures the physical therapist assistant may encounter when treating patients in any setting. Surgeries are performed to repair a structure (ie, a tendon or cartilage), remove part or all of a structure (ie, meniscus or lamina), reconstruct or replace a structure (ie, ACL reconstruction or hip replacement), realign or stabilize a joint or structure (ie, tighten the shoulder capsule or straighten the tibia), decompress a joint (ie, to create more space in the subacromial area), release a structure (ie, slit the fascia to release the muscles in the anterior compartment of the lower leg), or fuse or fix bony structures (ie, spinal fusion or fracture repair using plates and screws).

### Question for Thought

Do you know what these suffixes mean?

- -otomy: Making an incision (fasciotomy)
- -ectomy: Removing a structure (meniscectomy and laminectomy)
- -plasty: Reshaping or repairing or restoring a structure (chondroplasty and arthroplasty)

Familiarity with these suffixes is useful in understanding the type of surgical procedure.

The type of incision/surgical approach is used to describe surgical procedures. A large and deep incision is made during an open procedure so the surgeon can see and expose an entire area/joint. This type of procedure is most commonly used for total hip and knee arthroplasties. Arthroscopy is a minimally invasive surgical procedure in which several small incisions are made, allowing the surgeon to use special surgical tools and a camera to view and repair/remove structures in a joint. This procedure is commonly used in shoulders (ie, to repair rotator cuff tendons or decompress the subacromial space) and knees (ie, to repair ligaments or repair/remove part of a meniscus). The combination of arthroscopy and an open procedure is called a *mini-open procedure*. Rotator cuff repair procedures have been moving from mini-open to fully arthroscopic procedures as techniques and surgical outcomes continue to improve.[16]

## Common Orthopedic Surgical Procedures

Surgical procedures are used to repair tissues and bones. When a surgeon is replacing or reconstructing a ligament because the torn ends are unable to be approximated, a graft is used to stabilize the joint. There are 3 types of grafts used to replace ligaments. The ACL is commonly repaired by using an autograft or allograft. An **autograft** is tissue that is taken from one part of the patient and used elsewhere. Taking a part of the patient's patella tendon and inserting that tissue to replace the ACL is a common surgical procedure. An **allograft** is tissue that is taken from another donor (commonly a cadaver) and used to replace the damaged ligament. Allografts are the most commonly used grafts, and many surgeons prefer to use allografts or autografts vs synthetic grafts. Synthetic grafts are artificial ligaments; they tend to have a higher failure rate over time.[17]

Some fractures require surgical interventions and/or implants to stabilize bone fragments.[1] This procedure is called *open reduction and internal fixation*, and it is commonly used to stabilize wrist, hip, and tibia/fibula fractures. During the procedure, a surgeon may use metal rods, plates, pins, nails, and/or screws to align and secure the bony pieces to promote effective healing (Figure 3-1).

Hip, knee, and shoulder **arthroplasties** are performed to relieve pain and improve function for patients with severe arthritis or fractures; these are usually performed via an open procedure. Resurfacing is a less involved joint replacement procedure. During resurfacing, the surgeon trims the joint surface and caps the joint surface with a smooth metal covering. Joint repair can include resurfacing one or both articular surfaces of the bone(s) that form the joint. Another type of arthroplasty includes resecting the bone end(s) and then replacing them with implants on one (hemiarthroplasty) or both surfaces (total arthroplasty) to reshape the joint (Figure 3-2). One study determined that a total shoulder arthroplasty provided significantly better pain relief than a hemiarthroplasty in patients with shoulder osteoarthritis.[18]

The components used in joint replacements are either uncemented or cemented (using an acrylic type of cement). An uncemented component has a rough/porous surface that encourages natural bone to attach to secure the implant over time. A meta-analysis study reported that cemented total hip replacements performed better and longer than uncemented implants; however, the investigators noted that uncemented implant performance was improving.[19] The type of joint prosthetic (cemented vs uncemented) may affect the weight-bearing status that a physician prescribes for a patient postoperatively. The clinician will review weight-bearing orders in the postoperative physician orders.

A joint fusion or **arthrodesis** stabilizes an unstable or lax joint, and the fusion may be performed to reduce severe joint pain. This procedure is indicated when joint arthroplasties have failed and/or when the structures surrounding an unstable joint cannot provide adequate support. This procedure often results in a loss of function and mobility because of the decreased ROM at the fused joint. Arthrodesis is often a last-resort intervention because stabilizing one joint/segment leads to compensatory hypermobility at other joints/segments in the region, creating additional stresses on the body. Spinal fusion is an arthrodesis in the spine (more common in the cervical or lumbar region). The segments are often held together using a bony autograft (often harvested from the iliac crest) and screws, rods, and/or wires to stabilize the vertebrae and eliminate motion (Figure 3-3).

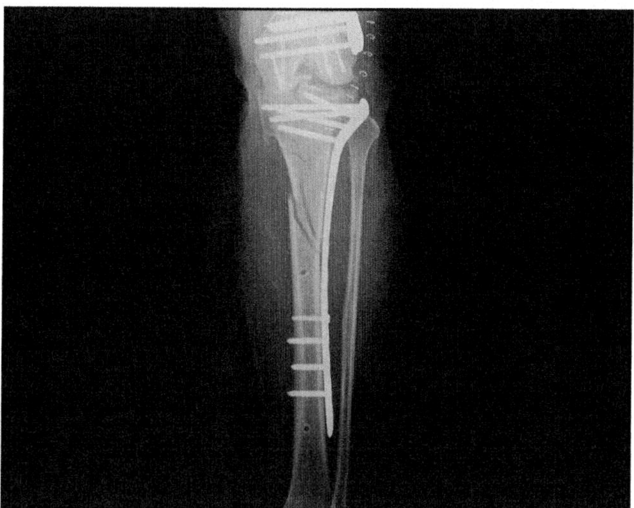

**Figure 3-1.** A photo of a distal femur and tibia fracture with open reduction and internal fixation (Yok_onepiece/Shutterstock.com).

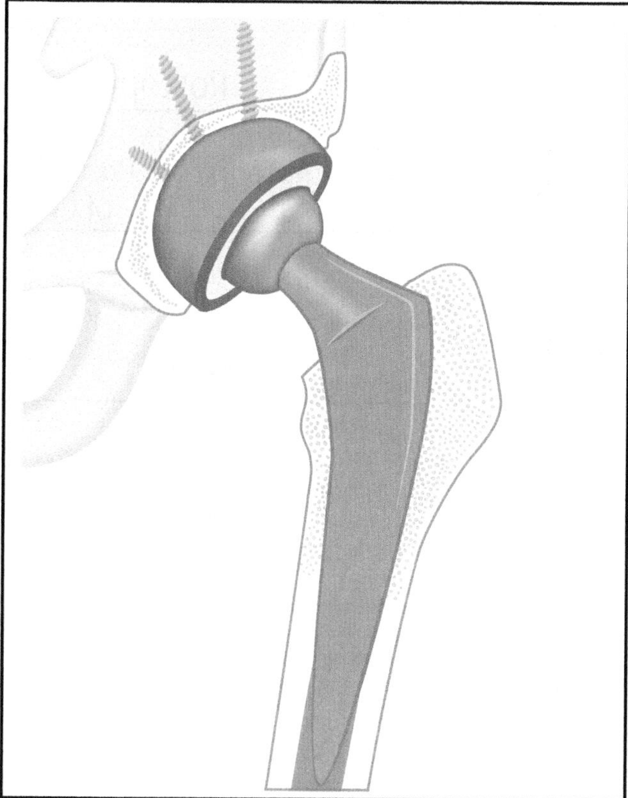

**Figure 3-2.** A photo of total hip arthroplasty (Aksanaku/Shutterstock.com).

Arthroscopic debridement is a procedure used to remove damaged cartilage or bone. This procedure is considered when a patient complains of significant pain, clicking, or catching in a joint when the patient moves. The shoulder and knee joints are commonly affected. The surgeon flushes out the joint to rid any debris floating in the joint (called *joint lavage*) and then surgically removes any fragments or rough areas that remain on the joint surfaces.

## *Postoperative Complications*

Physical therapist assistants should monitor patients for postoperative complications after all surgical procedures. Changes in patient presentation may indicate a change in medical status. Signs and symptoms due to complications can occur days, weeks, or months after the initial surgical intervention, so ongoing monitoring is essential. Prompt recognition and reporting of postoperative complications are imperative. This ensures that the patient receives timely and appropriate medical care.

Common postoperative complications that are more prevalent within the days/weeks postoperatively include atelectasis, infection, pneumonia, pulmonary embolism, and DVT. Many of these complications are associated with decreased mobility (ie, bed rest and venous stasis). Atelectasis (collapse of part of the lung tissue) is more common in patients after upper abdominal or thoracic surgeries. The risk of developing a DVT increases based on the surgical procedure, the presence of pelvic or lower extremity fractures, increased age, the use of oral contraception, cancer, and hereditary thrombotic disorders.[20] A DVT is the most common cause of a pulmonary embolism. Patients who have total knee or hip arthroplasties may be at greater risk for DVTs and pulmonary embolisms, so the physical therapist assistant must be able to recognize the signs and symptoms of all postoperative complications (Table 3-4). If a patient has a small pulmonary embolism, signs or symptoms may not be present. A large pulmonary embolism can be life-threatening. The clinician should review the patient's symptoms and presentation and then apply Wells' criteria to assess for the likelihood of a DVT or pulmonary embolism (refer to the Suggested Resources section at the end of the chapter for the DVT/pulmonary embolism risk calculator links). All findings should be reported to the medical team immediately.

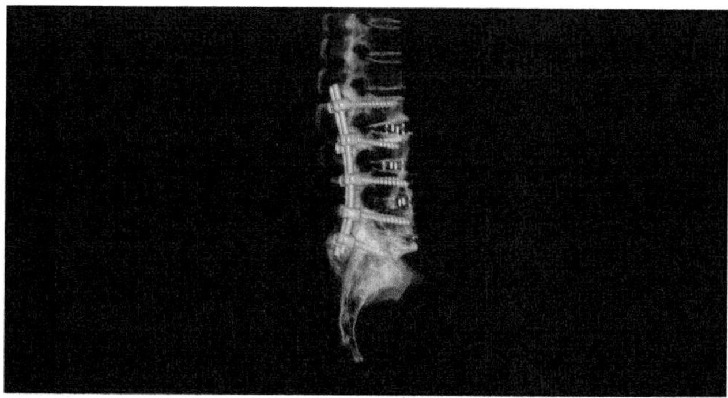

**Figure 3-3.** Lumbar fusion using screws and a rod. A computed tomography image of the spine showing pedicle screw fixation and decompression surgery in a patient with spinal canal stenosis (Yok_onepiece/Shutterstock.com).

**Table 3-4**

Postoperative Complications[a]

| Complications | Signs or Symptoms | Interventions to Promote Prevention of Complications | Time Frame of Occurrence | Action Step[a] |
|---|---|---|---|---|
| Atelectasis or pneumonia | Dyspnea, tachypnea, cyanosis, possible crackles, low oxygen saturation | Deep breathing exercises; standing and ambulation initiated as early as possible postoperatively | Early | Alert medical team immediately |
| Pulmonary embolism | Dyspnea, chest pain, cough, tachypnea (> 20 breaths/minute), crackles | Early ambulation/mobility, DVT prevention, careful monitoring of vital signs, monitoring for symptoms (can use Wells' criteria for pulmonary embolism) | Early/life-threatening | Initiate facility emergency response process, be prepared to initiate CPR, notify physician |
| DVT | Dull ache, tightness, pain and/or swelling (pitting edema) in the calf, increased leg/ankle skin temperature; may be asymptomatic<br>Presence of lower extremity DVT increases risk of developing a pulmonary embolism | Complete ankle pumps often, intermittent pneumatic compression, early ambulation, elevate legs when supine or seated, compression hose<br>Avoid: crossing legs, prolonged sitting/standing.<br>If patient complains of leg pain, do not massage legs.<br>Monitor for symptoms (use Wells' criteria for DVT) | Early/life-threatening | Notify physician/medical team immediately; stop therapy pending medical follow-up |
| Infection (local or systemic) | Pain/stiffness in a replaced joint that was functioning normally, swelling, warmth and redness around a joint/wound or drainage, fever, chills, night sweats | Requires physician referral and immediate care | Early/life-threatening (systemic) | Notify physician/medical team immediately; stop therapy pending medical follow-up |
| Loosening or failure of implants | Femoral pain (stem implant), groin or buttocks pain (acetabulum implant), pain with activity that goes away with rest | Requires physician referral and immediate care | Late | Notify supervising physical therapist and physician |

[a]The physical therapist assistant should complete necessary steps to maintain patient safety. The decision to initiate emergency medical response vs notifying supervising physical therapist, physician, or medical team member is based on the acuity of the presentation.
CPR = cardiopulmonary resuscitation.

Bacterial infections are less common, but they can occur days/weeks after the surgery or years later. Infections can occur in and around wounds or around implants. Signs and symptoms of infection can include redness, warmth, purulent wound discharge or odor, pain, and fever. If the infection affects the implant, a surgical intervention to remove it and place a joint spacer within the joint is performed. The patient will receive intravenous antibiotics for at least 6 weeks. Once the infection is resolved, the surgeon will perform a total joint revision (with a new implant).

Joint arthroplasty components can loosen over time. The most common cause of joint replacement loosening is related to wear on the implant surfaces, which weakens the surrounding bone. Osteolysis is the progressive destruction of bone surrounding the implant. The surrounding tissues may become irritated as the bone weakens and the implant shifts or moves. Investigators report the highest likelihood of loosening with cemented components, with loosening more likely for men, those who are overweight (greater than 25 kg/m$^2$), and younger patients. This may be due to the higher activity levels of these patients.[21] An additional sign associated with a hip component loosening may include the surgical leg being shorter and externally rotated compared with the nonsurgical limb.

After surgery, the incision is surgically closed. In typical healing, new collagen fibers form to mend the damage, which results in scar formation. Scar development is a normal step in the healing process after the dermis is disrupted. Abnormal scar formation is a complication that can result in regional restrictions of ROM and function. Hypertrophic scars are raised scars that develop within the borders of the incision or injury. Keloid scars are thick, raised scars that extend beyond the border of the incision or wound.

The physical therapist assistant should continually monitor each patient during each session to ensure patient safety. When changes in the patient's symptoms or presentation are present, the assistant should determine the necessary steps to take next. The decision to notify the supervising physical therapist, physician, or medical team member is based on the acuity of the presentation.

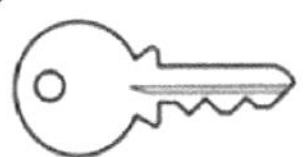

**Key Safety Considerations: The Postoperative Patient**

- Monitor vital signs.
- Monitor for any shortness of breath.
- Monitor for postoperative complications, including DVT.
- Monitor incision for signs/symptoms of infection.

## Conclusion

The physical therapist assistant is an integral member of the rehabilitation team. While working under the supervision of the physical therapist and within the therapist's POC, the assistant selects, implements, and advances therapeutic interventions. Understanding the physiology of healing allows the clinician to select appropriate interventions. Knowledge of common surgical techniques and complications guides the clinician in the development of appropriate treatment plans and the selection of the most appropriate patient monitoring to maintain patient safety.

## Review Questions

1. What is the correct term for degeneration of a tendon due to repetitive microtrauma without an inflammatory response?
2. A patient fell going down the stairs and reports hyperextending the left wrist. The patient reports moderate pain that increases with active movement. The physical therapist assistant observes visible localized swelling and some strength loss, and the patient's pain is greatly increased during passive stretching. Which grade of sprain/strain is this presentation most consistent with?
3. Which interventions are most appropriate during the inflammatory phase of healing?
4. Compare and contrast radiologic union and clinical union.
5. What education should the assistant provide to a patient to decrease the chance for postoperative complications?
6. List 3 therapy interventions that are appropriate to include in the minimal protection/return-to-function phase of healing.
7. List 2 advantages of participating in a prehabilitation program.
8. Describe the differences between an autograft and allograft.
9. List 3 risk factors for the development of DVT or pulmonary embolism.
10. Compare and contrast the healing times for muscles, tendons, ligaments, and bones.

## Suggested Resources

Wells P. Wells' criteria for DVT. MDCALC. Accessed January 24, 2023. https://www.mdcalc.com/wells-criteria-dvt

Wells P. Wells' criteria for pulmonary embolism. MDCALC. Accessed January 24, 2023. https://www.mdcalc.com/wells-criteria-pulmonary-embolism

# References


1. Brody LT. Soft-tissue and postoperative management. In: Brody LT, Hall CM, eds. *Therapeutic Exercise Moving Toward Function*. 4th ed. Wolters Kluwer; 2018:282-312.
2. Walsh W, ed. *Repair and Regeneration of Ligaments, Tendons, and Joint Capsule*. Humana Press; 2006.
3. Kisner C. Soft tissue injury, repair and management. In: Kisner C, Colby LA, Borstad J, eds. *Therapeutic Exercise Foundations and Techniques*. 7th ed. FA Davis; 2018:321-335.
4. Hauser RA, Dolan EE. Ligament injury and healing: an overview of current clinical concepts. *J Prolother.* 2011;3(4):836-846.
5. Thomopoulos S, Parks WC, Rifkin DB, Derwin KA. Mechanisms of tendon injury and repair. *J Orthop Res.* 2015;33(6):832-839. doi:10.1002/jor.22806
6. Fenwick SA, Hazleman BL, Riley GP. The vasculature and its role in the damaged and healing tendon. *Arthritis Res.* 2002;4(4):252-260. doi:10.1186/ar416
7. Moini J. *Anatomy and Physiology for Health Professionals*. 2nd ed. Jones and Bartlett Learning; 2016:84-100.
8. Woodley BL, Newsham-West RJ, Baxter GD. Chronic tendinopathy: effectiveness of eccentric exercise. *Br J Sports Med.* 2007;41:188-198. doi:10.1136/bjsm.2006.029769
9. Rooks DS, Huang J, Bierbaum BE, et al. Effect of preoperative exercise on measures of functional status in men and women undergoing total hip and knee arthroplasty. *Arthritis Rheum*. 2006;55(5):700-708. doi:10.1002/art.22223
10. Mayo N, Feldman L, Scott S, et al. Impact of preoperative change in physical function on postoperative recovery: argument supporting prehabilitation for colorectal surgery. *Surgery*. 2011;150(3):505-514.
11. Gillis C, Li C, Lee L, et al. Prehabilitation versus rehabilitation: a randomized control trial in patients undergoing colorectal resection for cancer. *Anesthesiology*. 2014;121(5):937-947.
12. Moran J, Guinan E, McCormick P. The ability of prehabilitation to influence postoperative outcome after intra-abdominal operation: a systematic review and meta-analysis. *Surgery*. 2016;160(5):1189-1201. doi:10.1016/j.surg.2016.05.014
13. Santa Mina D, Clarke H, Ritvo P, et al. Effect of total-body prehabilitation on postoperative outcomes: a systematic review and meta-analysis. *Physiotherapy*. 2014;100(3):196-207. doi:10.1016/j.physio.2013.08.008
14. Snow R, Granata J, Ruhil AV, et al. Associations between preoperative physical therapy and post-acute care utilization patterns and cost in total joint replacement. *J Bone Joint Surg Am*. 2014;96(19):e165.
15. Cabilan CJ, Hines S, Munday J. The effectiveness of prehabilitation or preoperative exercise for surgical patients: a systematic review. *JBI Database System Rev Implement Rep.* 2015;13(1):146-187. doi:10.11124/jbisrir-2015-1885
16. Ghodadra NS, Provencher MT, Verma NN, Wilk KE, Romeo AA. Open, mini-open, and all-arthroscopic rotator cuff repair surgery: indications and implications for rehabilitation. *J Orthop Sports Phys Ther.* 2009;39(2):81-89. doi:10.2519/jospt.2009.2918
17. Colby LA, Borstad J. Surgical interventions and postoperative management. In: Kisner C, Colby LA, Borstad J, eds. *Therapeutic Exercise Foundations and Techniques*. 7th ed. FA Davis; 2018:359-381.
18. Gartsman GM, Roddey TS, Hammerman SM. Shoulder arthroplasty with or without resurfacing of the glenoid in patients who have osteoarthritis. *J Bone Joint Surg Am.* 2000;82(1):26-34.
19. Morshed S, Bozic KJ, Ries MD, Malchau H, MColford J Jr. Comparison of cemented and uncemented fixation in total hip replacement. *Acta Orthop*. 2007;78(3):315-326. doi:10.1080/17453670710013861
20. Packel L. The respiratory system. In: Goodman CC, Fuller KS, eds. *Pathophysiology Implications for the Physical Therapist*. 4th ed. Elsevier; 2015:832-853.
21. Melloh M, Eggli S, Busato A, Rode C. Predictors of early stem loosening after total hip arthroplasty: a case-control study. *J Orthop Surg (Hong Kong)*. 2011;19(3):269-277. doi:10.1177/230949901101900301

Chapter 4

# Range of Motion and Manual Therapy Techniques

*Jacki Klaczak Kopack, PT, DPT and Karen A. Cascardi, PhD, MS, ATC, PTA*

**KEY TERMS** Active insufficiency | Capsular patterns | Closed-pack position | Contractures | Open-packed position | Passive insufficiency

## Chapter Objectives

1. Explain the types of range of motion (ROM).
2. Describe the continuum of mobility (hypomobility through hypermobility).
3. Identify physiologic factors that can impact available ROM.
4. Compare and contrast joint ROM vs muscle excursion.
5. List normative ROM values for each joint motion.
6. Explain active and passive insufficiency.
7. Differentiate normal and abnormal types of end feels.
8. Explain the indications, precautions, and contraindications for each type of ROM.
9. Describe the different types of manual therapy and their indications/contraindications.
10. Define joint mobilization and describe mobilization grades.
11. Given a case scenario, determine the most appropriate type of ROM program intervention.

For individuals to perform functional activities and mobility tasks, joints must move without restrictions, and the soft tissue must exhibit typical extensibility and contractile characteristics. ROM is defined as the amount of motion available in a given joint. ROM is measured using a goniometer, and restrictions in structures surrounding and/or within the joint (ie, joint capsule, articular cartilage, fibrocartilage, muscles, connective tissue, fascia, ligaments, blood vessels, nerves, and synovial fluid) can affect the range. These restrictions can lead to ROM limitations, reducing a person's ability to complete desired tasks/activities. Osteokinematics are the normal movements that occur between bones. Arthrokinematics refers to the motions that occur between joint surfaces (roll, spin, and glide) that allow normal joint motion. To achieve full, normal ROM against gravity, there must be normal arthrokinematics and osteokinematics, adequate soft tissue length, and appropriate muscle strength and coordination.

Clinicians can determine if ROM limitation is due to joint restriction(s) or a lack of musculotendinous extensibility. Muscle excursion or functional excursion is the measurable distance of a muscle from a maximal shortening



Kopack JK, Cascardi KA. *Principles of Therapeutic Exercise for the Physical Therapist Assistant* (pp 43-62).

to a maximal stretch. The amount of muscle excursion affects the available ROM in the joint(s) that the muscles cross. Muscle excursion is dependent on fiber arrangement and the number of joints the muscle crosses. Parallel muscle fiber alignment allows for the greatest amount of range/excursion compared with other fiber arrangements. Muscles that cross 2 or more joints (ie, the gastrocnemius) allow for greater muscle excursion compared with one-joint muscles (ie, soleus). When a muscle that crosses 2 or more joints (a 2-joint/multijoint muscle) contracts, the muscle will produce less tension when contracting across 2 joints compared with when it contracts and moves across only one joint. **Active insufficiency** occurs when a 2-joint or multijoint muscle agonist cannot complete full active motion at one joint when it is fully shortening (contracting) simultaneously over the second joint. **Passive insufficiency** occurs when a 2-joint muscle cannot be lengthened (stretched) simultaneously across both joints, which results in reduced ROM at each joint. As the muscle is stretched simultaneously across both joints, ROM at either joint is limited by the muscle's excursion.

ROM limitations can be a result of pathology affecting the joints (ie, osteoarthritis or ankylosing spondylosis), muscle tightness, spasticity, immobilization, lack of use, injury (ie, strains or sprains), or large muscle mass/muscle hypertrophy. Connective tissue changes occur during aging; there is a decrease in tissue composition and pliability in connective tissue structures, which can result in decreases in ROM.[1] Elbow and knee flexion are examples of joint motions in which the end ROM is limited by the bulk of the muscle mass of the biceps brachii and hamstrings/gastrocnemius, respectively. When soft tissue approximation limits the normal ROM, the joint end feel is a soft end feel.

ROM measurements are used to quantify joint movement. Active range of motion (AROM) and passive range of motion (PROM) are often measured during the physical therapy initial evaluation. When PROM and AROM are equally limited in one direction, this is often indicative of muscle guarding, tightness, or contractures. When the available PROM is greater than AROM, this is probably caused by muscle weakness. The amount of motion typically expected at a specific joint is called a *normative value*. Each joint and its respective available motion have been documented by several organizations; this text uses the American Academy of Orthopedic Surgeons values as a reference (Table 4-1).[2] The reader is referred to goniometry textbooks for in-depth information related to age- and sex-related variations in ROM normative values. It is important to observe the quality and quantity of the motion when measuring AROM. Physical therapist assistants should note if the movement is smooth and full (or complete) and if there is hesitation, difficulty, facial grimacing, or reports of pain during the motion. There may be audible sounds (ie, grinding or creaking) called *crepitus* as the joint surfaces move.

Patients may experience pain when moving joints through a range. Decreased quality in ROM, the presence of a painful arc, or hesitation when completing the range can occur for a variety of clinical reasons, including joint instability, muscle weakness, soft tissue guarding/inflexibility, inflammation, and/or arthritis. Observing, measuring, and documenting the quality and quantity of the motion accurately are important to track the patient's progress. Observing the quality/quantity of ROM provides necessary information that the physical therapist uses to develop an appropriate plan of care (POC) for the patient and that the assistant can use to guide intervention selection.

Excessive ROM beyond physiologic limits can be a cause of pain or dysfunction. Joint *hypermobility* is defined as ROM greater than the normative values. Hypermobility may not always be a concern as long as the increased mobility is paired with adequate muscle control, and it does not create harmful changes in joint biomechanics or pain. Instability can occur when hypermobility is paired with a lack of muscle control and/or joint laxity, increasing the risk of injury.

ROM occurs along a continuum, with hypermobility at one extreme and hypomobility and/or full loss of ROM at the other extreme. Hypomobility is motion that is less than the normative value for a given joint. There are numerous causes of hypomobility, including muscle tightness, adaptive shortening, contractures, and/or adhesions. Bone, joint, or soft tissue injury and/or surgical interventions and nonorthopedic surgical procedures (ie, cancer surgeries) can also result in hypomobility. Immobilization, which is often indicated to allow for structural healing (ie, bone fractures), and prolonged immobility (ie, bed rest) often result in a loss of ROM and an increased risk of adhesions and/or contracture formation, muscle atrophy, and slowed/sluggish circulation (due to decreased localized muscle pumping activity). Paralysis (due to spinal cord injury or stroke), joint diseases (eg, rheumatoid or osteoarthritis, ankylosing spondylitis, and adhesive capsulitis), and pain can result in ROM restrictions.

Muscle tightness or adaptive shortening can result from immobilizing a joint for several weeks. Immobilization in a long arm cast after a Colles fracture (distal radius fracture) typically occurs with the elbow positioned in about 80 degrees of flexion, which is a shortened position for the elbow flexors. Once the cast is removed, the patient may have difficulty extending the elbow due to the elbow flexors being positioned in this shortened state for a prolonged time. This is accompanied by stiffness and/or tightness that may be resistant to PROM when initially attempting to mobilize the elbow joint into extension. Adaptive shortening can also occur in patients with poor or faulty posture. When a patient assumes a forward head posture and rounded shoulders, the posterior trunk muscles (the rhomboid and middle trapezius muscles) become overstretched, and the anterior muscles (the pectoralis major and sternocleidomastoid muscles) become adaptively

**Table 4-1**

Normative Range of Motion Values According to the American Academy of Orthopedic Surgeons[2]

| Joint | Motion/Available Range of Motion (Degrees) | Joint | Motion/Available Range of Motion (Degrees) |
|---|---|---|---|
| Shoulder | Flexion = 0 to 180<br>Extension = 0 to 60<br>Abduction = 0 to 180<br>Adduction = 90 to 0<br>Internal rotation = 0 to 70<br>External rotation = 0 to 90 | Hip | Flexion = 0 to 120<br>Extension = 0 to 30<br>Abduction = 0 to 45<br>Adduction = 0 to 30<br>Internal rotation = 0 to 45<br>External rotation = 0 to 45 |
| Elbow | Flexion = 0 to 150<br>Extension = 150 to 0 | Knee | Flexion = 0 to 135<br>Extension = 135 to 0 |
| Forearm | Supination = 0 to 80<br>Pronation = 0 to 80 | Ankle | Dorsiflexion = 0 to 20<br>Plantar flexion = 0 to 50<br>Inversion = 0 to 35<br>Eversion = 0 to 15 |
| Wrist | Flexion = 0 to 80<br>Extension = 0 to 70<br>Radial deviation = 0 to 20<br>Ulnar deviation = 0 to 30 | | |
| Thumb | CMC flexion = 0 to 15<br>CMC abduction = 0 to 70<br>MCP extension/flexion = 0 to 50<br>Interphalangeal extension/flexion = 0 to 80 | Cervical spine | Flexion = 0 to 45<br>Extension = 0 to 45<br>Lateral bending = 0 to 45<br>Rotation = 0 to 60 |
| Fingers | MCP flexion = 0 to 90<br>MCP extension = 0 to 45<br>Proximal interphalangeal extension/flexion = 0 to 110<br>Distal interphalangeal extension/flexion = 0 to 90 | Lumbar spine | Flexion = 0 to 80<br>Extension = 0 to 25<br>Lateral bending = 0 to 35<br>Rotation = 0 to 45 |

CMC = carpometacarpal; MCP = metacarpophalangeal.

shortened. **Contractures** occur when the muscles and soft tissues shorten and become more fibrotic. This is often a result of increased tone and/or prolonged patient positioning in one posture or joint position. Contractures create high resistance to ROM and stretch, preventing the ability to achieve full motion at the joint(s). The formation of dense scar tissue or adhesions can occur because of injury, immobilization, or as a result of inadequate postoperative care, creating limitations in ROM. When adhesions develop between muscles and connective tissue (most commonly the fascia), ROM will be limited and very painful at the end of the patient's restricted available range. If a joint develops adhesions, the surgeon may perform a manipulation under anesthesia to help restore normal ROM.

### Clinical Tip

The physical therapist will screen all joints above and below the involved joint. Often, if motion at the involved joint is restricted, one or more of the surrounding joints may become hypermobile to allow for compensatory functional motion. This increase in mobility at the surrounding joint(s) may affect their normal biomechanics, predisposing the patient to future injuries or clinical issues. Effective treatment interventions will increase mobility at the restricted joints and increase stability at the surrounding hypermobile joints. The assistant should inform the supervising therapist of any adverse changes in ROM.

**Table 4-2**

**Impact of Immobilization Versus Tissue Mobilization for Various Tissues[3]**

| Tissue | Impact of Immobilization | Effect of Active Movement/ Mobilization of Affected Joint |
|---|---|---|
| Muscle | Muscle fiber atrophy<br>Loss of muscle mass<br>Deterioration in motor unit recruitment<br>Increased connective tissue and fat deposits | Gradual mobilization and use of full ROM activities over a prolonged period will promote restoration of muscle function |
| Tendon | Decreased number/size of collagen fibers<br>Decreased load tolerance<br>Decreased tensile strength<br>Collagen more disorganized | Gradual mobilization with controlled stress will increase tensile strength and minimize excessive scar formation (more organized collagen formation) |
| Ligament | Decreased collagen mass and strength<br>Decreased amount of load to failure<br>Ligament shortening<br>Increased ligament and joint stiffness and increased risk of avulsion<br>Bony resorption at attachment site | Gradual mobilization with controlled stress restores mechanical properties (may take longer than immobilization time) |
| Cartilage | Increased water content<br>Decreased cartilage thickness and stiffness<br>Collagen fiber splitting<br>Osteophyte development | Inappropriate and/or early loading postimmobilization can increase joint damage<br>Enhances synovial fluid movement |
| Bone | Decreased bone mass, synthesis, and trabecular bone volume | Effect of mobility depends on overall bone integrity<br>For otherwise healthy bone, controlled stress (resisted exercise, weight bearing) enhances bone health |

## Selecting Range of Motion Exercises

The primary purposes for performing ROM exercises include promoting soft tissue and joint mobility/flexibility and preventing the effects of immobilization (ie, adhesions, contractures, and atrophy). To maintain ROM, the joint and surrounding soft tissue structures must be moved through the available range regularly.

Selecting the type of ROM exercise depends on several factors, such as the phase of healing, the types/amount of tissues involved, the type/severity/complexity of injury and/or surgical repair, and the length of time a body part was immobilized. The impact of immobilization on various structures is listed in Table 4-2. Clinicians must determine if the ROM limitation is caused by joint restrictions, a lack of musculotendinous muscle excursion, or both. After a surgical repair, the type of ROM permitted may be driven by the physician's postoperative protocol.

In cases in which a patient is immobilized, a carefully controlled passive motion program may be initiated as long as the fracture site is stable (ie, plates, screws, or pins) and/or the soft tissue is securely repaired. The physician determines if ROM interventions are indicated based on several factors (ie, the severity of injury or repair, age, tissue health, and blood supply availability). If immobilization is prescribed, a carefully dosed plan for ROM activities for the joints above and below the immobilized area will be important to reduce the effects of immobilization on other joints and to promote the patient's ability to return to their prior function. Injury, immobilization, muscle guarding, and pain can lead to a self-perpetuating cycle of disability (Figure 4-1).

**Clinical Tip**

After immobilization, note that any surrounding structures that were also immobilized will be affected. The timing and dosage of ROM activities are critical to maximize the quality of healing tissues and to promote return to normal ROM and mobility.

ROM exercises create joint motion, which places tension on the surrounding tissues of the joint regardless of the type of ROM exercise. This tension (or load) can assist in maintaining the structural integrity of the soft tissues around the joint. The amount of tension/load varies with each type of ROM. The different types of ROM exercises a clinician can use include PROM, active assisted range of motion (AAROM), and AROM. There are indications, contraindications, precautions, limitations, and applications for each type of ROM (Table 4-3).

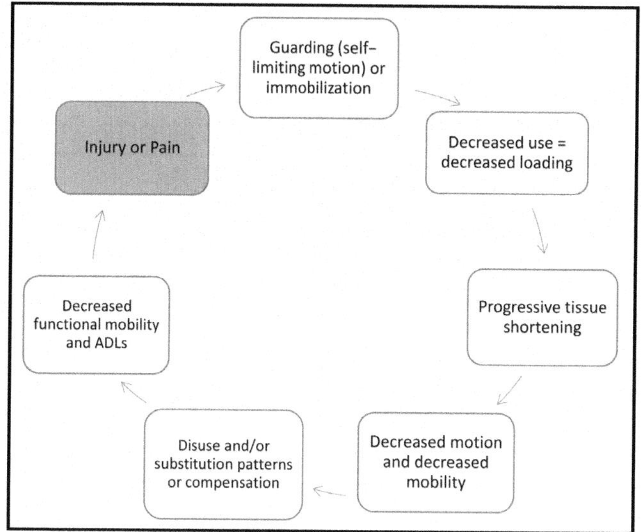


**Figure 4-1.** A self-perpetuating cycle of increasing disability. (ADLs = activities of daily living.)

## Range of Motion Contraindications and Precautions

Any type of ROM exercise is contraindicated if performing it will have an adverse effect on healing tissues. There are many benefits for performing ROM within a pain-free unrestricted range during the early stages of rehabilitation, but the presence of any of the cardinal signs/symptoms of inflammation (ie, heat, redness, edema, or resting pain) is a red flag and ROM exercises should be immediately terminated. AROM exercise is contraindicated for patients who have unstable cardiac conditions (ie, immediately after a myocardial infarction) until cleared by their physician.

The physical therapist assistant should review the medical record before treating any patient to verify that there are no contraindications, precautions, or physician protocols that could potentially restrict ROM exercise. Any questions or concerns should be discussed with the physical therapist before treating the patient.

## Passive Range of Motion

The movement of a body segment (ie, forearm or upper extremity) through an available, unrestricted, pain-free motion with total external assistance is called *PROM*. PROM exercises focus on moving a patient's limb, targeting motion at a specific joint; initially, it is performed in only one plane of motion (ie, sagittal, frontal, or transverse) at a time.

To perform PROM, the clinician must ensure that the patient is positioned comfortably in a position that allows full, unrestricted motion at the targeted joint. When a physical therapist assistant performs PROM with a patient, the clinician's grip and handling techniques take on increased importance. The clinician should use a firm grasp to fully support the entire affected limb (Figure 4-2A) but avoid grasping over any injured or tender areas. The clinician will fully explain the technique to decrease patient apprehension and use a quiet, calming voice as the patient's extremity is moved through their available ROM (Figure 4-2B). PROM is completed in a slow, rhythmic manner through the patient's pain-free available ROM as the clinician monitors the patient carefully throughout the intervention, modifying the technique as needed.

The assistant needs to be able to detect muscle guarding because the patient may involuntarily contract muscles to prevent further movement. If guarding occurs, the clinician should stop the movement, tell the patient to relax, and return the extremity to the initial starting position. For subsequent sets of PROM exercises, the limb should be moved through a lesser range to avoid further muscle guarding. The assistant should not feel any tissue resistance when performing PROM and may need to repeatedly cue the patient to relax the extremity to avoid active muscle contractions. The patient's limb should not be moved beyond the point of pain or beyond the current available ROM because it then becomes a stretching intervention and not a ROM intervention. When PROM is initiated, the assistant may only be able to move the limb a few degrees in any one direction (during the first few repetitions), but as the number of repetitions increase, the clinician may be able to gain more pain-free motion. The number of repititions and sets will depend on the therapy goals and should be adequate to meet the goals but not overstress healing tissues. It is suggested to start with lower repetitions (5 to 10 repetitions), assess patient status (ie, no increased symptoms), and then add an additional set if appropriate.

**Table 4-3**

Range of Motion Types: Indications, Contraindications, Precautions, Limitations, and Application[3]

| | PROM | AAROM | AROM |
|---|---|---|---|
| Indications | Use when AROM may disrupt healing or when AROM is contraindicated<br>ROM is desired without any muscle contraction<br>Patient is unable to complete AROM (physical or cognitive restriction, physician limitation)<br>To obtain relaxation<br>Assist with improving circulation | Patient is unable to complete motion through the full ROM because of weakness or some contraction throughout the available range is desired<br>Promote healing of connective tissue<br>Encourage proprioception, kinesthesia<br>Increases circulation | Contraction throughout the available range is desired<br>Promote connective tissue healing<br>Encourage proprioception, kinesthesia<br>Increase circulation<br>Prepares tissues for increased activity or aerobic conditioning |
| Contraindications | If motion will disrupt healing<br>Extreme pain at rest<br>If motion jeopardizes medical stability, significantly increases pain or inflammation, and acute cardiac conditions | Same as PROM | Same as PROM |
| Precautions | | | Acute cardiac diagnosis<br>If patient is unable to complete motion without substitution |
| Limitations | Does not increase ROM or strength<br>Does not prevent atrophy<br>Does not increase circulation as much as AROM does | Does not increase or maintain strength for muscles that are 3/5 or greater strength | Does not increase or maintain strength for muscles that are 3+/5 or greater strength<br>Develops skill/coordination *only* in practiced movement pattern |
| Application | The patient's limb is moved *only* by an external force (clinician, pulleys, CPM, gravity assisted, assisted through use of another limb)<br>Patient does not actively assist with motion | Patient actively completes motion but is assisted by external assistance<br>Performed using pulleys, ROM in gravity minimized (ie, sliding/powder board), cane, or self-assisted through use of another limb; clinician provides assistance | Patient completes desired joint motion against gravity |

CPM = continuous passive motion.

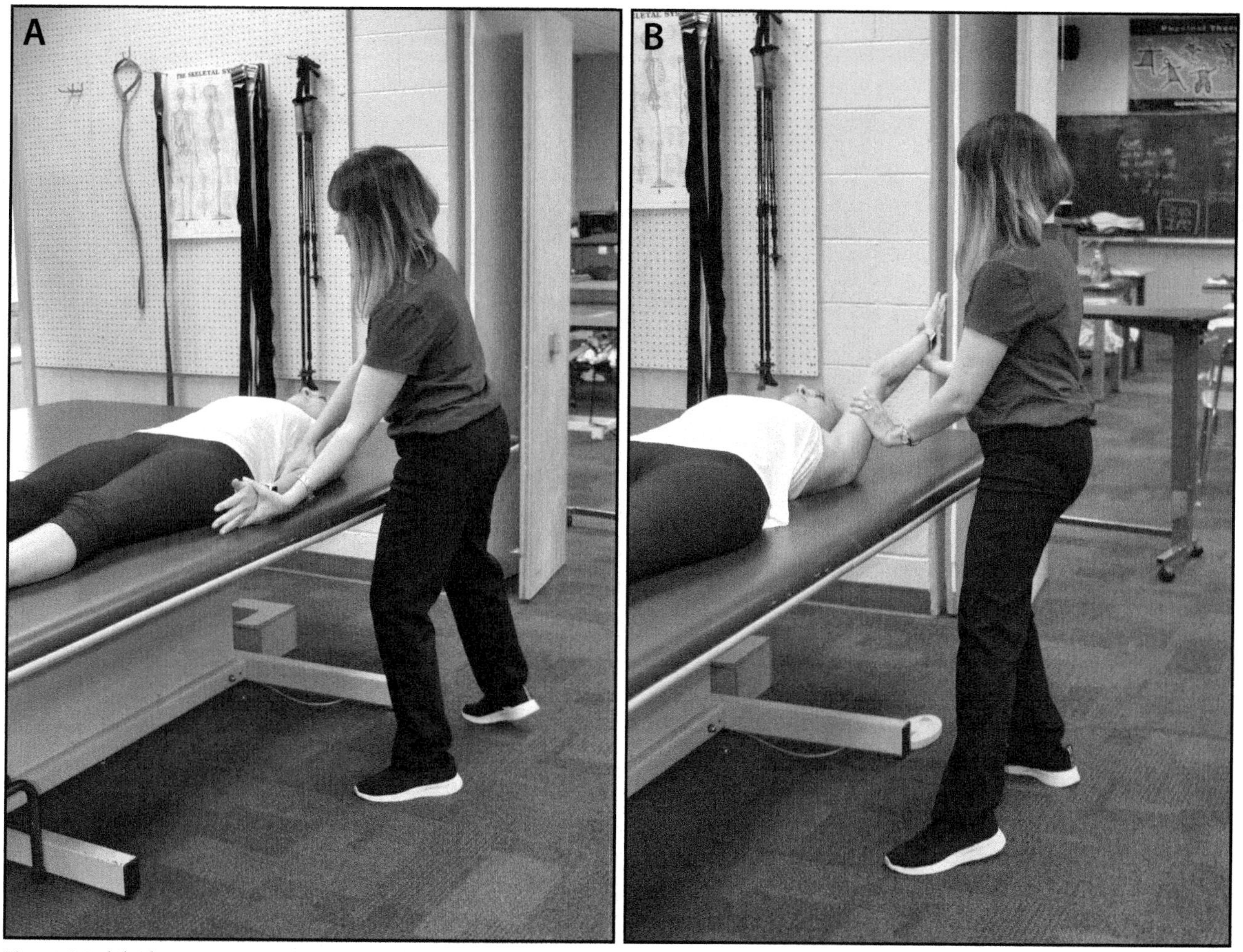

**Figure 4-2.** (A) The starting position before the clinician performs PROM shoulder flexion, firmly grasping the upper extremity. (B) The clinician performing PROM shoulder flexion while supporting the upper extremity and slowly moving through the available range.

The clinician should consider that a 2-joint muscle will have limited ROM at one joint if the muscle is already elongated over the second joint that it crosses (because of passive insufficiency). So, when a clinician performs PROM at one joint where a 2-joint muscle crosses, the second joint should be positioned so that the muscle is not in a lengthened state. For example, when performing hip flexion PROM, consider that the hamstrings cross both the hip and the knee. To prevent the hamstrings' length from restricting hip flexion, the knee must be flexed, keeping the hamstrings on slack as they cross the knee, thereby allowing full motion at the hip. It is challenging to control the motion and support the entire lower extremity (Figure 4-3A) when performing PROM, but the assistant must control and prevent knee hyperextension as the limb is moved from flexion into extension to avoid undue stress to the posterior knee (Figure 4-3B).

Other types of external assistance that can be used to assist the patient perform PROM include a CPM machine, which provides cyclical passive motion to a joint (Figure 4-4). The machine moves the joint through a controlled (preset) ROM. There are CPM machines made to fit most joints of the body. Pulleys can be used for PROM, but they are more typically used for AAROM interventions (described in the following section). The clinician should cautiously consider using equipment (ie, pulleys and straps) when applying PROM interventions because some patients are not able to fully relax to allow the intervention to be passive.

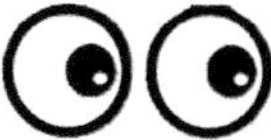

### Eye on the Research

Although there is some research that indicates that CPM use can be effective in increasing early ROM and recovery, there are additional studies with results that do not show clear benefits for the use of CPM machines, especially in terms of long-term outcomes.[3] Recent systematic reviews (based on evidence from 24 randomized trials) concluded that there is very little advantage of using a CPM machine after total knee arthroplasty.[4,5]

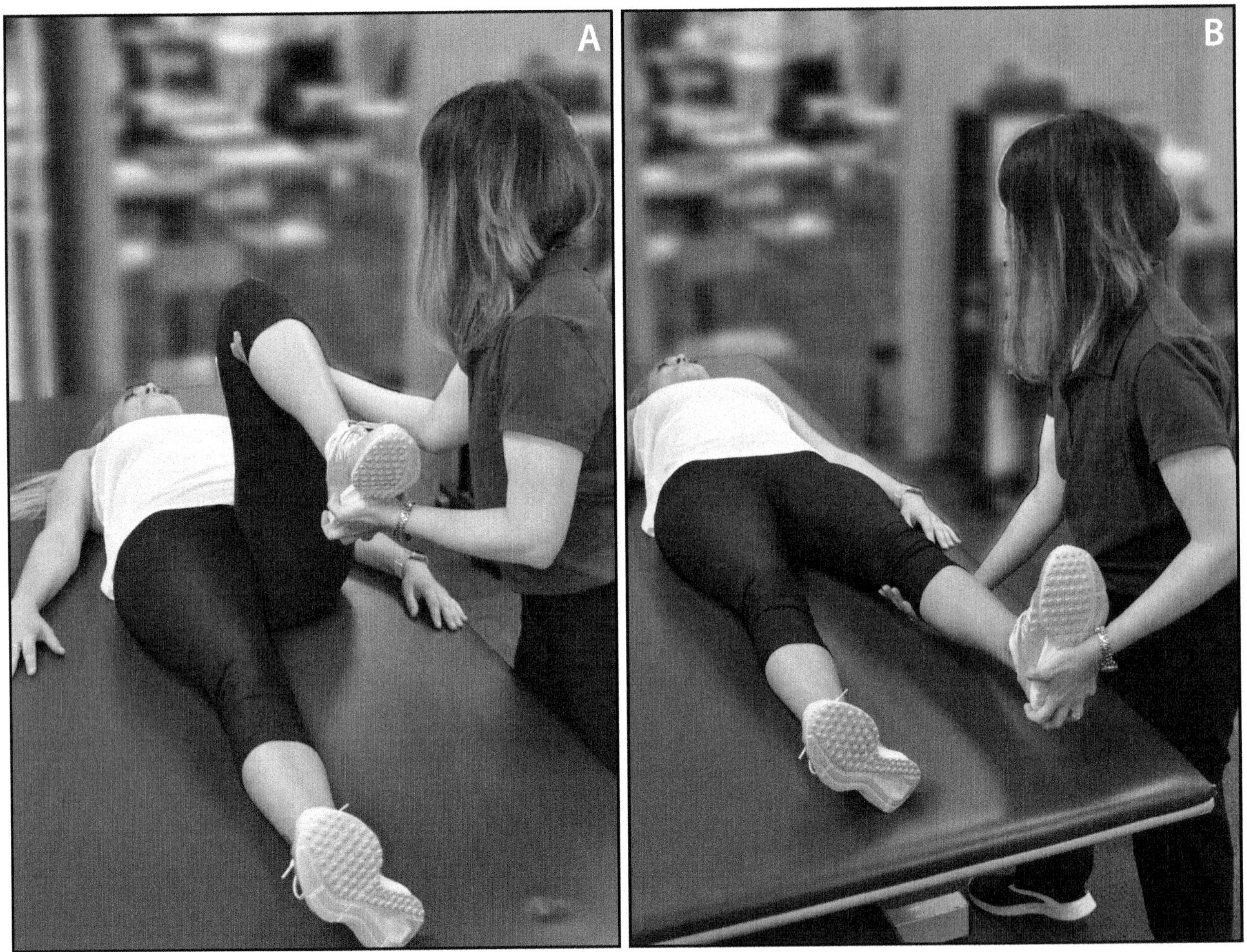

**Figure 4-3.** (A) The clinician supports the lower extremity (hip and knee) while performing PROM. The knee is flexed to avoid passive insufficiency of the hamstrings. (B) Notice how the clinician is protecting against knee hyperextension at the end of PROM.

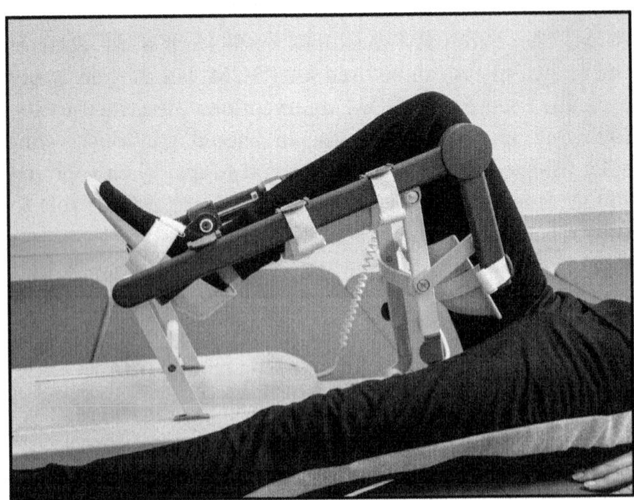

**Figure 4-4.** A photo of a CPM machine for the knee (Roman Zaiets/Shutterstock.com).

PROM is often performed during the acute phase (or maximum protective phase) of healing. The primary goals for initiating PROM include reducing the adverse effects of immobilization and inflammation, reducing pain, maintaining tissue mobility, improving circulation to the joints, and increasing synovial fluid movement to improve joint nutrition.

PROM may be indicated after certain musculoskeletal injuries or surgical interventions during the maximum protective phase of rehabilitation when AROM activities are contraindicated. Patients who are unable to move their extremities actively (ie, a coma, spinal cord injury, or stroke) can benefit from PROM. Performing PROM can help reduce the risk of contractures and is often paired with splinting for the best results.

Physical therapist assistants must understand that although PROM is beneficial, it does not reduce muscle atrophy or increase strength because no active muscle contractions should be occurring. Although it aids in improving circulation and synovial fluid movement, PROM is not as effective as the pumping action that occurs with active muscle contractions during AROM activities. PROM is not the same as stretching, and stretching is contraindicated during the acute stage of healing.

Other interventions such as joint mobilization (discussed later in this chapter) and stretching techniques (Chapter 5) are used to help restore normal joint arthrokinematics and full ROM once the patient is medically cleared for these activities. As the patient's healing progresses to the moderate protection and return-to-function phases, the tissues will be ready for additional stress/loads to increase strength and muscle endurance.

**Considerations for the Physical Therapist Assistant**

Stretching structures surrounding or supporting a joint is contraindicated during the maximum protection (or acute stage) phase of healing. PROM ≠ stretching. Care must be taken when performing PROM to ensure that the limb/joint motion that is occurring is within the patient's available pain-free ROM.

### Normal and Abnormal End Feels and Capsular Patterns

Recognizing and understanding normal and abnormal joint end feel (Table 4-4) and capsular patterns (Table 4-5) is necessary to perform PROM safely. When performing PROM, there is resistance felt by the clinician at the end of the available range that prevents further motion. This resistance is called the *joint end feel*. Each joint in the body has a typical/expected end feel for each motion the joint normally performs. The end feel for a specific joint may be different for different motions that occur at that joint (ie, the end feel for elbow extension is hard, but for flexion it is soft). The typical (normal) end feel of a joint is based on the properties of the tissues surrounding the joint.

Normal end feels include hard, firm, and soft. A hard end feel occurs when there is bone-to-bone contact at the end of ROM. A firm end feel occurs when the end feel is the result of a capsular, tendon, or ligament stretch, and a soft end feel occurs when the approximation of muscles limit further motion.

When the assistant assesses an end feel that is not typically expected for a joint, it is considered an abnormal end feel. An abnormal end feel can be hard, firm, soft, springy, or empty. Any of these can occur at a point (earlier or later) in the range than it would normally be expected. An empty end feel is recorded when the assistant does not feel any resistance, but the motion is limited by the patient's pain. A springy end feel indicates that a loose body (ie, torn cartilage) is limiting the ROM, and the clinician will feel a "bouncy" resistance. It should be noted that soft, firm, and hard end feels can also be considered abnormal if they occur prior in the range to where the end feel is normally expected. Any variation in end feel that is assessed during PROM may indicate a change in patient status, and the assistant should inform the supervising therapist.

**Capsular patterns** are joint-specific patterns of restrictions. Each joint has a specific pattern of restriction (see Table 4-5); the reader is referred to orthopedic physical therapy texts for lists that include smaller peripheral and vertebral joints. Arthritis, frozen shoulder (adhesive capsulitis), and immobilization (because of fractures or severe sprains) are common conditions that can result in joint motion restrictions. Patients with these conditions usually present with a firm end feel because of muscle guarding, capsule tightness, and/or soft tissue contractures. The loss of motion tends to be predictable and proportional.

Abnormal end feels and/or capsular patterns can affect normal joint arthrokinematics, thereby limiting PROM. These problems must be resolved in order to restore normal ROM. Interventions (ie, modalities, ROM exercises, and joint and soft tissue mobilization techniques) can be applied to restore pain-free ROM.

**Documentation Tip**

Record observations concisely but include all pertinent information. When recording PROM measurements, be sure to include the joint, motion, limb (right/left), measurement, joint end feel (if abnormal), and any variation from the recommended test position.

## *Active Assisted Range of Motion*

AAROM is joint motion that occurs when there is a combination of voluntary (active) muscular contraction and some external assistance. For example, AAROM occurs when a patient with upper extremity weakness poststroke completes clasped hand shoulder flexion or uses pulleys to assist with shoulder flexion.

**Clinical Tip**

A cane, pulleys, towel, sheet, or straps can be used to assist patients with self-PROM exercises as well as with AAROM.

When performing an AAROM exercise, the goal is to have the patient actively contract the target muscles through as much of the ROM as possible without pain. The physical therapist assistant should monitor and cue the patient to ensure that they are actively contracting the target muscles (without substituting with other muscles); the assistant will provide assistance through the range when needed. The amount of assistance is based on patient presentation and whether the limitation is caused by muscle weakness and/or

**Table 4-4**

Normal and Abnormal End Feel

| | End Feel | Possible Cause | Examples |
|---|---|---|---|
| Normal | Hard | Bone-to-bone contact | Elbow extension |
| | Firm | Capsular or ligament/tendon stretch | Shoulder external rotation, ankle dorsiflexion, hip internal and external rotation, forearm supination, finger extension |
| | Soft | Soft tissue approximation | Elbow flexion, knee flexion |
| Abnormal | Hard | Osteophyte | A hard resistance felt before the expected end ROM (ie, hard end feel at 30 degrees of hip external rotation) |
| | Firm | Spasticity, adhesive capsulitis | Resistance from tone; with adhesive capsulitis, a firm feel, much earlier than expected in the ROM |
| | Soft | Joint effusion | Knee extension with excessive edema, synovitis |
| | Springy | Loose body in joint | Medial meniscus tear |
| | Empty | Pain | Acute bursitis; pain limits motion due to joint inflammation |

**Table 4-5**

Capsular Patterns

| Peripheral Joints | Limitations/Restrictions (in Order From Most to Least Restrictions) |
|---|---|
| Ankle (talocrural) | Plantar flexion, dorsiflexion |
| Knee (tibiofemoral) | Flexion, extension |
| Hip | Flexion, abduction, internal rotation (all are limited) |
| Glenohumeral | External rotation, abduction, internal rotation |
| Humeroulnar | Flexion, extension |
| Humeroradial | Flexion, extension, supination, pronation |
| Wrist (radiocarpal) | Flexion, extension (equally limited) |

pain (ie, painful arc). The clinician may instruct the patient to complete self-AAROM exercises using equipment or the assistance of the contralateral extremity when performing a home exercise program. Equipment may include a cane/wand (Figure 4-5), pulleys (Figure 4-6), towel, and/or strap (Figure 4-7) to assist the patient in completing ROM. Self-AAROM knee flexion is illustrated in Figure 4-8. The seated patient puts their foot on the floor or a smooth surface with the knee slightly flexed. The use of a towel under the patient's foot reduces the friction, allowing the patient to actively contract the knee flexors with less effort and through as much of the range as possible. The patient can then use the opposite leg to assist with completing more motion when the hamstrings cannot perform additional motion because of weakness or pain.

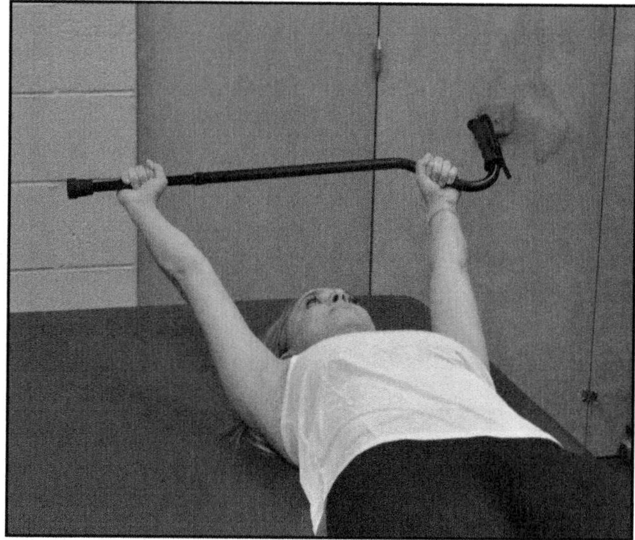

**Figure 4-5.** AAROM for right shoulder flexion using a cane.

**Documentation Tip**

If a patient completed 2 sets of 10 repetitions of the exercise depicted in Figure 4-7, this would be documented as follows: Supine: R LE heel slide self-AAROM with strap, 2 × 10 reps.

## *Active Range of Motion*

AROM occurs when movement at a joint is produced by active voluntary muscle contractions through an unrestricted range. AROM is necessary for performing ADLs, self-care tasks, and functional mobility activities.

AROM exercises are indicated for those joints above and below an affected joint that has been immobilized or following injury and/or surgical intervention. Physical therapist assistants must always be aware of multijoint muscles that cross the involved joint. AROM can be used as part of an aerobic exercise program, especially for persons with lower levels of fitness. If a patient is unable to complete AROM against gravity, the assistant can position the patient in a gravity-minimized position. Minimizing the impact of gravity serves to assist the patient in completing more of the ROM independently.

**Considerations for the Physical Therapist Assistant**

Some clinicians may document AROM completed in a gravity-minimized position as AAROM because the reduction of the impact of gravity serves as an assist; others may document this as AROM in a gravity-minimized position.

The goals for AROM are similar to those for PROM and AAROM, but the added benefits include developing stronger muscle contractions, increasing circulation through active muscle pumping actions (reducing risk for deep vein thrombosis), and improving coordination (in practiced movement patterns). If a patient is practicing AROM in one movement pattern (ie, shoulder flexion), the quality of motion, coordination, and muscle endurance may all improve but only in that specific direction or pattern. Performing AROM does not increase a patient's strength if their muscle strength grade is 3/5 (fair) or greater. However, if a patient was only able to perform AROM with gravity minimized (ie, muscle grade of 2/5) and progressed to performing the AROM against gravity, then strength gains were made.

Physical therapist assistants need to ensure proper joint mechanics are occurring when the patient is completing AROM. Poor arthrokinematics can occur because of pain, joint/soft tissue restrictions, poor joint stability, and/or muscle weakness and can increase injury risk. The assistant should carefully monitor the quality of movement to ensure that no muscle substitution patterns or compensatory motions occur as the patient moves through the range. Figures 4-9A and 4-9B illustrate good and poor shoulder joint arthrokinematics during shoulder abduction AROM. There are several possible causes for the substitution pattern depicted in Figure 4-9B, including poor inferior glide of the humeral head in the glenoid fossa (restricted capsular pattern), shoulder girdle muscle weakness, or poor glenohumeral/scapular rhythm. In this case, the assistant should check the therapist's evaluation to determine the possible cause of the compensatory motion. Any reductions in the patient's ROM or any new signs/symptoms should be reported to the supervising therapist.

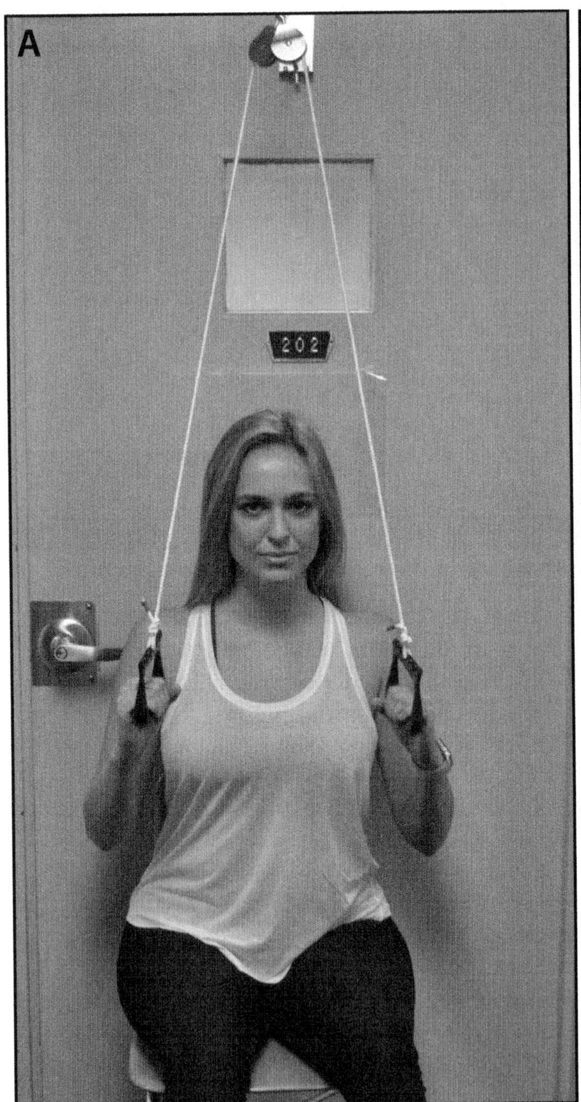


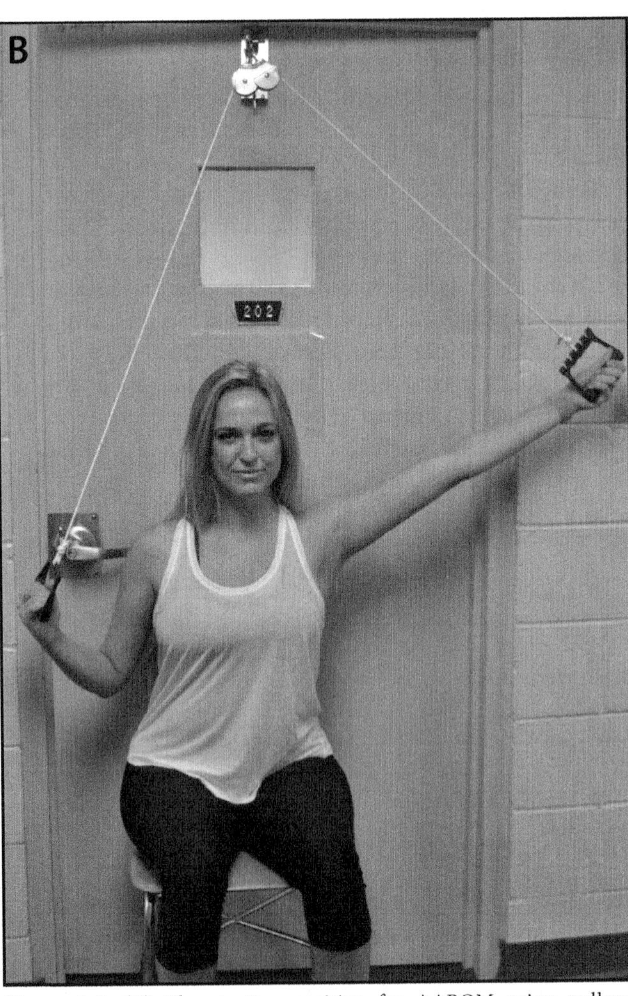


**Figure 4-6.** (A) The starting position for AAROM using pulleys. (B) Shoulder abduction using pulleys during AAROM.

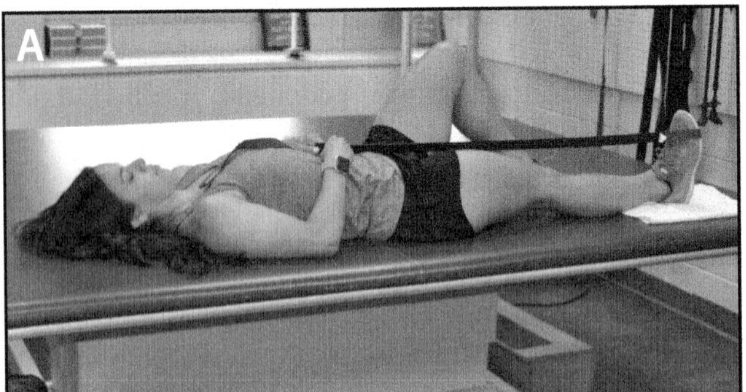


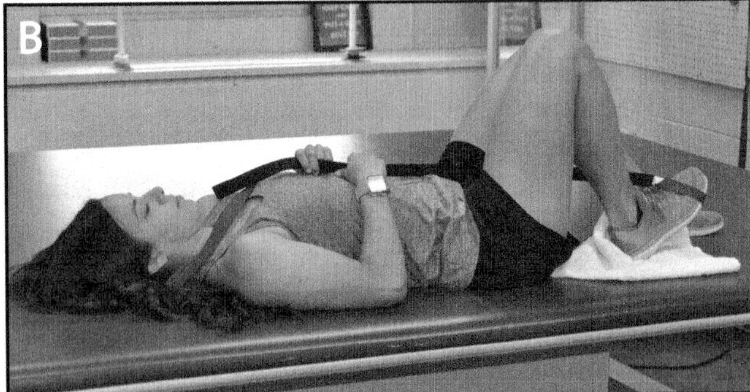


**Figure 4-7.** (A) The starting position using a towel and strap in preparation to perform AAROM hip and knee. (B) The patient pulls the strap to increase hip and knee flexion. The towel reduces friction and aids in AAROM.

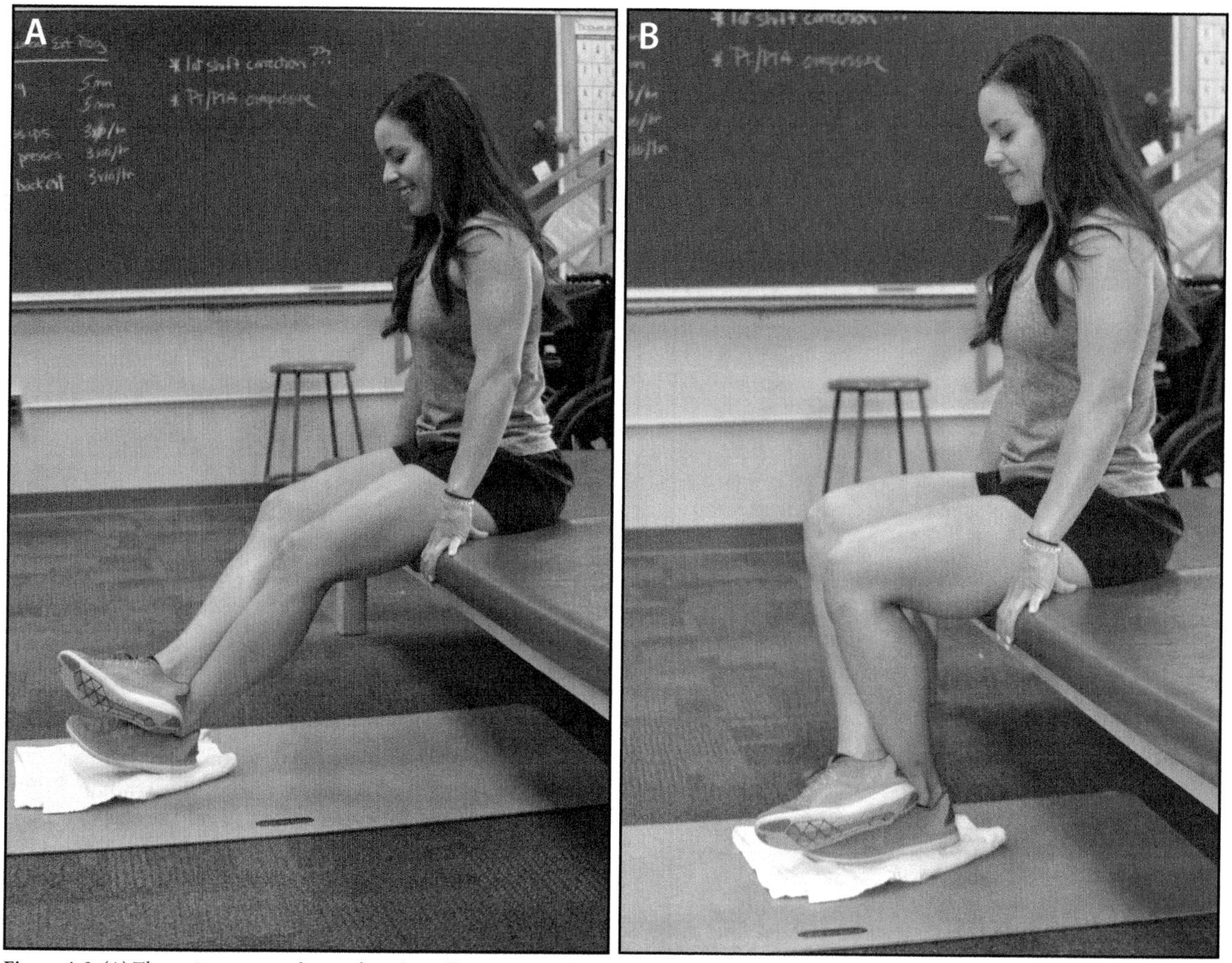

Figure 4-8. (A) The patient prepared to perform knee flexion AAROM. (B) The patient performs knee flexion actively until the muscles can no longer perform the motion, and then the contralateral leg moves to assist in gaining more motion.

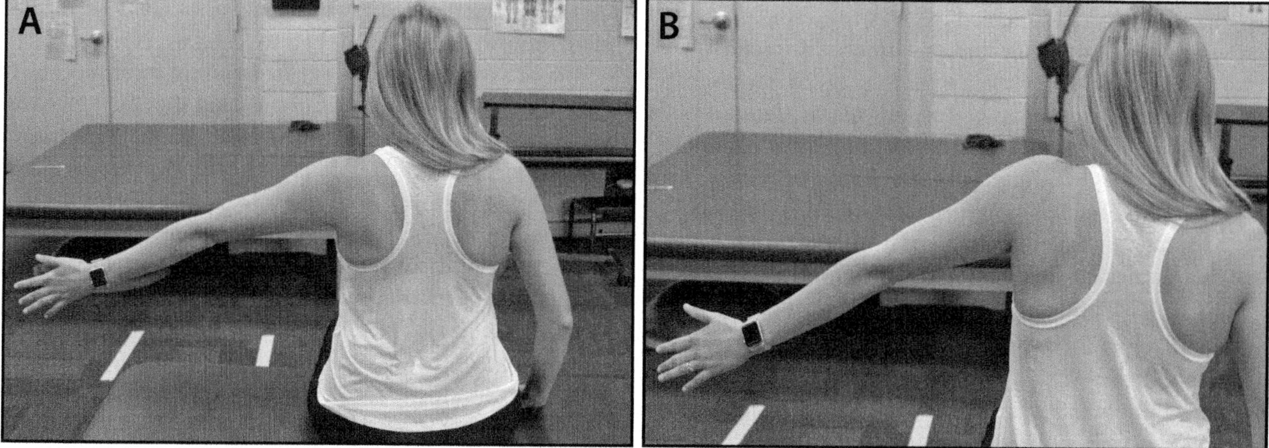


**Figure 4-9.** (A) Shoulder abduction with good joint arthrokinematics. (B) Shoulder abduction with faulty joint arthrokinematics (the patient leans to the right and the humeral head is elevated).

**Quick Class Activity**

How would you document the ROM that you observe in Figures 4-9A and 4-9B?

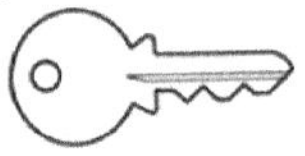

**Key Safety Considerations: Range of Motion**

- Consider the stage of healing if the patient is postinjury.
- Maintain compliance with all orthopedic precautions.
- Stop intervention and report to the physical therapist/ medical team if you note new signs/symptoms of inflammation, a significant increase in pain, an inappropriate change in vital signs or new cardiac signs/symptoms, or any significant changes in ROM.
- When medically appropriate and current exercises/ activities are pain free, progress to full available ROM and then increase the level of exercises (PROM, AAROM, AROM) as tolerated.
- Stop AROM if the patient is using substitution patterns or poor-quality movement.
- ROM occurs within the unrestricted available range; do not add stretching unless it is specifically ordered/ indicated.

# MANUAL THERAPY TECHNIQUES

According to the American Physical Therapy Association (APTA) *Guide to Physical Therapy Practice*:

> [M]anual therapy techniques are skilled hand movements and skilled passive movements of joints and soft tissue and are intended to improve tissue extensibility; increase range of motion; induce relaxation; mobilize or manipulate soft tissue and joints; modulate pain; and reduce soft tissue swelling, inflammation, or restriction. Techniques may include manual lymphatic drainage, manual traction, massage, mobilization/ manipulation, and passive range of motion.[6]

Joint and soft tissue mobilization are commonly used manual therapy techniques. The purpose of this section is to provide the physical therapist assistant student with entry-level knowledge and understanding about these techniques as well as indications and contraindications for their use (Box 4-1). There are areas of the country where the supervising physical therapist may delegate some of these techniques to the assistant. Delegation is based on the scope of practice (the legality of delegation is based on state laws and statutes/state physical therapy practice act) and the therapist's knowledge of and confidence in the skills of the assistant. Because joint mobilizations are not considered an entry-level skill for physical therapist assistants, those who are practicing in regions where joint mobilizations are included within the practice act can attend continuing education courses to increase their skills and knowledge.

**Box 4-1**

**Joint Mobilization Indications and Contraindications**

- Indications: Hypomobility, pain/muscle guarding, correction of a faulty bone position
- Relative contraindications/precautions: Inflammation,[a] swelling/effusion,[a] hypermobility,[a] total joint replacements, excessive pain, systemic connective tissue disease (ie, rheumatoid arthritis)
- Absolute contraindications: Malignancy, osteomyelitis, metabolic bone disease, unhealed fracture, fusion, ankylosis, infectious arthritis

[a]Joint mobilization techniques that increase ROM are definitely contraindicated, but gentle oscillations that do not stretch the capsule may be applied per the discretion of the evaluating physical therapist.

## *Joint Mobilizations*

Joint mobilizations are used to increase tissue extensibility, increase ROM, and/or help decrease pain. Joint mobilizations are included in the physical therapy POC based on the results of the initial examination. The APTA *Guide to Physical Therapy Practice* defines mobilization as "a manual therapy technique comprised of a continuum of skilled passive movements that are applied at varying speeds and amplitudes, including a small amplitude/high velocity therapeutic movement."[7]

It is important for physical therapist assistants to understand both the physiology and goals associated with joint mobilizations. There is an ongoing controversy specific to the role of assistants in the performance of joint mobilizations. In 2018, the APTA's position stated that only physical therapists can perform "spinal and peripheral joint mobilization/manipulation" because of the "immediate and continuous examination and evaluation."[8] Examination, evaluation, intervention, and clinical decision making are inseparable during the performance of mobilization/ manipulation. For this reason, the APTA states that it is inappropriate for a physical therapist to direct manual therapy procedures of joint mobilization/manipulation to the assistant under any circumstances.[7] However, an educational resource paper also published by the APTA states the following:

> The Commission on Accreditation in Physical Therapy Education (CAPTE) believes that the knowledge of an entry-level physical therapist assistant should include the rationale for manual therapy procedures such as soft tissue and non-thrust joint mobilization techniques. Furthermore, the Commission believes that it is *not* inappropriate to train assistants to perform

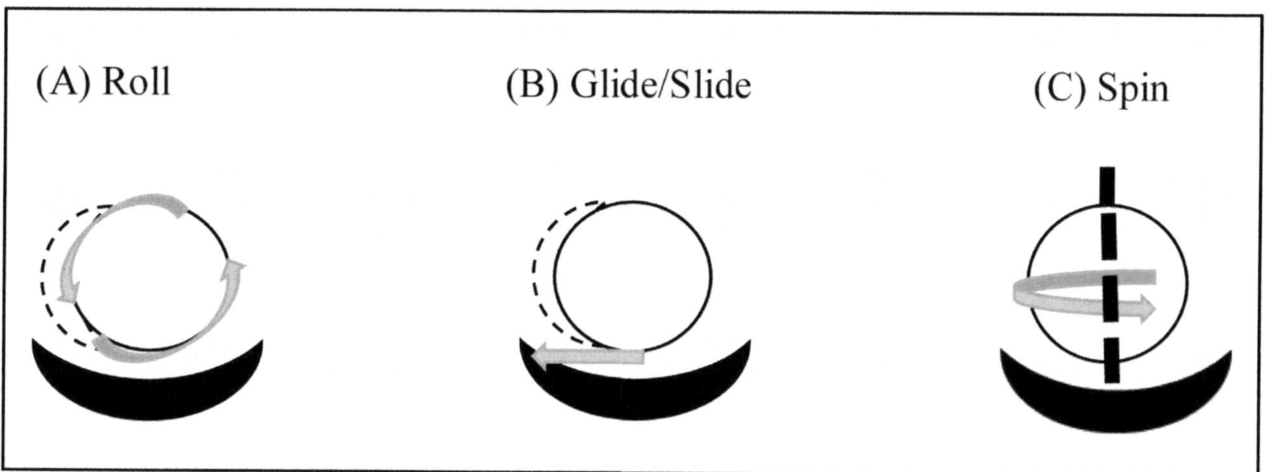


**Figure 4-10.** Joint arthrokinematics.

soft tissue mobilization or to manually assist the therapist in the delivery of peripheral joint mobilization procedures (i.e., assist with patient positioning, stabilization, or grade 1-2 movements). CAPTE expects educational programs to prepare physical therapy students to determine those components of interventions that may be directed to the physical therapist assistant. These considerations should include the level of skill and training required to perform the procedure, the level of experience/advanced competency of the individual assistant, the practice setting in which the procedure is performed, and the type of monitoring needed to accurately assess the patient's response to the intervention. In addition, acuity and complexity of the patient's condition and other clinical factors should be considered when directing assistants to safely and competently perform any intervention. CAPTE also expects physical therapist assisting educational programs to prepare physical therapist assistant students to recognize components of interventions that are beyond their scope of work.[9]

Some state practice acts allow physical therapist assistants to perform joint mobilization techniques. Physical therapist assistant programs put a varied emphasis on joint and soft tissue mobilization techniques based on the state practice act where the program is located. Performing joint mobilization skills are not considered entry-level skills, but understanding the theory and purpose for joint mobilization application is considered required entry-level knowledge for physical therapist assistants.

The assistant should know the contour of joint surfaces (convex or concave) that make up each joint, joint end feels, and how end feels and capsular patterns affect ROM. Assistants need to recognize the grades and types of mobilization techniques and the process for applying mobilization techniques to peripheral joints. This knowledge provides the assistant with insight as to what may be contributing to the patient's pain or limiting the patient's ROM so the information can be shared with the supervising therapist.

## Joint Mobilization: Theory, Terminology, and Techniques

Joint mobilizations provide passive motion as one bony surface moves over the other stable bony surface. Understanding normal joint arthrokinematics and the shape of each joint (articular) surface is needed to determine the direction of force that needs to be applied when performing joint mobilizations.

The normal joint arthrokinematics occurring at the joints include roll, spin, and glide (or slide) and are illustrated in Figure 4-10. Joint motions (arthrokinematics) occur as a result of the motion of the bones (osteokinematics) and are not voluntarily controlled by the patient. Rolling occurs when a new point of one surface contacts a new point of the other surface (ie, a tire moving on pavement). Gliding occurs when one joint surface moves parallel to the other, and spin occurs when one joint surface rotates around a fixed point on the other surface.

The type of motion that occurs between the bony articulations depends on the shape of the articulating bones. Synovial joints are either ovoid (condylar) or sellar (saddle joints). An ovoid joint has one bone with a concave surface and the other bone with a convex surface (ie, the glenohumeral joint). A saddle joint is convex in one direction and concave in the other (ie, CMC joint of the thumb).

The direction that a moving joint surface moves on a stable/fixed joint surface is based on the concave-convex rule (Figure 4-11). The concave-convex rule states that when a concave surface moves on a convex surface, there is gliding and rolling (or angular movement) in the same direction. When a convex surface moves on a concave surface, there is gliding and angular movement in opposite directions. The clinician needs to know the surface type (convex or concave) of the bone that is going to be mobilized because this determines the direction of the force to be applied.

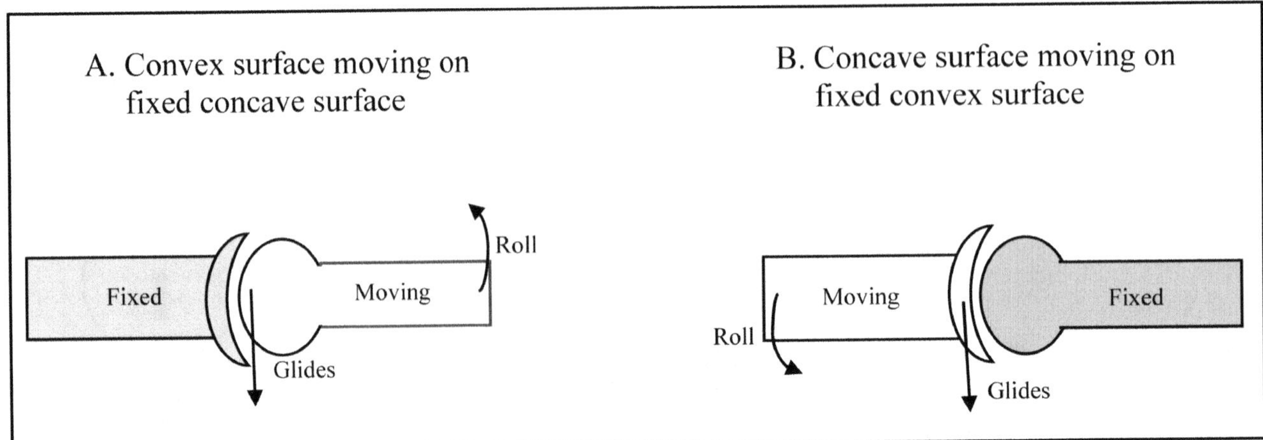


**Figure 4-11.** The convex-concave rule.

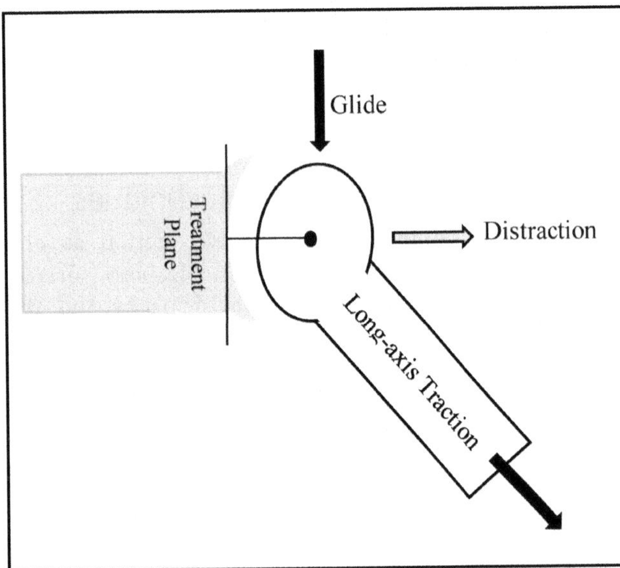


**Figure 4-12.** Treatment plane.

The physical therapist assesses the patient's available AROM, PROM, muscle strength in the available range, the quality of all joint motions, and joint play. Joint play is the amount of "give" or movement in the capsule and surrounding tissues between the bony segments forming the joint. Joints that are hypomobile usually have less joint play, resulting in ROM restrictions compared with normal or hypermobile joints. The assessment of joint play and initial joint mobilizations are typically performed in the open-packed position (resting position or loose-packed position) of the joint. The **open-packed position** is the position where the bone ends of the joint are least congruent and the greatest amount of joint play is possible because there is the least amount of pressure on the capsule and surrounding ligaments. The **closed-pack position** is the joint position where the joint surfaces are most congruent. Joint mobilizations should not be completed when a joint is in the closed-pack position. The open- and closed-pack positions for each joint are included in Chapters 12 and 13.

Low-amplitude joint mobilization improves nutrition to the joint by increasing the movement of synovial fluid, which improves nutrient distribution to joint surfaces. With more aggressive/larger-amplitude joint mobilizations, the joint capsule and surrounding tissues are stressed, causing plastic deformation of collagen. This stress on the collagen fibers may break up adhesions and promote realignment of the collagen fibers in the direction of the stress, resulting in increased ROM.

Two general types of joint mobilization are the oscillatory (Maitland) and sustained (Kaltenborn) techniques.[10] Terminology has traditionally distinguished mobilizations (nonthrust/lower-velocity passive motions) from manipulations (high-velocity thrust techniques). The APTA currently uses the terms *mobilization* and *manipulation* interchangeably, using the descriptor nonthrust or thrust to define the technique.

Clinicians must understand the rationale for including joint mobilization techniques in the treatment plan (ie, reducing pain and muscle guarding or increasing joint ROM). The purpose of treatment drives the selection of the specific mobilization grade, and then the clinician needs to determine the treatment plane. According to Kaltenborn, the treatment plane lies parallel to the concave joint surface and is perpendicular (90 degrees) to the center of the convex bone surface (Figure 4-12).[10] The treatment plane moves with the concave surface, and it remains stationary when the convex surface moves. Joint distraction or traction is the separating of the joint surfaces at a right angle (see Figure 4-12); these terms are often interchangeable. Long-axis joint traction is defined as pulling along the long axis (or shaft) of a long bone that is parallel to the concave joint surface or treatment plane. Gliding also occurs with long-axis traction.

There are various types of joint mobilization techniques (Figure 4-13) that can be used to either decrease pain and guarding or increase joint mobility. Maitland classified nonthrust mobilization using grades I through IV. Grade V was added to describe a high-thrust motion at the end of the available ROM. Grade V mobilizations are used to restore joint motion and are completed by the physical therapist only. Small-amplitude oscillations are rhythmic and rapid vibratory motions used during grade I and IV mobilizations. Large-amplitude oscillations are also rhythmic but are performed at a cadence of 2 to 3 oscillations per second through a larger portion of the ROM; these are used during grade II and III mobilizations.

Grade I mobilizations use small-amplitude oscillations applied gently at the beginning of the available ROM. Grade I mobilizations are used to reduce pain and muscle guarding/spasms and improve nutrient distribution to joint surfaces by increasing synovial fluid movement. Grade II large-amplitude oscillations are performed within the midpart of the available range and for the same purposes as grade I. If a patient reports pain with grade II, the clinician should slow the rate of oscillations and make sure the movements are smooth. Grade III large-amplitude oscillations apply stress to the tissues at the end of the available range to increase ROM. Grade IV small-amplitude oscillations are performed at the end of the available range, meeting tissue resistance to stretch the restricted tissues and capsule in order to increase ROM.

Sustained mobilization techniques (see Figure 4-13) are used specifically for joint play relevant to joint traction/distraction and gliding of joint surfaces. Nonthrust grade I sustained joint mobilization is used to reduce pain and muscle guarding/spasms and to improve nutrient distribution to joint surfaces by increasing synovial fluid movement. Grade II sustained techniques take up the tissue slack to determine the amount of available joint play. They are used as an initial test grade to determine the patient's tolerance to pain when determining the grade of mobilization that is most appropriate to use. Grade III sustained is a more aggressive stretching technique; it is used to reduce restricted hypomobile joint capsules and the surrounding ligaments and improve joint arthrokinematics to restore normal ROM and function. When applying pressure during a grade III sustained glide, a grade I distraction to separate the joint surfaces should be implemented first with one hand before initiating the glide (with the other hand), which will place significant stretch on the joint capsule and the surrounding tissues. To apply the force for a grade III mobilization, the clinician should first take up the slack and then continue to apply the force until the capsular tightness or restriction is felt. The force is maintained at that point because the goal of this technique is to increase ROM.

In states where physical therapist assistants are permitted to perform joint mobilizations, the assistant should consult with the supervising physical therapist before performing any joint or soft tissue mobilization technique. The contraindications and precautions should be reviewed and discussed with the therapist before initiating treatment (see Box 4-1).

Before initiating joint mobilization techniques, the patient is in a fully supported position, relaxed and draped appropriately. Provide a clear description of the intervention, the purpose of the intervention, and reassurance

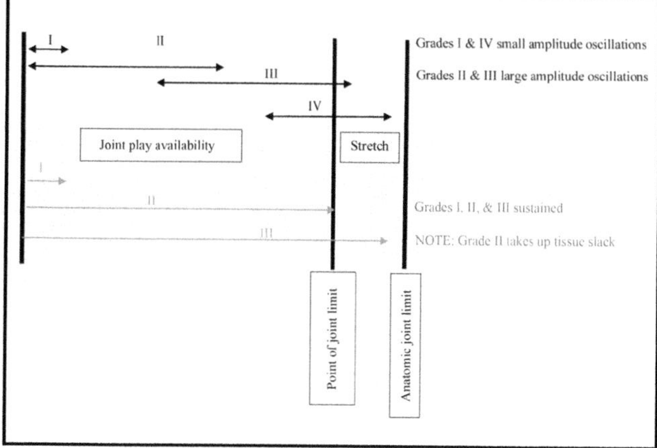


**Figure 4-13.** Joint mobilization grades.

about what can be expected. The joint and surrounding tissues should be heated (if not contraindicated) and the muscles relaxed (ie, appropriate education or massage). Apprehension or pain can cause muscle guarding, which can alter the effectiveness of the technique. The clinician should monitor for local muscle guarding and will verbally instruct the patient to relax before (and often during) the joint mobilization technique. Only one joint should be mobilized at a time.

The clinician will first identify the joint line and bony landmarks to ensure proper hand placement in relation to the direction of the force that is to be applied. Grasp should be firm (but not cause pain), and hand placement should be as close to the joint articulating surfaces (of the bones to be mobilized) as possible. The clinician should ensure one bone is truly stable and then apply a slight (grade I) traction force that is perpendicular to the treatment plane to the other bone to be mobilized. Mobilizations can be performed by using the clinician's hands or a mobilization belt. The clinician can proceed to more aggressive mobilization grades to gain ROM as appropriate. Figure 4-14 illustrates a clinician performing sustained grade III joint mobilization to improve shoulder abduction. The clinician should monitor their own body mechanics.

To maximize the benefit from vigorous joint mobilization interventions, the technique should be paired with stretching (by the patient or clinician) and followed by ROM and strengthening exercises within the newly gained range whenever possible to promote active control in the increased range.

## Other Types of Mobilization

Other types of mobilization include self-mobilization, mobilization with movement, and the use of muscle energy techniques. Self-mobilization techniques are performed by the patient and include a self-stretching intervention that uses traction or glides to a given portion of a joint capsule (Figure 4-15). Physical therapist assistants should instruct the patient on proper positioning and technique if these are performed as part of their home exercise program.

The clinician's left hand distracts the humerus and the right hand performs a grade III sustained inferior glide to the humeral head to increase the downward glide in order to improve shoulder abduction ROM.

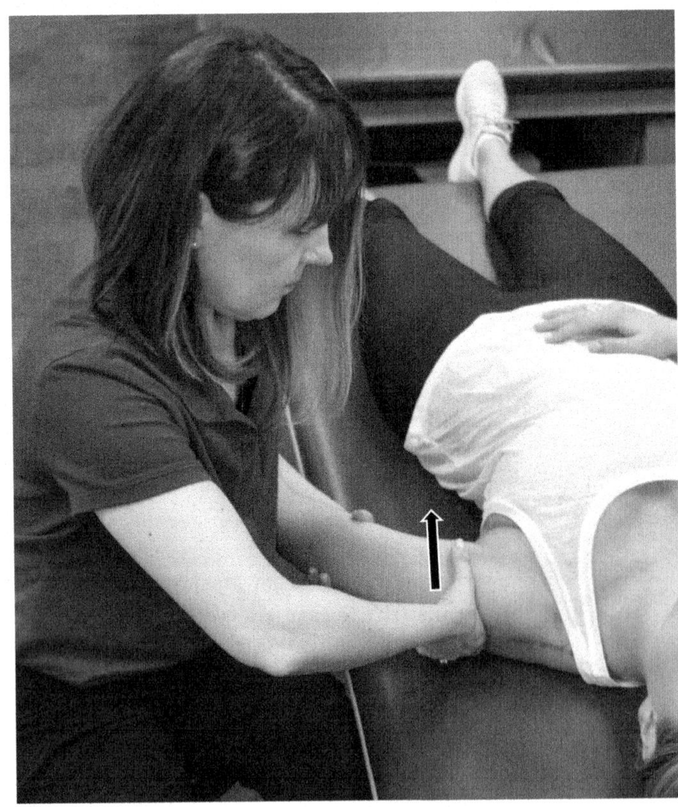

**Figure 4-14.** Joint mobilization.

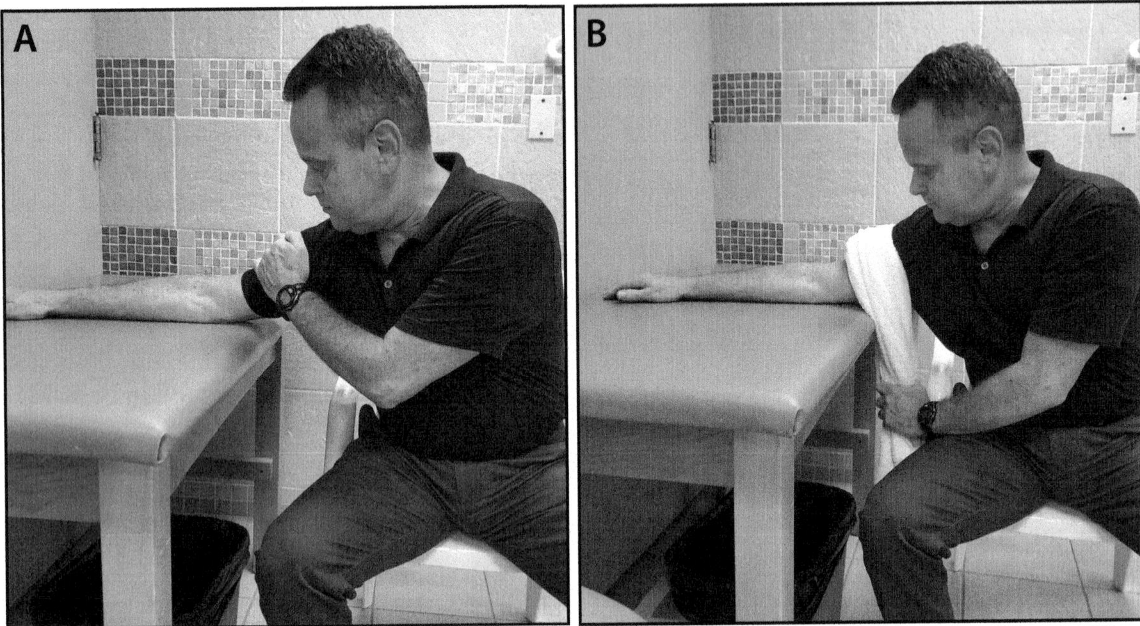


**Figure 4-15.** (A) A shoulder self-mobilization inferior glide to improve shoulder abduction. (B) Shoulder self-mobilization using a towel.

Mobilization with movement is a technique that was introduced by Brian Mulligan. It combines passive joint mobilization performed by a therapist with a specific active joint motion completed to end range by the patient. Muscle energy techniques are manual therapy techniques that target joint mobility and muscle extensibility. Muscle energy techniques are used to target accessory motions. The technique is used to assist in realigning joint surfaces (ie, sacroiliac joint) or to increase joint mobility (refer to Chapter 15). The patient is first positioned to best access the shortened muscle and instructed to perform an isometric muscle contraction (which creates accessory joint motion). After the contraction, the shortened muscle relaxes, resulting in an increase in ROM. The physical therapist assistant needs to stabilize the patient as well as resist the muscle contraction. This technique is based on similar treatment principles as reciprocal inhibition (discussed in Chapter 5). Additional knowledge of these techniques can be gained by attending continuing education courses.

There are situations in which a physician will perform a joint manipulation under anesthesia to break up adhesions that are limiting a patient's joint motion. Physical therapy is typically initiated very soon (that day or 1 to 2 days after) after the procedure is completed to maintain the newly gained ROM.

## Special Populations

### *Pediatric Considerations*

It is generally accepted that children exhibit greater flexibility than adults. When completing ROM with a developing child, clinicians will consider age-related norms, noting that there can be significant variability from child to child. As the child grows, flexibility usually decreases, approaching adult norms.

The clinician should recognize that certain pathologies are associated with changes in available ROM. For example, children with Down syndrome often present with increased flexibility compared with peers without the syndrome.[11] Children with arthrogryposis multiplex congenita present with a significant decrease in joint ROM and often benefit from orthopedic surgeries paired with physical therapy to improve ROM.[12] Regular ROM exercise is an important intervention for children who present with juvenile rheumatoid arthritis (JRA).[13] Children with JRA tend to have lower physical fitness levels than peers without JRA. Regular exercise has been shown to improve outcomes without increased joint damage or adverse results.[14] ROM exercises can be a gentle introduction to exercise for these patients.

### *Older Adult Considerations*

General functional decline and decreased activity levels can lead to hypomobility. Age-related changes in older adults include decreased water content in cartilage and decreased collagen synthesis, which can result in decreased ligament and tendon elasticity and strength and reduced joint capsule integrity. Regular ROM exercises/activities are useful for maintaining flexibility. The skin tends to become more fragile in older adults, and they are more prone to bruising and skin tears, so positioning and hand placement must be carefully considered when performing ROM with these patients.[15]

# Conclusion

Restoring and maintaining normal AROM and PROM can assist patients with sustaining functional mobility. ROM interventions are a commonly used physical therapy intervention across the continuum of care and with patients of all ages. The ability to differentiate between the types of ROM programs and to select the optimal type to help a patient meet their mobility goals is an important part of physical therapy practice. Safe and appropriate application of ROM and mobilization interventions will facilitate a patient's return to optimal levels of mobility and function.

# Review Questions

1. Compare and contrast AROM, AAROM, and PROM.
2. Differentiate between hypomobility and hypermobility.
3. What are 3 possible causes of hypomobility?
4. Differentiate joint ROM from muscle excursion.
5. For each of the following, state the normative value for PROM: shoulder external rotation, hip internal rotation, knee flexion, elbow flexion, cervical spine lateral bending, and wrist ulnar deviation.
6. Explain active insufficiency. Describe the joint motions that will produce active insufficiency in the hamstrings.
7. Define joint end feel, and list the types of normal joint end feels.
8. List the indications for performing a PROM exercise intervention.
9. What are the contraindications to performing AROM and PROM?
10. List and describe the grades of joint mobilization.

## Case Study 1

A patient presents 4 days status post a right femur fracture with an open reduction and internal fixation. The physician orders include AAROM right hip and knee and AROM right ankle, out of bed with assist, toe-touch weight bearing right lower extremity. The patient is being treated in a skilled nursing facility (estimated length of stay of 10 days), with goals of independent mobility with an assistive device and return home with spouse. Before onset, the patient was independent with all ADLs, instrumental ADLs, and ambulation without an assistive device.

1. Are there any red flags that the physical therapist assistant should consider?
2. Which type(s) of ROM are indicated and why?
3. Create an appropriate intervention plan for this patient.

## Case Study 2

A patient presents 1 day status post a left quadriceps contusion sustained during a soccer match. The physician orders include physical therapist evaluation and treatment, weight bearing as tolerated left lower extremity. The patient presents with pain with end ROM passive knee flexion and pain with AROM knee extension. The physical therapist's POC includes modalities, gait training with crutches (weight bearing as tolerated left lower extremity), patient education, and therapeutic exercise (progress ROM to stretching and initiate resisted exercises as appropriate).

1. Are there any red flags that the physical therapist assistant should consider?
2. Which type(s) of ROM are indicated and why?
3. Create an appropriate intervention plan for this patient.

## References


1. Levangie PK, Norkin C. *Joint Structure & Function: A Comprehensive Analysis.* 4th ed. FA Davis; 2005.
2. Norkin C, White D. *Measurement of Joint Motion.* 4th ed. FA Davis; 2009.
3. Kisner C. Range of motion. In: Kisner C, Colby LA, Borstad J, eds. *Therapeutic Exercise Foundations and Techniques.* 7th ed. FA Davis; 2018.
4. Chaudhry H, Bhandari M. Cochrane in *CORR*: continuous passive motion following total knee arthroplasty in people with arthritis (review). *Clin Orthop Relat Res.* 2015;473(11):3348-3354. doi:10.1007/s11999-015-4528-y
5. Harvey LA, Brosseau L, Herbert RD. Continuous passive motion following total knee arthroplasty in people with arthritis. *Cochrane Database Syst Rev.* 2014;2:CD004260. doi:10.1002/14651858.CD004260.pub3
6. American Physical Therapy Association. *Guide to Physical Therapist Practice.* American Physical Therapy Association; 2014. doi:10.2522/ptguide3.0_38
7. American Physical Therapy Association. Public Policy, practice and professional affairs unit. Physical therapists and direction of mobilization/manipulation: an educational resource paper. Updated July 14, 2016. Accessed January 24, 2023. https://www.apta.org/StateIssues/Manipulation/PTsDirectionofMobilizationManipulation/
8. American Physical Therapy Association. Interventions performed by physical therapists HOD P06-18-31-36. Accessed January 24, 2023. http://www.apta.org/uploadedFiles/APTAorg/About_Us/Policies/Practice/ProceduralInterventions.pdf
9. American Physical Therapy Association. CAPTE standards and required elements for accreditation of physical therapy assistant education programs. Revised December 7, 2017. Accessed January 24, 2023. http://www.capteonline.org/uploadedFiles/CAPTEorg/About_CAPTE/Resources/Accreditation_Handbook/CAPTE_PTAStandardsEvidence.pdf
10. Agarwal S, Raza S, Moiz JA, Anwer S, Alghadir AH. Effects of two different mobilization techniques on pain, range of motion and functional disability in patients with adhesive capsulitis: a comparative study. *J Phys Ther Sci.* 2016;28(12):3342-3349. doi:10.1589/jpts.28.3342
11. Parker AW, James B. Age changes in the flexibility of Down's syndrome children. *J Ment Defic Res.* 1985;29(Pt 3):207-218.
12. Fassier A, Wicart P, Dubousset J, Seringe R. Arthrogryposis multiplex congenita. Long-term follow-up from birth until skeletal maturity. *J Child Orthop.* 2009;3(5):383-390.
13. Doğru Apti M, Kasapçopur Ö, Mengi M, Öztürk G, Metin G. Regular aerobic training combined with range of motion exercises in juvenile idiopathic arthritis. *Biomed Res Int.* 2014;2014:748972. doi:10.1155/2014/748972
14. Takken T, Van Brussel M, Engelbert RH, Van Der Net J, Kuis W, Helders PJ. Exercise therapy in juvenile idiopathic arthritis: a Cochrane review. *Eur J Phys Rehabil Med.* 2008;44(3):287-297.
15. Fillit H, Rockwood K, Woodhouse K. *Brocklehurst's Textbook of Geriatric Medicine and Gerontology.* 7th ed. Elsevier; 2010.

Chapter 5

# Stretching and Flexibility

*Karen A. Cascardi, PhD, MS, ATC, PTA*

**KEY TERMS** Autogenic inhibition | Ballistic stretching | Flexibility | Reciprocal inhibition | Selective stretching | Static stretching | Stretch reflex | Stretching

## Chapter Objectives

1. Differentiate between flexibility and stretching.
2. Explain tissue adaptations that occur with stretching.
3. Differentiate between dynamic and passive flexibility.
4. Discuss the factors that can limit the effects of stretching.
5. List the benefits of stretching.
6. Differentiate between autogenic and reciprocal inhibition.
7. Define and demonstrate various types of stretching techniques and parameters.
8. Explain the indications, contraindications, precautions, and appropriate monitoring for a stretching program.
9. Given a case scenario or physical therapy plan of care, determine the most appropriate type of stretching exercise, parameters, and patient position.

## Introduction: Stretching and Flexibility

**Stretching** is a common intervention used in physical therapy. The ability to change and improve flexibility through the application of various stretching programs is well documented.[1,2] The purpose of stretching is to increase joint range of motion (ROM) and increase muscle-tendon extensibility. Normal ROM and good flexibility are necessary to perform basic activities of daily living. Improved flexibility may help reduce injury during sports or fitness training participation. Stretching is an important component of a plan to prevent poor postural habits associated with working long hours at the computer or endless texting (see Chapter 7). If stretching is performed incorrectly, injury can result, so it is important to pay attention to details and parameters when developing a stretching program.

**Flexibility** is defined as the ability of periarticular soft tissue (in conjunction with muscle deformation/lengthening) to allow a joint (or series of joints) to move in an unrestricted, pain-free ROM.[3-5] Decreased flexibility or



Kopack JK, Cascardi KA.
*Principles of Therapeutic Exercise for the Physical Therapist Assistant* (pp 63-80).

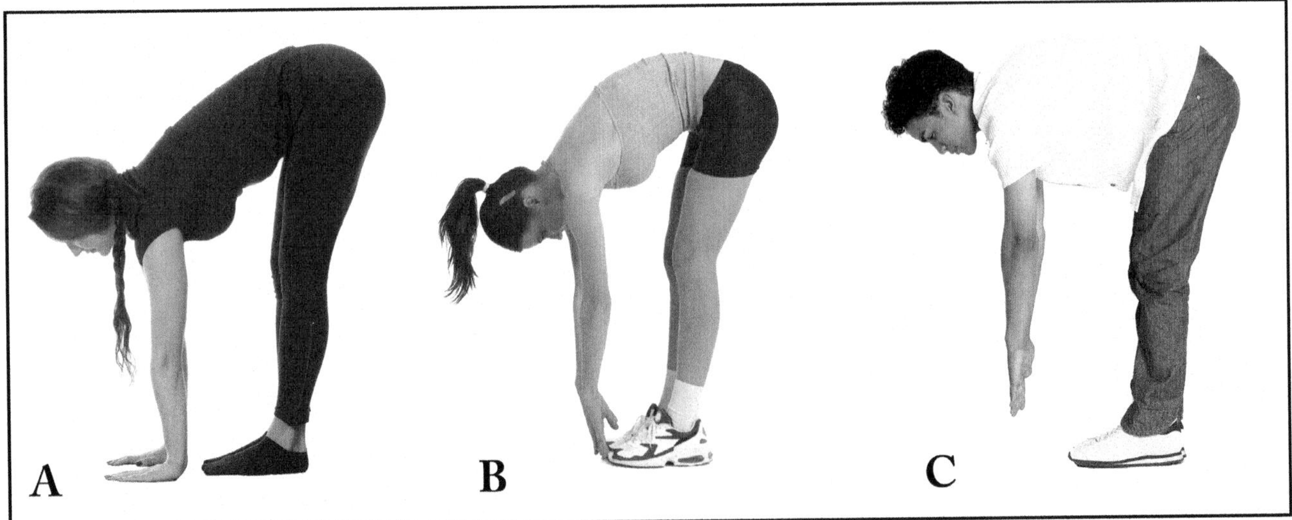


**Figure 5-1.** Hamstring length assessment. (A) This patient's hamstring length appears to be within normal limits (AleksZ Photo/Shutterstock.com). (B) The patient completes the task but appears to use increased thoracolumbar flexion mobility to compensate for limited hamstring length. Additionally, the knees are slightly flexed (Sean Nel/Shutterstock.com). (C) This patient may have both limited hamstring length as well as possible thoracolumbar ROM limitations (Image Source Collection/Shutterstock.com).

hypomobility results in a loss of ROM and can occur for any of the following reasons:

- Poor joint arthrokinematics
- Joint pain secondary to changes in articular surfaces (with or without joint effusion)
- Capsular or ligament tightness
- Prolonged immobilization
- Faulty postural alignment with associated muscle tightness and/or weakness
- Musculotendinous or joint injury
- Various musculoskeletal or neuromuscular conditions

To address flexibility, physical therapist assistants need to assess sequential joint movements and muscle excursion. The assistant must determine if the involved muscles performing the motions cross one or more than one joint. Muscle limitations or joint restrictions may result in the inability to complete normal ROM, which often presents with compensatory hypermobility at one or more adjacent joints. For example, a patient is instructed to touch the floor with their hands while keeping the knees straight (Figure 5-1). If the patient is unable to complete the task, the assistant needs to determine if the cause is due to hamstring tightness, back extensor tightness, joint limitation, or any combination of these causes. The clinician needs to ask the following questions to determine the cause of the limitation:

- Does the patient "fulcrum" or "hitch" (flex) at the hips when bending forward?
- Does the motion primarily occur at the hips?
- Do the hips reach 80 to 90 degrees of flexion?
- Is the patient's thoracic and lumbar spine flat or curved?

If the patient can perform the task with a straight spine (Figure 5-1A), there is adequate hamstring muscle excursion, but does the patient have back extensor tightness? Excessive thoracolumbar spine flexion can compensate for limited hamstring muscle mobility (Figure 5-1B). Limitations in hamstring length and thoracolumbar mobility result in an inability to touch the toes in standing (Figure 5-1C). In this scenario, the clinician must determine if the patient's inability to complete the task is due to a limitation in thoracolumbar flexion mobility, decreased hamstring length, or both. The answers to these questions help determine where the limitations are and guide the clinician in devising treatment interventions that target the involved structures.

Dynamic flexibility is the unrestricted ROM achieved during an active muscle contraction. Dynamic flexibility is synonymous with active range of motion (AROM). Passive flexibility is the ROM achieved when an external force moves a segment to the point of tissue resistance. Passive flexibility is synonymous with passive range of motion (PROM). Passive flexibility is dependent on the amount of muscle extensibility and the extensibility of the surrounding soft tissue. The amount of ROM also depends on whether the muscle being stretched crosses more than one joint and if the position of one of the joints creates an inability to stretch further over the second joint (passive insufficiency). During AROM, the muscle moves through a specific range, but during PROM the segment can be moved a small amount beyond the active range with the application of overpressure into this new range.[3] The available range of passive flexibility (PROM) is greater than dynamic flexibility (AROM).

Stretching is defined as the process of elongating a muscle or muscle group and their associated tendons and structures (capsular and/or nerve tissues) beyond the currently available ROM. Stretching techniques are used to either maintain or increase the normal resting length of a muscle. To increase joint ROM or muscle length, the muscle needs to be elongated (stretched) in the opposite direction from which it contracts. For example, a one-joint muscle that performs elbow flexion (ie, the brachialis) is elongated when the elbow joint is moved to the end range of elbow extension. The theory of passive insufficiency can be applied to effectively stretch a 2-joint muscle and increase its normal resting length. It is important to remember which muscles cross more than one joint.

In some specific situations, a patient may rely on the resting tightness of a muscle or muscle group to provide stability or function. In these situations, selective stretching will be performed, and traditional stretches for those structures must be modified. Selective stretching is commonly used when treating patients with spinal cord injuries and is discussed later in the chapter.

Other factors that can affect how the clinician modifies positioning and the selection of stretching parameters when designing a stretching program include patient activity level, age, sex, hormonal changes in pregnancy, phase of injury recovery, and the patient's medications. Certain medications can have an adverse effect on muscles and tendons (refer to the Medication Side Effects section in this chapter).

## Passive Insufficiency

Passive insufficiency occurs when a 2-joint (or multijoint) antagonist muscle cannot be lengthened simultaneously across both joints through the full ROM. This concept is important when creating an effective exercise to stretch a 2-joint muscle. The clinician must first stabilize one joint in a position that will adequately stretch the multijoint muscle and then passively move the second joint into the position needed to stretch the muscle. For example, to effectively stretch the rectus femoris, the hip needs to be placed in extension (ie, prone with the hip extended or supine similar to a Thomas Test position); then, the clinician passively moves the knee into flexion, effectively elongating the muscle across both joints (hip and knee) and creating a stretch.

## Neurophysiology and Proprioceptive Neuromuscular Facilitation Stretching

The normal resting length of a muscle is the actual length of that muscle without stresses or loads applied to it. Muscle excursion is the distance from maximal shortening to maximal lengthening. Muscles can contract to about one-half of their resting length and be stretched to approximately twice their resting length.[4]

As a muscle is stretched, tension increases in the direction of the force being applied. Stretching also occurs in the sarcomere. During a stretch, the overlap of the actin and myosin decreases (they move further apart) as the sarcomere lengthens, allowing the muscle fiber to elongate. Not all muscle fibers stretch at the same time, and the number of fibers being stretched determines the actual length of the muscle; the more fibers being stretched, the greater the muscle length. During a stretch, the surrounding connective tissue also stretches in the direction of the force.

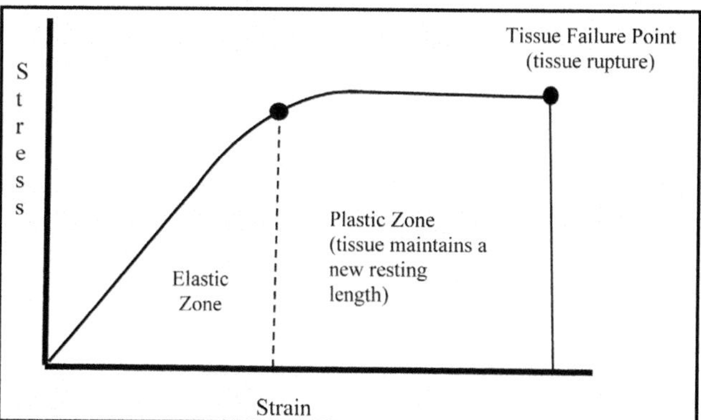

**Figure 5-2.** Stress-strain curve.

After injury or surgical intervention, stretching (initiated at the appropriate time) helps to realign scar tissue in an organized fashion, improving tissue healing and increasing desired tissue length. The healing cycle of the affected tissues determines the appropriate time to initiate stretching and the amount of intensity to use.

The tissues in the body undergo stress during mobility and activities of daily living. Contractility, excitability, elasticity, and extensibility are characteristics of muscle tissue. When performing a stretching exercise, the muscle gets longer (extensibility) and then returns to its original length (elasticity). Extensibility allows muscle tissue to be stretched when a force is applied, and elasticity is the muscle's ability to resume its normal resting length after the force is removed. Plasticity occurs when muscle tissue has been stretched and the muscle achieves an increase in resting length because of the forces applied.[4] This concept is based on the stress-strain curve. When a sustained load is placed on connective tissue, it can result in a permanent change in the length of the soft tissue. Overstretching can result in tissue failure that can occur from a strain/sprain or rupture (Figure 5-2).

Understanding the neurophysiology of muscles is helpful when applying proprioceptive neuromuscular facilitation (PNF) stretching techniques. "PNF stretching techniques, sometimes referred to as *active stretching or facilitative stretching*, integrate active muscle contractions into stretching maneuvers purportedly to inhibit or facilitate muscle activation and to increase the likelihood that the muscle to be lengthened remains as relaxed as possible as it is stretched"[4,p93]

Muscle spindles and Golgi tendon organs (GTOs) are sensory organs (mechanoreceptors) found in muscle tissue. The muscle spindles are dispersed in the belly of a muscle; they run parallel to the muscle fibers and are called *extrafusal fibers*. Within the muscle spindle, there are special fibers that are called *intrafusal fibers*. These fibers include afferent (sensory) and efferent (motor) fiber endings. When a muscle stretches, the muscle spindles stretch as well. Muscle spindles are sensitive to the amount of change and the rate of change in muscle length. The **stretch reflex** is a reflexive contraction in response to a quick stretch. When a muscle is stretched, the afferent or sensory fibers (located in skin and muscles) send a message to the posterior horn

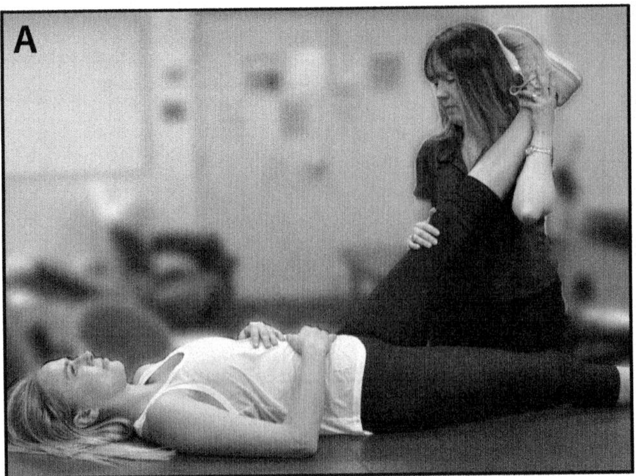


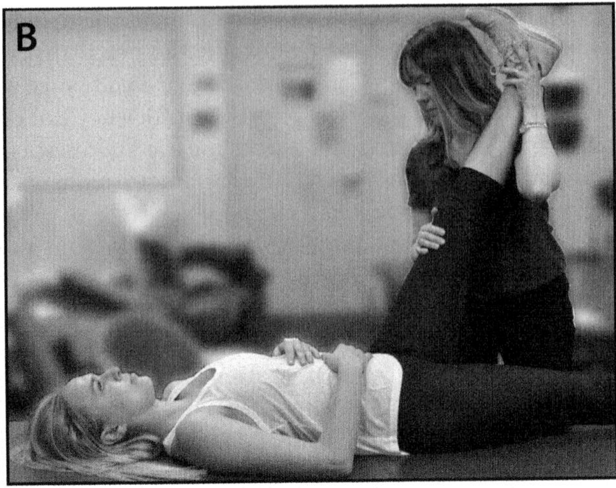


**Figure 5-3.** (A) Autogenic inhibition: The clinician moves the leg until a stretch is attained. The patient then performs a hamstring isometric contraction for 5 to 6 seconds. (B) The clinician then moves the leg into a new range, increasing the amount of hip flexion and creating a greater stretch of the hamstrings. GTO over-rides the muscle spindle.

of the spinal cord of the central nervous system (CNS). The CNS then sends a message to contract back to the muscle being stretched via the efferent or motor fibers to stop the stretch. A second message is sent to the antagonist muscles to relax (called *reflex inhibition*). This reflex is a protective mechanism to prevent muscle injury caused by overstretching.

GTOs are located at the musculotendinous junction. These sensory organs are responsive to passive stretching as well as muscle contractions. The GTO is sensitive to slight changes in tension and the rate of change in tension in a tendon. The GTO is activated when either a prolonged stretch or active muscle contraction creates tension in the muscle and tendon. The GTO sends a message to the CNS, which then sends a message back to the muscle directing that muscle to relax, thus allowing the muscle to be stretched further. GTO nerve fibers can over-ride impulses coming from the muscle spindle. When the hamstrings are put on a passive stretch (Figure 5-3A) and then followed by a submaximal isometric contraction (for about 5 to 6 seconds) of the hamstrings, there is an increase in tension in the tendons, which activates the GTOs and over-rides muscle spindle activity. This reduces tension in the hamstrings (antagonists) and allows the hip to be passively moved further into hip flexion (Figure 5-3B). This PNF stretching technique is called **autogenic inhibition**. This technique can be used for any muscle or muscle group (ie, quadriceps; hip flexors; gastrocnemius; or shoulder, elbow, and wrist flexors/extensors) whose shortened length prevents joint movement through its normal ROM. This PNF stretch is also referred to as a *hold-relax* or *contract-relax technique*.[4] Table 5-1 provides specific instructions when performing this stretching technique.

Autogenic inhibition also occurs when a muscle is suddenly stretched. For example, if a person's leg accidentally slips out from under them and the hamstrings are put on a quick stretch, the GTO acts protectively, causing a reflexive contraction of the muscles being stretched (antagonist) and a relaxation of the opposing hip flexors/knee extensors (agonist muscles). This reflexive response is an attempt to avoid injury.

**Reciprocal inhibition** is another PNF stretching technique that can be used to increase ROM. This type of PNF stretching technique is called *agonist contraction*. This stretching technique is a dynamic stretch. When agonist muscles concentrically contract, the antagonist muscles reflexively relax to allow for smooth motion. For example, when the elbow actively flexes, the biceps and brachialis muscles (agonists) concentrically contract to move the forearm, but this can only occur because the triceps (antagonists) reflexively relax. The GTO and muscle spindle responses signal the antagonist muscles (the triceps) to relax and the agonist muscles (the elbow flexors) to contract, allowing motion to occur. When using the reciprocal inhibition stretching technique, a physical therapist assistant passively moves the limb into a position where a tolerable stretch is placed on the antagonist muscle group (Figure 5-4A). After a short hold (about 10 seconds) in that position, the patient is instructed to actively contract the agonist muscles (in this case the hip flexors) into a new range (Figure 5-4B). This new position is then held by the clinician for about 10 to 15 seconds (Figure 5-4C). This increase in ROM is due to the synchronization of the opposing muscle groups (active movement of the agonists and reflexive relaxation of the antagonist muscles). Table 5-2 provides specific instructions when using reciprocal inhibition stretching. Using the combination of autogenic and reciprocal inhibition techniques is called *hold–relax–active contraction*, which is noted in Table 5-1. Several studies have shown that PNF stretching techniques increase ROM and flexibility,[6-9] whereas others found that these techniques are more effective at increasing ROM than static stretching exercises.[6,7,9]

**Table 5-1**

**Instructions Implementing Autogenic Inhibition Stretching**

1. Place the patient in a stable and comfortable position.
2. The clinician should support the patient's extremity and passively move it into the desired direction, putting the antagonist muscles on stretch.
   a. Say to the patient, "Tell me when you feel tension in the muscle; it may be slightly uncomfortable, but it should not be painful."
3. The clinician supports and stabilizes the limb in the newly gained position and prepares to resist a submaximal isometric contraction of the antagonist muscles. The clinician's body should be stable with the hands safely positioned to resist the patient's contraction.
4. The assistant should then instruct the patient to "push into me with moderate effort, and I am going to resist and hold you here." (The antagonist muscles are performing an isometric contraction as the assistant resists.)
5. The isometric contraction is held for 5 to 6 seconds. The assistant should count out loud, so the patient knows when to stop pushing. Following the contraction time, instruct the patient to slowly relax.
6. Once the patient relaxes, the clinician passively moves the extremity in the direction of the desired motion (the opposite direction of the isometric contraction) increasing the ROM.[a] This can be repeated up to 3 to 4 times.

[a]If the patient actively moves the limb into the new range following the antagonist's isometric contraction (vs the limb being passively moved), the stretch uses both autogenic and reciprocal techniques, which is called *hold–relax–active contraction.*

**Quick Tip: Remembering Proprioceptive Neuromuscular Facilitation Stretching Techniques**

Hold-relax: Uses autogenic inhibition; agonist is relaxed/antagonist contracts.

Agonist contraction: Uses reciprocal inhibition; agonist contracts/antagonist is relaxed.

Hold–relax–active contraction: Uses a combination of the 2 techniques. Agonist is relaxed/antagonist contracts followed by agonist contracts/antagonist is relaxed (hold-relax + agonist contraction).

## *Stretching Indications, Contraindications, and Precautions*

When designing a stretching program, physical therapist assistants must consider the type of tissues affected, the phase of healing the affected tissues are in, and the amount of allowable stress applied to healing tissues. The stretching program should be guided by tissue healing constraints and the patient's pain tolerance.

The main purpose of stretching is to increase ROM. Stretching is an indicated intervention to treat hypomobility (decreased ROM). Hypomobility can occur because of disuse, adhesions, or contractures and can result in limited function, leading to structural deformities and/or causing faulty postures. Faulty posture is often a result of muscle imbalances. Muscle imbalances arise when the muscles on one side are shortened (tight) and the opposing muscles are lengthened (or weak). Stretching shortened muscles and strengthening elongated muscles help restore function and decrease pain.

**Considerations for the Physical Therapist Assistant**

Flexibility is dependent on the skin, fascia, and surrounding tissue (ligaments, joint capsule, and nerve tissue) mobility, not just musculotendinous excursion.

There are situations when stretching is inappropriate or an unsafe intervention. Physical therapist assistants must know the contraindications and precautions for stretching (Table 5-3). Stretching hypermobile joints is contraindicated because it can create more joint instability. However, some athletes (ie, gymnasts) require greater ROM and flexibility than other athletes and far more range than the average person. This situation is an exception to the rule, as long as the muscles have the strength to control the excessive motions at these extreme end ranges.

Clinicians must know when stretching a muscle or a group of muscles is inappropriate. For example, it is contraindicated to stretch the low back extensors (erector spinae muscles) in a patient with a complete spinal cord injury because overstretching these muscles can affect their sitting stability. The clinician should also avoid stretching the wrist and finger flexors simultaneously for patients with tetraplegia who use tenodesis. Tenodesis relies on the normal resting length of the long finger flexors to achieve grasp during active wrist extension. Stretching the wrist and fingers

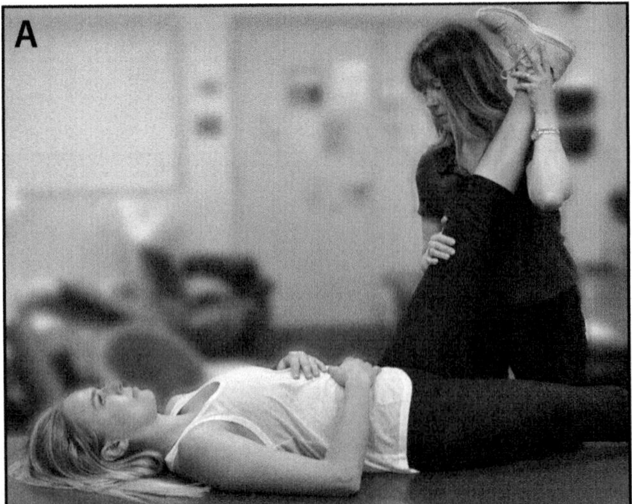


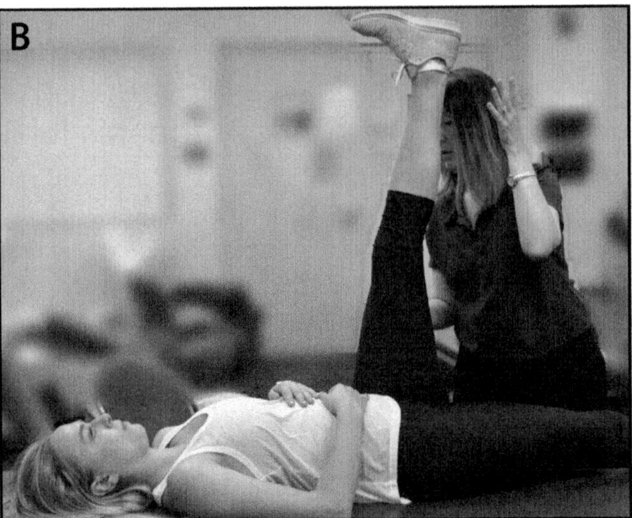


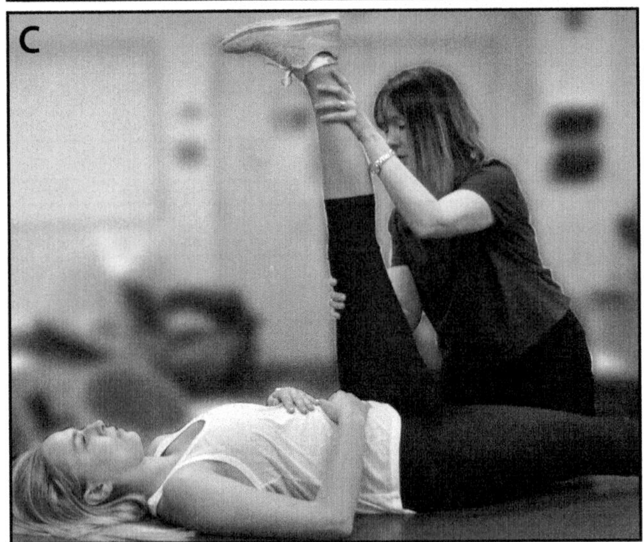


**Figure 5-4.** (A) Reciprocal inhibition; the patient is positioned supine. The clinician is assisting with the stretch. Notice how the leg is stabilized during the stretch. (B) The patient actively contracts the hip flexors as the hip extensors reflexively relax so the patient moves into a new increased ROM. (C) The clinician holds the patient's leg in the newly attained range for 10 to 15 seconds.

## Table 5-2

### Instructions Implementing Reciprocal Inhibition Stretching

1. Place the patient in a stable and comfortable position.
2. The clinician supports the patient's extremity and passively moves it in the desired direction, putting the antagonist muscles on stretch.
   a. Say to the patient, "Tell me when you feel tension in the muscle; it may be slightly uncomfortable, but it should not be painful."
3. After maintaining this position for a short period of time, instruct the patient to "see if you can move your leg/arm further into a new position. You should feel a stretch but not pain." The patient then contracts the agonist muscles, moving the limb into the new range. The assistant should maintain support and gently follow the patient's movement into the new range. Once in the new "tolerable" position, tell the patient "relax, and I am going to hold you here." The assistant holds this new stretching position for 10 to 15 seconds.
4. This technique can be repeated about 3 to 4 times as tolerated or if the limb no longer moves into a new range. The clinician should passively bring the patient's extremity back to the starting position (on the table) after the last repetition.

**Table 5-3**

Stretching Contraindications and Precautions

| Contraindications | Precautions |
|---|---|
| • Recent fracture, fracture not radiographically healed, or incomplete union<br>• Bony block (hard end feel)<br>• In the acute phase of healing<br>• Acute infection<br>• Sharp or sudden pain during the stretch<br>• Following a recent surgical procedure<br>• Joint effusion or tissue edema<br>• Stretching hypermobile joints<br>• Stretching structures that provide stability<br>• Osteoporosis (avoid stretches into trunk flexion)<br>• Bony metastases<br>• During an acute exacerbation of rheumatoid arthritis | • Avoid high-load stretching to recently healed fractures or long-term immobilized joints<br>• Do not stretch a joint beyond its normal range<br>• Limit interventions to gentle, pain-free stretching for patients with rheumatoid arthritis or osteoporosis (see contraindications) and monitor patients closely<br>• Check medication side effects before initiating a stretching program<br>• Avoid overstretching weak muscles<br>• Osteopenia |

into extension simultaneously overstretches these muscles, reducing the patient's ability to grasp. The clinician should modify the application of stretches for these patients (refer to Specialized Applications of Stretching section).

### Medication Side Effects

Some medications can affect the integrity of muscles and/or tendons. Physical therapist assistants should always review a patient's medical record and the physical therapy evaluation for a list of medications and any contraindications or precautions for stretching exercises. The assistant should consult with the physical therapist if there are any medication questions or concerns before treatment. Appendix E provides a list of medications commonly used in physical therapy.

Fluoroquinolones (FQs) or quinolones are strong antibiotics that can cause tendon or soft tissue damage or ruptures. Some common examples are Avelox (moxifloxacin), Levaquin (levofloxacin), and Cipro (ciprofloxacin). According to the Food and Drug Administration's Adverse Event Reporting System, there are reports of tendon ruptures associated with currently approved FQs, with the highest numbers occurring for levofloxacin, ciprofloxacin, and moxifloxacin. Risk factors for FQ-associated tendon rupture include increased age and concurrent corticosteroid use.[10]

The use of corticosteroids can cause myopathy. This muscle weakness is most commonly observed in proximal muscles of the upper and lower extremities and neck flexors.[11] Corticosteroids are commonly used to treat asthma, chronic obstructive pulmonary disease, rheumatoid arthritis, polymyositis, and other inflammatory diseases.[11] The assistant should notify the therapist of any medication changes or additions and any unusual patient responses or reports during treatment.

## *General Stretching Parameters*

Physical therapist assistants will need to select appropriate treatment parameters when incorporating stretching exercises in the rehabilitation program. Recalling muscle proximal and distal attachments and understanding if the muscle is a one-joint or multijoint muscle is important when targeting specific muscles to be stretched. The assistant must be able to determine the most appropriate patient position, stabilize the segment to be stretched, communicate what the patient should feel during the stretch, determine the stretch intensity, and determine how long (duration) the stretch should be maintained.

### Proper Positioning

Once the clinician identifies the structures/muscles to be stretched, the patient should be placed in a comfortable and supportive position, with the body aligned so that the structures can be stretched safely and efficiently. The patient's position should stress the muscle(s) using the maximal amount of tolerable tension. Proper positioning and support of adjacent joints/segments are also important. For example, there are several ways a physical therapist assistant can teach a patient to stretch the hamstring muscles. To stretch the hamstrings, the clinician knows that this muscle group crosses 2 joints. The patient can be positioned supine (Figures 5-5A and 5-5B), seated (Figure 5-5C), or standing (Figure 5-5D). If the assistant decides to have the patient seated, try the following quick class activity before reading on.

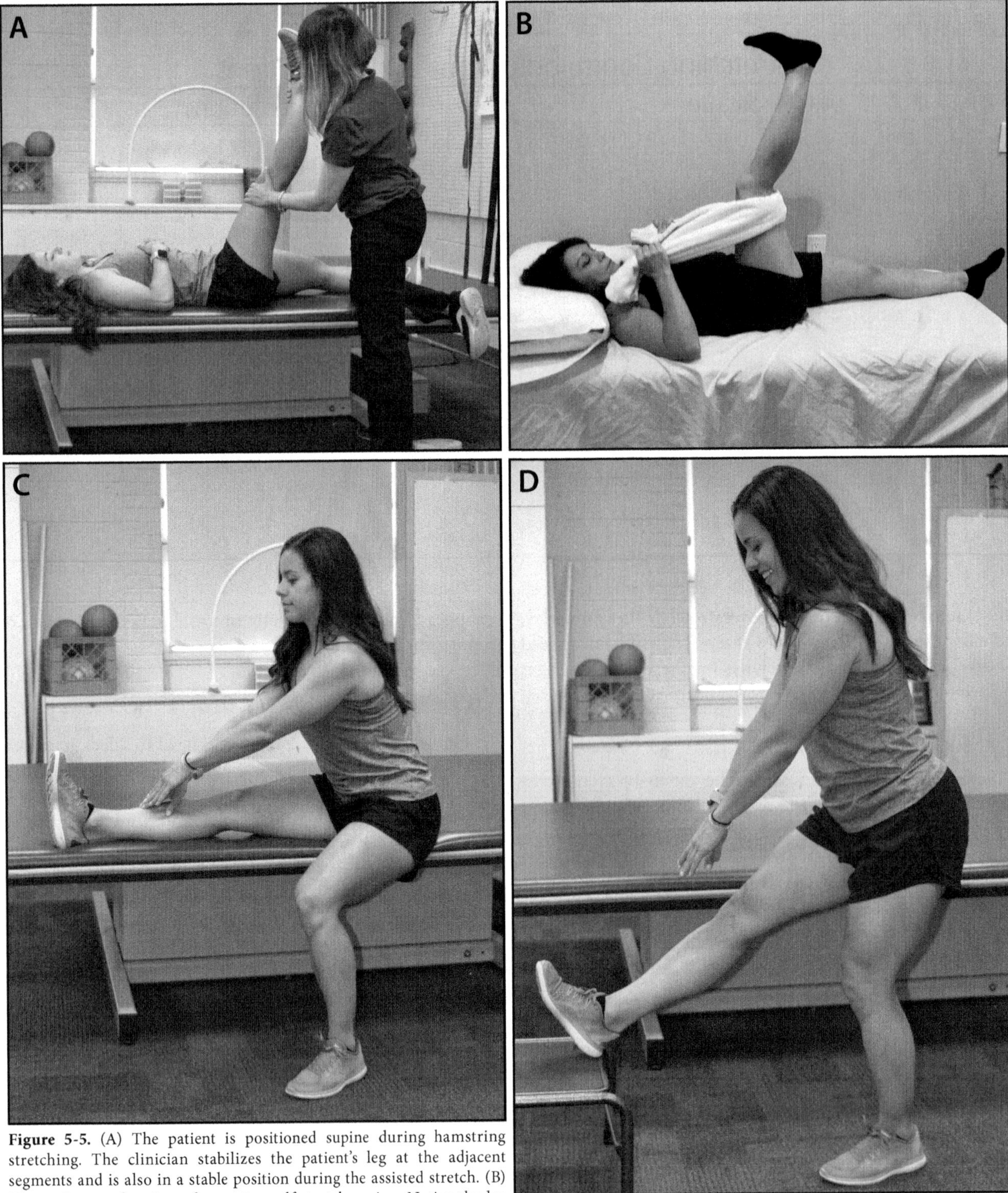


**Figure 5-5.** (A) The patient is positioned supine during hamstring stretching. The clinician stabilizes the patient's leg at the adjacent segments and is also in a stable position during the assisted stretch. (B) The patient performing a hamstring self-stretch supine. Notice the leg being stretched is stabilized using a towel around the thigh. (C) The patient performing a hamstring stretch. Notice the patient's straight spine position. (D) The standing hamstring stretch. Notice the patient is safely standing next to the treatment table.

> **Quick Class Activity**
>
> Hamstring stretch: Sit and place one leg on a plinth with the knee straight. First, slouch your back with the pelvis rotated into a posterior tilt. Then, sit up straight (rotate pelvis into an anterior tilt), and sit so you feel pressure on the ischial tuberosity. When do you feel the greatest stretch? Why?

Based on the class activity, you see why it is imperative to have the patient sit or stand with the pelvis tilted anteriorly and the spine straight. This position puts the greatest possible tension on the hamstring muscle group because the ischial tuberosity (hamstring proximal attachment) is positioned further away from the distal attachments of the muscles. If the assistant wants to target the biceps femoris, the patient should be instructed to roll the leg medially (internally rotate it), which places that muscle on a greater stretch because of its attachment on the fibula head. By externally rotating the thigh, the semimembranosus and semitendinosus are targeted because they attach more medially on the tibia.

## Proper Stabilization

The physical therapist assistant needs to determine which joint or muscle needs to be stabilized before the stretching activity. A structure can be stabilized by using a firm surface (eg, a plinth/table), the floor/wall, or manually by the patient or therapist (see Figure 5-5). The clinician or the patient can stabilize the appropriate structure distally (supporting the entire limb) or more proximally (supporting the proximal limb segment). Look at the hamstring stretch example that was performed in the Quick Class Activity again. The knee was straight, and the tibia and femur were fixed (stabilized by the plinth). The patient leaned forward from the hip joint, and the stretch was felt in the back of the leg. When standing (see Figure 5-5D), the patient stabilizes the distal end of the leg on a stool. The stretch can also be performed while sitting in a chair where the trunk, pelvis, and thighs (proximal segments) are supported while in short sitting. The patient can straighten the lower leg into knee extension as far as possible until the stretch is felt in the hamstrings. Both of these examples are performed by the patient and are called *self-stretches*. When the clinician performs the stretch passively, it is referred to as *manual or passive stretching*. Figure 5-5 illustrates both of these stretching techniques.

Many patients have both tight hamstrings and hip flexors, so, when stretching the patient's right hamstrings (for example), the left thigh may lift off the table slightly as the end range of the right hamstrings is reached. To maximize the effectiveness of the stretch, the clinician should also stabilize (or hold down) the left leg to prevent the pelvis from going into a posterior pelvic tilt.

## Stretch Intensity

The intensity of a stretch reflects the amount of force placed on the muscle. Low-load or low-intensity stretching is more comfortable, and it places less stress, thus reducing muscle guarding compared with high-load or high-intensity stretching. High-load stretching usually creates significant discomfort/pain. Low-intensity stretches applied for a prolonged duration have better outcomes than high-intensity, short-duration stretching.[4,12] This is most likely due to elastic deformation and plastic changes in the tissues.

In a large study examining stretch intensity, investigators summarized that gentle stretch intensity (between 30% and 60% maximal ROM) did not cause inflammation and that a painful stretch (90% of maximal ROM) did cause inflammation.[13] The researchers concluded that gentle stretching, stretching with discomfort by a therapist or machine, and maximal stretch with no pain with a therapist are beneficial.[13] The most effective technique combines a supported limb with a low-intensity force because it increases ROM while reducing the likelihood of triggering a stretch reflex and/or increasing the inflammatory response. Patients should be taught that a stretch should be taken to a point where it may cause discomfort or tightness, but it should not cause pain.[14]

## Stretch Duration (Time)

A clinician determines the duration and frequency of a stretching program. Stretches can be static (sustained) or ballistic. During static stretching, a muscle is placed on a stretch, and the duration is held for a set amount of time. The general recommendation for stretch duration is from 15 seconds[15] to 60 seconds[16]; the shorter the stretch duration, the higher number of repetitions that should be performed. A longer stretch duration with fewer repetitions is more effective at increasing AROM vs a program that includes shorter-duration stretches with more repetitions (when the total stretch time is the same between groups).[15] Research has shown that for older adults (65 years and older), holding a stretch for 60 seconds produces greater ROM than 15- or 30-second stretches.[16] Other researchers reported that static hamstring stretches held for 30 and 60 seconds were more effective than sustained 15-second stretching.[4,17] A 30-second sustained stretch of the hamstring was found to be more effective than self-stretching or PNF stretching for adults ages 21 to 35 years.[18] A stretch duration of 30 seconds is effective for improving ROM; however, in older adults, 60 seconds may be more beneficial.[16] Patient age and the duration of the sustained stretch should be considered when implementing a stretching program.

## Stretch Frequency

Frequency is determined based on the treatment goals and the type, duration, and intensity of the selected stretch. Lower-intensity, shorter-duration stretches should be repeated with greater frequency than high-intensity stretches.[4,13] General flexibility exercises should be completed at least 3 times a week, and daily performance is often preferred for the best outcome.[14]

**Table 5-4**

**Stretching Parameters According to the American College of Sports Medicine Recommendations and the FITT-VP Principle[14]**

- Frequency: Determined based on the treatment goals and the type, time, and intensity of the selected stretch. Lower-intensity, shorter-duration stretches should be repeated with greater frequency and are typically more appropriate than high-intensity stretches.
- Intensity: Research indicates that lower-intensity forces may be most appropriate to increase ROM while minimizing pain/inflammation.
- Type: Passive or manual, self-stretch, mechanical, dynamic, and PNF (ie, autogenic inhibition, reciprocal inhibition, or a combination).
- Time or duration: Should be selected and modified depending on the tolerated intensity and age of the patient. Lower-intensity stretches for longer durations are preferred.
- Manual and self-static stretches: Should be held for 15 to 60 seconds. Older adults benefit more from stretches held for 60 seconds.[16] Younger adults benefit from stretches held for 30 seconds.[17]
- Prolonged mechanical stretch: Can be applied for 15 minutes (ie, use of a weight) up to 8 to 10 hours (ie, Dynasplint [Dynasplint Systems, Inc]).
- Volume: Refers to the total stretching time; target a minimum of 60 seconds of stretching.
- Pattern: The number of repetitions to be performed for each stretch. Two to 4 repetitions of each selected stretch are recommended.

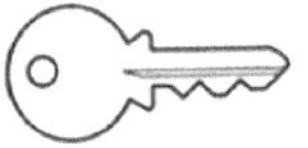

**Key Safety Considerations: Stretching Interventions**

- Review patient medications in the medical record.
- Check for stretching contraindications and precautions.
- Monitor patient response to activity (appropriate vs adverse response to the stretch).
- Monitor for signs/symptoms to terminate exercise (ie, cardiac).
- No pain during or after stretching; slight discomfort or tightness is acceptable during stretching.
- Monitor patient's breathing; avoid breath holding/Valsalva.
- Ensure the patient and muscles being stretched are both relaxed and supported.
- Check for appropriate patient positioning and proper form during the stretch.
- Physical therapist assistants should use good body mechanics and be stable.
- Verify stretching is appropriate given the stage of healing if postinjury or postsurgery.

The American College of Sports Medicine recommends using the FITT-VP (frequency, intensity, time, type, volume, progression) principle (Table 5-4) to determine optimal stretching parameters.[14] Before stretching, the clinician should complete any preprocedure measurements (ie, joint goniometric measurements), and the patient should complete a warm-up and/or relaxation activity (eg, light aerobic exercise or general muscle activity, moist heat, ultrasound). The clinician should implement the stretches and monitor the patient's response during the intervention. The patient should have no complaints of pain during stretching exercises and no reported pain/soreness lasting longer than 1 to 2 hours posttreatment. Slight discomfort or tightness is acceptable during the stretch. If symptoms worsen or the patient reports complaints of muscle soreness several hours after treatment, the stretching regimen must be adjusted accordingly; these symptoms indicate overstretching.

Following the stretching intervention, the patient should perform AROM into the newly gained ROM, and the clinician should complete a postmeasurement of AROM and PROM. The patient should use the new available ROM as much as possible to maintain the gains.

## Various Types of Stretching Techniques

Clinicians should consider many factors when selecting a stretching technique. Table 5-5 provides a list of things to consider when selecting a specific technique. Light aerobic (warm-up) activity should be performed before stretching (eg, walking, stationary bike, upper extremity bike performed for several minutes). The warm-up will increase a person's body temperature and overall circulation, which prepares the muscle(s) for stretching. The application of superficial heat will not penetrate deep enough to heat larger muscles but can be used for smaller joints or on patients with less adipose tissue. Deep heating modalities such as ultrasound are more effective than hot packs when used before stretching.[19]

**Table 5-5**

**Stretching Considerations**

- Identify target tissues to be stretched based on the physical therapist's evaluation/plan of care. Review ROM and muscle strength.
- Determine the phase of healing the patient is currently in (acute, subacute, chronic phase/return to sport).
- Are contraindications or precautions present?
- Check the patient's age and/or physical condition and other comorbidities.
- How is the stretching activity going to be performed (clinician, patient, both, or mechanical)?
- Which type of stretching is most appropriate for the patient at the current time (static/passive, PNF, self-stretch, or dynamic)?
- Is this the first stretching technique attempted or does the technique need to be modified due to progress based on increased ROM/flexibility or the lack thereof due to pain?
- Determine the most appropriate warm-up (about 5 minutes) to increase blood flow and tissue extensibility for larger muscle groups before stretching.

The types of stretching techniques include static, passive (manual), dynamic, self-stretching, and mechanical. Stretches can be performed actively, assisted by the patient, passively by a therapist, or mechanically (using a device or weight). Most of the stretches included in this chapter are performed as static self-stretches, but PNF techniques can also be applied to any of these exercises. Stretching exercises should be progressed from passive to more active techniques when appropriate to increase the patient's independence with the exercise (Figure 5-6).

**Static stretching** is a sustained hold of a muscle where some tension is created in one specific position for a predetermined length of time.

Passive (manual) stretching is initially performed by a clinician who manually moves the patient's extremity until tissue resistance is felt by the patient at the end of their available range. The therapist controls all of the parameters of the stretch. Manual or passive stretching is usually the initial technique used to increase ROM. As the patient progresses, the patient can be taught ways to complete the stretch as part of a home exercise program (HEP).

Mechanical stretching is used when a longer stretch duration is required (ie, joints with contractures). The duration of a low-load sustained stretch can be anywhere from 15 minutes to 8 to 10 hours.[4] The physical therapist may be responsible for ordering a mechanical stretching device. These devices provide a constant low-load stretch that is either preset or patient controlled. In the clinic, the physical therapist assistant may use a light cuff weight that is placed on the distalmost aspect of a patient's extremity for 5 to 15 minutes to obtain a stretch. The limb proximal to the joint/muscle being targeted for the stretch must be stabilized. An example of this is a stretch into knee extension (Figure 5-7). The patient is positioned prone with the thigh stabilized by the table, and a light cuff weight is placed around the patient's ankle. The combination of the cuff weight and the pull of gravity applies a low load, stretching the knee joint (hamstrings) into extension.

Dynamic stretching is performed actively by the patient. Muscles actively contract as close to the end range as possible with no hold time at end range. This technique uses momentum, but the range is more controlled than with ballistic stretching. Dynamic stretching is typically included in the last stage of a progression and is commonly included at the end of rehabilitation as a return-to-sport warm-up activity. Leg swings or large arm circles are examples of dynamic stretching.

Self-stretching is also a stretching technique performed by the patient. It can be performed passively or dynamically and can include static stretching and PNF techniques. It is usually included in the patient's HEP so that ROM gains obtained during treatment can be maintained. Physical therapist assistants should instruct patients on proper self-stretching techniques and provide written instructions so they can be continued correctly at home. Patients should demonstrate stretches correctly to the clinician before performing them independently at home. Examples of stretching exercises for various muscle groups in different positions are provided in Figures 5-8 to 5-17.

**Documentation Tip**

All parameters of the intervention provided should be documented. Manual stretch to a patient's hamstrings may be documented as follows: Manual R hamstring stretch: Patient supine, 3 reps 30 second hold. Increased R hip flexion PROM by 9 degrees post stretch. Patient instructed in long sitting self-stretch of R hamstring with anterior pelvic tilt and upright posture with verbal cues. Patient demonstrates exercise independently after instruction. A written copy of HEP was given to patient.

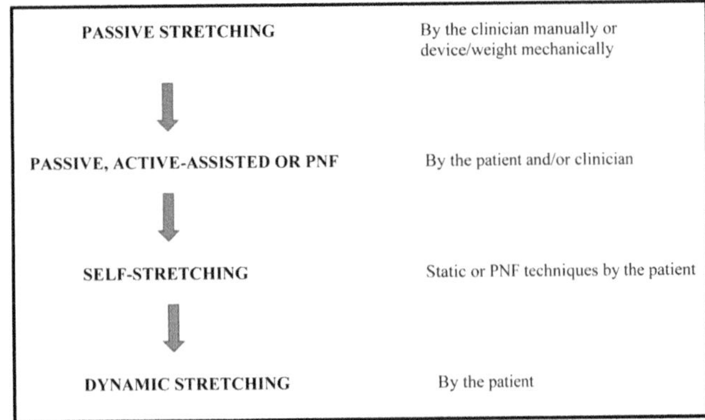


**Figure 5-6.** Stretching progression.

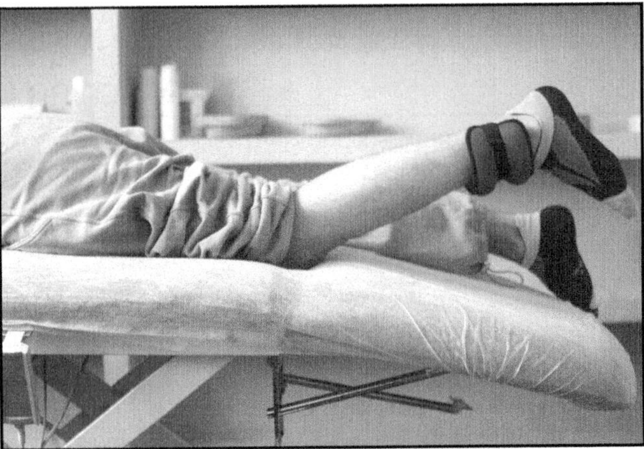

**Figure 5-7.** A photo of mechanical stretching. The patient's anterior aspect of the knee is in the space between the break in the table, which does not put pressure on the patella. A pillow could be placed under the thigh to relieve pressure on the patella if the table does not articulate (or move) and has a solid top (edwardolive/Shutterstock.com).

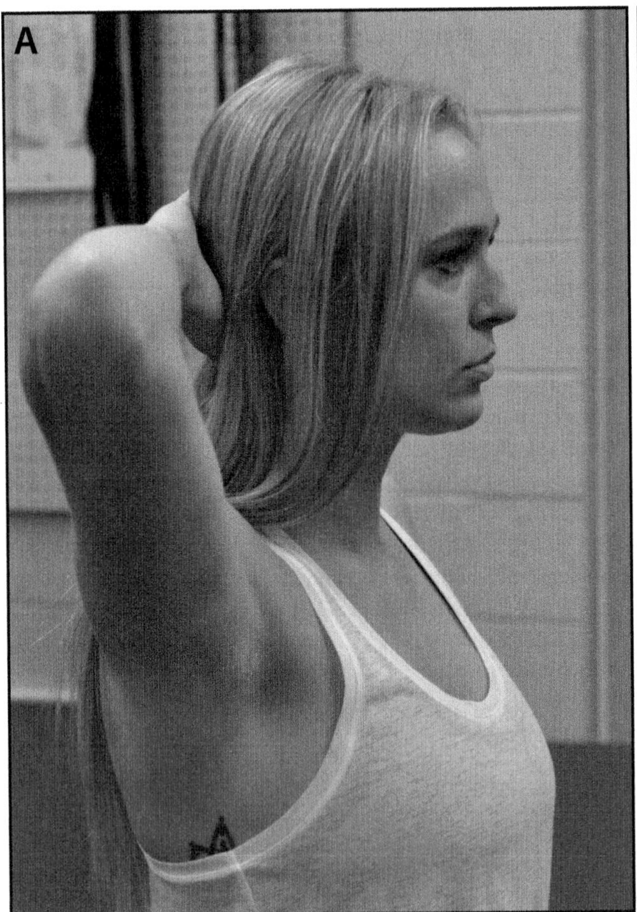


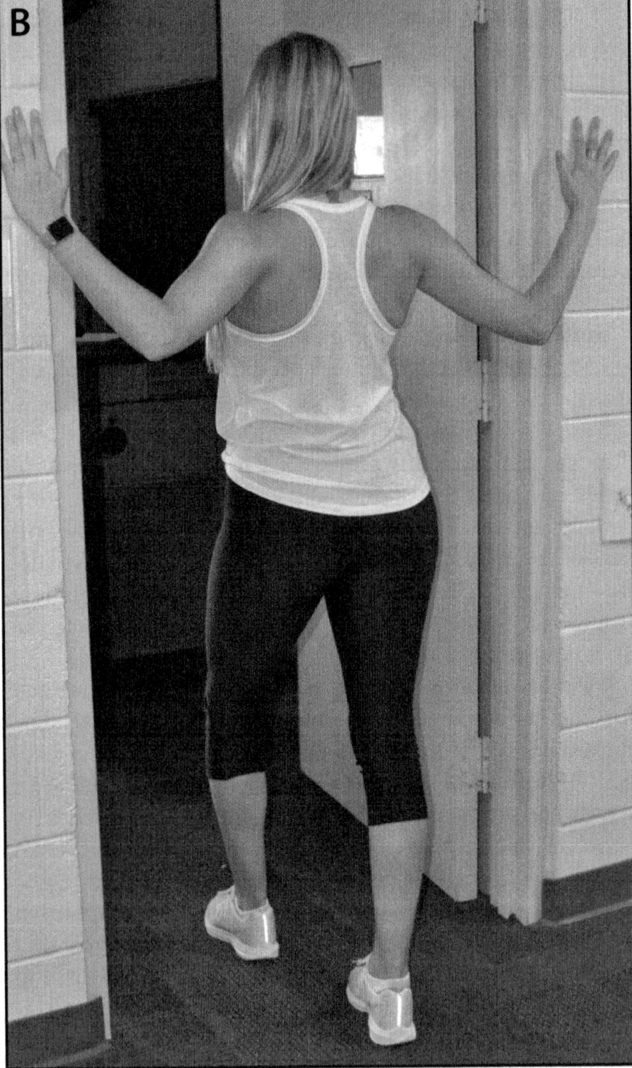


**Figure 5-8.** (A) The seated pectoralis major stretch. This is also a good position for a clinician to use autogenic inhibition PNF stretches. (B) Self-stretch for the pectoralis major muscle.

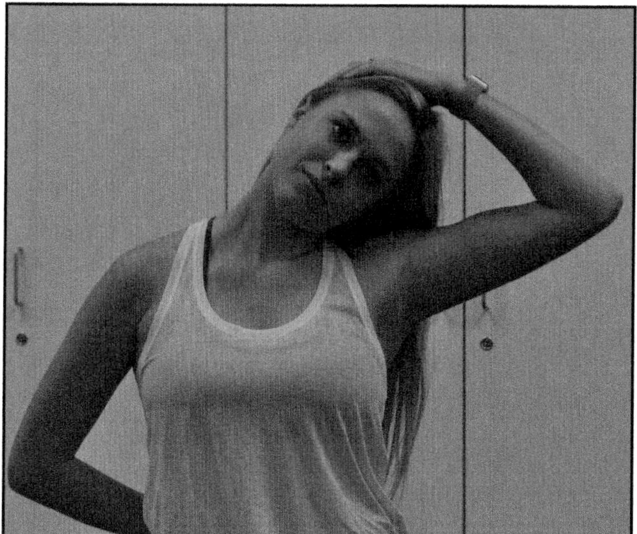

**Figure 5-9.** The upper trapezius stretch.

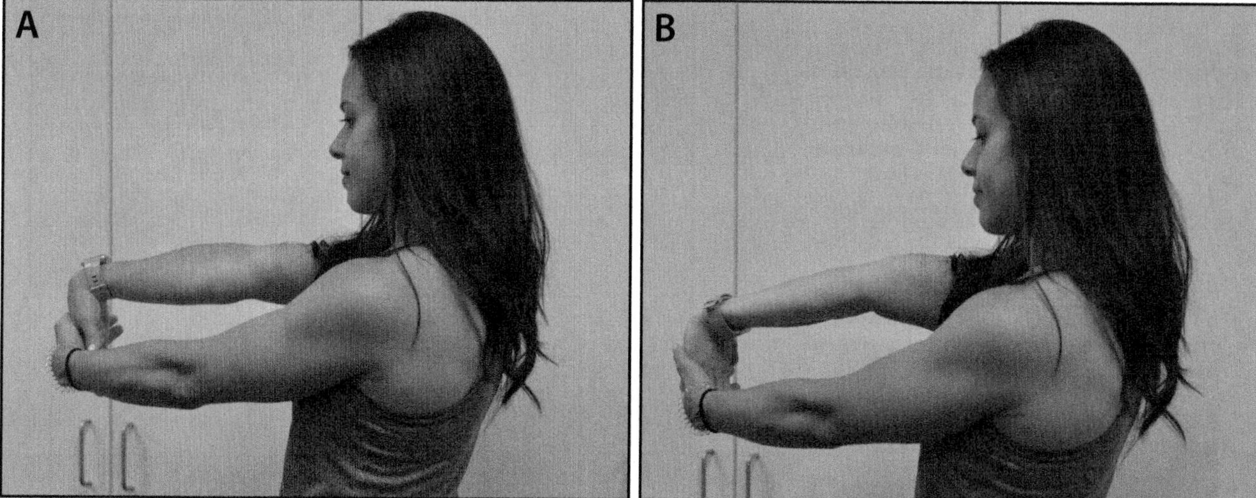


**Figure 5-10.** (A) The wrist extensor muscle stretch. (B) The wrist and finger flexor muscle stretch.

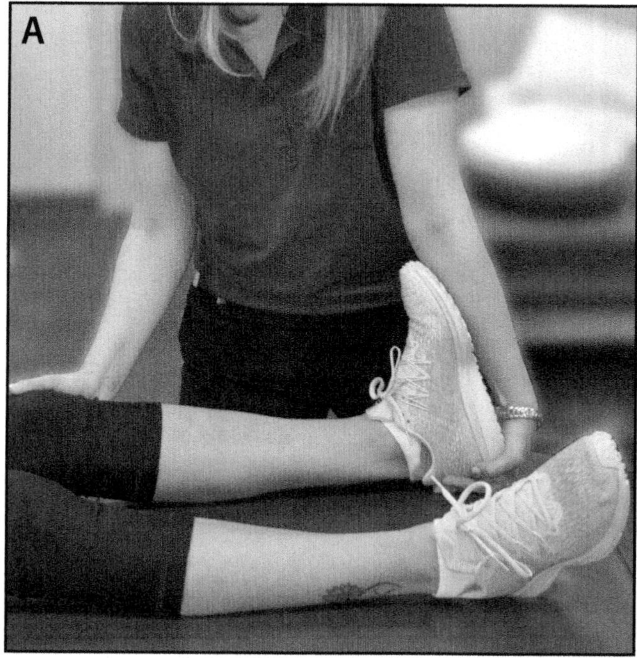


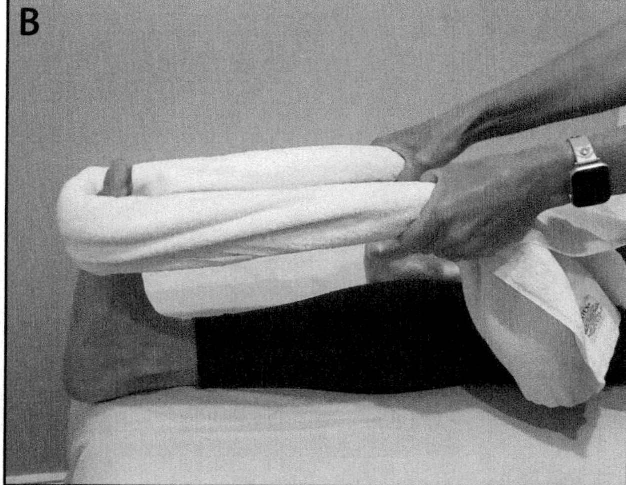


**Figure 5-11.** (A) The passive gastrocnemius stretch. (B) The towel stretch for the gastrocnemius. *(continued)*

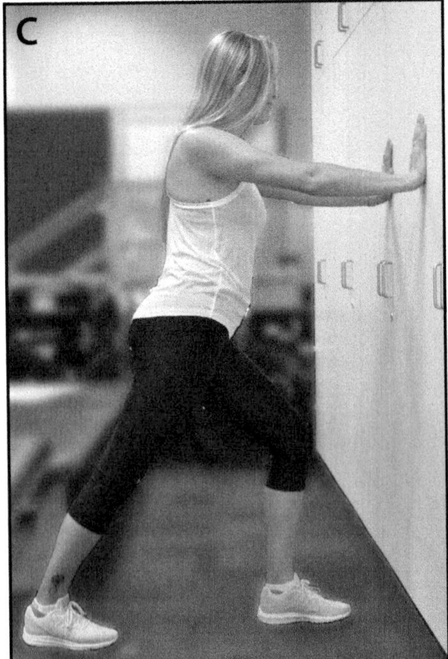


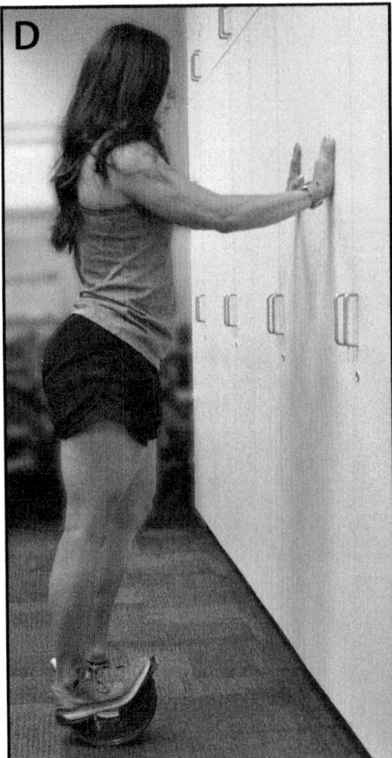


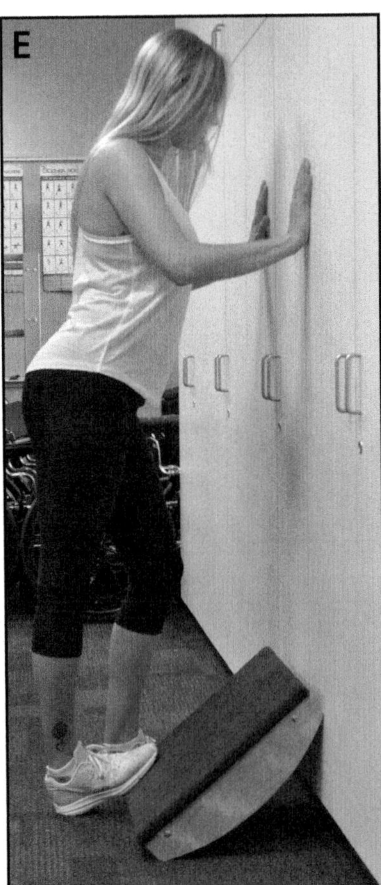


**Figure 5-11 (continued).** (C) The standing gastrocnemius stretch. (D) Gastrocnemius stretching using a foot rocker. (E) The standing gastrocnemius stretch using an incline board.

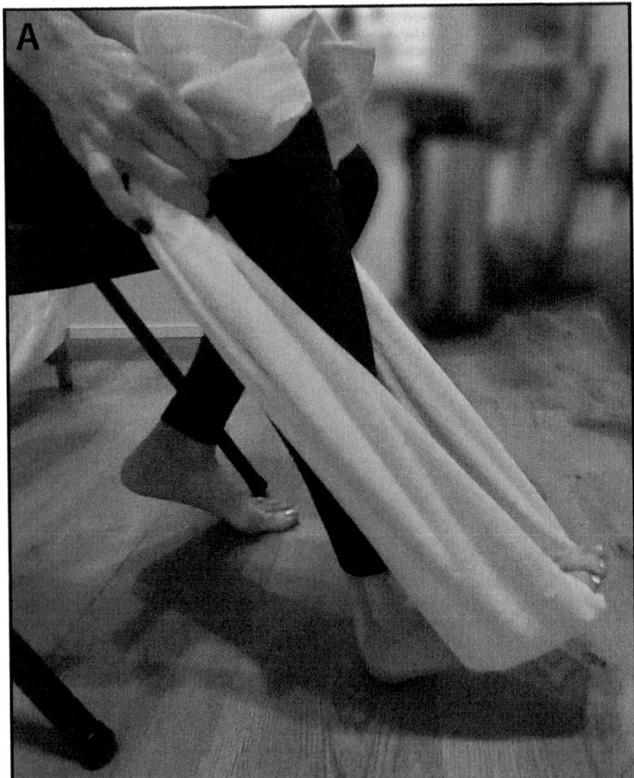


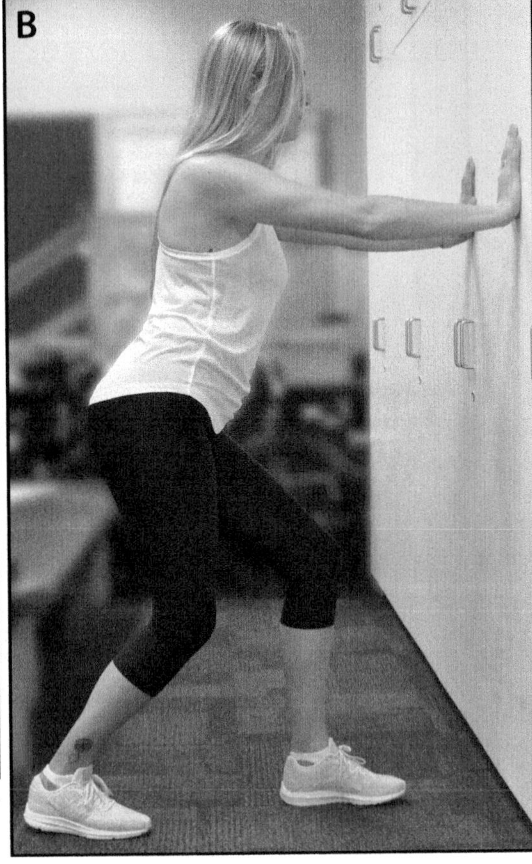


**Figure 5-12.** (A) The seated soleus stretch. (B) The standing soleus stretch; notice the flexed right knee.

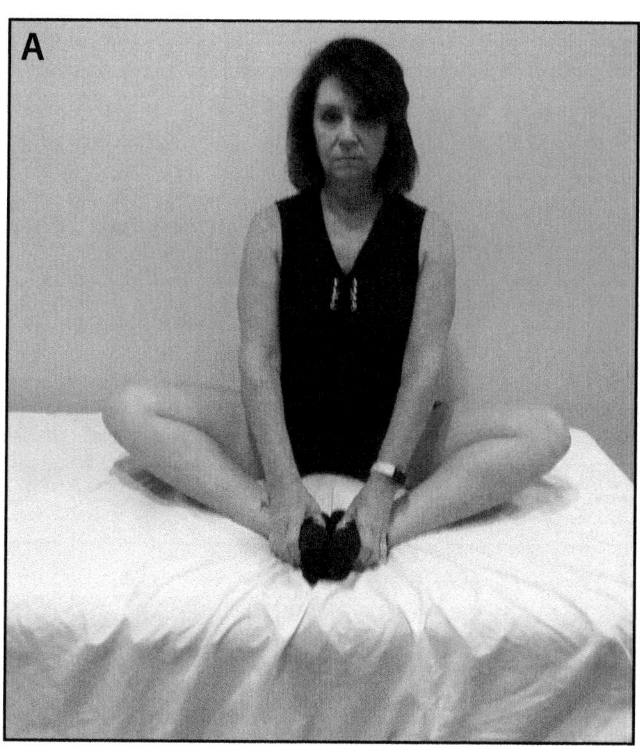


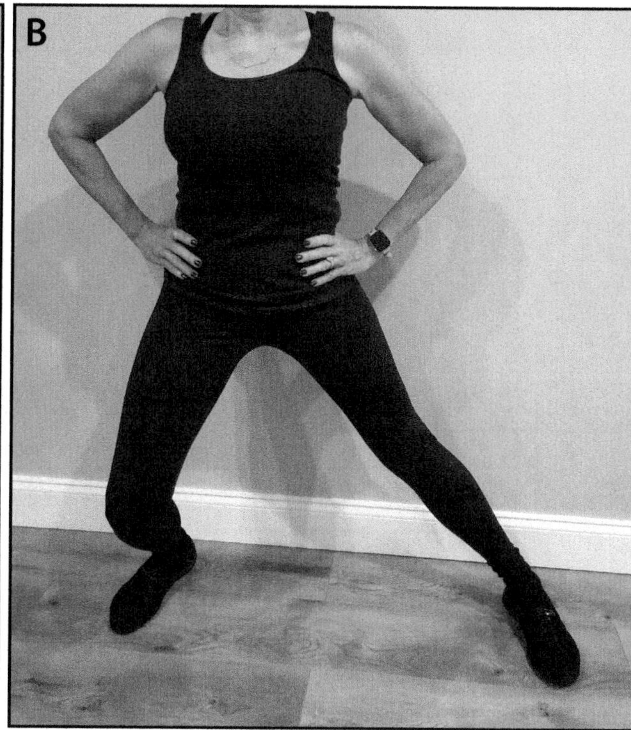


**Figure 5-13.** (A) The hip adductor stretch. (B) The standing hip adductor stretch.

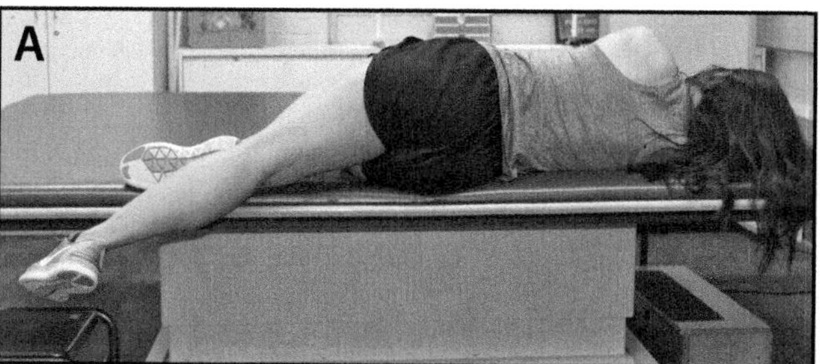


**Figure 5-14.** (A) The left hip abductor and tensor fascia latae stretch. (B) The standing right abductor and tensor fascia latae stretch.

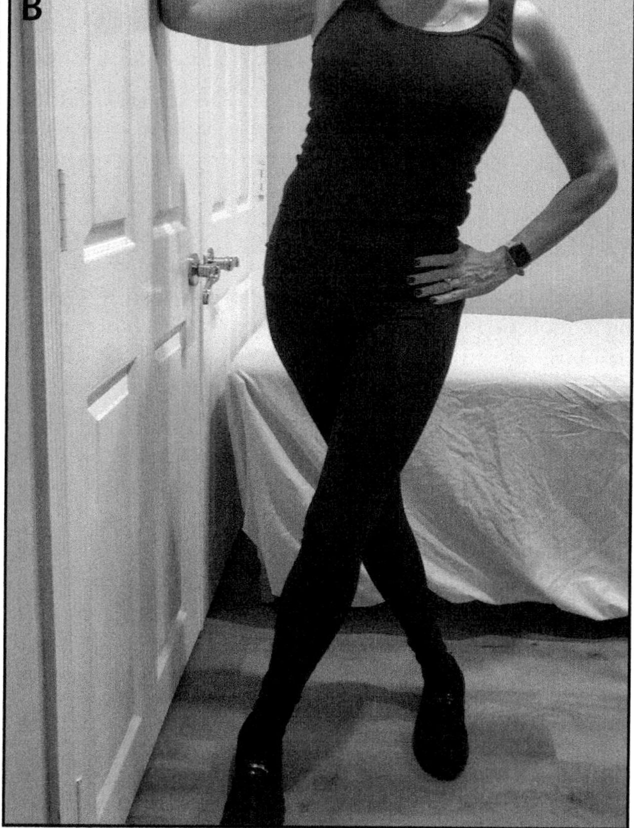

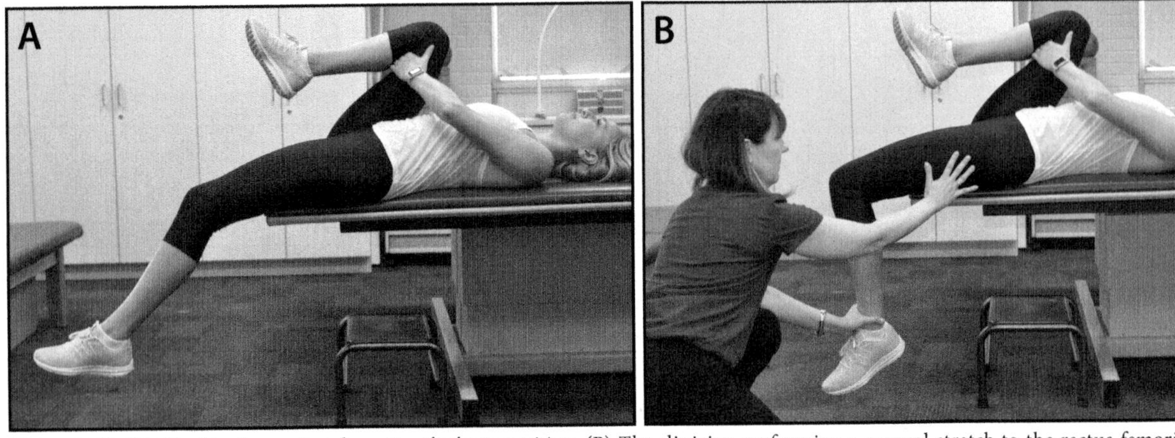


**Figure 5-15.** (A) The hip flexor stretch; notice the knee position. (B) The clinician performing a manual stretch to the rectus femoris (a 2-joint muscle).

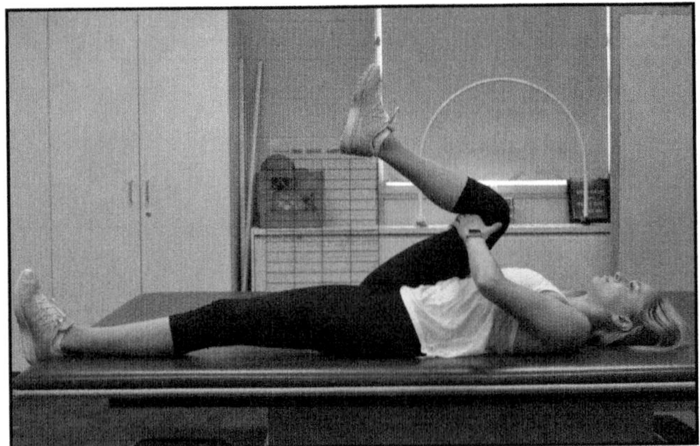

**Figure 5-16.** A single knee to the chest to stretch the gluteal and low back muscles.

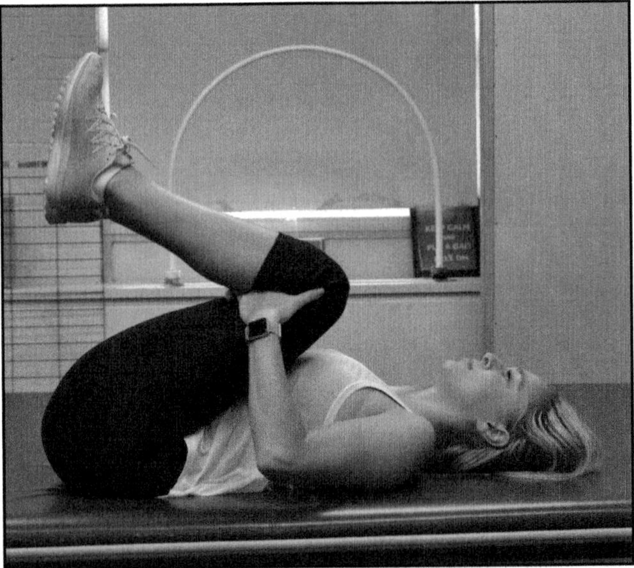

**Figure 5-17.** Double knees to the chest also stretch the gluteal and low back muscles.

## *Specialized Applications of Stretching*

**Selective stretching** is a technique in which positioning is modified to promote adequate joint flexibility while maintaining resting tension/length in a muscle. It allows for stretching of selected joints and muscles while maintaining restricted motion at others. Selective stretching is used in situations in which adequate muscle resting length is needed to provide either stability or compensatory functional movement patterns. As mentioned earlier, physical therapist assistants may use selective stretching for patients with tetraplegia or paraplegia. To selectively stretch the long finger flexors, the patient's wrist is maintained in a neutral position when fully extending the fingers. Persons with tetraplegia and paraplegia rely on the resting length of the lumbar erector spinae to limit their trunk flexion and provide stability when sitting. These patients need about 100 degrees of hip flexion (hamstring length) for mobility. To selectively stretch the hamstrings without overstretching the lumbar extensors, the assistant should manually stretch the hamstring muscles with the patient in a supine position. The patient's pelvic position should be monitored to ensure that the pelvis remains in a neutral position, avoiding posterior pelvic tilting during the stretch to minimize the tension on erector spinae muscles. Avoid seated hamstring stretches for these patients because the pelvis tends to move into a posterior pelvic tilt position during long sitting hamstring stretches, which results in overstretching the erector spinae muscles.

**Ballistic stretching** is a quick (high-intensity) repetitive bouncing movement that is completed in an attempt to increase flexibility beyond the currently available range. This is a lesser controlled type of motion than a static stretch. An example would be a standing repetitive trunk flexion (bouncing) exercise trying to touch the floor to increase hamstring length. According to Covert et al,[20] ballistic and static stretching increased hamstring length compared with a control group, but static stretching increased hamstring length more than the ballistic stretching group for patients 18 to 27 years old. Ballistic stretching is not commonly used in the rehabilitation interventions for sedentary and/or older patients or patients with healing and/or chronic musculoskeletal pathologies. This type of stretching can damage new healing tissue and/or chronic contractures.

## *Other Treatment Interventions and Stretching*

Other interventions are combined with stretching exercises to maximize effectiveness and maintain newly gained ROM. Manual therapy techniques, such as joint and soft tissue mobilizations, can decrease adhesions and muscle guarding or relax tissues before stretching. Before stretching, ultrasound can be used to heat soft tissue, or a prolonged cold application can be used on spastic muscles to reduce muscle tone. Biofeedback and deep breathing exercises can help with relaxation and reduce muscle tension, which can assist in attaining a more effective stretch.

It is important to incorporate strengthening of the muscles in the newly gained range and pain-free functional activities to maintain the gains achieved with stretching. Once a patient has increased shoulder PROM, AROM exercises into the new range should be added. Once the patient can move the arm actively against gravity with good joint mechanics, functional tasks using this new range should be added (ie, reaching into a cabinet). Early implementation of AROM and strengthening exercises is important to achieve functional improvement.

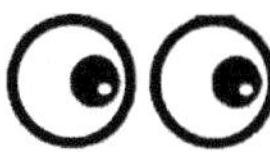

**Eye on the Research**

Instrument-assisted soft tissue mobilization (IASTM): IASTM techniques are used as an adjunct treatment to facilitate stretching and increase ROM. In a small systematic review,[21] researchers questioned if IASTM was beneficial in increasing shoulder ROM compared with static stretching techniques. They concluded that there was moderate evidence to support the use of IASTM to increase ROM in the glenohumeral joint. This is a newer treatment modality, and there is variability in the recommended treatment times and treatment intensity. The implementation of these techniques may require additional certification postlicensure.[21]

## *Limiting Factors*

Physical therapist assistants need to minimize the impact of any factors that could limit the effectiveness of a stretching program. The effectiveness of a stretch is diminished if the patient is unable to relax or resists the stretch. The presence of significant pain and/or increased muscle tone or guarding can limit the tissue's ability to stretch. Poor positioning and inadequate stretch duration can reduce the effectiveness of a stretch when attempting to increase ROM.

Stretching before or after workouts is sometimes recommended as a way to decrease workout-related pain. However, a recent systematic review concluded that stretching had little or no effect on delayed-onset muscle soreness when applied before, after, or before and after exercise in healthy adults.[22]

# Conclusion

An individualized stretching program can increase ROM and flexibility. To maximize the effectiveness of a stretching program, physical therapist assistants determine the muscles to be targeted, the type of stretching technique, appropriate patient positioning, and stabilization strategies that are most beneficial to achieve the patient's goals. The assistant needs to consider the healing process, tissue type, and indications/contraindications and use appropriate parameters to increase ROM and tissue extensibility while maintaining patient safety.

# Review Questions

1. What is the difference between passive and dynamic stretching?
2. Compare and contrast active and passive insufficiency.
3. Explain the difference between autogenic inhibition and reciprocal inhibition.
4. Describe the optimal parameters for a stretching program.
5. List 3 contraindications and 3 precautions for stretching exercises.
6. When is it appropriate to set up a self-stretching program?
7. Is ballistic stretching ever appropriate? If so, when/why?
8. Describe an appropriate stretching intervention for a person with an elbow flexion contracture of 10 degrees. List all parameters.
9. Which interventions can be implemented before a stretch to improve the effectiveness of a stretching exercise?
10. Which medications may affect the safety of a stretching program?

# Case Study

A 25-year-old man has been participating in a strength and conditioning program before the start of his basketball season. The exercises he is performing include squats with heavy weights, a leg press machine for the lower body, and strengthening the arms/chest using bench presses. Which stretching exercises should a physical therapist assistant recommend to complement the athlete's strengthening program?

1. Based on the scenario, which muscles are most likely to require stretching?
2. Select 2 appropriate lower extremity stretches and 2 upper extremity stretches.
3. Using the FITT (frequency, intensity, time, type) principle, select the appropriate parameters and describe optimal positioning and stabilization for the stretches selected.

## References


1. Page P. Clinical commentary: current concepts in muscle stretching for exercise and rehabilitation. *Int J Sports Phys Ther.* 2012:7(1):109-119.
2. Knudson D. The biomechanics of stretching. *J Exerc Sci Physiother.* 2016;2:3-12.
3. Prentice WE. Restoring range of motion and improving flexibility. In: Prentice WE, ed. *Rehabilitation Techniques for Sports Medicine and Athletic Training.* 6th ed. SLACK Incorporated; 2015:215-242.
4. Kisner C, Borstad J, Colby LA. Stretching for improved mobility. In: Kisner C, Colby LA, Borstad J, eds. *Therapeutic Exercise Foundations and Techniques.* 7th ed. FA Davis Company; 2018:82-126.
5. Bandy WD. Stretching activities for increasing muscle flexibility. In: Bandy WD, Sanders B, eds. *Therapeutic Exercise for Physical Therapist Assistants Techniques for Intervention.* 3rd ed. Lippincott Williams & Wilkins; 2013:87-116.
6. Sady SP, Wortman M, Blanke D. Flexibility training: ballistic, static or proprioceptive neuromuscular facilitation. *Arch Phys Med Rehabil.* 1982;63:261-263.
7. Davis DS, Hagerman-Hose M, Midkiff M, Newsome J, Williamson J. The effectiveness of 3 proprioceptive neuromuscular facilitation stretching techniques on the flexibility of hamstring muscle group. *J Orthop Sports Phys Ther.* 2004;34(1):A33-A34.
8. Sharman MJ, Cresswell AG, Riek S. Proprioceptive neuromuscular facilitation stretching mechanisms and clinical implications. *Sports Med.* 2006;36(11):929-939.
9. Feland JB, Myrer JW, Merrill RM. Acute changes in hamstring flexibility: PNF versus static stretch in senior athletes. *Phys Ther Sport.* 2001;2(4):186-193.
10. Arabyat RM, Raisch DW, McKoy JM, Bennett CL. Fluoroquinolone-associated tendon-rupture: a summary of reports in the Food and Drug Administration's adverse event reporting system. *Expert Opin Drug Saf.* 2015;14(11):1653-1660.
11. Foye PM. Corticosteroid-induced myopathy. Updated August 22, 2106. Accessed January 25, 2023. http://emedicine.medscape.com/article/313842-overview
12. Jacobs CA, Sciascia AD. Factors that influence the efficacy of stretching programs for patients with hypomobility. *Sports Health.* 2011;3(6):520-523. doi:10.1177/1941738111415233
13. Apostolopoulos N, Metsios GS, Flouris AD, Koutedakis Y, Wyon MA. The relevance of stretch intensity and position—a systematic review. *Front Psychol.* 2015;6:1128. doi:10.3389/fpsyg.2015.01128
14. Riebe L, ed. General principles of exercise prescription. In: Riebe L, ed. *ACSM's Guidelines for Exercise Testing and prescription.* 10th ed. Wolters Kluwer; 2018:167-173.
15. Roberts JM, Wilson K. Effect of stretching duration on active and passive range of motion in the lower extremity. *Br J Sports Med.* 1999;33:259-263.
16. Feland JB, Myrer JW, Schulties SS, Fellingham GW, Measom GW. The effect of duration of stretching of the hamstring muscle group for increasing range of motion in people aged 65 years or older. *Phys Ther.* 2001;81(5):1110-1117.
17. Nelson RT, Bandy WD. Eccentric training and static stretching of high school males. *J Athl Train.* 2004;39:31-35.
18. Davis DS, Ashby PF, McCale KL, McQuain, Wine JM. The effectiveness of 3 stretching techniques on hamstring flexibility using consistent stretching parameters. *J Strength Cond Res.* 2005;19(1):27-32.
19. Knight CA, Rutledge CR, Cox ME, Acosta M, Hall SJ. Effect of superficial heat, deep heat, and active exercise warm-up on the extensibility of the plantar flexors. *Phys Ther.* 2001;81(6):1206-2014. doi:10.1093/ptj/81.6.1206
20. Covert CA, Alexander MP, Petronis JJ, Davis DS. Comparison of ballistic and static stretching on hamstring length using and equal stretching dose. *J Strength Cond Res.* 2010;24(11):3008-3014.
21. Hussey MJ, Boron-Magulick AE, Valovich McLeod TC, Welch Bacon CE. The comparison of instrument-assisted soft tissue mobilization and self-stretch measures to increase shoulder range of motion in overhead athletes: a critically appraised topic. *J Sport Rehabil.* 2018;27(4):385-389. doi:10.1123/jsr.2016-0213
22. Herbert RD, de Noronha M, Kamper SJ. Stretching to prevent or reduce muscle soreness after exercise. *Cochrane Database Syst Rev.* 2011;7:CD004577. doi:10.1002/14651858.CD004577.pub3

Chapter 6

# Principles of Muscle Strengthening and Performance

*Jacki Klaczak Kopack, PT, DPT and Karen A. Cascardi, PhD, MS, ATC, PTA*

**KEY TERMS** Closed kinetic chain exercises | Concentric contraction | Delayed-onset muscle soreness | Eccentric contraction | Isokinetic exercise | Isometric contractions | Isotonic or dynamic contractions | Muscle endurance | Open kinetic chain exercises | Overload principle | Plyometrics | SAID (Specific Adaptation to Imposed Demands) principle | Strength, resistance, and weight training | Substitution patterns or compensation

## Chapter Objectives

1. Describe the common tissue adaptations that occur as a result of a strengthening program.
2. Differentiate between the various types of muscle contractions (concentric, eccentric, isometric, and isokinetic).
3. Compare and contrast strength, power, and endurance.
4. Discuss the importance of appropriate positioning, alignment, and stabilization when performing a strengthening exercise.
5. Explain the key components and program parameters a physical therapist assistant must consider when designing a resistance training program.
6. Discuss how proprioceptive neuromuscular facilitation (PNF) techniques can be used to facilitate a resistance training program.
7. Compare and contrast strengthening exercise protocols.
8. Select the exercises that are appropriate to perform for each of the phases of a rehabilitation program.
9. Identify 3 ways to prevent delayed-onset muscle soreness (DOMS).
10. Describe and perform the PNF techniques.

Staying strong is vital to maintaining good health across the life span, and adequate muscle performance is critical to maximizing function. International expert consensus recommends incorporating regular resistance training for people of all ages.[1,2] The American Physical Therapy Association recognizes the importance of a well-designed strengthening program for older adults to improve strength gains.[3] The World Health Organization and the American College of Sports Medicine (ACSM) recommend performing resistance training for all major muscle groups 2 to 3 times a week.[1,4]

The terms **strength, resistance, and weight training** are used interchangeably. Strength training is a physical conditioning program that uses isometric, isotonic, or isokinetic exercises to challenge, develop, and strengthen muscles. The physical therapy team is uniquely qualified to



Kopack JK, Cascardi KA.
*Principles of Therapeutic Exercise for the Physical Therapist Assistant* (pp 81-126).

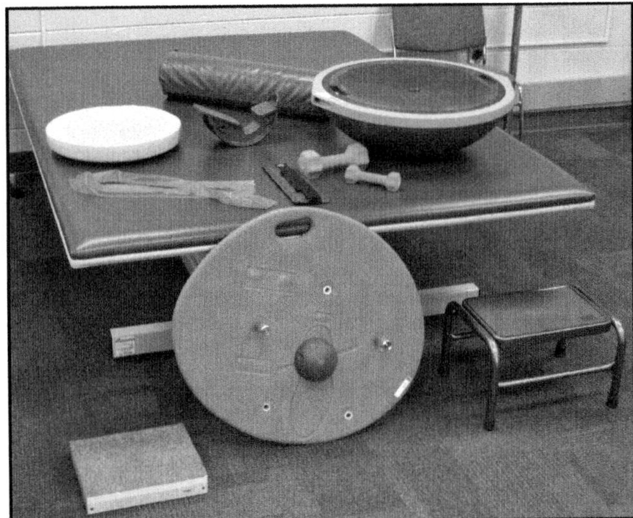

Figure 6-1. Exercise equipment.

develop strengthening programs across the continuum of care because of their comprehensive education in anatomy/physiology, therapeutic exercise training, and medical/health conditions across the life span. When designing a resistance exercise program that effectively increases strength and improves function, clinicians must have a clear understanding of muscle physiology and cardiopulmonary function as well as knowledge of exercise parameters, health conditions, and monitoring protocols. Physical therapist assistants must consider the patient's current level of function, phase of healing, health status, strength, and therapy goals when selecting exercises and implementing exercise protocols.

The clinician can select isometric, concentric, or eccentric exercises based on the treatment goals, level of acuity, and pathology. For example, isometrics may be appropriate in the early postoperative period (if a patient is not medically cleared for active range of motion [AROM]), whereas eccentric loading may be more appropriate when treating a patient with tendinopathy.[5] **Isometric contractions** produce muscle tension without joint motion. During a **concentric contraction**, a muscle's origin and insertion move closer together as the muscle shortens, and acceleration occurs. An **eccentric contraction** occurs during a controlled lengthening of a muscle (origin and insertion move apart), and deceleration occurs.

Common equipment used for resistance training includes free weights/dumbbells, resistance bands, cuff weights, a biomechanical ankle platform system (BAPS; Spectrum Therapy Products), and BOSU Balance Trainer (Figure 6-1) as well as isotonic machines with cable column systems (Figure 6-2) and isokinetic machines (Figure 6-3). The treatment environment (ie, the available space) and cost of equipment are factors that determine the type and amount of equipment found in a facility. A good clinician can create effective exercise interventions within the constraints of the environment and the equipment available.

The benefits associated with resistance training include improved motor performance, increased strength (muscle force), and increased muscle endurance.[6] Increased lean muscle mass reduces the risk of sarcopenia (ie, muscle wasting).[7-9] Sarcopenia is associated with an increased risk of functional decline in the aging population.[9] Resistance training can improve bone density and connective tissue strength, improve the ability to perform activities of daily living (ADLs), increase feelings of well-being, and reduce fall risk. Deconditioned individuals may also see improvement in aerobic capacity.[6] Resistance training postinjury can promote/improve tissue health, organize scar tissue formation, and increase the patient's ability to regain their prior level of function.

Frequency, intensity, and duration are the parameters used in a resistance exercise program to stimulate adaptive changes in muscle. It is also important to consider specificity, overload, and training velocity. The clinician considers all of these factors when developing a strengthening program. Although resistance training primarily affects skeletal muscle, other body systems (ie, the cardiac system) are affected when implementing any type of exercise program. The consideration of comorbidities and appropriate patient monitoring are important to ensure patient safety when completing any type of exercise intervention.

## Muscle Performance

Muscle performance is the capacity of a muscle or group of muscles to do work, including the ability to maintain posture, transition from sitting to standing, and participate in mobility tasks and/or recreational activities. Multiple body systems are activated during exercise; the patient must understand the activity (cognition), the nervous system generates impulses, the musculoskeletal system allows for joint movement and muscle contractions to complete activities, and the cardiac and pulmonary systems work together to provide oxygen to the muscles and organs.

Muscle performance is affected by the strength, power, and endurance of a muscle. Limitations in strength, power, or endurance can result in muscle imbalances, activity limitations, and increased injury risk. A well-designed exercise program should address these components. Clinicians must be able to differentiate between strength, muscle endurance, work, and power when developing a training program and should address these components based on the patient's goals.

Strength is defined as the maximal force a muscle can generate. A one-repetition maximum (1RM) is used to determine the strength in a muscle or muscle group. The 1RM is the maximal weight a person can lift with a single effort. For persons with comorbidities, a safer way to determine a muscle's 1RM is by using the Holten diagram (discussed later in this chapter). Adequate strength is required to perform tasks or skills efficiently. Strength is increased by using progressively heavier loads/weights with fewer repetitions.

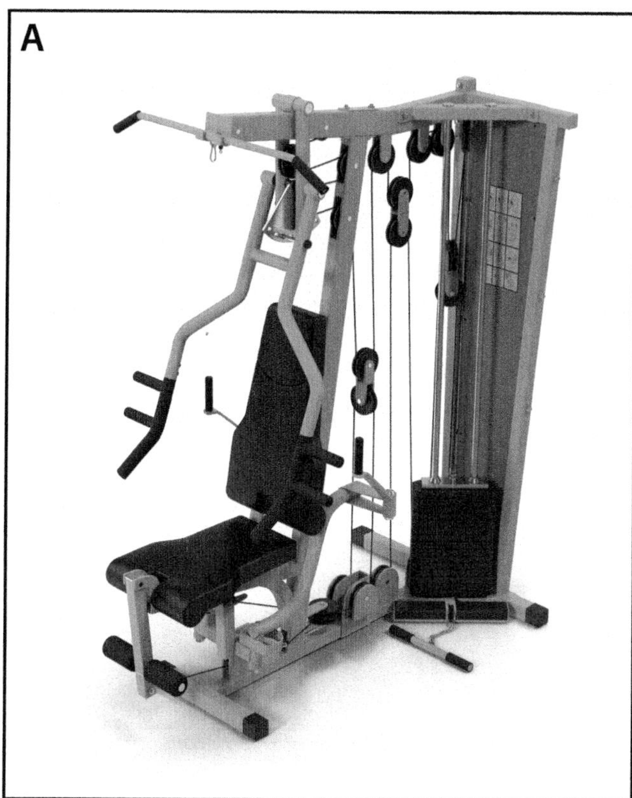


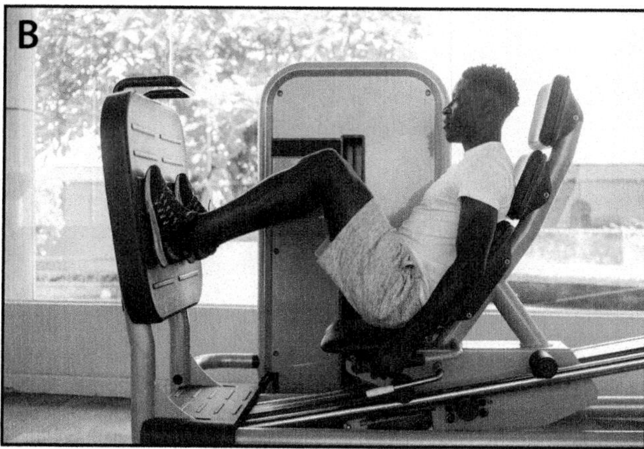


**Figure 6-2.** (A) Isotonic exercise: Weight column machine (3DMI/Shutterstock.com). (B) Isotonic exercise using leg press column weight machine with a mobile footplate (Twinsterphoto/Shutterstock.com).

**Muscle endurance** is the ability of a muscle to repeatedly contract over a period of time. Muscle endurance training is commonly associated with using light weights (or low resistance/load) and performing the exercise for a high number of repetitions or a prescribed period of time (seconds/minutes).

Work is defined as the amount of force it takes to move an object a certain distance. Work equals force times distance (W = F × D). For example, if a heavy book is sitting on top of a desk and it must be moved, it requires a specific amount of muscle force to slide the book a specific distance (ie, 2 feet [ft]); this effort is reflective of the work that has been expended. Power refers to the rate at which work is performed. Power is also described as the product of strength and velocity/speed (Power = Work ÷ Time [or Power = (Force × Distance) ÷ Time]). Because power has a speed and force component, it is possible to see increases in power as a result of strength training. Interventions to increase power include plyometric training, which requires high-intensity activity performed at increasing speeds (Figure 6-4).

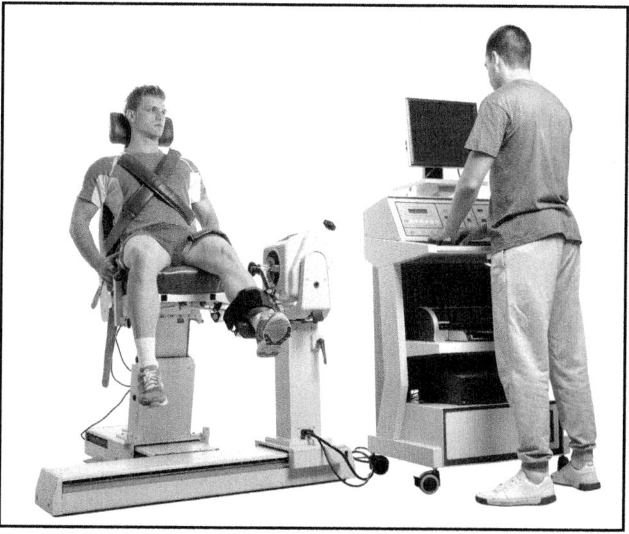

**Figure 6-3.** Isokinetic machine provides accommodating resistance and can be used for testing and exercise (cirkoglu/Shutterstock.com).

## Application Consideration: Body Size and Strength-to-Mass Ratio

Generally, when body size increases, muscle volume (and weight) tends to increase more than the muscle cross-sectional area (and muscle strength). When this occurs, a person must now move a larger mass (body size) with muscles whose strength have not increased proportionally. To effectively increase the muscle cross-sectional area and strength, the person must participate in a specific strengthening exercise program.

## *Muscle Characteristics and Performance*

A muscle's shape, size, and fiber orientation help determine the muscle's potential to produce force (strength). Larger muscles have the potential for greater strength than a muscle with a smaller cross-sectional area.

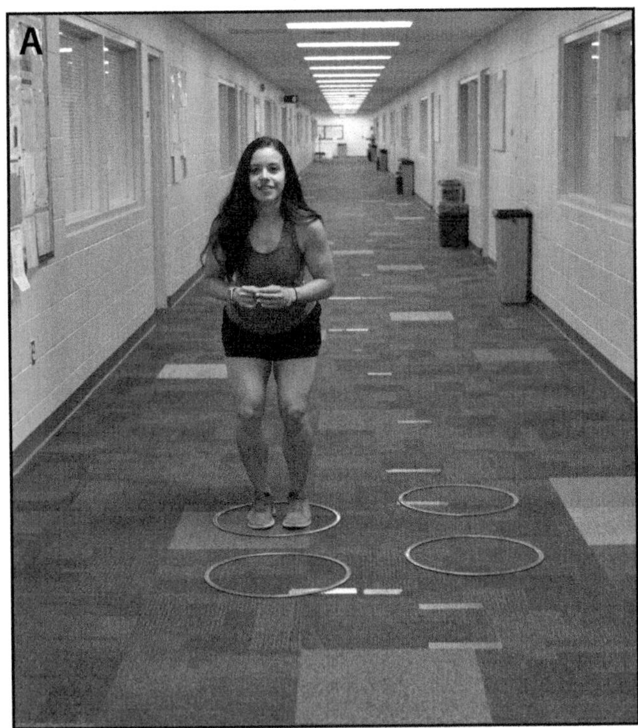


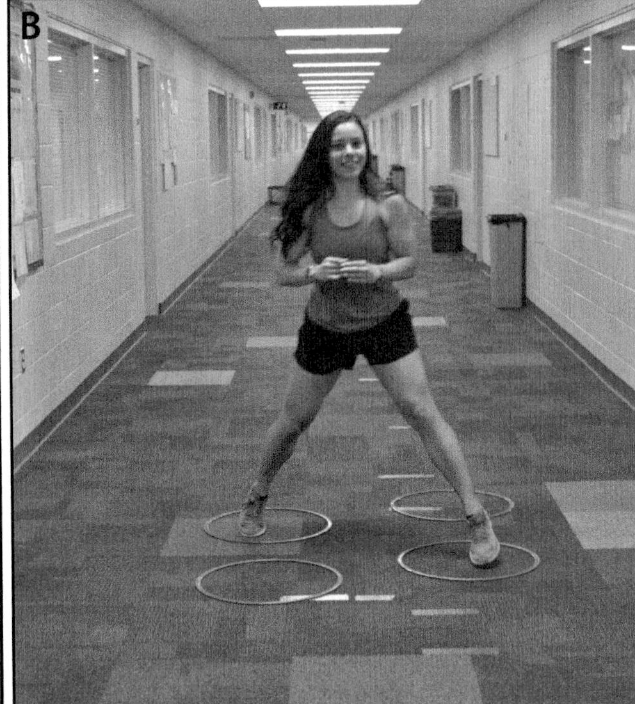


**Figure 6-4.** (A) Plyometric starting position. (B) The patient quickly and explosively pushes off to transition to another position. (C) Plyometric progression end.

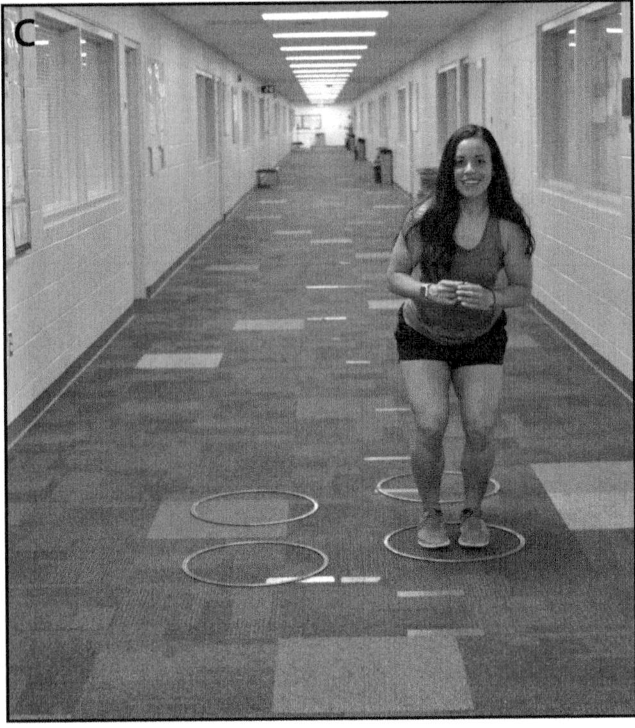

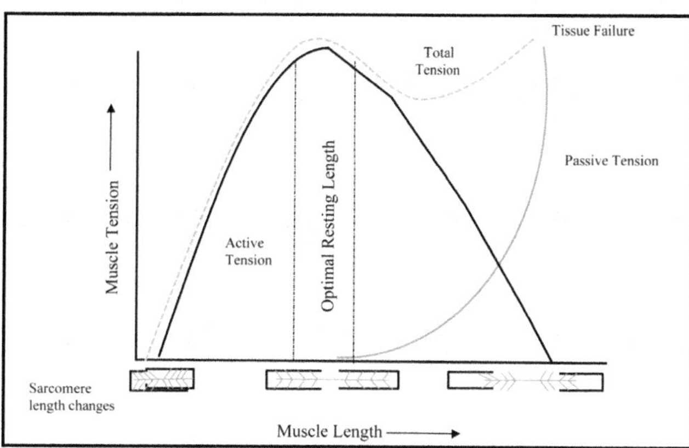


**Figure 6-5.** A length–tension relationship curve.

Muscle fibers are aligned in an oblique or parallel fashion. Pennate muscles have fibers that align at oblique angles to the muscle's tendon, and these muscles tend to be shorter in length than those with other types of muscle fibers. This oblique fiber orientation allows for greater force production than the other fiber alignments. Muscles can be multipennate (deltoid muscle), bipennate (rectus femoris), or unipennate (tibialis posterior). Strength training may alter fiber alignment (pennation angle), which can result in fiber hypertrophy and increased force production. Muscles with parallel orientation tend to produce less force but can generate greater velocity during contractions. Fusiform muscles have long fibers with a muscle belly and tapering at the ends. This type of muscle produces greater range of motion (ROM) compared with other muscles.

Neural control affects force production. Muscle fibers are organized as motor units within a muscle. Each motor unit includes a single motor neuron and all of the muscle fibers it innervates. The size of a motor unit is determined by the number of muscle fibers it innervates. Muscle force is greater when more motor units are recruited, motor units are larger, and they fire at a fast rate of speed. Small motor units are recruited for fine motor coordination. The initial improvement in strength is attributed to improved motor unit recruitment and firing (neural adaptation).

A muscle's potential to produce force is affected by biomechanics. There are contractile and noncontractile tissues that create active and passive tension in a muscle. The active length–tension curve is based on the length and strength of the muscle and the sliding filament theory (Figure 6-5). Based on this length–tension relationship, a muscle can generate the most force at its normal resting position. At the normal resting length of a sarcomere, actin and myosin filaments are aligned, allowing the greatest number of cross-bridges to be formed and therefore producing the greatest force. When a muscle is stretched beyond its normal resting length, fewer actin and myosin fibers are aligned, so fewer cross-bridges can be formed, resulting in fewer fibers contracting and less force production. Less force production occurs when a muscle is shortened beyond its normal resting length because the actin filaments already overlap the myosin, resulting in fewer cross-bridge formations.

Tension created by the noncontractile structures (passive force) depends on the position/amount of stretch of the muscle fibers. When the muscle is at its normal resting length, the passive structures are on slack (zero tension). As muscle length increases, passive tension increases, but when the muscle shortens (contracts), passive tension is released and decreases. For example, if a rubber band is stretched, passive forces build up, and when the rubber band is released at one end, the tension is released.

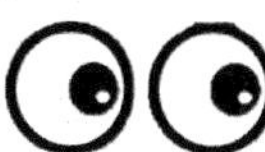

### Eye on the Research

The sliding filament theory was proposed by scientists Jean Hanson and Hugh E. Huxley in the 1950s. Their research led to the recognition of the role of the proteins actin and myosin and the mechanism of action resulting in muscle contraction. Newer research suggests that a possible third filament made up of an elastic protein (titan) has a similar and important role in muscle contractions, especially eccentric muscle contractions.[10-12]

Torque is the tendency of a force to create rotation around a joint or joint axis. The amount of torque a muscle produces will vary throughout the joint's available range. The amount of torque generated depends on the magnitude of the force and the length of the moment arm. The moment arm is the perpendicular line (or distance) from the muscle's line of pull (based on the muscle fiber configuration) and joint axis; the longer the moment arm, the greater the force that is produced. The muscle length–tension relationship varies as the muscle contracts and limb position changes, impacting torque. For example, the biceps brachii muscle produces the most torque when the elbow is flexed at 90 degrees because the moment arm's distance is at its greatest length at this point in the range. If biceps muscle strength is assessed at various points throughout the available range, it will test strongest when positioned at 90 degrees of flexion. As the angle of the elbow deviates above or below 90 degrees, the amount of torque decreases because the length of the moment arm also decreases (Figure 6-6). When the moment arm is zero, no torque can be produced.

### Quick Class Activity

To better understand torque, perform the following activity. Have your laboratory partner flex their elbow to 35, 90, and 135 degrees. Apply downward resistance (resisting the biceps) in each position. In what position was your laboratory partner the strongest? That is the position where the greatest amount of torque is created.

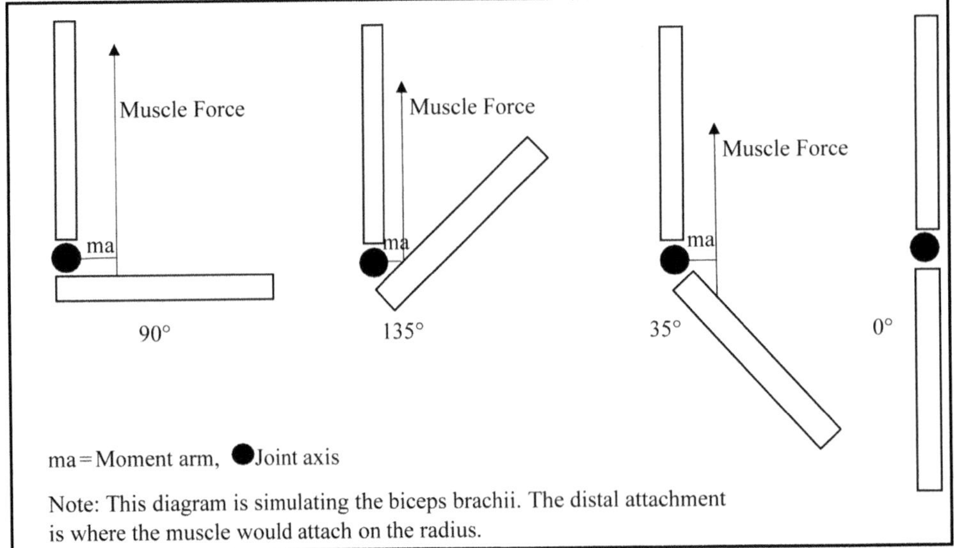


**Figure 6-6.** Torque and moment arms.

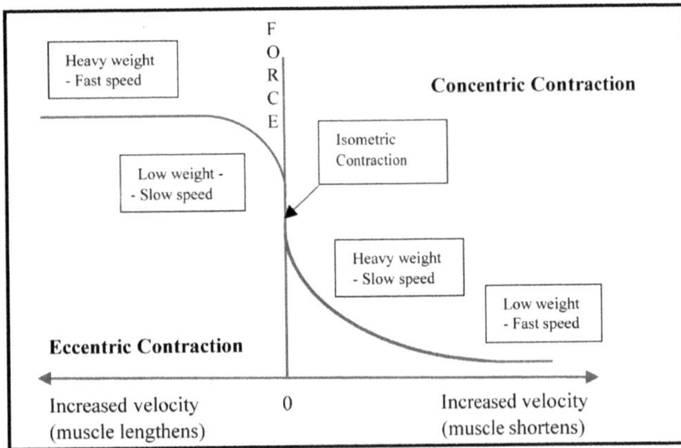


**Figure 6-7.** A force–velocity curve.

Torque production is impacted by muscle length, and muscle length changes occur in both the active and passive structures in patients who present with variations from normal alignment. For example, a habitually forward flexed thoracic posture (kyphosis) results in areas of tightness as well as areas where structures are lengthened. Tissues become adaptively shortened or lengthened, requiring stretching or strengthening to restore the muscles back to their normal resting length. In this example, the rhomboids are in a lengthened state as a result of the kyphosis and scapular protraction. The rhomboids will test weaker than expected because the proper test position tests them in a (relatively) shortened length.

The type and speed of muscle contractions affect force production. This force–velocity relationship is illustrated in Figure 6-7. The speed at which a muscle shortens (or concentrically contracts) is inversely related to the load it moves. In other words, if the load/weight is heavy, there will be an increase in muscle tension, but the velocity (or speed) of the contraction will be decreased/slower. There is less muscle tension buildup when moving a lighter weight; thus, the velocity/speed of the concentric contraction can be quicker. The best way to increase tension during a concentric contraction is to perform the activity at a slower speed with a heavier weight because this allows for more time to build up tension in the muscle. Concentric contractions generate the least amount of force followed by isometric contractions, and eccentric contractions produce the greatest amount of force. During an isometric contraction, there is no movement, so the velocity is equal to zero. The greatest amount of force occurs when muscles contract eccentrically at higher speeds (velocity) moving heavier weights (there is a greater opposing force). However, it should be noted that there is a quick leveling off of muscle tension/force; this is a protective response to the quick deceleration of the muscle.[13]

## Muscle Fiber Types and Their Role in Functional Activity and Exercise

Skeletal muscle is made up of 2 distinct types of muscle fibers: slow-twitch (type I, aerobic) and fast-twitch (type II, anaerobic) fibers. Muscle fiber characteristics are described in Table 6-1. There is some variation in the preferred terminology regarding the subtypes. Type I fibers primarily generate energy aerobically. They resist fatigue well and are used to power endurance-type activities/work. Type I fibers are called *slow oxidative fibers*, referring to their slow contraction speed and reliance on oxygen to fuel their energy production. These fibers are also referred to as *tonic fibers*; they are found in postural muscles that contract for extended periods of time to maintain upright posture. Type II fibers include subtypes IIa, IIx, and IIb. Fast-twitch fibers rely on the glycolytic system for energy production rather than oxygen. These fibers are capable of rapid transmission of electrical signals (action potentials) and have a rapid calcium release and uptake, allowing quick and forceful muscle contractions. Fast-twitch fibers produce short-term, large-force muscle contractions. Fast-twitch fibers are also referred to as *phasic fibers*, and they quickly fatigue.[14]

**Table 6-1**

Muscle Fiber Characteristics[14]

| Fiber Type | I Aerobic, Slow Oxidative | IIa Anaerobic, Fast Oxidative, Glycolytic | IIx (Previously Named IIb) Anaerobic, Fast Glycolytic | The New IIb Subtype |
|---|---|---|---|---|
| Contraction speed | Slow | Moderately fast | Fast | Very fast |
| Size of motor neuron (larger motor neurons allow nerve impulses to operate more quickly) | Small | Medium | Large | Very large |
| Activity used for | Endurance | Short (but longer-term anaerobic), 2 minutes | Very short maximal intensity exercise | Short maximal intensity exercise |
| Resistance to fatigue | High | Fairly high | Intermediate | Low |
| Efficiency (higher efficiency does not burn as much fuel but may not produce as much force) | High | Intermediate | Low | Low |
| Number of mitochondria (located in muscle fibers; these produce energy aerobically) | High | High | Medium | Low |
| Capillary density (capillaries transport oxygen and nutrients to muscles and remove waste products) | High | Intermediate | Low | Low |
| Oxidative capacity (the capacity of the muscle fiber to use oxygen for energy production) | High | High | Intermediate | Low |
| Glycolytic capacity (the fiber's capacity to store and break down glycogen as a high-intensity energy source) | Low | High | High | High |
| Maximum duration of use | Hours | 30 minutes | 5 minutes | 1 minute |

The proportion of each type of muscle fiber varies from muscle to muscle depending on the muscle's function. The proportion of fiber types also varies from person to person. The ratio of fiber types in most muscles is determined by genetics and sex (which dictates hormone production levels), but proper training can enhance the function of both types of fibers. Muscle fiber training is impacted by the types of activities performed. This reflects the theory of specificity of training (ie, practice of a task/skill is necessary to develop improvement in that specific task/skill). When performing endurance (aerobic) activities, type I fibers are slow to fatigue; they are stressed more, and their function will improve. Likewise, when participating in weight-lifting activities (short duration, large-force production), increased efficiency in the muscle's fast-twitch fibers (type II) occurs. Sports such as rugby, field hockey, and soccer, which require short bursts of energy and force production, rely on the fast-twitch fibers, but the longer duration running throughout the game relies on the slow-twitch fibers. These athletes need to work on both aerobic and anaerobic activities to improve the function and efficiency of both types of muscle fibers.[14]

## *Tissue Adaptation and Strengthening Exercises*

Tissue adaptations occur as a result of strengthening programs. A muscle's ability to increase force production is a result of increased muscle fiber size (hypertrophy) and improved efficiency of the muscle's ability to recruit motor units (neural adaptation).[15] Skeletal muscle adaptation to strength training begins shortly after initiating a training program, as long as the load is adequate to stress the muscles. If the load is not sufficient to overload muscles, then no adaptation occurs. Strength gains and hypertrophy occur approximately 4 to 8 weeks after a moderate- to high-intensity strengthening program.[14] Connective tissue (ie, tendons and ligaments) and bone adaptations also occur, but these changes take longer. Collagen initially degrades with the initiation of a strength program, but subsequent collagen synthesis rates increase significantly, resulting in increased tensile strength of tendons and fascia. Bone mineral density increases, although it can take months to see measurable changes in bone density.[16]

Resistance training also has a beneficial effect on cardiovascular function. Heart size and chamber volume both increase as a result of exercise training. These changes result in a more effective heart rate and blood pressure response during strenuous activity and improvements in resting vital signs. As a result of training, the resting heart rate and blood pressure may be lower than the pretraining values.[6,16] Resistance training programs can also result in lower lipid and glucose profiles,[17-19] increased lean body mass, and reduced body fat.[6,14]

Training must occur with appropriate intensity and frequency for adaptations to occur. With typical aging, there is a decrease in the lean muscle mass and resting metabolic rate with each added decade of life. The addition of resistance training can mitigate these changes.

## Strength Training Principles

Training principles that affect tissue adaptations and result in improved function include overload, specificity, progression, and transfer of training. The **overload principle** states that in order for muscle strength to increase, a resistance or external force must be greater than the normal stresses placed on a muscle. As muscles are challenged, they respond to these increased demands with increases in strength. Overload can be created by increasing load/resistance; increasing frequency, intensity, and duration (time/repetitions); decreasing the rest periods; or any combination of these parameters. If muscles are not continually challenged beyond what they are accustomed to, then tissue adaptation or increases in strength will not occur.[6] Clinical judgment and patient education are vital to ensure that a patient does not "overdo it" when creating an overload.

Knowing a patient's current physical/medical status, level of fitness, and goals is important when determining the exercise intensity. Intervention planning and program development for an athlete who wants to return to competitive sports will be very different than a program designed for an older adult whose goal is to play golf or garden. Clinicians should develop an individualized plan based on the patient's goals. If the primary goal is to increase strength, then the plan should focus on progressively increasing loads/weights. If the goal is to improve muscle endurance, then the focus shifts to progressively increasing the time/duration of the exercise. A patient's perception of exertion provides a subjective estimate of exercise/activity intensity. Combining the use of the Borg rating of perceived exertion score and vital sign monitoring can help determine the patient's tolerance to the exercise.[20] If the vital sign response appears inconsistent with the patient's rating of perceived exertion report, the patient should be assessed further.

The **SAID (Specific Adaptation to Imposed Demands) principle** states that the body will adapt to those demands placed on it. This is true for all body systems, and it helps clinicians determine appropriate exercise parameters when creating a treatment program. The muscles, movement patterns, speed of the movements (addressing type I and/or II fibers), and types of contraction should all be addressed. Incorporating specificity of training (ie, practicing specific tasks/skills) will result in improved performance of that specific skill/task. This is true for simple (eg, going up or down stairs) and complex tasks (eg, throwing a ball). For example, if a soccer goalie wants to improve their ability to quickly transition in and out of making diving saves to prevent a goal, then this particular task must be practiced at the speed and intensity and in the directions that will be used in game situations. The intensity of the training must be systematically increased over time in order to make gains. This is called the *progression principle*. In this scenario, the skill first needs to be broken down into 2 components. The goalie needs to perform multidirectional changes first and then practice the dive (without a ball and then with a ball) and get back up. Practice initially starts at slower speeds and then progresses to faster speeds and more responsive/reflexive movements. The 2 tasks are finally combined and performed as one skill, simulating game situations. Practicing any skill (simple or complex) is an important component for successful, efficient performance. Practice instills confidence when performing the skill or task.[6]

The transfer of training principle describes the potential for carryover of training effects from one task or exercise to another. Tasks that are very different do not tend to have a lot of transfer of training (ie, strengthening using lower extremity [LE] plyometric drills will not result in significant improvement in a person's freestyle swim stroke). Training at one speed (ie, slow speed) may not translate into improved strength/performance when completing the task at a higher speed.[6]

Overtraining refers to the longer-term decrease in performance/function or strength that is associated with excessive overloading combined with inadequate rest or recovery time. This is preventable and should be avoided at all costs. The restoration of full function can take weeks of recovery after overtraining occurs. A common presentation of overtraining includes a decrease in performance, excessive fatigue, and an increased sense of effort during training.[6] Careful implementation and progression of an appropriate-intensity exercise program paired with

**Table 6-2**

Manual Muscle Testing Grades

| Grade | Score | Description |
|---|---|---|
| 5 | Normal | Patient can hold position against maximum resistance. Patient has full ROM. |
| 4 | Good | Patient can hold position against moderate resistance. Patient has full ROM. |
| 3+ | Fair + | Patient can hold position against mild resistance. Patient has full ROM. |
| 3 | Fair | Patient can tolerate no resistance but can move through full ROM. |
| 2+ | Poor + | Patient has full ROM in the gravity-eliminated position and can hold against mild resistance. |
| 2 | Poor | Patient has full ROM in the gravity-eliminated position. |
| 2– | Poor – | Patient can complete partial ROM in gravity-eliminated position. |
| 1 | Trace | Examiner can palpate or visually detect some contractile activity. |
| 0 | Zero | No visible or palpable contraction. |

adequate recovery times, careful monitoring, and consistent patient education lower the risk of overtraining.

The reversibility principle, in layperson's terms, is described as "use it or lose it." Training effects are transient. Strength gains are lost once resistance training is stopped; this loss of strength is referred to as *detraining*. Detraining can begin as early as 1 week after the discontinuation of the exercises or failure to maintain the current level of intensity of functional activities.[4] Patients should be encouraged to continue exercising after discharge from physical therapy as a lifelong goal.

## Measuring Muscle Strength

It is important to assess a patient's muscle strength before determining the exercises most appropriate for the patient. Muscle strength can be quantified in a number of ways including dynamometry, isokinetic testing, functional strength testing, or manual muscle testing (MMT). MMT is widely used by therapists, and the generally accepted grading scale is listed in Table 6-2. The primary advantage to using MMT is that there is no equipment required. A disadvantage is the fact that extensive time and practice are required to ensure that the clinician's results are as accurate and reliable as possible. The patient must be positioned/aligned and stabilized properly to test the targeted muscle, and clinicians should observe for muscle substitution or compensatory movements. Most MMT techniques test strength isometrically. Therefore, the MMT results truly only determine the strength in the testing position; they do not capture weakness in other parts of the range.

Determination of the 1RM is another tool used to measure muscle strength. One concern when using this method is the potential effect muscle fatigue has on the results. It can be difficult to select the correct weight when trying to determine the 1RM; having the patient perform multiple trials can lead to diminished reliability of test results if the muscle is fatigued. This method is most appropriate to use with athletes or healthy adults. An alternate method (appropriate for many patients) is called the *submaximal repetition test* using the Holten diagram (or method). Oddvar Holten (a physical therapist) developed the theory of medical exercise therapy as a method for determining training intensity. The Holten diagram (Figure 6-8) allows the clinician to select a moderate weight and have the patient perform the exercise as many times as they can correctly through the full ROM. Based on the number of repetitions performed, a percentage of intensity can be determined using the diagram, and the 1RM can be calculated using the equation on the bottom of Figure 6-8.[21,22] For example, if a patient can lift 10 pounds (lb) for 16 repetitions, that is equivalent to 75% of a 1RM. So, the 1RM is equal to 13.3 (calculated as [10.0 lb × 100%] ÷ 75% = 13.3 lb). The results can help therapists select the most appropriate weight to improve strength or muscle endurance. To increase strength, a weight closer to the calculated 1RM (13.3 lb) should be selected, and the patient will perform fewer repetitions. To increase muscular endurance, a weight slightly lighter than 10 lb should be selected, and the patient will perform a higher number of repetitions.

## Considerations for the Physical Therapist Assistant

Clinicians often develop strengthening programs for older patients that are not challenging enough to result in adaptation and increased strength. The Holten curve method allows a clinician to safely estimate a 1RM and develop an appropriate individualized resistance program. For example, a patient's 1RM for knee extension was 15 lb (determined during the initial evaluation). To address strengthening, the clinician asks the patient to perform an exercise at 60% to 80% (or 9 to 12 lb) of the 1RM (determination of the actual percentage is individualized and based on factors that include the presence of comorbidities and the overall fitness level). In this instance, the exercise prescription will start with 2 to 3 sets of 6 to 12 repetitions of knee extension (long-arc quadriceps) using 12 lb. The clinician will modify the activity based on patient tolerance.

## Documentation Tip

Using the 1RM example, the documentation could state the following:

O: Strengthening Ex: LAQ (long-arc quadriceps) with 12 lb 2 × 10 repetitions with verbal cue for proper breathing and 2-minute rest between sets. Fatigue reported after the second set.

A: Strengthening program initiated, and patient required verbal cue to prevent Valsalva. Increased knee extensor strength will promote progression to improve ability to climb flight of stairs at home.

P: Assess patient's report of symptoms at start of next session. Add third set if indicated based on a negative symptom report.

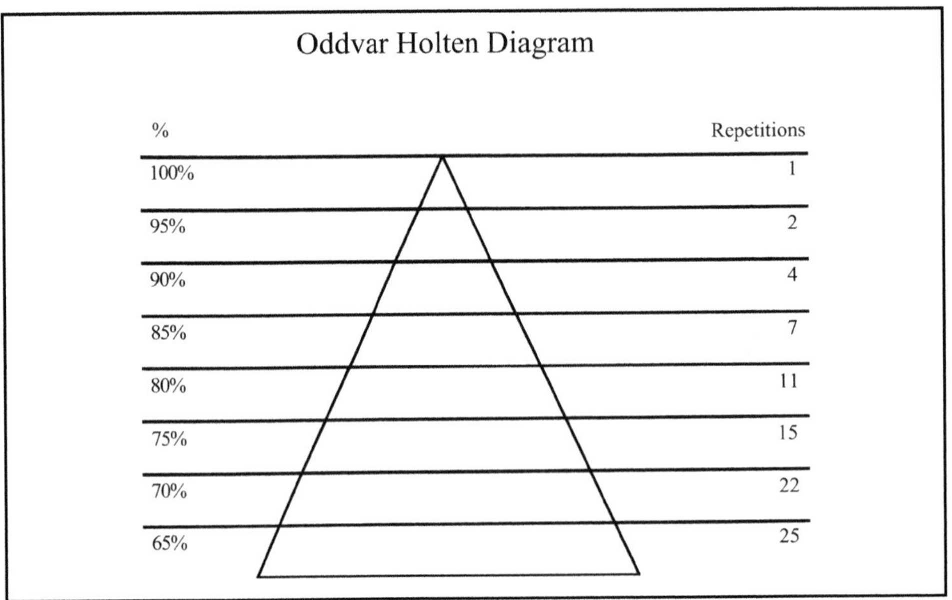


**Figure 6-8.** An Odvar Holten curve. (Reproduced with permission from Oostdam N, van Poppel MNM, Eekhoff EMW, Wouters MGAJ, van Mechelen W. Design of FitFor2 study: the effects of an exercise program on insulin sensitivity and plasma glucose levels in pregnant women at high risk for gestational diabetes. *BMC Pregnancy Childbirth*. 2009;9:1. doi:10.1186/1471-2393-9-1)

A dynamometer is a common tool used in occupational and physical therapy to objectively quantify grip strength (Figure 6-9). Decreased grip strength is associated with a greater likelihood for the development of disability, an increased risk of complications/prolonged length of stay after hospitalization or surgery, and an overall increased risk of premature mortality.[23] Grip strength may be useful as a baseline assessment for all middle-aged and older adults.[23]

Isokinetic testing assesses strength, torque, and power.[24] Isokinetic machines (see Figure 6-3) provide an accommodating resistance; the speed is selected by the clinician, and the patient is instructed to move the limb segment as hard and fast as possible. If the patient experiences pain or is unable to meet the selected speed, the resistance the patient feels will be minimal. Isokinetic testing is an objective, valid, and reliable method of testing muscle strength (using slower speeds of 30 to 60 degrees per second) and muscle endurance (using higher speeds of 240 to 360 degrees per second) for UEs and LEs. Isokinetic machines are expensive and have a large footprint; therefore, a number of outpatient facilities may not have this equipment. They are computerized so that testing and exercise bouts can be saved and compared with previous test results.

## Muscle Contractions and Various Resistance Exercises

Resistance exercise is a type of active exercise in which a muscle contraction is resisted by an outside force.[24] The types of muscle contractions are isometric, concentric, and eccentric. An outside force can be applied manually or mechanically; can use the effect of gravity; and includes various equipment, weights, or resistance bands. There are static and dynamic types of exercises, and the resistance or force can be constant or variable. Dynamic/resistance exercise is commonly referred to as *progressive resistive exercises* (PREs). The goal of PRE programs is to gradually increase the resistance as a person's strength improves in order to improve muscle function, coordinated movement, and skill. Clinicians must recognize when it is appropriate to make an exercise more challenging to meet the patient's goals. To help physical therapist assistant students with problem solving, the strengthening problem-solving algorithm is presented in the Conclusion of this chapter.

### *Isometric Contractions and Exercises*

Isometric contractions are static contractions and the amount of tension produced varies based on the amount of voluntary effort that is exerted by the patient to create the muscle contraction. Numerous activities that people perform require some isometric component. For this reason, proximal stabilization exercises and core stability exercises that incorporate isometric contractions are often included in early portions of many exercise programs. Adequate proximal muscle stability is needed to allow for distal mobility.

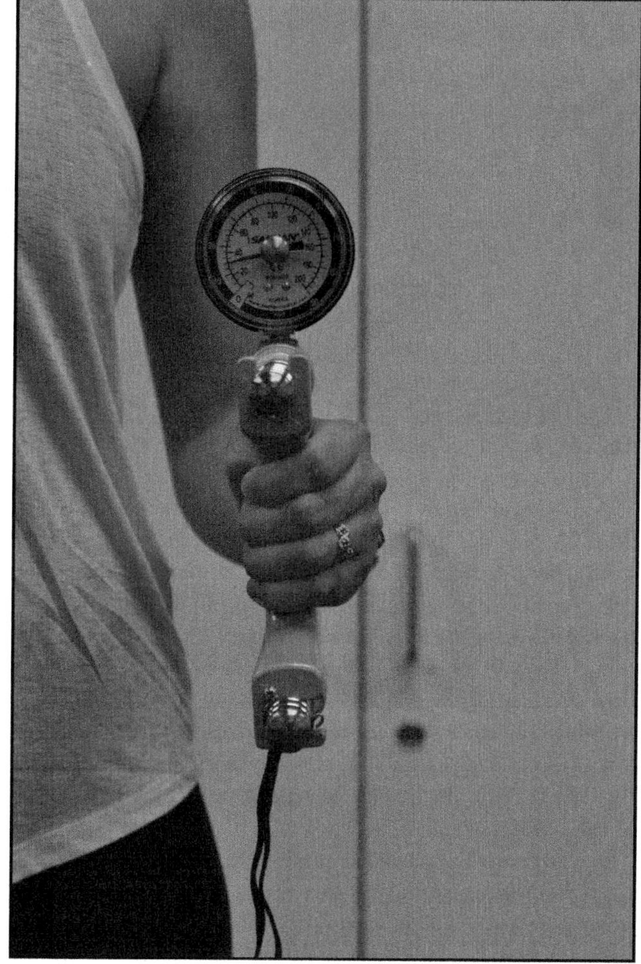

**Figure 6-9.** A dynamometer.

Isometric exercises are useful to prevent atrophy, develop joint or postural stability, create static strength at selected points in joint ROM (typically those needed for a given task performance), increase circulation, and facilitate muscle contraction. Additionally, isometrics can be used (if medically approved) to minimize atrophy when joint motion is not permitted (ie, cast or splint) and in the early stages of soft tissue healing before joint motion is permitted. An isometric program is often initiated before any other exercise program (ie, before completion of active assisted ROM or AROM).

There are different types of isometric exercises. Muscle setting is a type of submaximal, low-intensity isometric exercise that can be performed in the acute stage of healing (ie, scapula/shoulder blade squeezes after rotator cuff injury/surgery). No resistance is applied during the activity, and the patient is asked to contract the targeted muscles without moving the local joints. Muscle setting exercises can help reduce muscle guarding, promote relaxation of the surrounding muscles (ie, upper trapezius and levator scapulae), and prevent atrophy of the contracting muscles. Common setting exercises used in the LE include quadricep, gluteal, and hamstring sets (called *quad sets*, *glut sets*, and *ham sets*, respectively). Quadriceps setting exercise is pictured in Figure 6-10. Progression from muscle setting to submaximal or multiangle isometrics is dependent on the stage of healing and based on the physician protocol for postoperative patients.

Submaximal isometrics are similar to muscle setting, but the clinician applies manual resistance while the patient is performing these exercises. This exercise is performed with an effort/contraction that does not cause pain. Communication with the patient is very important when first initiating submaximal isometrics. The therapist can use a percentage scale to help grade the patient's ability to perform the isometric. For example, the clinician may instruct the patient to use 20% effort when performing the isometric. If there are no complaints of pain or if the patient reports it is too easy, the clinician can have the patient attempt the exercise with more force (ie, 50% effort) and/or progress to a multiangle isometric exercise. The goal is to have the patient perform isometric contractions with greater than 75% effort/force effort pain free. A minimum of 60% intensity of a muscle contraction will increase strength.[13] Submaximal isometrics should be performed in various points within a pain-free available ROM. These exercises are initially used for muscle re-education and facilitation.

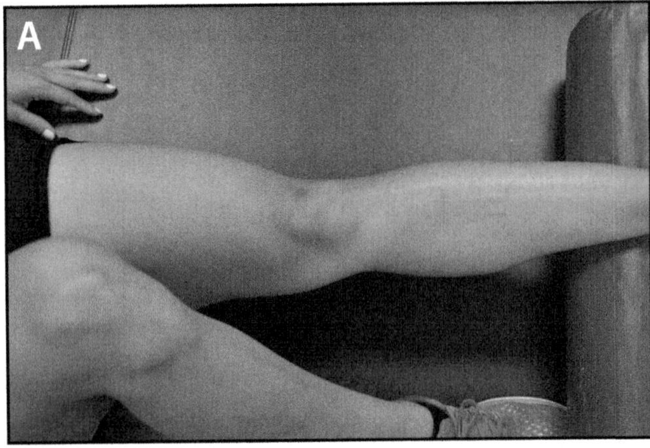


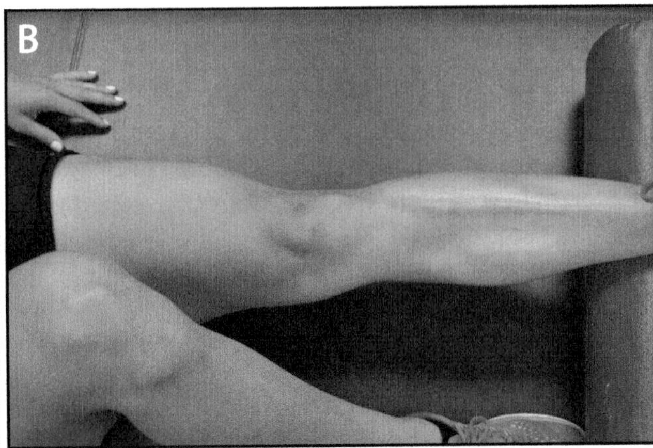


**Figure 6-10.** (A) Quadriceps set start; the vastus medialis is relaxed. (B) Quadriceps set contraction; the muscle is visible when it contracts.

Multiangle isometrics incorporate isometric contractions at multiple points throughout the ROM. Isometric strengthening is joint angle specific, so performing the exercise at numerous points in the range will increase strength throughout the range. At least 4 to 6 points in the range should be selected because there is a minimal overflow of strength benefits (10 degrees or less).[6,25] Patients who have a painful arc when performing AROM can perform isometric exercises at various points above and below the painful arc; the goal is to reduce or eliminate the size of the painful arc.

Isometric stabilization is used to facilitate joint or postural stability. Alternating isometrics, rhythmic stabilization, core stabilization (transverse abdominal isometrics), and segmental stabilization (multifidus isometrics) are examples of various types of isometric stabilization exercises (refer to Chapter 15). These exercises can be performed in open kinetic chain (OKC) or closed kinetic chain (CKC) conditions.

Alternating isometrics and rhythmic stabilization exercises are PNF techniques that can be used to improve upper extremity (UE), LE, and/or trunk stability. To perform alternating isometrics (also referred to as *stabilizing reversals*), the clinician applies manual resistance in one direction or plane and instructs the patient to resist the force for a short period of time. Then, the clinician applies the resistance in the opposite direction repeating the instructions. Rhythmic stabilization uses muscular cocontractions applying resistance in different directions simultaneously and is usually performed in CKC positions. Rhythmic stabilization can be applied as a manual technique by the clinician or facilitated by using a piece of equipment and cuing the patient in selected motions. Stabilization and cocontraction exercises can be static or dynamic. An isometric ball push (Figure 6-11A) is an example of a static closed chain stabilization exercise, and having a patient push into a therapy ball and make small circles on the wall is dynamic (Figure 6-11B). Both exercises target the muscles of the shoulder and shoulder girdle.

### Considerations for the Physical Therapist Assistant

Patients usually require instruction regarding how to activate weak muscles without contracting accessory muscles. Once the patient is able to isolate the appropriate muscles, then strengthening can begin. The assistant needs to monitor for muscle fatigue; muscle substitution is more likely to occur when muscles are fatigued.

## Parameters for Isometric Exercise Implementation

The type of resistance, duration of the contraction, and number of repetitions are important considerations. The joint angles and intensity of the muscle contractions must be documented. The type of resistance that may be used when performing isometric exercises includes manual resistance by the therapist or the patient (self-resisting), pushing into a wall or doorframe, or a therapy ball. Isometric shoulder external rotation performed in different positions is depicted in Figure 6-12.

The duration of an isometric contraction should be at least 6 seconds but no longer than 10 seconds during the initial phase of strengthening because the muscle will fatigue quickly. The exercise can be performed a few times throughout the day. The patient's response (ie, DOMS or pain) should be monitored and the program modified as indicated. Patient positioning and limb stabilization are also monitored to prevent substitution patterns.

### Clinical Tip: Rule of 10s for Isometric Contractions

The assistant should remember: A 10-second contraction followed by a 10-second rest for 10 repetitions. Instruct the patient to complete a 2-second gradual increase in muscle contraction intensity followed by a 6-second hold and then a slow 2-second release of the contraction (for a total of 10 seconds). Each contraction is followed by a 10-second rest and performed for 10 repetitions.[13]

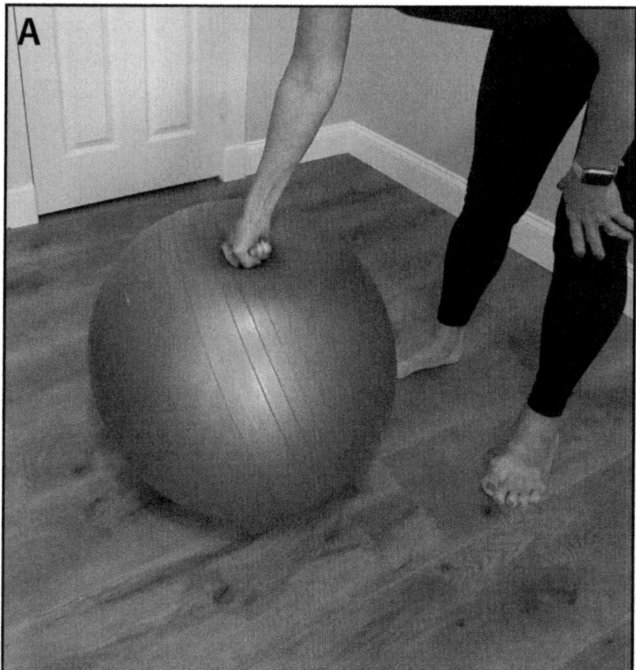


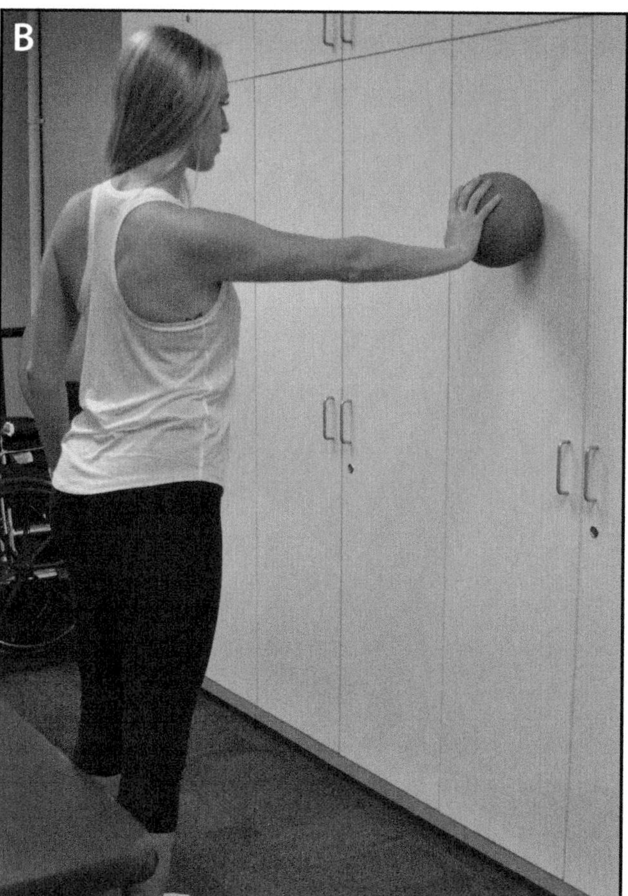


**Figure 6-11.** (A) Ball push isometrics is a closed chain activity to facilitate both shoulder and scapula muscle contractions. (B) Shoulder dynamic stabilization. The patient makes small circles while pushing the ball into the wall.

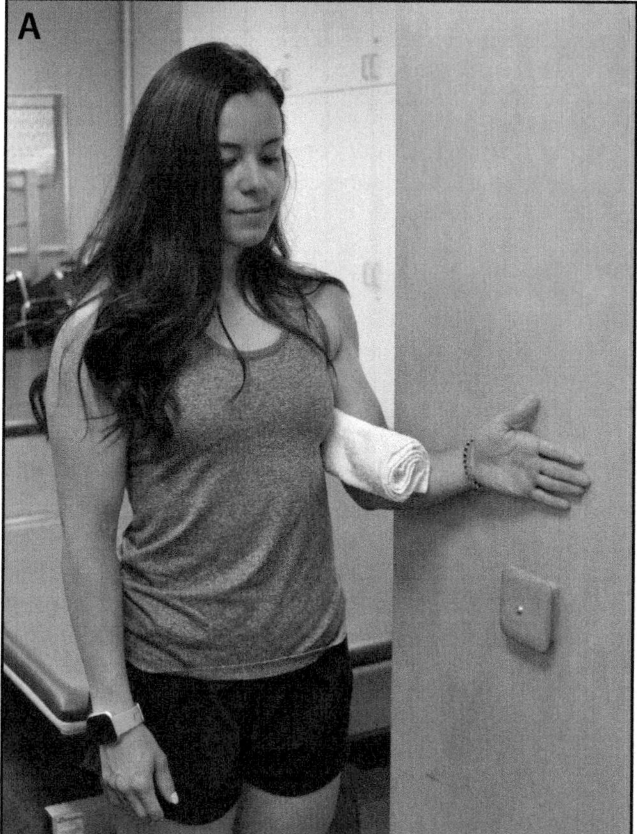


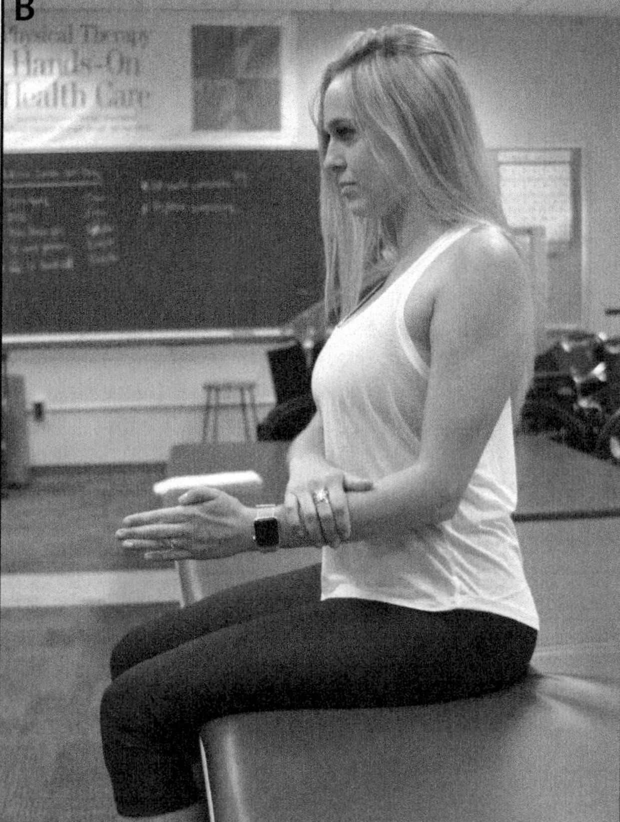


**Figure 6-12.** (A) Shoulder external rotation isometric at wall. (B) Shoulder external rotation isometric self-resistance.

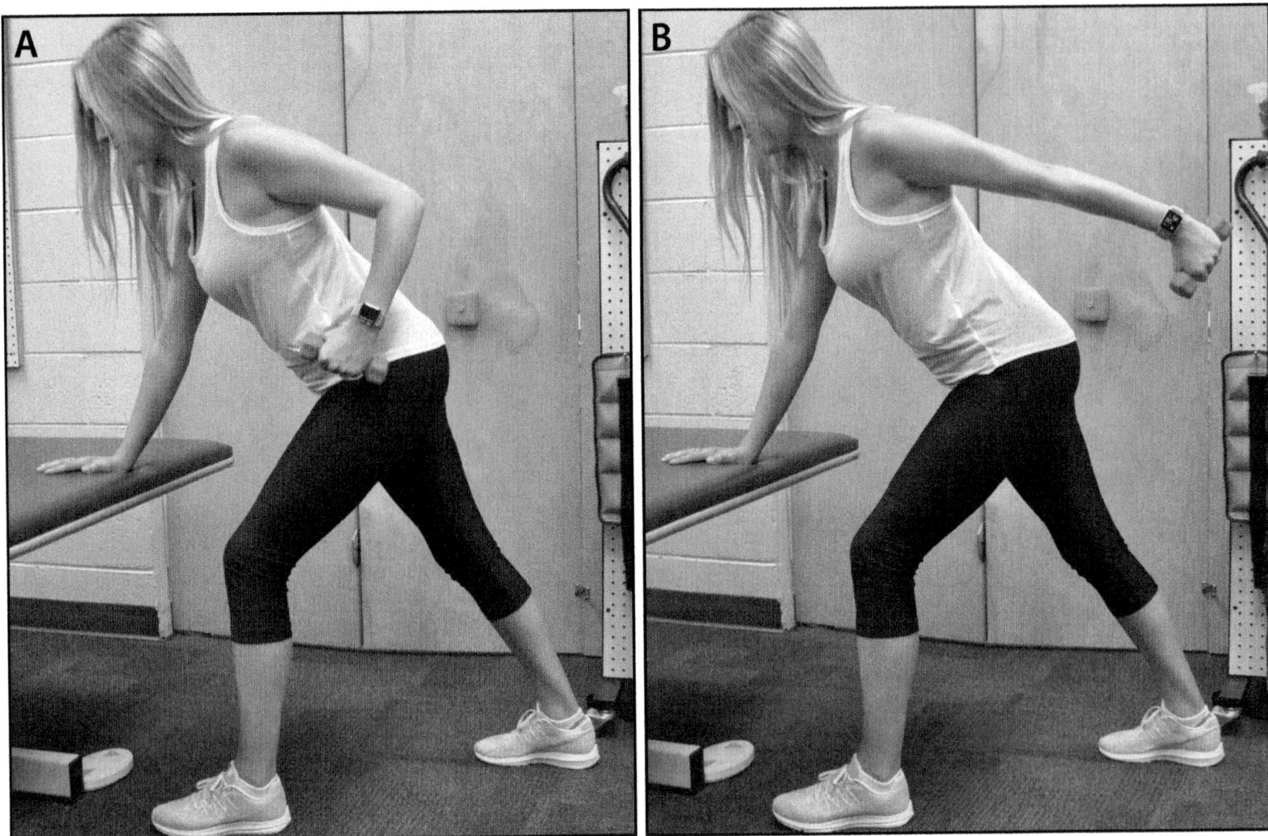


**Figure 6-13.** (A) Concentric triceps contraction start position. (B) Concentric triceps contraction end position.

### Precautions and Contraindications

Physical therapist assistants should monitor patients to ensure they do not hold their breath when performing isometrics (this is especially important for patients with cardiac considerations). Holding the breath (with a closed glottis) and then forcefully exhaling is called the *Valsalva maneuver*. Performing the Valsalva maneuver is followed by a transient increase in cardiac output/blood pressure that can be dangerous for many patients. The Valsalva maneuver should be avoided at all costs when performing any exercise. It is important that patients exhale while holding isometric contractions. It is helpful to have the patient count out loud when performing the contraction. High-intensity isometric training is contraindicated for any person with a history of cardiac disease. Additional contraindications and precautions regarding strength training are discussed later in this chapter and should be incorporated during all types of resistance training.

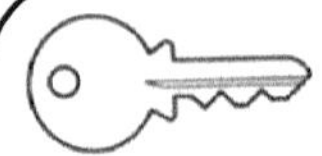

**Key Safety Considerations**

Avoid the Valsalva maneuver at all times when patients are performing any type of resistance exercises.

## *Isotonic Contractions and Progressive Resistance Exercises*

Concentric and eccentric contractions occur when performing most functional activities. Strength training must be specific to the types of contractions that are needed to complete a task; to improve function, strength training programs should include both types of contractions.

### Isotonic Contractions

**Isotonic or dynamic contractions** include concentric and eccentric muscle contractions. During isotonic contractions, the resistance (or load) remains constant throughout the motion, but the tension that the muscle generates to lift a load varies as the joint angle changes. The ability to lift/move a load through the entire ROM will always be limited by the point in the range where the muscle creates the least amount of torque. During concentric contractions, the muscle shortens, and acceleration occurs. Concentric contractions require more force (at a fixed load) than eccentric exercise, making it feel harder to lift a heavy weight than to lower it down. Figure 6-13 depicts a concentric contraction of the triceps.

Eccentric contractions create tension in a muscle and produce force while the muscle is lengthening and decelerating during a "controlled lowering" as the muscle resists gravity (Figure 6-14). There are situations when performing slow controlled eccentric exercises are indicated. Eccentric exercises are most appropriate in situations when pain is

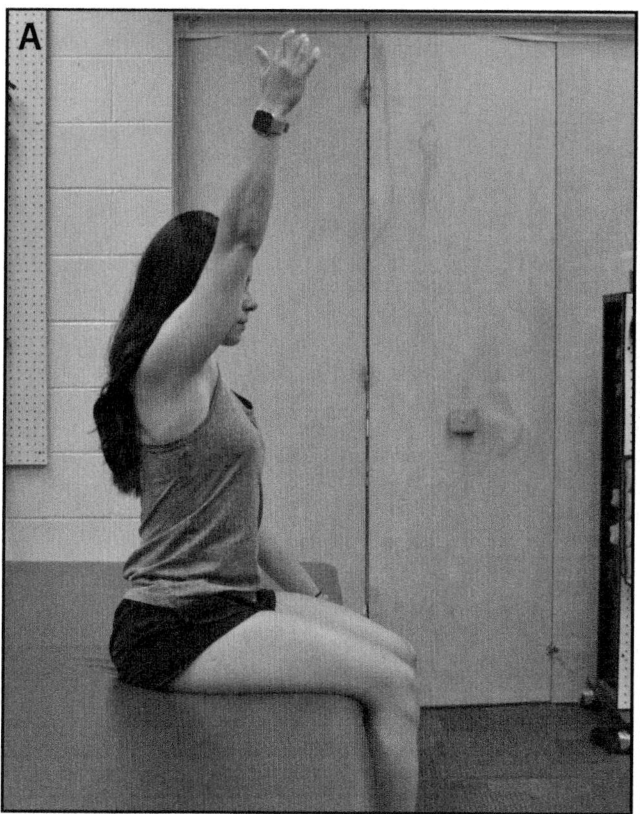


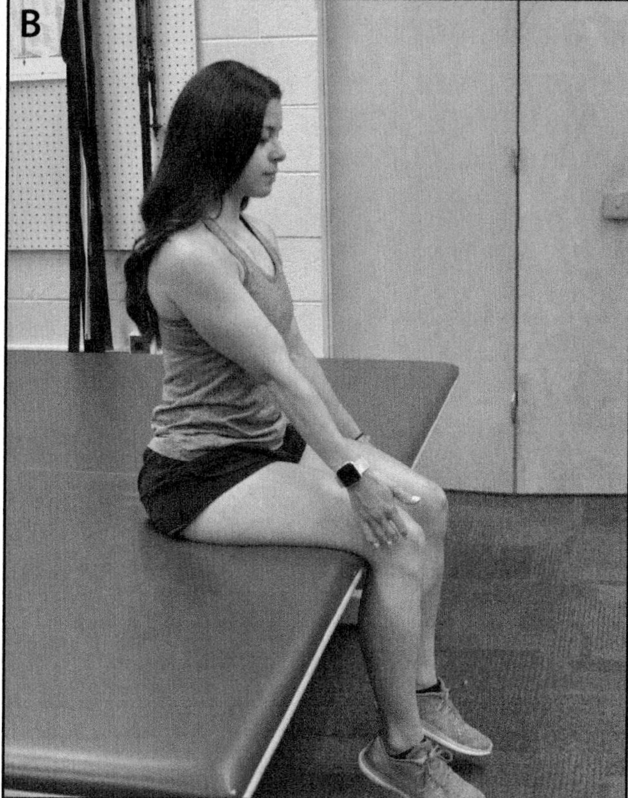


**Figure 6-14.** (A) Anterior deltoid eccentric contraction start position. (B) Anterior deltoid eccentric end position.

elicited during a concentric contraction, a patient complains of joint crepitus or a painful arc when performing an exercise against gravity, or the patient has a diagnosis of tendinitis. Eccentric training can also be used later in the rehabilitation phase to improve athletic performance.

Training adaptations are greater with maximal eccentric exercise than with maximal concentric exercise. However, the risk for **DOMS** is higher with unaccustomed high-intensity eccentric exercise than with concentric exercise. The development of DOMS indicates that the resistance or treatment parameters are too high and must be adjusted.[13]

> **Considerations for the Physical Therapist Assistant**
>
> If a patient experiences pain when performing concentric contractions against gravity, try having the patient perform the exercise gravity minimized or eccentrically and monitor their pain.

## *Types of Resistance and Dynamic Exercises*

When performing progressive dynamic resistive exercises, the resistance is either constant or variable. The type of resistance selected is determined based on the stage of healing, patient presentation (current strength, abilities, and impairments), the physical therapy goals, and the plan of care (POC). Constant resistance refers to a specific weight or load. Constant resistance includes free weights (ie, cuff weights, dumbbells, and weighted balls) and some simple pulley machines. Even with a static/constant load (ie, a 5-lb dumbbell), the tension the muscle must develop to move the load varies at different points in the range. This is a result of the changes in moment arm distance (torque) and the length–tension relationship. Types of variable resistance include isokinetic exercise, manual resistance, elastic resistance bands/tubing, and weight stacked or hydraulic resistance machines.

### Isokinetic Exercise

With **isokinetic exercise**, the speed or velocity of the motion remains constant regardless of the amount of force applied to overcome the resistance. This constant, fixed speed is accomplished using a rate-limiting computerized dynamometer. Examples of isokinetic equipment include Biodex, Kin-Com (Chattanooga Group), and Cybex (Lumex, Inc; see Figure 6-3). The speeds of these machines can be preset. There are slow speeds (30 to 60 degrees per second), medium speeds (90 to 180 degrees per second), and fast speeds (240 to 360 degrees per second). Isokinetic exercise is called *accommodating resistance* because it accommodates for the amount of effort the muscles can exert. For example, if a patient is unable to move a limb fast enough to meet the set speed of the machine, the patient will not encounter any resistance. However, when the patient moves harder and faster, the machine will provide resistance directly related to the speed the limb is moving.

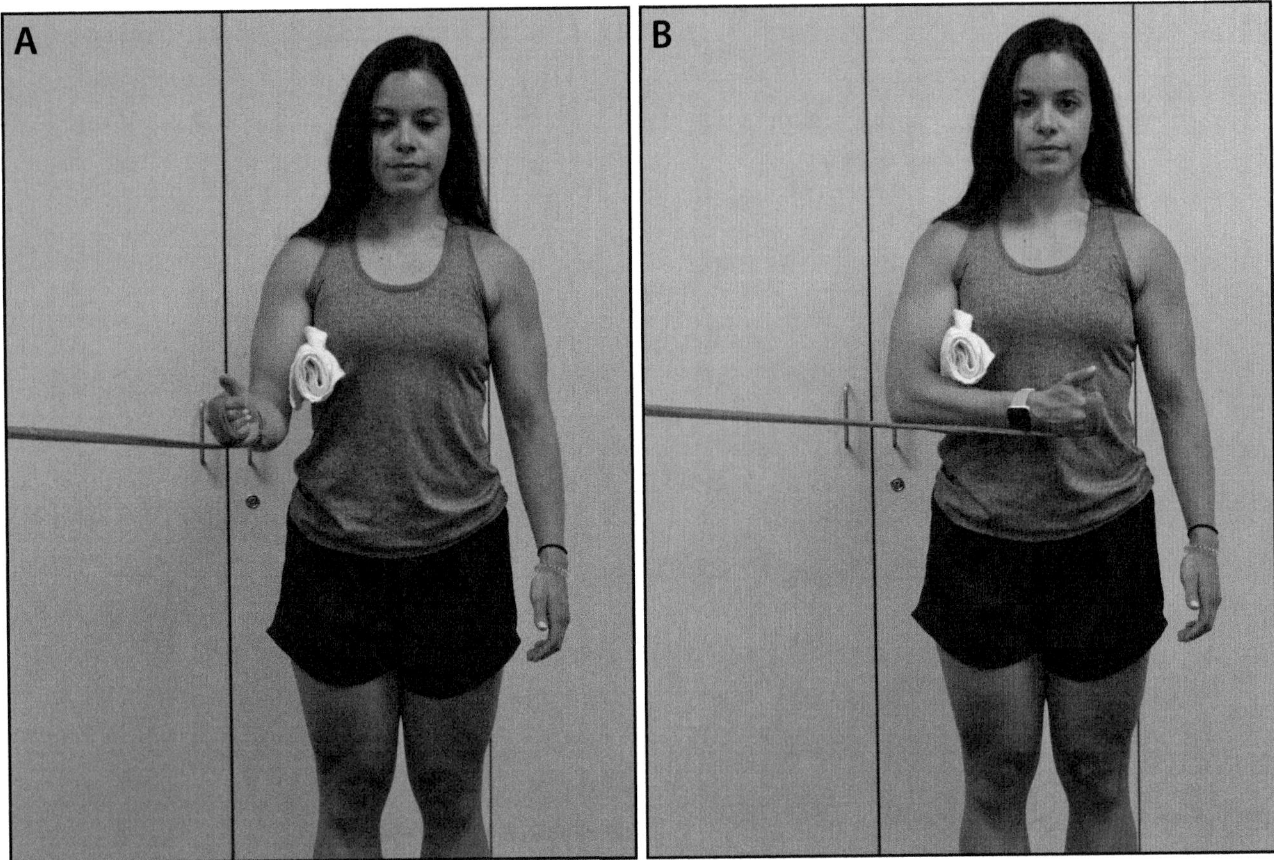


**Figure 6-15.** (A) Elastic band resistance for shoulder internal rotation: Starting position. (B) Concentric contraction: End position. When returning back to the starting position, an eccentric contraction of the internal rotators occurs.

Isokinetic exercise machines provide resistance based on the amount of force the limb can produce throughout the entire range. If the patient is stronger at one point in the range, the resistance will be greater, and, conversely, if the patient is weaker in another part of the range, the resistance will be less.

## Manual Resistance

Manual resistance is a type of exercise in which a physical therapist assistant provides a force resisting a muscle contraction either statically (isometric contraction) or dynamically throughout a patient's available range. Manual resistance can be a safe way to initiate resistance exercises because the clinician can apply force at different intensities at various points in a range based on the patient's ability to resist. Assistants can initially apply light resistance so the patient can perform multiangle submaximal isometric contractions in a pain-free range. Resistance can be applied during single-plane motions (ie, sagittal, frontal, or transverse) and progressed to multiplane motions (ie, diagonal patterns). Manual resistance is often used early in the rehabilitation process when muscles are weaker (4/5 or less) and strengthening is not a contraindication. The clinician must control the ROM and adjust the amount of resistance based on the stage of healing of the affected tissues and patient tolerance.

There are some limitations to using manual resistance. First, manual resistance is time intensive and physically intensive for the clinician. The forces to be applied are limited by the therapist's strength and ability to maintain good body mechanics, making this technique less appropriate to use for resisting large/strong muscles. Manual resistance is not appropriate as a part of a home exercise program (HEP) because the amount and timing of the resistance require the skill of a trained clinician.

## Elastic Resistance Bands or Tubing

Elastic resistance bands or tubing provide a type of variable resistance. There are several companies that make these items; Theraband (Theraband) is the most recognized brand. Each band or tubing is color coded, with each color representing a different level of resistance. Theraband bands/tubing range from yellow (the easiest) to red, green, blue, black, and silver (the most difficult). The patient in Figure 6-15 is demonstrating shoulder internal rotation using an elastic band for strengthening. Familiarity with the levels of resistance of each band/tube and knowledge of application and safety considerations are useful to the clinician. This equipment is very versatile and is used in clinics and for HEPs.

Elastic band/tubing resistance increases based on the amount the band is stretched. When the tubing is not on stretch (the resting length), there is no resistance, but as

**Table 6-3**

**Theraband Percentage of Elongation/Strain and Corresponding Resistance in Pound Equivalent[a]**

| Color | 25% | 50% | 100% | 150% | 200% | 250% |
|---|---|---|---|---|---|---|
| Yellow | 1 | 2 | 3 | 4 | 5 | 6 |
| Red | 1.5 | 2.5 | 4 | 5 | 6 | 7 |
| Green | 2 | 3 | 5 | 6.5 | 8 | 9.5 |
| Blue | 2.5 | 4.5 | 7 | 9 | 11 | 13.5 |
| Black | 3.5 | 6.5 | 9.5 | 12.5 | 15 | 17.5 |
| Silver | 5 | 8.5 | 13 | 17 | 21 | 25.5 |

[a]These are estimated pound values.

Adapted from Page P, Labbe A, Topp R. Clinical force production of Thera-Band elastic bands. *J Orthop Sports Phys Ther.* 2000;30(1):47-48.

## Box 6-1

### Safety Guidelines for Resistance Tubing/Band Use

- Check all resistance tubing for drying, cracking, or fraying before use every session. Discard if damaged; it is at risk for breaking.
- Make sure handles are securely attached to the ends of the tubing. If handles are not used, make loops at each end of the tubing (large enough for the patient's hand/foot) to simulate handles.
- When only one end of the tubing is used for an exercise, make sure the other end is safely secured so it will not break loose and snap back toward the patient.
- Instruct patients to wear safety goggles/protective eyeglasses to prevent eye injury.
- Patient instructions to secure tubing for home use: Have the patient stand on one side of a bathroom door and secure one end of the tubing on the opposite side of the door around the knob. Close the door securely (ensure tubing is not interfering with the door latch and lock door).
  - If both handles are to be used, place the middle of the tubing on the doorknob on the opposite side of the door where the patient is standing. Have the patient hold both ends of the tubing and securely close the door (stay clear of the latch).
- Do not allow the patient to step on the tubing to secure it.

the tubing gets stretched, the resistance increases. The tubing can be strained (stretched) to approximately 250% of its resting length.[26] Each colored band has a percentage of strain (or elongation) from 25% to 250% that corresponds to resistance in pounds. For example, if the resting length of a yellow band is 3-ft long, 50% strain would be equivalent to the band being stretched 1.5 ft (total length = 4.5 ft), and the estimated force is equal to 2 lb. Table 6-3 provides information to guide the color selection of the band to use and how much the band/tubing should be stretched to provide the desired level of resistance.[27]

Some advantages for using elastic resistance include versatility (they can be used for upper or LE and trunk strengthening in various movement patterns), portability, and inexpensive cost. It is safe to use these at various velocities depending on the desired effects (ie, slow, medium, or fast). Some disadvantages include difficultly comparing the resistance of the tubing to free weight pounds and the risk of band/tube failure (snapping), which can create an injury risk. Make sure patients wear glasses or protective eyewear to reduce eye injury risk. Some products contain latex; the clinician must be aware of any latex allergies or sensitivities.

It is important to adhere to safety guidelines when using resistance bands/tubing during treatment (Box 6-1). The assistant should provide safety training to the patient when the exercises are given as part of their HEP.

### Considerations for the Physical Therapist Assistant

When using resistance bands/tubing, muscles may fatigue more quickly as exercises work the targeted muscle both concentrically and eccentrically.

### Weight Training Machines

Weight machines found in fitness centers and outpatient clinics usually provide a variable resistance. There are 2 types of resistance training machines that are most commonly seen: weight stacked (more common) or hydraulic. A cable attached to a weight stack passes over an elliptical-shaped item called a *cam*, which effectively varies the amount of weight experienced by the targeted muscle group throughout the range. Different machines target different muscle groups. The individual in Figure 6-2B is performing a leg press exercise for hip/knee extension strengthening, targeting the hip and knee extensors concentrically during knee extension and eccentrically when controlling the return to the starting position.

Weight machines are often used during the later phases of rehabilitation to improve muscular strength and endurance. It is suggested that a patient should have a muscle strength grade of 4/5 (good) before using some of these machines. There are times when variable resistance machines can be used sooner, but the physical therapist assistant should consult with the physical therapist before initiating the use of weight machines because of healing tissue constraints.

There are a number of advantages to selecting variable weight machines. The first time a patient uses a weight machine, an objective baseline is established so that strength gains can be recorded over time. Patients can perform strengthening exercises on machines at heavier loads than a therapist can manually resist. Once properly instructed on their use, patients can use these machines independently, and they can be a part of a fitness program after discharge from physical therapy.

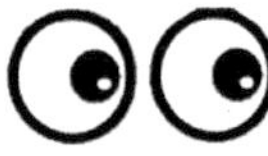

**Eye on the Research**

Lima et al[28] compared the effectiveness of resistance training using weight machines with elastic resistance tubing in healthy middle-aged to older adults. They determined that both groups had similar, significant positive effects on muscle force and functional exercise capacity after exercising for 3 times a week for 12 weeks.

**Question for Thought**

If a patient is performing a leg press exercise, is that considered an OKC or CKC activity?

### Open Kinetic Chain Exercises: Utilization and Justification

**OKC exercises** challenge muscles during a single-joint motion and are performed in a nonweight position. When a patient performs an elbow flexion exercise (Figure 6-16), the elbow joint is the only joint in motion, and the elbow flexors are the muscles performing the action. However, depending on the position of the forearm (supinated, pronated, or neutral), the biceps (palm up/supinated), brachialis (palm down/pronated), or brachioradialis (thumb up/forearm neutral) can specifically be targeted. When resistance is needed to challenge the muscle, it is typically placed at the distal end of the moving segment (ie, a cuff weight around the wrist or a handheld dumbbell).

The clinician must monitor for substitution or compensatory patterns when a patient is performing exercises. **Substitution patterns or compensation** occur when muscles other than those normally responsible for creating the motion assist when completing a desired movement. Substitution patterns often occur because of joint pain or weakness and/or fatigue in the primary muscles that typically complete the desired action. One area a clinician may see a compensatory or substitution pattern occur is during the completion of shoulder abduction. If a patient experiences pain or has weakness in the rotator cuff/scapulothoracic muscles, the patient may hike the shoulder or laterally bend the trunk when trying to complete shoulder abduction compared with normal joint mechanics and muscle strength (Figure 6-17).

**Clinical Tip**

Having patients perform exercises while looking in a mirror provides feedback while the physical therapist assistant provides appropriate cuing and corrections to compensatory motions.

## *Open and Closed Kinetic Chain Exercise*

OKC exercises are performed when the distal segment of a limb is moving freely (ie, shoulder flexion and seated knee extension). OKC activities have traditionally been categorized as activities that are non–weight bearing. CKC exercises are performed when the distal segment of a limb is fixed (ie, squats and push-ups). CKC activities have traditionally been categorized as activities that are weight bearing. There is controversy as to what truly defines OKC or CKC activities, but both OKC and CKC exercises have specific purposes, and both are important to use throughout the rehabilitation process.

Once muscle substitution is observed, the clinician should support or stabilize the patient's joint or proximal segment so the desired muscles can fire and motion can occur. This allows the muscles to be better isolated while completing the exercise. When performing OKC exercises, patients usually have better control of a specific movement when only one joint is involved.

OKC exercises can increase the strength of isolated muscles and can increase ROM, but the clinician must be cautious because these exercises can generate shearing forces on healing tissues. They can also increase compression forces. For example, when performing a seated long arc

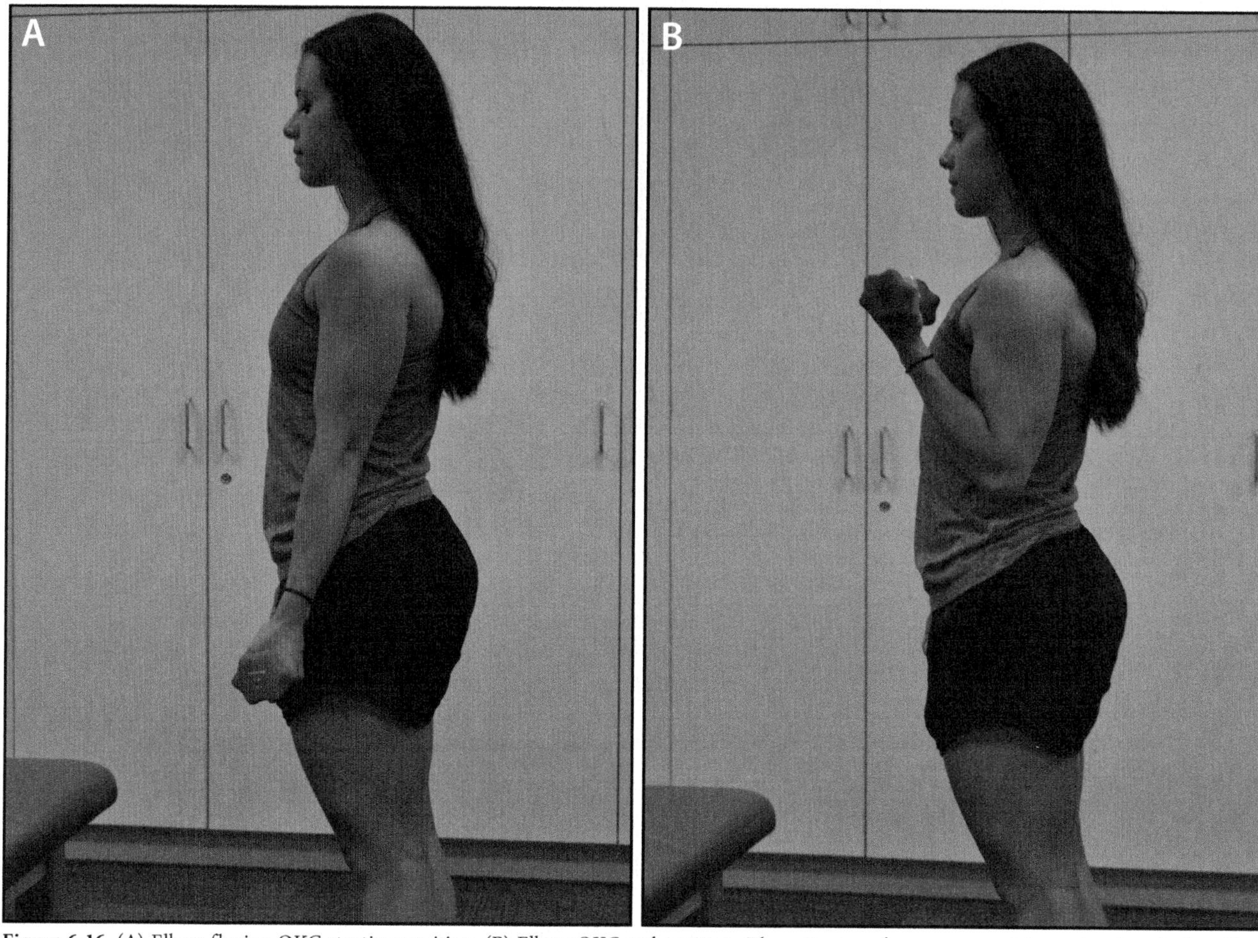


**Figure 6-16.** (A) Elbow flexion OKC starting position. (B) Elbow OKC end position. The patient performs a concentric contraction during elbow flexion and an eccentric contraction as the weight gets lowered back to the starting position.

quadriceps knee extension exercise with resistance, there is an increase in tibiofemoral shear and patellofemoral compression, making this exercise inappropriate for some patients (ie, certain patients with anterior cruciate ligament repair or patellofemoral conditions depending on the level of acuity, injury history, and/or postoperative procedures).

### Closed Kinetic Chain Exercises: Utilization and Justification

**CKC exercises** can be used when joint approximation (compression), increased joint stability (static and dynamic), and weight-bearing activities are indicated. During CKC exercises, several joints typically move, and multiple muscles contract to complete the activity. For example, when performing a partial squat, hip flexion/extension, knee flexion/extension, and ankle dorsiflexion/plantar flexion all need to occur to complete the exercise (Figure 6-18). Because several muscles and joints have to contract to control the movement pattern, CKC activities reduce shearing forces on healing tissues and increase joint proprioception and sensory input. If joint stabilization is a treatment goal, CKC activities are an excellent option. These exercises can be used early in the rehabilitation process as long as the patient does not have a weight-bearing restriction on the affected extremity. CKC activities facilitate cocontractions of agonist and antagonist muscles. For example, if a patient has rotator cuff weakness and instability problems, pushing into a therapy ball (see Figure 6-11A) for 20 to 30 seconds will create joint approximation and facilitate muscle firing safely.

If patients have balance issues or postural instability, CKC exercises should be included in therapeutic interventions because they target stabilizing muscles. It should be noted that there are instances when CKC exercises are either contraindicated or performed with extreme caution for patients with weight-bearing restrictions, decreased ROM, and increased swelling or pain.

## *Plyometrics*

**Plyometrics** are intense, ballistic, power-generating activities that are often required for patients who participate in sports or physically demanding work. These exercises are typically added at the end of a sports/work-specific training program to prepare patients for a safe return to full activity. Because plyometrics include high-velocity, ballistic motions, they are not appropriate to implement until tissue healing is complete. The patient should demonstrate

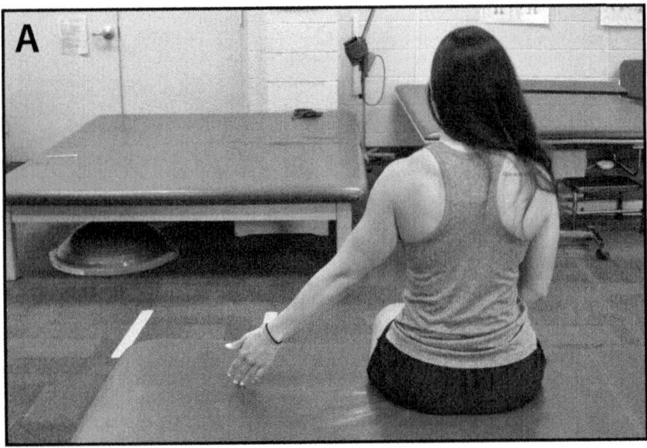


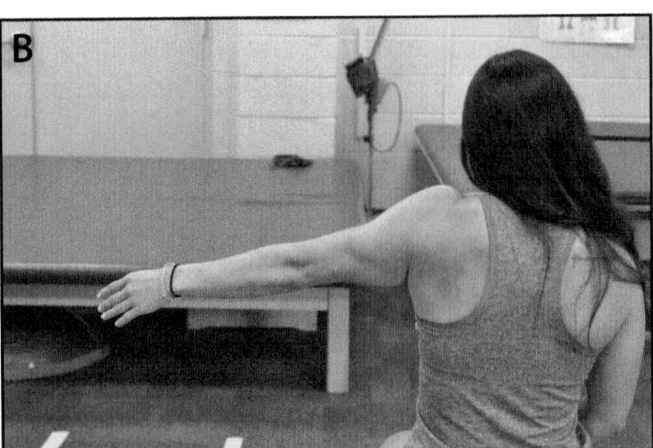


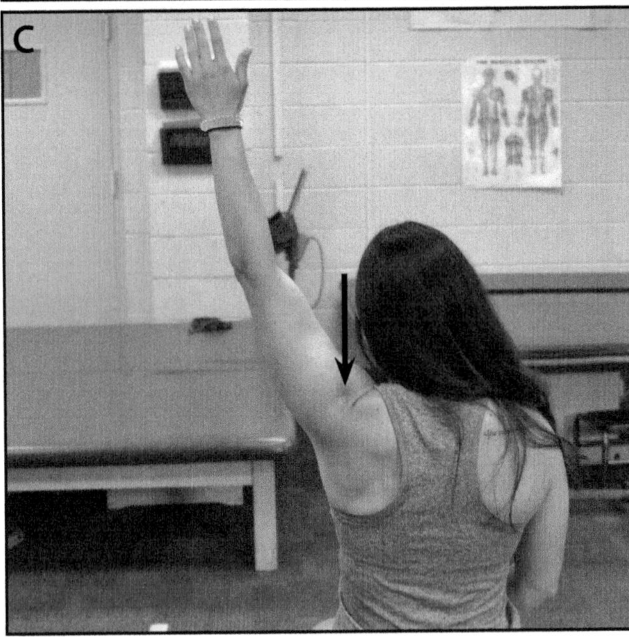


**Figure 6-17.** (A) Normal shoulder abduction is initiated. (B) During abduction, notice the shoulder joint elevation substitution pattern in midrange, which is commonly observed due to pain or muscle weakness. (C) Shoulder abduction close to end range with good joint mechanics. Note the glenohumeral depression indicated by the arrow.

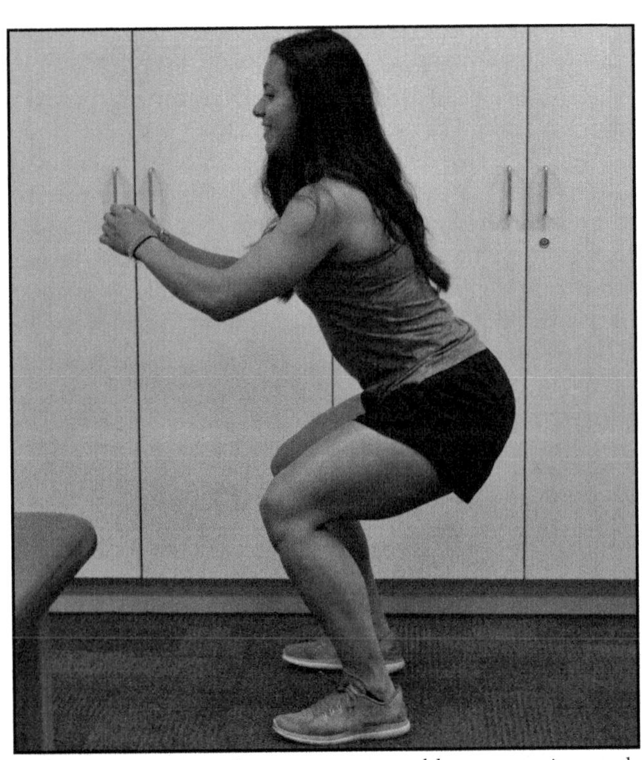

**Figure 6-18.** CKC partial squat targets several lower extremity muscle groups.

full AROM and muscle strength (5/5) in the involved areas before integrating plyometric exercises. The goal of plyometrics is to increase the speed and strength of muscle contractions. When performing plyometric exercises, there is a rapid eccentric loading of the muscle followed by a rapid concentric contraction of the same muscle. In other words, there is a quick prestretch of the target muscle followed by a rapid, strong shortening of the same muscle. Some examples of plyometrics include swinging a weighted object (ie, an axe or sledgehammer); jumping up/down onto a box; throwing and catching a weighted ball (about 2 to 3 lbs) against a mini-trampoline; and quick starts, stops, and directional changes on command. Plyometric exercise performance using directional jumps is illustrated in Figure 6-4. Plyometrics retrain the neuromuscular system's response to quick, ballistic movements. They are progressive in nature and skill/sport specific. For LE programs, the patient must typically have normal balance and the ability to complete the single-limb stance safely. For UE programs, patients must demonstrate good joint stability, static and dynamic strength, and muscle endurance. Initially, plyometrics should be completed on a surface with adequate shock-absorbing qualities to protect joints, but

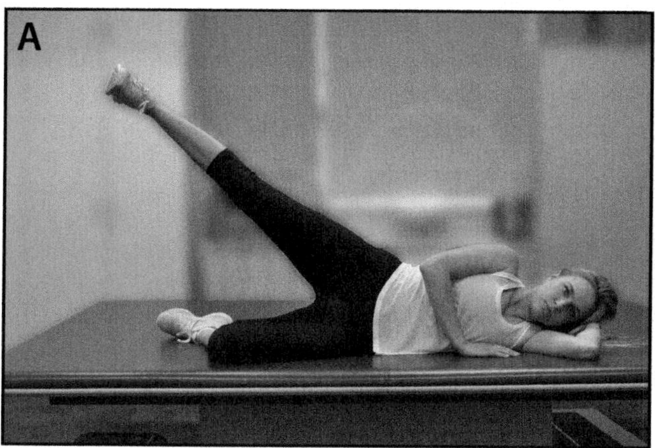


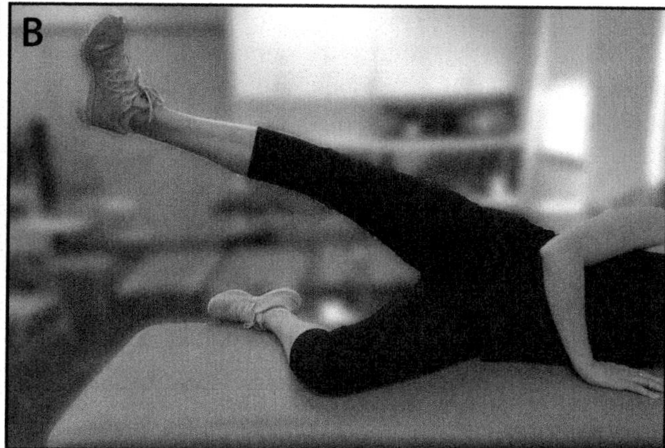


**Figure 6-19.** (A) The gluteus medius muscle is targeted when the hip is not rotated, and the toes point straight ahead. (B) The tensor fasciae latae muscle is targeted when the hip is externally rotated.

training should be progressed to surfaces similar to those used during work or sport activities. Not all patients need to participate in plyometric training.

## Key Components of a Progressive Resistance Exercise Program

Before designing a PRE training program, clinicians need to review the patient's goals. Typically, PRE programs are developed for rehabilitative purposes to maximize strength (so that ADLs can be performed more easily and efficiently), for injury risk reduction, for prevention/management of chronic health conditions and diseases (ie, type 2 diabetes mellitus, obesity, and osteoporosis), or to improve overall fitness levels. Factors considered when implementing a PRE program include age, overall health status, medications, prior and current level of function, cognition, and muscle impairments or limitations.[4,29] Patients' input regarding treatment goals increases the likelihood of patient compliance with exercise programs.

The ACSM's evidence-based guidelines create a framework to guide exercise program development; these guidelines incorporate the FITT-VP (frequency, intensity, time, type, volume, progression) principle. Frequency describes how often the exercise is performed each week. Intensity refers to how hard the exercise is, and time describes the exercise duration. Type is the mode of exercise, volume refers to the total amount of exercise, and progression describes how exercise activities and programs are advanced. Every resistance program should address all of the guidelines, but the parameters should be individualized to the patient.[4]

### *Positioning, Alignment, and Stabilization*

After determining appropriate exercise parameters, the clinician needs to consider the patient's position, joint/limb alignment, and stabilization of adjacent structures. Proper positioning and stabilization decrease the potential for compensatory movement patterns or muscle substitution.

When targeting a specific muscle for strengthening, appropriate patient positioning and stabilization ensure good joint position and proper muscle fiber alignment, which promote efficient muscle action and line of pull. Stabilization can be performed by an external force (ie, a therapist, strap, or treatment table) or by proximal adjacent muscle contraction (internal force). Figure 6-19 illustrates how positioning, stabilization, and the line of pull affect muscle performance. Just a slight shifting of the position or performing movements in a different plane can shift the strengthening focus to a different muscle. Look at the difference between Figures 6-19A and 19-B. When performing hip abduction, the pelvis should be in neutral with the hip in slight extension so that the gluteus medius muscle fibers are better aligned (line of pull) and are recruited (see Figure 6-19A). In Figure 6-19B, the pelvis is still in neutral, but the femur is slightly flexed and externally rotated. In this position, the tensor fasciae latae muscle fibers are better aligned to perform the muscle action. In both examples, the pelvis is stabilized by trunk muscle contractions and the table, which also supports the opposite LE. If the patient was unable to perform hip abduction against gravity (because of weakness), changing the patient's position to supine or standing would allow the patient to perform the exercise while minimizing the effect of gravity. Muscle strength is a determinant that influences a clinician's selection for patient positioning and the method of stabilization. The clinician's goal is to determine the position that will best align the patient so that the targeted muscle's line of pull creates an efficient and effective contraction.[14,15] Patients with chronic conditions (ie, osteoporosis or spinal stenosis) may need to be positioned and stabilized differently to accommodate for their comorbidities while still optimizing the targeted muscle's line of pull.

### *Exercise Frequency*

As a general rule, the ACSM recommends that the frequency of resistance training for all major muscle groups should be 2 to 3 days per week with at least 48 hours of rest between sessions that address the same muscle group. The intensity, number of repetitions, and sets performed will determine how much rest is needed for recovery. Those who perform high-intensity eccentric exercises should typically perform these less frequently to reduce the risk of DOMS or overtraining.

There are different ways to structure a fitness program. A whole-body program includes exercise for all of the major muscles in one session. This program should occur 3 days per week with 1 day of rest between each session. A split program addresses selected muscle groups (ie, upper body or lower body). In a split program, the patient may exercise more days per week because of the alternating days targeting different muscle groups or body parts.[4,30] Both programs are effective, but the clinician should work with the patient to select the one that is likely to promote compliance. As a general rule for fitness training, exercises for large muscle groups and multijoint muscles should be completed first followed by smaller and single-joint muscle exercises. Alternating between exercises that work opposing muscle groups (agonists and then antagonist muscles) is beneficial.[30]

Goals for rehabilitation programs are different than those for fitness programs. Early postoperative or postinjury rehabilitation programs often include a small number of exercises that are performed several times a day every day at a low intensity (ie, muscle setting) to prevent muscle atrophy and reduce muscle guarding. As the patient progresses through the phases of rehabilitation, exercise resistance and repetitions are modified to address muscular strength and endurance goals. The frequency of exercise performance is changed to several times a week or every other day to allow for muscles to recover as intensity is increased.

## Exercise Intensity, Time, and Duration

Intensity reflects the workload used during training and includes the amount of weight/resistance and the number of repetitions performed; these are inversely related. Determination of the amount of resistance or the number of repetitions is based on the treatment goals. If the goal is to increase muscle strength and power, then heavier resistance and lower repetitions are indicated; these are often considered high-intensity exercises. If the goal is to increase muscle endurance, then lighter resistance and a higher number of repetitions are appropriate (low-intensity exercises). Clinicians should determine the intensity of the exercise(s) that is appropriate for the patient. The patient's age, tissues involved, stage of healing, exercise goal (strength vs muscle endurance), and the patient's familiarity with the selected exercise(s) must be considered.

Low-intensity exercises are appropriate for patients when the healing tissue needs to be protected (early during the acute stage of healing). Muscle setting and submaximal isometrics are often selected early in the rehabilitation process to prevent atrophy of supporting muscles and to reduce muscle guarding. When instructing patients on exercises they are not familiar with, begin without using resistance, and use a low number of repetitions. Physical therapist assistants will monitor patient performance for accuracy and patient tolerance. Once the patient performs the exercise correctly, heavier weights/resistance can be introduced when it is clinically appropriate, if increasing strength or power are specific goals.

Higher-intensity exercises are used by those patients who have to meet the demands of rigorous sport or work conditions. These are implemented later in the rehabilitation process as the patient progresses toward their prior level of function. Care is taken to increase intensity only as clinically appropriate; increasing intensity too early in the healing process can result in injury.

There are no evidence-based guidelines to define time, but it is generally recognized that each resistance training session should be less than 45 to 60 minutes. A high-intensity session may only last 20 minutes.[4]

## Exercise Types and Mode

There are different types of exercise and equipment that can be selected (ie, free weights, exercise bands, exercise equipment/machines, and body weight resistance); these are sometimes referred to as the *mode* or *method*. Clinicians need to determine if an exercise type/mode will include OKC or CKC exercises; static or dynamic activities; manual or mechanical resistance; and/or include isometric, isotonic, or isokinetic activities. A patient's body weight can also be used as a type of resistance. The resistance can be varied based on the position assumed by the patient. For example, a patient can perform a push-up against a wall, on an incline, with the knees flexed or straight, using one arm, placing the hands further apart or closer together, and progressing to an unstable surface. Each of these variations alters the level of difficulty. Figure 6-20 illustrates a series of push-ups as a progression, increasing in difficulty. Exercise selection is based on muscle strength and observing the patient's form for correctness when completing the exercise. Evidence of muscle substitution/compensation or the inability to complete the exercise with good form indicates that the activity is too advanced for the patient. The clinician should either modify the exercise or select another exercise that is lower in intensity.

## Volume: Using Repetitions and Sets

The exercise volume includes the total number of repetitions and sets of an exercise. Repetitions are defined as the number of times the specific exercise is performed consecutively. A set is a specific number of repetitions of the same exercise performed together. For example, if a patient performs 15 biceps curls, they have completed 15 repetitions.

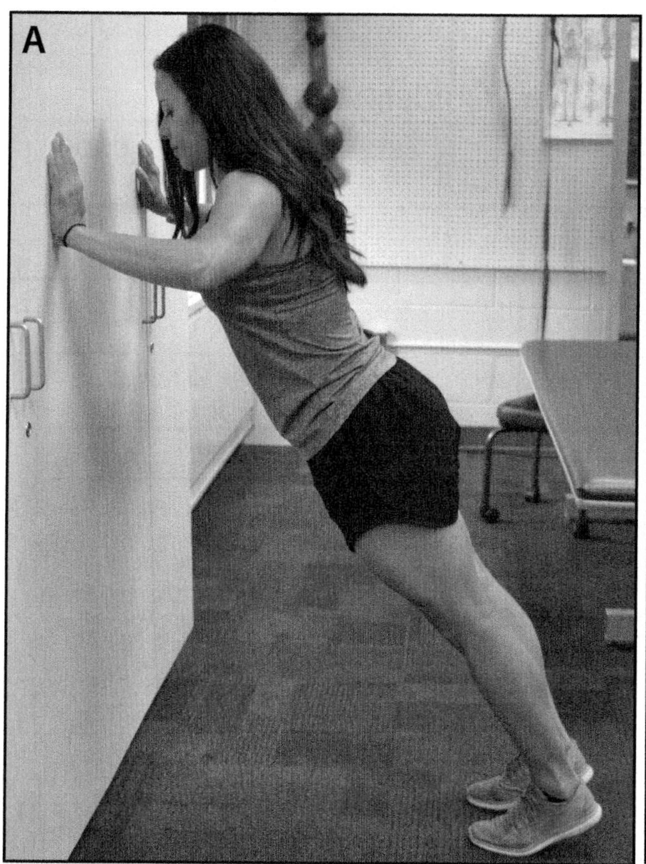


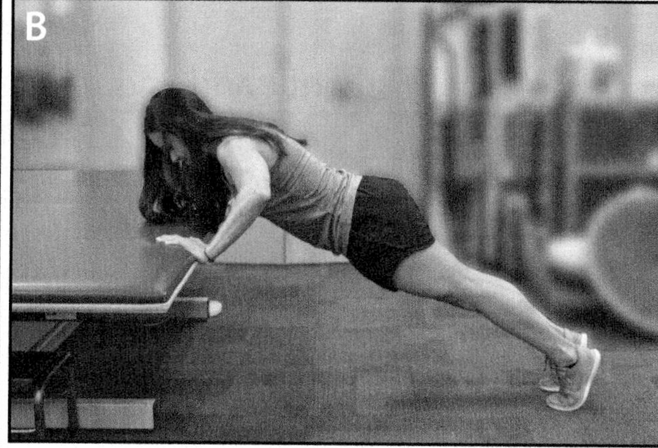


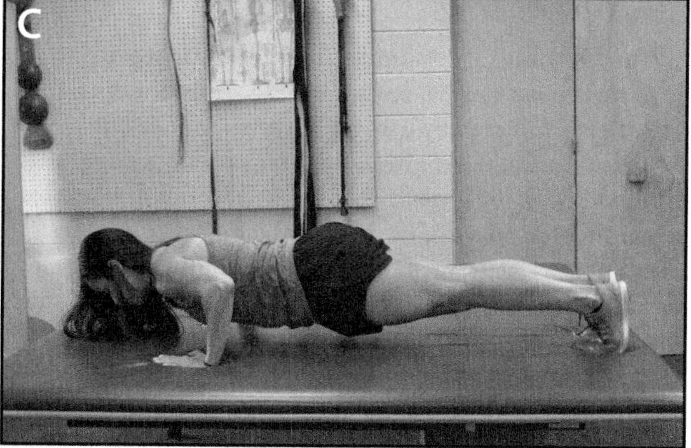


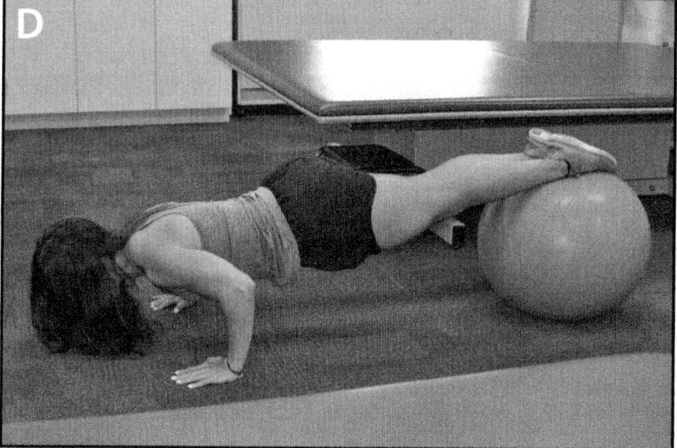


**Figure 6-20.** Push-up progressions. (A) A push-up against the wall. (B) A push-up on an incline. (C) A push-up with legs straight. (D) A push-up with feet on the ball (compliant surface).

If the patient performs another 15 repetitions of biceps curls after a short rest period (1 to 2 minutes), they have completed 2 sets of 15 repetitions. When documenting sets and repetitions, the number of sets is usually written times the number of repetitions. In the previous example, it would be documented as 2 × 15.

Determining the number of sets and repetitions is dependent on patient presentation and their treatment goals. A goal to increase strength or power is best achieved when using higher resistance and fewer repetitions (Table 6-4). Using a resistance at 70% to 80% (a moderate load) of a 1RM and performing 1 to 3 sets for 6 to 12 repetitions creates muscle fatigue and will produce strength gains.[16,30,31] Meta-analytical data have shown that using 60% of a 1RM resistance produces the largest effect/strength increases in novice individuals.[16] Using loads at 85% of a 1RM is most effective for developing maximal dynamic strength but is more typically reserved for athletes or persons late in the rehabilitation program with goals to return to high levels of function/sport.[16,30] The amount of resistance needs to be increased once the exercise can be performed without fatigue in order to continue making strength gains. A goal of increasing muscle endurance will be best met by using more repetitions (20 to 40 for 3 to 5 sets) with a submaximal load.[31] Using low- or light-resistance bands or submaximal isometric contractions with increased hold times can also be effective ways to increase muscle endurance.

**Table 6-4**

Strength and Endurance Training Guidelines[4,6,13]

| Exercise Goal | Recommended Resistance | Repetitions | Sets | Rest Period |
|---|---|---|---|---|
| Increase muscle strength | 60% to 85% of 1RM | ≤6 | 2 to 6 | 2 to 5 minutes |
| Increase muscle endurance | ≤67% of 1RM | ≥12 | 1 to 2 | <30 seconds |
| Increase muscle power | 80% to 90% | 1 to 2 | 3 to 5 | 2 to 5 minutes |

When beginning a training program to improve power, the patient must have at least normal strength. Improving strength is addressed by using a heavy resistance and slower rates of contraction to improve force production, but this is only one part of improving power. Additional exercises should include training at both light and medium resistance/intensity at fast speeds, targeting multijoint muscles to increase force at these greater speeds. Suggested parameters for this second component of power training include resistance exercises (0% to 60% of a 1RM for lower body exercises and 30% to 60% of a 1RM for upper body exercises) performed at a fast contraction velocity. According to the ACSM 2009 position statement, 3 to 5 sets with 3 to 5 minutes of rest between sets for high-velocity exercises is advised to improve power.[16] It is suggested that performing more complex total-body power training exercises should be completed first followed by less complex exercises (ie, squats).[30]

The ACSM recommends training each muscle group for 2 to 4 sets of either the same exercise or a different exercise that targets the same muscle(s). For persons who are deconditioned, training benefits can be seen with as few as one set of resistance exercises.

### Student Activity: Tabulate a Patient's Strengthening Exercise Parameters

A patient's POC includes right elbow flexor strengthening, and the patient was able to perform 11 repetitions using 8 lb. Determine the weight needed and parameters to increase the patient's strength. What weight and parameters best target muscle endurance? Which specific muscles need to be targeted? (Note: Do not forget patient positioning.) Write a SOAP (Subjective, Objective, Assessment, and Plan) note for this activity.

### Documentation Tip

Clearly document all parameters of each exercise. Include information that validates that skilled intervention is occurring and include any modifications made based on the patient's performance.

O: Patient instructed in R hip exercises to increase R hip strength to improve standing balance, reduce pain with ambulation, and reduce compensatory motions during gait. Patient performed R hip: Abduction side lying 2×8 and 1×4 with 3 lb, prone extension 3×8 with 3 lb, and supine R SLR [straight leg raise] 3×8 with 5 lb. Gait training 3×60 ft with 15-second rest between sets.

A: R hip strength improving; patient now able to complete exercises with increased weight of 1 lb today compared to last treatment. Patient able to complete third set of SLR and hip extension for first time but only able to complete 4 reps of hip abduction in third set due to gluteus medius fatigue. Pelvic control during gait improved with decreased Trendelenburg during midstance on R, with decreased report of hip pain. Patient demonstrated increased ambulation distance compared to last week. Progressing toward long-term goal of return to pain-free community level ambulation.

P: Increase hip extension and SLR resistance next session. Initiate standing balance exercises and weight shift activities to increase standing and gait tolerance; monitor pelvic control.

## *Progression*

Exercise progression depends on the strength training principles discussed earlier in this chapter (ie, overload principle and SAID principle). To progress an exercise program, the clinician can increase the resistance/load, increase the volume (ie, repetitions and sets), increase the speed of the contractions, or decrease rest periods. Only one of these variables should be modified at a time, and all increases should be gradual to lower the risk of overtraining.[4,16]

# Other Considerations Influencing Muscle Performance

A proper warm-up and cooldown will prepare the patient and lower injury risk. Rest, recovery, fatigue, and DOMS are other factors that can affect muscle performance.

## Warm-Up and Cooldown

The purpose of a warm-up program is to increase core temperature and blood flow to help prepare muscle tissue for more strenuous exercise. The warm-up should be performed for 5 to 10 minutes. Low-intensity activities such as walking on a treadmill or using a stationary bike will prepare the LE muscles for exercise, whereas using an upper bike ergometer or arm/shoulder exercises (ie, arm circles) will prepare the UEs. Warm-up activities typically target multiple joints and larger muscles. Stretching is safer to perform after a warm-up because the muscles are more pliable and will respond better to the stretch.

A cooldown after a PRE program may reduce the severity of DOMS. The exercises are similar to those performed in a warm-up program. The exercises should be light and followed by gentle stretching.

## Rest and Recovery Periods

Rest periods should be scheduled between sets as well as between training sessions. Proper rest is critical for safe and appropriate exercise progression. Inadequate rest and recovery periods increase the risk of injury, muscle fatigue, DOMS, and/or overtraining. A 48-hour rest period after a strength training session is necessary to allow for muscle recovery. The physiologic changes that occur during the recovery period include restoring oxygen, glycogen, and energy stores and removing lactic acid. Glycogen may take days to be replenished, lactic acid removal occurs within an hour, and the other physiologic changes occur rapidly.

The amount of rest will depend on the parameters of the exercise. Longer rest periods of 2 to 3 minutes are recommended between sets for exercises specifically selected to increase strength. When the goal is to improve muscular endurance, rest periods should be shorter. A 1- to 2-minute rest period between sets is recommended for 15 to 20 or more repetitions and less than a 1-minute rest between sets of 10 to 15 repetitions. When the goal is to improve power, 3- to 5-minute rest periods are recommended after multijoint exercises.[16,30] While a patient is resting an agonist muscle or muscle group (the ones that just completed an exercise), the opposing muscle (antagonist) of the same extremity or a muscle group on the opposite extremity can complete an exercise. Older adults and patients with chronic conditions and/or comorbidities tend to fatigue easily and may require longer rest periods (more than 3 minutes) between sets. Obtaining feedback from patients about symptoms occurring during and/or after exercise as well as at the next visit will help the clinician determine if modifications to exercise parameters or rest periods are indicated.

## Muscle Fatigue

Muscle fatigue is a temporary, decreased ability of a muscle to generate force as a result of rigorous or repetitive muscle contractions during resistive exercise. This is a normal and reversible physiologic response to muscle overload. Clinicians typically recommend that an exercise should be completed to the point of muscle fatigue; the patient should feel as if it is a struggle to complete the next repetition, but it should still be completed with good form.

Signs and symptoms of muscle fatigue include the inability to perform the exercise smoothly (ie, jerking or cogwheel motion) through the full or available ROM, using substitution patterns or compensatory motions to help complete the exercise, or completing the exercise at a slower speed compared with the initial repetitions. Visible shaking or trembling as the muscle contracts during the exercise and/or complaints of pain, muscle burn, or cramping can also indicate muscle fatigue.[14] If any of these signs or symptoms occur, either the load needs to be reduced or the exercise terminated for that set so that the muscle can rest.

## Exercise-Related Acute- and Delayed-Onset Muscle Soreness

Muscle soreness is common in individuals who have started a PRE program and who are not accustomed to performing these types of exercise. Acute muscle soreness occurs during the exercise or immediately after the exercise (when muscles have fatigued). The ache or muscle burn dissipates very quickly during the rest period after terminating the exercise because oxygen, energy stores, and blood supply are rapidly replenished. Performing a low-intensity exercise (ie, stationary bike at approximately 25% intensity) or a cooldown after the exercise bout has been shown to reduce blood lactate levels, which can further reduce cramping and soreness.[32] Mild soreness may persist after exercise.

DOMS is a possible outcome when exercise intensity is increased too aggressively. There is a higher risk of developing DOMS when high-intensity eccentric exercises are incorporated in an exercise program. The most severe symptoms of DOMS occur because of high-intensity, high-speed eccentric training. Diffuse muscle soreness and stiffness, tenderness with palpation along the musculotendinous junction and/or in the muscle belly, inflammation (localized swelling and warmth), and reduced ROM are signs and symptoms of DOMS. Patients usually experience increased soreness with active concentric contractions or passive muscle lengthening. These signs and symptoms generally appear 12 to 24 hours after the exercise session and peak 48 to 72 hours postexercise followed by a gradual reduction in symptoms over the next 48 to 72 hours.[14] DOMS can be differentiated from an acute muscle strain by the absence of a specific incident that resulted in the pain. Physical therapist assistants are responsible for collecting data and details about the patient's symptoms and presenting this information to the physical therapist.

There is no consensus on consistently effective treatments for DOMS.[33,34] General recommendations for treatment include the use of nonsteroidal anti-inflammatory drugs, rest, or gentle exercise (reduced intensity and duration) for 1 to 2 days after onset. Cryotherapy and stretching have demonstrated no significant effect on the alleviation of muscle soreness or other DOMS symptoms.[33,34] Massage appears to have some benefit, but the results are inconsistent.[34]

The best approach to prevent DOMS is implementing a gradual progressive, individualized exercise program. To decrease the likelihood of developing DOMS, gradually increase exercise intensity and volume (repetitions and sets) and limit the introduction of eccentric training and new exercises at the start of a training period.[33] Performing a multijoint/muscle low-intensity warm-up and cooldown and gentle stretching before and after rigorous resistance exercise are generally accepted as tools that may help reduce the severity of DOMS, but there is little evidence to support this claim.[34] Some clinicians use "soreness guidelines" as parameters to adjust and progress the intensity of training programs. These guidelines were created specifically as guidelines for resistance training and were adapted as guidelines for walking/running programs after anterior cruciate ligament repair.[35] The soreness guidelines include the following[35]:

- Soreness during the warm-up that continues during the session = 2 days off; drop down a level
- Soreness during the warm-up that goes away = stay at that level
- Soreness during the warm-up that goes away but redevelops during session = 2 days off; drop down a level
- Soreness the day after (not muscle soreness) = 1 day off; do not advance program
- No soreness = advance 1 level once there is no soreness for 3 consecutive attempts at that level

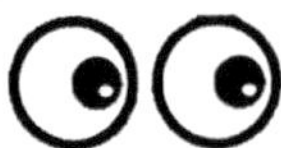

### Eye on the Research: Performance, Delayed-Onset Muscle Soreness, and Foam Rolling Techniques

Foam rolling is an intervention touted to alleviate muscle fatigue and soreness and to improve muscular performance. In a very small study (n = 8), Pearcey et al[36] concluded that foam rolling substantially improved DOMS by a moderate to large amount and led to improvements in sprint time and dynamic strength and endurance outcomes. Macdonald et al[37] concluded that foam rolling was beneficial in decreasing DOMS and that participants who completed foam rolling demonstrated improved vertical jump height, muscle activation, and passive and dynamic ROM in comparison with a control group. Romero-Moraleda et al[38] compared the immediate effects of a neurodynamic mobilization treatment with foam roller treatment after DOMS and determined that both treatments were effective in reducing the perception of pain after DOMS; only participants who did foam rolling showed improvements in posttreatment strength. Peacock et al[39] found that self-myofascial release using a foam roller was more effective at improving power, agility, strength, and speed compared with a full-body dynamic warm-up routine.

### Considerations for the Physical Therapist Assistant

The assistant is responsible for creating a therapeutic exercise plan that is both effective and safe and based on the solid principles of strength training. Treatment interventions should be selected based on the physical therapist's POC and the patient's goals to facilitate improvement in their functional performance.

## Maximizing Patient Safety During Exercise

Monitoring of vital signs pre- and postexercise is indicated for all patients. Every patient should be educated pretreatment regarding cardiac signs/symptoms that would warrant exercise termination and physical therapist notification. These signs include chest pain, left jaw or arm pain, sudden shortness of breath, dizziness, midscapular pain (women), and/or profuse sweating. Physical therapist assistants should monitor patients during all aspects of the strengthening program, observing for any potential signs of a change in status. To maximize patient safety, the therapy team ensures that the patient is completing the exercise safely in a controlled manner and using appropriate form for maximum benefits. Patients should be instructed to exhale during the concentric phase of the exercise and inhale during the eccentric phase to avoid the Valsalva maneuver.

**Table 6-5**

DeLorme Program

| Set Number | Number of Repetitions | Weight as a Percentage of a 10RM |
|---|---|---|
| 1 | 10 | 50 |
| 2 | 10 | 75 |
| 3 | 10 | 100 |

**Table 6-6**

Oxford Technique

| Set Number | Number of Repetitions | Weight as a Percentage of a 10RM |
|---|---|---|
| 1 | 10 | 100 |
| 2 | 10 | 75 |
| 3 | 10 | 50 |

A resistance training program should begin with a low-intensity warm-up (5 to 10 minutes) and end with a gradual decrease in the intensity cooldown period followed by gentle stretching. Clinicians should ensure that the program includes training for both agonist and antagonist muscles so that muscle imbalance does not occur because this could increase the potential for injury. The exercise program should be balanced to build a proper ratio of strength between the agonist and antagonist muscle groups.

## Resistance Exercise Protocols

The determination to use a specific exercise protocol is based on the patient's presentation, diagnosis, stage of healing, comorbidities, and treatment goals. There are many types of resistance training protocols, but there are 3 primary protocols that are used in physical therapy: the DeLorme, Oxford, and daily adjusted progressive resistance exercise (DAPRE) programs.

### *DeLorme and Oxford Protocols*

The first step in both the DeLorme and Oxford programs is to determine a 10-repetition maximum (10RM) for the muscle group to be strengthened. The 10RM is the maximum weight that can be lifted for 10 repetitions.

The DeLorme program (Table 6-5) includes a built-in warm-up set because the program starts with submaximal muscle contractions. For the first set, the patient completes 10 repetitions at one-half (50%) of the 10RM. For the next set, 10 repetitions are completed at 75% of the 10RM. For the third/final set, 10 repetitions are completed with 100% of the 10RM weight. The patient should rest briefly between each set.[40]

The Oxford technique (Table 6-6) is theorized to take advantage of applying resistance as a muscle fatigues. When the Oxford technique is implemented, the patient first completes 10 repetitions at 100% of the 10RM weight, then 10 repetitions using a weight equal to 75% of the 10RM, and for the third set the patient performs 10 repetitions at 50% the 10RM. There should be a rest period between each set for the muscles to recover. With both the DeLorme and Oxford programs, the weight/resistance can be increased weekly. There is not a prescriptive/recommended increase.[41]

### *Daily Adjusted Progressive Resistance Exercise Program*

The DAPRE program formulated by Dr. Kenneth Knight allows for a more objective progression of resistance. The sets are adjusted during the current PRE session and then readjusted for the next session based on the number of repetitions completed by the patient. The DAPRE program is highly individualized and considers the various rates of the patient's progression. Close patient supervision by the clinician is recommended.[42] First, the patient's 6-repetition maximum (6RM) is determined. DAPRE includes 4 sets of a selected exercise in each session (Table 6-7). In the first set, the patient performs 10 repetitions at 50% of the 6RM and 6 repetitions at 75% of the 6RM for the second set. During the third set, the patient completes as many repetitions as possible using 100% of the 6RM weight to the point of fatigue. Based on the number of repetitions performed during the third set, an adjusted working weight is calculated for the fourth set as shown in Table 6-8. The patient then completes as many repetitions as possible in the fourth set using the adjusted weight. Based on the number of repetitions performed during the fourth set, an adjusted working weight is calculated for the next session as the new 100% 6RM.

**Table 6-7**

Daily Adjusted Progressive Resistive Exercise Program[42]

| Set Number | Number of Repetitions | Weight as a Percentage of a 1RM |
|---|---|---|
| 1 | 10 | 50 |
| 2 | 6 | 75 |
| 3 | Maximum repetitions performed | 100 |
| 4 | Maximum repetitions performed | Adjusted weight based on set 3 repetitions in Table 6-8 |

**Table 6-8**

Daily Adjusted Progressive Resistive Exercise Program Weight Adjustments Based on the Repetitions Performed[42]

| Number of Repetitions Performed in the Third Set | Weight Adjustment to be Performed in the Fourth Set | Weight Adjustment to be Used for the Next Session |
|---|---|---|
| 0 to 2 | Decrease 5 to 10 lb | Decrease 5 to 10 lb |
| 3 to 4 | 0 weight change to decrease 5 lb | Use same weight |
| 5 to 6 | Use same weight | 0 weight change to increase 10 lb |
| 7 to 10 | Increase 5 to 10 lb | Increase 5 to 15 lb |
| 11 or greater | Increase 10 to 15 lb | Increase 10 to 15 lb |

## *Circuit Training*

Circuit training uses a sequence of exercises to improve muscular strength and/or endurance and promotes general fitness. A typical circuit training protocol usually includes 8 to 10 exercise stations, and the circuit can be repeated several times. There are typically 1 or 2 exercises targeting each body part. The patient completes a very brief rest (30 seconds or less) between sets as they move from one exercise station to another depending on the goals. The stations can include a variety of types of exercises, such as weight training (free weights or machines), calisthenics (ie, jumping jacks and lunges), dynamic/static stretching exercises, and/or short aerobic bouts of exercise (ie, jumping rope, stationary bike, and treadmill running).[13]

When designing a circuit weight training program, it is important to incorporate exercises that alternately target muscle groups and/or body areas. For example, select an exercise to address a LE muscle group (ie, squats, knee extension, calf raises, or hamstring curls), one for an UE muscle group (ie, chest press, latissimus pull downs, or bicep curls), and one for the trunk or core muscles (ie, sit-ups or plank extensions). This allows each muscle group an adequate rest period and recovery.

Circuit training can be used at the end of the rehabilitation process as a return-to-sport component if the rehabilitating muscles are included in the program. An athlete could begin circuit training earlier in the rehabilitation process to improve or maintain overall fitness levels, but exercises that target healing structures would not be included in the circuit. This program does not typically allow for maximal resistance training but does challenge both the anaerobic and the aerobic energy systems.

# Neuromuscular Training Concepts: Proprioceptive Neuromuscular Facilitation

Neuromuscular training interventions are targeted approaches that use the patient's nervous system to facilitate motor responses to promote skill acquisition. These interventions include the use of facilitation techniques to improve motor patterns and postural control. They are based on the work and research of Dr. Kabat, Maggie Knotts, and Dorothy Voss. Interventions focus on progression from the development of mobility (ROM) and stability (postural and joint stabilization) to controlled mobility (the ability to weight shift and move within a posture) and skill (the ability to easily move in and out of varied postures/movement patterns).

PNF is a neuromuscular training technique that was initially developed for use with patients with neurologic diagnoses or tone differences and/or those with difficulty completing developmental skills or ADLs. PNF incorporates functional movement patterns. PNF focuses on the importance of promoting proximal stability first and then

**Table 6-9**

**Upper Extremity Proprioceptive Neuromuscular Facilitation Diagonal Motion Patterns (Ending Positions)[42]**

| UE End Positions | Shoulder | Scapula | Forearm | Wrist | Fingers, Thumb | |
|---|---|---|---|---|---|---|
| UE D1 flexion (Figures 6-21A and 6-21B) | Flexion, adduction, external rotation | Elevation, abduction, upward rotation | Supination | Flexion, radial deviation | Flexion, adduction | The elbow (middle joint) can be in flexion or extension when performing any of these patterns. |
| UE D1 extension (Figures 6-22A and 6-22B) | Extension, abduction, internal rotation | Depression, adduction, downward rotation | Pronation | Extension, ulnar deviation | Extension, adduction | |
| UE D2 flexion (Figures 6-23A and 6-23B) | Flexion, abduction, external rotation | Elevation, abduction, upward rotation | Supination | Extension, radial deviation | Extension, abduction | |
| UE D2 extension (Figures 6-24A and 6-24B) | Extension, adduction, internal rotation | Depression, adduction, downward rotation | Pronation | Flexion, ulnar deviation | Flexion, adduction | |

Each PNF pattern direction is named for the end position of the proximal joint in the pattern. For example, when performing the UE D1 flexion PNF pattern, the starting position for the UE (see Figure 6-21A) is the end position for D1 extension (see Figure 6-22B).

progressing to distal mobility. Proprioceptive cuing is used to facilitate the movements and is paired with motor learning strategies (ie, task practice and the use of feedback) to promote improved function.[13,43,44]

These techniques are useful to incorporate with patients who have voluntary control of the limb or are regaining neurologic return postinjury. PNF is used to train a patient in the acquisition of skills needed for controlled, coordinated motion and to facilitate normal movement patterns. These strategies and techniques are useful for increasing joint stability and controlling developmental postures, and moving in and out of postures can facilitate and improve function in patients. Incorporating key strategies typically used in a PNF program can be useful when creating strengthening programs. PNF training techniques can be modified for use throughout the stages of healing. Contraindications for PNF are the same as those for resistance exercise training.

## *Proprioceptive Neuromuscular Facilitation Movement Patterns*

PNF interventions are based on the use of specific movement patterns and specific sensory cues to facilitate a motor response. The movement patterns used in PNF are based on synergistic patterns of motion performed on a diagonal and incorporate motions at each joint in a limb. Each pattern is multijoint and multiplanar motion. These patterns mirror movement patterns used in many daily activities or functional tasks. There are 2 pairs of diagonal patterns (D1 and D2) for both the UE and the LE. Each diagonal movement pattern is named for the moving limb (UE or LE), the diagonal PNF pattern (D1 or D2), and the motion (flexion or extension) of the most proximal joint.

Tables 6-9 and 6-10 describe the end positions for each joint during the specific PNF patterns for the UEs and LEs. When a patient is performing a PNF pattern (ie, UE D1 flexion), the patient's starting position (in this case, UE D1 extension) is going to be in the opposite position from where they end (UE D1 flexion). In this example, the patient will be placed in shoulder extension, abduction, and internal rotation while the forearm is positioned in pronation, the wrist in extension and ulnar deviation, and the fingers extended (see Figure 6-21A). From this starting position, the motions are first initiated distally, and then the next more proximal joints will move. Therefore, finger flexion, wrist flexion, and radial deviation will occur first followed by the other joint motions until the end position is achieved (see Figure 6-21B). Figures 6-21 through 6-28 provide pictures of starting and end positions for each UE and LE PNF pattern.

**Table 6-10**

**Lower Extremity Proprioceptive Neuromuscular Facilitation Diagonal Motion Patterns (Ending Positions)[13,43]**

| LE End Positions | Hip | Ankle | Toes | |
|---|---|---|---|---|
| LE D1 flexion (Figures 6-25A and 6-25B) | Flexion, adduction, external rotation | Dorsiflexion, inversion | Extension | The knee (middle joint) can be in flexion or extension when performing any of these patterns. |
| LE D1 extension (Figures 6-26A and 6-26B) | Extension, abduction, internal rotation | Plantar flexion, eversion | Flexion | |
| LE D2 flexion (Figures 6-27A and 6-27B) | Flexion, abduction, internal rotation | Dorsiflexion, eversion | Extension | |
| LE D2 extension (Figures 6-28A and 6-28B) | Extension, adduction, external rotation | Plantar flexion, inversion | Flexion | |
| Each PNF pattern direction is named for the end position of the proximal joint in the pattern. For example, when performing the LE D1 flexion PNF pattern, the starting position for the LE (see Figure 6-25A) is the end position for D1 extension (see Figure 6-26B). | | | | |

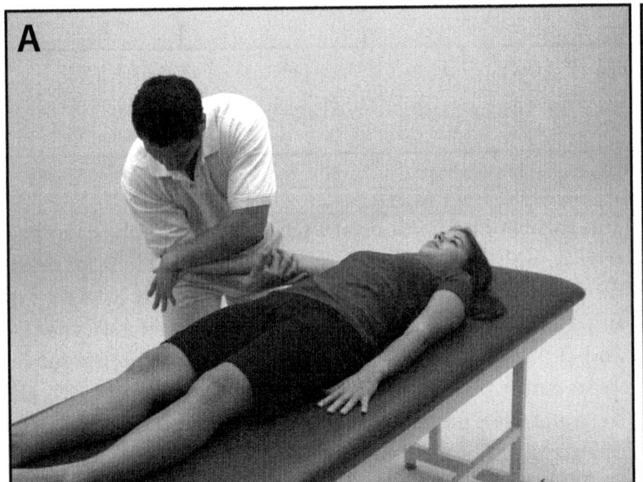


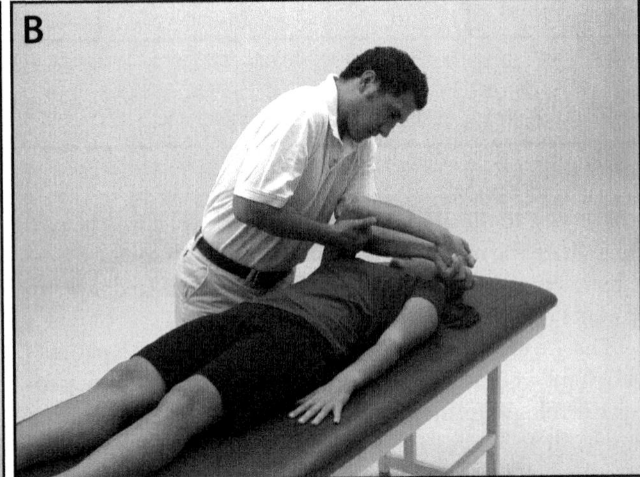


**Figure 6-21.** (A) PNF UE D1 flexion: Starting position. The patient's shoulder is abducted, extended, and internally rotated with the elbow straight with forearm pronation, and the wrist extended with ulnar deviation with the fingers extended. The clinician's left hand is on the patient's palmar aspect of the hand to resist elbow flexion, forearm supination, and wrist and finger flexion. The right hand is on the medial and anterior surface of the elbow to resist shoulder flexion, adduction, and internal rotation. Instruct the patient to pull up and across. (B) The PNF UE D1 flexion end position is the same as the UE D1 extension starting position as shown in Figure 6-22A. (Reproduced with permission from Prentice WE. *Rehabilitation Techniques for Sports Medicine and Athletic Training.* 6th ed. SLACK Incorporated; 2015.)

PNF patterns can be applied to one limb (unilaterally) in one direction (flexion or extension) or as a coordinated flow from one direction to the opposite direction (ie, flexion to extension or extension to flexion). PNF patterns can be performed bilaterally (to both UE or both LE limbs simultaneously). When patterns are performed bilaterally, they can be applied symmetrically (performing the same pattern on both extremities [ie, D1 flexion of both UEs]), asymmetrically (different pattern in the same direction to both UEs or LEs [ie, right UE D1 flexion and left UE D2 flexion at the same time]), or reciprocally (using the same pattern in opposing directions on each extremity [ie, right UE D1 flexion and left UE D1 extension]). Bilateral patterns are typically used to facilitate specific trunk motions for postural control and/or to encourage mobility. For example, performing bilateral UE symmetrical D2 flexion facilitates trunk extension and may be selected to facilitate postural extension in patients for whom flexed posturing is an issue (ie, patients with Parkinson disease). This can be a useful adjunct to a traditional extensor muscle PRE program.[13,43,44]

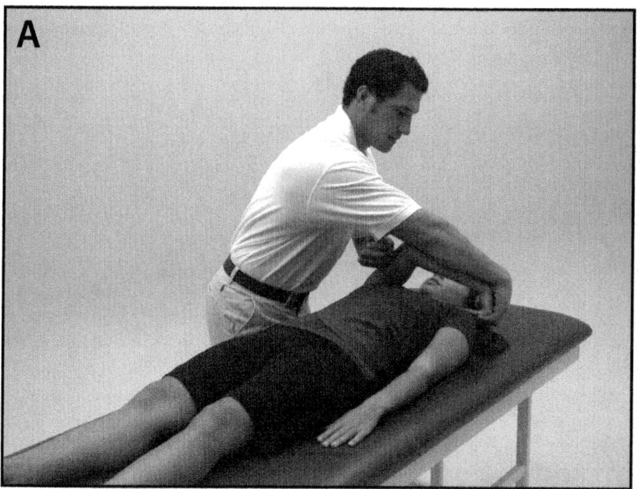


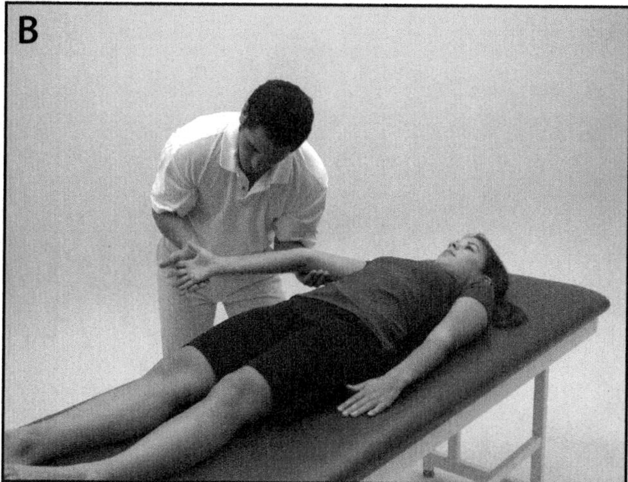


**Figure 6-22.** (A) PNF UE D1 extension: Starting position. The patient's shoulder is flexed, adducted, and externally rotated with the elbow flexed, the forearm supinated, and the wrist flexed and radially deviated with the fingers flexed. The patient's arm is across the midline, and their hand is by the ear on the opposite side. The clinician's right hand is on the dorsal surface of the patient's hand to resist forearm pronation and wrist and finger extension. The left hand is placed on the posterior humerus to resist shoulder abduction, extension, and internal rotation. Instruct the patient to push down and away. (B) The PNF UE D1 extension end position. (Reproduced with permission from Prentice WE. *Rehabilitation Techniques for Sports Medicine and Athletic Training*. 6th ed. SLACK Incorporated; 2015.)

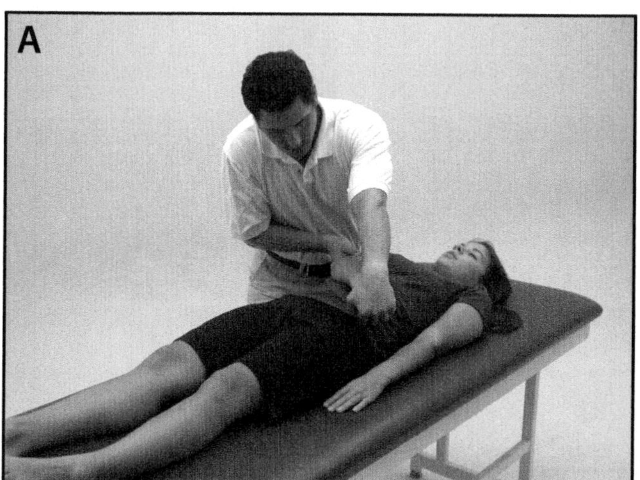


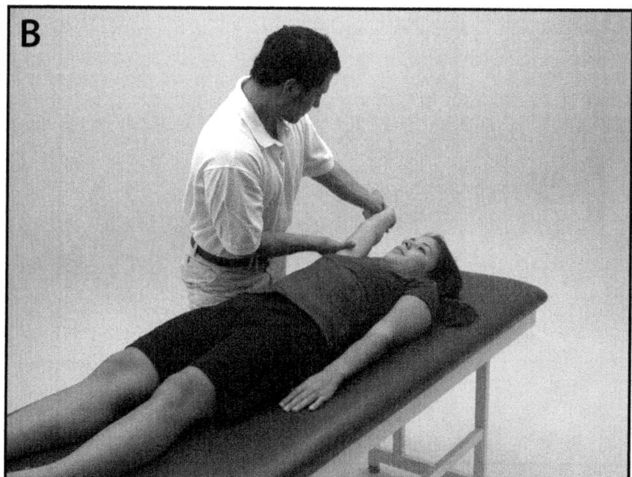


**Figure 6-23.** (A) PNF UE D2 flexion: Starting position. The patient's arm is in shoulder adduction and internal rotation across the midline with the elbow flexed, the forearm pronated, and the wrist flexed with ulnar deviation with the fingers flexed. The clinician's right hand is on the posterior aspect of the humerus to resist shoulder flexion, abduction, and external rotation. The left hand is placed on the dorsal surface of the patient's hand to resist forearm supination and wrist and finger extension. (B) The PNF UE D2 flexion end position is the same as the UE D2 extension starting position as shown in Figure 6-24A. (Reproduced with permission from Prentice WE. *Rehabilitation Techniques for Sports Medicine and Athletic Training*. 6th ed. SLACK Incorporated; 2015.)

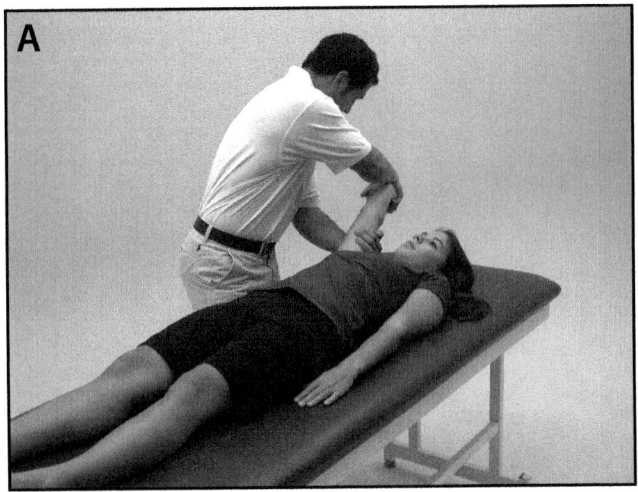


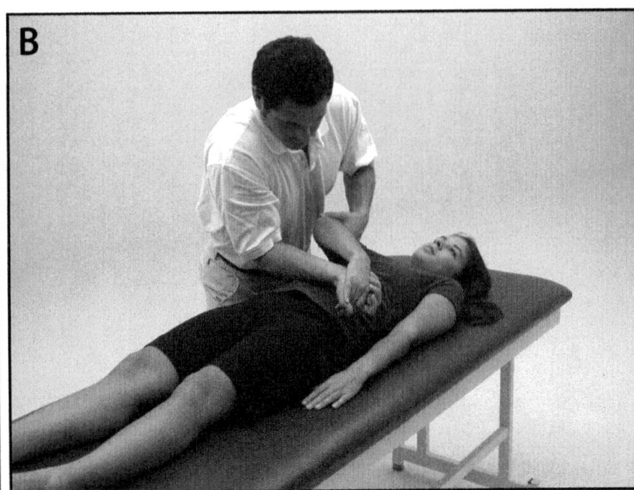


**Figure 6-24.** (A) PNF UE D2 extension: Starting position. The patient's arm is in full shoulder flexion, abduction, and external rotation; the elbow is straight with the forearm supinated; and the wrist is extended and radially deviated with the fingers extended. The clinician's hand positions are the same for UE D1 flexion, but the right hand is on the palmar aspect of the patient's hand and the left hand in the crease of the elbow to resist shoulder extension, adduction, and internal rotation. (B) The PNF UE D2 extension end position. (Reproduced with permission from Prentice WE. *Rehabilitation Techniques for Sports Medicine and Athletic Training.* 6th ed. SLACK Incorporated; 2015.)

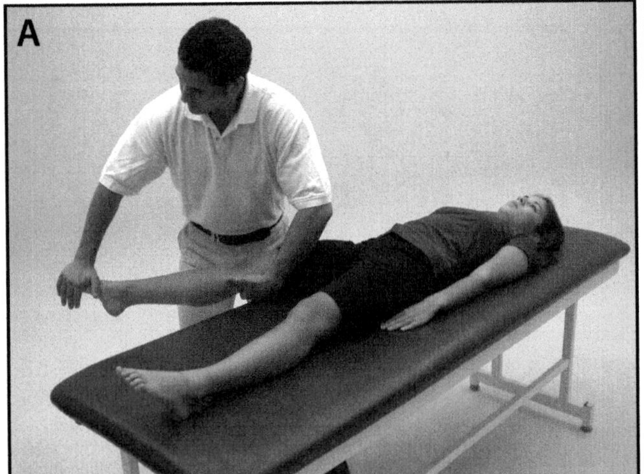


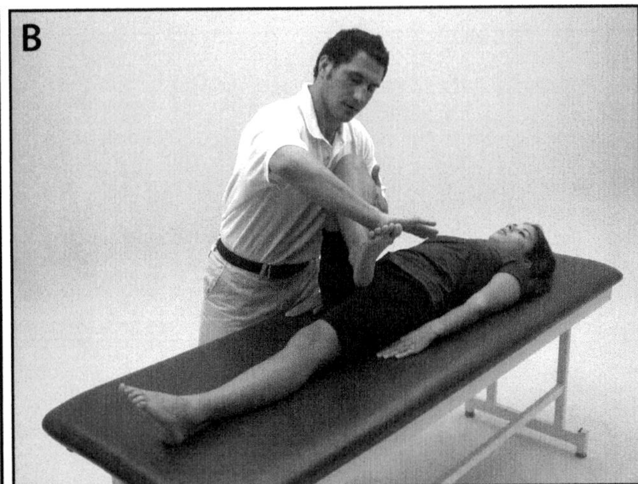


**Figure 6-25.** (A) PNF LE D1 flexion: Starting position. The patient's hip is extended, abducted, and internally rotated; the knee is extended; and the ankle plantar is flexed and inverted with the toes flexed. The clinician's right hand is positioned on the dorsal aspect of the foot with the finger around the arch to resist ankle inversion, dorsiflexion, and toe extension. The left hand is on the medial aspect of the knee and distal femur to resist hip flexion, adduction, and external rotation. (B) The PNF LE D1 flexion end position is the same as the starting position for LE D1 extension as shown in Figure 6-26A. (Reproduced with permission from Prentice WE. *Rehabilitation Techniques for Sports Medicine and Athletic Training.* 6th ed. SLACK Incorporated; 2015.)

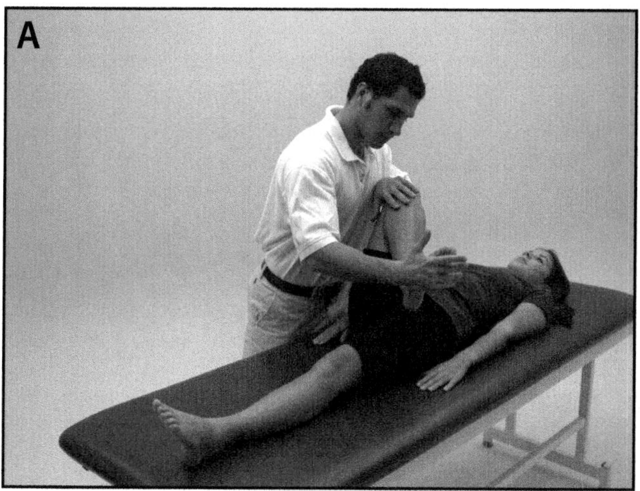


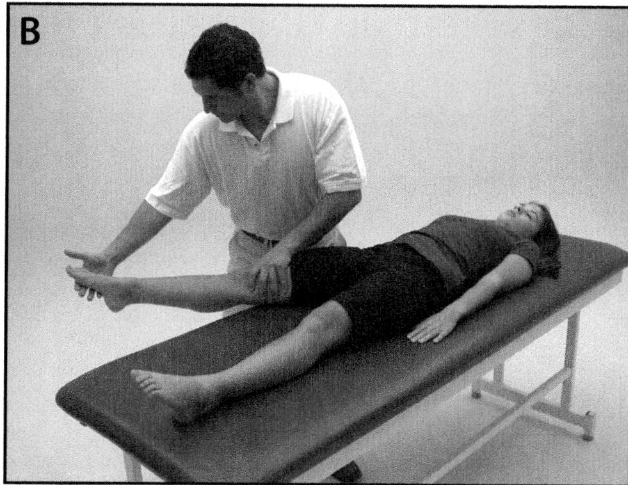


**Figure 6-26.** (A) PNF LE D1 extension: Starting position. The patient's hip is flexed, adducted, and externally rotated; the knee is flexed; and the ankle is dorsiflexed and inverted. The clinician's right hand is on the lateral and plantar surface of the foot to resist plantar flexion, eversion, and toe flexion. The left hand is placed in the popliteal space on the posterolateral aspect to resist hip extension abduction and then moved more medially to resist internal rotation. (B) The PNF LE D1 extension end position. (Reproduced with permission from Prentice WE. *Rehabilitation Techniques for Sports Medicine and Athletic Training*. 6th ed. SLACK Incorporated; 2015.)

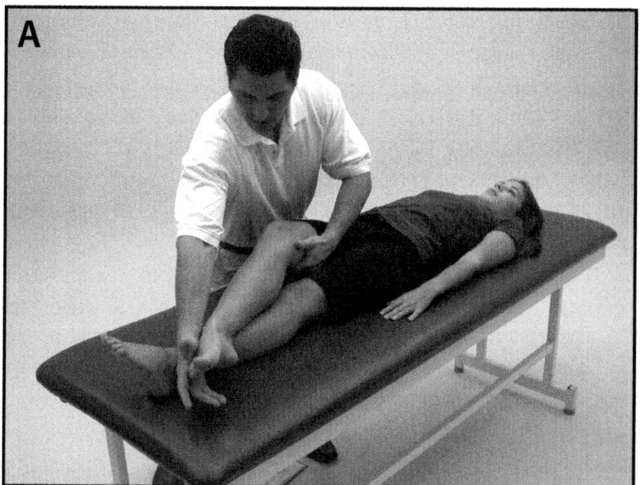


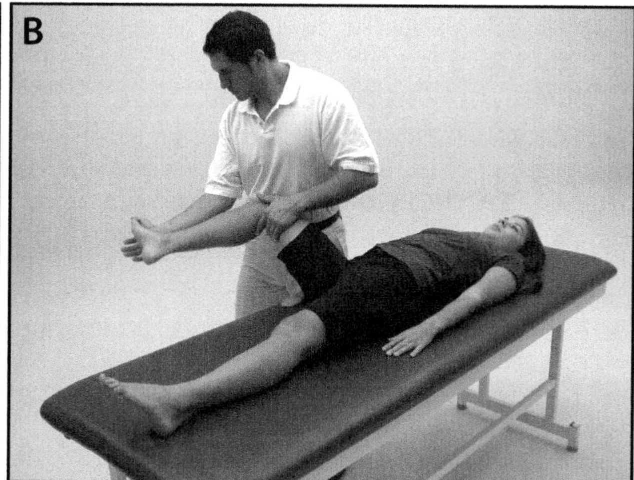


**Figure 6-27.** (A) PNF LE D2 flexion: Starting position. The patient's hip is extended, adducted, and externally rotated, and the knee is straight with the ankle plantar flexed and inverted and the toes flexed. The clinician's right hand is placed on the dorsal and lateral aspect of the foot to resist knee flexion, ankle dorsiflexion, eversion, and toe extension. The left hand is placed on the anterior and lateral aspect of the knee and distal femur with the fingers extended medially to resist hip flexion, abduction, and internal rotation. (B) The PNF LE D2 flexion end position. (Reproduced with permission from Prentice WE. *Rehabilitation Techniques for Sports Medicine and Athletic Training*. 6th ed. SLACK Incorporated; 2015.)

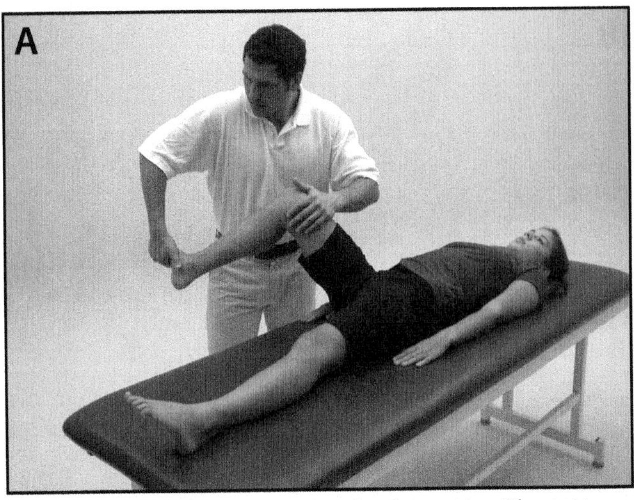


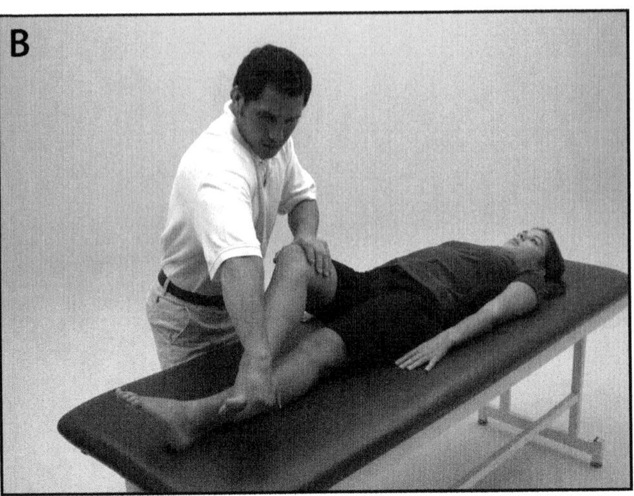


**Figure 6-28.** (A) PNF LE D2 extension: Starting position. The starting position is the same as the end position for LE D2 flexion (see Figure 6-27A). The clinician's right hand is placed on the plantar surface of the foot with the palm of the hand around the arch and the fingers toward the toes to resist plantar flexion, inversion, toe flexion, and knee extension. The heel of the left hand is placed on the anterolateral aspect of the knee and distal femur with the fingers extended medially to resist hip extension, adduction, and external rotation. (B) The PNF LE D2 extension end position. (Reproduced with permission from Prentice WE. *Rehabilitation Techniques for Sports Medicine and Athletic Training*. 6th ed. SLACK Incorporated; 2015.)

### Sensory Cue Application and Proprioceptive Neuromuscular Facilitation Treatment Principles

Patient–clinician interaction and the proper use of sensory cues are vital to effective implementation of PNF techniques. Table 6-11 provides a description of treatment principles used when applying PNF techniques.[13,43,44]

**Clinical Tip**

The ability to effectively provide PNF sensory cues and facilitation while verbally guiding and manually resisting a patient's limb during movement in a diagonal pattern requires a significant amount of coordination from the physical therapist assistant. These techniques typically require considerable practice to gain competence.

PNF techniques can be used to increase postural stability and control, to facilitate patient control of movement patterns, and to promote increased functional use of an extremity. These techniques can promote cocontraction and joint stability as well as increased motor coordination, control, and strength. Table 6-12 provides an overview of PNF techniques.

## Resistance Exercise Progression Guidelines

Goals of a rehabilitation PRE program after an injury or surgical procedure are to improve a patient's strength, muscular endurance, and/or power by gradually challenging the involved muscles. Effective exercise progressions are designed to overload the muscles so they will adapt to the imposed demands, resulting in increased strength. Each exercise program should be individualized based on the goals outlined in the initial physical therapy evaluation. Physical therapist assistants should always prioritize orthopedic restrictions (ie, weight-bearing status or restricted ROM). Some physicians have specific postoperative protocols that must be followed. Questions or concerns about a patient's ability to progress through a postoperative protocol should be discussed with the supervising therapist and then shared with the surgeon.

The healing stages of tissues and the rehabilitation phases must be considered and respected when applying/progressing PRE. This chapter provides general strength training guidelines related to the stages of healing. The orthopedic chapters in Section II provide specific guidance regarding intervention and progression programs for various joints.

### *Exercise Progressions for Strength Training Across the Rehabilitation Phases*

Physical therapists and physical therapist assistants treat patients with various musculoskeletal injuries (ie, sprains, strains, and dislocations). Sprains and strains are classified depending on the severity of the damage (refer to Chapter 3). A clinician who understands the physiology of healing will find it easier to develop appropriate exercise programs. Healing tissues should not be overstressed; however, appropriately controlled stresses should be applied to healing tissues to promote optimal healing and to encourage the return to full function.[6] The determination of appropriate controlled stresses is based on the stage of healing and tissue type; each tissue heals at different rates (see Chapter 3). The assistant should recognize characteristic presentations and contraindications associated with each stage of healing (refer to Chapter 3). Box 6-2 provides a reference for selecting proper PREs across the rehabilitation phases. Questions or concerns regarding exercise progression and/or healing constraints should be deferred to the physical therapist and/or physician.

## Table 6-11

### Proprioceptive Neuromuscular Facilitation Treatment Procedures/Principles of Treatment[13,43,44]

| Procedure/ Principle | Indication for Use | Description |
|---|---|---|
| Manual contacts | Tactile cues used to apply resistance and facilitate the desired motions | Where and how the clinician places their hands to enhance the motion. Typically, contact is over the agonist muscle belly/tendon. |
| Verbal commands | Guide and direct movement; enhance strength | Commands are typically high volume, staccato, and timed with the desired motion to facilitate a response. |
| Patterns of motion | Enhance motor performance | PNF diagonal movement patterns occurring in synergistic patterns; encourage firing of all of the muscles within the pattern. |
| Timing | Promote coordinated movement; facilitate neuromuscular control | Extremity motion occurs with distal muscles firing before proximal. The distal component should complete the movement pattern before the proximal portion. Functional activities will require proximal stabilization before distal motion. The clinician will cue and adjust the timing based on movement pattern/mobility intervention. |
| Resistance | Facilitate contraction of all muscles within the pattern | Resistance is adjusted throughout the pattern to allow the maximal contraction that the patient can achieve smoothly and without pain. |
| Approximation | Stimulate cocontraction; improve postural control and dynamic stability | The patient can be placed in a weight-bearing posture, and the clinician can add overpressure to the joints if indicated; approximation facilitates sensory feedback from joint receptors. |
| Traction | Decrease pain; facilitate motion | A slight separation of the joint surfaces can decrease pain and allow increased motion. |
| Visual input | Increase coordination and proper execution and improve contraction | The patient is asked to follow the motion of the limb with their eyes to promote self-correction of movement patterns. |
| Irradiation and reinforcement | Enhance strength of contraction of weaker muscles in pattern | Resistance applied to stronger muscles in the pattern can create overflow to weaker muscles. The clinician needs to gauge the appropriate amounts of resistance to maximize overflow. |
| Quick stretch | Facilitate muscle contraction | Applying a quick stretch to the agonist muscle before movement is used to stimulate the stretch reflex and increase contraction. |
| Patient position | Enhance contraction; maximize stability | Placing the patient in neutral alignment in a supported position allows for optimal participation. |
| Therapist position | Allow patient unrestricted movement through movement pattern; decrease therapist fatigue | The clinician should stand aligned with the direction of the diagonal pattern to be completed and should pivot their body using good body mechanics. Appropriate positioning allows the clinician to use their body weight to apply resistance (vs just the arms). |

**Table 6-12**

Various Proprioceptive Neuromuscular Facilitation Techniques[13,43,44]

| Application Technique | Indication for Use | Technique Description |
|---|---|---|
| ***These Techniques Are Used to Increase Muscle Force/Strength and/or Coordination.*** | | |
| Rhythmic initiation | Hypertonicity, difficulty initiating motion, apraxia | The patient is instructed to relax. Then, the assistant first moves the patient through the motion passively; then using active assisted ROM, cuing the patient to assist; and then AROM, progressing to resisted ROM. |
| Prolonged hold | Weakness | Resistance is applied isometrically to the target muscle (usually a proximal muscle that is contracting inappropriately) until the muscle fatigues, allowing the core/stabilizing muscles to begin to contract and stabilize. |
| Reversal of antagonists: Dynamic reversals (isotonic reversals, slow reversal, slow reversal hold) | Strengthen weak muscles in the pattern; promote improved reciprocal contraction of the agonist and antagonist | Ask the patient to concentrically contract the stronger muscle (agonist) followed by a contraction of the weaker motion pattern (antagonist). If an isometric contraction is used, the patient is asked to hold it at the end of the ROM before reversing the motion. |
| Reversal of antagonists: Stabilizing reversals, alternating isometrics, isometric reversals | Improve strength, stability | The clinician applies resistance (the patient is typically in a weight-bearing posture) in a uniplanar direction, alternating the direction of the force. |
| Rhythmic stabilization | Promote stability, especially of core and proximal muscles | Progression of alternating isometrics: The clinician applies resistance (the patient is typically in a weight-bearing posture) in a diagonal (multiplane) direction, alternating the direction of the force. |
| Repeated contractions (repeated stretch) | Strengthen the agonist | Repeated quick stretches are applied to the weak agonist as it completes the movement pattern to elicit a quick stretch and reflexive contraction. |
| Combination of isotonic exercises (reversal of agonists) | Weak postural muscles, inability to eccentrically control a motion | The clinician resists a motion concentrically, asks the patient to hold the contraction isometrically at end range, and then the clinician resists the motion eccentrically ("Slowly let it move, control it"). |
| Timing for emphasis | Weakness, decreased coordination | Alter the timing of a movement pattern by increasing resistance to a muscle in the pattern (typically a stronger muscle to encourage irradiation). |
| Resisted gait progression | Decreased LE coordination with gait, decreased endurance | Clinician applies gentle resistance to the trunk with gait (manual or with resistance band) without disrupting the patient's momentum. |

*(continued)*

**Table 6-12 (continued)**

Various Proprioceptive Neuromuscular Facilitation Techniques[13,43,44]

| Application Technique | Indication for Use | Technique Description |
|---|---|---|
| ***This Technique Is Generally Used to Decrease Tone.*** | | |
| Rhythmic rotation | Promotes relaxation, decreased tone | Clinician applies slow, rotational ROM proximal to distal, paired with slow gentle cues ("Just relax, let me move you.") |
| ***These Techniques Are Used to Increase ROM.*** | | |
| Contract-relax (autogenic inhibition) | Increase ROM | Clinician moves the patient to the end of the available ROM and asks the patient to isometrically contract the range limiting antagonist. The patient then relaxes, and the clinician moves the patient into a new range. |
| Hold-relax (reciprocal inhibition) | Increase ROM | Clinician moves the limb to the end of the available ROM and asks the patient to contract the agonist muscle, moving it into a new range. |

Box 6-2

**Strengthening Exercises During Various Phases of Rehabilitation**

**Maximum Protection Phase**

- Muscle setting[a]
- Pain-free submaximal isometrics
- Strengthening muscles that cross other joints or on the opposite extremity

**Controlled Mobility Phase**

- Submaximal isometrics with greater intensity or duration
- Multiangle isometrics
- Exercises to facilitate cocontractions and proximal joint stability
- OKC low-intensity pain-free isotonic exercises
- Progress to controlled CKC exercises

**Return-to-Function Phase**

- Increase exercise intensity and volume
- Progress from single-plane to multiplane exercises
- Progress from static to dynamic strengthening
- Address power; begin plyometrics later in this phase

[a]This is not a strengthening exercise; it reduces muscle guarding and prevents atrophy.

Important note: The selection of exercises is based on the stage of healing as well as patient presentation. Signs or symptoms of inflammation may warrant downgrading exercises to those in an earlier phase or terminating the activity pending follow-up with the physical therapist. These general exercises are the ones typically used; physician postoperative protocols override these general guidelines.

## Maximum Protective Phase of Rehabilitation (Acute Stage of Healing)

This stage often lasts 2 to 3 days and typically not longer than a week, but the duration depends on the severity of the injury or if surgical intervention was performed. During this phase, protection, rest, ice, compression, and elevation are indicated. The goals in this phase are to limit potential adverse effects from immobilization, promote healing, and decrease pain and inflammation. General treatment interventions that are indicated during the maximum protection phase usually include patient education; protection, rest, ice, compression, and elevation; joint protection (ie, restricted weight bearing and use of splints/braces and/or assistive devices; modalities for pain and swelling control; pain-free passive ROM; and, in some situations, grade I or II joint mobilizations or gentle massage.

Strengthening the involved muscles is contraindicated during this phase, but it is important to initiate muscle setting and/or gentle submaximal isometrics as tolerated to reduce muscle guarding and help prevent atrophy. Generally, it is acceptable to include strength training for those muscles in joints proximal and/or distal to the injured area. Clinicians must be aware of, and avoid strengthening of, 2-joint muscles that cross the involved joint. For example, if a patient has a shoulder injury, it is safe to perform wrist/finger strengthening as long as the UE is supported. However, it may not be appropriate to perform elbow flexion with the forearm supinated because the biceps cross both the elbow and the shoulder. It may be acceptable to perform elbow flexion with the forearm pronated or in neutral (as long as the limb is appropriately stabilized) because these positions target muscles that only cross the elbow joint. In this case, strength training of the opposite extremity and the LEs should be encouraged.

If a patient wants to engage in aerobic conditioning while an injured limb is healing, the clinician must determine which type of aerobic equipment is most appropriate. The aerobic exercise should not stress the injured limb, and the clinician must also consider if the patient is a fall risk. For patients rehabilitating from a UE injury/surgery, a stationary bike, recumbent bike, or NuStep (NuStep, Inc) may be the safest equipment to use because there is a reduced fall risk compared with using a treadmill or elliptical. If the patient experienced an LE injury, then UE strengthening and/or aerobic exercise using an upper bike ergometer is more appropriate.

## Controlled Mobility Phase (Subacute Stage of Healing)

Typically, this phase lasts less than 3 to 4 weeks but may last longer depending on the severity of the injury and the type of tissue involved. The introduction of gentle stresses in the direction of normal loading and in line with healing tissue fiber alignment (active assisted ROM or AROM) is appropriate during this phase. New healing connective tissue tends to be randomly aligned, whereas normal connective tissue fibers are longitudinally aligned; carefully introducing graded stresses promotes an organized fiber alignment and strengthens the newly formed connective tissue fibers. Diminishing signs and symptoms of inflammation, pain that no longer occurs with active motion (except at the end of available ROM), muscle weakness and decreased function are typical presentations during this phase. Patients begin to feel better, so it is important that they understand that overdoing activities or exercise can lead to increased injury because of the frailty of the healing tissues.

General treatment interventions during the moderate protection phase include AROM as tolerated through a pain-free range and progressing to concentric and eccentric exercises through the full ROM. AROM is not considered a strengthening exercise. Initiating activities at a slower pace allows the patient to better control the activity and increases their ability to perform the motion correctly. Gentle stretching progressions and soft tissue mobilization can place stresses on healing tissues safely. Progressive submaximal and multiangle isometric strengthening exercises are appropriate as long as pain is minimal. These exercises should be performed only at those angles that do not elicit pain. It is advised to perform the isometrics above and below the painful points. Simple CKC exercises (see Figure 6-11A) may be indicated to facilitate joint approximation and stability if they do not produce pain. Joint approximation creates muscle cocontractions that improve joint stability in a controlled manner. For example, closed chain terminal knee extension reduces shear forces on the knee joint. OKC exercises isolate one joint, allowing targeted contraction of a specific muscle or muscle group. Low-intensity isotonic exercises can be introduced later in this phase as long as pain or other symptoms are not exacerbated. Targeting proximal stabilizing muscles (ie, scapula muscles and trunk muscles) is crucial to improve joint mobility and proper joint mechanics (ie, scapulothoracic rhythm). Postural muscles need to work against gravity throughout the day, so it is important to address muscle endurance for these muscles.

**Considerations for the Physical Therapist Assistant**

Remember that proximal stability is needed for distal joint mobility.

## Return-to-Function Phase (Chronic Stage of Healing)

As the patient progresses to the return-to-function phase, the tissues continue to heal, and collagen fibers realign in response to the stresses that are placed on them. This phase can last for months to more than 1 year depending on the severity of the injury and/or surgical intervention and the type of tissue(s) involved. Characteristic presentation during this phase includes pain (only with normal end-range stretching), reduced muscular strength, endurance, and decreased neuromuscular control. In some cases, adhesions or contractures may have developed during the healing process and need to be addressed. Patients should have no signs or symptoms of inflammation. The focus remains on patient education regarding safe and appropriate progressions, the importance of rest and appropriate exercise intensity, the use of ice, and activity modification as needed to prevent pain and/or reinjury.

General treatment goals during this phase include full ROM and normal strength (5/5); adequate muscle endurance and coordination when performing ADLs (early in this phase); and increasing muscular strength, endurance, and neuromuscular control for returning to the prior level of function or sport (later in this phase). General exercises should progress from single-plane to multiplane exercise patterns, from simple static to more dynamic complex strengthening, and from slower to higher velocity with dynamic activities.

Tissue loading is still indicated, but patients may experience acute muscle soreness with PREs as muscles adapt to the new demands and continue to increase muscle strength and endurance. Clinicians should try to prevent or limit DOMS. Athletes should focus on gradual eccentric loading, power training, and plyometric progressions during the mid to later phase to address treatment goals.

## Box 6-3

### Strength Training Myths

- "No pain, no gain." When performing strength training exercises with proper form and intensity, they should *not* cause pain.
- "The type of equipment makes a difference." Selecting the type/mode of equipment is dependent on meeting the needs, goals, and tolerance level of the person exercising. There is no one "best" type of equipment.
- "Patients are too old (or too young) for a strength training program." Resistance training is beneficial for young and older populations.
- "If some is good, more is better." There is increased risk of injury when exercising at too high of an intensity or with inadequate rest/recovery time built into the program.
- "I'll look too bulked up if I do strengthening exercises." There will be some increase in muscle size, but a person is limited (by genetic makeup) as to how much muscle bulk will increase.

# Medical Considerations, Contraindications, Precautions, and Myths

When initiating a PRE program, physical therapist assistants should review the physical therapist's initial evaluation for any pathologies that might be considered a contraindication or precaution. Box 6-3 provides a list of common myths that patients may express to the assistant. This is an opportunity for the assistant to educate patients.

Physical therapist assistants should review the medical record to check for medications the patient is taking because some of these warrant additional patient monitoring during exercise. For example, statins (ie, Lipitor [atorvastatin], Crestor [rosuvastatin], and Zocor [simvastatin]) are used by tens of millions of people to lower cholesterol; yet, they can reduce the body's magnesium levels.[45,46] Approximately one-quarter of statin users who exercise may experience unusual onset of muscle pain, muscle fatigue, aching, cramping, and weakness that is progressive. Approximately 0.1% of statin users develop rhabdomyolysis, which is a rare yet life-threatening side effect.[45,46] It is of critical importance for the assistant to notify the evaluating therapist of any medication changes or additions and any unusual patient responses or reports during treatment sessions. Exertional rhabdomyolysis is discussed in Chapter 23.

As a general rule, patients in the acute stage of an injury (inflammatory stage) should not perform PREs. In the following situations, resistance exercise programs are generally considered to be contraindicated:

- Significant pain that does not decrease with lower load/resistance[13]
- Patients with inflammatory neuromuscular disease (ie, Guillain-Barré syndrome, polio myositis, or dermatomyositis)[13]
- Acute joint inflammation[13]
- Acute congestive heart failure, uncontrolled hypertension or arrhythmias, or severe valve disease[4]
- Eccentric exercise for persons with Duchenne muscular dystrophy[47,48]
- Severe osteoporosis[47,48]
- In the area of bony metastasis[47,48]
- Lower limb lymphedema postgynecologic cancer[4]

Additional medical conditions that require specific clarification from the physician before the implementation of a strengthening program include after a fracture, osteoporosis, and cancer (the presence of bony metastasis located at other sites). If the physician clears these patients for a strengthening program, all activities should be completed at a submaximal level with careful and ongoing monitoring. The initial focus of the program should be on core and postural stability.

Clinicians should educate all patients on strategies to avoid using a Valsalva maneuver when performing resistance exercise, especially during the initial lifting of a weight or load. Patients should exhale during the exertion phase of the lift; counting repetitions out loud during the concentric phase of isotonic exercises also helps ensure that patients are exhaling at the proper time. When patients are performing isometric exercises, counting the "hold" time aloud prevents breath holding during this activity. These techniques are important to monitor, especially for patients with high blood pressure.

# Special Considerations for Various Populations or Conditions

Progressive resistance exercise programs can be safe and effective for children, older adults, and those with chronic diseases, but clinicians must ensure proper form and technique are maintained to avoid muscle imbalances and risk of injury. Refer to Chapter 23 for considerations for athletes related to injury prevention and safe return to sport.

## Children

Resistance exercise for children can be safe and effective.[4,6,49] The resistance training program should be carefully supervised, adhere to established training guidelines, and include appropriate monitoring and medical clearance before initiating the program. Whenever possible, activity recommendations should be met through regular participation in sport and play activities. Formalized strength training is not recommended until at least 7 to 8 years of age to allow for the development of postural support and balance reactions.[49] Warm-up and cooldown are strongly advised, and strength training should begin with light weights with an emphasis on proper form/technique and controlled lifting and lowering while targeting all major muscle groups and core stabilizers. Strength training equipment is often designed for adults and is not always adjustable to accommodate smaller sizes, in which case free weights or resistance bands/tubing may be more appropriate. The amount of resistance should not be increased by more than 10% at a time.[49] Resistance should only be increased once the child can lift 8 to 15 repetitions with good form with reports of less than moderate fatigue.[4]

Although high-impact activities that occur during unstructured play are appropriate for children, incorporating plyometric training for children is a concern. Plyometric training usually includes multiple repetitions of near maximal effort completed repeatedly, raising the concern of unnecessary stress placed on unclosed epiphyseal plates, which can pose a risk of injury or overtraining.[49-51]

## The Adolescent Client

Adolescents can perform resistance training using submaximal loads. The American Academy of Pediatrics does not endorse using maximal lifts or resistance for strength training.[49] Single maximal lifts are not recommended until skeletal maturity is attained. Adolescent strength training programs should incorporate a variety of resistance types and exercises to target the major muscle groups, balancing the flexors and extensors in the upper and lower body.[49] Preventive exercise (prehabilitation) is appropriate. These programs should focus on strength training those muscle groups that are subjected to overuse in the specific sport (eg, strengthening rotator cuff and scapular muscles for swimmers and baseball/softball players, strengthening the hamstrings and quadriceps for football players, and LE strengthening and plyometrics for soccer players).[49] Chapter 23 provides additional considerations for adolescent athletes.

## The Older Adult Client

Resistance training is safe and effective to increase muscle mass and strength in older adults. Results of resistance training programs for older adults include significant gains in muscular strength, endurance, and power with a reduction in sarcopenia (muscle wasting). Research has shown that higher-intensity exercise is more effective than low-intensity exercise in eliciting adaptions in both older and younger populations. A meta-analysis reported a positive correlation between intensity and strength gains in older adults.[7] The optimal intensity varies based on a patient's overall condition and mobility; research indicates that high-velocity resistance training using low weights can provide similar improvements in muscle power and physical performance compared with using higher loads in mobility-limited older adults.[8]

PRE programs for an older adult need to be individualized, just as for any other patient. Medical clearance and supervision are indicated to ensure safe patient participation. A fitness program that includes strength, flexibility, balance, and aerobic exercises is recommended for this population. The principles for developing a training program found in this chapter should be followed, but modifications may be needed based on comorbidities and the overall level of fitness/conditioning.

## Persons With Chronic Illness

Clinicians must consider the following factors when working with patients with chronic illness:

- Accessibility: Clinicians must address a patient's individual barriers to exercise, including the ability to access a gym, limitations based on a patient's size/girth, fall risk, and overall limitations in functional mobility.
- Patients with chronic disease are often unaccustomed to exercise. Start slow with low-intensity activities; encourage patients to continue to participate.
- Patients need to see results. Build a program that provides early evidence of success to encourage compliance and reinforce motivation. Reward small gains.
- Individualize patient goals. What is the patient's primary focus (improved function, quality of life [QOL], or preventing further deconditioning)?
- Patient anxiety or fear that they "can't work out" or society's perception that patients with chronic disease are "too sick" to exercise. Those diagnosed with chronic illness can be good candidates for a PRE program; resistance training may be an additional way to improve function and QOL for these patients.

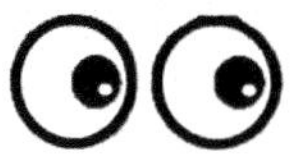

## Eye on the Research: Chronic Diseases and Exercises

Current estimates indicate that at least half of all Americans are living with at least one chronic disease (including, but not limited to, type 2 diabetes mellitus, chronic obstructive pulmonary disease [COPD], and/or heart disease), and 25% of Americans are living with 2 or more chronic illnesses.[52,53] Exercise programs (and treatment plans) for patients with chronic diseases are complex and require strong clinical decision making, knowledge of pathology, and the ability to appropriately monitor patient presentation and performance.

To implement appropriate and safe exercises for these patients, clinicians must have knowledge of exercise principles, an understanding of the patient's pathology, and a willingness to explore new research. A systematic review of 18 articles reported that PRE is safe and effective for patients with orthopedic (ie, musculoskeletal injuries, osteoarthritis, or osteoporosis) or cardiopulmonary (ie, hypertension or COPD) conditions as well as type 2 diabetes mellitus, neuromuscular conditions (cerebral palsy or stroke), and geriatric patients. PREs should be designed to increase force production and follow the principles of using a load that allows for performing 8 to 12 repetitions until fatigue, allowing adequate rest between exercises or sets, and increasing resistance when appropriate to increase muscle strength/force.[54]

Recent research summarized that small to moderate favorable effects in pain reduction severity and improvement in physical function were achieved in persons with chronic pain after exercise (although the results were not consistent across all studies). Investigators concluded that there was preliminary support for incorporating physical activity and exercise as interventions to improve pain levels, physical function, and QOL. Few adverse effects were reported, but there is a need for additional research addressing longer-term results.[55]

Patients with type 2 diabetes mellitus can benefit from regular resistance training. Studies demonstrate a decrease in cardiovascular risk factors and increased muscle strength.[56] Aerobic and resistance exercises are beneficial for patients with type 2 diabetes.[57] Strength training improves glycemic control, especially in early stages of type 2 diabetes mellitus.[58]

Exercise is beneficial for people with multiple sclerosis. There is evidence of the positive effect of resistance training on improving muscle strength.[59] There is less evidence indicating improvements in functional capacity, balance, fatigue, and QOL for patients with multiple sclerosis.[59] Prolonged resistance training improves strength as well as functional capacity for these patients.[59,60] The benefits of exercise are only obtained with regular participation in an exercise program, but limited exercise compliance is a risk with these patients. Learmonth et al[61] determined that a HEP with additional support including exercise videos, instruction, and access to coaching support increased HEP completion and compliance (Appendices C and D).[61]

Patients with Parkinson disease benefit from resistance training, with increases in strength and function.[62,63] Newer research highlights a potential benefit of combining resistance training with instability-inducing activities, noting even greater gains in functional performance when destabilizing tasks are added to the resistance exercise program.[64] Resistance training exercise has been shown to decrease dyspnea, increase strength, and play a role in decreasing the mortality rate in people with COPD.[65,66]

An increased awareness and understanding of medical treatments, medications, and their side effects are very important when working with people with chronic disease. Exercise progressions should follow the general principles of resistance training program development but should be modified to address individual presentations and disease progression.[47,48,67]

## *Athletes and Periodization*

Specific sports training programs require a detailed analysis of sport-specific demands (consider ROM, strength, endurance, and aerobic and power requirements). Once a patient has progressed to the last stage of the rehabilitation process, sport-specific analysis should be a primary focus of the training program. The clinician prioritizes exercises that target sport-specific skills (consider strength, endurance, and the power of muscle groups critical to effective performance).

One approach to sports training is called *periodization*. Periodization is a program that varies the training intensity and volume of exercises in a thoughtful and scheduled way. Periodization is often created over a yearlong cycle schedule that is built around the individual's sport competition schedule.[14] The goal is to vary the training so that peak performance coincides with major competitions. Periodization more effectively improves training adaptions and strength compared with traditional PRE programs.[68] Periodization relies on a schedule broken into the following phases: a preparation phase, first transition (strength development) phase, competition phase, and second transition (active recovery) phase.[14] Exercise intensities, volumes, frequencies, and rest periods are modified based on the athlete's current periodization phase. The primary advantage to periodization includes program variation (ie, exercise intensity, frequency, and volume), which is created to prevent overtraining. The variety is also beneficial in maintaining motivation and enhancing preparation for competition.

## The Role of Therapeutic Modalities and Alternative Training Interventions

Therapeutic modalities may be used to augment or support physical therapy programs. Common modalities include electrical stimulation, biofeedback, therapeutic taping, and the use of compression garments. The use of blood flow restriction techniques during strength training programs is being researched as a way to potentially improve strength training program outcomes.

Neuromuscular electrical stimulation (NMES) is used to stimulate innervated muscle and can be a useful adjunct to a strengthening program.[69] NMES is typically used in the early stages of rehabilitation to initiate strengthening (postoperatively, after immobilization) and is used to elicit submaximal muscle contractions. The strength of a muscle contraction created by NMES is typically limited by the patient's sensory/pain tolerance. Biofeedback is an electrotherapeutic device that can be used to enhance the contraction of weak muscles or reduce tension in tight or guarded muscles to improve function.[69] Therapeutic taping is used clinically to support other physical therapy interventions, including strength training programs. The goal of taping is often to produce a stabilizing force or to reduce pain. Recent studies indicate that therapeutic taping may not be as effective in reducing pain or promoting increased strength or ROM as early proponents have reported.[70,71] Further research is needed to better define the most appropriate indications for taping.

Compression garments compress and stabilize muscles, assist muscles during the performance of explosive/power moves during training, facilitate venous return, and clear postexercise metabolites from muscles. Some researchers have found positive benefits in both the recovery of symptoms and performance.[72,73] Recent systematic reviews suggest that compression garments may improve postexercise recovery.[74,75] Although research shows mixed results in terms of effectiveness with regard to improving performance, there is no evidence that the use of these garments is harmful; if the garments are comfortable for the wearer, there does not appear to be a reason not to wear them.

Blood flow restriction training is a technique that uses a cuff or wrap placed around an extremity during resistance exercises. The purpose of this technique is to maintain arterial inflow to the muscle while preventing venous return. Early research indicates that this technique may be effective.[76] Utilization of this technique requires training beyond entry-level schooling; clinicians must be properly trained in implementing this technique before adding it to a training regimen.

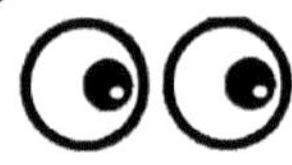

### Eye on the Research: Blood Flow Restriction Training

In a small study of patients with persistent muscle weakness and/or the inability to complete high-resistance exercises, patients completed exercise using blood flow restriction therapy at low loads (20% of a 1RM). All of the patients demonstrated posttraining improvement in quadriceps and hamstring peak torque, average power, and total work.[76] A meta-analysis review of 20 blood flow restriction studies reported similar results when comparing traditional low-load resistance training to low-load training with blood flow restriction.[77] Both studies reported that blood flow restriction training is more effective and tolerable than traditional resistance training, and researchers suggest that blood flow restriction should be considered as a viable rehabilitation tool.

## Conclusion

The ability to develop, implement, monitor, and modify resistance training exercises and programs is a vital skill for physical therapist assistants. The assistant must apply knowledge of the physiology of healing when developing an exercise program to appropriately grade activities as a patient moves through the rehabilitation phases postinjury. Exercises play a role in a person's rehabilitation protocol, and several types (isometric, isotonic, PNF, isokinetic, and/or plyometrics) can assist the patient in reaching their goals of improving function and returning to the highest feasible level of activity. Selecting optimal exercise parameters (FITT-VP principle) will help patients achieve their goals effectively while minimizing injury risk and the risk of developing DOMS. Physical therapist assistants should be able to create individualized, safe, and effective resistance training programs for various populations. An algorithm to guide the selection of appropriate strengthening exercises is provided in Figure 6-29.

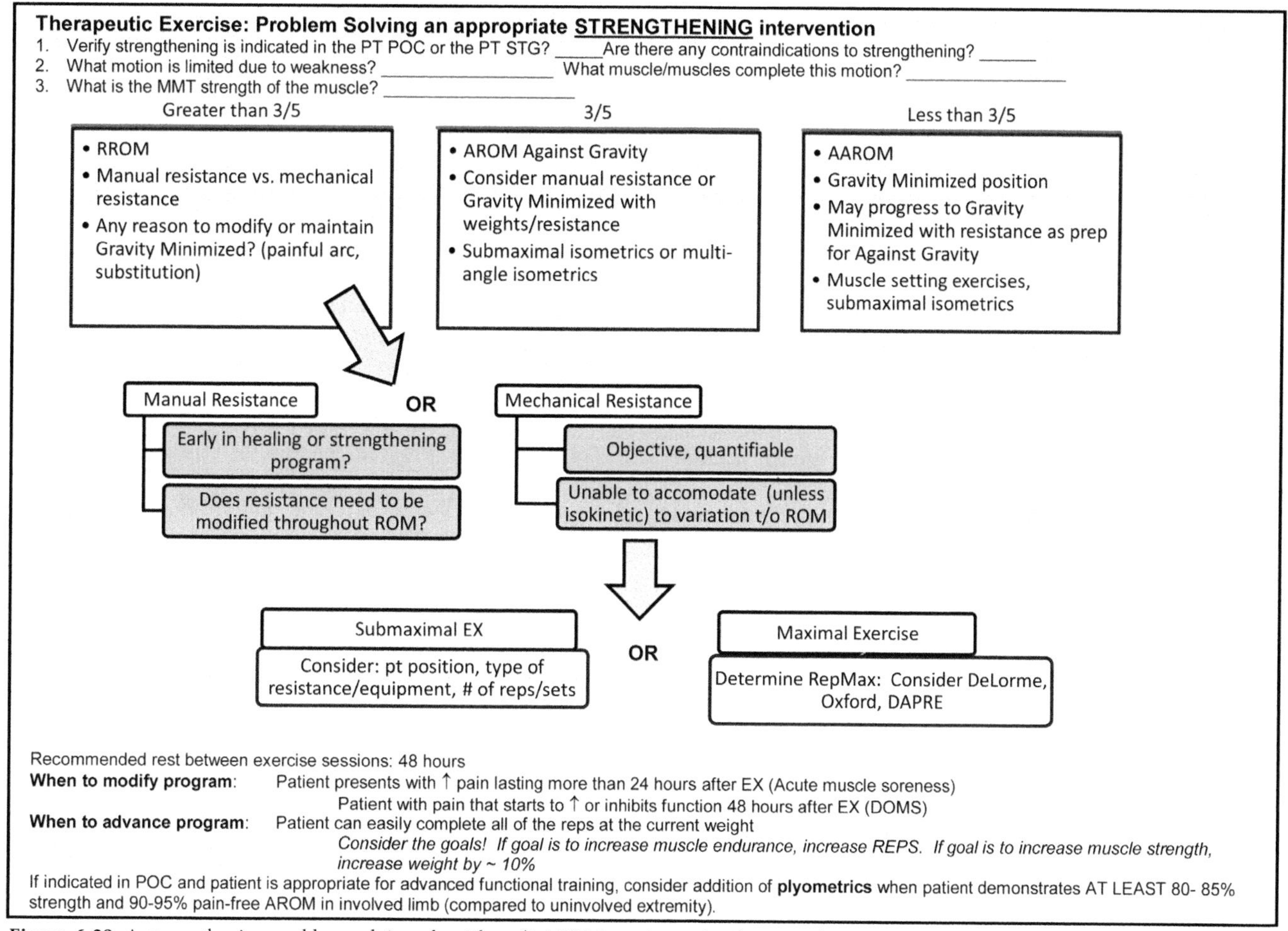


**Figure 6-29.** A strengthening problem-solving algorithm. (AAROM = active assisted range of motion; EX = exercise; RROM = resistive range of motion.)

## Review Questions

1. Define a repetition maximum. Describe at least 2 different ways to determine a patient's 1RM.
2. Define what each exercise parameter in the FITT-VP acronym represents.
3. Describe the role of rest in a resistance training program.
4. Compare and contrast concentric and eccentric contractions. Give an example of each.
5. What is an advantage to the selection of manual resistance vs mechanical resistance? What is a disadvantage?
6. List 2 principles of the PNF training philosophy that could be used to enhance a patient's response during strengthening exercise.
7. State at least 3 contraindications to resistance training.
8. Is performing the Valsalva maneuver an appropriate way to improve a patient's response to resistance training? Why/why not?
9. List at least 2 ways to decrease the likelihood of a patient developing DOMS.
10. Describe what a compensatory movement pattern is and provide at least 2 examples of how to prevent compensatory patterns during a resistance training program.

## Case Study

A 23-year-old patient had a right grade II inversion ankle sprain 2 days ago. The patient is wearing an air splint and is ambulating with crutches weight bearing as tolerated. The right knee/hip AROM and strength are within normal limits. The right ankle AROM is as follows: dorsiflexion 5 degrees with discomfort, eversion 0 degrees, and plantar flexion 0 to 5 degrees with pain; inversion was not tested because of acuity and pain. The patient has tenderness with palpation over the anterior talofibular ligament. According to the Ottawa ankle rule, the patient is negative for fracture.

1. Develop an appropriate exercise program for this patient based on the current presentation.
2. List any additional monitoring that is indicated.
3. Are there any contraindications for treatment?
4. Create an exercise progression plan for this patient for the subacute/controlled motion phase and for the return-to-function phase of healing.

## References


1. Lloyd RS, Faigenbaum AD, Stone MH, et al. Position statement on youth resistance training: the 2014 International Consensus. *Br J Sports Med*. 2014:48(7):498-505.
2. World Health Organization. *Global Recommendations on Physical Activity for Health*. World Health Organization; 2010. https://apps.who.int/iris/bitstream/handle/10665/44399/9789241599979_eng.pdf?s
3. American Physical Therapy Association. Choosing Wisely. September 15, 2014. Accessed January 26, 2023. http://www.choosingwisely.org/clinician-lists/american-physical-therapy-association-under-dosed-strength-training-for-older-adults/
4. American College of Sports Medicine. *ACSM's Guidelines for Ex Testing and Prescription*. 9th ed. Wolters Kluwer/Lippincott Williams &Wilkins; 2014.
5. Frizziero A, Vittadini F, Fusco A, Giombini A, Masiero S. Efficacy of eccentric exercise in lower limb tendinopathies in athletes. *J Sports Med Phys Fitness*. 2016;56(11):1352-1358.
6. Haff G, Triplett N, eds. *Essentials of Strength Training*. 4th ed. National Strength and Conditioning Association; 2016.
7. Murlasits Z, Reed J, Wells K. Effect of resistance training frequency on physiological adaptations in older adults. *J Exerc Sci Fit*. 2012;10:28-32.
8. Reid KF, Martin KI, Doros G, et al. Comparative effects of light or heavy resistance power training for improving lower extremity power and physical performance in mobility-limited older adults. *J Gerontol A Biol Sci Med Sci*. 2015;70(3):374-380. doi:10.1093/gerona/glu156
9. Björkman M, Jyväkorpi SK, Strandberg TE, Pitkälä KH, Tilvis RS. Sarcopenia indicators as predictors of functional decline and need for care among older people. *J Nutr Health Aging*. 2019;23:916-922. doi:10.1007/s12603-019-1280-0
10. Herzog W. The role of titin in eccentric muscle contraction. *J Exp Biol*. 2014;217:2825-2833. doi:10.1242/jeb.099127
11. Myhre JL, Pilgrim D. A titan but not necessarily a ruler: assessing the role of titin during thick filament patterning and assembly. *Anat Rec*. 2014;297:1604-1614. doi:10.1002/ar.22987
12. Nishikawa KC, Monroy JA, Uyeno TE, Yeo SH, Pai DK, Lindstedt SL. Is titin a "winding filament"? A new twist on muscle contraction. *Proc Biol Sci*. 2012;279(1730):981-990. doi:10.1098/rspb.2011.1304
13. Colby LA, Borstad J. Resistance exercise for impaired performance. In: Kisner C, Colby LA, Borstad J, eds. *Therapeutic Exercise Foundations and Techniques*. 7th ed. FA Davis; 2018:166-245.
14. McArdle WD, Katch FI, Katch VI. *Essentials of Exercise Physiology*. 5th ed. Lippincott, Williams & Wilkins; 2016.
15. Kenney W, Wilmore J, Costill DL. *Physiology of Sport and Exercise*. 6th ed. Human Kinetics; 2015.
16. Ratamess NA, Brent AA, Evetoch TK, Housh J, Kibler, BK, Kraemer WJ, Triplett NT. ACSM position stand. Progression models in resistance training for healthy adults. *Med Sci Sports Exerc*. 2009;41(3):687-708. doi:10.1249/MSS.0b013e318191567
17. Tomeleri CM, Ribeiro AS, Souza MF. Resistance training improves inflammatory level, lipid and glycemic profiles in obese older women: a randomized controlled trial. *Exp Gerontol*. 2016;84:80-87. doi:10.1016/j.exger.2016.09.005
18. Simpson KA, Mavros Y, Kay S, Meiklejohn J, et al. Graded Resistance Exercise And Type 2 Diabetes in Older adults (The GREAT2DO study): methods and baseline cohort characteristics of a randomized controlled trial. *Trials*. 2015;16:512. doi:10.1186/s13063-015-1037-y
19. Ishiguro H, Kodama S, Horikawa C, Fujihara K, et al. In search of the ideal resistance training program to improve glycemic control and its indication for patients with type 2 diabetes mellitus: a systematic review and meta-analysis. *Sports Med*. 2016;46(1):67-77. doi:10.1007/s40279-015-0379-7
20. Rush TC. *Prevention Practice: A Physical Therapist's Guide to Health, Fitness and Wellness*. SLACK Incorporated; 2007:44-46.
21. Oostdam N, Van Poppel MN, Eekhoff EM, Wouters MG, Van Mechelen W. Design of FitFor2 study: the effects of an exercise program on insulin sensitivity and plasma glucose levels in pregnant women at high risk for gestational diabetes. *BMC Pregnancy Childbirth*. 2009;9:1. doi:10.1186/1471-2393-9-1
22. Lorenz DS, Reiman MP, Walker JC. Periodization: current review and suggested implementation for athletic rehabilitation. *Sports Health*. 2010;2(6):509-518. doi:10.1177/1941738110375910
23. Bohannon RW. Hand-grip dynamometry predicts future outcome in aging adults. *J Geriatr Phys Ther*. 2008;31(1):3-10.
24. Ratamess N. *ACSM's Foundations of Strength Training and Conditioning*. Wolters Kluwer/Lippincott Williams & Wilkins; 2012.
25. Lindh M. Increase of muscle strength from isometric quadriceps exercises at different knee angles. *Scand J Rehabil Med*. 1979;11(1):33-36.
26. Patterson RM, Stegink Jansen CW, Hogan HA, Nassif MD. Material properties of Thera-Band Tubing. *Phys Ther*. 2001;81(8):1437-1445. doi:10.1093/ptj/81.8.1437
27. Page P, Labbe A, Topp A. Clinical force production of Thera-Band elastic bands. *J Orthop Sports Phys Ther*. 2000;30(1):47-48.
28. Lima FF, Camillo CA, Gobbo LA, et al. Resistance training using low cost elastic tubing is equally effective to conventional weight machines in middle-aged to older healthy adults: a quasi-randomized controlled clinical trial. *J Sports Sci Med*. 2018;17(1):153-160.
29. Evans WJ. Exercise training guidelines for the elderly. *Med Sci Sports Exerc*. 1999;31:12-17.
30. Kraemer WJ, Ratamess NA. Fundamentals of resistance training progression and exercise prescription. *Med Sci Sports Exer*. 2004;36(4):674-688. doi:10.1249/01.MSS.0000121945.36635.61
31. Stone WJ, Coulter SP. Strength/endurance effects from three resistance training protocols with women. *J Strength Cond Res*. 1994;8(4):231-234.
32. Corder KP, Potteiger JA, Nau KL, Figoni SE, Hershberger SL. Effects of active and passive recovery conditions on blood lactate, rating of perceived exertion and performance during resistance training. *J Strength Cond Res*. 2000;14(2):1551-1556.
33. Cheung K, Hume P, Maxwell L. Delayed onset muscle soreness: treatment strategies and performance factors. *Sports Med*. 2003;33(2):145-164.

34. Torres R, Ribeiro F, Alberto Duarte J, Cabri JM. Evidence of the physiotherapeutic interventions used currently after exercise-induced muscle damage: systematic review and meta-analysis. *Phys Ther Sport.* 2012;13(2):101-114. doi:10.1016/j.ptsp.2011.07.005
35. Adams D, Logerstedt DS, Hunter-Giordano A, Axe MJ, Snyder-Mackler L. Current concepts for anterior cruciate ligament reconstruction: a criterion-based rehabilitation progression. *J Orthop Sports Phys Ther.* 2012;42(7):601-614. doi:10.2519/jospt.2012.3871
36. Pearcey GE, Bradbury-Squires DJ, Kawamoto JE, Drinkwater EJ, Behm DG, Button DC. Foam rolling for delayed-onset muscle soreness and recovery of dynamic performance measures. *J Athl Train.* 2015;50(1):5-13. doi:10.4085/1062-6050-50.1.01
37. Macdonald GZ, Button DC, Drinkwater EJ, Behm DG. Foam rolling as a recovery tool after an intense bout of physical activity. *Med Sci Sports Exerc.* 2014;46(1):131-142. doi:10.1249/MSS.0b013e3182a123db
38. Romero-Moraleda B, La Touche R, Lerma-Lara S, et al. Neurodynamic mobilization and foam rolling improved delayed-onset muscle soreness in a healthy adult population: a randomized controlled clinical trial. *PeerJ.* 2017;5:e3908. doi:10.7717/peerj.3908
39. Peacock CA, Krein DD, Silver TA, Sanders GJ, Carlowitz KA. An acute bout of self-myofascial release in the form of foam rolling improves performance testing. *Int J Exerc Sci.* 2014;7(3):202-211.
40. DeLorme TL, Watkins AL. *Progressive Resistance Exercise.* Appleton-Century-Crofts; 1951.
41. Zinovieff AN. Heavy-resistance exercises the "Oxford technique." *Br J Phys Med.* 1951;14(6):129-132.
42. Knight KL. Guidelines for rehabilitation of sports injuries. *Clin Sports Med.* 1985;4(3):405-416.
43. O'Sullivan S. Proprioceptive neuromuscular facilitation. In: O'Sullivan ST, Schmitz TJ, eds. *Improving Functional Outcomes in Physical Rehabilitation.* 2nd ed. FA Davis; 2018:262-267.
44. Prentice WE. *Rehabilitation Techniques for Sports Medicine and Athletic Training.* 6th ed. SLACK Incorporated; 2015:255-259, 371-377.
45. Torres PA, Helmstetter JA, Kaye AM, Kaye AD. Rhabdomyolysis: pathogenesis, diagnosis, and treatment. *Ochsner J.* 2015;15(1):58-69.
46. Mendes P, Robles PG, Mathur S. Statin-induced rhabdomyolysis: a comprehensive review of case reports. *Physiother Can.* 2014;66(2):124-132. doi:10.3138/ptc.2012-65
47. Goodman C, Helgeson K. *Exercise Prescription for Medical Conditions Handbook for Physical Therapists.* FA Davis; 2011.
48. Goodman C, Fuller K. *Pathology: Implications for the Physical Therapist.* 4th ed. FA Davis; 2014.
49. American Academy of Pediatrics Council on Sports Medicine and Fitness; McCambridge TM, Stricker PR. Strength training by children and adolescents. *Pediatrics.* 2008;121(4):835-840. doi:10.1542/peds.2007-3790
50. Faigenbaum AD, Myer GD. Pediatric resistance training: benefits, concerns, and program design considerations. *Curr Sports Med Rep.* 2010;9(3):161-168. doi:10.1249/JSR.0b013e3181de1214
51. Faigenbaum AD, Kraemer WJ, Blimkie CJ, et al. Youth resistance training: updated position statement paper from the national strength and conditioning association. *J Strength Cond Res.* 2009;23(suppl):S60-S79. doi:10.1519/JSC.0b013e31819df407
52. Ward BW, Black LI. State and regional prevalence of diagnosed multiple chronic conditions among adults aged ≥18 years - United States, 2014. *MMWR Morb Mortal Wkly Rep.* 2016;65(29):735-738. doi:10.15585/mmwr.mm6529a3
53. Ward BW. Multiple chronic conditions and labor force outcomes: a population study of U.S. adults. *Am J Ind Med.* 2015;58(9):943-954. doi:10.1002/ajim.22439
54. Taylor NF, Dodd KJ, Damiano DL. Progressive resistance exercise in physical therapy: a summary of systematic reviews. *Phys Ther.* 2005;85(11):1208-1223.
55. Geneen LJ, Moore RA, Clarke C, Martin D, Colvin LA, Smith BH. Physical activity and exercise for chronic pain in adults: an overview of Cochrane Reviews. *Cochrane Database Syst Rev.* 2017;4:CD011279. doi:10.1002/14651858.CD011279.pub3
56. Hsieh PL, Tseng CH, Tseng YJ, Yang WS. Resistance training improves muscle function and cardiometabolic risks but not quality of life in older people with type 2 diabetes mellitus: a randomized controlled trial. *J Geriatr Phys Ther.* 2018;41(2):65-76.
57. Yang Z, Scott CA, Mao C, Tang J, Farmer AJ. Resistance exercise versus aerobic exercise for type 2 diabetes: a systematic review and meta-analysis. *Sports Med.* 2014;44(4):487-499. doi:10.1007/s40279-013-0128-8
58. Ishiguro H, Kodama S, Horikawa C, et al. In search of the ideal resistance training program to improve glycemic control and its indication for patients with type 2 diabetes mellitus: a systematic review and meta-analysis. *Sports Med.* 2016;46(1):67-77. doi:10.1007/s40279-015-0379-7
59. Kjølhede T, Vissing K, Dalgas U. Multiple sclerosis and progressive resistance training: a systematic review. *Mult Scler.* 2012;18(9):1215-1228. doi:10.1177/1352458512437418
60. Kjølhede T, Vissing K, de Place L, et al. Neuromuscular adaptations to long-term progressive resistance training translates to improved functional capacity for people with multiple sclerosis and is maintained at follow-up. *Mult Scler.* 2015;21(5):599-611. doi:10.1177/1352458514549402
61. Learmonth YC, Adamson BC, Kinnett-Hopkins D, Bohri M, Motl RW. Results of a feasibility randomised controlled study of the guidelines for exercise in multiple sclerosis project. *Contemp Clin Trials.* 2017;54:84-97. doi:10.1016/j.cct.2016.11.012
62. Chung CL, Thilarajah S, Tan D. Effectiveness of resistance training on muscle strength and physical function in people with Parkinson's disease: a systematic review and meta-analysis. *Clin Rehabil.* 2016;30(1):11-23. doi:10.1177/0269215515570381
63. Lima LO, Scianni A, Rodrigues-de-Paula F. Progressive resistance exercise improves strength and physical performance in people with mild to moderate Parkinson's disease: a systematic review. *J Physiother.* 2013;59(1):7-13. doi:10.1016/S1836-9553(13)70141-3
64. Silva-Batista C, Corcos DM, Roschel H, et al. Resistance training with instability for patients with Parkinson's disease. *Med Sci Sports Exerc.* 2016;48(9):1678-1687. doi:10.1249/MSS.0000000000000945

65. Loprinzi PD, Sng E, Walker JF. Muscle strengthening activity associates with reduced all-cause mortality in COPD. *Chronic Illn.* 2017;13(2):140-147.
66. Liao WH, Chen JW, Chen X, et al. Impact of resistance training in subjects with COPD: a systematic review and meta-analysis. *Respir Care.* 2015;60(8):1130-1145. doi:10.4187/respcare.03598
67. Ciccolo J, Nosrat S. Resistance training and chronic disease. *ACSM Health Fit J.* 2016;20(5):44-49.
68. Harries SK, Lubans DR, Callister R. Systematic review and meta-analysis of linear and undulating periodized resistance training programs on muscular strength. *J Strength Cond Res.* 2015;29(4):1113-1125. doi:10.1519/JSC.0000000000000712
69. Behrens BJ, Beinart H. *Physical Agents Theory and Practice.* 3rd ed. FA Davis; 2014.
70. Kalron A, Bar-Sela S. A systematic review of the effectiveness of Kinesio Taping--fact or fashion? *Eur J Phys Rehabil Med.* 2013;49(5):699-709.
71. Parreira Pdo C, Costa Lda C, Hespanhol LC Jr, Lopes AD, Costa LO. Current evidence does not support the use of Kinesio Taping in clinical practice: a systematic review. *J Physiother.* 2014;60(1):31-39. doi:10.1016/j.jphys.2013.12.008
72. Jakeman JR, Byrne C, Eston RG. Lower limb compression garment improves recovery from exercise-induced muscle damage in young, active females. *Eur J Appl Physiol.* 2010;109(6):1137-1144. doi:10.1007/s00421-010-1464-0
73. Hill J, Howatson G, van Someren K, et al. The effects of compression garment pressure on recovery from strenuous exercise. *Int J Sports Physiol Perform.* 2017;12(8):1078-1084. doi:10.1123/ijspp.2016-0380
74. Marqués-Jiménez D, Calleja-González J, Arratibel I, Delextrat A, Terrados N. Are compression garments effective for the recovery of exercise-induced muscle damage? A systematic review with meta-analysis. *Physiol Behav.* 2016;1(153):133-148. doi:10.1016/j.physbeh.2015.10.027
75. Born DP, Sperlich B, Holmberg HC. Bringing light into the dark: effects of compression clothing on performance and recovery. *Int J Sports Physiol Perform.* 2013;8(1):4-18.
76. Hylden C, Burns T, Stinner D, Owen J. Blood flow restriction rehabilitation for extremity weakness: a case series. *J Spec Oper Med.* 2015;15(1):50-56.
77. Hughes L, Paton B Rosenblatt B Gissane C, Patterson SD. Blood flow restriction training in clinical musculoskeletal rehabilitation: a systematic review and meta-analysis. *Br J Sports Med.* 2017;51:1003-1011. doi:10.1136/bjsports-2016-097071

Chapter 7

# Posture, Pregait, and Gait Training Interventions

*Karen A. Cascardi, PhD, MS, ATC, PTA*

**KEY TERMS** Dynamic posture | Gait cycle | Kyphosis | Limb advancement | Lordosis | Scoliosis | Single-limb stance | Static posture | Weight acceptance

## Chapter Objectives

1. Describe static and dynamic posture.
2. Differentiate between good and faulty posture.
3. Explain the contributing factors associated with faulty posture.
4. Describe the landmarks during static sitting and standing postural assessments.
5. Identify specific muscle imbalances that are associated with faulty posture.
6. Select the appropriate exercises to correct postural deviations.
7. Identify the components necessary to facilitate a sit-to-stand transfer.
8. Demonstrate techniques that help facilitate safe and efficient sit-to-stand transfers for patients.
9. Describe the various phases/periods and tasks of the gait cycle.
10. Describe gait distance and time parameters.
11. Identify compensatory gait patterns and their associated causes.
12. Describe the appropriate interventions to facilitate a normal gait pattern.
13. Discuss the outcome tools that can be used to assess gait.

## Introduction to Posture

Posture can be defined as any positions in which all body segments are appropriately aligned. **Static posture** is the ability to maintain body segments at rest (ie, lying down, sitting, or standing). **Dynamic posture** is the ability to maintain the alignment of the body while in motion (ie, walking or running). Clinicians continually observe patients' ability to maintain static postures and how they dynamically transition from any one position to another. Individuals need to maintain and transition between various postures while performing upper/lower extremity tasks (eg, reaching overhead and climbing stairs), activities of daily living (ADLs), and/or participating in sport or work activities.

Physical therapist assistants must recognize the difference between good and faulty posture. Good posture



Kopack JK, Cascardi KA.
*Principles of Therapeutic Exercise for the Physical Therapist Assistant* (pp 127-159).

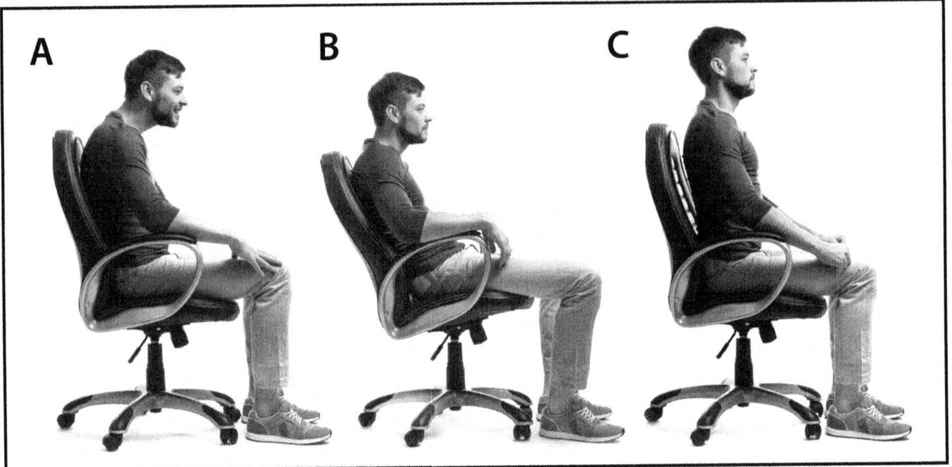


**Figure 7-1.** Faulty and good sitting postures. (A) Increased thoracic kyphosis and forward head. (B) A slumped posture and forward head. (C) Good erect posture (Africa Studio/Shutterstock.com).

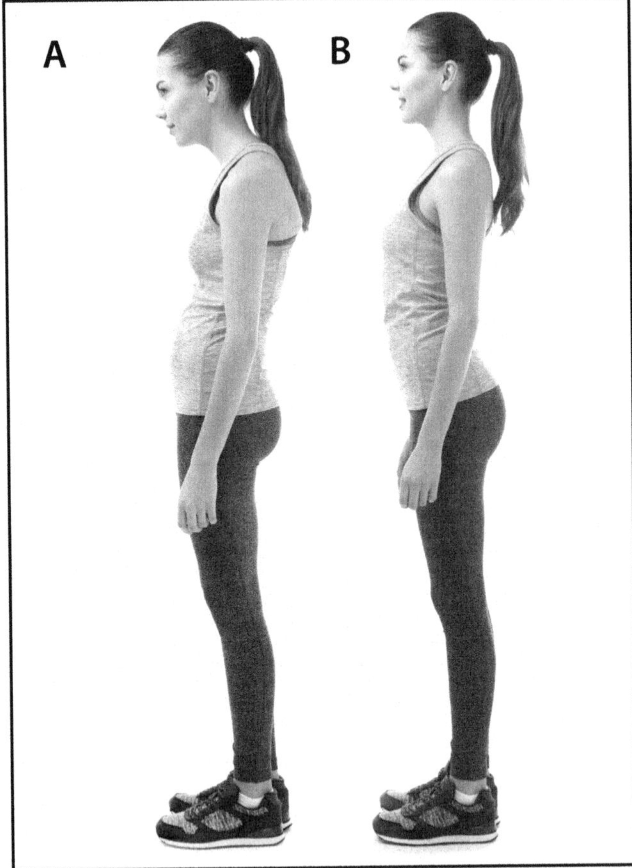


**Figure 7-2.** Faulty and good standing postures. (A) Faulty posture with a forward head promotes an increase in flexion of the thoracic spine and rounded shoulders. (B) Good erect posture is balanced and requires less energy (Africa Studio/Shutterstock.com).

is achieved when bones and joints are properly aligned; this alignment creates the opportunity for the optimal length–tension relationship of muscles (as long as good muscular strength and flexibility are maintained). In order to maintain good posture against gravity, one must have normal joint range of motion (ROM), proper bony alignment, good flexibility, and good muscular strength and endurance. There must be a balance between flexor and extensor muscles to allow the musculoskeletal and neuromuscular systems to function efficiently. Good standing posture allows the body to maintain equilibrium with the least amount of effort or energy.[1] Good sitting and standing alignment reduces prolonged stress/strain on static structures, maintains optimal muscle length and efficiency, and helps prevent overuse syndromes and/or pain.

Figures 7-1 and 7-2 compare faulty and proper sitting and standing postures. The position of one joint can have a direct effect on the positioning of another joint. Maintaining prolonged poor spinal alignment for long durations can affect static structures (bones and ligaments) and dynamic structures (muscles), altering the cervical, thoracic, and lumbar curves, which can result in compensatory responses at other joints. This increases the risk for muscle imbalances. Faulty postural positions can create numerous health issues across the life span.[2] Postural malalignment can limit a patient's ROM, preventing the safe and efficient performance of tasks. Impairments caused by prolonged faulty posture can include low back pain with or without radicular symptoms, neck pain leading to headaches, breathing problems, and arthritic changes at various joints that can result in balance and mobility changes. Treatment interventions and patient education should focus on the importance of maintaining good posture while targeting involved tissues that need to be stretched and/or strengthened. Postural muscles work against gravity over long periods of time, so muscular endurance is of primary concern. The physical therapist completes a postural assessment as a part of the initial evaluation.

> **Quick Class Activity**
>
> Sit in a slumped position and flex both arms over your head as high as possible. Note the ROM. Next, sit up straight and flex both arms over your head as high as possible again. What is the difference between the 2 activities? What is the difference between the 2 postures? What are the functional implications of these differences?

## Contributing Factors Affecting Posture

Generally, there are 2 categoric factors that may contribute to faulty posture: habitual positioning (functional) and structural problems. Although habitually assuming poor posture can lead to structural problems, oftentimes these habits can be corrected. Structural causes of faulty posture include deformities caused by congenital issues, trauma, or disease. Physical therapy interventions typically cannot correct postural faults that result from structural causes. Abnormal structural postures may require various external supports or surgical corrections to improve or maintain comfortable positioning.

Poor sitting or standing postures are the most common factors that lead to pain, muscle imbalances, and adaptive changes. For example, persistent slouching in a chair for long periods of time or prolonged standing looking down at your phone constantly can lead to neck, shoulder, and back pain. Common postural deviations include forward head, thoracic spine kyphosis, increased/decreased tilting of the pelvis, increased/decreased lumbar spine angles, and/or bilateral shoulder protraction and internal rotation. Over time, musculature can become adaptively shortened and tight or lengthened and weak. These tissue adaptions affect posture and function.

There are also a number of diseases or conditions that can affect posture. Osteoporotic compression fractures, spinal degenerative disease, stenosis, or spondylolisthesis can result in changes in the vertebral curves/postural changes in adults. Certain diseases result in postural changes, including Scheuermann disease (thoracic kyphosis) and ankylosing spondylitis (decreased lumbar lordosis and spinal ossification). Muscular dystrophy, cerebral palsy, and progressive neuromuscular diseases present with decreased neuromuscular control, resulting in poor spinal alignment and postural control impairments. Many patients have comorbidities that can affect postural control. Patients who have permanent postural changes caused by structural issues or disabilities (ie, tetraplegic patients, severe cerebral palsy, or myelomeningocele) benefit from the use of postural support systems to maintain proper positioning and comfort.

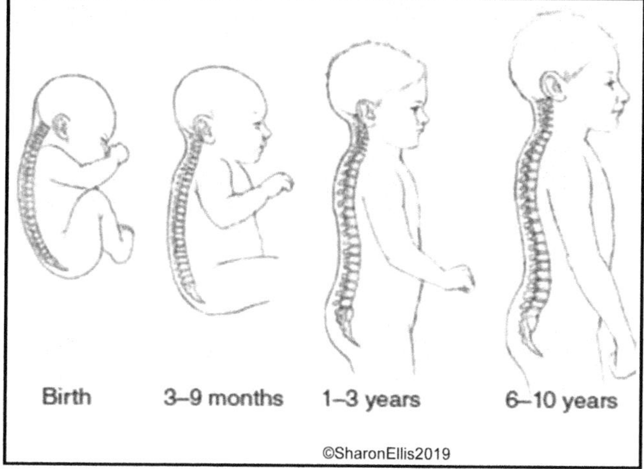


**Figure 7-3.** Primary and secondary curves. (Reproduced with permission from Sharon Ellis.)

## Posture Across the Life Span

As a newborn, an infant's spine is flexed (concave). The thoracic spine and sacrum maintain flexed curves into adulthood and are called *primary curves.* As infants age and are able to lift and hold their head up (at about 3 to 4 months), maintain a seated posture, and finally progress to standing (at 6 to 9 months), the cervical and lumbar curves become lordotic. The cervical lordotic curve develops earlier than the lumbar spinal curve; these curves are considered *secondary curves* (Figure 7-3).

At the time a child begins to stand and walk (at about 10 months to 1 year), the foot is initially flat, with approximately 8 degrees of calcaneal valgus. As the child grows, the valgus decreases by 1 degree for each year of age until neutral alignment is achieved, typically by age 8 years. The intrinsic muscles of the foot strengthen as the medial longitudinal arch becomes more prominent and stable by approximately the same age. The type of shoes worn and the child's sex may have some effect on this development.[3] Infants are usually born with genu varum (bow legs), and as they age, it commonly self-corrects by 18 months. Between the age of 2 and 3 years, the knees appear with a valgus angle (knock knees), which continues to progress until the age of 4 to 5 years. Once the child reaches 6 to 7 years of age, the knees align more vertically, and by age 12 years the knees will typically assume and maintain their actual vertical alignment (Figure 7-4).[4]

Young children (4 to 6 years) tend to have an exaggerated lordotic curve, which may be caused by weaker abdominals.[5] There is a high prevalence of postural deviations in children and adolescents, which may be attributed to growth spurts as well as environmental issues. Boys between the ages of 7 and 9 years may have an increased incidence of scapula winging compared with girls of the same age. Because the maturation process begins earlier for girls than for boys, girls typically reach their maximum muscle force earlier than boys.[6]

Slouched sitting or standing postures as well as other extrinsic factors, such as carrying heavy backpacks or

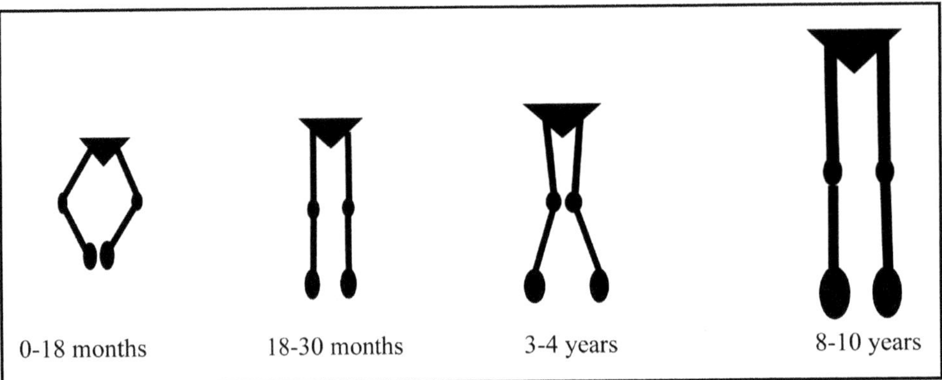


**Figure 7-4.** Knee development from birth to age 8 years.

carrying young children on the same side over a prolonged period of time (months and years), may all contribute to postural syndromes. Thoracic kyphosis and shoulder protraction are more common in women during adolescence because of breast development and perceived body image.[6] Teenagers tend to have a higher prevalence of forward head posture, which may be due to texting and performing frequent computer-related tasks.[7] These postural bad habits are common. It is important to make changes early through physical therapy interventions and patient education to prevent progression into more significant problems. Because of the increased use of mobile phones, tablets, and computers by all individuals, no one is exempt from the risk of developing postural syndromes.

During pregnancy, postural changes are inevitable. The spine becomes more lordotic, and the abdominal muscles lengthen to accommodate for the increased weight and size of the fetus. These changes increase weight-bearing loads on the facet joints, which can contribute to low back pain. Research indicates that there are many benefits associated with exercising during pregnancy (see Chapter 21). Research completed by Dumas et al[8] indicated that regular exercise during pregnancy did not have a detectable effect on posture nor did it result in postural improvements. However, the researchers acknowledged that the exercise protocols may not have been completed at an adequate intensity to result in changes, and they recommend additional research investigating exercise parameters and the effect of postural exercises initiated earlier during pregnancy.[8]

Older adults may develop thoracic kyphosis as they age; this is commonly a result of arthritic spinal changes (wedging), disk degeneration, osteoporosis, and/or stenosis. According to the Framingham longitudinal study, there were a number of functional impairments associated with poor posture in women 72 to 96 years old.[9] Some of these impairments included difficulty walking, standing longer than 15 minutes, and completing instrumental ADLs.[9] Other studies found that increasing ROM, strength, balance, and coordination can have a direct effect on improving posture and reducing falls in older women.[10,11]

## Static and Dynamic Postural Assessments

Appropriate postural alignment promotes equal weight distribution through the spine, allowing efficient transfer of the weight of both the upper body and any objects a person is carrying or using into the base of support (BOS).[12] Performing a postural assessment on patients helps determine their ability to maintain specific positions, change positions, and perform tasks in various environments. The clinician observes vertical spinal alignment, the segmental relationship of the 3 curves, and the size and position of the BOS in static and dynamic postures. The way a patient sits, stands, and moves provides a wealth of information regarding the postures they typically assume and the movement patterns they repetitively perform.

### *Static Postural Assessments: Sitting and Standing*

A static postural assessment is performed when a patient is stationary to identify any asymmetries. Sitting and standing postures must be observed and assessed from lateral, anterior, and posterior views to determine if any postural deviations are present (Table 7-1). Deviations with rotational components can be observed in all planes. If deviations/abnormalities are observed during a static assessment, then the ability to change positions or initiate and maintain specific gait patterns may be inefficient. Maintaining postural deviations for long durations or performing abnormal movement patterns repetitively increases a person's risk of injury.

A patient's posture can be recorded and graded using the postural assessment chart found in the Suggested Resources section at the end of this chapter. There are tests that can also provide valuable information regarding a patient's standing (or sitting) posture, including the vertical compression test, the elbow flexion test, and the lumbar protective mechanism (see the Static Standing Postural Assessments section).[12,13]

**Table 7-1**

**Landmarks for Sitting and Standing Postural Assessments**

| Positions/ Views to Be Observed | Lateral View | Posterior View | Anterior View |
|---|---|---|---|
| Sitting posture | • External auditory meatus<br>• Bisect acromion process, shaft of humerus<br>• Through or slightly posterior to greater trochanter<br>Note: PSIS should be level with or slightly higher than ASIS. | • Bisects the head<br>• Shoulders level (acromion processes)[a]<br>• Bisects spinous processes<br>• Scapulae equal distance from spinous processes<br>• Through the gluteal cleft<br>• Iliac crests should be level | • Bisect the nose (check for head rotation or tilting)<br>• Bisect sternum<br>• Shoulders level[a]<br>• Iliac crests level<br>• Knees equal distance from the plumb line |
| Standing posture | • External auditory meatus<br>• Slightly posterior to cervical spine<br>• Slightly anterior to thoracic spine<br>• Bisect acromion process, shaft of the humerus<br>• Through the vertebral bodies of lumbar spine<br>• Through the greater trochanter<br>• Just posterior to patella<br>• Just anterior to lateral malleolus | • Bisects the head<br>• Shoulders level (acromion processes)[a]<br>• Inferior angles of the scapulae equal<br>• Bisects the spinous processes<br>• The scapulae equal distance from the spinous processes<br>• Through the gluteal cleft<br>• Equal height for iliac crests, PSISs, gluteal folds, and greater trochanters<br>• Knee vertically aligned (no genu varus/valgus)<br>• Knee popliteal folds are equal<br>• Bilateral calcaneus in neutral (no varus or valgus) | • Bisect the nose (check for head rotation or tilting)<br>• Bisect the sternum<br>• Shoulders level[a]<br>• Equal distance from the plumb line: Bilateral ASISs, medial knee joints, and medial malleoli<br>• Tibial tubercle facing anteriorly (no rotation)<br>• Navicular height equal from the floor |

[a]Dominant shoulder may be slightly lower than the nondominant shoulder.
ASIS = anterior superior iliac spine; PSIS = posterior superior iliac spine.

## Static Sitting Postural Assessments

Ideally, when an individual sits, the BOS should support a balanced spinal alignment; this minimizes stress on the joints and lowers muscle energy expenditure. The sitting postures an individual can assume include supported erect, supported slouched (using a chairback for support), unsupported active erect, unsupported relaxed erect, and unsupported slumped (Figure 7-5). The clinician should observe active and relaxed unsupported sitting postures when assessing sitting posture. Assess unsupported relaxed sitting first to view the posture that the individual naturally assumes. After viewing the patient in the relaxed position, instruct the patient to sit up as straight as possible to view unsupported active sitting. This position requires muscle activity of the back extensors and core muscles.

To complete a static seated postural assessment, observe the posture from a lateral, anterior, and posterior view (Figure 7-6) while using a plumb line to represent the line of gravity (LoG). The support surface should be firm and without back support. The patient should be seated with the hips positioned slightly less than 90 degrees in relation to the knees and the knees flexed to 90 degrees with the feet flat on the floor.

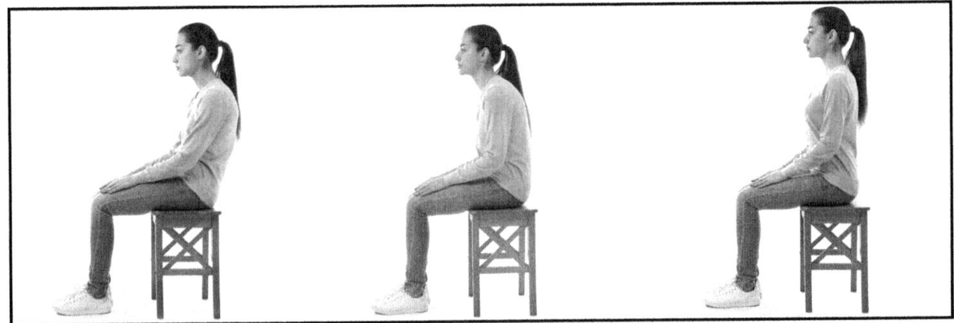

**Figure 7-5.** Various unsupported sitting postures (AfricaStudio/Shutterstock.com).

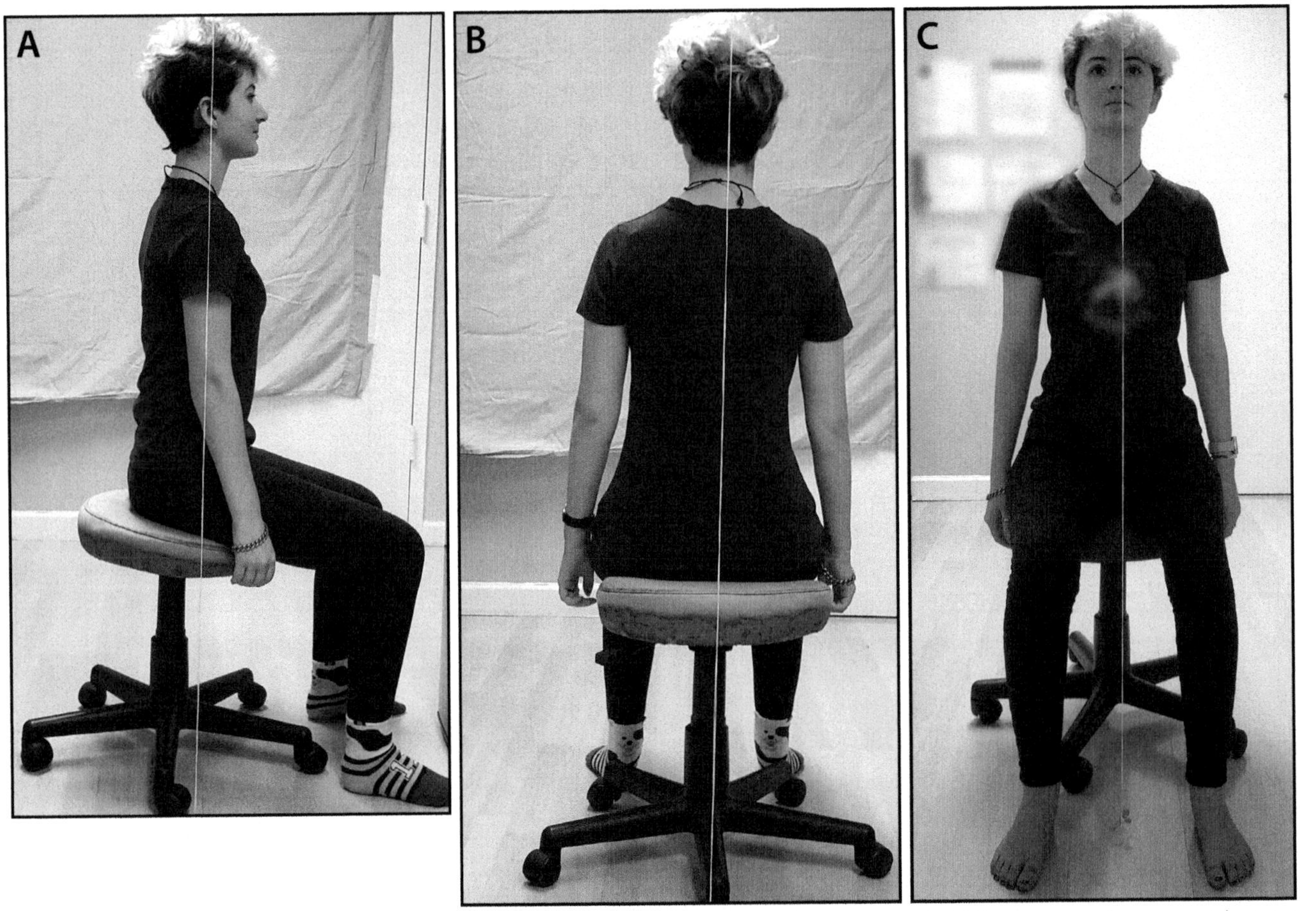

**Figure 7-6.** (A) Sitting postural assessment (lateral view). (B) Sitting postural assessment (posterior view). (C) Sitting postural assessment (anterior view).

View the patient laterally (see Figure 7-6A). Observe if the shoulders are rotated or protracted. The head should be directly over the hips with the LoG directly through the hip joint during relaxed erect posture and slightly posterior to the hip joint during active erect posture. The pelvis is the key to good sitting postural alignment. The PSIS should be level or slightly higher (or no less than a 1-inch [in] difference) in relation to the ASIS. This positions the pelvis in a slight anterior pelvic tilt. If there is normal alignment, the LoG (plumb line) passes through the landmarks presented in Table 7-1.

Next, observe the posterior (see Figure 7-6B) and anterior (see Figure 7-6C) views. The LoG should bisect the trunk. From the front, check the head position, shoulder symmetry, alignment at the hips and knees, and the position of the feet. From behind, check the position of the scapulae and their distance from the spinous processes; determine if lateral curvatures of the spine are present. Weight distribution should be equal on both ischial tuberosities. Refer to Table 7-2 for common malalignment issues and the common muscle imbalances associated with each postural deviation.

## Static Standing Postural Assessments

When assessing standing posture, have the patient stand comfortably with the feet positioned approximately 4 to 6 in apart. To determine the "ideal" posture, refer to the anatomic landmarks for all 3 views in relation to the plumb line

**Table 7-2**

**Sitting Postural Assessment Malalignment Issues and Muscle Involvement**

| Body Part | Possible Malalignment Issues | Possible Muscle Involvement |
|---|---|---|
| Head and thoracic spine | Forward head | Tight cervical extensors and weak deep neck flexors |
| | Lateral head tilt or rotation | Tight sternocleidomastoid if lateral flexion on same side with rotation to opposite side, tight splenius capitis if flexed and rotated to same side (may present with headaches), and tight scalenes if flexed to the same side |
| | Increased kyphosis of the thoracic spine | Weak/lengthened thoracic paraspinals, tight pectoralis major and internal rotators |
| Pelvis and lumbar spine | Significant posterior tilt resulting in flat lumbar curve (sacral sitting) | Tight hamstrings and weak lumbar paraspinals; abdominals may be weak |
| | Anterior tilt resulting in lordosis | Tight lumbar paraspinals and possibly hip flexors, weak abdominals |
| Hips | Excessive external (lateral) hip rotation and abduction | Tight hip rotators and abductors |
| | Unequal weight bearing on ischial tuberosities | Quadratus lumborum tightness on one side |

Note: Structural problems may not be correctable through exercise. Proper support systems such as cushions should be used to maintain better postural positions and avoid further deformities.

(see Table 7-2). Observe for deviations based on the plumb line location relative to each of the anatomical landmarks.

Begin the observation from a lateral view (Figure 7-7A) with the plumb line positioned just anteriorly to the lateral malleolus. Record any deviations, and then progress to a posterior view (Figure 7-7B). Posteriorly, the LoG should divide the head into equal halves; pass straight down between the scapulae along the vertebral column and through the gluteal cleft; and be equidistant from the PSISs, the medial knee joints, and the medial malleoli. The shoulders should be fairly level; however, it is common for a person's dominant shoulder to be slightly lower than their nondominant side. In this case, there may be a slight thoracic and/or lumbar compensatory curvature as well as an elevated hip noted on the dominant side. If the PSISs are not level, there may be a leg length discrepancy, which may result in scoliosis. The clinician can check scapulae positioning in relation to the thoracic spine by measuring the distance using a tape measure. The typical measurement from the spine of scapula to the spinous process of T4 should be approximately 8 cm (3.2 in). The inferior angles of scapulae should be level, and the measurement from the inferior angle of the scapula to T9 should be 9 cm (3.5 in). Abnormal scapular positions at rest have been associated with cervical and shoulder impairments and pain.[14]

From the anterior view (Figure 7-7C), the plumb line should bisect the body through the midsagittal plane. The plumb line should pass through the middle of the forehead, nose, and chin; along the sternum through the umbilicus; and equidistant between the ASIS, medial knee joints, and medial malleoli. The tibial tubercles should be facing forward and the tibia vertical with the feet in subtalar neutral.

**Considerations for the Physical Therapist Assistant**

If a patient is right-handed, that is considered their dominant side. Often the dominant shoulder will present lower than the nondominant side. There may be a slight compensatory thoracic curvature to the left, and the right hip may be slightly higher if the person is right-side dominant.

Three static tests can provide helpful information to clinicians. The vertical compression test assesses spinal alignment and weight distribution through the ischial tuberosities when seated and spinal alignment down to the floor when standing. The elbow flexion test provides information regarding the patient's ability to appropriately initiate sequential muscle firing of the local/deep (transverse abdominis, erector spinae, and multifidus) and global/superficial (rectus abdominis and internal/external obliques) muscles while maintaining good postural alignment. These tests should be performed while the patient is in their normal relaxed postural positions. If a patient presents with any diagnosis or clinical presentation in which resistance or compressive forces through the spine or upper extremities are contraindicated, these tests are contraindicated.

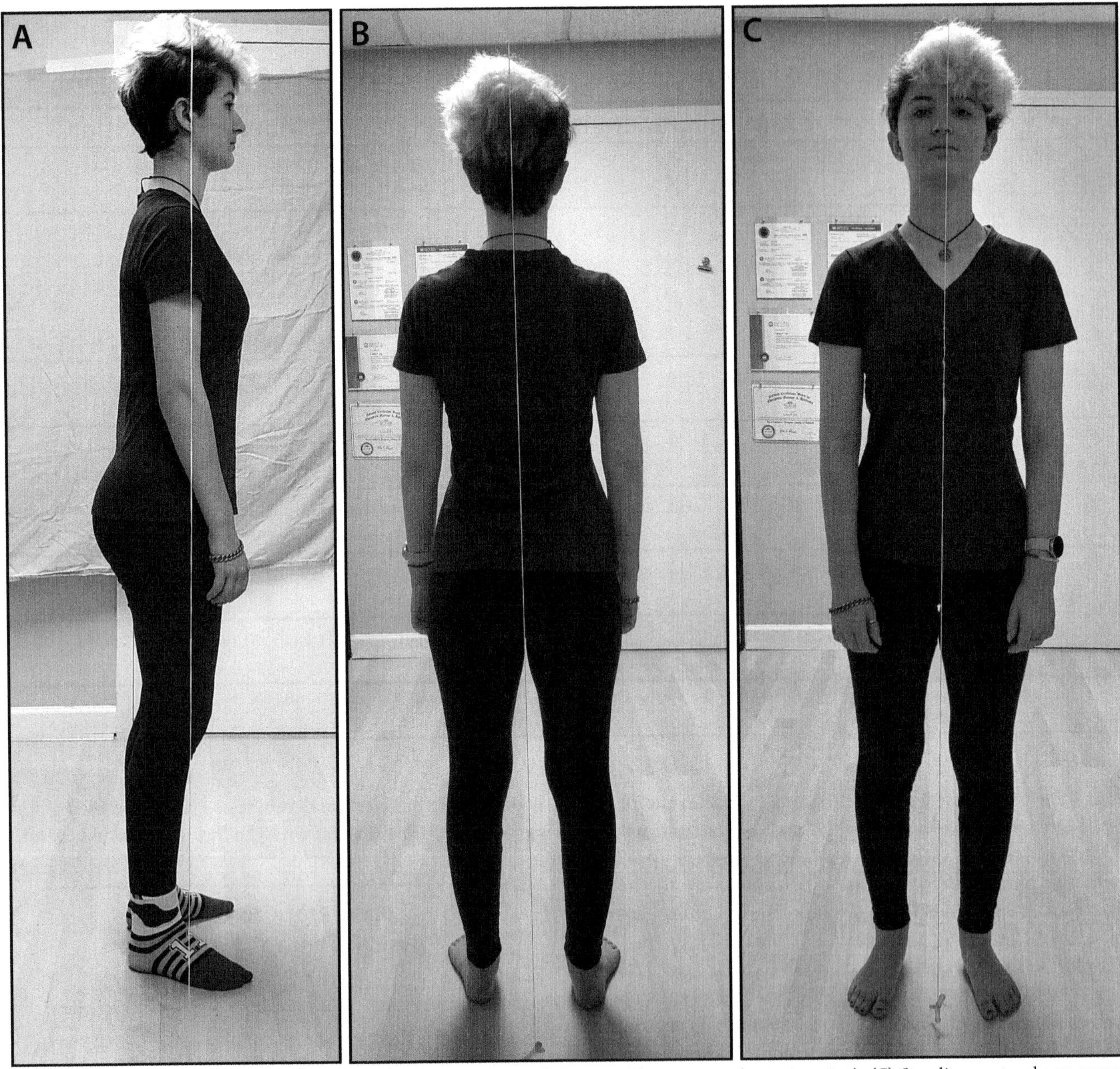


**Figure 7-7.** (A) Standing postural assessment (lateral view). (B) Standing postural assessment (posterior view). (C) Standing postural assessment (anterior view).

The vertical compression test (Figure 7-8) is a part of the Saliba Postural Classification System to assess posture.[12,13] This test has substantial intra- and inter-rater reliability and good validity.[12] This test can be performed while sitting and/or standing. The clinician stands behind the patient (see Figure 7-8A), on a stool if necessary, and places one hand on the top of each shoulder (see Figure 7-8B) over the acromion process and first rib. The clinician pushes straight down (vertically) with a gradual amount of increasing pressure (see Figure 7-8C). A pressure grade of 1 would be gentle, when the clinician feels pressure on the thenar eminences. The pressure grade of 2 is doubling that pressure, grade 3 triples the pressure, grade 4 quadruples the pressure, and grade 5 is full pressure. If the clinician feels any "give" or buckling of the patient's spine (most commonly into extension), the test is positive (see Figure 7-8D). A positive test indicates a postural deviation or spinal instability, and the patient often reports pain at that spinal segment.[13] Once the patient feels the buckling, they can better understand that their faulty posture is contributing to their pain. When patients understand the cause of their pain, they are usually more willing to make changes to improve their posture and participate in the rehabilitation process.

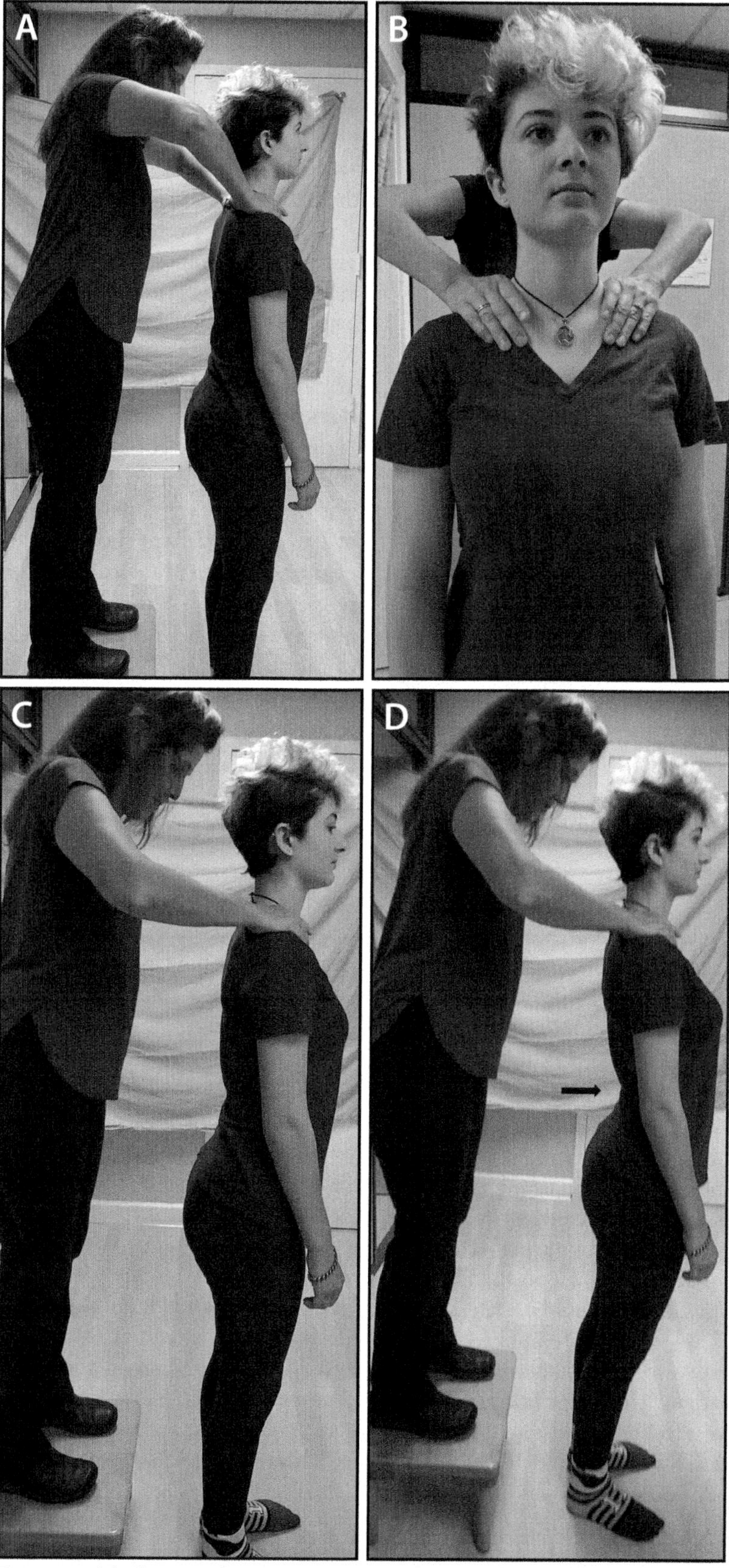


**Figure 7-8.** (A) The vertical compression test. (B) Hand placement for the vertical compression test. (C) The patient is able to maintain a stable upright posture during the vertical compression test. (D) A positive vertical compression test. Observe the increased spinal extension with downward force.

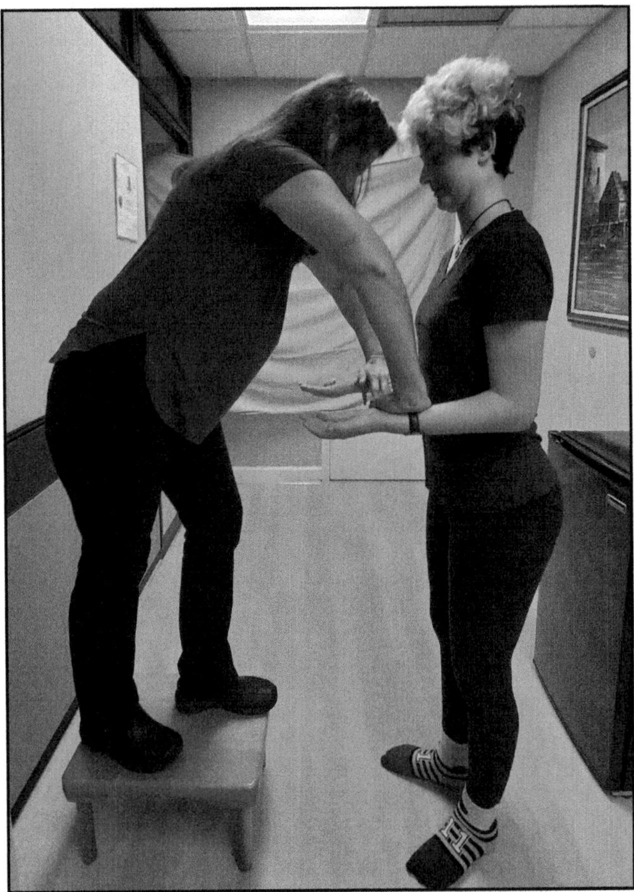

**Figure 7-9.** The elbow flexion test.

The elbow flexion test assesses the timing of muscle recruitment to determine if there is appropriate recruitment of local vs global muscles in response to an external force.[13] The clinician instructs the patient to stand normally, with the upper arms resting at the sides and the elbows flexed to 90 degrees with the palms facing upward (Figure 7-9). The clinician stands in front of the patient, placing one hand on the distal end of each forearm. The patient is instructed to remain stable while maintaining the elbow position. The clinician assumes a staggered stance and tells the patient "Do not let me straighten your arms." The clinician then gradually pushes straight down on the forearms with increasing pressure (grades 1 through 5). Determining a grade depends on the level of pressure applied when a postural deviation or change in their stable base occurs. During the test, ask the patient "How hard is it to resist my force?" and "Where did you feel the most strain or pain?" The clinician should observe for any changes in trunk position and determine if the local/deep muscles engaged first to maintain a stable base. The transverse abdominis should be the first to react followed by the abdominals to stabilize the trunk. The scapula stabilization muscles should engage next followed by the shoulder and arm muscles.[13] The clinician should document if the patient was stable, lost their balance, or flexed forward. The clinicians should ensure the patient's safety by using proper guarding as needed.

The lumbar protective mechanism test is used to determine if a patient is able to maintain alignment when an anterior or posterior external force is applied.[12,13] The patient is instructed to stand with one foot forward and one back, and the clinician assumes the same staggered stance. The clinician places one hand on the lateral half of each clavicle at the level of the second and third ribs as shown in Figure 7-10A. The clinician tells the patient to "Hold steady and do not let me move you" and then applies a slow posterior force with a gradual buildup of pressure from a grade of 1 to 5. The patient should be able to maintain a vertical posture and fire the local and then the global muscles in proper sequence. A test is positive (Figure 7-10B) if there is poor core muscle initiation or endurance, rotation, posterior (or lateral) weight shifting, loss of balance, or reports of pain. This test should be repeated from a posterior position with the application of an anterior force.

## Dynamic Sitting and Standing Assessments

There are numerous dynamic sitting and standing postural assessments available to assess the patient's ability to perform skills or tasks. Dynamic assessments provide information about a patient's ROM, muscle strength and endurance, and ability to maintain postural control and good alignment.

There are seated dynamic tests that are more suited for patients who are wheelchair bound or have limited walking ability. The Seated Reach Test and the Function in Sitting Test can be used for these patients.[15,16] The Sitting Balance Assessment Tool can be used for a variety of patients; it challenges a patient's balance under numerous conditions.[17]

Tests that combine sitting and standing static and dynamic tests include the Berg Balance Test and the Performance-Oriented Mobility Assessment (Tinetti). Links to these assessment tools are included in the Suggested Resources section at the end of this chapter. Postural issues may contribute to balance deficits, and when postural issues are corrected, the patient's balance can be addressed (Chapter 8).

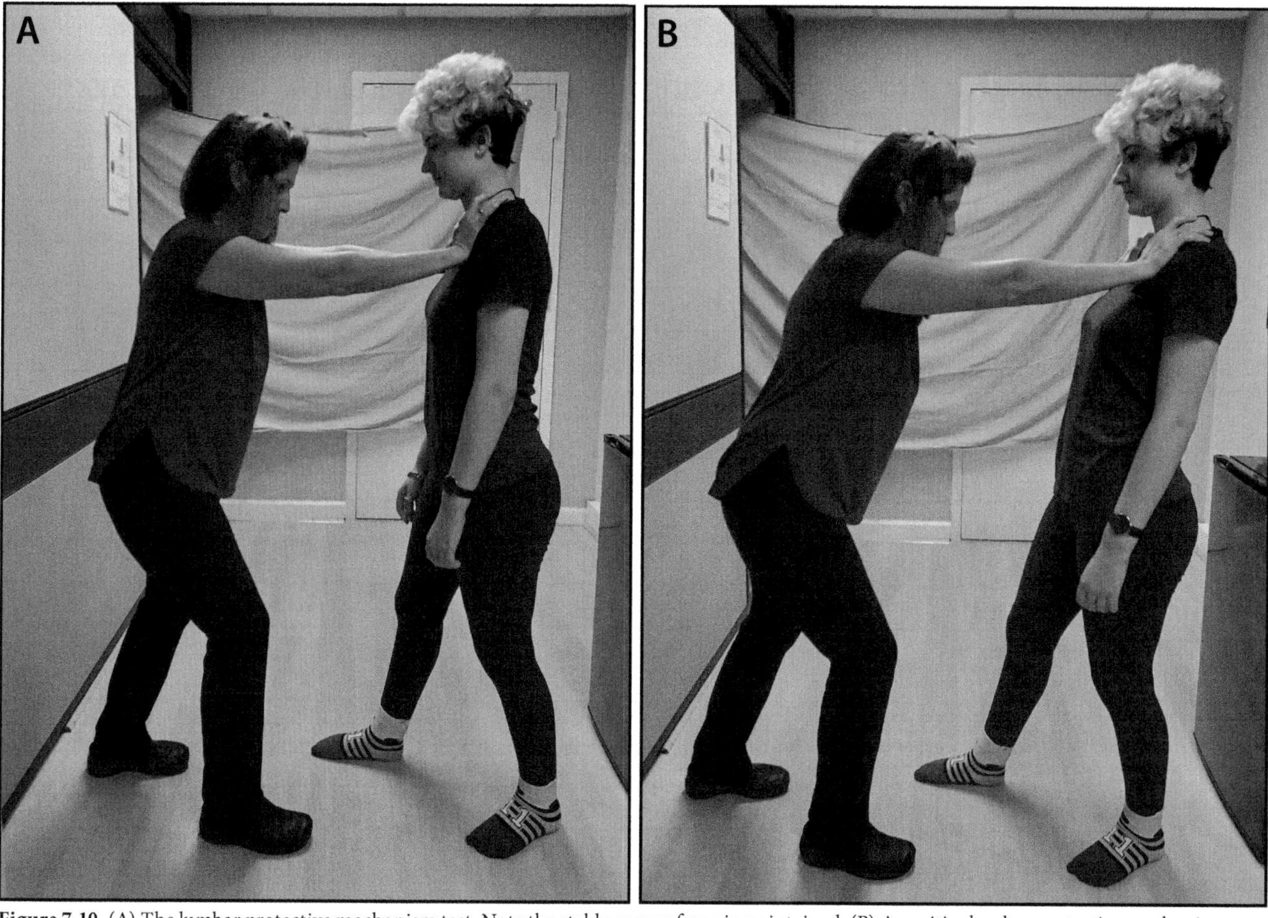


**Figure 7-10.** (A) The lumbar protective mechanism test. Note the stable core as force is maintained. (B) A positive lumbar protective mechanism test. Note the posterior lean of the patient as force is applied.

## *Spinal Deviations or Malalignment Issues*

Spinal deviations can be observed during sitting (see Table 7-2) or standing (Table 7-3) postural assessments. Common postural deviations are described later and are illustrated in Figure 7-11.

Forward head posture is an exaggerated upper cervical lordosis (increased extension) with a flattening (increased flexion) of the lower cervical joints. It is the most common postural deviation, affecting between 66% and 90% of the population.[18] It is often present with other postural deviations, such as thoracic kyphosis and lumbar lordosis. To understand one of the reasons why faulty posture may increase pain, note that for every inch of a forward head excursion, there is an increase of about 10 pounds of pressure placed on the neck.[18]

**Lordosis** is an exaggerated anterior curvature of the spine; it is most common in the cervical or lumbar spine (see Figure 7-11A). The lumbosacral angle is a measure of lumbar lordosis. It is the angle formed between the top of the sacrum and the horizontal plane; the normal value is 30 degrees (Figure 7-12A).[19] Lumbar lordosis is associated with an increased lumbosacral angle (greater than 30 degrees; Figure 7-12B) and an increase in hip flexion.

Lordotic posture is different than swayback posture. With swayback posture, the entire pelvis translates anteriorly (but maintains a neutral tilt position), resulting in the lower thoracic spine flexing (kyphosis) on the upper lumbar spine, which creates lower lumbar (L5-S1) lordosis in order to maintain a relatively upright position (see Figure 7-11D). The flexing of the thoracic spine on the lumbar spine causes hip extension and knee hyperextension. Swayback posture also is often associated with forward head posture and protracted shoulders.[19]

In flat back posture, there is decreased lumbar lordosis and associated posterior pelvic tilt (see Figure 7-11C). The lumbosacral angle is less than 30 degrees (Figure 7-12C). This posture is commonly observed in patients who tend to slouch when they sit or stand.

**Kyphosis** is an exaggerated flexed curvature of the spine that is most commonly noted in the thoracic spine (see Figure 7-11B). This rounded upper back posture is usually accompanied by a forward head, protracted scapulae, and internal (medial) rotation of the shoulders.

**Table 7-3**

Standing Postural Assessments and Possible Compensatory Deviations

| View | Body Part | Possible Deviations |
|---|---|---|
| Lateral | Head | Forward head |
| | Cervical spine | Lordosis or flat curvature |
| | Thoracic spine | Flat or kyphotic curve |
| | Scapulae | Protracted scapulae, glenohumeral sulcus |
| | Shoulders | Internal (medial) rotation of humerus |
| | Lumbar spine | Lordosis or flat curvature |
| | Pelvis | Anterior or posterior tilt (ASIS to PSIS level > 1 in) |
| | Hips | Flexed, extended, internal/external rotation |
| | Knees | Recurvatum or flexed |
| Posterior | Head | Laterally flexed or tilted |
| | Thoracic spine | Lateral curvature (scoliotic) |
| | Shoulders | Unequal height (Note: Dominant shoulder may be slightly lower), internal (medial) rotation of humerus |
| | Scapulae | Unequal distance from vertebral border to spinous processes |
| | Lumbar spine | Lateral curvature |
| | Pelvis | Unequal PSIS height, pelvis rotated anteriorly/posteriorly |
| | Knees | Genu valgus or varus |
| | Feet | Calcaneal varus or valgus, pes planus or cavus |
| Anterior | Head | Laterally flexed or rotated |
| | Shoulders | Humerus appears internally (medially) rotated |
| | Hands | Dorsal surface facing anteriorly |
| | Pelvis | Iliac crest heights unequal |
| | Knees | Tibial torsion, patellae location lateral/medial/alta/baja |
| | Feet | Excessive toe out/toe in, hallux valgus, pes planus or cavus |

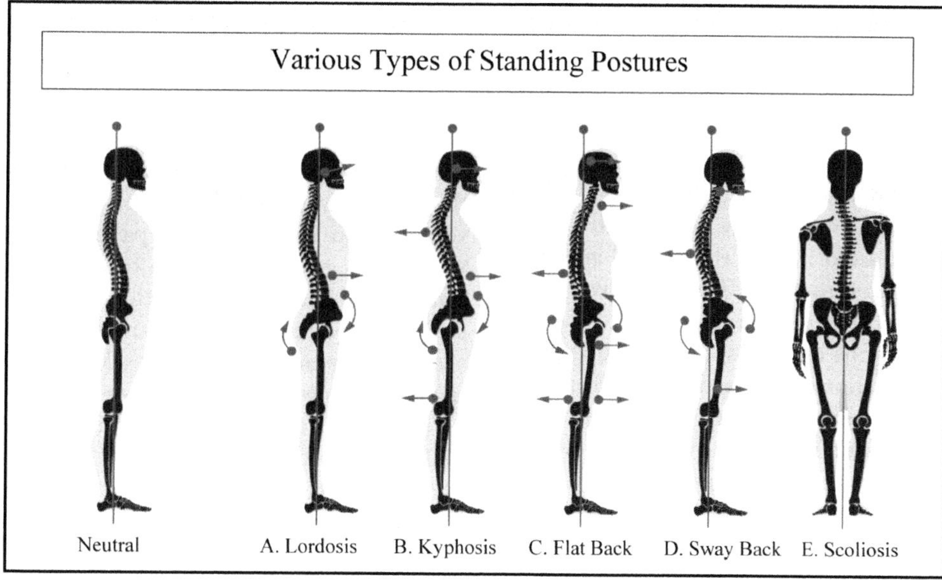


**Figure 7-11.** Various types of standing postures (handmadee3d/Shutterstock.com).

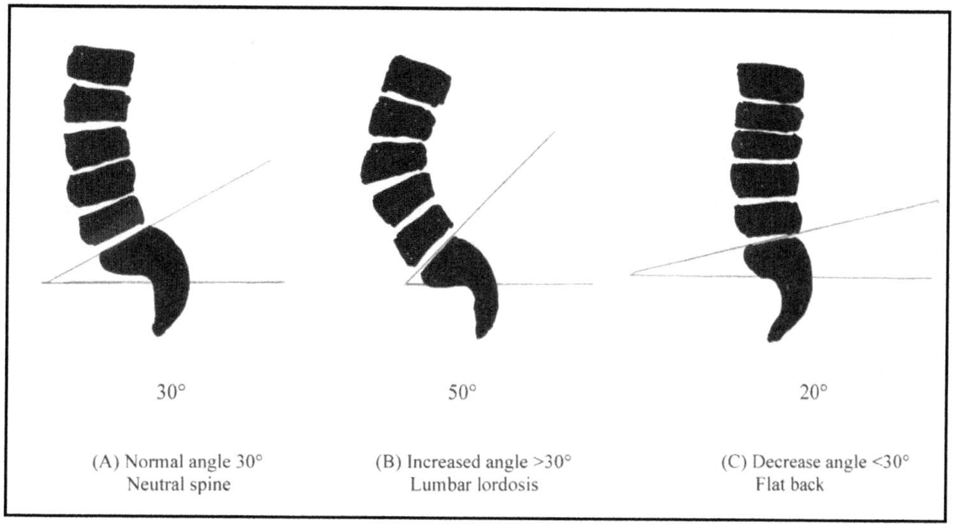


**Figure 7-12.** Lumbosacral angles and the corresponding lumbar curves.

**Scoliosis** is a lateral curvature of the spine, affecting the thoracic and/or lumbar spines (see Figure 7-11E). The scoliosis is described as "C" shaped if it affects one spinal area. "S"-shaped curves affect both the thoracic and lumbar spines. Scoliosis can be structural (fixed) or functional (nonstructural). Structural scoliosis is a lateral curvature that is irreversible. Structural scoliosis can be idiopathic (a result of unknown causes), or it can be a result of other disorders/diseases, such as connective tissue disease (Marfan syndrome), neuromuscular disease (ie, cerebral palsy, Duchenne muscular dystrophy, or spinal muscular atrophy), or birth defects (hemivertebrae). The ribs and vertebrae in the thoracic spine rotate toward the convex side of the curve, so when the patient bends forward, a rib hump appears on the convex side. Functional scoliosis is a lateral curve that is reversible. When the patient bends forward or to one side, it disappears. This type of scoliosis can be corrected by correcting the pelvic position, strengthening/stretching muscles, or accommodating for a leg length discrepancy.

## Considerations for the Physical Therapist Assistant

A deviation in one area of the body can cause compensatory deviations in another area. This is because of the close links between the head, trunk, spine and pelvis, and extremities. For example, a patient with thoracic kyphosis usually has a forward head; the forward head is compensatory, allowing the head to remain upright.

Problem-solving opportunity: Stand on a 1-in book with one foot and keep the other on the floor. How does this simulated leg length discrepancy affect the joints up and down the kinetic chain (ie, foot, pelvis, and spine)?

## Exercise Interventions to Improve Posture

Before considering stretching or strengthening exercises to improve a patient's posture, it is important to understand the differences between tonic (or postural) and phasic muscles. Tonic muscles are slow-twitch muscles (for endurance). They are primarily flexors and are prone to hypertonicity and contractures. They are involved in performing repetitive activities and less likely to atrophy. Phasic muscles (mostly the extensors) tend to work eccentrically against gravitational forces and atrophy easily (resulting in slouched posture). Phasic muscles are prone to being weak or inhibited.[5] Changes in muscle tone can lead to muscle imbalances commonly associated with postural malalignments, which ultimately result in movement dysfunction and pain. It is important to address the cause of the patient's pain and not just the source of their pain. Table 7-4 provides a list of various postural deviations and the associated compensated structures; this information will help guide the physical therapist assistant in developing the patient's exercise program. Assistants should review the patient's initial evaluation for the results of the postural assessment (identifying deviations) and other tests and measures (eg, ROM, muscle strength/endurance, flexibility) performed by the physical therapist. The assistant will use this information to determine appropriate treatment interventions to address the patient's impairments and the plan of care (POC).

### Clinical Tip

The patient should understand the importance of good posture and how to correct any deviations. Correctly performing postural exercises and practicing them while maintaining proper posture are necessary so that the patient does not revert back into bad postural habits. To increase patient compliance and reinforce good postural habits, suggest that the patient relate the postural corrections to a commonly completed task or event (eg, "Every time a commercial comes on TV, correct your sitting posture" or "Every time you walk through a doorway, correct your head and upper back posture").

After the physical therapist assistant reviews the physical therapist's POC, the following questions should be considered before treating the patient:

- Are the patient's limitations structural (requiring the use of external supports) or functional (caused by poor habits)?
- What is causing/creating the patient's instability, limitations, and/or pain?
- Does proximal stability cause patient limitations with distal mobility?
- Which muscles need to be stretched?
- Which muscles need to be strengthened?
- What other interventions are indicated to improve postural stability?

After answering these questions, the assistant can use the treatment guidelines in Table 7-5 to develop an intervention plan to improve the patient's posture and stability. Patients can be taught to recognize and correct their impaired posture using stretching, strengthening, and sensorimotor and/or neuromuscular training. Clinicians should use practice and feedback techniques to facilitate motor learning and to positively reinforce good posture so patients can automatically assume, maintain, and correct their posture independently (refer to Chapter 2). Chapters 14 and 15 discuss exercises that target the trunk and cervical muscles.

### Considerations for the Physical Therapist Assistant

To correct faulty postural positions, the shortened/tight muscles need to be stretched first and then strengthened in their new optimal, efficient position. Phasic muscles must be strengthened to work against gravity more effectively and to create a good muscle balance between tonic and phasic muscles.

To better understand this, consider the following example. A physical therapist assistant is treating a patient who presents with a forward head. The assistant should start by stretching the tight upper cervical extensor muscles and cuing the patient to contract the deep neck flexor stabilizers in the supine position (ie, chin tucks or nods). Initially, the assistant can provide visual feedback using a mirror and tactile cues so the patient can differentiate between faulty and proper head positions. Progress the patient by having them correct and maintain proper head position in sitting and standing positions without feedback. Strengthen the weak muscles and also the previously tight muscles in their new available ROM so these muscles can maintain the corrected posture for prolonged periods of time. When patients assume a more upright posture and improved head position, they may initially state that they feel like they are falling, feel off balance, or feel as if they are leaning backward when standing unsupported. This occurs because the sensorimotor systems (vision, somatosensory, and vestibular systems) have to adjust and adapt to this new "vertical" position. As the patient assumes their new vertical position, the spinal and head alignment is different, and the patient's weight-bearing position may also change. The patient should now have more centered/equalized weight bearing in both sitting and standing positions. They will experience a slight anterior shift over the arches of the feet vs being back on the heels during standing. Once the patient adjusts

**Table 7-4**

**Various Postural Deviations, Associated Compensatory Structures, and Muscle Adaptations[19]**

| | Condition | Structures Involved | Shortened/Tight Muscles (Tonic/Postural) | Lengthened/Weak Muscles |
|---|---|---|---|---|
| Head and shoulders<br><br>Thoracic spine | Upper cervical hyperextension and lower cervical flexion with thoracic kyphosis: Posterior curvature of the thoracic spine with a forward head and protracted and internally rotated shoulders | Stresses to anterior longitudinal ligaments and facet compression in the upper cervical spine due to hyperextension and posterior longitudinal ligaments due to excessive flexion of lower cervical spine/upper thoracic spines; protracted and internally rotated shoulders | Suboccipital/neck extensors (upper cervical); anterior thoracic and scapula muscles attaching to the head (pectoralis major and minor, serratus anterior, SCM, scalenes, levator scapula, upper trapezius), subscapularis | Deep neck flexors (upper cervical capital flexors, longus capitis and colli); lower cervical extensors, thoracic erector spinae, scapula retractors (rhomboids, middle and lower trapezius), shoulder external rotators |
| Lumbar spine | Lordosis: Anterior curvature of the lumbar spine with an increased lumbosacral angle | Stresses anterior longitudinal ligaments; compresses facet joints; decreases intervertebral foramen; anterior pelvic tilt | Lumbar extensors (erector spinae); hip flexors (iliopsoas, rectus femoris) | Abdominals (rectus and transverse abdominis; internal/external obliques) |
| Lumbar spine | Flat back: Decreased lumbar lordosis, lumbosacral angle, and posterior pelvic tilt; slight decreased thoracic curve with a slight forward lean; increased axial extension (flexion of the occiput on the atlas) and flattening of the cervical lordosis curve | Stresses posterior longitudinal ligaments; compresses anterior aspect of lumbar disks; hips and knees in slight extension | Trunk flexors (rectus abdominis); hip extensors (hamstrings); ankle plantar flexors (gastrocnemius); sub-occipital/neck extensors | Lumbar extensors (erector spinae); hip flexors (iliopsoas, rectus femoris); lower cervical extensors and thoracic erector spinae |
| Thoracic and/or lumbar spine | Scoliosis: Lateral curvature of the thoracic and/or lumbar spine | Thoracic and/or lumbar spine; can be structural or functional | The muscles on the concave side of the curvature are tight. | The muscles on the convex side are lengthened and weak. |

SCM = sternocleidomastoid.

**Table 7-5**

**Treatment Guidelines to Improve Posture and Stability**

1. Reposition the patient into a proper postural alignment without pain (promote kinesthetic self-awareness).
   a. Initially use a mirror for patient feedback; clinician uses tactile and verbal cues to make corrections.
   b. Make sure the patient understands and can correct their posture throughout the day. Patient postural education is essential.
   c. Inaccurate somatosensory awareness of "true" vertical results in decreased postural stability. Patients need to know and feel their weight bearing is truly centered (in sitting or standing).
2. Restore normal muscle balance and/or muscle length.
   a. Stretch all muscles that are shortened using manual stretches, self-stretching exercises, and other techniques to maintain proper alignment and increase ROM.
3. Restore normal muscle balance and tone: Strengthening and balance
   a. First, work on segmental stability. Cervical spine: Activate the deep neck flexors ("nodding yes"); use a mirror for feedback. Perform supine and then progress to isometrics in other positions and then add chin tuck head lifts supine. Lumbar spine: Work on core stability; perform abdominal bracing and/or drawing-in maneuver for transverse abdominis and multifidi isometrics for spinal stability (refer to Chapters 14 and 15).
   b. Strengthen weak global muscles next, including, but not limited to, the erector spinae, rectus abdominis, and internal/external obliques. Once patients achieve proper alignment and can activate and coordinate segmental stabilizers and global muscles, add extremity movements using proprioceptive neuromuscular facilitation techniques in various positions (ie, kneeling and quadruped).
      i. Increase reaction time and muscle endurance by using alternating isometrics and rhythmic stabilization of the trunk in sitting and standing. Add rotational resistance and perturbations.
   c. Initiate coordinated movements/activities (ie, break down tasks); target both stabilizing and global muscles. Some muscles need to stabilize, whereas distal ones need to create movements and contract quickly. Use resistance bands/weights to increase strength and muscle endurance.
4. Increase overall muscular endurance while performing coordinated movements in various environments (stable/unstable surfaces) and with unpredicted reactions (eg, ball tosses, balloon hits on foam, or half roll). Vary the BOS.
   a. Make corrections; watch for substitution patterns as muscles fatigue. For postural muscles, remember muscle endurance is more important than strength. Perform exercises with low intensity and longer duration/repetitions.
   b. When walking, change surface types and speed during activities to adapt to real-world environments (eg, walk on grass, go up/down curbs).
5. To maximize the potential for success:
   a. Clinicians must address patient goals while keeping patients motivated and engaged. Exercises should focus on and target specific patient issues. Explain why selected exercises are important for patients to perform at home.
   b. Patients must understand that performing these exercises will have positive results/effects. When patients understand the why and how their exercises are beneficial, they are more compliant with their home program.

to and is able to maintain their new postural position, their reports of pain should decrease, and an increase in standing stability should occur. The patient should be challenged in various positions (sitting, kneeling, and standing) with changes in BOS (wide, narrow, and single-leg standing) and surfaces (firm or uneven) so that ADLs and instrumental ADLs can be resumed while maintaining proper posture without a conscious effort.

## Pregait Activities

Pregait activities help prepare patients for walking (Box 7-1). In order to walk, patients must be able to maintain an upright standing position while weight bearing through both lower extremities, weight shift from side to side, and advance one lower extremity at a time while maintaining their balance.

## Box 7-1

### Purpose of Pregait Activities

- To increase ROM, strength, and coordination (strengthening/stretching muscles should address specific deficits)
- To improve postural stability and balance in sitting and then standing before initiating gait activities (ie, use perturbations in alternating directions at various speeds, intensities, and durations)
- To increase the ability and efficiency to transition from one position to another (supine to sit and sit to stand)

## *Improving Patient Sit-to-Stand Transfers*

Before addressing a patient's ability to transition from sitting to standing efficiently, physical therapist assistants should determine their ability to complete each of the following subtasks: (1) assume and maintain their sitting BOS with good trunk alignment, (2) shift their weight forward, (3) tolerate lower extremity weight bearing, and (4) maintain standing balance (with/without an assistive device) after the transfer.

Chair height, armrest use, and foot position can influence a patient's ability to transfer from sit to stand.[15] If a chair is too low, the patient has to use more strength because the trunk, knees, and ankles have to move through a greater range and the muscles are not at a mechanical advantage to contract efficiently to stand. The patient's center of mass has to be shifted forward more to compensate for the lower height. "The minimum height for successful rising for [older adults] (community-dwelling and nursing home residents 64-105 years of age) with chair rise difficulties appears to be 120% of the lower leg length."[15]

Traditionally, clinicians learn to instruct patients to scoot to the edge of the chair, lean forward ("nose over toes"), and push up. This takes a tremendous amount of energy and may not be the most efficient way to transition from sitting to standing. The assistant can consider using an alternate method, which may be easier and more efficient. Patient positioning before the start of a transfer is extremely important to increase the efficiency of the sit-to-stand transfer. Ideally, the patient's pubic symphysis should be situated 2 to 3 in (5 to 8 cm) from the front edge of the chair with the hips slightly higher than the knees, the knees flexed, and the feet staggered (but can be parallel) on the floor (Figure 7-13A).[13] The patient positions their hands with the palms on the front part of the armrest (not on the top), facing toward the back of the chair. This allows the patient to push away from the chair when standing and propel the body forward on an angle instead of straight up.

There are 3 exercises that specifically mimic the components of this task and that activate the trunk, hip, and knee muscles that must contract during the transfer. These quick and easy exercises should be performed just before executing the transfer, with the patient positioned as if preparing to perform the sit-to-stand transfer. These exercises facilitate contraction of the specific muscles needed for the transfer and provide neuromuscular feedback to the patient. The exercises only need to be performed a couple of times/repetitions. The clinician cues the patient to complete each of the following exercises in order:

- Active forward trunk flexion: Flexing at the hips with a straight back and head up (Figure 7-13B). Cue the patient to feel the core muscles engage when rocking forward.
- Resisted trunk isometrics (see Figure 7-13B): When the patient is positioned in slight trunk flexion, the assistant places one hand on the patient's sternum applying a posterior force and states "Do not let me move you." This facilitates a stronger transverse abdominal muscle contraction to stabilize the core.
- Hip extension isometrics: Have the patient push each foot down into the floor to facilitate the hamstrings and gluteus maximus (Figure 7-13C) while the assistant resists and feels for the extensors to contract. The patient's buttocks should slightly lift off the chair. This helps the patient understand how to initially drive with the legs using the hip/knee extensors.

It is important to note that the isometric exercises promote a cocontraction of the abdominals and back extensors to produce a stable trunk and a cocontraction of the gluteal, hamstring, and quadriceps muscles to propel the patient on a slight angle forward into standing. Remember that proximal stability of the trunk allows for the efficient distal mobility of the legs to propel them to stand. Monitor and cue patients to breathe to ensure they do not hold their breath (Valsalva) during the transfer.

During the exercises, make sure patients feel the neuromuscular response of the abdominal muscles stabilizing the trunk when the spine is properly aligned and the hip extensors contract to initially propel the body forward to stand before the transfer is attempted. The patient and clinician should be positioned as shown in Figure 7-13D. The key points the patient must understand before performing the actual transfer are to effectively maintain a straight spine and to drive the motion with the legs (Figures 7-13E and 7-13F). To better facilitate the transfer, the clinician can use the following instructions:

- "Scoot to the edge of the chair."
- "Stagger your feet."
- "Rock forward (hitch/bend) from the hips."
- "Drive with the legs; push back and away with the hands."
- "Take off like a jet (not like a helicopter)."

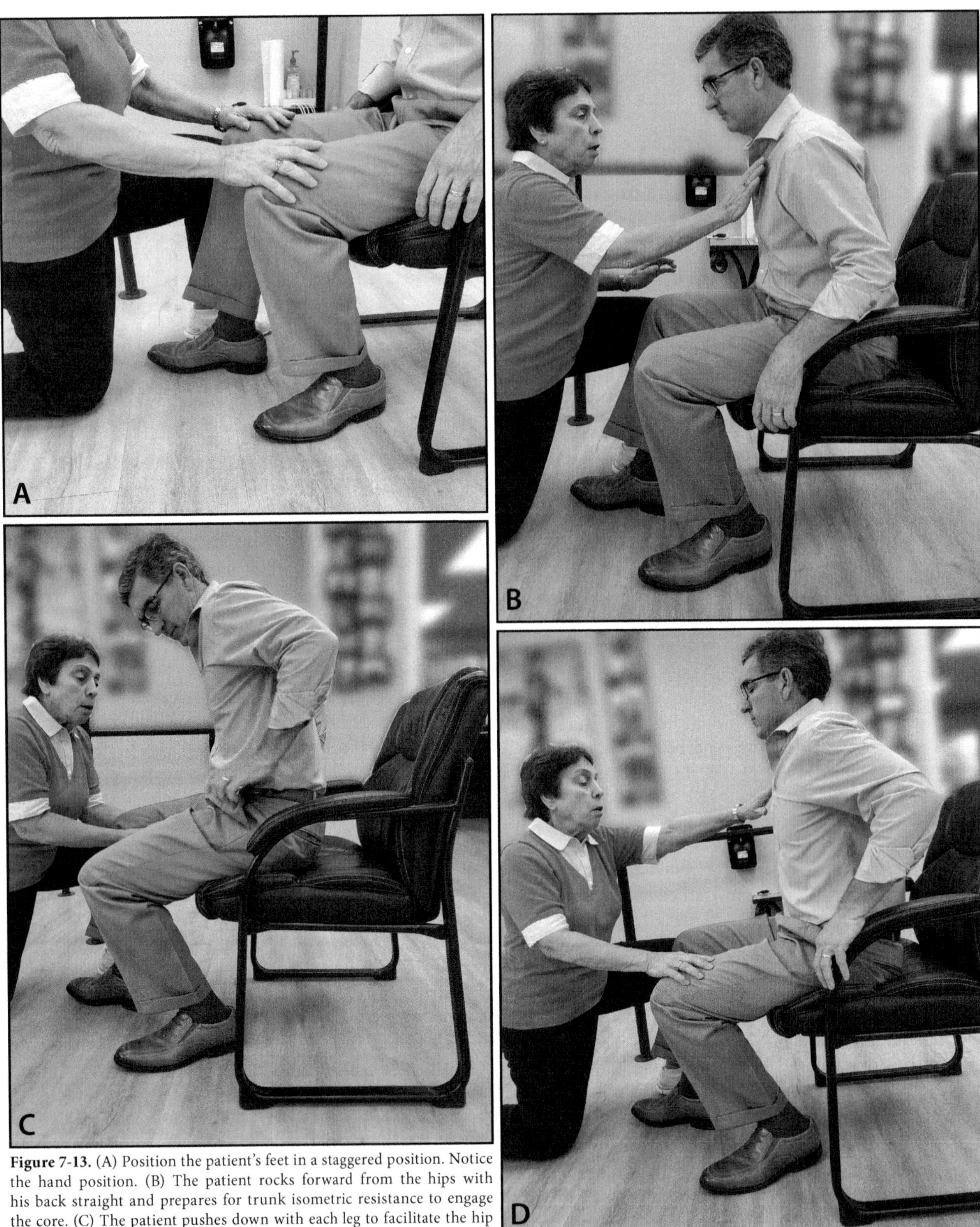

**Figure 7-13.** (A) Position the patient's feet in a staggered position. Notice the hand position. (B) The patient rocks forward from the hips with his back straight and prepares for trunk isometric resistance to engage the core. (C) The patient pushes down with each leg to facilitate the hip extensors. The clinician resists and feels for contraction. (D) The patient positioned in preparation for the transfer. *(continued)*

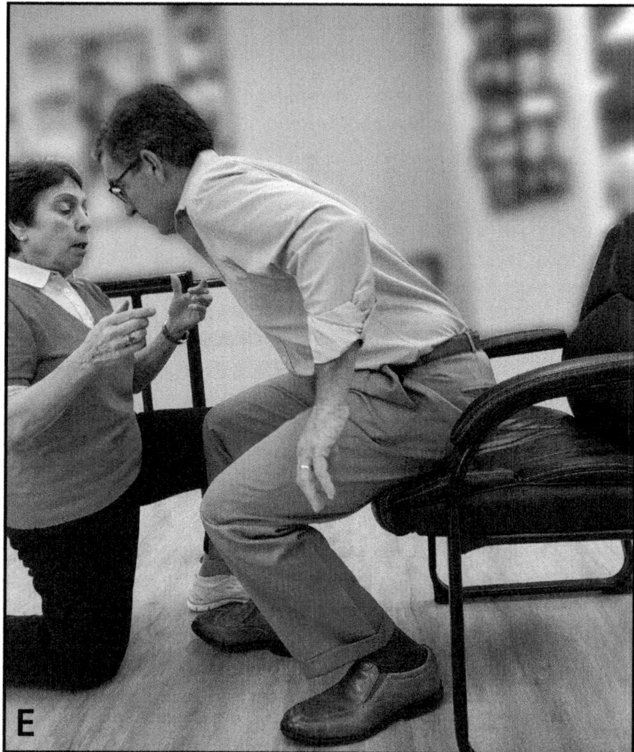


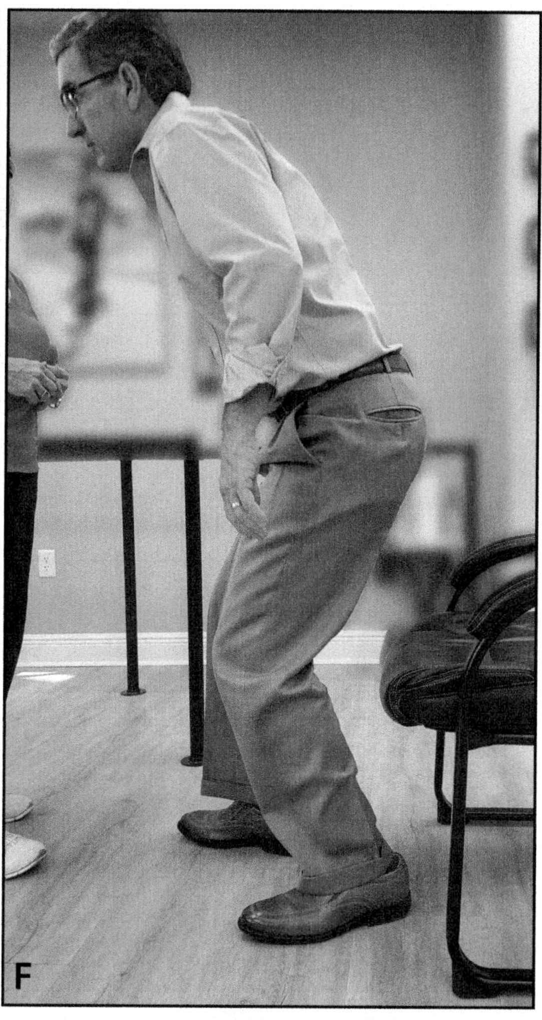


**Figure 7-13 (continued).** (E) Notice the good spinal alignment as the patient performs the transfer. The assistant is positioned in front of the patient for safety. (F) The patient is able to complete the transfer maintaining a stable trunk and staggered base.

The clinician is positioned in front of the patient for safety reasons and to reduce the patient's fear of falling forward as they lean anteriorly during the transfer.

### Quick Class Activity

Sit with a slightly slumped posture and rock forward from the hips. Now sit up straight with your chest and head up (back straight) and rock forward from the hips again. When did you feel the abdominal muscles engage? Next, perform a sit-to-stand transfer with a slumped posture and then with a straight back posture. Which was easier? Why?

To track a patient's progress objectively, the clinician can have the patient perform a 30-second Sit-to-Stand Test or a 5 Times Sit-to-Stand Test. Testing procedures and norms for various age groups or persons with various diseases are located in the American Physical Therapy Association Test and Measures link found in the Suggested Resources section at the end of this chapter.

## Normal Gait, Gait Deviations, and Interventions

The ability to walk is important for independence and quality of life. Normal walking allows efficient movement from place to place, requiring less energy expenditure than the use of an abnormal gait pattern. Normal gait patterns require joint integrity, joint mobility, muscle flexibility and strength, motor control, and balance. Normal walking incorporates forward propulsion and a smooth transfer of weight from one lower extremity to the other.

Health conditions such as osteoarthritis, Parkinson disease, stroke, and lower extremity amputation(s) can affect a patient's gait mechanics, making it difficult to walk normally. Pain, muscle tightness, and muscle weakness can also contribute to abnormal gait patterns. Understanding normal gait mechanics and abnormal gait compensations allows the assistant to select specific treatment interventions (stretching, strengthening, or neuromuscular facilitation or inhibition techniques) to improve patient functional mobility and to correct pathological gait patterns.

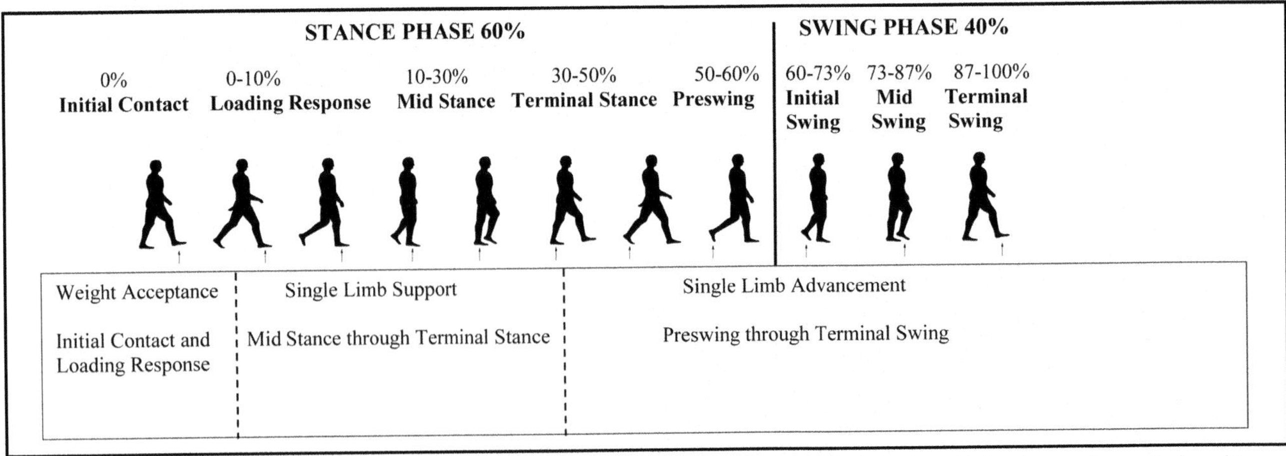


**Figure 7-14.** The gait cycle on the right leg. Note that double-limb support occurs twice on one limb (at the initial contact and preswing), making up about 20% of the stance phase (Carboxylase/Shutterstock.com).

## Box 7-2

### Gait Cycle Periods

**Stance Phase**

Initial contact (heel strike): When the foot hits the floor (preferably the heel) as the other foot is in preswing. (Double-limb support is occurring.)

Loading response (foot flat): Occurs as the foot absorbs the shock until it is flat on the floor.

Midstance: Occurs as the body moves over the supported limb into a single-leg stance.

Terminal stance (heel off): Occurs as the heel lifts off the floor in preparation to push off.

Preswing (toe off): From toe off of the stance leg with initial contact of the opposite leg. A transfer of weight during this phase as double-limb support occurs again.

**Swing Phase**

Initial swing (acceleration): When the foot leaves the floor and the swinging foot is even with the foot on the stance side.

Midswing: Occurs at the end of the initial swing until the tibia is vertical. This corresponds to midstance on the opposite leg.

Terminal swing (deceleration): The final swing phase. This period begins at the point of a vertical tibia and ends immediately before the initial contact (or heel strike).

Locomotion activities can take place in a variety of environments. The clinician may initiate training in the parallel bars on a smooth surface (floor) and/or progress onto compliant surfaces (on carpet or outside on grass/sand), up/down curbs or stairs, ramps, or on a treadmill. Body weight support systems can assist patients to move with less fear.

## *Normal Phases of the Gait Cycle*

There are 2 terminology systems used to describe the phases of the **gait cycle**: Ranchos Los Amigos and traditional. One gait cycle is the period from ipsilateral heel strike to ipsilateral heel strike. The gait cycle has 2 general phases: the stance phase and the swing phase (Figure 7-14). The stance phase occurs when the foot is in contact with the ground, and the swing phase occurs when the limb is off the ground. Approximately 60% to 62% of the gait cycle occurs in the stance phase and 38% to 40% in the swing phase.[19-24] There are also periods when a double stance period occurs (both legs are in contact with the ground).

The 2 phases are further broken down into 8 periods (or subphases) of the gait cycle. Ranchos Los Amigos describes the subphases of the gait cycle as follows (traditional terms are identified in parentheses): the stance phase includes the initial contact (heel strike), loading response (foot flat), midstance (midstance), terminal stance (heel off), and preswing (toe off), and the swing phase includes the initial swing (acceleration), midswing (midswing), and terminal swing (deceleration).[19-21] Box 7-2 provides descriptions of each subphase.

Normal walking includes the patient's ability to demonstrate (1) prepositioning of the foot/ankle at the initial contact, (2) general stability during the stance phase, (3) the ability to clear the foot when progressing from the preswing through the swing phase, (4) taking an adequate step with each leg, and (5) energy conservation with walking.[24]

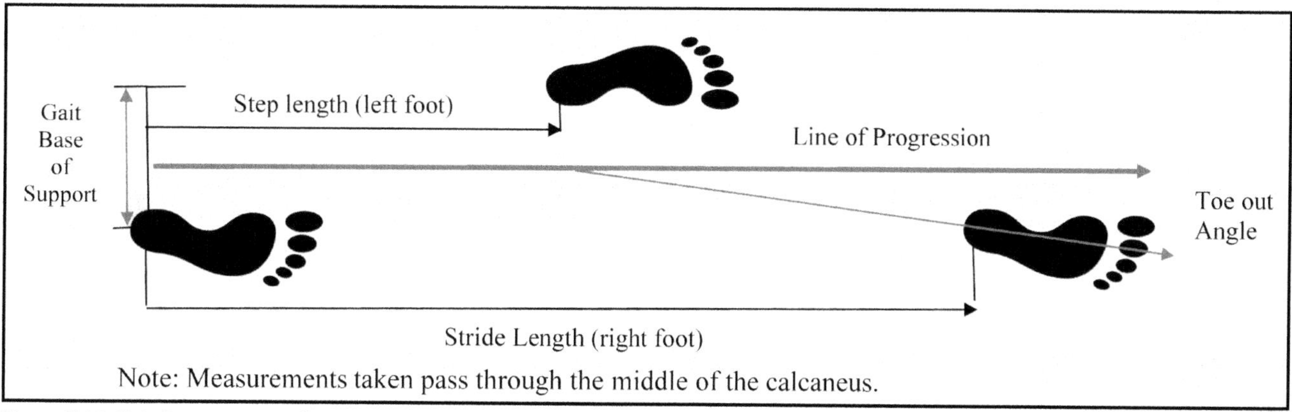


**Figure 7-15.** Gait distance terminology.

## Box 7-3

### The Parameter Descriptions During Gait

Cadence: The number of steps per minute (average is 90 to 120 steps per minute)[19]

Speed: Distance/time. The velocity of the gait (average about 3 miles per hour). Velocity depends on cadence and stride length.[19,24]

Swing time: The time one leg spends during the swing phase of the gait cycle.

Stance time: The amount of time spent standing on one leg. If there is increased stance time on one leg, there is a decrease in the swing time on the opposite leg.

Double-limb support time: The amount of time that both feet are on the ground. As gait speed decreases, double-limb support time increases. There is no double-limb support when running.

## Common Gait Cycle Distance and Time Parameters

The gait cycle can be described in terms of time and distance. Distance parameters (Figure 7-15) include step length and stride length. Step length is the distance from the heel strike of one foot (ipsilateral) to the heel of the other foot (contralateral), and stride length is the distance from the heel of one foot to the heel of the same foot (ipsilateral heel strike to ipsilateral heel strike). These parameters can highlight variations from normal (ie, if a step length is not equal to the opposite foot in terms of distance). The patient's gait BOS during walking/running is the distance widthwise between 2 feet. A normal gait BOS width during normal walking is about 2 to 4 in (~5-10 cm). The clinician observes the BOS to see if the patient's feet are too close together or too far apart when they are walking.

The time parameters used to describe gait include cadence, speed, stance time, swing time, and double-limb support (Box 7-3). If a patient walks with an antalgic gait (a limp), there is a shorter stance time on the involved leg compared with the swing time (which is increased).

### Clinical Tip

Walking speed is an easy way to assess patient progress. The clinician can time a patient who is walking a predetermined distance. Walking speed tests ranging from 5 to 10 meters in length provide reliable results and are easy to administer in many settings.

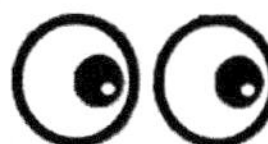

### Eye on the Research

Walking speed is a valid and reliable tool for assessing and monitoring functional status. It can be an indicator of overall health in a wide range of populations, and some researchers suggest it should be included as a "sixth vital sign." Walking speed is predictive for a range of outcomes, including the response to treatment, the risk of functional dependence, frailty, falls, mobility disability, institutionalization, cardiovascular-related events, and mortality. There are walking speed values associated with functional ability and walking speed predictive for mobility-related risks. A self-selected walking speed greater than 0.1 meters/second is associated with a healthy adult population with a lower risk of health events. A self-selected walking speed less than 0.6 meters/second is associated with an increased risk of functional and cognitive decline, institutionalization, and mortality.[25]

## Muscle Activation During Gait Cycle Tasks

During each gait cycle, 3 tasks occur: **weight acceptance,** single-limb support, and **limb advancement** (see Figure 7-14). Joints need to move through typical ROMs, and muscles must contract appropriately during each phase (Table 7-6) for normal walking to occur.

Weight acceptance occurs as body weight transfers onto one limb during the initial contact (heel strike) and the loading response (foot flat). This is a demanding task because the lower extremity is absorbing the shock associated with the ground reaction forces.

During the initial contact, the ankle is in neutral, the knee is extended, and the hip is flexed 25 degrees. The anterior tibialis, extensor hallucis, and extensor digitorum contract to maintain the neutral ankle position as the quadriceps and hamstrings control the knee position. The gluteus maximus contracts eccentrically to control the hip, preventing excess hip flexion.[23] To absorb shock efficiently during the loading response, the quadriceps eccentrically contract to control the knee as it flexes to 15 degrees. At the beginning of this phase, the gluteus maximus and adductor magnus isometrically contract so the hip remains in 25 degrees of flexion in the sagittal plane, and the gluteus medius isometrically contracts to prevent the pelvis from dropping in the frontal plane.[20] With the transition into the loading response, the ankle rapidly moves into 10 degrees of plantar flexion controlled by a strong eccentric contraction of the dorsiflexors.

The beginning of midstance through terminal stance (deceleration) is called *single-limb support*. A fixed foot supports the lower extremity as the body progresses forward.[20] During single-limb support, the hip, pelvis, and trunk need to be stable because motion is limited in the sagittal and frontal planes. Sufficient ankle dorsiflexion ROM is needed so the tibia can move anteriorly as body weight is shifted toward the forefoot.

During midstance, the ankle moves from a slightly plantar flexed position to 10 degrees of dorsiflexion by the end of this period, and motion is primarily controlled by an eccentric contraction of the soleus. Gastrocnemius, posterior tibialis, flexor hallucis longus, flexor digitorum longus, and peroneus (fibularis) longus and brevis also eccentrically contract to control dorsiflexion,[20,23] whereas the knee fully extends and the tibia becomes more vertical as the body continues its forward progression. There is minimal quadriceps activity because of the LoG falling vertically through the lower extremity.[20,23] Forces occurring at the hip are the greatest during midstance because a lateral shifting (about 2 cm) of the body over the leg occurs. During this time, the gluteus medius on the stance leg contracts to prevent a pelvic drop on the contralateral leg during the swing phase. The gluteus maximus is active to provide hip stability during slow walking, and it becomes significantly more active (concentrically contracting) with a faster pace or walking up an incline.[24]

During terminal stance, the heel raises off the ground as the body weight shifts over the metatarsal heads. Initially, the knee is extended, and the ankle moves from 10 degrees of dorsiflexion to 5 degrees of plantar flexion by the end of this period. The soleus and toe flexors continue to contract eccentrically to control ankle dorsiflexion as the tibia moves forward in preparation for heel rise at the beginning of terminal stance. During late terminal stance and early preswing, the plantar flexor muscles begin to concentrically contract to propel the lower extremity forward as the posterior tibialis and peroneal muscles stabilize the ankle joint.[19,23] The hip passively moves to about 10 degrees of hyperextension by the end of this phase. No active hip extension or hip abduction occurs at this point.[22]

By the end of preswing (heel off), the limb completes 20 degrees of passive ankle plantar flexion and 40 degrees of knee flexion as momentum moves the body forward. As this motion occurs, the stance leg becomes less stable in preparation for the initial swing phase.[23] The hip moves to neutral from its hyperextended position as the iliopsoas and rectus femoris contract.[20] At this point, the metatarsal phalangeal joints are extended about 60 degrees.

Preswing (heel off), initial swing (toe off), midswing, and terminal swing (deceleration) make up the final task of the gait cycle called *swing limb advancement*.[23] During this task, there is a transition from unloading the foot during preswing to allowing foot clearance to occur as the limb moves into the swing phases of the gait cycle. There is a quick transfer of weight from the preswing (heel off) limb to the opposite limb, which is moving into the initial contact (heel strike). Because both feet are on the ground simultaneously, double stance occurs.

Most energy expenditure (or acceleration) occurs during the last 2 stance phases. During the swing phases, less energy is expended because momentum advances the leg.[20] During the initial swing (toe off) period, the hip moves from neutral at the end of preswing to quickly flexing 20 degrees as the iliopsoas concentrically contracts with assistance from the adductor longus, gracilis, and sartorius.[23] The knee flexes to approximately 60 degrees, creating foot clearance. This is achieved mostly because of the momentum and is assisted by the biceps femoris (short head), gracilis, and sartorius.[23] The ankle dorsiflexors and toe extensors contract to move the ankle from 20 degrees of plantar flexion to neutral dorsiflexion, initiating foot clearance at the end of preswing.[20,23] Foot clearance is also dependent on the amount of hip and knee flexion that is achieved.

By midswing, when the maximal amount of active hip flexion of 30 degrees is reached, the hamstrings quickly eccentrically contract to decelerate hip flexion. There is a passive extension of the knee to 30 degrees by the end of midswing as a result of momentum as the leg continues to move forward. At this point, the tibia is vertical, the ankle is in neutral, and the dorsiflexors concentrically contract to maintain dorsiflexion.

**Table 7-6**

Muscle Involvement and Tasks During the Phases of the Gait Cycle

| | Initial Contact | Loading Response | Midstance | Terminal Stance | Preswing | Initial Swing | Midswing | Terminal Swing |
|---|---|---|---|---|---|---|---|---|
| Hip Muscles | Gluteus maximus (E), hamstrings (E) | Gluteus maximus (C), hamstrings (C) | Gluteus maximus (C), iliopsoas (E), gluteus medius (E) to prevent pelvic drop on OKC side | Psoas (E) | Psoas (E), rectus femoris (E) | Psoas (C), adductor longus (C) | Psoas (C) | |
| Knee Muscles | Quadriceps (E) | Quadriceps (E initially but C at foot flat) | | Gastrocnemius (C) to initiate knee flexion | | Gracilis (C), sartorius (C) | Hamstrings (E) | Hamstrings (E), quadriceps (C) |
| Ankle/Foot Muscles | Dorsiflexors (C) | Dorsiflexors (E) to slow plantar flexion | Plantar flexors (E) | Initially soleus and toe flexors (E), but C at end of the phase | Plantar flexors (C) until foot leaves the floor | Dorsiflexors (C), toe extensors (C) | Dorsiflexors (C) | Dorsiflexors (I) |
| **Tasks** | | | | | | | | |
| | Weight acceptance | Weight acceptance | Single-leg Stance | Single-leg stance | Limb advancement | Limb advancement | Limb advancement | Limb advancement |

C=concentric contraction; E=eccentric contraction; I=isometric contraction; OKC=open kinetic chain.

The limb advancement task ends with terminal swing, which occurs just before weight acceptance and the initial contact (heel strike). By the end of this period, the knee should be extended and the ankle positioned correctly for the calcaneus to touch down. During this period, the limb decelerates as the hamstrings continue eccentrically contracting to slow hip flexion (to 25 to 30 degrees), preventing knee hyperextension. Knee extension to neutral occurs as the quadriceps are active, and ankle neutral is maintained with isometric dorsiflexion in preparation for the initial contact.[20]

### Other Important Movement Considerations During Normal Walking

During normal walking, the body moves up and down in the sagittal plane in a rhythmic fashion. The highest point occurs during midstance, and the lowest point occurs during double-limb support (preswing and initial contact). There is about a 2-in vertical displacement between the highest and lowest points.[22]

Pelvic motion occurring about the hip is important to observe during normal walking. The largest displacement of the center of mass laterally occurs toward the midstance limb as the contralateral limb is in midswing. During midstance, there is a slight hip adduction on the stance phase side controlled by the hip abductors on that limb. The gluteus medius on the stance limb contracts to control the pelvis to ensure a minimal pelvic drop on the swing phase side. The paraspinals, latissimus dorsi, and quadratus lumborum muscles are active on the swing phase side to resist downward movement of the pelvis. Normal pelvic rotation occurs in the transverse plane; this contributes to step length during swing limb advancement. During terminal stance, the pelvis is posteriorly positioned, and the hip is externally rotated. From this point through terminal swing, the pelvis then rotates forward as the fixed femur internally rotates during the weight acceptance phase.[22]

## Common Gait Deviations

Patients may display abnormal gait patterns for numerous reasons, including lower extremity injury, muscle weakness, contractures, or other pathologies. Patients create subconscious compensations as they walk to accommodate for pain or weakness. Common gait deviations occur as a result of orthopedic causes. For example, a gluteus maximus gait pattern (or gluteal lurch) is a result of gluteus maximus muscle weakness, and the patient will demonstrate a posterior trunk lean during weight acceptance. A compensated or uncompensated Trendelenburg gait results from a weak gluteus medius muscle. When a patient leans their trunk over the weak lower extremity during stance phase, they are compensating for the pain/weakness of the muscle. However, when the patient displays a pelvic drop on the open kinetic side during the swing phase, they have not compensated for gluteus medius pain/weakness on the (closed chain) stance phase limb.

A circumducted gait pattern occurs during the swing phase as a result of a leg length discrepancy, decreased knee ROM, or hip flexor or dorsiflexor weakness in the swinging limb. A vaulting gait pattern occurs when the ankle, in a **single-limb stance** phase, excessively plantar flexes to create foot clearance for the limb in the swing phase. This can result from a leg length discrepancy, decreased knee ROM, or hip flexor or dorsiflexor weakness in the swinging limb. A hip hike gait results from weak hip flexors and is observed when the pelvis on the weak side hikes upward (the quadratus lumborum contracts) during the swing phase. Knee buckling or excessive hip flexion in weight acceptance (or forward lurch) is commonly caused by quadriceps weakness. Quadriceps weakness can also result in genu recurvatum during the loading response. An antalgic gait results from pain with weight bearing and is characterized by a decreased stance time on the affected limb.

Gait deviations commonly noted in patients with a neurologic diagnosis include a scissoring gait, festinating gait, hemiplegic gait, cerebellar ataxia, foot slap, and steppage gait. A scissoring gait is characterized by the affected limb crossing the midline; this is often observed in patients with spasticity (ie, cerebral palsy) with lower extremity limb flexion, increased hip adductor tone, and decreased neuromuscular control. A festinating gait is associated with Parkinson disease and is characterized by small shuffling steps, a narrow BOS, and an anterior trunk lean (shifting their center of gravity forward, creating an anterior momentum).

Changes in gait patterns can also occur as a result of the aging process. Geriatric gait deviations may include slow cadence, decreased step length, shuffling gait (increased double stance time), decreased heel strike (during the initial contact), decreased push-off during terminal swing and preswing, and a posterior pelvic tilt posture.

The fear of falling contributes to the increased fall risk in older adults and can cause gait deviations. Increased double-limb support and a forward flexed posture are very common in this population. The ability to correct gait deviations can depend on a number of factors. One of the most important things that a physical therapist assistant can do is to display confidence in their intervention skills. Often, patients are more willing to be challenged when they trust the clinician. Begin with small challenges, and as successes are achieved, the patient will feel more confident with their abilities, and their fear of falling will decrease. When patients feel more stable with their standing and walking abilities, their confidence significantly increases (fear of falling decreases).

### *Interventions to Promote a Normal Gait Pattern*

Many gait deviations can be improved through stretching tight structures, strengthening weak ones (Table 7-7), and/or with balance training (refer to Chapter 8). Older adults tend to use their hip flexors instead of hip extensors when walking, so facilitating lower extremity extensor muscles can improve their gait mechanics and efficiency. The physical therapy team needs to determine the best treatment interventions to achieve a more normalized gait pattern.

**Table 7-7**

**Various Gait Deviations During the Gait Cycle: Causes and Treatment Suggestions by Body Segment**

| Body Segment | Deviation | Period of the Gait Cycle Occurrence | Cause/Signs | Treatment Suggestions |
|---|---|---|---|---|
| Trunk | Ipsilateral lean toward the stance side (compensated Trendelenburg; O) | Loading response ⇨ terminal stance | Gluteus medius weakness on the stance side, may be due to hip pain also | Strengthen gluteus medius (side lying, side stepping with/without resistance) |
| | Extension lean/gluteal lurch (E) | Initial contact ⇨ loading response | Gluteus maximus weakness (most common), hip flexor weakness or contracture (difficulty bringing swing leg through) | Stretch hip flexors and strengthen gluteus maximus prone or standing with/without resistance |
| | Crouch gait (N), common in cerebral palsy patients | | Excessive hip and knee flexion and plantar flexion during stance phase; hamstring contractures contribute to deviation | Lower extremity stretches |
| | Festinating gait, common in Parkinson disease (N) | | Patients have difficulty initiating gait, take small quick steps, and have difficulty stopping | Rhythmic weight shifting, lower extremity stretching, and work on taking longer steps on both legs |
| Pelvis | Pelvic drop on OKC side during swing phase (uncompensated Trendelenburg; O) | Drop on uninvolved side when involved side is in stance phase | Gluteus medius weakness on the stance side | Strengthen gluteus medius (ie, side lying, side stepping with/without resistance) |
| | Hip hiking of the pelvis on open chain side; ipsilateral lean on closed chain side (compensated Trendelenburg; O) | Loading response ⇨ terminal stance | Gluteus medius weakness on the stance side | Strengthen gluteus medius (ie, side lying, side stepping with/without resistance) |
| | Hip hiking unrelated to gluteus medius weakness | Swing phase | Hip/knee flexor and ankle dorsiflexion weakness on OKC side or decreased hip/knee ROM | May also need to strengthen hip/knee flexors/dorsiflexion and stretch quadratus lumborum |
| Hip | Scissor or diplegic gait (N), common in cerebral palsy patients | Swing phase; narrow BOS with toe drag | Hip adductor spasticity | Stretch hip adductors and strengthen hip abductors |
| | Ataxic (cerebellar lesions; N) | | Poor balance and staggering uncoordinated gait | Work on balance issues (refer to Chapter 8) |
| | Circumducted gait pattern (E) | Swing phase | Swings leg out to the side to compensate for weak hip flexors and/or knee flexors | Strengthen hip adductors and hip/knee flexors and stretch hip abductors |

*(continued)*

**Table 7-7 (continued)**

Various Gait Deviations During the Gait Cycle: Causes and Treatment Suggestions by Body Segment

| Body Segment | Deviation | Period of the Gait Cycle Occurrence | Cause/Signs | Treatment Suggestions |
|---|---|---|---|---|
| Upper leg | Forward lean of trunk (E) | Initial contact ⇨ midstance | Quadriceps weakness | Strengthen quadriceps |
| | Knee hyperextension (genu recurvatum; E) | Terminal swing ⇨ midstance | Poor hamstring control or weakness and quadriceps paralysis or Plantar flexion contracture | Strengthen hamstrings eccentrically, strengthen quadriceps, and stretch plantar flexion |
| Lower leg/ foot | Drop foot (E) | Initial contact (forefoot contacts the floor first) | Plantar flexion contracture or dorsiflexion weakness; can also be due to compensatory heel pain or shorter leg on involved side | Stretch plantar flexion, strengthen dorsiflexion, and issue orthotic |
| | Foot slap (E) | Loading response | Lack of control of ankle plantar flexion due to tibialis anterior muscle weakness | Strengthen dorsiflexion |
| | Foot slap (E) | Initial contact (excessive hip flexion then quickly extends knee at terminal swing) | Commonly a peripheral nerve involvement (deep peroneal nerve) or other neurologic conditions | Strengthen dorsiflexion and/or patient to wear ankle-foot orthosis |

E=either orthopedic or neurologic; N=neurologic reason; O=orthopedic reason may be due to ROM limitations or muscle weakness.

Interventions that target common deficits include lower quarter stretching (ie, calf, hamstring, and hip flexor stretches). Strengthening exercises may include resistance exercises that target the gluteus maximus and medius, knee extensors, and ankle dorsiflexors. The most appropriate exercises are determined based on the type of abnormal gait pattern (and its cause) and which phase(s) of the gait cycle the deviation appears. Exercises to target the lower extremity muscles are discussed in Chapter 13.

The clinician can incorporate other techniques, such as resisted walking, to help patients normalize their gait. Resisted walking facilitates contraction of the hip extensor muscles during the loading response and midstance and the ankle plantar flexors at the end of terminal stance and the beginning of preswing. When performing resisted walking, the physical therapist assistant carefully places their hand on the patient's sternum, just below the sternal notch with the thumb and index fingers just below the clavicles, as seen in Figure 7-16. Be extremely careful if the patient is osteoporotic. Instruct the patient to stand up straight and tell them to "Lean into my hand as if you are walking against a strong wind." As the patient takes each step, instruct them to push with their legs and feet. Maintain steady resistance. The neuromuscular system should respond to the resistance and help correct the step length and speed. The clinician can incorporate cues, equipment, and resistance. Instructing the patient to walk with a purpose can facilitate longer steps and increase gait speed. Verbal cues (ie, "heel, toe, away we go") can encourage the patient to make heel contact with the ground first. Facilitate arm swing with cues during resisted walking (the patient may automatically initiate reciprocal arm swing as they push against your resistance). If that does not occur, use 2 poles (one in each hand) to facilitate reciprocal arm swing (Figure 7-17).

## Devices That Can Assist Patients to Improve Walking Mechanics

Patients with some orthopedic conditions are prescribed weight-bearing restrictions by their physician to protect a surgical (ie, implant) or injury (ie, fracture) site and to facilitate tissue healing. Physical therapist assistants can train patients to adhere to limited weight bearing when walking. Common ways to educate patients so they comply with maintaining the prescribed weight-bearing status include tactile feedback and scales (ie, to determine the specific number of pounds allowed on the injured leg). Patients must understand what it feels like to bear the appropriate amount of weight on their involved extremity. Unfortunately, these methods are not effective when converting static weight-bearing status to walking.[25]

Biofeedback devices and force plates are more accurate at providing patients constant feedback on weight-bearing status when walking. Portable biofeedback devices are available. Sensors are placed inside the patient's shoe and connected to a small portable device. F-Scan (Tekscan Inc) and SmartStep (Andante Medical Devices) devices have been shown to be reliable and valid in their accuracy and effectiveness in improving patient compliance with maintaining appropriate weight-bearing status.[26,27]

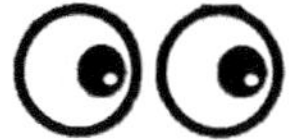

### Eye on the Research: Body Weight–Supported Treadmill Training and Robotic-Assisted Gait Training

Body weight–supported treadmill training can be used as part of a rehabilitation program for patients with neurologic conditions (ie, spinal cord injury, stroke, or traumatic brain injury) to help normalize walking and increase endurance. A harness is suspended on a track from the ceiling or from a metal frame positioned over a treadmill. Body weight–supported treadmill training often requires more than one therapist; one to assist the patient with foot placement and another to facilitate pelvic weight shifting. The support system allows the clinician to increase weight bearing on the lower extremities (as a percentage of body weight) as the patient improves their ability to maintain an upright posture and balance.

A 2018 single-blind randomized controlled pilot study completed on patients who were status poststroke compared 3 treatment groups: an isolated body weight–supported treadmill training group (45 minutes twice a week), a combined training group (included conventional therapy 5 days a week along with body weight–supported treadmill training for 45 minutes twice a week), and a conventional training group (for 5 days a week). The combined training group had significantly better outcomes in balance, mobility, and fear of falling compared with the other groups. The body weight–supported treadmill training group (performed at a lower intensity of exercise) was as effective as the conventional training group performing at a higher intensity.[28]

Robotic-assisted walking devices (Figure 7-18) have a weight support system but also have foot plates that are automated and can move the patient's legs independently without clinician assistance. This allows for more gait consistency and longer repetitive practice periods compared with clinician-assisted gait training with body weight–supported treadmill training. The ability to accurately control other variables, such as gait speed and step length, and to normalize joint movements during the gait cycle provides crucial feedback (ie, movement quality and muscle activity) for spinal cord input and output.[29]

A 2017 Cochrane review of (electromechanical) robotic-assisted training for walking after a stroke concluded that patients who received this type of gait training along with physical therapy were more likely to walk independently than those patients who participated in gait training without electromechanical assistance. Those patients who were not able to walk in the first 3 months after a stroke appeared to benefit the most from this intervention.[30]

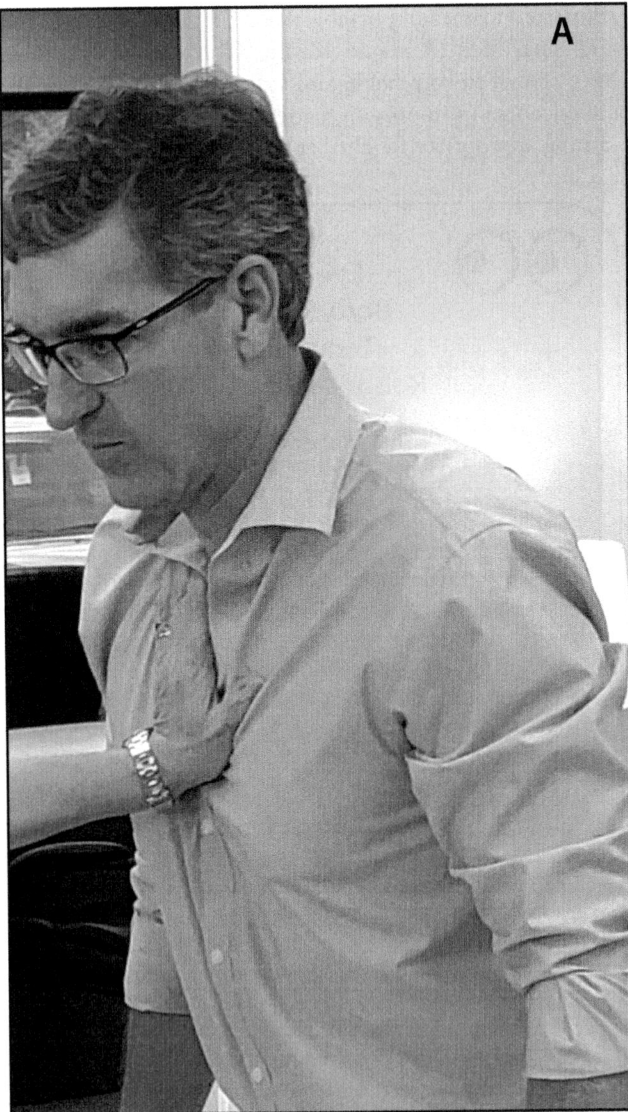

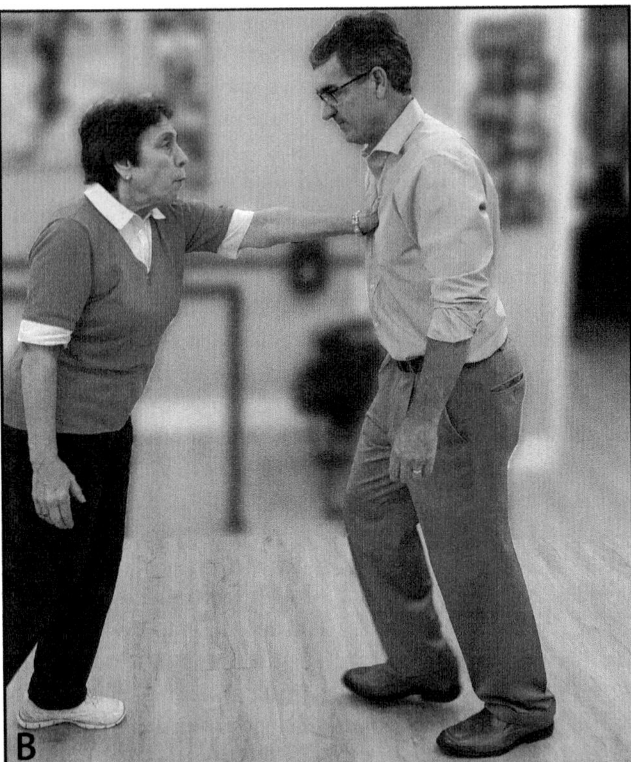

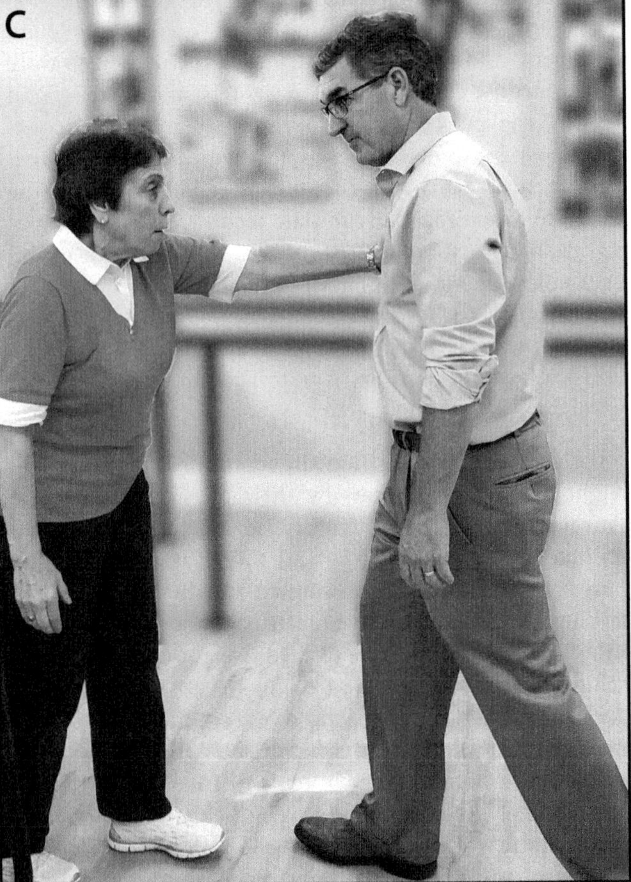

**Figure 7-16.** (A) Hand placement for resisted walking. (B) Start from a standing position; instruct the patient to take a step as the clinician provides resistance. (C) Resisted walking encourages the patient to use hip extensors and plantar flexors to improve gait mechanics.

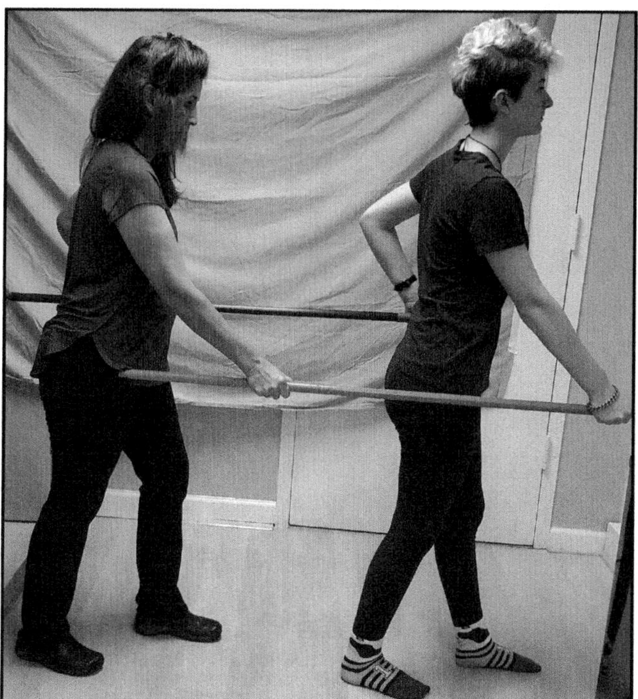

**Figure 7-17.** The clinician stands behind the patient to facilitate reciprocal arm swing.

Robotic technology continues to advance, and more portable rigid exoskeleton (external braces that are battery operated and computer driven) devices are now available; these may increase patient independence and quality of life.

## *Common Balance and Gait Tests*

Physical therapist assistants use various tests to assess gait and balance because these tools provide objective data that can be used to determine a patient's baseline status and to track patient progress. The physical therapist will typically assess a patient's static and dynamic balance, functional balance reactions, and gait. The Berg Balance Scale, Sit-to-Stand Test, the 10-Meter Walk Test, and the Timed Up and Go (TUG) Test are tools that are used in both inpatient and outpatient clinical environments. These tests have normative values, and many have thresholds or cutoff scores to determine a patient's risk for falling. The assistant should be able to perform these tests with good inter-rater reliability with the evaluating therapist.

The TUG assesses a patient's ability to move from sitting to standing, walk, and return to sitting. A score greater than 30 seconds indicates a patient has a significant mobility impairment and is at a high risk for falling. For frail patients or patients with disabilities, scores of 11 to 20 seconds are considered acceptable.[31]

Faster walking speeds have been associated with a decreased fall rate and increased survival rate in older adults.[32,33] Because gait speeds of older adults tend to be slower than younger adults, including a timed walking test is important to assess function.[34] The 10-Meter Walk Test is a quick and easy way to determine a patient's gait speed.

Other assessment tools that physical therapist assistants may find useful include the Tinetti Performance-Oriented Mobility Test, dual-task tests (Walking While Talking test), and the Functional Gait Assessment.

### Documentation Tip

Include interpretation of the clinical significance of balance/functional test results in the assessment portion of your note. Include a concise description of the impact of the treatment interventions on the patient's previous vs current performance and on long-term functional outcomes. For example, if a patient's TUG performance was assessed, the following information could be noted in the patient's documentation.

O: TUG completed with the use of rolling walker with close supervision in 20 seconds. No loss of balance.

A: Patient's TUG score has improved from 60 seconds at physical therapy evaluation. Patient has improved and regained ability to ambulate to/from bathroom with supervision (from minimal assist at evaluation). TUG score continues to indicate increased fall risk. Balance and gait training continues to promote progress to long-term goal and to return patient to their prior level of function (independent ability to toilet and independent ambulation community level with rolling walker).

P: Progress gait training activities per physical therapist's POC and include timed gait speed tasks with cues for increased cadence and ambulation endurance activities. Per physical therapist's POC, progress to advanced standing dynamic balance tasks, including dual-task activities that address functional demands of community-level ambulation.

## Conclusion

Physical therapist assistants will participate in postural and gait assessments. Recognizing faulty postural positioning and gait patterns allows the assistant to determine which body structures are likely weak or tight. The assistant will use that knowledge to develop and implement treatment plans that target these weak/tight structures. Appropriate stretching and strengthening interventions, when paired with postural retraining, transfer, and gait training, will improve patient function and independence.

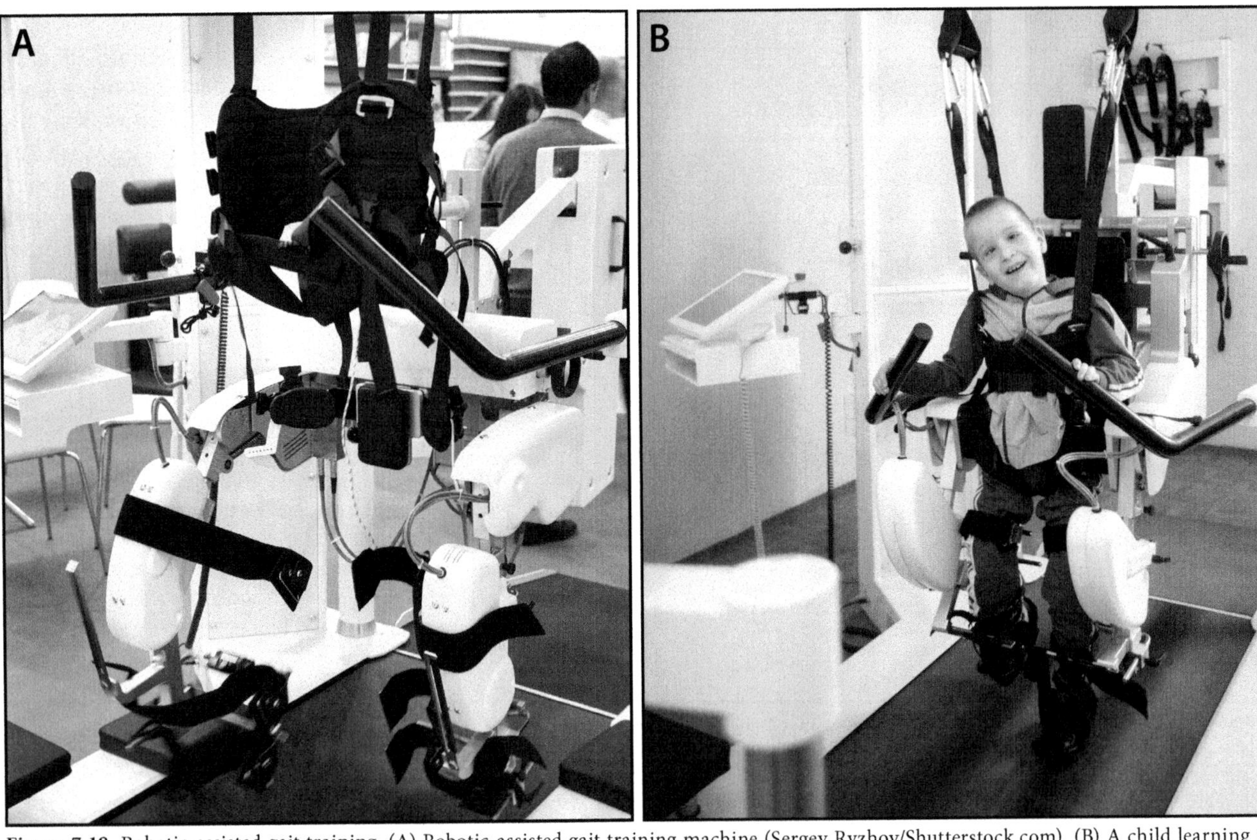


**Figure 7-18.** Robotic-assisted gait training. (A) Robotic-assisted gait training machine (Sergey Ryzhov/Shutterstock.com). (B) A child learning to walk using an assisted gait training robotic machine (Olesia Bilkei/Shutterstock.com).

## Review Questions

1. List 2 contributing factors that can cause faulty posture.
2. Where should the plumb line fall indicating normal standing posture when observing a patient from the side?
3. From a posterior view, the physical therapist assistant notices the patient's head is laterally flexed to the right with a rotation to the left. Which muscles could cause this deviation? Which muscle needs to be stretched, and which muscle needs to be strengthened?
4. When observing a patient's posture from a lateral view, the patient displays an anterior pelvic tilt with an increased lumbar lordosis and protruding abdomen. Which muscles are likely responsible for creating these deviations?
5. If a patient has right thoracic scoliosis, which muscles should the physical therapist assistant expect to be tight? What exercises would strengthen the weak muscles?
6. What could cause a patient to have a forward trunk lean during the loading response?
7. A person has left gluteus maximus weakness. Name and describe the gait pattern(s) a physical therapist assistant would expect to see. List one open and closed kinetic exercise that would address this weakness.
8. Describe 3 interventions/techniques that an assistant can implement to improve a patient's sit-to-stand transfer.
9. What is cadence? What is the clinical significance of a very slow walking speed?
10. Which gait deviations are likely to be present for a patient with anterior tibialis strength of 1/5?

## Case Study

A 72-year-old woman has been writing children's books for 30 years. The patient complains of neck and thoracic pain and is unable to sit and write for more than 1 hour before complaining that her pain is 7 out of 10. The patient reports difficulty reaching up into cabinets at eye level because of bilateral shoulder pain. The physical therapist's initial evaluation reveals forward head, increased kyphosis, protracted scapula, and shoulder internal rotation. A vertical compression test and elbow flexion test are both positive. The evaluation indicates muscle weakness in the abdominals, erector spinae, scapula retractors, shoulder external rotators, and deep neck flexors. The tight muscles include the suboccipital muscles, upper trapezius, levator scapulae, and pectoralis major and minor. The patient has a slow gait pattern with decreased step length and increased double stance time. The physical therapist assistant observes that the patient has diminished push off during terminal stance bilaterally.

1. Based on the patient's postural assessment and additional test results, select 2 stretching and 2 strengthening exercises for the involved muscles to improve posture and muscle balance.
2. Which muscles need to be strengthened to improve the patient's core stability (refer to Chapter 15 for assistance)? Provide one exercise to address local muscles and one to address global muscles.
3. Which muscles need strengthening to improve the patient's ability to push off during the terminal phase of the gait cycle? What exercise and intervention will help the patient improve her gait pattern?

## Suggested Resources

American Physical Therapy Association. Tests and Measures. 2022. Accessed January 26, 2023. https://www.apta.org/patient-care/evidence-based-practice-resources/test-measures

Postural Assessment Chart (Figure 7-19)

Saliba Johnson S. The Sabila Postural Classification System: a valid and reliable approach to improving functional alignment. Septmber 23, 2017. Accessed January 26, 2023. https://cdn.ymaws.com/www.tptatn.org/resource/resmgr/2017_Meetings/Fall/Handouts/Saliba_Postural_Outline.pdf

Shirley Ryan Ability Lab. Berg Balance Test. Updated June 30, 2020. Accessed January 26, 2023. https://www.sralab.org/rehabilitation-measures/berg-balance-scale

Shirley Ryan Ability Lab. Function in Sitting Test. Updated November 27, 2012. Accessed January 26, 2023. https://www.sralab.org/sites/default/files/2017-07/fist_score_sheet.pdf

Shirley Ryan Ability Lab. Functional Reach Test/Modified Functional Reach Test. Updated December 4, 2013. Accessed January 26, 2023. https://www.sralab.org/rehabilitation-measures/functional-reach-test-modified-functional-reach-test

Shirley Ryan Ability Lab. Tinetti Performance-Oriented Mobility Assessment. Updated January 31, 2014. Accessed January 26, 2023. https://www.sralab.org/rehabilitation-measures/tinetti-performance-oriented-mobility-assessment

Sitting Balance Assessment Tool: https://www.sralab.org/rehabilitation-measures/function-sitting-test

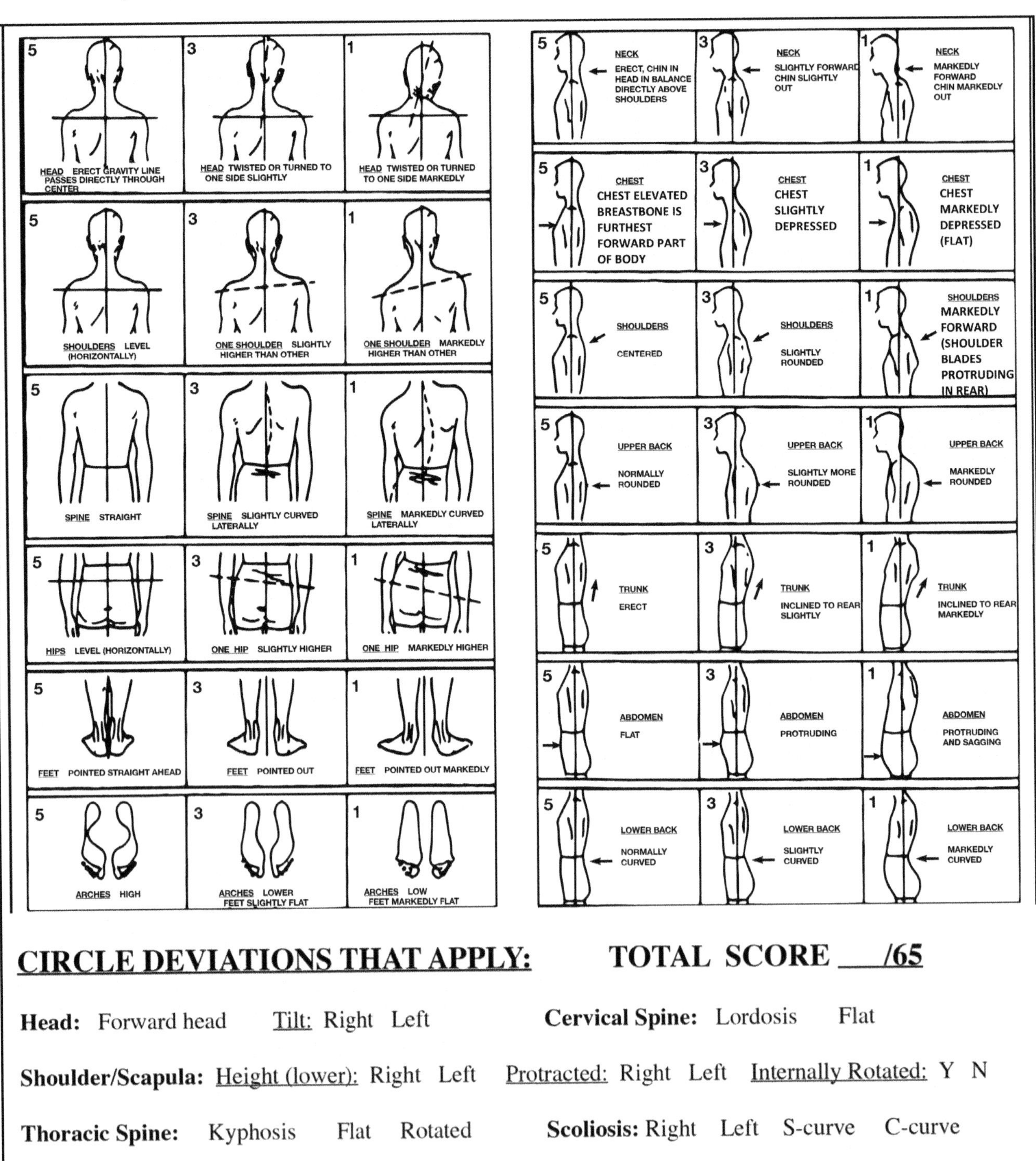


**CIRCLE DEVIATIONS THAT APPLY:** **TOTAL SCORE ___/65**

**Head:** Forward head Tilt: Right Left **Cervical Spine:** Lordosis Flat

**Shoulder/Scapula:** Height (lower): Right Left Protracted: Right Left Internally Rotated: Y N

**Thoracic Spine:** Kyphosis Flat Rotated **Scoliosis:** Right Left S-curve C-curve

**Pelvis:** Height (lower): Right Left Tilt: Ant Post **Lumbar Spine:** Lordotic Swayback Flat

**Knee(s):** Valgus Varus Recurvatum **Ankle (calcaneus):** Valgus Varus

**ADDITIONAL COMMENTS:**________________________________________

**Figure 7-19.** Postural assessment chart. (Both reproduced by permission of the State Education Department, The University of the State of New York, Albany, NY.)

# References


1. Kritz MF, Cronin J. Static posture assessment screen of athletes: benefits and considerations. *Strength Cond J.* 2008;30(5):18-27.
2. Novak CB. Upper extremity work-related musculoskeletal disorders: a treatment perspective. *J Orthop Sports Phys Ther.* 2004;34(10):628-637.
3. Tong TJ, Kong PW. Medial longitudinal arch development of children aged 7 to 9 years: longitudinal investigation. *Phys Ther.* 2016;96(8):1216-1224.
4. Hale JM, Doyle SM. Bowlegs and normal growth and development of the legs and knees. January 19, 2012. Accessed January 26, 2023. https://www.hss.edu/conditions_bowlegs-and-normal-growth-development-legs-knees.asp
5. Magee DJ. Assessment of posture. In: Magee DJ, ed. *Orthopedic Physical Assessment.* 6th ed. W.B. Saunders; 2014:1017-1053.
6. Batistão MV, Moreira RF, Coury H, Salasar LE, Sato TO. Prevalence of postural deviations and associated factors in children and adolescents: a cross-sectional study. *Fisioter Mov.* 2016;29(4):777-785.
7. Gillespie RM. The physical impact of computers and electronic game use on children and adolescents, a review of current literature. *Work.* 2002;3(18):249-259.
8. Dumas GA, Reid JG, Wolfe LA, Griffin MP, McGrath MJ. Exercise, posture, and back pain during pregnancy. *Clin Biomech (Bristol, Avon).* 1999;10(2):98-103.
9. Edmond S, Kiel D, Samelson E, Kelly-Hayes M, Felson D. Vertebral deformity, back symptoms, and functional limitations among older women: the Framingham Study. *Osteoporosis Int.* 2005;16(9):1086-1095.
10. Carter ND, Khan KM, McKay HA, et al. Community-based exercise program reduces risk factors for falls in 65- to 75-year-old women with osteoporosis: randomized controlled trial. *CMAJ.* 2002;167(9):997-1004.
11. Britnell S, Cole JV, Isherwood L, et al. Postural health in women: the role of physiotherapy. *J Obstet Gynaecol Can.* 2005;2(5):493-500.
12. Saliba VL, Johnson GS. *Back Education and Training.* The Institute of Physical Art Functional Manual Therapy; 2010;112-118.
13. Collins CK, Johnson VS, Godwin EM, Pappas E. The reliability and validity of the Saliba Postural Classification system. *J Man Manip Ther.* 2016;24(3):174-181. doi:10.1080/10669817.2016.1138599
14. Nijs J, Roussel N, Struyf F, Mottram S, Meeusen R. Clinical assessment of scapular positioning in patients with shoulder pain: state of the art. *J Manipulative Physiol Ther.* 2007;30:69-75.
15. Janssen GM, Bussmann HBJ, Stam HJ. Determinants of the sit-to-stand movement: a review. *Phys Ther.* 2002;82(9):866-879.
16. Gorman SL. *Function in Sitting Test (FIST) Training and Instruction Manual.* May 20, 2011. Accessed January 26, 2023. https://www.pogoe.org/sites/default/files/FIST%20Training%20Manual%20v1-5.pdf
17. Sitting balance assessment tool (SitBAT). Accessed January 26, 2023. www.pichealth.com/uploads/1/0/3/4/10347770/sitbat_sitting_balance_1-7-21.pdf
18. Kage V, Patel NY, Pai MP. To compare the effects of deep neck flexors strengthening exercise and McKenzie neck exercise in subjects with forward neck posture: a randomised clinical trial. *Int J Physiother Res.* 2016;4(2):1451-1458. doi:10.16965/ijpr.2016.117
19. Dutton M. Gait and posture analysis. In: Dutton M, ed. *Dutton's Orthopaedic Examination, Evaluation and Intervention.* 3rd ed. McGraw Hill; 2012:260-307.
20. Rose J, Gamble JG. Gait analysis: clinical decision making. In: Rose J, Gamble JG, eds. *Human Walking.* 3rd ed. Lippincott Williams & Wilkins; 2006:165-169.
21. Bogey P. Gait analysis. Accessed January 26, 2023. http://emedicine.medscape.com/article/320160-overview#a3
22. Perry J, Burnfield JM. Phases of gait. In: Perry J, Brunfield JM, eds. *Gait Analysis: Normal and Pathological Function.* 2nd ed. SLACK Incorporated; 2010:3-16.
23. Perry J, Burnfield JM. Total limb function and bilateral synergistic relationships. In: Perry J, Brunfield JM, eds. *Gait Analysis: Normal and Pathological Function.* 2nd ed. SLACK Incorporated; 2010:137-160.
24. Mansfield PJ, Neumann DA. Fundamentals of human gait. In: Mansfield PJ, Neumann DA, eds. *Essentials of Kinesiology for the Physical Therapist Assistant.* 2nd ed. Elsevier; 2014:344-360.
25. Middleton A, Fritz SL, Lusardi M. Walking speed: the functional vital sign. *J Aging Phys Act.* 2015;23(2):314-322. doi:10.1123/japa.2013-0236
26. Hustedt JW, Blizzard DJ, Baumgaertner MR, Leslie MP, Grauer JN. Current advances in training orthopaedic patients to comply with partial weight-bearing instructions. *Yale J Biol Med.* 2012;85(1):119-125.
27. Hustedt JW, Blizzard DJ, Baumgaertner MR, Leslie MP, Grauer JN. Is it possible to train patients to limit weight bearing on a lower extremity? *Orthopedics.* 2012;35(1):e31-e37. doi:10.3928/01477447-20111122-14
28. Mustafaoğlu R, Erhan B, Yeldan İ, Ersöz Hüseyinsinoğlu B, Gündüz B, Razak Özdinçler A. The effects of body weight-supported treadmill training on static and dynamic balance in stroke patients: a pilot, single-blind, randomized trial. *Turk J Phys Med Rehabil.* 2018;64(4):344-352. doi:10.5606/tftrd.2018.2672
29. Palmer E. Clinical review: gait training, robotic-assisted. January 5, 2018. Accessed January 26, 2023. https://www.ebscohost.com/assets-sample-content/RRC-Robotic-Assisted-Gait-Training-Clinical-Review.pdf
30. Mehrholz J, Thomas S, Werner C, Kugler J, Pohl M, Elsner B. Electromechanical-assisted training for walking after stroke. *Cochrane Database Syst Rev.* 2017;5:CD006185. doi:10.1002/14651858.CD006185.pub4
31. Schmitz, TJ, O'Sullivan SB. Examination of coordination and balance. In: O'Sullivan SB, Schmitz TJ, Fulk GD, eds. *Physical Rehabilitation.* 7th ed. FA Davis Company; 2019:188-219.
32. Ambrose AF, Paul G, Hausdorff JM. Risk factors for falls among older adults: a review of the literature. *Maturitas.* 2013;75(1):51-61.
33. Studenski S, Perera S, Patel K, et al. Gait speed and survival in older adults. *JAMA.* 2011;305(1):50-58. doi:10.1001/jama.2010.1923
34. Middleton A, Fritz SL, Lusardi M. Walking speed: the functional vital sign. *J Aging Phys Act.* 2015;23(2):314-322. doi:10.1123/japa.2013-0236

Chapter 8

# Balance Training and Vestibular Rehabilitation

*Karen A. Cascardi, PhD, MS, ATC, PTA and Jacki Klaczak Kopack, PT, DPT*

**KEY TERMS** Balance | Benign paroxysmal position vertigo | Epley maneuver or canal repositioning techniques | Limit of stability | Postural control | Vertigo

## Chapter Objectives

1. Describe the 3 systems that must provide input to allow normal balance reactions.
2. List the age-related changes that affect balance and that can affect the vestibular system.
3. Identify the intrinsic and extrinsic factors that increase fall risk.
4. Differentiate between the various vestibular tests and balance tests.
5. Explain the difference between vestibular rehabilitation and balance training.
6. Discuss the common treatment interventions used to treat patients with various types of **benign paroxysmal positional vertigo (BPPV)**.
7. Compare and contrast the vestibular interventions including adaptation, habituation, and substitution exercises.
8. Given patient-specific considerations, select the most appropriate balance or vestibular exercises appropriate for varied patient diagnoses.

Falls are one of the leading causes of mortality and morbidity in older adults.[1,2] In 2014 in the United States alone, about 27,000 people died after experiencing a fall, and 2.8 million adults 65 years and older were treated for fall-related injuries in hospital emergency departments.[1] According to the Centers for Disease Control and Prevention (CDC), direct Medicare costs related to falls are estimated at $31.3 billion; this is expected to increase by approximately 55% by 2030.[1]

There are numerous factors that increase fall risk. Intrinsic factors that affect fall risk include increased age, decreased strength, impaired gait or balance, visual impairments, cognitive changes, and the presence of neurologic and chronic diseases (ie, diabetes, cardiovascular, and Parkinson disease).[2] According to the CDC, the "rate of fall-related injuries for adults 85 and older was almost four times that for adults between 65 and 74 in the U.S."[2] The probability of falling increases with age and the presence of additional risk factors. Extrinsic factors include home and environmental issues (ie, slippery floors, throw rugs, low lighting, and inappropriate footwear) and medication usage. The side effects of several drugs can cause dizziness, and the number of medications (polypharmacy)



Kopack JK, Cascardi KA.
*Principles of Therapeutic Exercise for the Physical Therapist Assistant* (pp 161-196).

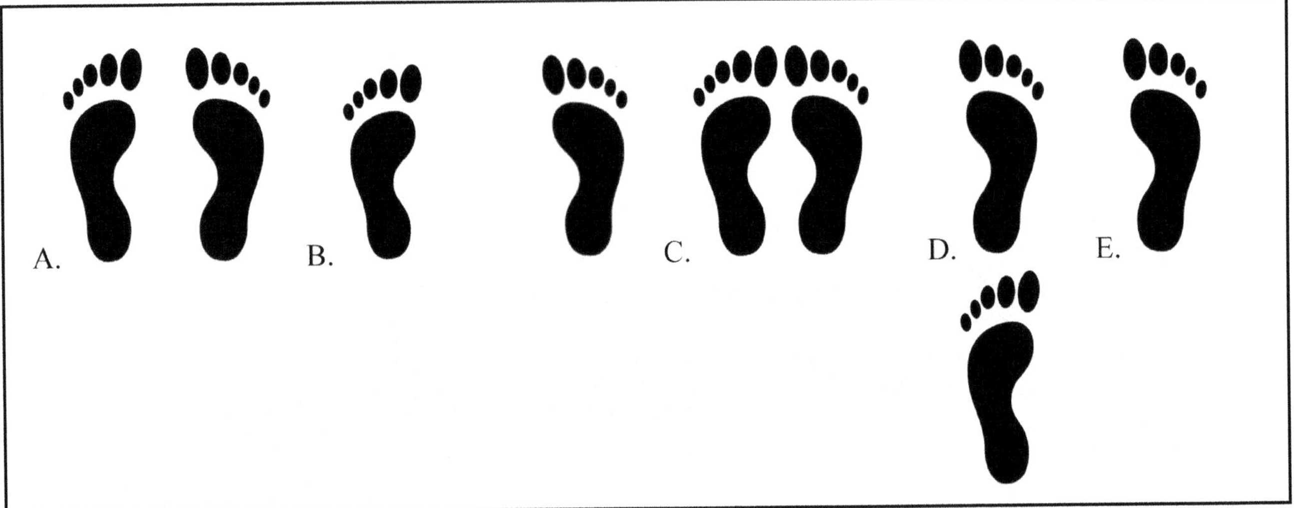


**Figure 8-1.** Varied BOS positions during standing. (A) Quiet stance, (B) wide BOS, (C) Romberg, (D) tandem or sharpened Romberg, and (E) single-leg stance.

older adults take can also increase the likelihood of falls. (Appendix E includes the side effects of commonly used medications.[2]) Vestibular disorders can cause dizziness, vertigo, and poor balance, which can increase fear of falling in older adults; the presence of these disorders is also a predictor for falling in active older adults.[3,4] Patients with vestibular disorders and/or fear of falling tend to reduce their normal activity and become more sedentary. These patients avoid turning their head, which may decrease participation in normal and/or recreational activities, leading to decreased strength, flexibility, and endurance and an increase in a fear of falling, reducing one's quality of life (QOL). Patients with postural deviations or unilateral lower extremity pain may be unaware of where their true center of balance is. These patients may increase weight bearing on the nonpainful limb side or stand with their weight shifted posteriorly (back on the heels); these compensatory postures can increase the risk of falling.

Exercise is an effective strategy for reducing falls in community-dwelling older adults.[4,5] Physical activities specifically designed to address a patient's deficit and level of fall risk are important when designing a program.[4] Weight-bearing exercises have been shown to improve both stepping reaction times and the 6-Minute Walk Test.[6] Current research indicates that fall prevention exercise programs are effective but that community implementation of these programs could be more collaborative in order to increase success.[7]

Vestibular rehabilitation therapy (VRT) and balance training are integral parts of physical therapy interventions for reducing falls and improving function. Physical therapist assistants must be able to understand the results of vestibular and balance tests that the physical therapist performs during the initial evaluation. The assistant may repeat these tests during the episode of care to determine patient progress. It is the assistant's responsibility to keep the physical therapist informed of any changes observed during treatment sessions.

## Balance and Postural Control

The goals of balance training and VRT include improving static and dynamic stability. Balance is achieved through integrated sensory input and motor output via the central nervous system (CNS). The physical therapy team considers sensory input, sensory integration, and musculoskeletal components when treating patients with balance deficits and/or vestibular diagnoses. After reviewing the physical therapy initial evaluation, the assistant selects interventions based on the patient's presentation and plan of care (POC) developed by the physical therapist. Interventions should gradually become more challenging based on patient progress with balance responses.

By definition, **balance** is the ability to maintain one's center of mass (COM) over a base of support (BOS).[8] **Postural control** is the ability to maintain one's body in a stable manner with normal alignment of the body segments and body under various conditions. The body must be able to respond to various challenges that arise from the environment and quickly make corrections. Maintaining postural control is crucial when performing tasks. Consider the following example: A patient wants to pick up a briefcase that weighs 10 pounds from the floor. The patient has to reach out of their BOS, leaning to the side and reaching down to grab the handle and then transitioning into an upright position. To perform this task, the patient uses sensory input (information from the visual, vestibular, and somatosensory systems) to create and modify the movements (motor output).

A person's BOS is the area where the body contacts the support surface in a given position. Figure 8-1 provides illustrations of various BOS positions during standing. **Limit of stability (LOS)** is the maximal sway angle from a vertical position in any given direction that can be achieved without loss of balance (LOB; Figure 8-2). The distance and the speed (velocity) at which a person can lean or sway about the ankles in any one direction is important, and

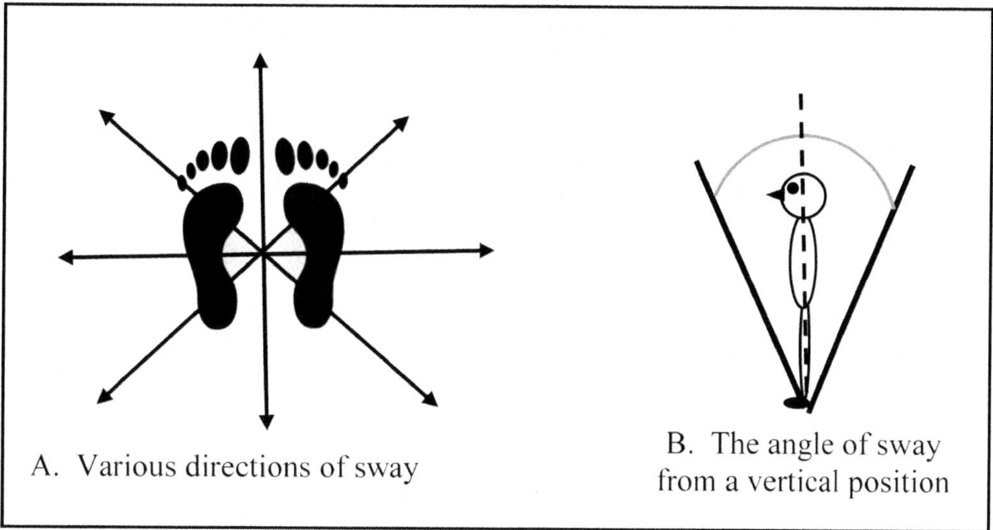


**Figure 8-2.** LOS.

**Table 8-1**

**Functional Balance Grades**[8]

| Grade | Description |
|---|---|
| Normal | Static: Patient maintains a steady balance without upper extremity support.<br>Dynamic: Patient accepts maximal challenge and can weight shift easily in all directions, maintaining balance at maximal limits of stability. |
| Good | Static: Patient maintains a steady balance without upper extremity support; limited observable sway.<br>Dynamic: Patient accepts moderate challenge; maintains balance while picking objects up off the floor. |
| Fair | Static: Patient maintains a steady balance with upper extremity support; may require occasional minimal assistance.<br>Dynamic: Patient accepts minimal challenge; maintains balance while turning head/trunk. |
| Poor | Static: Patient requires upper extremity support and moderate/maximal assistance to maintain balance.<br>Dynamic: Patient is unable to accept challenge or move without LOB. |

there are several factors that can affect one's LOS, including postural alignment, foot length, BOS width, body height, ankle flexibility, and strength.[8,9]

Normal functional mobility requires normal static postural control (or static balance) and dynamic postural control (or dynamic balance). Static balance is the ability to maintain one's balance when the body is at rest (ie, sitting or standing). Dynamic balance is the ability to maintain one's center of gravity (COG) over the BOS while other body parts are in motion (ie, weight shifting, reaching, bending, running, and walking).[9] The physical therapist assesses a patient's static and dynamic balance during the evaluation and then documents the patient's functional balance grades (Table 8-1). These grades describe balance in sitting, in normal standing (quiet stance), in Romberg (feet together), in tandem standing, or during single-leg standing. A minimal amount of muscle energy is required to maintain an upright position when individuals are able to sustain normal postural alignment.

To maintain upright posture (or COM over the BOS), the musculoskeletal system needs to respond quickly to various challenges. These musculoskeletal responses to a disturbance can vary from simple to complex, and the timing and intensity of the contractions will vary depending on the severity or size of the disturbance. There are 3 postural strategies that can be used to maintain balance (Table 8-2). The ankle strategy (Figure 8-3A) is very effective when responding to small balance disturbances. This strategy uses an anterior/posterior movement about the ankles; this strategy is critical for sensitive vestibular reactions. It uses a distal to proximal muscle activation pattern, and the head stays in line (or in phase) with the hips. A hip strategy (Figure 8-3B) allows for control of the body's COM during larger disturbances, when the BOS is small (ie, Romberg, sharpened Romberg, or single-leg standing), and/or when standing on a compliant surface (when an ankle strategy is inadequate to keep the body upright). When using this strategy, there is an anterior/posterior translation (flexion

**Table 8-2**

**Automatic Postural Strategies/Motor Strategies to Maintain Balance**

| Strategy | Perturbation | Muscle Activation |
|---|---|---|
| Ankle | Response to small or slow speed perturbations | Distal to proximal muscle activation.<br>• With perturbation in the anterior direction (from posterior), the gastrocnemius/soleus fires first (with support if needed from the hamstrings and then the paraspinals).<br>• With perturbation in the posterior direction (from anterior), the anterior tibialis fires first (with support if needed from the quadriceps and then the abdominals). |
| Hip | Response to larger/faster disturbance to COG or when standing with a smaller BOS | Proximal pattern of muscle activation. Based on the direction of perturbation or shift of COG, the abdominal muscles and hip flexors fire or paraspinals and hamstrings fire. If the shift of COG is lateral, the hip abductors will fire first. |
| Stepping | Response to very fast/large perturbations | Incorporates stepping as well as protective/reactive motions of upper extremities. |

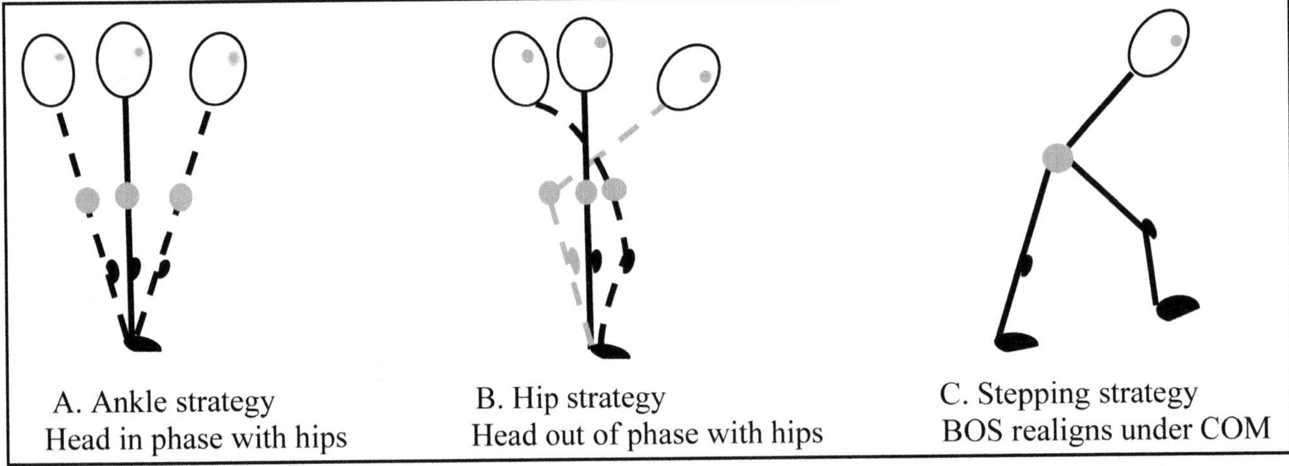


**Figure 8-3.** Postural strategies: Strategies used to maintain balance.

or extension) of the hips because a proximal to distal muscle activation pattern is used. The hip strategy is most effective with larger anterior/posterior or lateral disturbances. When larger disturbances occur, the head and hips move in opposite directions (or are out of phase) in order to restore balance. Ankle and hip strategies are considered in-place strategies. Older adults tend to rely more on hip strategies rather than ankle strategies, which can increase their risk for falls. Neuropathy and reduced ankle flexibility and/or weakness are some causes for increased reliance on the use of a hip strategy. A stepping strategy (Figure 8-3C) is used when the in-place strategies become ineffective, and one must take a step to prevent a fall. The disturbance is usually large and quick, requiring realignment of the BOS under the COM. If someone is standing behind you and pushes you unexpectedly, you would probably need to take a step forward to prevent falling. Postural malalignments (discussed in Chapter 7) can alter a patient's COM in a specific direction, which can increase the risk of falls and affect a patient's ability to perform tasks safely and efficiently.

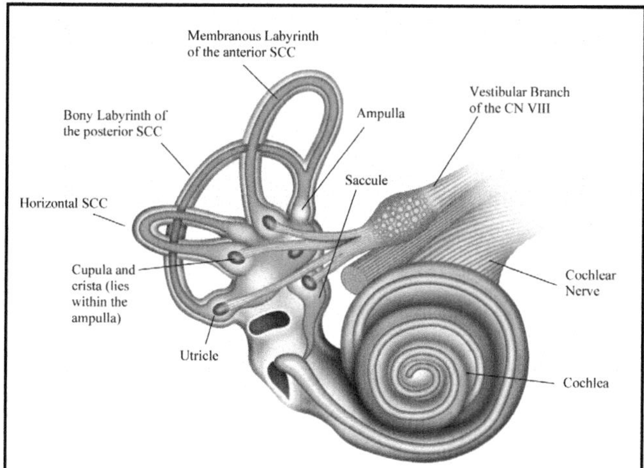


**Figure 8-4.** Peripheral vestibular system anatomy (ilusmedical/Shutterstock.com).

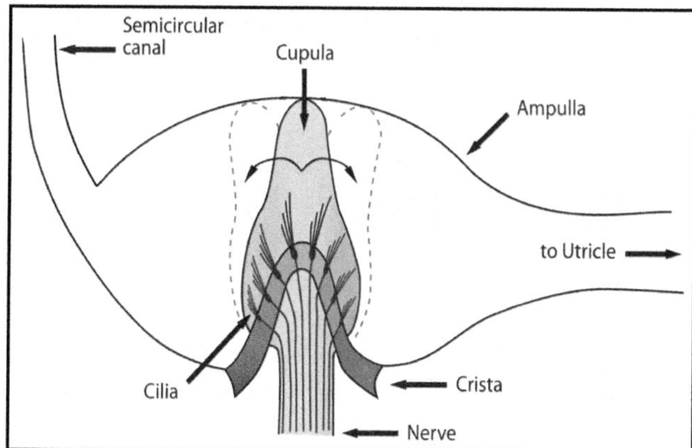


**Figure 8-5.** The cupula. If the cupula moves to the right, the long cilia is stimulated. If it moves left, it is inhibited. (Reproduced with permission from Plishka CM. Balance systems. In: Plishka CM. *A Clinician's Guide to Balance and Dizziness Evaluation and Treatment.* SLACK Incorporated; 2015: 2-44.)

# Anatomy and Physiology of the Vestibular System

The vestibular system is responsible for maintaining postural control and balance. The vestibular system relays incoming sensory information about head position and movement (the body's perceived orientation in space) to the CNS, and this information is used to modify motor responses to maintain one's balance. The vestibular system detects the direction of gravity and orients the body and head in line with the vertical plane. It also keeps vision stable during motion. For example, when a person jogs, the vestibular system maintains clear (unjumpy) vision. It coordinates eye and head movement, especially during quick head movements. When someone calls your name and you quickly turn your head, the vestibular system works to allow you to focus on that person (without seeing a blur as you rotate your head) without losing your balance. The system is extremely sensitive, and it makes rapid corrections to maintain postural control. Impairments affecting the vestibulocochlear nerve (cranial nerve [CN] VIII) and/or the vestibular system can result in vertigo, vomiting/nausea, postural instability, and impaired balance; in cases of damage to the CN VIII, there may also be associated hearing loss.

The 3 parts of the vestibular system (ie, the peripheral vestibular system, central processor system, and motor output) work together to keep the body upright and functioning normally in the environment.[10] Sensory input is provided by the peripheral vestibular system located in the inner ear. The central processor system interprets incoming sensory information from the peripheral vestibular system (received via CN VIII) and provides output to various reflexes, which generate motor and eye responses.

## *Peripheral Vestibular System*

The peripheral vestibular system (Figure 8-4) is composed of the vestibular branch of CN VIII, 3 semicircular canals (SCCs), and 2 otolith organs (saccules and utricles) located in each inner ear. These structures have specialized sensory structures that relay information about movement and head position.

### Semicircular Canals

The SCCs are named for their location (ie, anterior [superior], posterior [inferior], and horizontal [lateral]). They are aligned approximately at right angles to each other. Each SCC works in a coplanar pair with the opposite side; the left anterior SCC works with the right posterior SCC and the left posterior canal with the right anterior canal. The horizontal canals also work as a coplanar pair; they are positioned approximately 30 degrees upward and are perpendicular to the anterior and posterior canals. The horizontal canals are sensitive to motion in the transverse plane, and the anterior/posterior canals sense rotational movements in the sagittal and frontal planes. The SCCs provide sensory information about head angular velocity for short rotational periods only (not prolonged spinning).

Perilymph fluid lies between the bony and membranous labyrinth. The SCCs are filled with endolymph fluid that moves freely within the canals and is slightly denser than water (see Figure 8-4).[10,11] At the end of each SCC, there is a widening of the canal called the *ampulla*. The cupula is a projection in the ampulla surrounded by endolymph fluid. There are specialized sensory hair cells (cilia) that extend from the ampulla embedded in the crista and extend into the base of the cupula. The cupula has hair cells that connect to nerves providing information about angular head movements to the CNS.[11] When the head moves, the endolymph shifts, bending the hair cells of the coplanar pair in opposite directions. When the cupula moves toward the kinocilia (the long cilia), that specific canal gets stimulated, but when the cupula moves away from the kinocilia, that canal becomes inhibited (Figure 8-5). For example, when the head rotates to the right, the endolymph fluid in the right horizontal SCC moves in the opposite direction (left), whereas the fluid in the left horizontal SCC deflects the

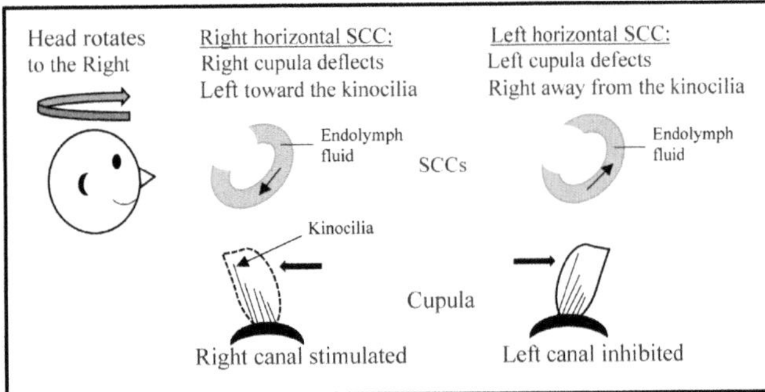


**Figure 8-6.** The push-pull mechanism.

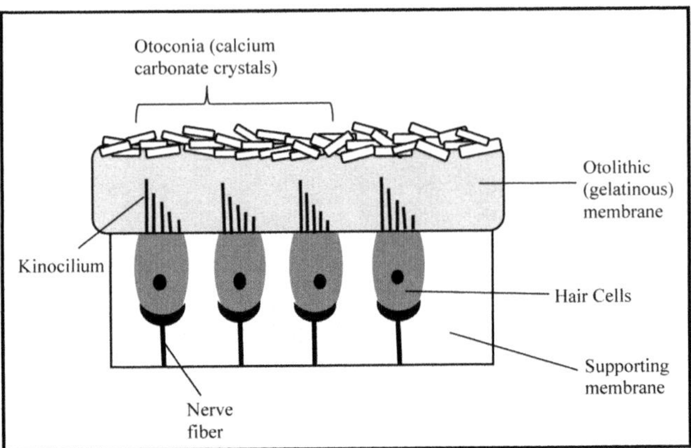


**Figure 8-7.** A diagram of the macula.

cupula to the right (Figure 8-6). In this example, the right horizontal SCC is stimulated, and the left SCC is inhibited. This is called the *push-pull mechanism*.[12] The amount of endolymph shift/displacement is proportional to the speed of rotary head motion; this supplies the CNS with information related to head motion speed.[11] If the input from one canal is disrupted, the input from the other canal is still sent to the CNS. The transmission of incomplete information can result in inaccurate processing of the information by the CNS, resulting in vestibular symptoms including the inability to maintain stable vision, dizziness, and/or feeling off-balance.

### Interesting Fact

Cupula deflection is slightly delayed because of a lag in the endolymph fluid motion when the head initially rotates. During prolonged rotation, the cupula gradually returns to its original upright position, which signals to the brain that the person is stationary. If the eyes are closed, the person feels as if they are not moving, but if the eyes are open, the person perceives continued motion. Ice skaters who perform several high-speed rotations avoid dizziness by using their eyes to "spot" or fixate on stationary objects. They rely on visual input because the vestibular input from the SCCs and cupula becomes ineffective.[10]

### Otolith Organs

The otolith organs (utricles and saccules) are responsible for responding to/relaying information about linear head movement (ie, acceleration or deceleration) and static head tilt in relation to gravity. The macula is contained within the saccules and utricles and is composed of otoconia (microscopic calcium carbonate crystals) that rest on a layer of gelatinous material (Figure 8-7). The sensory hair cells are mechanoreceptors embedded in a supporting membrane; they are stimulated when the head tilts or when linear acceleration occurs.

The utricles (Figure 8-8) are horizontally oriented, and the saccules are vertically oriented. The saccules sense acceleration and deceleration vertically (ie, going up and down an elevator).[11] The saccules also respond to motion in anterior-posterior directions, so they react during an activity like cervical flexion/extension. The utricles sense acceleration/deceleration laterally (side to side) and in anterior-posterior directions, and they respond to lateral head tilts. Consider these examples. Imagine sitting at a stoplight, and it turns green; you step on the gas and increase your speed. In this instance, the otoliths provide information to the CNS (via CN VIII) that you are accelerating. The utricles detect the change in the velocity. In a second example, consider flying in a plane cruising at a constant speed; you cannot detect how fast you are going, but as the plane starts to descend, the otoliths (which are gravity dependent) detect the tilt of the plane and deceleration in speed. In the second example, during the descent, there is a change in speed, which results in the otoliths responding. The otoconia drag and move across the otolithic membrane, which stimulates those sensory hair cells to send signals to the CNS regarding the direction of the linear movement as well as the change of velocity.

## Central Vestibular Processing and Neuropathways

Sensory information about head movement is sent from the SCCs and otolith organs and relayed to a central processor (the vestibular nuclei complex and cerebellum) via the vestibular portion of CN VIII. The input is processed and then relayed to the eye muscles and spinal cord. The vestibular nuclei receive and process vestibular information and simultaneously process afferent visual and somatosensory (proprioception) information.[10,11] The vestibular nuclei connect to the extraocular muscles to coordinate eye and head movements, and they also transmit information to the muscles to maintain postural control and balance.

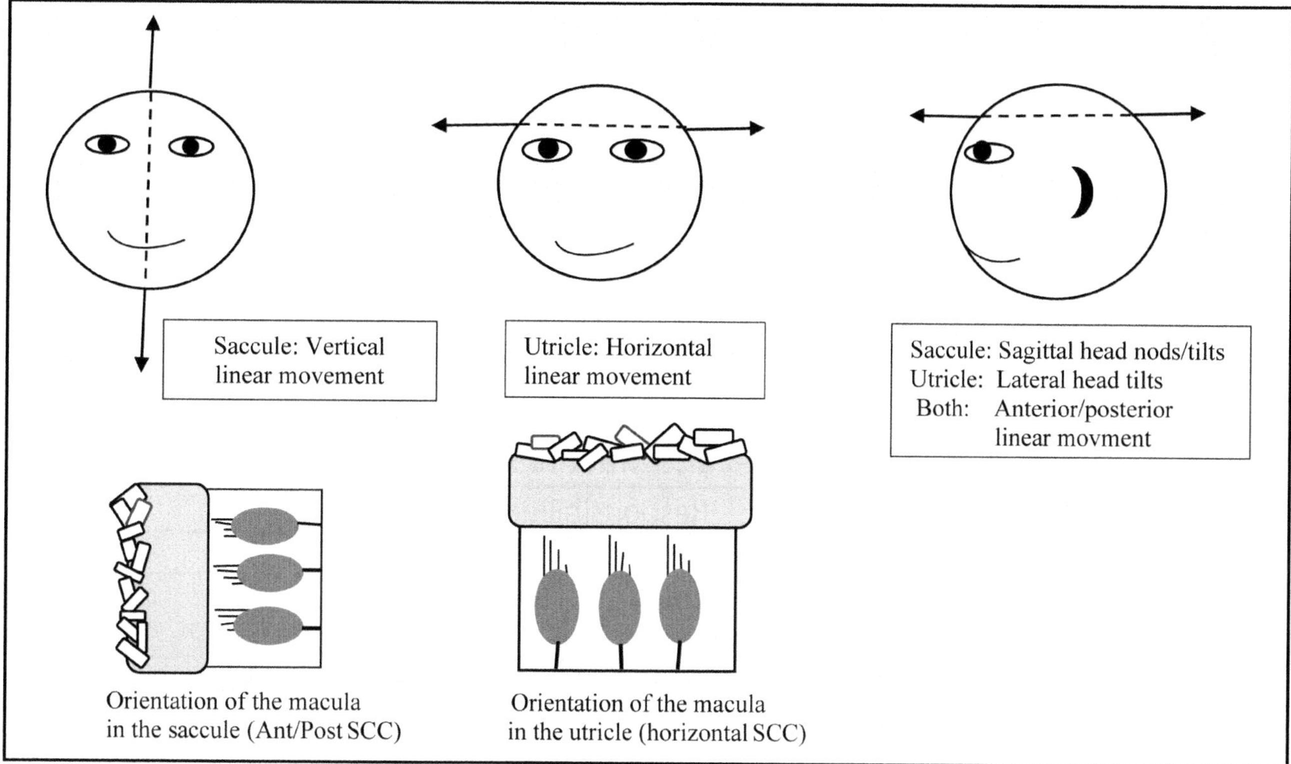


**Figure 8-8.** The utricle and saccule related to linear head movement and orientation.

The extraocular eye muscles are arranged in pairs. Each pair of SCCs is connected to a single pair of muscles and innervated by a specific nerve (Table 8-3). A summary of the vestibular nuclei actions is found in Table 8-4. The ascending tracts control eye movements, and the descending tracts transmit impulses to muscles to maintain upright postures and postural responses.[8]

The cerebellum assists with static/dynamic balance, limb coordination, and visual stabilization by using information that it receives from the vestibular nuclei and the peripheral nervous system to modulate these activities.[10] The cerebellum integrates and prioritizes this information when there is a conflict between any of the systems providing input. The cerebellum provides direction to the muscles of the body to adjust movements or movement patterns based on the input received and body position (eg, sitting, standing, or walking).[11] Cerebellar lesions can affect the VSR, resulting in ataxia and trunk instability. Without cerebellar input, the vestibular reflexes become ineffective.

The vestibular nuclei relay messages to the extraocular muscles to help coordinate eye movements with head movements to stabilize gaze or vision. The vestibular nuclei generate nerve impulses that stimulate 3 reflexes that are important to maintaining a normal vestibular system: the vestibulo-ocular reflex (VOR), the vestibulospinal reflex (VSR), and the vestibulocollic reflex (VCR).[10,11]

The VOR maintains clear vision during head movement in all planes. To maintain clear vision, the VOR provides rapid compensatory eye movements in the opposite direction of head movement. The speed of head and eye movements should be equal but in opposite directions (ie, the head moves right and the eyes move left). The ratio of eye movement to head movements is called the *VOR gain*, and the ratio should equal 1. The timing of eye to head velocity (measured in degrees/second) is called the *VOR phase*.[12] If there is a 2 degree/second difference or greater between eye to head velocity, the vestibular nuclei must respond to correct the error.[10] There are 2 components of the VOR: an angular and linear component. The SCCs provide information about angular motion; this is called *angular VOR*. This reflex creates compensation as the head rotates side to side, stabilizing the gaze and allowing vision to remain focused on an object. In this scenario, the horizontal canals are responsible for keeping vision clear. Figure 8-9 illustrates the pathways from the SCC to the extraocular muscles as the head turns.

## Quick Class Activity

Draw an X on a piece of paper and hold it about 2 to 3 feet (ft) away from your lab partner at their eye level. You should observe their eyes staying on the X. Tell them to flex their head down about 20 to 30 degrees. Have them focus on the X, and tell them to shake their head side to side in small amplitudes (eg, saying "no") quickly while keeping their eyes focused on the letter. Time them for 30 seconds as you watch their eyes. Do they stay focused on the letter? What direction did the eyes move in relation to the head?

**Table 8-3**

**Canal Pairing With Extraocular Muscles and Nerve Innervations**

| Canal | Extraocular Muscles | Cranial Nerve |
|---|---|---|
| Posterior | Inferior and superior obliques | Trochlear CN IV |
| Anterior | Superior rectus | Oculomotor CN III superior branch |
| Horizontal | Medial rectus<br>Lateral rectus | Oculomotor CN III inferior branch<br>Abducens CN VI |

**Table 8-4**

**Vestibular Nuclei and Tract Responsibilities**

| Vestibular Nucleus | Responsibilities of the Nucleus |
|---|---|
| Superior | Relays information for the VOR and VCR based on SCC input. |
| Lateral | The VSR sends information via the lateral vestibular descending tract and transmits impulses that create adjustments in postural responses by activating the antigravity (extensor) muscles to keep a person upright. |
| Medial | Relays information for the VOR and VSR (coordinates eye and head movements). |
| Descending | Connects all other nuclei and the cerebellum. |

VCR = vestibulocollic reflex; VOR = vestibulo-oculomotor reflex; VSR = vestibulospinal reflex.

Patients who report that they lose their balance or feel dizzy (vertigo symptoms) when they rotate their head quickly may experience a problem with their angular VOR. These patients totally avoid turning their head when they walk because this provokes symptoms. The activity described in the Quick Class Activity (called *times 1 [×1] viewing*) is an exercise commonly given to these patients to stimulate the VOR. Once the VOR is "jump-started," it is important to incorporate other tasks that include head movements so that the patient can maintain head/trunk disassociation and good VOR function. Gaze stabilization exercises are used to improve VOR function.

Linear motion is controlled by the otolith organs and is called *linear VOR*. Linear VOR is important when the head moves at high velocities and when viewing close objects (ie, grocery shopping). Vertical linear acceleration is detected by the saccules, and horizontal acceleration is detected by the utricles. The cerebellum modulates VOR function.[10]

The VSR works with the vestibular system to coordinate head position in relation to body position and in sending impulses to skeletal muscles to control limb and trunk movement (static and dynamic). The VSR is responsible for keeping the head vertical when stationary or moving and compensates for head tilting (Box 8-1), body tilting, and perturbations.

Three cervical reflexes also play a role in maintaining balance. The cervico-ocular reflex (COR) interacts with the VOR and stabilizes vision in response to slow cervical rotation; it is not as effective during rapid head motions. Patients who have bilateral vestibular lesions (BVLs) do not have VOR function on either side and rely on their COR. The cervicospinal reflex works with the VSR, sending sensory information received from the cervical spine to the limbs to alter positions to maintain balance.[10] The cervicocollic reflex responds to cervical proprioception by contracting cervical muscles to stabilize the head on the body.[10,11]

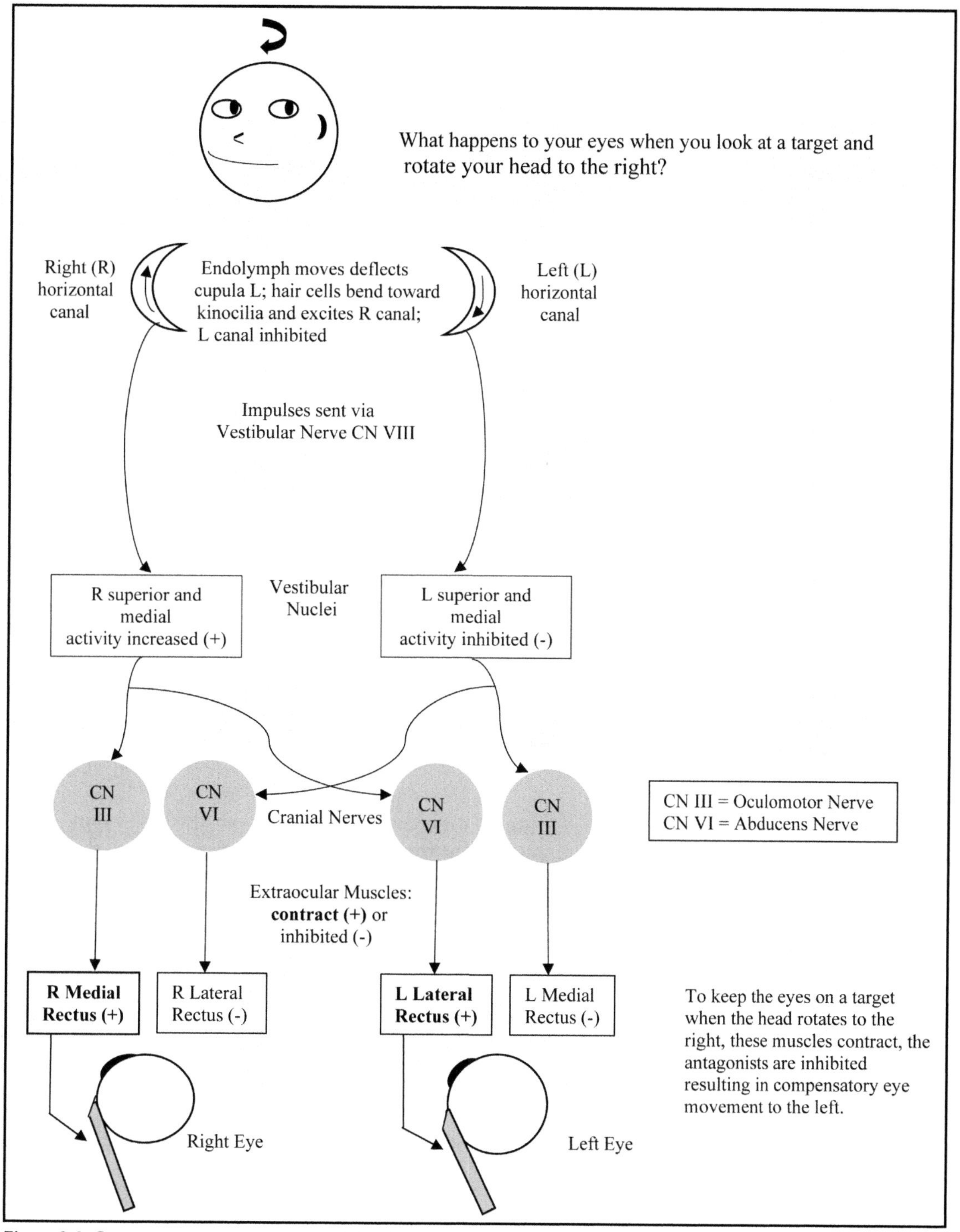

What happens to your eyes when you look at a target and rotate your head to the right?

Right (R) horizontal canal

Endolymph moves deflects cupula L; hair cells bend toward kinocilia and excites R canal; L canal inhibited

Left (L) horizontal canal

Impulses sent via Vestibular Nerve CN VIII

R superior and medial activity increased (+)

Vestibular Nuclei

L superior and medial activity inhibited (-)

CN III

CN VI

Cranial Nerves

CN VI

CN III

CN III = Oculomotor Nerve
CN VI = Abducens Nerve

Extraocular Muscles: **contract (+)** or inhibited (-)

**R Medial Rectus (+)**

R Lateral Rectus (-)

**L Lateral Rectus (+)**

L Medial Rectus (-)

To keep the eyes on a target when the head rotates to the right, these muscles contract, the antagonists are inhibited resulting in compensatory eye movement to the left.

Right Eye

Left Eye

**Figure 8-9.** Compensatory eye movement with head rotation.

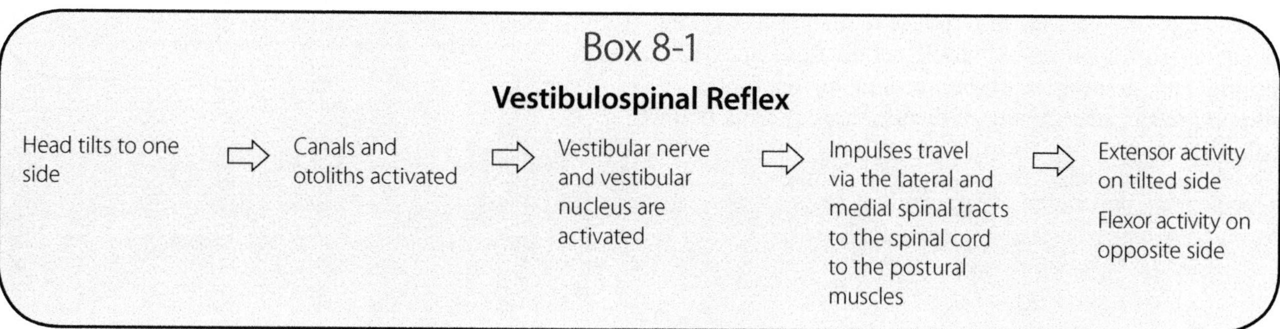

Box 8-1

**Vestibulospinal Reflex**

Head tilts to one side ⇨ Canals and otoliths activated ⇨ Vestibular nerve and vestibular nucleus are activated ⇨ Impulses travel via the lateral and medial spinal tracts to the spinal cord to the postural muscles ⇨ Extensor activity on tilted side

Flexor activity on opposite side

## Sensory Integration and Postural Control

Maintaining balance while performing tasks or activities requires appropriate interactions between the somatosensory, visual, and vestibular systems and the environment. Sensory integration is the ability to organize and use sensory information effectively. Maintaining one's balance is a multifactorial interaction between the motor, sensory, and visual systems (Figure 8-10). Impairments affecting the somatosensory, visual, or vestibular systems or in sensory integration result in an increased risk of LOB and/or falls.

The somatosensory system collects information from the sensory receptors such as pain, temperature, touch, position, and vibration. Input provides information to the CNS about pressure felt on the bottom of the feet and the surface where one is standing as well as information about body position and motion with respect to the support surface and other body segments (joint proprioception and kinesthesia). This system also provides input to the CNS about COM movement and conscious and subconscious perception of stability. It allows the CNS to differentiate whether a body is flexing at the neck or flexing at the waist. It provides the fastest and most sensitive response to balance disturbances.

The visual system provides information about head and body movement with respect to the surrounding environment. It determines head and eye movement/position in relation to the surroundings. It provides information about slow movements or static tilts of the head and relays information about stabilizing vision (VOR) and maintaining gaze (VSR). Visual information is relayed more slowly than somatosensory information. Individuals tend to be more reliant on their vision input, even when the information is inaccurate. Consider what happens when you are sitting in a car waiting at a stoplight and a truck is stopped next to you. If the truck begins to roll back slowly, what is your response? It is likely that you will push harder on the brake pedal because you feel like you are moving forward. The visual input created the perception of movement; yet, you were stationary, and the truck was actually moving.

As stated earlier, the vestibular system is both a sensory and motor system. The musculoskeletal element is the motor system that responds to various changes or disturbances in one's balance. The motor responses (simple or complex) include selecting an appropriate postural strategy (ankle, hip, or stepping) in response to disturbances. The sequencing of appropriate muscle contractions and their timing and grading must be accurate to appropriately respond to the size/amount of disturbances and maintain balance.

### Quick Class Activity

Stand quietly with your feet in a comfortable position on the floor with your eyes open. Feel the floor with your feet. Have your lab partner observe you from the side. Report what you are feeling to your lab partner. Now repeat the activity with your feet together. Then, stand normally again but with your eyes closed. Try each activity while standing on foam. Have your partner record your verbal responses and their visual observations. (Safety first—ensure proper guarding during this activity!)

Answer the following questions: In which situation do you feel that you relied more on your vision vs the feedback from your feet? In which situation did you feel more sway? In which situation did your partner observe the most sway? In which situation did you think you used your vestibular system the most?

Consider another example. A person walks along a smooth cement path, and the path ends at the start of a soft sandy beach. The person must adapt to the change in surface as they continue walking. To make a smooth transition, the visual and sensory information from their eyes and feet (about the surface change) is relayed to the CNS, which then makes motor output modifications. These modifications allow the muscles to adapt to the surface change and keep the body vertically aligned and stable. If the person in this example was texting when initially stepping onto the sand, the responses could have been quite different. In this variation, the CNS would not have had the immediate visual input to pair with the somatosensory information, creating a much less complete picture of what was occurring. The lower extremity muscles would have probably contracted more intensely, and perhaps both arms may have moved (ie, throwing the arms up/out) to maintain balance because the CNS would have had inaccurate (or minimal) input from the visual system. The visual input could have helped to determine the depth of the sand or surface change.

### Questions for Thought

What if the person in this example had neuropathy in both feet and was texting while walking? Would this increase or decrease the person's risk of falling? Why? Which system has to keep the person upright and solve any internal conflicts between systems? Do you think the person with neuropathy would be walking with a wider or narrower BOS?

An individual with an impaired somatosensory system will be more reliant on their vision. If the person with neuropathy was not watching where they were walking (ie, texting), the somatosensory and visual inputs are unreliable. Effective function and integration of all 3 systems are vital to maintaining static and dynamic balance. Impairment in one or more systems increases the risk for balance impairments and falls.

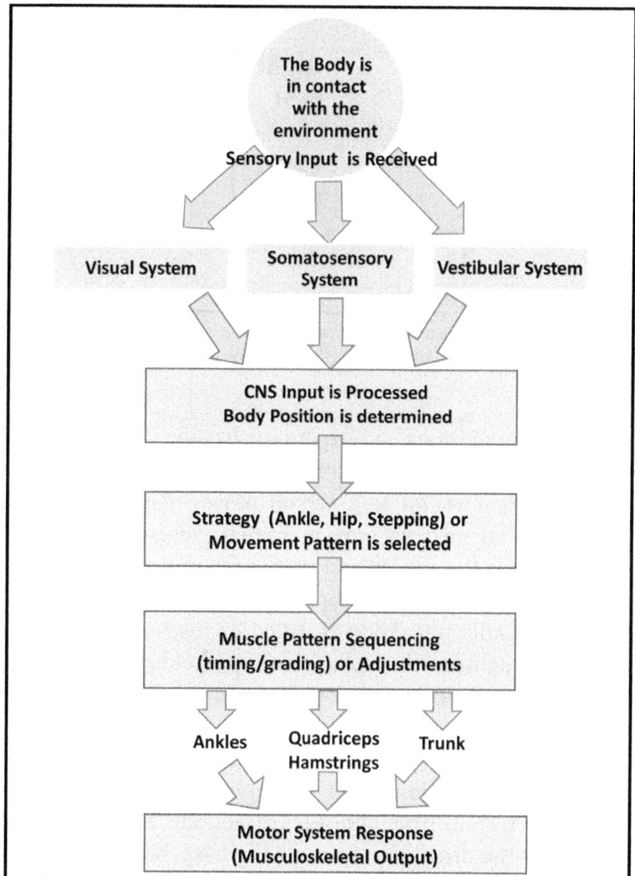


**Figure 8-10.** System integration and interactions.

## Age-Related Changes

Physiological changes associated with aging can affect balance. Knowledge of these changes guides physical therapist assistants in selecting interventions that improve balance and reduce fear of falling. Decreases in range of motion, flexibility, strength, and reaction times have direct effects on posture and mobility. Common gait changes such as slow cadence, increased double stance time, increased width of gait BOS, and a decrease in step length may be due to fear of falling, poor postural control, and/or a decrease in ankle flexibility or lower extremity strength. Older adults often experience a decline in vision, somatosensory feedback, and vestibular function. These changes are also associated with a fear of falling and increased fall risk.[2,4,8,11,13] Cognitive impairments or dementia also can increase one's risk for falls.[2]

Older adults may experience vision changes and have difficulty adjusting to glare or light intensity and/or a delayed response transitioning from bright light to darkness or vice versa. This can cause diminished vision for a couple of minutes until the eyes adjust to the changes. Cataracts (cloudy lenses or blurring vision) affect contrast sensitivity and are common in adults 55 years and older. Macular degeneration affects near and far central vision in some older adults. Low vision occupational therapy programs can be helpful for these patients.[11,14] Patients who wear bifocal/trifocal glasses are at an increased risk of falling because of depth perception problems. These patients should be instructed to look through the top part of the lens when stepping off curbs or descending stairs.

As discussed in the previous examples, older adults tend to rely on visual input for balance, but if vision is impaired, there will be an increased reliance on the somatosensory and vestibular systems. The patient will have more difficulty if these systems are impaired. The function of these systems usually remains stable until age 79 years, but there can be a significant rate of deterioration if they are not continually challenged.[15]

Dizziness and LOB are very common in older patients. Research indicates that older adults have lower VOR gain (lower than normal ratio of head to eye movement) at higher head velocities (greater than 2 Hz) than younger subjects because of degenerative changes in both the peripheral and central vestibular systems.[11,14] BPPV is the most common cause of dizziness in adults aged 65 years and older.[16,17] Decreases in cutaneous sensation and a decline in proprioception in older adults create increased instability. Postural sway also increases with age and is worse in people who have previously fallen vs those who have not. Knee joint proprioception is more accurate during full weight-bearing activities because of receptor activation.[17] There is a strong association between patients who have peripheral neuropathy and increased fall risk.[18]

Studies have shown that fear of falling increases with age, and it is more prevalent in women, which often results in functional limitations. One does not have to experience a fall to have a fear of falling.[19] It is helpful to determine the reason behind the patient's fear. The physical therapy interventions need to challenge a patient's balance enough for the patient to be slightly uncomfortable, but the clinician needs to ensure that the patient trusts their ability to keep them safe. As the patient's balance improves and they feel more stable, balance confidence also tends to improve.

There is strong evidence that physical activities/exercises are effective ways to improve function and reduce fall risk.[2,8,11,18] Research also indicates that VOR training may also improve postural control and reduce falls.[20]

## Understanding Nystagmus

When a vestibular pathology is present, atypical eye movements occur as a result of the CNS receiving inaccurate information and trying to compensate for movement that is not occurring. This results in nystagmus, which is a

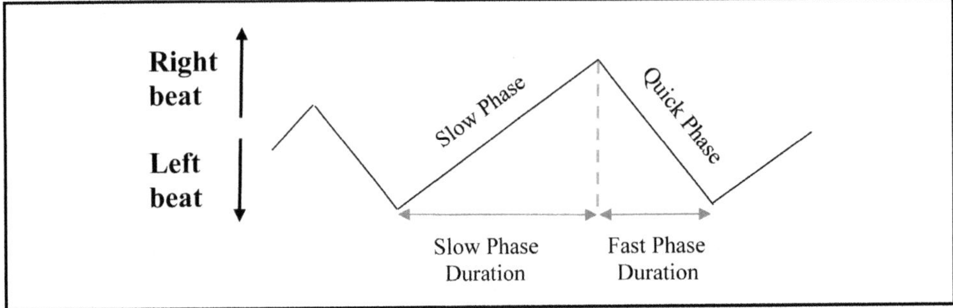


**Figure 8-11.** Understanding nystagmus. The beat is named by the quick (or fast) phase and, in this case, is called a *left-beating nystagmus*. The pathology is on the slow phase side (in this example, the right side).

rhythmic involuntary movement of the eyes. Physiological nystagmus is a normal occurrence that helps the VOR maintain clear vision as a person moves. Pathologic nystagmus is abnormal eye movement that causes a blurring of vision and/or the perception that surrounding objects are moving (eg, spinning or jumping). The illusion of "jumpy" vision or oscillating vision is called *oscillopsia*. The direction of nystagmus helps determine if pathology is related to a central or a peripheral lesion. Physical therapist assistants should document the direction of the observed nystagmus.

Abnormal nystagmus has 2 phases: a slow drift of the eyes in one direction (slow phase) and rapid movement (quick phase) in the opposite direction. Nystagmus is named for the direction of the quick phase. Nystagmus can be vertical, horizontal, or a combination of vertical and left or right rotational component. The direction of the nystagmus provides vital information regarding the type and location (central or peripheral) of the vestibular problem. For example, if a patient has a right-sided vestibular problem, the quick phase would be to the left (called *left-beating nystagmus*), and the slow phase would be to the right as shown in Figure 8-11.

Spontaneous nystagmus occurs when there is a vestibular imbalance in either the peripheral or central system, resulting in eye oscillation without any precipitating motion. The direction of the nystagmus (horizontal, vertical, or torsional) and the ability to suppress the nystagmus (or not) helps the physical therapist determine whether the central or peripheral system is involved. The physical therapist assistant's understanding of vestibular pathology and patient presentation will help the assistant to develop and/or implement treatment interventions to accurately address the therapy diagnosis.

### Other Eye Movements

There are 4 basic types of eye movements: VOR, saccades, smooth pursuit, and vergence. VOR stabilizes one's vision in relation to the environment. Rapid corrective eye movements to focus on a target are called *saccades*. These eye movements can be small (eg, while reading this book) or larger (eg, when one looks around a room). If a person is asked to focus on a target and either undershoots or overshoots it before getting focused, the target is abnormal and may denote a central problem. Smooth pursuit is the ability of the eyes to complete slow tracking movements when following an object as it moves from side to side (or up and down).

> **Quick Class Activity**
>
> Get a strip of striped material about 18 inches (in) long or a piece of lined notebook paper (color in every other line with a black marker until you have 10 colored lines). Hold it about 2 ft away from your partner's face and tell them to count the dark-colored stripes as you slowly move the material from the right to the left. What did you observe? This is an example of physiological (optokinetic) nystagmus and is a combination of smooth pursuit (slow) and corrective saccades (quick).

During most eye movements, both eyes will move in the same direction, but if the eyes move in opposite directions, that is called *vergence*. Convergence occurs when both eyes move inward (eg, when moving a pen toward a person's nose and asking them to track the object). Divergence occurs when the eyes move outward and then back to a normal position (eg, when tracking the pen as it moves away from a person's nose/face).

## Vestibular Pathologies

Central and peripheral pathologies or lesions can result in various vestibular conditions/presentations. Intrinsic causes refer to pathologies that arise from within the vestibular system, and extrinsic factors refer to causes external to the vestibular system.

### *Central Vestibular Pathologies*

Extrinsic factors that can affect vestibular system function include ototoxic drugs, cardiac issues (eg, orthostatic hypotension or atrial fibrillation), viral or bacterial infections, dehydration, cervical spine trauma, orthopedic issues, and anxiety.[2] Patients with orthostatic hypotension or anxiety may also report feeling dizzy, but they are usually experiencing light-headedness or a fainting feeling. The assistant should have the patient specifically describe the symptoms they are feeling; this helps ensure that the terminology selected is an accurate descriptor of the patient's symptoms.

Intrinsic factors that can affect vestibular function include damage to the CNS or central neural pathways (vestibular nuclei, cerebellum, and/or the cerebrum). Damage to these structures can affect sensory integration processing. Cerebellar degenerative conditions cause approximately 20% of cases, and 38% of cases are idiopathic.[21]

Vertical nystagmus is most common with central vestibular lesions. Patients who experience cerebellar disorders tend to exhibit a downbeat (quick phase) nystagmus and patients with brainstem lesions exhibit an upbeat (quick phase) nystagmus. Patients with central vestibular lesions cannot suppress spontaneous nystagmus even when focusing on an object. Direction-changing nystagmus can be seen in patients with either cerebellar or brainstem lesions.[21]

## Peripheral Vestibular Pathologies

Pathologies affecting the peripheral vestibular apparatus include damage to the SCC, otolith organs, or CN VIII. Damage can be bilateral (BVLs) or unilateral (unilateral vestibular lesions [UVLs]). Patients with unilateral involvement usually complain of dizziness or vertigo. **Vertigo** describes the illusion of movement. Patients report the perception that either the room is spinning or that they are spinning. This perception of movement occurs because the system on one side is working and the other side/system is not, creating an imbalance between the 2 push-pull dynamics of the 2 vestibular systems. Patients with UVL pathologies have difficulty stabilizing the gaze during head movements and difficulty with static and dynamic postural stability. They inappropriately rely on ankle strategies, even with large perturbations or standing with a narrow BOS. They need to learn how to use hip strategies during these activities. Those with bilateral hypofunction commonly complain of feeling off-balance (also known as *disequilibrium*) as opposed to complaints of vertigo. They have difficulty walking on uneven surfaces and in dark rooms, and moving their head quickly affects their static and dynamic balance.

Intrinsic peripheral pathologies include vestibular neuritis (neuronitis), labyrinthitis, Meniere disease, and perilymph fistula. Some of these pathologies may cause temporary or permanent hearing loss. Most peripheral disorders occur suddenly, and the patient can recall when the onset of symptoms occurred. BPPV is the most common cause of vertigo, and it can affect any of the SCCs. Patients with BPPV usually report dizziness, and they can identify the specific positions that provoke symptoms. The most common complaints occur when rolling over in bed ("When I roll to the right the room spins.") or sitting up from a supine/side-lying position. They may also complain that looking up overhead or bending over to look into a lower cabinet provokes symptoms. These patients tend to avoid the specific head position(s) that recreate symptoms. Patients who have experienced whiplash or minor head trauma may also experience BPPV. BPPV commonly affects older adults, and idiopathic BPPV is most prevalent.

BPPV is classified as either cupulolithiasis or canalithiasis. Cupulolithiasis occurs when the otoconia adhere to the cupula, whereas canalithiasis occurs when the otoconia are floating in one of the SCCs. The posterior canal is most frequently affected with BPPV, and canalithiasis is more common than cupulolithiasis.[22] The primary characteristics of canalithiasis and cupulolithiasis are described in Table 8-5. BPPV associated with an anterior or posterior canal has a vertical and torsional (rotational) component (Table 8-6) that indicates canal involvement. The nystagmus responses are observable when the patient is positioned in the provoking position. Nystagmus associated with BPPV in the horizontal canals is classified as *geotropic* or *apogeotropic*. Geotropic describes nystagmus with a downbeat toward the ground when the involved side is facing the floor. Apogeotropic describes nystagmus with an upbeat toward the ceiling. If BPPV patients are taking Antivert (meclizine), nystagmus is not observable because medications suppress nystagmus.

### Considerations for the Physical Therapist Assistant: Cupulolithiasis Versus Canalithiasis

There is an immediate onset of symptoms with cupulolithiasis because the weight of the otoconia deflects (bends) the cupula and it stays in that position, so symptoms do not usually fatigue quicky. When a patient has canalithiasis, there is a delay in the onset of symptoms up to 30 seconds, and these symptoms fatigue faster.

Upon reviewing the physical therapist's initial evaluation and POC, the assistant should recognize the signs and symptoms of peripheral or central pathologies and discuss test results performed with the therapist. In-depth discussion of vestibular pathologies is beyond entry-level practice expectations. The Balance and Vestibular Intervention section provides general treatment guidelines for BPPV, UVLs, and BVLs. The list of Suggested Resources at the end of the chapter provides more in-depth information, and physical therapist assistants can attend continuing education courses to advance their knowledge and proficiency in this practice area.

**Table 8-5**

**Benign Paroxysmal Positional Vertigo Characteristics of Canalithiasis and Cupulolithiasis**

| Canalithiasis | Cupulolithiasis |
|---|---|
| • Delayed onset of vertigo (about 3 to 30 seconds)<br>• Increasing to decreasing intensity of nystagmus (fatigues)<br>• Nystagmus disappears after about 1 minute<br>• Complaints of vertigo and nystagmus latency are equal<br>• Very common | • Immediate onset of vertigo<br>• Complaints of vertigo and nystagmus latency are equal<br>• Nystagmus is persistent (> 1 minute) due to cupula deflection<br>• Not as common |

**Table 8-6**

**Canal Involvement and Nystagmus Response to Benign Paroxysmal Positional Vertigo**

| Canal Involvement | Nystagmus Response |
|---|---|
| • Right posterior | • Upbeat and to the right |
| • Right anterior | • Downbeat and to the right |
| • Left posterior | • Upbeat and to the left |
| • Left anterior | • Downbeat and to the left |
| • Horizontal canal | • Geotropic (toward the ground) |
| • Horizontal canal (cupula) | • Apogeotropic (toward the ceiling) |

## Vestibular and Balance Testing

The physical therapy examination may include oculomotor testing, positional testing for BPPV, and balance testing. These tests assess a patient's ocular motor system function, balance, sensory integration, and/or postural control. Ocular motor tests are used to differentiate central and peripheral dysfunctions, and these tests are repeated during the episode of care to determine the patient's progress. Positional testing is used to assess for BPPV, and it can include the Dix-Hallpike Test, Semont liberatory maneuver, and the roll test. Table 8-7 lists the common tests used to differentiate peripheral problems from central problems. Based on test results, the assistant should select interventions that target the impaired systems.

Tests that can assess the input and responses of the vestibular system and the resultant impact on balance include perturbations, LOS testing, the Clinical Test of Sensory Interaction on Balance (CTSIB), the Modified Clinical Test of Sensory Interaction on Balance (mCTSIB), and the Sensory Organization Test (SOT). Perturbation testing is used to assess reactive responses (the ability to regain COM over BOS) and sensory strategies with expected and unexpected pushing at the hips and sternum. LOS testing is usually performed on a stationary balance platform that can quantify (and record) various movements associated with the participant's ability to voluntarily sway as far as possible in an indicated direction and maintain balance briefly. The platform records data on reaction time, distance or excursion of the lean/sway, and directional control (Figure 8-12).

The SOT is performed on a computerized balance platform, and it measures postural sway in 6 conditions (Figure 8-13). The platform and walls (the visual surround) can move, creating various conditions in which vision and somatosensory input are conflicting. There are 3 conditions in which the platform is stationary: with the patient's (1) eyes open, (2) eyes closed, and (3) visual surroundings moving up and down. The platform moves during the last 3 conditions: with the patient's (4) eyes open, (5) eyes closed, and (6) eyes open with the visual surroundings moving up and down. The patient has to respond correctly to the varied visual and somatosensory information in order to maintain balance. This test identifies how well sensory input is processed by the CNS.[8] The information provided from this test is used to select the appropriate vestibular and balance training protocols.

**Table 8-7**

**Central and Peripheral Ocular Motor and Benign Paroxysmal Positional Vertigo Testing**

| Test Name | Central Problem | Peripheral Problem |
|---|---|---|
| Spontaneous nystagmus | Cannot suppress nystagmus when focused on fixed object | Can suppress nystagmus when focused on fixed object |
| Smooth pursuit | Consistent saccades | |
| VOR cancellation | Results should match smooth pursuit | |
| Saccade test | Look for over/under shoot | |
| Head shake test | Vertical nystagmus | Horizontal nystagmus |
| Head impulse test | | Corrective saccades |
| Dynamic visual acuity | | > 3-line difference (usually BVL) |
| Dix-Hallpike test (Figure 8-16) | | BPPV anterior/posterior canal |
| Alternate test: Side lying (Figure 8-17) | | BPPV anterior/posterior canal |
| Semont liberatory maneuver (Figure 8-18) | | BPPV canalithiasis or cupulolithiasis |
| Roll test (Figure 8-19) | | Horizontal canalithiasis or cupulolithiasis |

The CTSIB is a modified version of the SOT that can be performed without the expensive computer system. The CTSIB assesses balance in the same 6 conditions as the SOT. The mCTSIB is an abbreviated version of the CTSIB that assesses sway in only 4 positions: the eyes open on a firm surface, eyes closed on a firm surface, eyes open on foam, and eyes closed on foam (conditions 3 and 6 are omitted). The mCTSIB can be performed on a stationary balance platform with recorded results (Figure 8-14) or on the floor (Figures 8-15A through 8-15D) using a stopwatch to measure time. This test provides information about how a patient maintains balance with varied visual or sensory input.

## *Benign Paroxysmal Positional Vertigo Testing*

The physical therapist obtains the patient's history of symptoms to determine which canal is most likely involved and which test is most appropriate to perform. The Dix-Hallpike test (see Figure 8-16) is used to test the anterior or posterior canals. The patient is instructed to bend their knees to protect their back before being lowered from a sitting to a supine position by the clinician. This test places the involved posterior/anterior canal in a gravity-dependent position. This position will elicit vertigo as the otoconia move along the canal. If the therapist observes upbeat and torsional nystagmus to the side of the down-positioned ear, the posterior canal is affected. If downbeating nystagmus is observed with torsion toward the involved ear, the anterior canal is affected.

If a patient cannot tolerate the Dix-Hallpike test, a side-lying test can be performed.[22] This test is more commonly used for patients who are obese or have neck and/or back issues. The patient's head is rotated 45 degrees to the opposite side to be tested before moving down into a side-lying position. For example, if the patient turns their head to the right, the patient then assumes a left-side–lying position (see Figure 8-17). The nystagmus seen in this test for a left posterior canal would be upbeat and to the left; a downbeat to the left would denote a left anterior canal (see Table 8-6). If the nystagmus starts immediately and lasts longer than 1 minute, the patient may have cupulolithiasis, and the Semont liberatory maneuver is indicated. To perform the Semont liberatory maneuver, the patient is seated on the edge of the table (see Figure 8-18A). The clinician turns the patient's head to the left (to treat a right posterior or left anterior cupulolithiasis) and then quickly brings the patient down into a right-side–lying position (see Figure 8-18B) and waits for 1 minute or until symptoms subside. Then, quickly move the patient all the way to the other side to the final position nose down and wait for 1 minute or until symptoms subside. The patient is moved into each position as quickly as possible to deflect the cupula violently. These tests only need to be performed a few times.

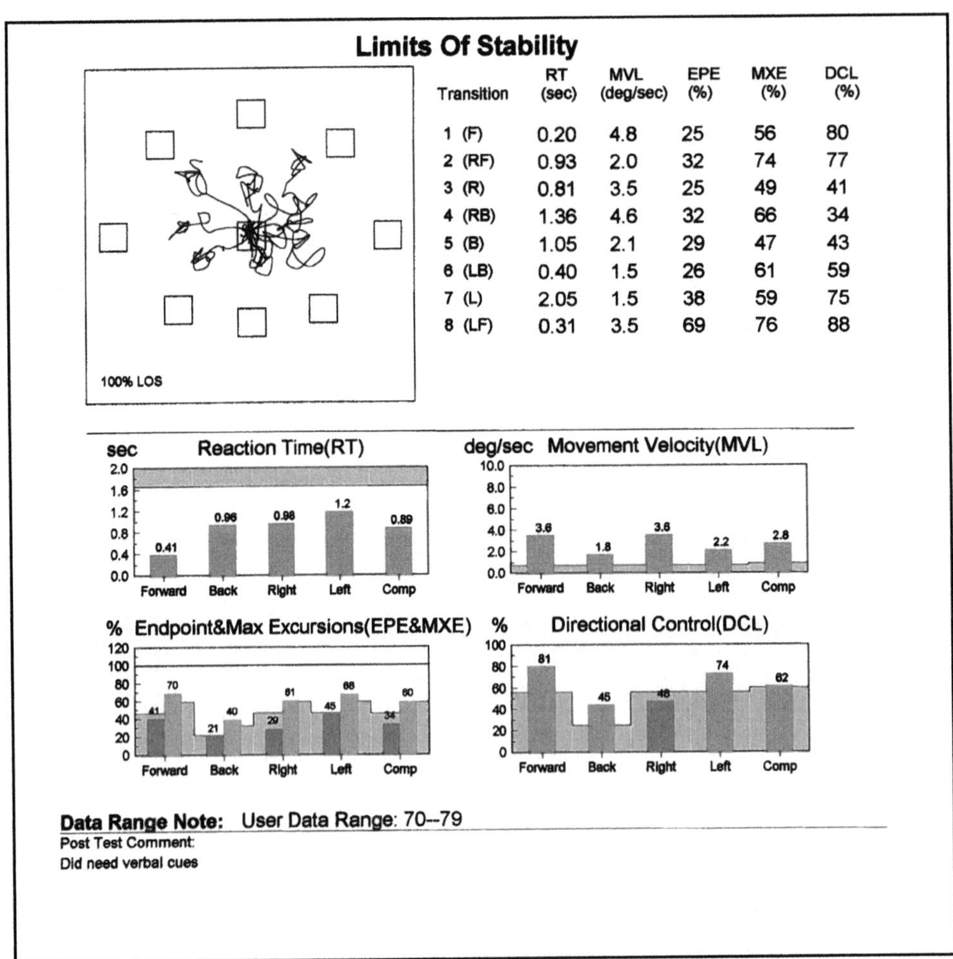

**Limits Of Stability**

| Transition | RT (sec) | MVL (deg/sec) | EPE (%) | MXE (%) | DCL (%) |
|---|---|---|---|---|---|
| 1 (F) | 0.20 | 4.8 | 25 | 56 | 80 |
| 2 (RF) | 0.93 | 2.0 | 32 | 74 | 77 |
| 3 (R) | 0.81 | 3.5 | 25 | 49 | 41 |
| 4 (RB) | 1.36 | 4.6 | 32 | 66 | 34 |
| 5 (B) | 1.05 | 2.1 | 29 | 47 | 43 |
| 6 (LB) | 0.40 | 1.5 | 26 | 61 | 59 |
| 7 (L) | 2.05 | 1.5 | 38 | 59 | 75 |
| 8 (LF) | 0.31 | 3.5 | 69 | 76 | 88 |



**Figure 8-12.** The LOS test. This graphic depicts actual results of an LOS test. These results indicate that this patient did not shift their weight very far in any direction, and weight shift to the right was most limited. These results are actual patient test results on a NeuroCom Balance Master (NeuroCom International, Inc).

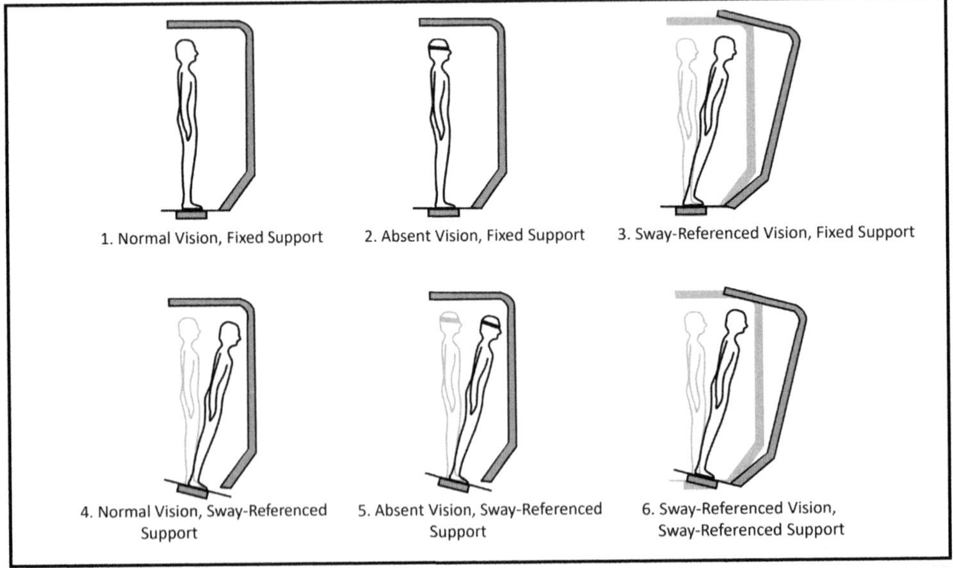



**Figure 8-13.** The SOT. There are 3 conditions in which the platform is stationary: (1) the eyes are opened, (2) eyes are closed, and (3) visual surrounding moves up and down. For the last 3 conditions, the platform moves in 3 different conditions: (4) with the patient's eyes open, (5) patient's eyes closed, and (6) patient's eyes open with the visual surrounding moving up and down. (Graphic created by Jimmy Kopack.)

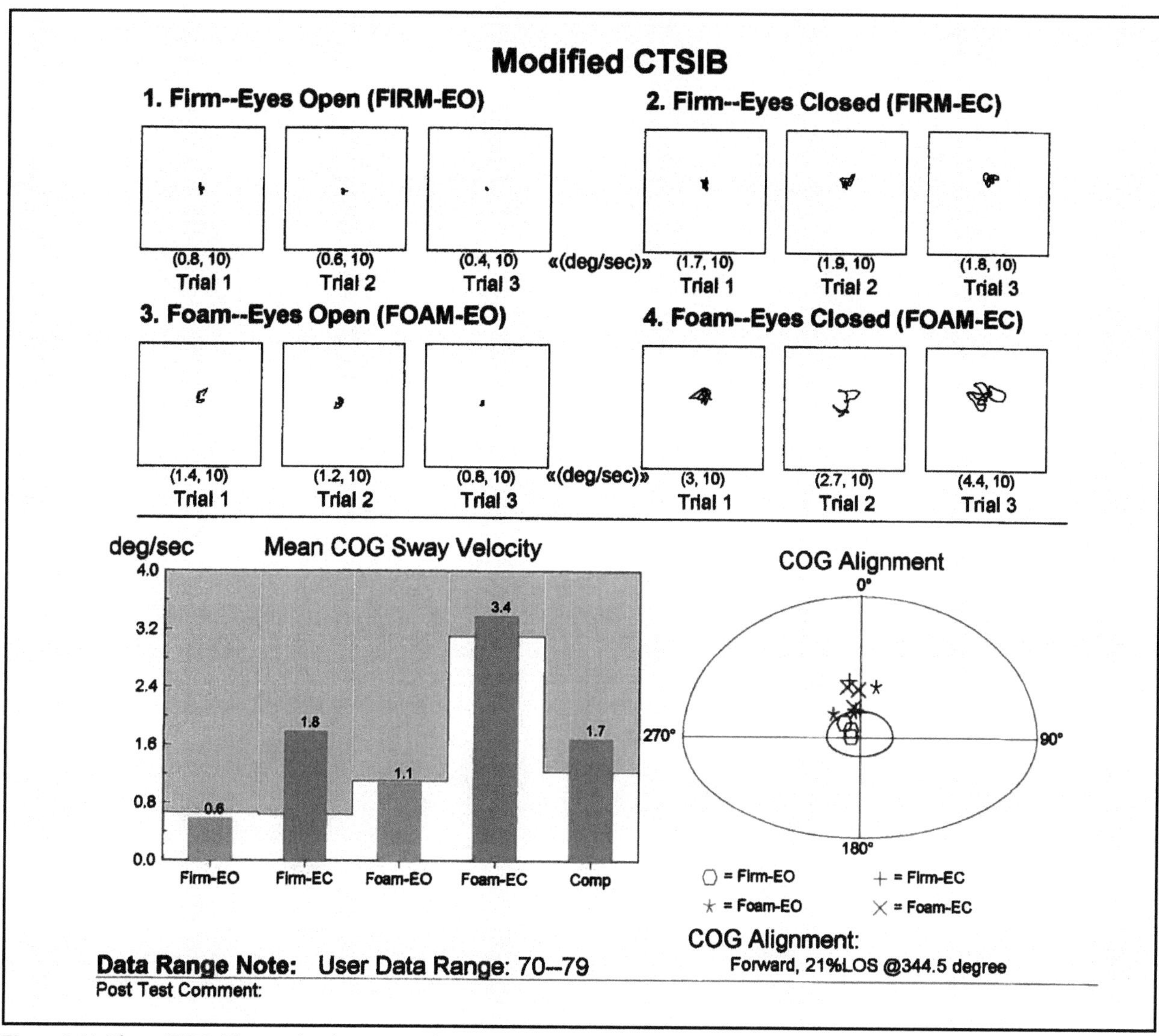


**Figure 8-14.** The mCTSIB. This graphic depicts actual results of an mCTSIB performed on a platform that recorded the results. These test results reveal that the patient is weight bearing more through the left lower extremity than the right and has significant sway with the patient's eyes closed on the floor and on the foam. These results are actual patient test results on a NeuroCom Balance Master (NeuroCom International, Inc).

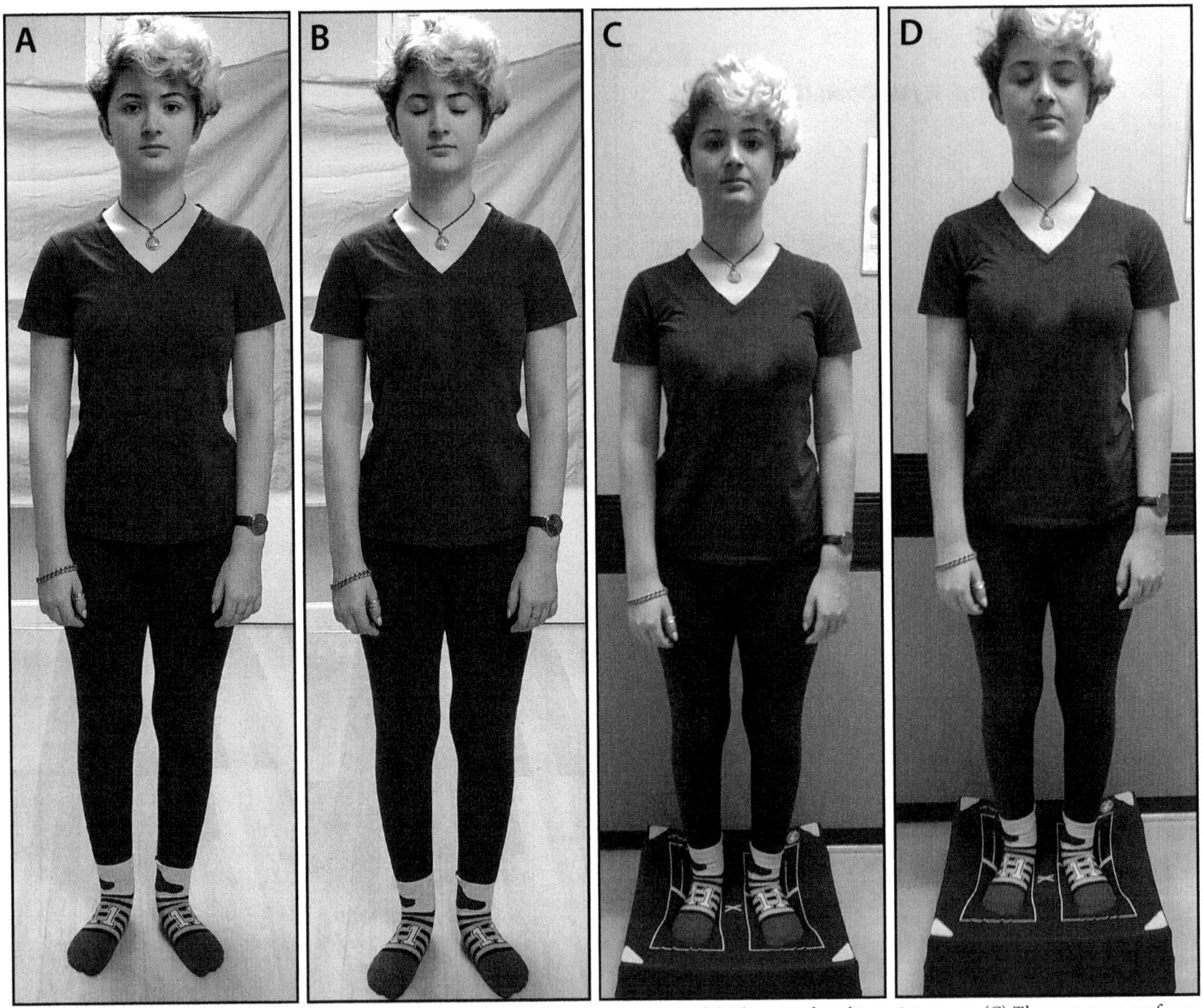

**Figure 8-15.** (A) The mCTSIB without using a platform. The eyes open in quiet stance. (B) The eyes closed in quiet stance. (C) The eyes open on foam. (D) The eyes closed on foam.

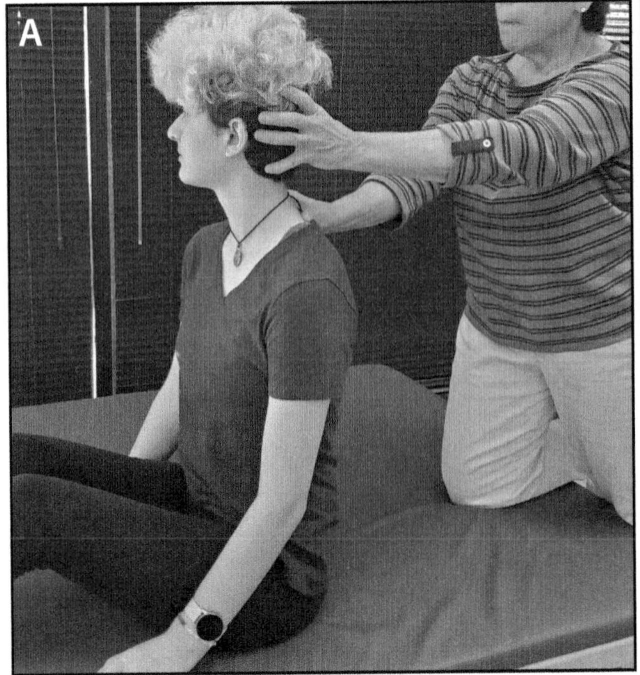


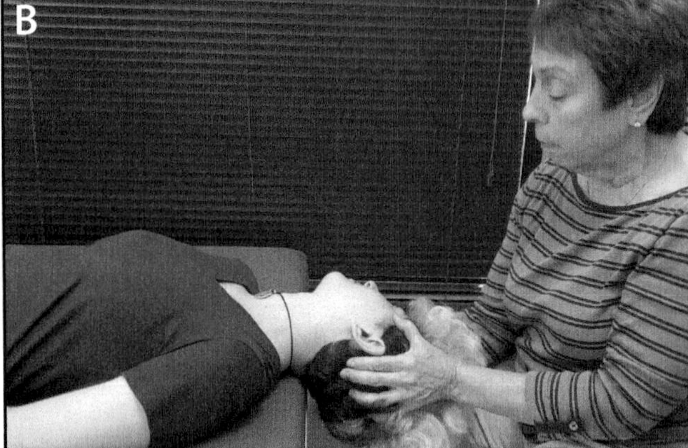


**Figure 8-16.** (A) The Dix-Hallpike test for the right posterior canal starting position. (B) The Dix-Hallpike end position. The clinician is looking at the patient's eyes to determine right anterior or posterior SCC involvement.

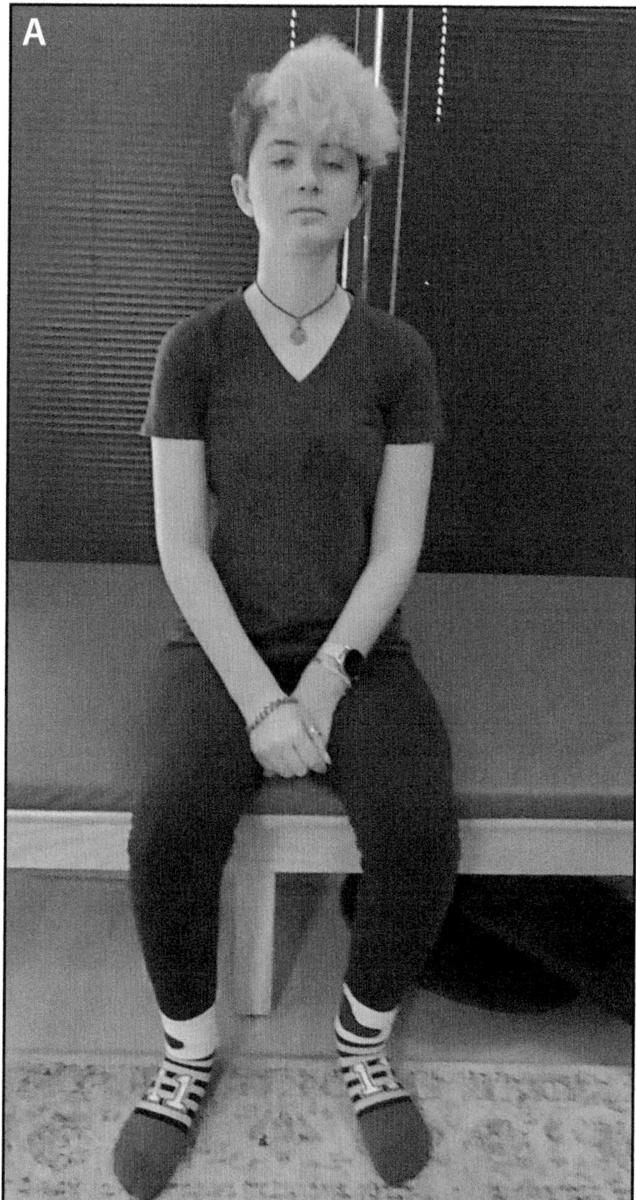

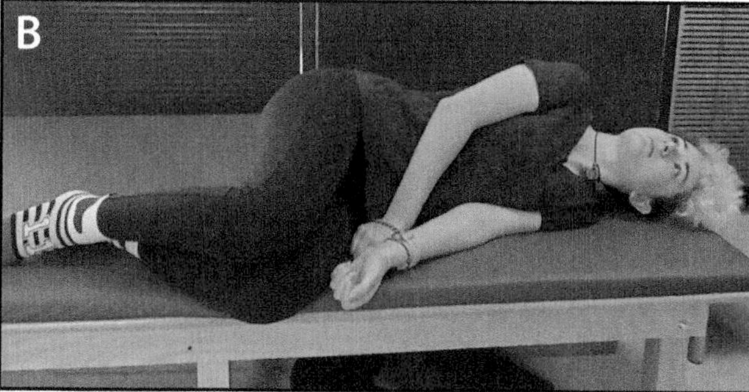

**Figure 8-17.** (A) The starting position for the side-lying test. Remind the patient to keep their eyes open during the test. (B) The side-lying test for the left SCC (end position) can be used in place of the Dix-Hallpike test.

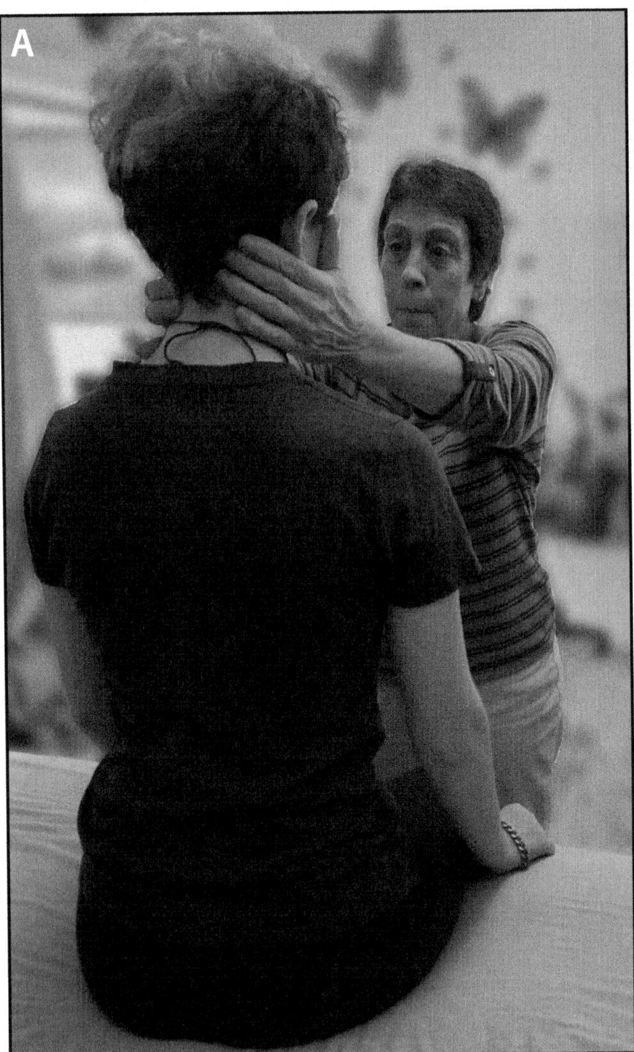


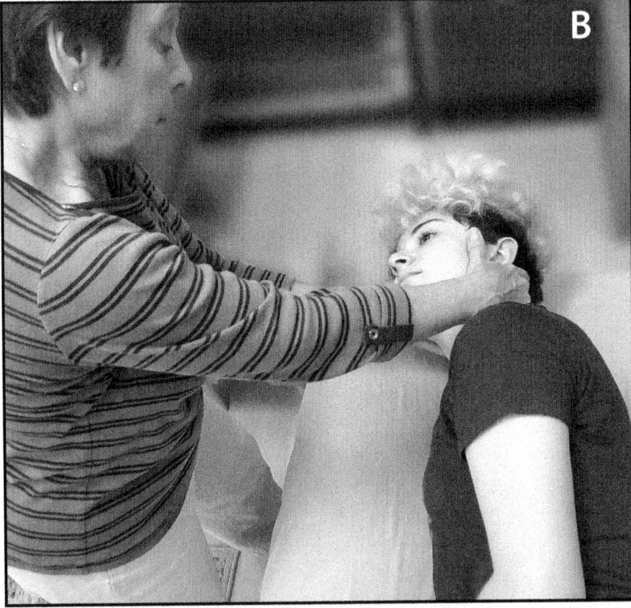


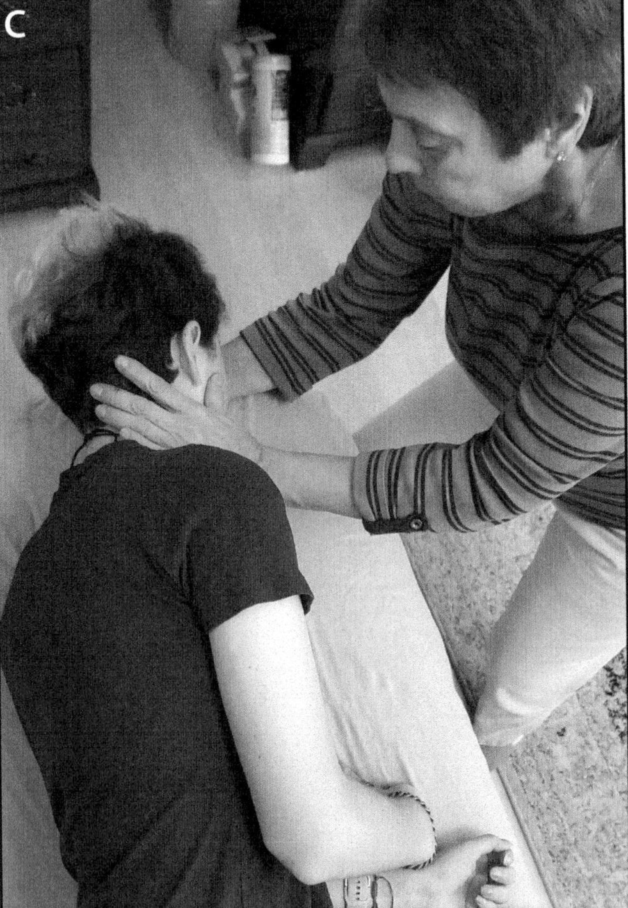


**Figure 8-18.** (A) The starting position for the Semont liberatory maneuver. Support the neck and rotate the head left. (B) Bring the patient down quickly with the nose up to treat right posterior cupulolithiasis. (C) The final position for the Semont liberatory maneuver.

If the Dix-Hallpike test or side-lying test does not provoke vertigo or observable nystagmus, the roll test (see Figure 8-19) can be performed to test the horizontal canals. The nystagmus observed will be either geotropic (toward the floor) or apogeotropic (toward the ceiling). The head must be slightly flexed about 10 degrees before rotating the head to the left or right. Horizontal canalithiasis will produce geotropic nystagmus, and horizontal cupulolithiasis produces apogeotropic nystagmus. BPPV treatment intervention is initiated immediately after the nystagmus is observed and it fatigues. The Dix-Hallpike and the roll test procedures serve as the beginning of the actual treatment intervention. Because the replication of testing procedures is part of the treatment intervention, assistants need to be familiar with the testing procedures and the results.

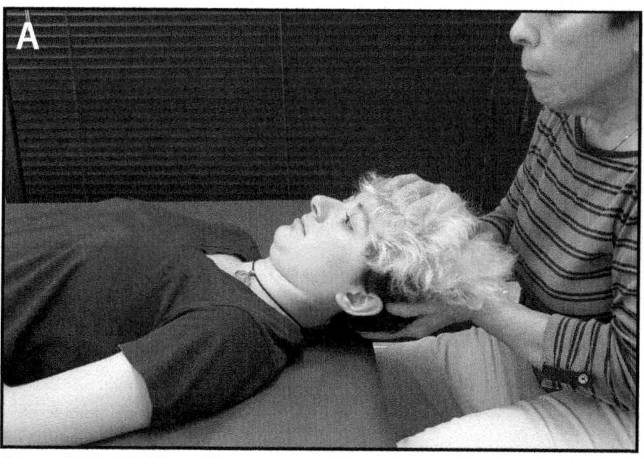


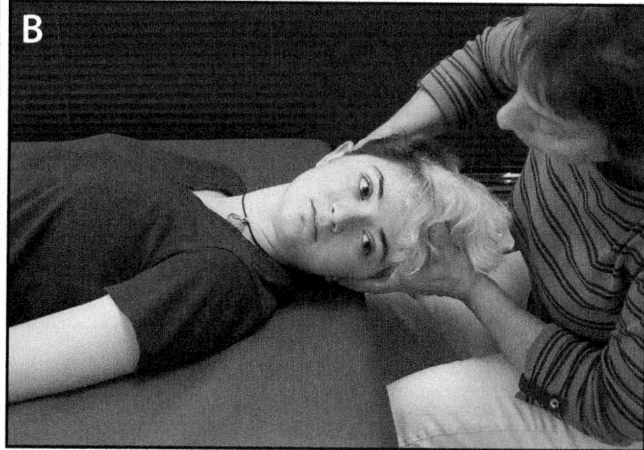


**Figure 8-19.** (A) The roll test to assess horizontal SCC involvement. Notice the patient's head is held in slight flexion so the canals are more in line with gravity. (B) The roll test to assess the left horizontal SCC. The clinician is looking for geotropism (canal involvement) or ageotropism (cupula involvement) during the test.

### *Functional Balance Tests*

Balance and gait tests are used to collect objective data that describe a patient's baseline status and are used to quantify their progress. The Romberg Test, single-leg stance (SLS), Functional Reach Test, and the Berg Balance Scale are useful tools to assess functional balance; these are commonly used in both inpatient and outpatient clinical environments. Many functional tests have thresholds or cutoff scores to determine if a patient is at risk for falling (Table 8-8). The assistant should be proficient with grading patient performance on these tests; good inter-rater reliability with the supervising therapist increases the reliability of the results.

The Dynamic Gait Index assesses changes in gait speeds, direction changes, stepping over and around objects, gait with horizontal and vertical head movements, and stair climbing capabilities. The Berg Balance Scale and the Dynamic Gait Index have a moderate correlation for patients with vestibular and balance conditions.[8]

Tools that assess a patient's fear of falling or balance confidence can provide useful information. The Activities Specific Balance Scale is a commonly used self-report tool that ranks a patient's balance confidence. Physical therapist assistants should consider the reliability and validity of available clinical tools that assess balance or fall risk. Additional tools that are used to assess balance include (but are not limited to) the Timed Up and Go (TUG) Test and the 10-Meter Walk Test (refer to Chapter 7), the Balance Evaluation Systems Test, the Mini Balance Evaluation Systems Test, the Brunel Balance Assessment, the Star Excursion Balance Test (more commonly used to determine readiness to return to sport), the Tinetti Performance-Oriented Mobility Assessment, and the Timed Single-Limb Stance Test.

## Balance and Vestibular Interventions

Balance training and vestibular rehabilitation can effectively help reduce fall risk and the fear of falling and improve QOL. Balance retraining is used to improve and enhance motor coordination and movements related to maintaining COM over the BOS during static and dynamic activities. BPPV and gaze stabilization exercises, adaptation, habituation, and substitution are vestibular rehabilitation interventions that reduce vertigo symptoms, improve gaze stability, and improve postural control responses. With increasing access to and affordability of technology, there may be better access to technological tools in the clinic that facilitate balance assessment and treatment, such as computerized balance scales, virtual reality, and Dynavision (Dynavision International).

### *Balance Training*

Balance activities are used to improve a patient's steadiness with static or dynamic balance under various conditions (ie, reaching, performing dual tasks, or walking on uneven surfaces). It is important to challenge the patient's balance so they have to work at maintaining their balance, but balance training must be performed in a controlled and safe environment. The use of a body weight support harness or a gait belt during training activities can provide additional support during early treatment. Initial treatment interventions should focus on improving the patient's static balance and correctly selecting an appropriate balance strategy in response to COM movements (ankle, hip, or stepping strategy). Balance skills are highly task/context specific, so interventions should reflect the patient's individual presentation, functional needs, and goals.

**Table 8-8**

Balance and Gait Tests[8]

| Test | Assesses | Scoring Parameters |
|---|---|---|
| Berg Balance Scale | Static and dynamic balance, fall risk | Maximum score of 56<br>Fall risk with score ≤45 |
| SLS | Balance | < 10 seconds = balance problem<br>≤5 seconds = fall risk |
| Dynamic Gait Index | Dynamic balance and fall risk | Maximum score of 24<br>≤19 indicates fall risk |

### Considerations for the Physical Therapist Assistant

Initiating balance training can be scary for patients, especially initially. To decrease anxiety and promote patient engagement, thoroughly explain the task to the patient, provide encouragement, and provide the needed physical support/assistance. The clinician should provide support initially, but be prepared to decrease this support as soon as possible to challenge balance and promote active control by the patient.

Clinicians should select training interventions that address the patient's deficits and goals. General guidelines when selecting balance training interventions include answering the following questions:

- Does the patient demonstrate equal weight bearing, or do they sit or stand shifted to one side? The goal is to obtain symmetrical weight bearing.
- Does the patient use the proper strategy (ankle, hip, or stepping) that matches the size of the perturbation? The goal is utilization of the appropriate strategy.
- How safe is the patient when performing an activity in sitting or standing (static postures)? The goal is independent and safe ability to maintain static postures and safe completion of each activity.
- How stable is the patient in sitting on a solid surface or compliant (foam cushion or ball) surface? The goal is for the patient to be able to maintain balance during activities of daily living (ADLs) and mobility; consider household seating options.
- How stable is the patient in standing on a solid surface? A compliant (ie, foam or sand/grass) surface? The goal is for the patient to be able to maintain balance during ADLs and mobility; consider household flooring. Can the patient maintain balance by varying the size of the BOS (ie, from normal stance to progressing to single-leg standing)? The goal is for the patient to be able to maintain balance within varied size BOS positions.
- Can the patient maintain their balance while moving? Can the patient walk on the floor or a compliant surface (ie, grass or carpet) and pair ambulation with an activity/motion (ie, turn their head while walking)? The goal is for the patient to be able to maintain balance on whichever surfaces they are routinely performing ADLs and mobility on with movement transitions and during dual tasks.

It is important to select the appropriate exercises to promote the desired postural strategy (ie, ankle or hip). To promote the proper utilization of ankle strategies (Figure 8-20), it is appropriate to include exercises such as weight shifting laterally and controlled anterior/posterior sway; partial step-ups; or standing on a BOSU Balance Trainer or rocker board, a mini-trampoline, or foam. Using a small BOS promotes a hip strategy utilization. Activity progressions include standing with feet together (Romberg), modified tandem stance (modified sharpened Romberg), tandem stance (sharpened Romberg), and single-leg standing (Figures 8-21A through 8-21D). The patient should be able to demonstrate ankle strategies with light or small perturbations and hip strategies with larger ones. Once the patient is able to use the desired strategy and maintain balance in that position with control, the assistant can make the activity more challenging by changing the surface, adding upper extremity tasks, changing the size of the BOS, and/or initiating dynamic activities. Some dynamic activities include standing on a half roll, walking on a balance beam (or on a line taped/painted on the floor), walking on uneven surfaces, walking while tossing or kicking a ball, and other stepping activities. The goal is for the patient to be able to make reflexive decisions and use the appropriate strategy based on the size of the balance disturbance; use an ankle strategy first for small disturbances and then a hip strategy for larger in-place disturbances. If disturbances are too large for in-place strategies, the patient should be able to take a reflexive step to maintain their balance and avoid falling.

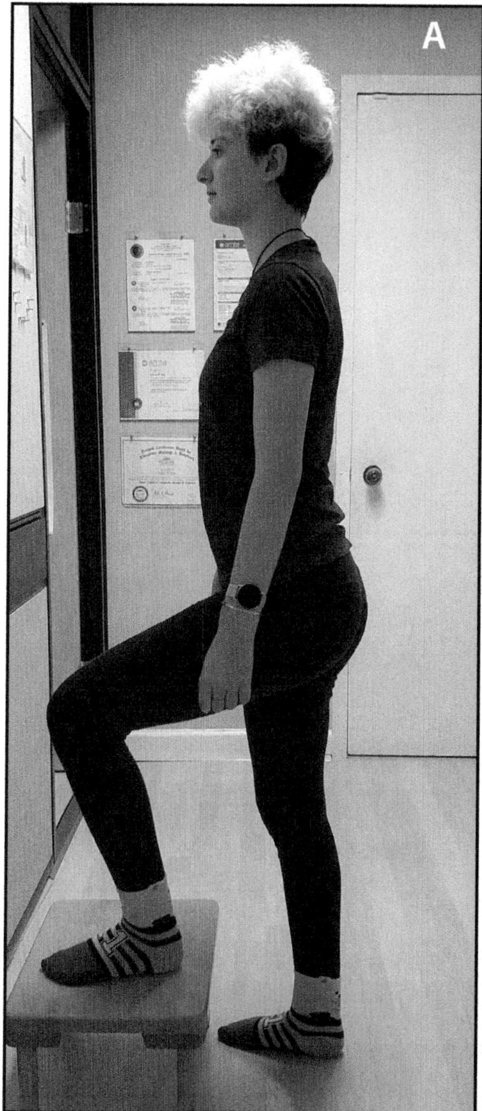

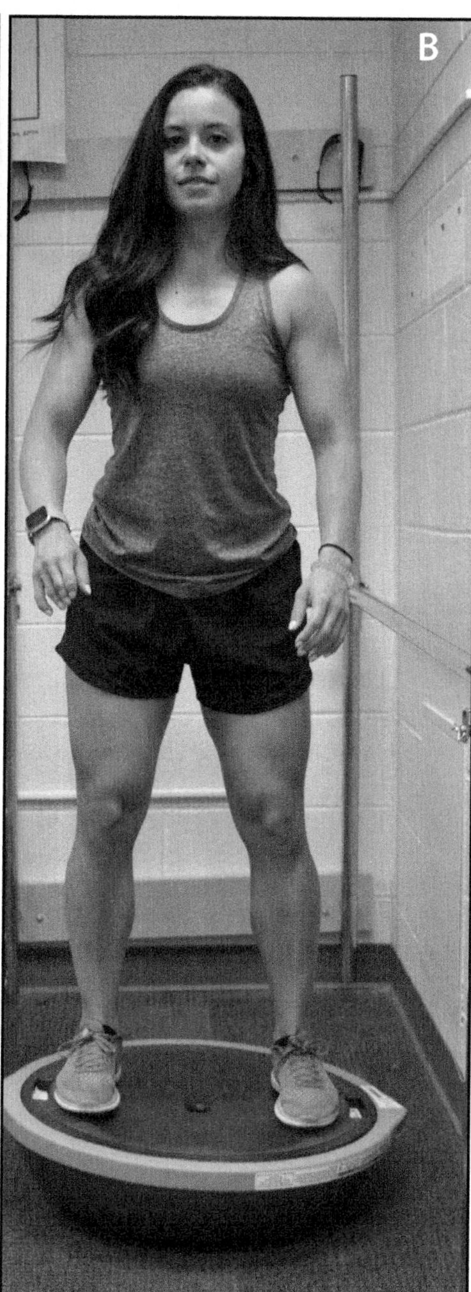

**Figure 8-20.** (A) A partial step-up to promote ankle strategy on the right leg. (B) BOSU Balance Trainer or a wobble board facilitates an ankle strategy.

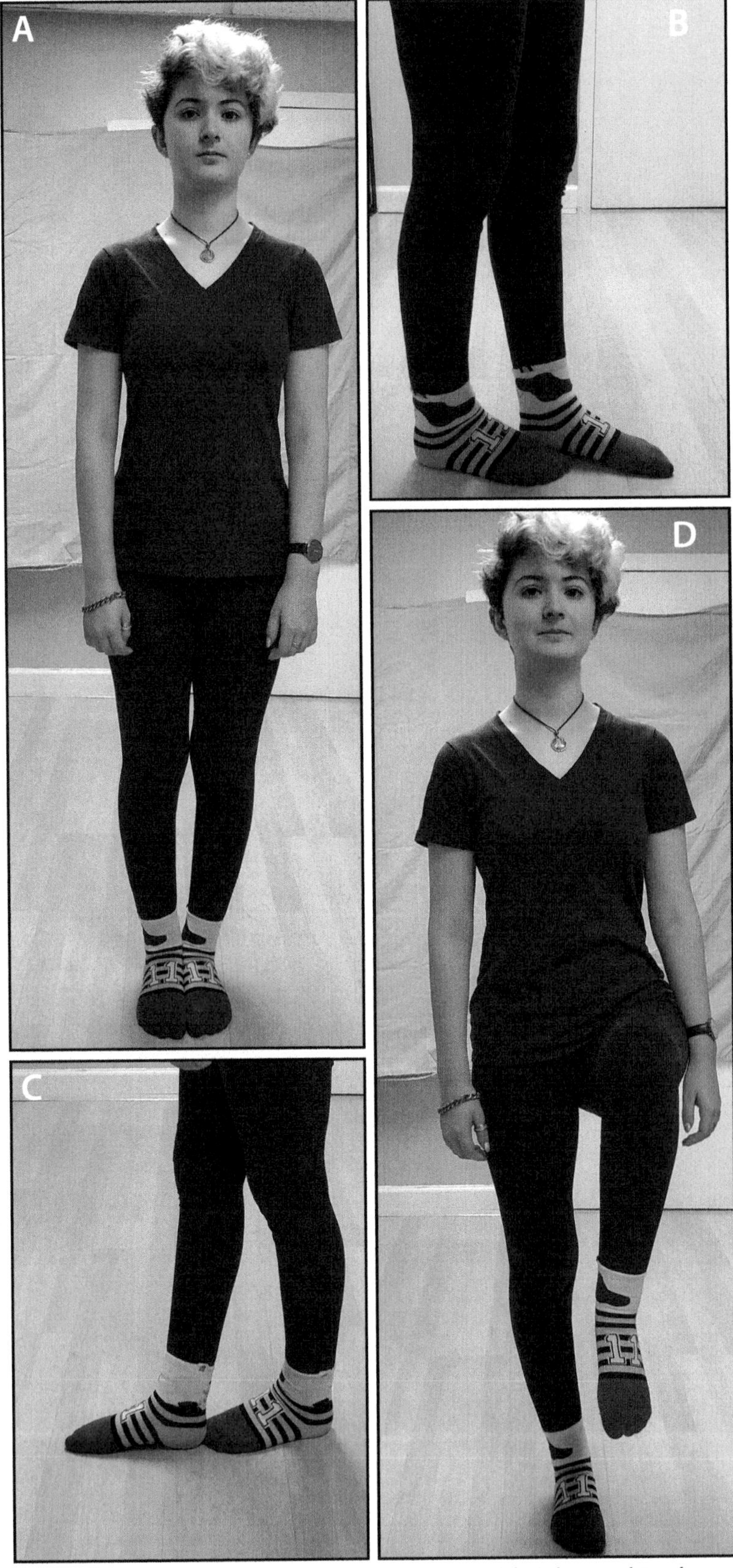


**Figure 8-21.** (A) Romberg with the eyes open. (B) The modified sharpened Romberg or tandem standing promotes hip strategies to maintain balance. (C) Sharpened Romberg or tandem standing to promote hip strategy. (D) Single-leg standing.

**Table 8-9**

## Static Balance Exercise Progressions

Ensure that the environment is safe, that the clinician is guarding appropriately, and that the tasks are challenging but not too advanced given the patient's current level of function.

### Sample Progressions: Sitting

- Static sitting with clinician support ⇨ progress by decreasing support provided while increasing the time that the clinician maintains the posture
- Static sitting with bilateral upper extremity support ⇨ unilateral upper extremity support ⇨ no upper extremity support
- Static sitting with eyes open ⇨ eyes closed
- Static sitting on level surface ⇨ foam pad ⇨ physioball
- Static stance with widened BOS ⇨ narrow BOS

### Sample Progressions: Standing

- Static standing with clinician support ⇨ progress by decreasing support provided while increasing the time that the clinician maintains the posture
- Static standing with bilateral upper extremity support ⇨ unilateral upper extremity support ⇨ no upper extremity support
- Static stance with eyes open ⇨ eyes closed
- Static stance on level surface ⇨ foam pad ⇨ wobble board
- Static stance with wide BOS ⇨ narrow BOS ⇨ feet together ⇨ semi-tandem ⇨ tandem ⇨ SLS

Physical therapist assistants typically address sitting balance first and advance interventions to challenge the patient based on their response (Table 8-9). Static balance interventions are typically progressed by increasing the time that a patient can maintain the initial posture without assistance. Progressions are listed in Table 8-9.

As static balance improves, the clinician will initiate and progress dynamic balance training interventions to promote the patient's return to maximal independence (Table 8-10). Dynamic interventions are initiated after the patient can statically maintain a posture without assistance with limited postural sway. Activities that promote weight shifts within the BOS are progressed to weight shifts/motions that shift the COM outside of the BOS. Additional progressions include decreasing the use of upper extremity support, decreasing the BOS, moving from a solid surface to a compliant surface, and moving from eyes open to eyes closed. The general goals of dynamic balance training are to increase consistency, range, and speed of self-initiated motions while encouraging symmetry. The clinician uses varied tasks while gradually decreasing assistance/support and progressively increasing challenges to retrain the patient's automatic balance reactions and protective responses. Training progresses from a closed to an open environment and, finally, to environments and tasks that simulate those needed for ADLs, independent ADLs, and recreational/community level function. Clinicians can incorporate sensory stimulation techniques and timed task training to improve response times.

### Documentation Tip

Document all parameters of balance training interventions that are included in a treatment session, including task description, surface, use of upper extremity support, need for assistance, and time/repetitions completed. For example, documentation that states "Dynamic balance exercises completed for 8 minutes" is inadequate; it does not justify that skilled care was provided nor does it aid with continuity of care (the next clinician cannot determine the specific exercise/activity the patient performed). Appropriate documentation includes the following:

O: Static balance on foam surface eyes open × 2 minutes × 3 reps with close S and no LOB. Standing balance activities, including weight shifts anterior/posterior with 3-second hold at end of LOS no UE support × 2 minutes × 3 reps with close S with LOB 1 × on last rep requiring VC to regain balance. Functional reach activities for cones with no UE support with CG and VC for weight shifting to regain balance (required during reaching tasks that result in shift of COG).

A: Patient's static balance has improved from last week, with less sway on foam. Weight shift now occurs without assistance and with increased distance during weight shift to end of LOS using ankle strategy, indicating improvement. The LOB on last rep was associated with fatigue. Patient's improved ability to complete reaching tasks is needed for return to I with ADLs.

P: Progress dynamic balance training activities: Attempt eyes closed on foam and increase practice time duration with weight shifts, add variable perturbations to address appropriate strategy selection, and increase excursion of functional reach activities.

**Table 8-10**

Dynamic Balance Exercise Progressions

| Ensure that the environment is safe, that the clinician is guarding appropriately, and that the tasks are challenging but not too advanced given the patient's current level of function. Not all patients will be able to progress through/complete all levels. |
|---|
| **Early/Beginner Interventions** |
| • Start with widened or normal stance, eyes open<br>• Progress from bilateral upper extremity support to light touch to unilateral upper extremity light touch support to no use of upper extremities for support<br>• Suggested task progressions<br>○ Weight shifts (small excursion within BOS to larger excursions approaching LOS)<br>○ Head rotations; progress to head and trunk rotations<br>○ Head tilts<br>○ Heel/toe raises<br>○ Hip circles<br>○ Gait |
| **Intermediate-Level Tasks** |
| • Sit to stands (vary surface height: Elevated with progression to lower height, speed, with upper extremity support to no upper extremity support)<br>• Exaggerated arm swings<br>• Functional reaching<br>• High marches<br>• Partial squats<br>• Partial lunges<br>• Gait with narrowed BOS<br>• Gait with wide turns<br>• Side stepping (progress from upper extremity support to no upper extremity support) |

*(continued)*

## Compensatory Interventions and Environmental Adaptations

Some patients may not improve their balance enough to be safe for independent household and/or community-level function. In these situations, clinicians need to assess individual situations and create recommendations to maximize the patient's safety at their current level of function. Providing training that incorporates compensatory strategies can help patients return to some activities. These strategies include wearing appropriate footwear (ie, sneakers/shoes with nonslip soles and no flip-flops or high heels), using an assistive device, using a wider BOS and decreased speed during turning, and using a wider BOS with a lower COM when performing activities in less stable situations.

The physical therapy team plays an important role in fall prevention. Fall prevention education is indicated for patients and older adults in the community setting. Educational resources have been developed by the American Physical Therapy Association and the CDC to target fall prevention (see Suggested Resources). Clinicians should educate patients regarding the following basic environmental modifications that can decrease fall risk:

- Ensure there is adequate lighting (ie, add night-lights to ensure rooms are well lit and use a minimum of 60-watt light bulbs in lamps).
- Make sure light switches are easily accessible, or suggest lights be put on timers.
- Remove throw rugs; ensure all carpets/rugs are firmly tacked down.
- Create open pathways around furniture; remove clutter.
- Use chairs that are at appropriate heights and firmness.
- Provide adequate lighting and marking on stairs (consider the use of contrast tape); install handrails if needed.
- Install grab bars in bathrooms, use nonskid mats in shower/tub area, or use a shower chair.

**Table 8-10 (continued)**

## Dynamic Balance Exercise Progressions

| Advanced-Level Tasks |
|---|
| • Single-limb stance (progressions: With heel/toe raises on weight-bearing limb, partial squats on weight-bearing limb, alphabet trace with unweighted limb, ball kicks with unweighted limb)<br>• Dual-task activities (bouncing/catching/throwing ball, balloon toss/hit with paddle, Walkie-Talkie test)<br>• Games: Bowling, shuffleboard, Wii (Nintendo)<br>• Picking objects up in squat<br>• Lunges to half kneel (progress from upper extremity support to no upper extremity support)<br>• Floor-to-stand transfers<br>• 4-way gait (eyes open/eyes closed)<br>• Tandem gait<br>• Gait with head turns<br>• Braiding, line dancing<br>• Gait with small turns<br>• Walking in circles, figure 8<br>• Quick starts/stops<br>• Treadmill training (progress by increasing speed)<br>• Heel/toe walking<br>• Walking over ladder rungs<br>• Obstacle courses<br>• Step-ups (forward, backward, lateral)<br>• Steps/ramps/curbs<br>• Community activities: Opening doors/pushing carts/car and bus transfers/carrying items, getting on/off escalator/elevator, crossing street |

Recommendations for modifications should be individualized to the patient. A home environmental assessment allows the clinician to create individualized/specific recommendations to maximize patient safety.

## Vestibular Rehabilitation

Vestibular rehabilitation promotes compensation for vestibular deficits using specific exercises to address those deficits while promoting optimal use of the vestibular, visual somatosensory, and motor systems. Exercises are designed to reduce dizziness and/or vertigo, stabilize one's vision during static and/or dynamic activities (using gaze stabilization exercises), and improve postural stability. The order of treatment intervention is very important with vestibular rehabilitation. There is moderate to strong evidence that vestibular rehabilitation is a safe and effective intervention to manage vestibular disorders.[23]

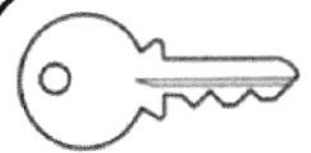

**Key Safety Considerations**

Patients must have a stable vestibular lesion before initiating vestibular rehabilitation exercises.

### Benign Paroxysmal Positional Vertigo Interventions

The order of treatment is very important, and treating the patient's dizziness/vertigo or BPPV (if present) must occur first. Before testing and treatment, the clinician should explain the procedure and inform the patient that they will likely experience dizziness during the treatment and they might be nauseous, but symptoms should significantly resolve after the treatment. Before performing the initial examination, the physical therapist obtains the patient's consent and then completes the appropriate screening (ie, the vertebral artery test) to ensure that it is safe/appropriate to proceed. Once cleared and with the affected canal identified, the clinician can proceed to treating the dizziness.

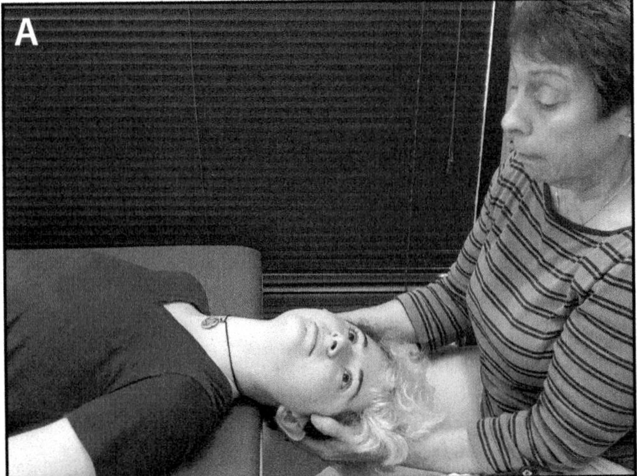


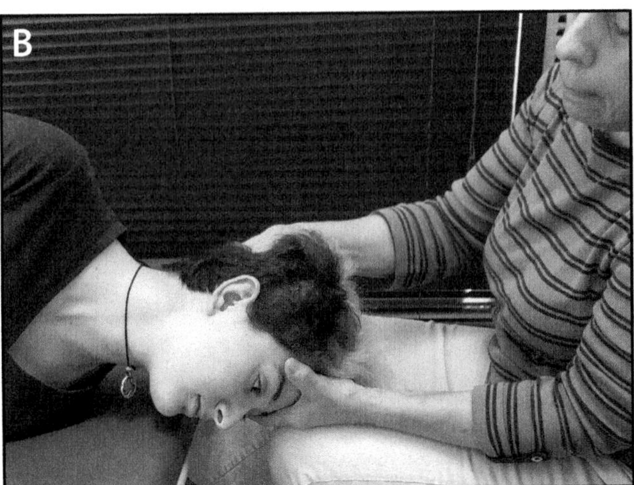


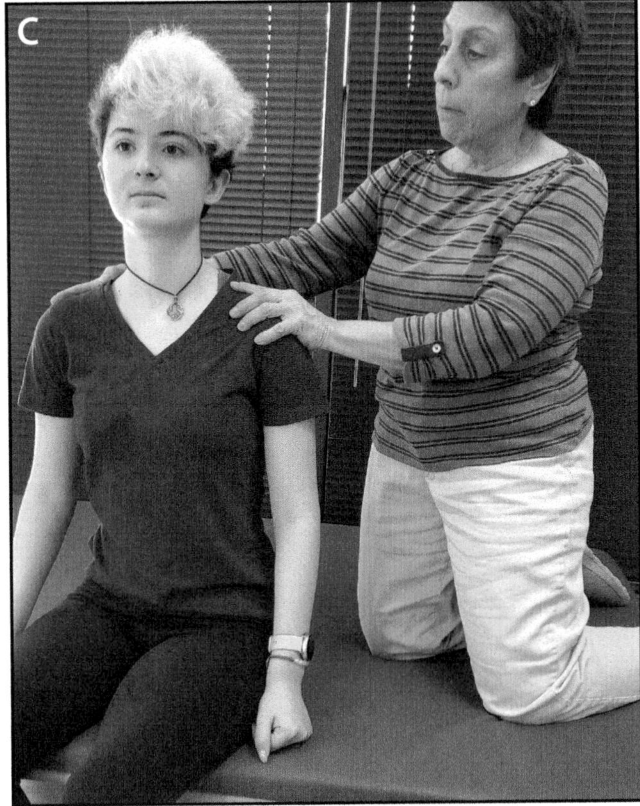


**Figure 8-22.** (A) The CRT follows the Dix-Hallpike test. For a right posterior canal, the head is rotated to the left 90 degrees. Notice the head is maintained in 10 degrees of extension. (B) The patient's head is supported in a slight nose down position, and the clinician's forearm rests on her thigh and acts as a stabilizer. (C) The patient is brought into sitting and supported by the clinician.

The **Epley maneuver or canal repositioning techniques (CRTs)** and Semont liberatory maneuver are commonly used to move the debris from the canal(s) and/or off the cupula and back into the otolith organ.[12,22] Because the posterior canal is most commonly affected, the Dix-Hallpike test (see Figure 8-16) is performed with the involved ear down during the test (in the case depicted in the figure, the right posterior SCC). The test position should be held until the torsional nystagmus fatigues (or is longer than 1 minute) and/or the patient reports the dizziness has stopped. The clinician will assess the results of the Dix-Hallpike test to determine if CRT or the Semont liberatory maneuver is indicated.

After bringing the patient down into the Dix-Hallpike maneuver (see Figure 8-16), the patient is then put through the movement sequence described in Figures 8-22A through 8-22C. The clinician should remind the patient to keep their eyes open during the entire procedure so nystagmus can be observed. The patient usually tells the clinician when their spinning starts and when it decreases or has stopped. The patient can be moved to the next sequential position once symptoms have resolved for about 20 seconds. During the final step of the procedure, the clinician should support the patient, who may experience dizziness upon returning to the sitting position (see Figure 8-22C). It is ideal to have another clinician in front of the patient to observe for any torsional nystagmus when returning to sitting. After waiting a few minutes, the clinician assesses the patient's symptoms and repeats the Dix-Hallpike test to see if the canal has been cleared. If nystagmus is still noted, the clinician may repeat the CRT one more time only. If no or minimal reports of dizziness are reported or there is no

## Box 8-2

### Instructions for Patients After the Canal Repositioning Technique for Benign Paroxysmal Positional Vertigo

- Sleep on an incline at about 30 degrees or in a recliner for 1 to 2 nights after the treatment.
- Stay as upright as possible. Avoid bending forward (eg, picking things off the floor, looking in a low cabinet or reaching into an overhead cabinet) for 1 to 2 days.
- Avoid tilting the head forward or backward (eg, washing your hair, brushing your teeth).
- Avoid moving the head quickly in any direction because symptoms may not be tolerated.
- Expect some episodes of slight dizziness or feeling for balance for up to 1 to 5 days.
- If symptoms still occur, return to physical therapy.

observable nystagmus, the clinician assists the patient back into sitting and gives the patient written instructions for home following the treatment (Box 8-2).

If the therapist determines that the Semont liberatory maneuver (see Figure 8-18) is indicated because of cupulolithiasis, the clinician should complete 2 to 3 repetitions of the maneuver before repeating the Dix-Hallpike test. Based on the results of the Dix-Hallpike test, the therapist will either proceed with the CRT treatment or determine that the treatment is complete.

There are different treatments that can be used to treat horizontal canalithiasis, and the Gufoni maneuver is one example (Figure 8-23). For this maneuver, the patient quickly moves down toward the uninvolved side while continuing to look straight ahead, then holding that position for approximately 1 to 2 minutes (Figure 8-23A). The patient then quickly rotates the head downward toward the floor and holds that position for 1 to 2 minutes (Figure 8-23B) prior to returning back to a sitting position (Figure 8-23C).[22] When treating horizontal cupulolithiasis, the position hold times are the same, but the patient moves toward the involved side looking straight ahead and then rotates the head up toward the ceiling before returning to a sitting position.

After any BPPV treatment, the clinician should have the patient rest for about 15 to 20 minutes before leaving the facility, and it is strongly recommended that the patient have transportation to and from the facility for safety reasons. The patient should demonstrate understanding of the written instructions provided by the clinician for home use. The clinician should explain to the patient that intermittent episodes of slight dizziness may occur the following day, but they should not be intense and should subside with static sitting. A follow-up session is recommended to reassess the patient to ensure that the BPPV has resolved.

There are other techniques used to treat BPPV, and the reader is referred to the Suggested Resources listed at the end of the chapter. Physical therapist assistants interested in treating patients with BPPV and other vestibular pathologies will need to continue their education in this specialty practice area.

## Vestibulo-Ocular Reflex Adaptation

There are 3 treatment modes used in vestibular rehabilitation: adaptation (where the vestibular system learns to adapt to error signals), habituation, and substitution. Once dizziness is resolved, the clinician prescribes gaze stabilization exercises to reduce the illusion of movement during eye and head movements and to improve VOR function. It is important to educate patients to move their head. Symptoms may be worse initially because patients tend to avoid head movements (for fear of getting dizzy or having blurred vision), but this should resolve as they continue to perform the exercises over time. The neuroplasticity of the vestibular system responds and accommodates quickly to the exercises. Those activities/motions that make the dizziness worse should be practiced first. When patients perform these exercises, they should experience moderate complaints of symptoms (dizziness). This assists the CNS in making corrections and adapting (to the stimulus that makes them dizzy), and, eventually, the symptoms will disappear. The purpose of gaze stabilization exercises is to improve VOR function by focusing on a target as the head moves. This action creates a retinal slip as the image of the target moves off the retina. A retinal slip is an error signal that occurs, signaling the CNS to adapt and thereby improving the VOR's ability to stabilize vision.[12] The key to stabilizing vision is to make sure the head is moving quickly enough (either horizontally and/or vertically) to keep the target in focus while provoking moderate symptoms and creating the retinal slip signal. If the patient reports severe symptoms of nausea or dizziness, then the head is moving too quickly, and the clinician should educate the patient, cuing them to modify the speed of the movement.

If the patient has a peripheral UVL (and the lesion is stable), the patient will perform specific eye/head movement exercises that allow the CNS to make corrections and adapt to the imbalanced signals coming from the impaired peripheral sensory receptors. There are 2 common exercises to improve VOR function: ×1 viewing and times 2 (×2) viewing. Figure 8-24 illustrates a ×1 viewing exercise, in which a letter is written on a card and held at arm's length or placed on a blank wall (ie, on a sticky note). The patient is instructed to slightly tilt the head down (about 20 degrees

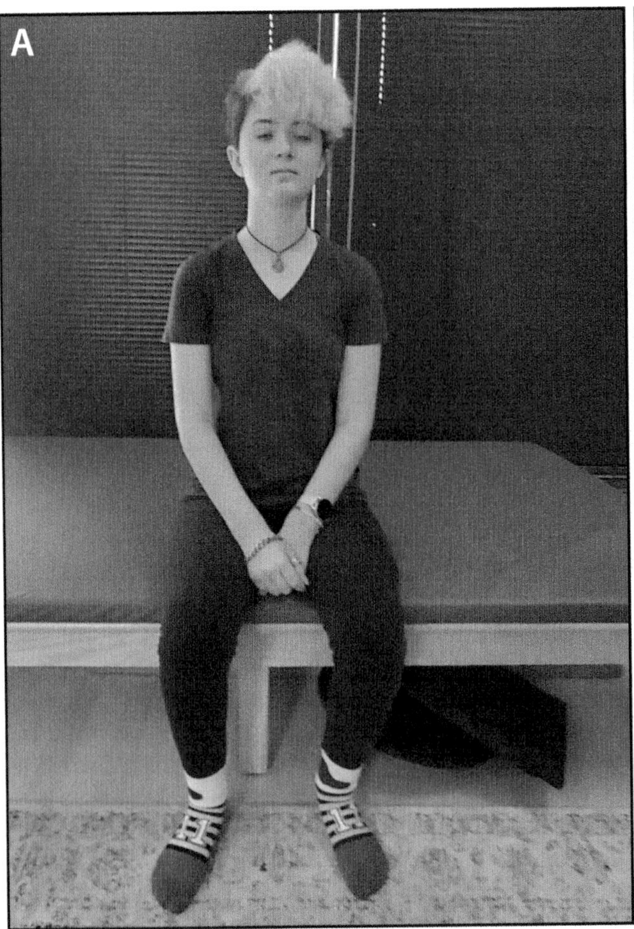


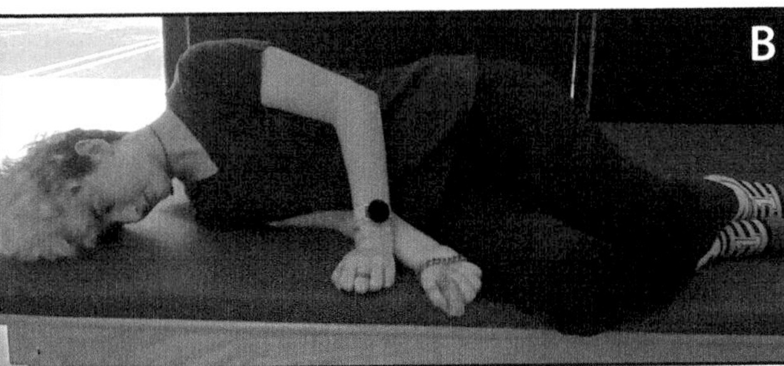


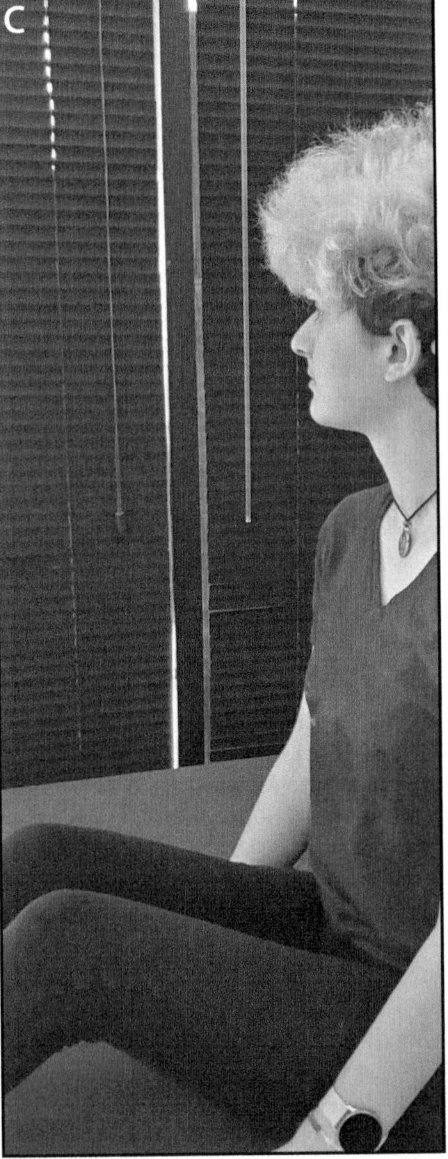


**Figure 8-23.** (A) Starting position for Gufoni maneuver—left horizontal SCC then quickly move onto the right (uninvolved side) keeping the head facing forward and hold for 1 to 2 minutes. (B) Quickly rotate head downward and hold for 1 to 2 minutes. (C) Return to sitting with head rotated right, and once upright, turn head forward facing.

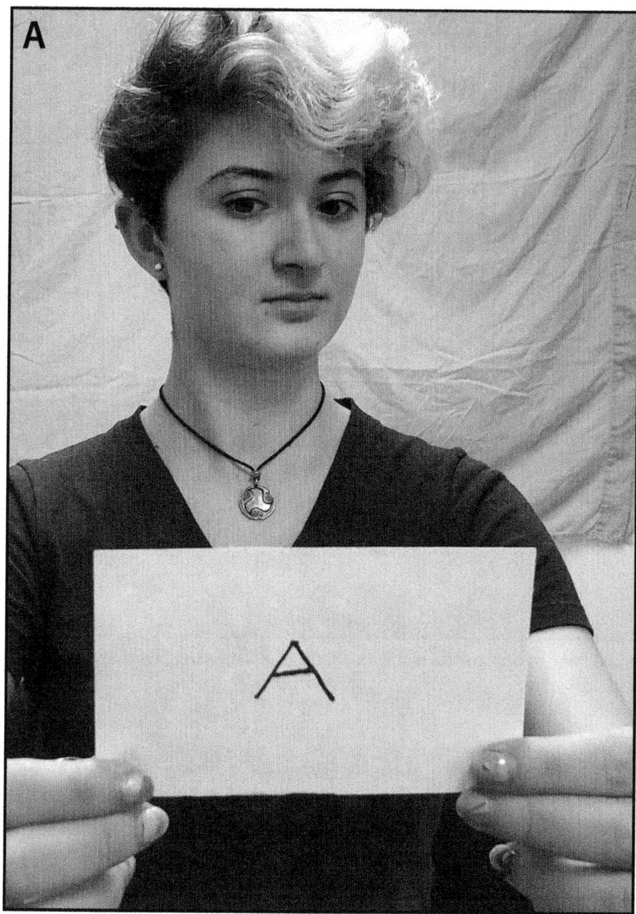


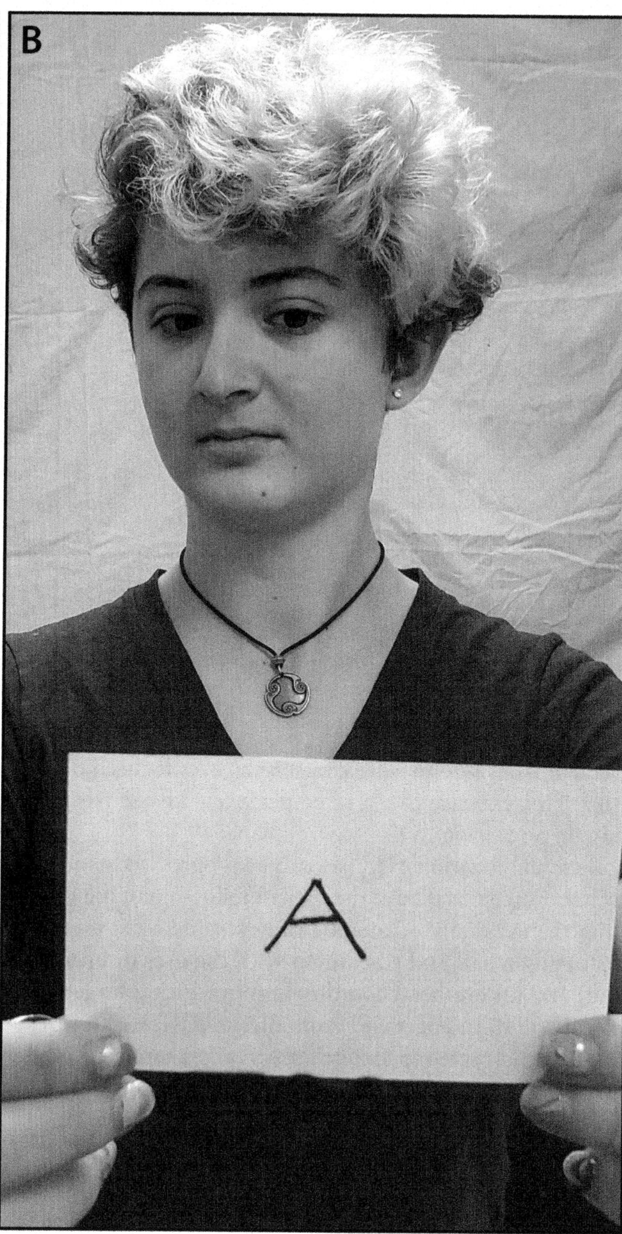


**Figure 8-24.** (A) VOR × 1 viewing. Starting with the head turned to the left and the eyes looking right staying on the target. (B) VOR × 1 viewing. Notice as the patient stays on the target as the head moves.

to bring the horizontal SCC in the correct position) and then move their head side to side in small amplitudes (about 30 degrees, like saying "no") or up and down (like saying "yes") as quickly as possible, keeping the letter in focus. The head should move back and forth at about 2 cycles per second (120 times per minute). Motion direction (horizontal or vertical) is based on which motion makes the patient feel the dizziest. The clinician monitors the length of time that the patient performs the exercise. The goal is 1 minute. When the patient's symptoms increase beyond a tolerable level, head oscillations become erratic, or the patient reports that the letter is blurred, the exercise is stopped, and the duration/time is documented. As patient tolerance increases, the clinician can advance the training by having the patient perform the exercise under various conditions such as standing 3 to 6 ft away from the target or changing the patient's BOS or surface type (ie, foam). Changing the background of the target from a blank wall to a checkerboard will also make the exercise more challenging.

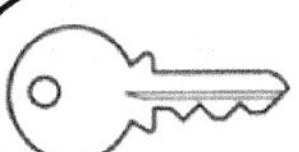

**Key Safety Considerations**

The vestibular system can fatigue, so "more" is not always better. The exercises need to be challenging, but listening to the patient's report of symptoms and close monitoring of the patient's responses are key to creating a proper exercise dosing schedule. Resting 2 to 5 minutes between exercise bouts so the patient's vestibular system can recover is advised.

When performing the × 2 viewing exercise, the patient uses the same card, but the head and card move in opposite directions simultaneously. The patient is instructed to hold the card in the right hand and place the arm approximately 30 degrees to the right of center (Figure 8-25). Instruct the patient to turn the head quickly to the left while still focusing on the letter. The patient is instructed to move the head

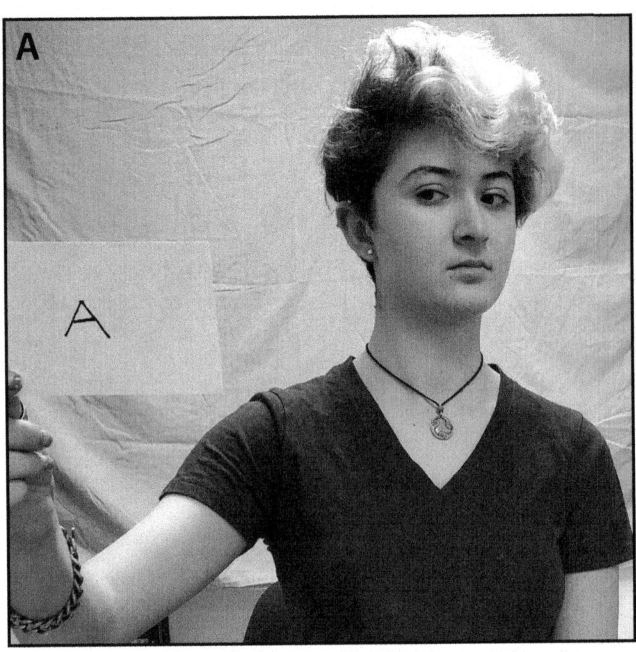


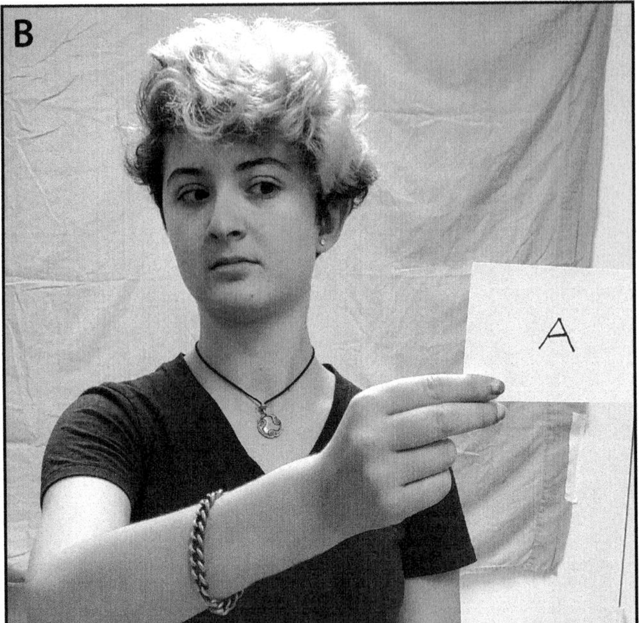


**Figure 8-25.** (A) VOR × 2 viewing starting position. Notice how the eyes and head are in opposite directions. (B) VOR × 2 viewing. The card is moved across the body, and the eyes follow the card as the head rotates in the opposite direction.

and arm from side to side, keeping the eyes focused on the letter. This exercise can also be performed by moving the head up and down in the sagittal plane.

Gaze stabilization exercises can be progressed to include 2 other exercises: (1) have the patient follow a moving target using the eyes only or moving the eyes and head together (ie, tossing a ball and tracking it with the eyes or eyes and head) and (2) eye-head coordination in which 2 targets are held about 18 in apart (horizontally or vertically) and the patient is instructed to focus the eyes on the target and then turn the head toward the target as quickly as possible. With all of these exercises, the goal is for the patient to be able to perform the exercises for at least 1 minute. It is acceptable for the patient to complain of mild to moderate dizziness while performing the exercises; this should decrease over time. Reports of severe dizziness/nausea indicate that the head is moving too quickly. If patients do not report any symptoms above their baseline, then the head is moving too slow, and the speed needs to be increased. Clinicians should adjust the intervention and provide cuing based on the patient's symptoms. Clinicians may also observe that the patient's head movements may be less synchronized at the end of the exercise compared with the movements at the beginning of the exercise. If this occurs, instruct the patient to stop the exercise and rest.

To assess the effectiveness of exercise performance, ask the patient to grade their level of dizziness before the start, during, and at the end of the exercise. Symptoms should subside after a few minutes, so continual monitoring of the time and level of dizziness after exercise should be recorded. A 0-to-5 or 0-to-10 scale can be used to assess the level of dizziness. These exercises can be performed 2 to 3 times a day.[24] Continue to monitor and assess as the patient progresses.

Once vision is stable, the treatment focus shifts to sensory integration and balance or postural control training. The key to successful treatment is to promote optimal use and integration of the vestibular, visual, and somatosensory systems so that patients can return to their normal activities.

## Habituation and Substitution

Patients with UVL tend to rely more on somatosensory input rather than vestibular input.[25] These patients tend to use the ankle strategy to maintain balance and underuse the hip strategy. They can be observed using the ankle strategy when they stand in Romberg stance or tandem stance and/or perform heel-toe walking. A normal postural response to a narrow BOS is the use of a hip strategy. These patients benefit from retraining to use the correct strategy in the appropriate situation. Habituation and substitution exercises are used to address UVL and BVL dysfunction.

Habituation exercises decrease dizziness using several repetitions of specific movements or positions that exacerbate patient symptoms. The Motion Sensitivity Quotient Test is a list of 16 different positions that the patient can perform to determine which positions make the patient dizziest. The test is scored based on the duration of the symptoms and the patient's report on the severity of symptoms (both based on a 0-to-5 scale).[26] The test positions include sitting, supine, and sitting; sitting, side lying, and sitting to the left and right; the Dix-Hallpike test; head tilting toward each knee/foot and return to sitting; and head turns in both directions. This test has good validity and reliability.[27] Once the positions that cause the most severe symptoms are determined, only 3 to 4 positions (maximally) should be given to the patient to perform at home. For example, if a patient complains of dizziness when they bend down to tie the right shoe but not the left, the exercise down to the right should be given to the patient to perform

**Table 8-11**

**Times 1 and Times 2 Viewing Progression: Improve Vestibular Oculomotor Reflex Function and Gaze Stabilization**

| Exercise Parameter | Exercise Progression |
|---|---|
| Positions | Sitting ⇨ standing normally ⇨ progressively narrow the BOS ⇨ vary surface (firm to compliant) |
| Speed of head movements (the goal is at least 2 hertz [Hz] or 120 back and forth motions/minute) | Begin with slower head oscillations and progress to faster speeds as long as (1) the target stays in focus, (2) head oscillations are consistent, and (3) no more than moderate dizziness is reported. No report of nausea! |
| Duration | Continue exercises as long as dizziness remains at a tolerable level. The goal is to maintain the activity for 1 to 2 minutes. |
| Background | Begin exercises using a solid background; progress to patterned/busier background (eg, checkerboard, striped/patterned wrapping paper) |
| Target distance | Start at arm's length and then move target farther away until it is 5 to 6 ft away |
| Incorporate balance training (see Table 8-10) once gaze and VOR function has improved. | |

repetitively (about 10 repetitions) at home. The repeated exposure to that (noxious) stimulus should result in the reduction of symptoms over time. The patient may have increased dizziness during the first few repetitions (ie, 1 to 4), get less dizzy for repetitions 5 to 7, and then experience an increase of the symptoms again for the last few repetitions due to vestibular system fatigue. The clinician should explain to the patient that they should have mild/moderate temporary dizziness and should wait until symptoms subside back to their baseline (or wait about 15 seconds) before changing positions again. Over time, the severity of symptoms will become less and eventually disappear during repetitions in those position(s) as the system adapts to the exercise (or noxious stimulus).

Patients with BVL need to use other systems to maintain balance and avoid falls because the vestibular systems on both sides are impaired. Substitution exercises are used when both systems are damaged, and a compensatory approach is needed. These patients are more dependent on visual input; this is a concern when the visual system provides inaccurate information. Patients with BVL often report fear of falling, difficulty walking, and feeling off balance. Their gait pattern tends to be slow with a wide BOS and no head motion because they recognize that head motion affects their balance. They have trouble walking in the dark and on uneven surfaces. Clinicians should instruct the patient to use night-lights at home and to consider using a walker or cane for safety when in crowds or walking community distances.

Patients with BVL must rely on the COR and smooth pursuit eye movements only to maintain gaze during slow head movements. These patients cannot perform quick head movements because the VOR on both sides is not functioning. The interventions in Table 8-11 must be modified to substitute slower × 1 viewing (approximately 1 cycle per second or 60 cycles per minute) and the performance of seated trunk moving on head rotations while focusing on a target. These patients benefit from performing smooth pursuit and saccadic exercises with head movements.[24] These exercises are part of an adaptive strategy substituting for the lack of VOR function.[25] To improve the patient's eye-head movements, place 2 cards about shoulder width apart and have the patient look at one target and slowly turn the head toward that target and then look at the other target and rotate the head toward that target. Patients can also perform target imagery exercises. To perform this exercise, the patient focuses on a target and then closes their eyes and rotates the head, attempting to keep the eyes on the target. Then, the patient opens their eyes to see if they are looking at the target. The head speed can also be increased as accuracy improves. This exercise is progressed from completion in sitting to completion in standing. As with VOR training, speed is dependent on the target staying in focus and the amount of dizziness the patient reports. Start slow and progress to the patient's tolerance. Their dizziness should not last for more than 5 or 10 minutes before returning back to their baseline. If the symptoms exceed these parameters, the next session should include a decrease in speed and/or repetitions.

Patients who have BVL deficits can improve their balance, but it takes longer (compared to those with UVL), and they do not usually return to their prior level of function.

These patients experience disequilibrium and gait instability (ataxia), so patients with BVL need to work on visual stabilization with head movements to tolerance (slow to faster) and using somatosensory input more efficiently. Initially, standing and/or walking exercises should have a wider BOS and slowly progress to a narrower BOS as balance improves. Also, instruct these patients to always use night lights and tactile cuing (eg, touching walls) when walking in the dark for safety since their vision is reduced.

## Treatment Summary

The focus of vestibular treatment interventions is to eliminate the patient's vertiginous symptoms first. The appropriate selection of CRT (for BPPV) for those experiencing dizziness, adaptation (for patients with a depressed VOR), habituation exercises for position-sensitive patients, or substitution for BVL patients is critical. Once the vertigo resolves, the physical therapist assistant addresses gaze stabilization (VOR function) and postural control. Successful treatment results from appropriate challenges to the affected systems that reduce dizziness, stabilize gaze, improve static/dynamic stability, reduce the fear of falling, and improve QOL. General muscle stretching and strengthening are included in the rehabilitation process when appropriate.

### Quick Reference for Indications for Vestibular Rehabilitation Treatment Protocols

- Gaze stabilization: Indicated for patients with UVL (use ×1 and ×2 exercises), BVL, and central lesions (use smooth pursuit and saccades)
- Habituation: Indicated for patients with UVL or those who are position sensitive
- Substitution: Indicated for patients with BVL
- Postural stabilization: Indicated for patients with UVL, BVL, or central lesions

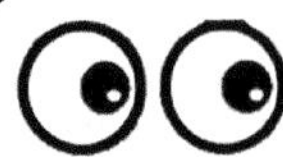

### Eye on the Research: Fear of Falling

Physical therapy interventions can significantly reduce the fear of falling and low balance confidence in persons with and without a history of falling. Fear of falling can be more debilitating than falling and can lead to activity and participation restrictions for patients.

Gait and balance training, tai chi, and yoga can be effective in reducing fear of falling and in improving balance confidence in persons with type 2 diabetes.[28] When creating intervention programs to reduce falls in persons with arthritis, researchers summarized that physical and psychological factors (especially fear of falling) should be addressed.[27] Additionally, research has determined that when considering the relationship between personal perceptions of falls and confidence of self-management in falls (CSMoF), fear of falling was the most predictive factor of CSMoF among older persons.[29] One's fear of falling affects CSMoF and can result in physical function limitations. Fall prevention programs for older adults include interventions that address modifiable subjective factors of fall perceptions/fear of falling.[29] Programs that include multifactorial interventions (including exercise prescription) have the highest likelihood of reducing fall rates in older people.[30]

The physical therapy team is often involved in addressing falls and in fall prevention programs and education. The STEADI (Stopping Elderly Accidents, Deaths, and Injuries) and Otago programs are fall prevention initiatives that reduce falls in older community-dwelling adults. The CDC recommends asking 3 simple questions of patients: Have you fallen in the past year? Do you feel unsteady when standing or walking? and Do you worry about falling? If the patient responds yes to any of these screening questions, the CDC recommends further assessment.[31] Clinicians can include targeted balance exercises, task-specific training, environmental safety assessment, and patient education to reduce fall risk that specifically addresses fear of falling to create a comprehensive fall prevention program.

## Conclusion

The physical therapy team plays an important role in treatment interventions that can improve a person's balance, decrease fall risk, and improve functional mobility. The assistant incorporates appropriate interventions to address static and dynamic balance exercises while training patients to select the best balance strategies (ankle, hip, or stepping). Interventions that challenge the visual, somatosensory, and/or vestibular system are included in programs to address an individual's specific deficits. Interventions that target the vestibular system can reduce a person's dizziness, stabilize vision, reduce noxious stimuli (through habituation), or provide substitution strategies to improve safe functional activities. Effective balance responses are important for patients to maintain optimal functional mobility and to maximize function.

## Review Questions

1. What are the 3 systems that provide input for normal balance reactions?
2. List 3 risk factors for falling.
3. Describe the difference between the SCCs and otolith organs specific to input they provide to the CNS.
4. Describe the balance grades.
5. Describe the relationship between compensatory eye movement and head movement. Why is this important?
6. Compare and contrast the difference between smooth pursuit, saccadic eye movements, and gaze stabilization.
7. Describe the common treatment interventions for BPPV.
8. Give an example of an adaptation exercise, a habituation exercise, and a substitution exercise.
9. List and describe 3 objective tests that can be used to provide objective data about a person with balance deficits.
10. List at least 3 balance exercises/interventions that are appropriate for a person with the following:
    - Fair static sitting balance
    - Good dynamic standing balance
    - Poor static standing balance

## Case Study 1

A 67-year-old patient presents with resultant mild right hemiparesis 5 weeks after a left ischemic cerebral vascular accident. The physical therapist's initial evaluation indicates the following: (1) The patient has 4/5 strength in the right upper extremity and 4/5 strength in the right lower extremity, except the ankle, which has right dorsiflexion of 3/5; (2) static sitting balance is normal and dynamic sitting balance is good; (3) static standing balance is good and dynamic standing balance is fair; (4) the patient is independent with bed mobility and independent with transfers but requires increased time and the use of the upper extremity to push up; (5) the patient ambulates 120 ft with a rolling walker with decreased step length on the left and increased time in double stance; (6) the TUG (completed with rolling walker) is 27 seconds; and (7) the SLS test on the left lower extremity is 4 seconds, and the patient is unable to complete the SLS test on the right lower extremity without upper extremity support.

The physical therapist's POC includes patient/caregiver education, therapeutic exercise, balance training, neurofacilitation interventions, bed mobility/transfer/gait training, and stair training; progress as appropriate. The standard treatment goals were to improve right lower extremity strength to 5/5 to improve patient ability to participate in mobility training tasks, improve sitting and standing balance by one grade to decrease the risk of falls, improve TUG and SLS to increase safety with functional mobility and ADLs, and progress gait to independent with a single-point cane to 500 ft to promote the safe return to community-level function.

1. Select at least 5 exercises that can address strength and motor control for the lower extremity.
2. Create an appropriate intervention plan (with progressions) to target sitting balance for this patient.
3. Create an appropriate intervention plan (with progressions) to target standing balance for this patient.
4. List interventions that can be included to promote progress to the physical therapy goals of improving gait for this patient.
5. Are the goals for strengthening and balance important to meeting the goal of improving balance? Gait? Why/why not?

## Case Study 2

A 68-year-old male patient reports "feeling like the room spins" when he rolls to his right side before sitting up when he attempts to get out of bed. He lives at home with his spouse. His prior level of function included walking independently and playing golf with his friends 3 times per week. He states he feels off balance when he walks but not dizzy. The patient's prime goal is to reduce his fear of falling and to get back to playing golf again.

The physical therapist's initial evaluation indicated that the patient had a past medical history of total knee arthroplasty 3 years ago and was taking vitamins and Aleve (naproxen) as needed. The patient's tests and measurements were as follows: (1) Vital signs were within normal limits; (2) lower extremity strength was within normal limits, but bilateral ankle dorsiflexion range of motion was 10 degrees; (3) cervical rotation left and right is decreased by 35%; (4) positive Dix-Hallpike for the right SCC; and (5) Dynamic Gait Index of 19/24. The patient uses a straight cane with a very slow gait, a wide BOS, and increased double-stance time. The patient looks down at the floor when walking and does not move the head when turning.

1. What should the assistant suspect when the Dix-Hallpike is performed? the quick phase is upbeat, and to the right nystagmus is observed after 10 seconds that reduces in intensity?
2. The patient has been seen for 2 visits and comes into therapy for the third session still using the cane. The patient reports no dizziness when getting out of bed anymore. What should the assistant address first to improve the patient's balance? Why?
3. List 5 other interventions the assistant should complete with this patient during the third physical therapy session.
4. The patient is attending his eighth treatment visit and states his confidence has improved and he is able to walk around the house without the cane but still does not feel he can play golf. Based on your responses in question 3, how would you progress each of those activities to address the patient's goals?

## Suggested Resources

American Physical Therapy Association. The value of physical therapy in reducing the risk of falling and injuries from falls. Updated Septmeber 21, 2020. Accessed January 27, 2023. https://www.apta.org/patient-care/public-health-population-care/balance-and-falls/research-on-falls

Centers for Disease Control and Prevention. STEADI: stopping elderly accidents, deaths, and injuries. Reviewed July 26, 2021. Accessed January 27, 2023. https://www.cdc.gov/steadi/index.html

Herdman SJ, Clendaniel RA. *Vestibular Rehabilitation*. 4th ed. FA Davis Company: 2014.

Physiopedia. Category:Outcomes Measures. Accessed January 27, 2023. https://www.physio-pedia.com/Category:Outcome_Measures

Plishka CM. *A Clinician's Guide to Balance and Dizziness Evaluation and Treatment*. SLACK Incorporated; 2015.

## References


1. Bergen G, Stevens MR, Burns ER. Falls and fall injuries among adults aged ≥ 65 years-United States, 2014. September 23, 2016. Accessed January 27, 2023. https://www.cdc.gov/mmwr/volumes/65/wr/mm6537a2.htm
2. Ambrose AF, Paul G, Hausdorff JM. Risk factors for falls among older adults: a review of the literature. May 2013. Accessed January 27, 2023. http://www.sciencedirect.com/science/article/pii/S0378512213000546?via%3Dihub
3. Tuunainen E, Rasku, Pirkko J, Ilmari P. Risk factors of falls in community dwelling active elderly. February 2014. Accessed January 27, 2023. http://www.sciencedirect.com/science/article/pii/S0385814613001211
4. Rose DJ. The role of exercise in preventing falls among older adults. *ACSMs Health Fit J*. 2015;19(3):23-29.
5. Gillespie LD, Robertson MC, Gillespie WJ, et al. Interventions for preventing falls in older people living in the community. *Cochrane Database Syst Rev*. 2012;9:CD007146. doi:10.1002/14651858.CD007146.pub3
6. Lord SR, Castell S, Corcoran J, et al. The effect of group exercise on physical functioning and falls in frail older people living in retirement villages: a randomized controlled trial. *J Am Geriatr Soc*. 2003;51(12):1685-1692.
7. Li F, Eckstrom E, Harmer P, Fitzgerald K, Voit J, Cameron KA. Exercise and fall prevention: narrowing the research-to-practice gap and enhancing integration of clinical and community practice. *J Am Geriatr Soc*. 2016;64(2):425-431.
8. Schmitz TJ, O'Sullivan SB. Examination of coordination and balance. In: O'Sullivan SB, Schmitz TJ, Fulk GD, eds. *Physical Rehabilitation*. 7th ed. FA Davis; 2019:188-219.
9. O'Sullivan SB. Strategies to improve motor function. In: O'Sullivan SB, Schmitz TJ, Fulk GD, eds. *Physical Rehabilitation*. 7th ed. FA Davis; 2019:361-392.
10. Hain TC, Helminski JO. Anatomy and physiology of the normal vestibular system. In: Herdman SJ, Clendaniel RA, eds. *Vestibular Rehabilitation*. 4th ed. FA Davis; 2014:2-18.
11. Plishka CM. Balance systems. In: Plishka CM, ed. *A Clinician's Guide to Balance and Dizziness Evaluation and Treatment*. SLACK Incorporated; 2015:2-44.
12. Schubert MC. Vestibular disorders. In: O'Sullivan SB, Schmitz TJ, Fulk GD, eds. *Physical Rehabilitation*. 6th ed. FA Davis; 2019:918-940.
13. Kanekar N, Aruin AS. Aging and balance control in response to external perturbations: role of anticipatory and compensatory postural mechanisms. *Age (Dordr)*. 2014;36(3):9621. doi:10.1007/s11357-014-9621-8
14. Whitney SL, Marchetti GF. Physical therapy management of the older person with vestibular dysfunction. In: Herdman SJ, Clendaniel RA, eds. *Vestibular Rehabilitation*. 4th ed. FA Davis; 2014:480-503.
15. Li C, Layman AJ, Geary R, et al. Epidemiology of vestibulo-ocular reflex function: data from the Baltimore Longitudinal Study of Aging. *Otol Neurotol*. 2015;36(2):267-272. doi:10.1097/MAO.0000000000000610
16. Liu D-H, Kuo C-H, Wang C-T, et al. Age-related increases in benign paroxysmal positional vertigo are reversed in women taking estrogen replacement therapy: a population-based study in Taiwan. *Front Aging Neurosci*. 2017;9:404. doi:10.3389/fnagi.2017.00404
17. Iwasaki S, Yamasoba T. Dizziness and imbalance in the elderly: age-related decline in the vestibular system. *Aging Dis*. 2015;6(1):38-47. doi:10.14336/AD.2014.0128
18. Sturnieks DL, St George R, Lord SR. Balance disorders in the elderly. *Neurophysiol Clin*. 2008;38(6):467-478. doi:10.1016/j.neucli.2008.09.001_
19. Hatch J, Gill-Brody KM, Portney LG. Determinants of balance confidence in community-dwelling elderly people. *Phys Ther*. 2003;83(12):1072-1079.
20. Smith PF. Age-related neurochemical changes in the vestibular nuclei. *Front Neurol*. 2016;7:20. doi:10.3389/fneur.2016.00020
21. Dietrich M, Brandt T. Chapter 5: vestibular lesions of the central vestibular pathways. In: Herdman SJ, Clendaniel RA, eds. *Vestibular Rehabilitation*. 4th ed. FA Davis; 2014:59-84.
22. Plishka CM. Chapter 5: benign paroxysmal positional vertigo (BPPV). In: Plishka CM, ed. *A Clinician's Guide to Balance and Dizziness Evaluation and Treatment*. SLACK Incorporated; 2015:111-189.
23. McDonnell MN, Hillier SL. Vestibular rehabilitation for unilateral peripheral vestibular dysfunction. *Cochrane Database Syst Rev*. 2015;1:CD005397. doi:10.1002/14651858.CD005397.pub4
24. Hall CD, Herdman SJ, Whitney SL, et al. Vestibular rehabilitation for peripheral vestibular hypofunction: an evidence-based clinical practice guideline: from the American Physical Therapy Association neurology section. *J Neurol Phys Ther*. 2016;40(2):124-155. doi:10.1097/NPT.0000000000000120
25. Han BI, Song HS, Kim JS. Vestibular rehabilitation therapy: review of indications, mechanisms, and key exercises. *J Clin Neurol*. 2011;7(4):184-196. doi:10.3988/jcn.2011.7.4.184
26. Akin FW, Davenport MJ. Validity and reliability of the motion sensitivity test. *J Rehabil Res Dev*. 2003;40(5):415-421. doi:10.1682/jrrd.2003.09.0415
27. Byun M, Kim J, Kim M. Physical and psychological factors affecting falls in older patients with arthritis. *Int J Environ Res Public Health*. 2020;17(3):1098. doi:10.3390/ijerph17031098
28. Hewston P, Deshpande N. Fear of falling and balance confidence in older adults with type 2 diabetes mellitus: a scoping review. *Can J Diabetes*. 2018;42(6):664-670. doi:10.1016/j.jcjd.2018.02.009
29. Li Q, Mpofu E, Yin C, Turner KW. Perception of falls and confidence in self-management of falls among older adults. *Int J Environ Res Public Health*. 2019;16(24):5054. doi:10.3390/ijerph16245054
30. Hopewell S, Copsey B, Nicolson P, Adedire B, Boniface G, Lamb S. Multifactorial interventions for preventing falls in older people living in the community: a systematic review and meta-analysis of 41 trials and almost 20 000 participants. *Br J Sports Med*. 2020;54(22):1340-1350. doi:10.1136/bjsports-2019-100732
31. Centers for Disease Control and Prevention, National Center for Injury Prevention and Control. STEADI-older adult fall prevention. Accessed January 27, 2023. https://www.cdc.gov/steadi/index.html

Chapter 9

# Aerobic Conditioning

Jacki Klaczak Kopack, PT, DPT

**KEY TERMS** Aerobic or cardiorespiratory endurance | Cardiac rehabilitation | Graded exercise tests | Metabolic equivalent task | Physical activity | Physical fitness | Rate of perceived exertion

## Chapter Objectives

1. Describe physical activity, fitness, conditioning, and aerobic exercise.
2. Explain the key components of an aerobic exercise program, and describe parameters that will be modified based on the patient's diagnosis and presentation.
3. Discuss the indications, contraindications, and reasons to terminate an aerobic exercise program.
4. Correctly identify the expected acute and adaptive responses to aerobic exercise.
5. Given a patient case scenario and plan of care, appropriately create and define progressions of an aerobic exercise program.
6. Describe cardiac rehabilitation.
7. Discuss the treatment goals and intervention parameters of a cardiac rehabilitation program.
8. Summarize the indications to progress, modify, or terminate a cardiac rehabilitation program.
9. Explain the modifications and additional monitoring that are indicated based on cardiac pathology/procedure or medication usage.
10. Describe additional monitoring and modifications that are indicated when a patient presents with selected medical diagnoses.
11. Describe the impact medications can have on physiological responses to exercise and how to ensure safe and appropriate patient monitoring.

*If we had a pill that contained all of the benefits of exercise, it would be the most widely prescribed drug in the world.*

—Ronald M. Davis, MD
American Medical Association Past President

Many patients referred to physical therapy have a goal to increase fitness or functional mobility. **Physical fitness,** which is defined as the characteristics that provide a person the ability to perform physical activity, has 2 components.[1] Health-related fitness components include cardiorespiratory endurance, muscle strength, muscle endurance, flexibility, and body composition (ie, the percentage of the body made up of muscle, bone, and fat). Skill-related fitness components include agility (the ability to change position with speed and accuracy), coordination (the ability to use



Kopack JK, Cascardi KA.
*Principles of Therapeutic Exercise for the Physical Therapist Assistant* (pp 197-221).

sensory input to create motion that occurs with appropriate timing, force, and accuracy), balance (maintaining equilibrium), power (the rate of doing work), reaction time (the time between introducing a stimulus and the beginning of the reaction to it), and speed (the ability to perform movement within a short period of time).[1] **Physical activity** is any movement that results in a substantial increase in energy expenditure (compared with resting energy expenditure). Regularly planned physical activity is part of a conditioning program that is geared to improve fitness.[1] Adequate **aerobic or cardiorespiratory endurance** is defined as the ability of the circulatory and pulmonary systems to provide oxygen during sustained physical activity.

Participation in regular fitness activities and conditioning programs results in a lower mortality risk compared with a sedentary lifestyle.[2] Regular exercise can decrease the risk of developing stroke, heart disease, type 2 diabetes, and some forms of cancer.[2,3] Additional benefits of regular exercise include improved feelings of well-being, improved quality of life (QOL), more energy, and a decreased risk of cognitive decline.[4] The US government recognizes the importance of physical activity and exercise and created the *Physical Activity Guidelines for Americans* and the Healthy People 2030 report.[2,3,5] Despite the strong evidence that increased physical activity is important for health, many Americans are less active than ever. Weekly hours of physical activity continue to drop, and rates of obesity continue to rise.[6,7]

In 2018, the Centers for Disease Control and Prevention reported only 54% of Americans met the minimum activity recommendations determined by the *2008 Physical Activity Guidelines for Americans*, and less than 40% met the criteria for high aerobic fitness levels. Many patients are starting exercise programs at lower levels of fitness. This provides physical therapist assistants with an opportunity to develop programs that will help patients improve their overall health status and QOL.[7] Physical therapy clinicians can play an important role when an aerobic exercise or conditioning program is prescribed for a patient. It is helpful for physical therapist assistants to know typical physiological responses to conditioning exercises because understanding "normal" responses assists the therapist in recognizing and responding when a patient's response is not consistent with what is expected. The assistant must incorporate appropriate monitoring with all patients. The most accurate way to assess a patient's physiological responses is via vital sign measurements. The importance of regular and consistent monitoring of vital signs for all patients regardless of diagnosis, treatment setting, or age is emphasized throughout the chapter. Vital signs are vital; they should be assessed on every patient during every session.

## Cellular Metabolism

When a person moves from a resting state to an exercising state, the muscles that are responsible for the exercise respond first followed by increased activity of the heart and lungs. The musculoskeletal, cardiac, and respiratory systems must respond appropriately to allow for an effective and efficient increase in activity. Calories and nutrients from (food) digestion provide the energy required for muscle activity. The body must have adequate access to energy sources (fats, carbohydrates, and proteins) and nutrients for normal metabolism to occur. Carbohydrates are the preferred fuel source for cells during most activities. The central nervous system can only use glucose (carbohydrate) as an energy source. Carbohydrates are the fuel source for anaerobic metabolism (the primary source of energy production at the initiation of activity). Carbohydrates are converted into glucose and are stored in the liver as glycogen. Fat and protein are also available as energy sources, but they are not as efficient a source compared with carbohydrates. Fat metabolism requires significant oxygen for lipolysis (ie, the breakdown of triglycerides for energy) and is generally not the body's preferred energy source during high-intensity exercises. Protein is used as a fuel source in periods of extreme energy depletion and extended endurance exercise but is not the body's preferred energy source under normal conditions.[8-10]

The conversion of food into fuel required for activity provides the energy a cell needs to perform work. Food is broken down during digestion, and the by-products of digestion will be used in the 3 metabolic pathways that the body uses to create adenosine triphosphate (ATP). ATP is the cell's basic energy source, and it is stored in the cells in small amounts. Once the cells use up this stored ATP, additional ATP can be produced using one of the following pathways: the phosphagen or adenosine triphosphate-phosphocreatine (ATP-PC) system, the glycolytic system, and the oxidative system (cellular respiration). Muscles typically rely on anaerobic sources of energy during the first 2 to 3 minutes of high-intensity work (ATP-PC and glycolytic systems). This allows the cardiac and pulmonary systems time to increase function and meet the increased demands of the body in preparation for using the oxidative system.[9-11]

During very short bursts of activity, the ATP stored within the cell is broken down, releasing its energy. The cells use phosphocreatine (available in limited supplies in the muscle) to resynthesize ATP inside the cell, providing energy for work during the first 30 seconds of activity.[11] This immediate response relies on the anaerobic energy producing processes supplied by ATP and phosphocreatine within the cells and the surrounding muscle fibers. This response yields enough energy for an additional 3 to 15 seconds of work. The ATP-PC system is replenished when the muscle is rested. Replenishment typically takes about 3 times longer than the burst of activity.[8-10]

The next phase of ATP production is provided by the glycolytic system, which provides energy to continue to work from about 30 to 90 seconds of activity.[11] This anaerobic system relies on stored glycogen, which is released from the liver, for energy production. This system uses enzymatic reactions to break down the glucose and produce ATP. A by-product of these reactions is the production of pyruvic acid, which converts into lactic acid. This lactic acid buildup in the muscles causes them to fatigue and prevents further muscle contractions, limiting this pathway's ability to produce energy to short durations.[8-10]

The oxidative system (cellular respiration) requires oxygen and glucose to produce sustained energy/work. Aerobic activity is the completion of sustained large muscle activity over a period of time; adequate oxygen and glucose availability is required to perform aerobic activity. The cells rely on aerobic cellular respiration processes (the Krebs cycle) to produce energy for sustained aerobic activity. Aerobic cellular respiration produces significantly greater amounts of ATP for the cells (compared with the anaerobic process). This oxidative system is the primary system used by the muscles to produce energy after the first 2 minutes of activity.[8-10]

Understanding the role of each metabolic pathway allows the clinician to select the most appropriate exercise(s). These roles are as follows:

- ATP-PC system: Short-term activity (10 to 15 seconds) and bursts of intense activity (eg, short sprints, powerlifting, shot put); every second of work requires 10 to 12 seconds of rest.
- ATP-PC and glycolytic systems: Intense activity that lasts 1 to 2 minutes with repeated bouts of activity (ie, lifting weights for short periods and high-intensity interval training [HIIT]) and followed by rest (or low-intensity work).
- Aerobic system (ATP-PC, glycolytic, and oxidation systems): Longer submaximal activity duration (exceeding 4 to 5 minutes) and activities that intersperse repeated bursts of higher-intensity large muscle activity with periods of lower-intensity work (eg, cycling, walking, running, swimming).

Adequate nutrition (including macronutrients) contributes to a person's ability to exercise. Carbohydrates provide glucose for ATP conversion and are the most efficient energy source for all 3 pathways. The aerobic pathway uses carbohydrates and fats for energy during prolonged activity.[8] Individuals who are not ingesting an adequate amount of each type of macronutrient (carbohydrates, fats, and protein) or calories may have difficulty exercising effectively at maximal performance.[12] This is relevant when considering trendy diet recommendations; consider the implications of a high-protein/low-carbohydrate diet on energy requirements of sustained aerobic activity. There are numerous reference texts available for a reader who wants to further explore the impact of diet on fitness training.

## Defining Exercise Intensity Based on Energy Usage

The relative intensity of energy expenditure can be quantified based on the amount of oxygen used by the body when completing an activity. Common ways to measure energy use include the measurement of oxygen consumption, kilocalories (5 kcal = 1 L oxygen consumed), or the use of **metabolic equivalent of task (MET)** levels.[11] MET levels describe the relative intensity of work/activity. One MET is defined as the oxygen consumed per kilogram of body weight per minute and is equivalent to the oxygen used in a resting state (or 3.5 mL/kg).[11] Higher MET levels indicate the increased oxygen/energy used during activity compared with the oxygen needed at rest; the higher the MET level, the higher the intensity of the activity (Table 9-1).

Light physical activity is defined as activity requiring less than 3 METs, moderate activity requires 3 to 5.9 METs, and vigorous activity requires equal or greater to 6 METs.[13] These are relative values; they must be individualized as needed for each patient based on fitness and skill level. For example, a fit patient will not require as much oxygen during the 2 MET activity of walking at 1.5 mph, but a very deconditioned patient requires more oxygen to complete that same task. A MET level activity chart is useful, but activity selection must be based on the individual patient's presentation, not just a standardized value for a task. There are several reference sources that have compiled comprehensive lists of activities and their relative intensity.[2,13,14]

## Defining Exercise Intensity Using a Rate of Perceived Exertion Scale

Subjective reports of the **rate of perceived exertion (RPE),** the respiratory response to exercise, and the exertional heart rate (HR) are physiologically related. HR is the most objective measure of exercise intensity, but for patients for whom medications or the presence of medical conditions alter HR response, RPE is a preferred means of monitoring/measurement. There are 2 RPE scales that are widely used. The RPE scale ranging from 6 to 20 is based on the linear relationship between HR and the level of exertion. The 0-to-10 RPE scale is based on the nonlinear relationship between ventilation and exertion and is well suited for use with patients with pulmonary dysfunction.[4]

In healthy patients, a high correlation exists between a person's RPE × 10 (using the Borg 6 to 20 scale) and their actual HR during physical activity.[15] Borg determined that if a patient's RPE during exercise is 14, then 10 × 14 = 140 is the calculated estimated HR of 140 beats/minute.[15] The actual HR may vary from the estimate depending on the patient's age and physical condition.[16] Recent research indicates that although the validity of the Borg RPE Scale may be lower than originally reported, it remains a useful tool, especially for patients whose HR response may be impacted by medications.[17]

RPE can be calibrated to an individual's respiratory response using the talk test, which is a simple way to measure relative exercise intensity. During moderate-intensity activity, a person can talk but not sing during the activity. During vigorous-intensity activity, a person cannot say more than a few words without pausing for a breath.[18]

**Table 9-1**

**Metabolic Equivalency of Activities of Various Intensity[13]**

| | | |
|---|---|---|
| Light Activity, < 3 Metabolic Equivalent Task | 1 MET | Lying or sitting quietly |
| | 1.5 MET | Seated: Eating, playing cards, talking, bathing |
| | 2.0 MET | Walking < 2 miles per hour (mph)<br>Standing food preparation, washing dishes<br>Grooming (seated) |
| | 2.5 MET | Playing musical instrument, childcare (seated), dressing |
| Moderate Activity, 3 to 5.9 Metabolic Equivalent Task | 3 MET | Walking at 3 mph, vacuuming, heavy cleaning, slow dancing |
| | 4 MET | Bicycling (< 10 mph), video exercise workouts (moderate effort), stair climbing (slow pace) |
| | 5 MET | Hiking, walking using crutches, walking 4 mph (brisk pace) |
| Vigorous Activity, ≥ 6 Metabolic Equivalent Task | 7 to 9 MET | Brisk walking (uphill) |
| | 7 to 8 MET | Jogging |
| | 8 to 23 MET | Running (12 minutes/mile to 4.3 minutes/mile) |
| | 6 to 12 MET | Basketball, tennis, football |

## Normal Physiological Responses to Increased Activity

As the physical demands on the body increase and the body produces work, the heart and lungs must respond by increasing activity. As activity increases, the cardiovascular system delivers the oxygen extracted by the lungs to the body by increasing the rate of delivery (HR) and/or by increasing the volume of blood that is pumped out of the heart (stroke volume [SV]).[9] Understanding the normal/expected physiological response to activity allows the clinician to compare a patient's actual response to determine if the response is normal or if modification or termination of the activity is indicated.

A person may exhibit an atypical vital sign response during exercise as a result of medication use, a cardiac or pulmonary pathology, environmental temperature, and/or the activity intensity. The physical therapist assistant should monitor and record vital signs before, during, and after exercise. It is important to monitor vital signs during the recovery period for at least 6 minutes postexercise or until vital signs return to close to baseline. This can yield additional information regarding cardiopulmonary function.[19]

The amount of blood that the heart pumps out per minute is called the *cardiac output* (CO).[20] CO is the product of SV (SV is the volume pumped out of the ventricle in one heartbeat) and HR (CO = SV × HR).[20] CO should increase as activity increases. HR (beats/minute) increases linearly with an increase in activity level.[19] The typical HR increase is approximately 10 beats/minute (± 2) per MET level of activity for less active patients.[21] SV increases with increased activity (up to 40% to 60% of the resting value).[22] The increase in CO tends to be linear because of the increases in HR and SV. During high-intensity exercise, after the maximal possible increase in SV is achieved, further increases in CO are achieved with increases in HR.[19] Peak HR capacity is often diminished in persons with cardiac and/or pulmonary disease, so the clinician must modify exercise activity accordingly to maintain patient safety.[23]

HR should plateau as the intensity of exercise plateaus and decrease as exercise intensity decreases.[19,21] HR drops rapidly (at least 12 beats/minute) in the first minute postexercise and should return to close to baseline shortly after exercise is discontinued.[24,25]

Systolic blood pressure (SBP) should increase as the intensity of exercise increases, plateau as intensity plateaus, and decrease as exercise intensity decreases. After exercise, SBP typically returns to baseline within the 6-minute recovery period and may drop below the pre-exercise levels for several hours.[19] An inadequate increase in SBP with exercise has been tied to an increased mortality risk.[26,27] Typically, SBP increases as a reflection of the MET level of activity. The SBP typically increases approximately 7 to 10 mm Hg per MET level of activity.[21,28,29] The diastolic blood pressure (DBP) should not usually change during exercise, and any significant change in DBP (greater than 10 mm Hg) should be discussed with the physical therapist.[21]

The normal respiratory rate (RR) is 12 to 20 breaths/minute, which should increase with exercise. The maximal RR with exercise is typically 35 to 45 breaths/minute.[30] At higher RRs, there is less time for adequate air exchange.

The mean arterial pressure (MAP) is an indicator of blood perfusion to the organs. A normal MAP reading is between 70 and 110. As MAP levels decrease, there is less blood and oxygen perfused to the organs. MAP can only be measured directly by invasive monitoring, but it can be estimated using the following formula: the sum of (DBP × 2) + SBP divided by 3. Blood pressure and MAP parameters are determined by the physician based on the underlying medical diagnosis, and the physical therapy team will treat the patient within those medical parameters.[31]

As exercise intensity increases, the amount of oxygen extracted by the muscles increases, and there is a higher percentage of blood shunted directly to the muscles. This results in increased oxygen availability for working muscle cells.

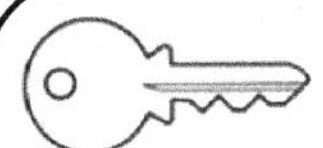

**Key Safety Consideration**

Increased blood shunting to the muscles explains one of the reasons that physical therapy may be "held" for certain patients (ie, a patient in the intensive care unit [ICU] who is not hemodynamically stable). Performing exercises in this situation increases the cardiac strain and diverts an already limited supply away from the organs to the working muscles. MAP levels less than 65 are representative of decreased perfusion and may indicate that therapy should be held.[32]

# Monitoring for an Appropriate Response

Physical therapist assistants monitor each patient to ensure they are responding appropriately to exercise. Appropriate responses include flushed face; increased perspiration; and an appropriate increase in RR, HR, and SBP. Signs and symptoms of an inappropriate response to exercise include inadequate HR or SBP increase based on exercise intensity, a drop in HR or SBP, a change in DBP greater than 10 mm Hg, or an increase in DBP greater than 115 mm Hg. New onset of angina, severe shortness of breath, pale or cold skin or cyanosis, confusion or vertigo, claudication pain, and severe fatigue are inappropriate responses that warrant the termination of exercise (Table 9-2) and additional monitoring/treatment.[21,33]

# Physiological Adaptations to Regular Exercise

Important physiological adaptations that occur with regular aerobic exercise include increases in maximal oxygen uptake and a decrease in myocardial oxygen cost during submaximal exercise. The resting HR and blood pressure will lower, and the exercise HR and blood pressure will be lower than pretraining values at submaximal exercise intensities. Skeletal muscle capillary density will increase, and there is less buildup of lactate in the blood (due to increased muscle efficiency). These adaptations lead to increased exercise tolerance. Aerobic conditioning often allows the patient to complete higher levels of activity before the onset of pathology-specific signs/symptoms (ie, angina and intermittent claudication).[21] Regular exercise increases the average life expectancy and improves overall health by reducing the risk of chronic disease development.[34] Structured endurance exercise can improve maximal oxygen consumption and lower the resting HR (2 key indicators of fitness), even when initiated later in life. These improvements provide evidence of a training effect and have been noted for people of all ages, including those who begin to exercise after the age of 40 years.[35,36]

# Regular Aerobic Physical Exercise: Benefits, Indications, Contraindications, and Safety Considerations

## *Benefits*

There are many benefits associated with participating in regular physical activity in addition to the physiological adaptations discussed previously. Serum triglyceride levels decrease, high-density lipoprotein cholesterol increases, body fat may be reduced (especially intra-abdominal fat), and there is a decreased need for insulin as the body's glucose tolerance improves. The overall risk for cardiovascular disease, coronary artery disease, stroke, type 2 diabetes, osteoporosis, certain cancers, and metabolic syndrome decreases with regular exercise. Additional benefits include a decrease in anxiety and depression, an enhanced ability to complete activities of daily living, improved cognition, improved ability to maintain function and independence, a reduced risk of falls, and improved performance in recreational activities.[21,37,38]

Research shows that large amounts of time spent doing sedentary activities and very low levels of physical activity

**Table 9-2**

Absolute Reasons to Terminate Exercise[48]

| |
|---|
| • SBP decreases > 10 mm Hg with workload increase<br>• SBP does not increase with increased workload/exercise intensity<br>• DBP > 110 mm Hg<br>• New or increased chest pain<br>• Abnormal changes on electrocardiography (EKG), including, but not limited to, ventricular tachycardia (sustained), ST elevation, or significant change<br>• Dizziness, ataxia<br>• Cyanosis or pallor<br>• Patient requests to stop |
| The following relative reasons indicate that exercise should be terminated based on the patient's clinical presentation. Any of the following changes warrant follow-up with the medical team and physical therapist before continuation.<br>• Arrhythmias (premature ventricular contractions, premature ventricular contraction triplets, heart block, bradyarrhythmia)<br>• Report of fatigue, leg cramping, or wheezing<br>• SBP > 250 mm Hg or DBP > 115 mm Hg<br>• Bundle branch block |

increase mortality risk.[39,40] Excessive time watching TV (3 or more hours per day) correlates with increased mortality risk. High levels of moderate-intensity physical activity (ie, 60 to 75 minutes per day) seem to eliminate the increased risk of death associated with prolonged sitting time. Increased exercise levels neutralize (but do not fully eliminate) the increased risk associated with high TV viewing time.[39] Increasing overall daily activity (eg, household chores, lawn and garden work, and daily walking) is beneficial, especially for persons with low levels of fitness.[40]

The known benefits should provide an incentive to exercise regularly and decrease the time spent in sedentary activities (especially TV watching) each day; this dual focus provides the best likelihood of decreasing the risk of cardiovascular disease.[41] Physical therapist assistants can gather information from patients regarding their daily habits, including exercise time, general physical activity, and time spent in sedentary pursuits (ie, watching TV, cell phone use, and sitting at a desk). This creates a baseline from which to set activity goals for each patient.

## *Indications*

The Exercise is Medicine Initiative was launched by the American College of Sports Medicine (ACSM) and the American Medical Association in 2007 to emphasize the importance of regular exercise and the role it can play in preventing mortality. The Exercise is Medicine Initiative recommends that physical activity be monitored as a vital sign and that prescribing physical activity should be a regular part of routine medical care.[42,43]

The recommended minimal weekly physical activity level is 150 minutes of moderate to vigorous physical activity (per the World Health Organization). Persons reporting activity below the weekly target physical activity level should be prescribed physical activity and/or referred to a health professional for guidance and support in initiating a program.[42,44] Early studies indicate small but clinically significant improvements for patients when physicians asked about exercise as a vital sign question. These 2 questions include "On average, how many days per week do you engage in moderate to strenuous exercise (like a brisk walk; 0 to 7 days)?" and "On average, how many minutes do you engage in exercise at this level?" Minutes are recorded in blocks of 10 (0, 10, 20, 30 … to 150 or greater). Researchers noted that when health care practitioners regularly documented physical activity levels in the medical record, they offered more exercise counseling. These practice changes were associated with improved patient outcomes, including greater relative weight loss in overweight patients and a decline in hemoglobin A1c levels in patients with diabetes.[45,46]

## *Contraindications and Related Risks*

Exercise does not typically provoke cardiovascular events in healthy individuals with normal cardiovascular and pulmonary system function.[19,21] The risk of a cardiac event for a person without a cardiac history is 1 in 400,000 to 800,000 hours of exercise; for those with a cardiac history, an event can occur an average of 1 every 62,000 exercise hours.[19] For this reason, pre-exercise screening is important.

There are occasions when the risks of completing aerobic exercise outweigh the potential benefits. Typically, patients who are considered at risk will complete pre-exercise testing. Contraindications to aerobic exercise and pre-exercise testing include unstable angina, uncontrolled arrhythmias, recent myocardial infarction (MI) or an acute cardiac event, symptomatic severe aortic stenosis, active endocarditis, decompensated symptomatic heart failure, acute pulmonary embolus, an acute medical disorder that may be aggravated by exercise (ie, renal failure, liver failure, or infection), acute myocarditis, and acute pericarditis.[19]

In situations in which a higher risk is associated with exercise program participation, the risks and benefits should be clearly discussed between the patient and the physician. The therapy team must ensure that the patient clearly understands the risks and benefits and freely offers informed consent before starting a test or a new exercise program.

### Safety Considerations

Each patient should have a medical checkup before starting a new exercise program because certain diseases may warrant modifications from a standard program. Each program should start at a low but appropriate intensity, and the intensity should be gradually increased when the patient's response indicates a training effect. Each program should be individualized to a person's fitness level and medical condition.[21,33,47,48] Isometrics may overload the heart muscle, especially for older patients and patients with cardiovascular disease, and should be used only when the benefit is determined to outweigh the risk.[21,33,47,48]

## Pre-Exercise Screening, Fitness, or Graded Exercise Testing: Which Is Indicated?

Clinicians will review the patient's overall medical status, medical history, age, risk factors for cardiovascular disease, and resting vital signs before initiating an exercise program. Each person should be screened or tested based on their medical presentation and risk factors before starting a new exercise program. The American Association of Cardiovascular and Pulmonary Rehabilitation (AACVPR) and the American Heart Association (AHA) recommend screening for the presence of cardiovascular disease.[24,49,50] The ACSM has created a set of recommendations that incorporate appropriate screening while minimizing the barriers to adopting a healthier lifestyle and increasing fitness.[21] Adverse events from exercise can occur as a result of activity or disease-related risks, and although they cannot be completely eliminated, they can be minimized.[21,49]

Activity-related risks are minimized by selecting appropriate activities and exercise intensities and following basic safety precautions. Basic safety precautions include compliance with equipment safety, the use of appropriate footwear, and using an appropriate progression of activity. Disease-specific risks are minimized by prescribing exercise intensity that is appropriate and monitoring vital signs. The risk of an exercise-related event (ie, cardiac arrest) is highest for persons who are unaccustomed to performing vigorous activity. The risk of an exercise-related event for persons with cardiovascular disease during light to moderate exercise is approximately the same as the risk of experiencing such an event when the patient is at rest.[21]

### Preparticipation Health Screening

The goals of preparticipation health screening are to appropriately identify the presence of medical risk and health conditions, maintain patient safety during exercise/testing, and act as a guide for developing a safe exercise program for each patient. A physician or physical therapist screens for the presence of cardiovascular pathologies, pulmonary disease, metabolic disorders, and health status changes (pregnancy, musculoskeletal, or orthopedic diagnoses). The therapist will communicate to the referring physician any information that indicates the presence of contraindications to exercise or any response to activity that warrants further medical evaluation or exercise testing.

Preparticipation health screening can include any or all of the following: self-assessment of physical fitness, a cardiovascular disease risk assessment by the physician, a full medical examination, and/or exercise test (exercise stress test). Oftentimes a stress test is completed by an exercise physiologist with a cardiologist present. A commonly used self-assessment form is the Physical Activity Readiness Questionnaire.[51] This tool includes a decision tree to minimize unnecessary referrals for medical follow-up for healthy adults, removing barriers to starting an exercise program.[52]

### Fitness Testing and Graded Exercise Testing

Pre-exercise testing can be divided into 2 categories: fitness testing for the healthy population and stress testing or exercise testing of persons at high risk, with known cardiovascular disease, or with significant comorbidities.

#### Fitness Testing

Fitness testing for healthy clients/patients includes the use of field tests, treadmill testing, cycle ergometer testing, or step tests. Commonly used tests include the Cooper 12-Minute Test (run/walk the greatest possible distance in 12 minutes) or the 1.5-Mile Test for Time (where one runs the distance as fast as possible). The 6-Minute Walk Test and the 1-Mile Walk Test (also known as the *Rockport 1-Mile Fitness Walking Test*) are appropriate for low-risk patients with lower initial levels of fitness. The Bruce Protocol is the most commonly used treadmill test. In each stage of this protocol, a prescribed increase in speed and percent of incline occurs every 3 minutes, resulting in large increases in energy expenditure; a modified protocol may

**Table 9-3**

**Key Safety Considerations With Fitness Testing in a Healthy Population[21]**

- Individuals complete a warm-up prior.
- Monitor HR, blood pressure, and RPE at rest and at least twice during each stage of testing.
- If HR is > 110 beats/minute, a second HR in that stage should indicate a steady state is reached before increasing intensity.
- Observe patients for signs/symptoms of inappropriate response.
- Test should be terminated if patient reaches 85% of maximal HR, requests to stop, or demonstrates any adverse response to testing.
- Cooldown must be completed after testing.
- Monitor vital signs at least 5 minutes after activity or until vital signs stabilize.

be indicated for individuals who are less fit. The most commonly used cycle ergometer test is the Astrand-Rhyming Test. The YMCA Step Test Protocol is another tool to determine a fitness baseline in a healthy population.[21] During fitness testing with healthy adults, the clinician should monitor the list of safety considerations listed in Table 9-3.

## Maximal and Submaximal Graded Exercise Testing

**Graded exercise tests (GXTs)** are also called *exercise tolerance tests, exercise stress tests,* or *stress tests.* These tests assist with detecting heart disease, predicting patient response/risk and maximal exercise intensity, and monitoring a patient's response to an exercise program.[21] GXTs are not categorically indicated for persons at low risk (men or women less than 55 years old or with one risk factor) who are planning to participate in moderate or vigorous exercise. Risk factors include a family history of heart disease, high cholesterol, obesity, impaired fasting glucose, cigarette smoking, and a sedentary lifestyle. GXTs are typically recommended before starting an exercise program for persons at moderate risk (men more than 45 years old or women more than 55 years old with 2 or more risk factors) if they are planning to begin a vigorous exercise program.[21,24,49] Persons are high risk if they have 2 or more major risk factors or signs or symptoms that are consistent with cardiac, pulmonary, or metabolic disease. GXTs are recommended before beginning moderate or vigorous exercise for this population.[11,24,49]

GXTs can assist with determining the severity of cardiovascular disease as well as determining functional/aerobic capacity (this is useful for providing education about physical activity recommendations and limitations).[21] GXTs can be maximal or submaximal tests. Maximal GXTs (symptom-limited exercise tests) are often used with young active or healthy sedentary persons. During a maximal GXT, a person seeks to perform their maximum workload, progressing through stages of increasing intensity levels until they either ask to stop the test or demonstrate abnormal signs/symptoms. The use of maximal GXTs (ie, the Bruce Protocol Test) can screen for abnormal responses that are not evident at lower levels of activity. This test protocol establishes more precise activity recommendations than submaximal testing. However, for most healthy people, similar physiological information can be obtained with submaximal stress testing. Submaximal testing is often preferred because it eliminates physical discomfort and considerable stress that maximal testing may trigger.[11] A submaximal GXT typically uses a treadmill or a cycle ergometer and avoids large, unequal increases in intensity, allowing a more uniform increase in the physiological response to activity.[21] Common submaximal GXTs include the modified Balke-Ware Test (for normal sedentary adults) and the Modified Naughton Test (for very sedentary adults).

All GXTs should begin with a warm-up and start at an initial exercise intensity level (usually low intensity) that progresses by increasing the intensity at each stage (of a predetermined time) of testing. The duration of a stress test is typically 8 to 12 minutes and is limited by the patient's tolerance. There is no significant benefit reported with longer duration testing.[24,49]

Clinical exercise testing is generally considered to be safe, but the risk of an adverse event does exist. To maximize safety, GXTs are typically performed by a qualified health professional (commonly an exercise physiologist or physician assistant) under the direct supervision of a physician. Patient monitoring during a GXT includes the use of 12-lead EKG monitoring; HR and blood pressure monitoring; patient observation; and subjective monitoring of angina pain, RPE, and perception of dyspnea. Submaximal GXT is recommended by the AHA for patients post-MI before hospital discharge (2 to 6 days post-MI depending on the severity and individual presentation) to assist with creating activity and exercise recommendations.[49]

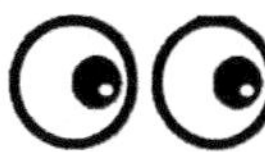

**Eye on the Research**

According to the ACSM, "aerobic capacity may be one of the single best prognostic markers in all individuals regardless of health status."[21] Aerobic training and GXTs can play a role in prognosticating adverse effects and postsurgical risks. In one systematic review, researchers noted that lung cancer patients who underwent lung resection and whose presurgical treatment included moderate-intensity aerobic exercise achieved greater improvements in functional capacity and a reduction in postoperative morbidity compared with patients who only received postoperative rehabilitation.[53] Decreased preoperative aerobic capacity in patients before liver transplantation was associated with higher mortality rates and longer postoperative hospital stays.[54] Low preoperative cardiorespiratory fitness tolerance (less than 5 METs) was associated with higher operative and 30-day mortality after coronary artery bypass graft surgery.[55] For patients postesophagostomy, there was a higher risk for postoperative pulmonary complications in persons who had lower preoperative physical activity tolerance.[56] Researchers determined that targeting physical activity preoperatively could result in fewer postoperative pulmonary complications.[56]

# Aerobic Exercise Program Parameters

Effective conditioning programs are individualized to a patient's current physical abilities and fitness level yet must provide adequate workload/intensity to challenge the patient to promote improved status. The principles of specificity and overload are important when developing an aerobic exercise program.

The theory of specificity states that the patient will experience improvement in function that is specific to the type of activity they are completing. Aerobic activity uses large muscles and cyclical motions for long durations to promote increased cardiorespiratory endurance. Activities such as swimming and running improve overall cardiorespiratory status and overall endurance, but a swimming program will better improve a person's swimming endurance than it will for running.

A person must work at an adequate intensity to challenge the cardiorespiratory system, which is consistent with the overload principle.[21] Work completed at a lower intensity will not result in significant changes/improvement in cardiorespiratory function. Persons who are fit need to exercise at a higher intensity to challenge their systems and to see a training effect compared with those who are less fit. An effective aerobic training treatment plan will address the FITT-VP (frequency, intensity, time, type, volume, progression) principle.[57]

## *Aerobic Training Program Components*

Aerobic training programs include a warm-up period, the conditioning or training activity, and a cooldown period.[21] A warm-up activity consists of light to moderate large muscle endurance activities completed for 5 to 10 minutes. The patient's HR should gradually increase to within 20 beats/minute of the target HR during the warm-up. The warm-up prepares the muscles and body for exercise and reduces injury risk. The aerobic conditioning phase includes 20 to 60 minutes of large muscle endurance work; the patient's HR should remain elevated at/near the target HR. A cooldown for 5 to 10 minutes consists of large muscle movements at a decreasing intensity. The cooldown allows a gradual return to pre-exercise resting vital signs and helps regulate blood flow, which prevents the dizziness and lightheadedness associated with rapid exercise termination. Typically, all vital signs should return close to pre-exercise resting (baseline) values within 5 minutes after exercise.

## *FITT-VP Principles*

The FITT-VP principles are derived from research and physiology studies and apply generally when creating an exercise program. Cardiorespiratory programs address the frequency, intensity, time, and type of exercise and consider volume and progression to create an optimal training program.[57] Clinicians consider the patient's presentation and medical status when individualizing these parameters during exercise program development.

The recommended frequency of an aerobic exercise program is 3 to 5 times per week. Recommendations for moderate-intensity aerobic exercise are 5 times per week; high-intensity exercise is recommended to occur 3 times per week. Performing high-intensity exercise more than 3 times per week increases the risk of musculoskeletal overuse injuries. "Weekend warrior"–type exercise activities (exercising once or twice per week at moderate to high intensity) are not recommended because the risk of injury and cardiovascular events is higher when a person unaccustomed to regular activity engages in vigorous exercise.[21,57]

Exercise intensity can be estimated using target HR formulas and/or RPE. The maximal HR ($HR_{max}$) is tabulated as $220 - \text{age}$ and should not be exceeded during exercise. Newer research indicates that alternate formulas may be more accurate when prescribing exercise for the healthy population (ie, $HR_{max} = 207 - [0.7 \times \text{age}]$).[58,59] $HR_{max} = 220 - \text{age}$ is still commonly used in physical therapy clinics, especially for patients with comorbidities.

The target HR reflects the level at which the heart is beating with moderate to high intensity; sustained exercise at this pace can improve endurance. The target HR is sometimes tabulated for fit/athletic individuals by multiplying $HR_{max}$ by the percentage of exercise intensity desired (target HR = $HR_{max}$ × exercise intensity %), but this formula may lead to an over- or underestimation of the target HR. To improve the accuracy of the target HR tabulation, the heart rate reserve (HRR) or Karvonen's formula can be used to tabulate the target HR. The HRR formula is as follows: target HR = ([$HR_{max}$ − $HR_{rest}$] × exercise intensity %) + $HR_{rest}$.[60]

A person with a lower level of fitness, a person who has not had an exercise test, or a person just beginning an exercise program should begin a program at a lower intensity (ie, 2 to 4 MET level activity, 11 to 13 RPE, or 40% to 60% exercise intensity using the HRR formula).[50,61] Low-intensity activities include walking, aquatic exercise, and cycling at a leisurely rate. As the person acclimates to increased activity, the clinician can gradually increase the intensity and duration of the activity. A healthy adult can begin exercising at more moderate intensity (60% to 75% intensity using the HRR formula), and an athletic population may complete aerobic exercise at a more vigorous intensity (70% to 85% intensity using the HRR formula).

The recommended exercise time/duration is 30 to 60 minutes per day of moderate exercise (at least 150 minutes per week) or 20 to 60 minutes per day of vigorous exercise (at least 75 minutes per week). Persons who are very deconditioned may still benefit from exercising for shorter periods of time; shorter bouts of exercise (at least 10 minutes each) can also have a beneficial effect cumulatively when completed over a day.[21,57]

## Clinical Tips

"I don't have time" is a common statement made by patients when considering initiating exercise. Physical activity accumulated in bouts of at least 10 minutes at a time can improve a variety of health-related outcomes. Bouts of moderate to vigorous physical activity (of any duration) contribute to improved health.[3] Patients should be encouraged and reminded that moderate to vigorous physical activity of any duration will be beneficial.

The types of aerobic exercise vary but typically include rhythmic exercises of the large muscles of the body. Because the body adapts according to the SAID (Specific Adaptation to Imposed Demands) principle, the activity should reflect the patient's fitness goals. The type of exercise is selected with consideration of the person's overall fitness level, abilities, and goals. An individual who is less fit may benefit from a walking program, whereas a person who is more fit may benefit from an aerobics class, a spin class, or time on a rowing machine or elliptical. Persons with balance deficits may benefit more from aerobic exercise in a fully supported position (ie, a recumbent bike or a NuStep cross trainer [NuStep, Inc]). Commonly used types of aerobic exercise equipment are pictured in Figure 9-1.

The volume of exercise is important, especially if the patient has a specific goal of weight loss or body composition change. The greater the participation in physical activity, the more overall health and fitness levels will improve. Exercise volume can be tabulated in MET minutes as follows: (number of METs) × (time in minutes) × (number of days per week) = total MET minutes a week. For example, if a patient runs 4 mph (6 METs) for 30 minutes 4 days per week, the total MET minutes is equal to 720 (6 METs × 30 minutes × 4). The advantage of determining MET minutes is that it can provide a standardized manner of reporting activity regardless of the activity type. The targeted weekly exercise volume should be between 500 and 1000 MET minutes a week.[21,57]

## Documentation Tip

Record all aspects of treatment and clinical observations thoroughly but concisely. When recording aerobic activity, be sure to include vital signs; RPE (if indicated); and all parameters of warm-up, cooldown, and the aerobic exercise. For example, if the patient completes aerobic exercises on the NuStep, the documentation would be recorded as follows: vital signs (rest): blood pressure 126/72 mm Hg, HR 76 beats/minute, 12 RR; warm-up: patient completed 5 minutes treadmill @ 2 mph; vital signs: blood pressure 136/72 mm Hg, HR 88 beats/minute, RR 12, RPE 9/20 followed by NuStep 20 minutes (workload 4); vital signs: blood pressure 152/72, HR 124 beats/minute, RR 16, RPE 13/20; and cooldown: 5 minutes treadmill @ 2 mph with vital signs: blood pressure 134/72 mm Hg, HR 90 beats/minute, RR 12, RPE 9/20. Vital signs returned to resting values within 5 minutes following activity.

Once a patient is able to tolerate the aerobic exercise intensity, the physical therapist assistant must determine when (and how much) to increase the intensity of the exercise to progress the program. Persons exercising at a low intensity will benefit from increasing the duration of exercise by 5 to 10 minutes every 1 to 2 weeks until the patient can tolerate 20 to 30 minutes of continuous activity; at that point, the assistant can increase the intensity of activity by 5% of exercise intensity (using the HRR formula) every 1 to 2 weeks. The increase in duration and intensity progresses at a slower rate for persons who are very deconditioned, and the assistant should monitor each patient (symptoms and vital signs) for adverse reactions as the activity level is increased.[21]

An exercise session should be modified (decrease intensity) if the patient is having difficulty exercising at a new, higher intensity. Other reasons to decrease the intensity or terminate exercise include inappropriate vital sign responses, excessive fatigue, or excessive dyspnea on exertion. Clinicians and patients should be aware of the reasons to terminate an exercise program (Box 9-1). Patients are instructed that if any of these symptoms occur, the patient should contact the therapist or call 911 depending on the severity of the symptoms.

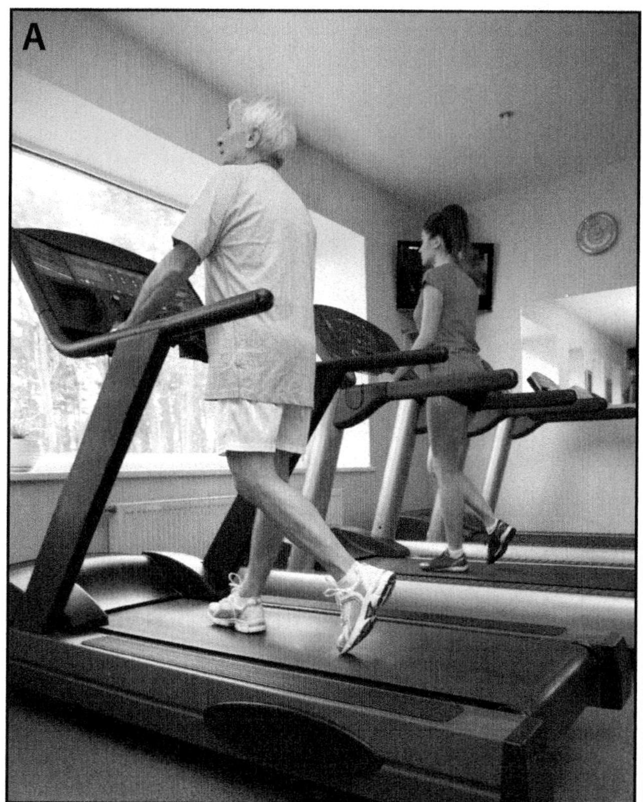


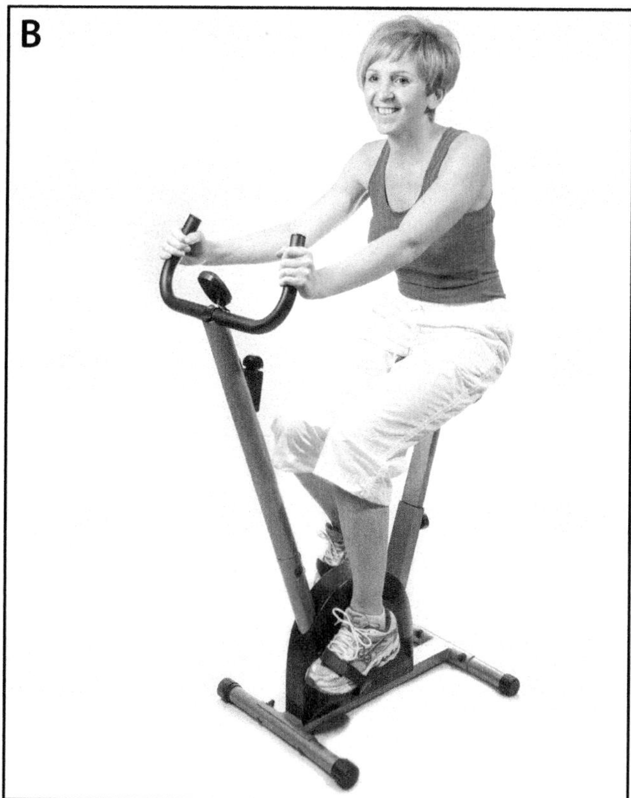


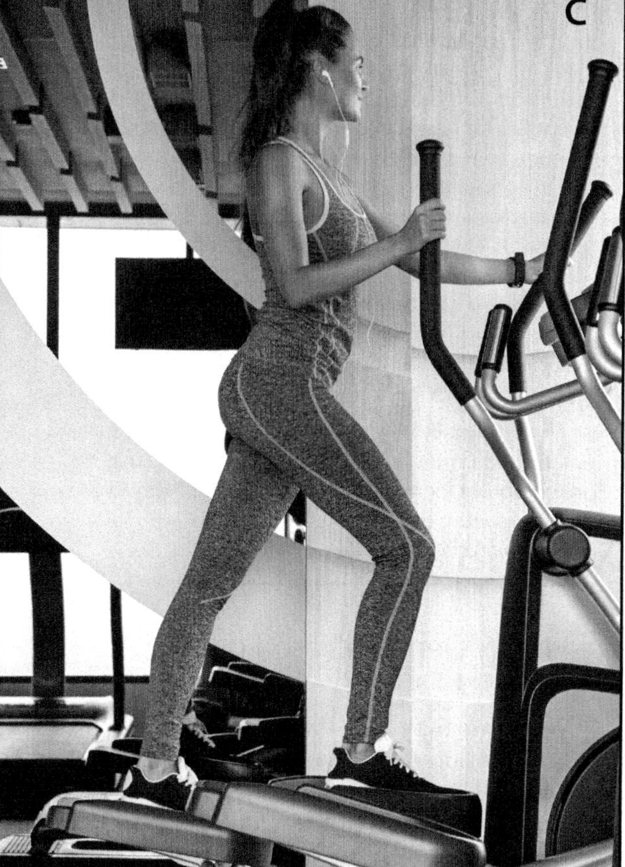


**Figure 9-1.** Commonly used aerobic equipment: (A) Treadmill (Nejron Photo/Shutterstock.com). (B) Stationary bike (Slawomir Kruz/Shutterstock.com). (C) Elliptical (BLACKDAY/Shutterstock.com). *(continued)*

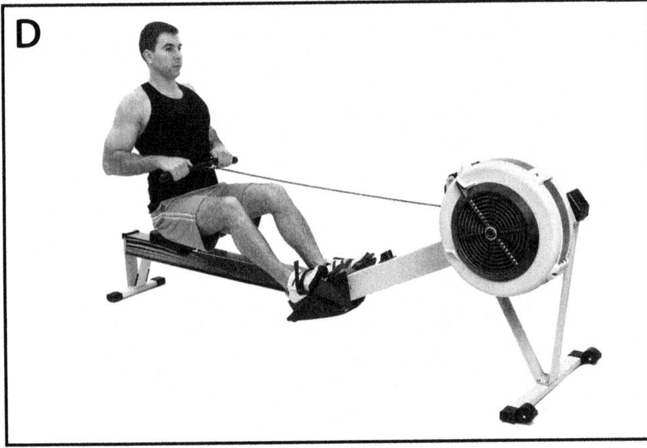


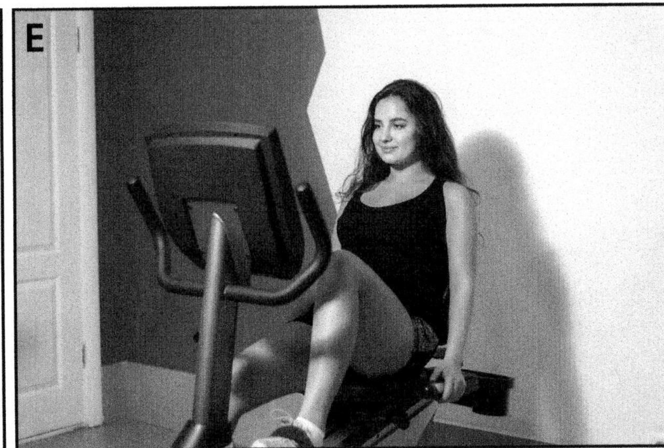


**Figure 9-1 (continued).** (D) Rowing machine (Serghei Starus/Shutterstock.com). (E) Recumbent bike (Olek Lu/Shutterstock.com).

## Box 9-1

### Reasons to Terminate an Exercise Program (Cardiac Signs/Symptoms)[21,48]

- Severe dyspnea on exertion
- Chest pain
- Left arm pain
- Jaw pain
- Dizziness
- Pallor
- Excessive sweating
- Midscapular pain or excessive fatigue (women)

Note: Patients should be educated on these signs and symptoms. Providing education at the start of each session when completing vital signs is a great habit to incorporate as standard care.

Once patients/clients have reached the desired level of fitness, they can transition to a maintenance program. The recommended level of weekly activity is at least 150 minutes per week of moderate exercise or greater than 75 minutes per week of vigorous exercise or a combination of the 2 for a total greater than 500 MET minutes a week. To maximize compliance, it is recommended that the patient participate in various types of activities to decrease boredom.[3,21]

Participation in a maintenance program is critical to maintaining fitness levels and overall health. The fitness level decreases significantly within the first month of discontinuing exercise. Cardiorespiratory training effects and metabolic and musculoskeletal adaptations are also reversed after exercise has ceased.[62] Clinicians should encourage and educate patients regarding the benefits of long-term fitness and maintaining a healthy lifestyle. If a patient misses a couple of sessions, they should be encouraged to restart as soon as possible. Regular exercise is important. Remember—use it or lose it.

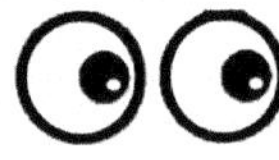

### Eye on the Research: High-Intensity Interval Training

HIIT is promoted in the general media as a new "super technique" for optimizing fitness. HIIT programs include aerobic exercise performed at a high intensity interspersed with active or passive recovery periods. Proponents claim greater fitness benefits (in less time) than a traditional moderate-intensity cardiovascular training (MICT) program. A systematic review reported that HIIT was more effective than MICT at improving brachial artery vascular function and that it had a tendency to positively influence chronic renal failure, traditional cardiovascular disease risk factors, vascular function, oxidative stress, inflammation, and insulin sensitivity.[63] Reichert et al[64] compared MICT and interval training in an aquatic environment and noted that although both groups of patients demonstrated improvement in function and outcomes, only the interval training group experienced a decrease in blood pressure. Sawyer et al[65] completed a small study with obese adults and determined that both HIIT and MICT appeared to produce improvements and vascular adaptations but that HIIT required 27.5% less total exercise time and about 25% less energy expenditure than MICT.

HIIT has generally been shown to be an effective training intervention, but the high-energy expenditure may be inappropriate for many patients until the fitness levels have improved using an initial training program with submaximal training options.

## Energy Demand Based on Mode of Exercise

Upper extremity and lower extremity exercises elicit different physiological responses. The oxygen and energy demands are higher for upper extremity work than lower extremity work. Thus, arm exercise is less efficient than leg exercise. At similar intensities, arm exercises use more oxygen, create more lactic acid, and require higher myocardial oxygen consumption. With the demand for greater myocardial oxygen, the workload on the heart is higher for arm exercises vs leg exercises at similar intensities.[11,66,67]

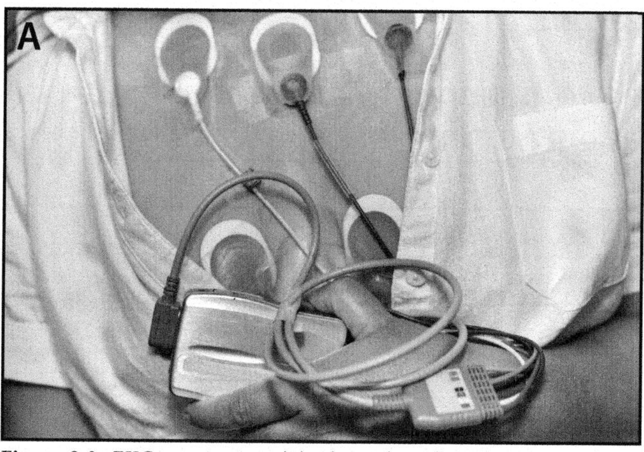


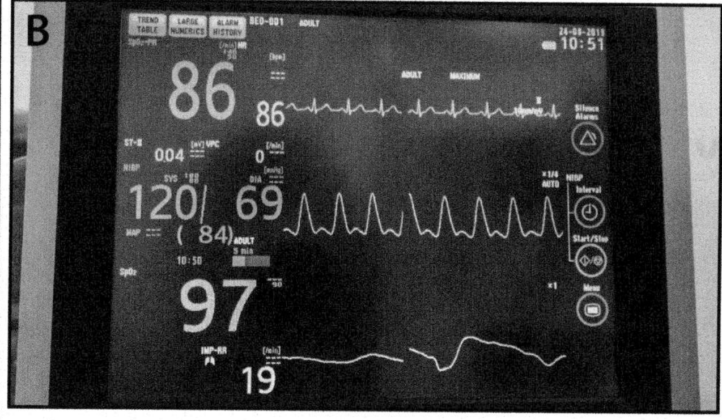


**Figure 9-2.** EKG monitoring. (A) Electrodes adhered to the patient (NAOWARAT/Shutterstock.com). (B) Telemetry monitor (Pixels Studio/Shutterstock.com).

**Considerations for the Physical Therapist Assistant**

Patients with a cardiac history may develop cardiac symptoms at a lower workload with arm exercises. These patients may be able to complete more work or work at higher intensities when incorporating leg exercises.

# Cardiovascular Disease and Cardiac Rehabilitation

There are many known risk factors for cardiovascular disease, and an increasing number of Americans are at risk for cardiovascular disease. Risk factors include age (men more than 45 years old and women more than 55 years old), a family history of MI or sudden death (men less than 55 years old and women less than 65 years old), smoking, obesity, prediabetes, dyslipidemia, hypertension, and a sedentary lifestyle.[50]

When a patient presents with cardiovascular disease due to atherosclerosis, it is possible that the patient may also have atherosclerotic deposits in vessels elsewhere in the body, increasing the risk of angina or MI, a cerebrovascular accident, and peripheral arterial disease (PAD). PAD indicates the presence of vascular occlusion (in peripheral arteries), and angina is characterized by cardiac vascular occlusion. Although angina can indicate an increased risk of MI, some patients who sustain MI do not report symptoms before the heart attack. Patients who sustain an acute cardiac event require emergent care for survival. Research indicates that the most important predictor of survival is the early use of an automated external defibrillator.[68] Physical therapist assistants should be trained in cardiopulmonary resuscitation and should have knowledge of where the closest automated external defibrillator is located within the workplace.

**Box 9-2**

**Diagnoses and Indications Appropriate for Cardiac Rehabilitation[50,60,62]**

- Stable angina
- Stable post-MI
- Coronary artery bypass graft surgery
- Percutaneous transluminal coronary angioplasty
- Stable heart failure (controlled congestive heart failure/chronic congestive heart failure)
- Valvular heart surgery
- PAD
- Patients at risk for coronary arterial disease
- Persons with diabetes mellitus, dyslipidemia, hypertension, or obesity

## *Cardiac Rehabilitation*

**Cardiac rehabilitation** is a formal, coordinated intervention with the goal of decreasing the morbidity and mortality associated with cardiac diseases/procedures. The AHA reports that participation in cardiac rehabilitation decreases the incidence of cardiac events, death from cardiac events, and hospital readmissions.[69] Oversight of a cardiac rehabilitation program is typically provided by a physician, with direct patient care provided in the acute care/inpatient setting by nursing and the physical therapy team. Patients are monitored via telemetry using EKG monitoring as depicted in Figure 9-2. Diagnoses that benefit from participating in a cardiac rehabilitation program are listed in Box 9-2. Patients must be medically stable before participating in a cardiac rehabilitation program, and contraindications include unstable angina, severe symptomatic valve stenosis or regurgitation, certain categories of congenital heart disease, and uncontrolled arrhythmia.[21,50]

**Table 9-4**

**Routine Safety Checklist Before Treating Patients in Acute Care/Inpatient Setting**

| | |
|---|---|
| ✓ | Check the patient's medical record. |
| | Any new or revised physician orders? |
| | Any new test results (laboratory values, magnetic resonance imaging, radiograph, etc)? |
| | Any changes noted in patient's overall medical status? |
| | Review physical therapist's evaluation and most recent therapy notes (goals and current status). |
| ✓ | Check with nursing. |
| | Any changes in patient status since last therapy session? |
| | Current medical status? |
| | Any current concerns or additional monitoring in place? |
| ✓ | Check the patient's: |
| | Appearance |
| | Vital signs |
| ✓ | If all looks good, proceed. If any questions remain after review, discuss with the supervising therapist before initiating treatment. |

Cardiac rehabilitation protocols typically have 3 or 4 phases (dependent on regional practice patterns). Generally, 3-phase programs include the inpatient/acute phase (phase 1), an outpatient phase (phase 2), and a maintenance phase (phase 3). Programs with 4 phases typically include the inpatient/acute phase (phase 1), 2 outpatient phases (phases 2 and 3 are monitored with telemetry and phase 3 includes higher-intensity exercise), and a maintenance phase (phase 4). Because of the variability in phase terminology, an overview of the typical progressions is described later without numerical phasing applied.

With advances in medical care and monitoring (and depending on regional practice patterns), a patient post-MI may be in acute care as few as 3 to 5 days. After uncomplicated percutaneous transluminal angioplasty, patients may be discharged home as early as 24 hours after surgery.

After a cardiac event or surgery, patients may receive medical care in a cardiovascular ICU or ICU setting. The AACVPR and the AHA developed criteria that assess the risk of exercise and activity based on medical presentation; the medical team considers these criteria when determining the patient's plan of care. If medically appropriate, the physician initiates orders for a physical therapy evaluation.[50] The physical therapist completes the evaluation and determines if the patient is appropriate to delegate to the physical therapist assistant based on acuity and presentation.[50]

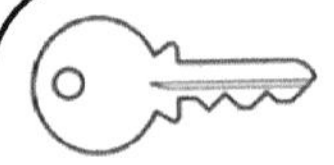

**Key Safety Consideration**

Comply with all postoperative mobility restrictions as per the physician's orders. For cardiac patients after open heart surgery, this may include the use of sternal precautions.

Patients typically remain in a cardiovascular ICU/ICU or a cardiac step-down unit for 2 to 3 days with telemetry monitoring and medical care. Table 9-4 provides a sample of a safety checklist that a physical therapist assistant should complete before initiating treatment with a hospitalized patient. Activities are typically limited to 2 MET level activities, and the physician may also write orders that contain activity restrictions based on HR and/or blood pressure response (ie, limit activity to ensure SBP does not increase to greater than 20 mm Hg and HR does not increase greater than 20 beats/minute above the resting value).

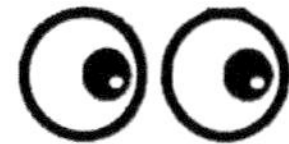

## Eye on the Research: Sterna l Precautions

Sternal precautions are routinely prescribed to patients after open heart surgery (with median sternotomy) to prevent sternal complications. Sternal precautions typically include restricted arm motion (shoulder flexion limited to 90 degrees; avoid shoulder abduction and horizontal abduction), restricted lifting, and avoiding pushing/pulling with the arms for 6 to 8 weeks postoperatively. These restrictions can make it very difficult for some patients to complete activities of daily living, transfers, and bed mobility. Sternal precautions can exacerbate loss of independence, and, in some cases, this decreased mobility may prevent a patient from returning home directly after hospital discharge.

There is no consistent support indicating that the benefits of using sternal precautions outweigh the risks for postoperative complications associated with decreased independence.[70] More recent research suggests that less restrictive sternal precautions may improve physical function, pain, fear of movement, and health-related QOL. "Keep your move in the tube" is demonstrating improved patient outcomes and compliance without a significant increase in complications.[71] These recommendations are evolving; clinicians should regularly review evolving research.

Appropriate activities in this early phase of treatment include assisted ambulation, transfers, bed mobility, self-care, and range of motion exercises. All exercise and activity should occur at an intensity below the patient's threshold for symptoms, and activity should be terminated with any abnormal cardiac response. Routine monitoring of vital sign response, patient symptoms, and RPE relative to actual activities performed is indicated. Patient activities and exercise intensity are typically increased in small increments (ie, 0.5 MET level per day) as long as the patient responds appropriately to the activity. Therapy typically begins with 3 to 5 minutes of activity, allowing rest as indicated by the patient's presentation (ie, symptoms, RPE, vital signs, and/or telemetry responses). Patients are often seen by physical therapy once or twice a day, and time out of bed is encouraged. If the patient is performing at a high level of physical mobility (walking with minimum assistance or less), nursing may also add additional walking times with the patient. The goal is to increase activity time while gradually decreasing the rest time required between each activity. Rest should be permitted when indicated by the patient's presentation, symptoms, or request.[50]

The therapy team completes mobility training, supervises activity progressions, monitors vital sign status, and educates the patient regarding safe activity. Patient education emphasizes the benefits of exercise and regular activity, safe exercise progressions, and a home exercise program (HEP). Clinicians typically provide input to the medical team regarding a patient's safety with functional mobility tasks (ambulation, bed mobility, and stair negotiation), and this information is used to determine if a patient is safe to return home or requires additional therapy before returning home. The goal is typically to discharge a patient directly to home (initially with home care or directly to an outpatient cardiac rehabilitation program). Patients who are more medically fragile or have difficulty regaining the level of function required for safe return home may require extended therapy. This therapy is often provided in a subacute/skilled nursing setting. Patients who are discharged home should receive written instructions regarding vital sign monitoring, cardiac signs/symptoms, progression of a walking program, an HEP (if indicated), reasons to terminate exercise, and reasons to initiate the emergency medical system (EMS [911]).

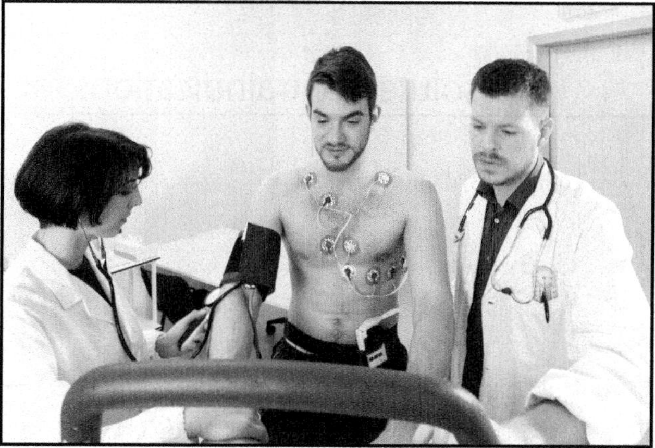

**Figure 9-3.** A cardiac stress test (Serafino Mozzo/Shutterstock.com).

In the outpatient setting, cardiac rehabilitation programs can be provided/monitored by a physical therapist, a physical therapist assistant, or an exercise physiologist. Patients with cardiac pathology may complete an exercise stress test as depicted in Figure 9-3. The absolute contraindications for stress testing cardiac patients are listed in Table 9-5. Some patients who are unable to physically complete an exercise stress test may complete a pharmacologic stress test.

Many practicing therapists can recall when outpatient cardiac rehabilitation programs included a minimum of a 12-week phase that included EKG monitoring and formal exercise stress testing. This was typically followed by a supervised exercise program (without telemetry monitoring) in a gym or a group setting. In the present medical landscape, the length of treatment is often dictated by insurance providers. The physical therapy team will advocate for appropriate care. If the duration of insurance-approved care does not ensure that the patient is at a safe/appropriate level for discharge, then the physical therapy team will complete an appeal to insurance providers requesting additional treatment time.

**Table 9-5**

## Absolute Contraindications for Stress Testing Cardiac Patients[50,62]

- Acute MI (within 2 days)
- High-risk unstable angina
- Uncontrolled cardiac dysrhythmias
- Active endocarditis
- Severe symptomatic aortic stenosis
- Decompensated heart failure
- Acute pulmonary embolus
- Acute noncardiac conditions that may be exacerbated by exercise (ie, infection and renal failure)
- Acute myocarditis or pericarditis
- Inability to obtain consent

### Box 9-3

**Goals for Outpatient Cardiac Rehabilitation[21,50]**

- Monitor for any abnormal cardiac responses while gradually increasing activity/participation level.
- Promote positive changes to exercise and lifestyle habits.
- Promote secondary prevention/prevention of an additional event.
- Facilitate return to premorbid level of function and activity (or higher if indicated).

The goals for an outpatient cardiac rehabilitation program are listed in Box 9-3. Telemetry monitoring is used so that any abnormal cardiac changes can be addressed during this phase. At the start of each session, physical therapist assistants will check resting vital signs, RPE, and oxygen saturation; review cardiac signs and symptoms; and obtain a pain and dyspnea on exertion rating from the patient at rest. The assistant will also ask if there have been any changes in patient status, medical diagnosis, medications, or symptoms. Any change in status should be discussed with the physical therapist before initiating treatment. Ongoing education is a vital activity during the outpatient phase, and new healthier habits are pivotal to the patient's long-term success.

Patients benefit from psychosocial support by meeting, exercising, and interacting with other persons in similar situations or with similar medical conditions. Cardiac rehabilitation patients often support and encourage each other. Patients may be apprehensive about restarting familiar activities or increasing physical activity because of fear of experiencing another cardiac event. The ability to gradually increase activity while being monitored by a medical team trained to deal with emergencies is reassuring to many patients.

As with all exercise programs, a warm-up and cooldown are important components of an outpatient cardiac exercise program. Circuit training or interval training on different pieces of equipment may be a better option than a timed program on one piece of equipment. This allows the patient to complete as little as 2 to 4 minutes on a particular machine (ie, a recumbent bike) before transitioning to the next activity (ie, a treadmill or ergometer). After warm-up, the initial exercise session is often 15 to 20 minutes of light-intensity exercise. During exercise, the clinician monitors appropriate vital sign responses and checks the patient's tolerance to the activity, verifying that there are no increased symptoms.

At some point during this phase, the patient will undergo an exercise stress test. The test results and the patient's presentation and response to the activity will guide the intensity progressions (and limitations) of subsequent activities. Patients will exercise below the GXT threshold results and below the ischemic/angina threshold (maintaining an exercise intensity at least 10 beats/minute lower than their anginal threshold). The RPE should not exceed 16. If GXT results are not available, the clinician can start a patient's program at 40% to 60% of HRR (using Karvonen's formula) provided this is appropriate based on the patient's presentation.[50] Regardless of the recommended intensity or patient-reported RPE, the onset of any abnormal vital sign response or cardiac sign or symptom is an indication to decrease exercise intensity/terminate the session and complete further medical assessment (as indicated by the situation).[50] The exercise program can be progressed when there is an appropriate vital sign response to activity and the absence of symptoms. Although there is no standardized prescription for progression, the progression should be gradual and individualized based on the patient's tolerance. Cardiac disease is dynamic, and a patient's presentation and symptoms can change rapidly; therefore, the clinician should verify that the patient is appropriate for treatment by reviewing medications, vital signs, and signs/symptoms every session.

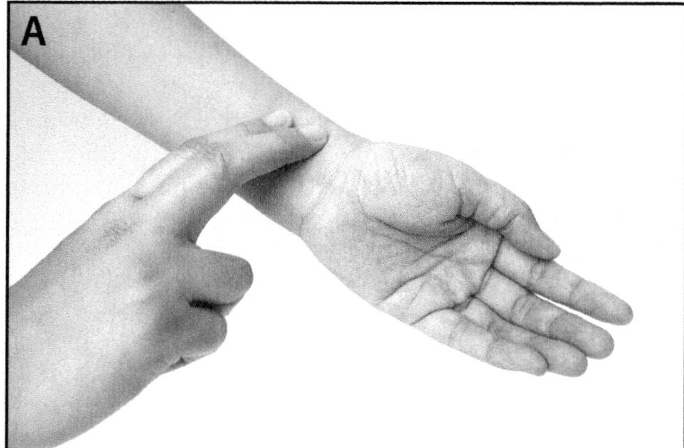


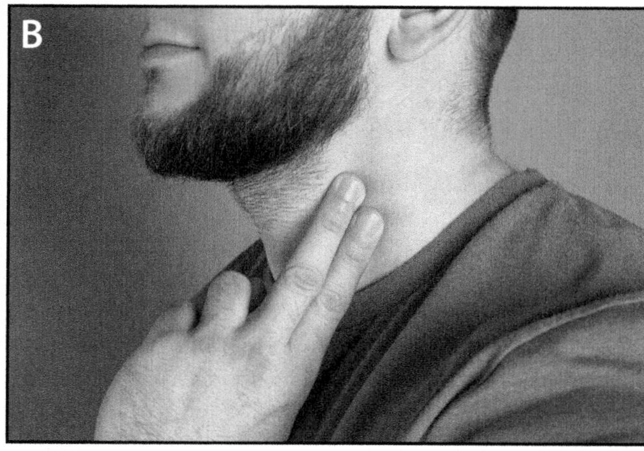


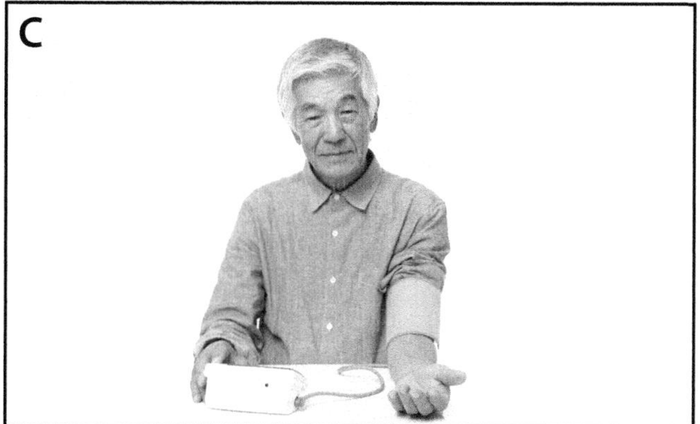


**Figure 9-4.** Self-monitoring of vital signs. (A) Radial pulse (Ratchanee Sawasdijira/Shutterstock.com). (B) Carotid pulse (New Africa/Shutterstock.com). (C) Self-monitoring of blood pressure using an automatic blood pressure machine (UV70/Shutterstock.com).

After completing an outpatient cardiac rehabilitation program, patients who are low risk (based on the AACVPR stratification system) can transition to a group or gym exercise program. Patients are encouraged to select the options that they are most likely to be compliant with. Patients who are considered moderate or high risk will benefit more from an ongoing supervised program.[50]

An often unspoken consideration in every care decision is the cost and availability of services. If insurance coverage or service availability are barriers to appropriate patient care, the physical therapist team member should discuss options with the physician, social worker/case manager, and the patient/caregiver. There is not one recommended solution to address these issues. A solution may require selective research by team members. The physical therapist team member should consider any reasonable option afforded by emerging technology. Is remote (internet-based) consultation an option? Is the completion of a video exercise program with remote telemetry monitoring available? Are group sessions in the home environment with physical therapist/assistant supervision via a web-based interactive platform available? What level of supervision is required to maximize safety for this particular patient? New options for access continue to emerge.

## When Is a Patient Ready to Be Discharged With a Home Exercise Program?

Patients are considered for discharge with an HEP once they consistently demonstrate an appropriate response to exercise/activity. The patient should exhibit appropriate vital sign response during exercise and normal EKG responses with activity. Patients should be able to self-monitor their vital signs (Figure 9-4) and independently verbalize the cardiac signs/symptoms and appropriate response/actions if they experience any symptoms. Patients should also be able to list the risk factors associated with worsening of disease and how to monitor medications. The patient should not experience cardiac signs/symptoms at rest or with activity; the resting HR and blood pressure should be stable.[50,60] Refer to Appendices C and D for guidance in structuring an HEP.

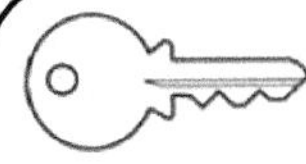

**Key Safety Consideration**

Many patients with cardiac diagnoses are prescribed cardiac medications. Certain cardiac medications will blunt HR and/or blood pressure response to exercise (see Appendix E). For this reason, it is important to monitor RPE, vital signs, and shortness of breath. Cardiac rehabilitation may be the most appropriate initial intervention for persons diagnosed with angina. An extended warm-up and cooldown are indicated. Avoid isometric exercises and the Valsalva maneuver for persons with a cardiac diagnosis.

# Aerobic Conditioning Considerations for Special Populations and Situations

The assistant should incorporate additional monitoring and awareness of precautions to maintain safety when a patient presents with increased frailty, significant health issues, and/or comorbidities. New research and medical advances occur regularly. The information included is an overview of the additional monitoring indicated for persons with selected conditions. Novice physical therapist assistants should be aware of facility protocols; physician orders; and current patient status including current vital signs, results of recent medical/diagnostic tests, and laboratory values before initiating treatment. Physical therapist assistants should never hesitate to ask for assistance/guidance from the supervising physical therapist or medical team when faced with any situation that is new or more complex than they are comfortable performing. The standard of care for all complex patients includes regular vital sign monitoring as well as a more gradual and longer warm-up/cooldown. Any abnormal response to activity warrants terminating the activity and follow-up with the supervising physical therapist.[21,48]

## *Various Types of Special Populations*

Physical therapist assistants will treat patients with various conditions across the life span. Knowledge of various pathologies, normal/abnormal laboratory values, normal/abnormal patient responses and tolerance to exercise, and the ability to recognize changes in patient presentations are important skills for assistants to have; these skills are especially important when treating persons with multiple comorbidities.

### Patients With Chronic Illness or Deconditioning

When treating patients who are deconditioned and/or have been diagnosed with a chronic illness, the physical therapist assistant should review laboratory value results before starting a therapy session (refer to Chapter 2 for laboratory values). It is best to start an activity at the patient's self-selected walking speed with a duration that the patient can tolerate. Consider using the 2-Minute or 6-Minute Walk Test as a baseline outcome measurement. If medically appropriate, gradually increase the exercise time to meet the goal of 30 minutes per day. Once the time is increased, gradually increase intensity. Patients may not tolerate moderate-intensity or high-intensity exercise, and these patients will benefit from a longer warm-up and cooldown.[21]

### Patients Who Are Obese

Patients who are obese can benefit from aerobic and strength training programs. Walking is considered a moderate- to high-intensity activity because of their increased weight; bicycling, water exercise, simple calisthenics, and strength training may be better treatment options. Patients may be at increased risk for low back and joint pain, so the program may need to be modified to address these issues. Careful consideration of patient-specific barriers to exercise should be discussed and addressed.[21]

### The Older Adult Population

Older patients are at an increased risk for comorbidities and polypharmacy, so a thorough review of medical history is indicated. The assistant should review the results of gait speed, balance tests, and functional assessments (ie, Timed Up and Go Test, Berg Balance Scale, and the 6-Minute Walk Test) to assess for fall risk and implement fall precautions as indicated. Combining aerobic conditioning with strength training can improve the results.[21] Adequate nutrition (protein intake) and hydration are key to optimizing exercise results; clinicians should review these factors with the medical team (especially if the patient is struggling to achieve goals).[34,72]

### The Pediatric Population

When working with young patients, allow increased time for heat acclimatization and limit exercise in hot, humid environments while ensuring proper hydration. Children who are overweight should gradually increase activity and may not initially tolerate the 60 minutes per day recommended by the ACSM. Limit the time spent in sedentary activities and work to increase activities that encourage fitness (eg, walking and cycling).[21]

## *Environmental Considerations: Exercising in the Heat, Cold, and High Altitudes*

The environmental temperature creates safety risks for patients who are exercising. During cold-related exercise conditions, early signs/symptoms of hypothermia include shivering, increased blood pressure, poor judgment, and ataxia. Fatigue, lack of sleep, low blood sugar, immersion in water/wet clothing, the presence of infection, and recent trauma increase the risk of hypothermia. Tolerance to cold diminishes with aging. Early symptoms of frostbite include feeling "numb" or a "wooden" sensation in extremity.

To minimize the risk of cold-related injury, educate patients to wear appropriate clothing and dress in layers and to minimize exercise and activity in the cold (especially if it is raining or the wind chill is low). Although persons with asthma and cardiovascular disease can exercise in the cold, they should be monitored more closely. The risk of a cardiac event may be elevated when exercising in cold water because angina signs and symptoms are under-reported by patients in water temperatures less than 77 °F (25 °C). If hypothermia or frostbite is suspected, remove the patient from the cold environment and institute medically monitored rewarming. If moderate or severe hypothermia or frostbite is suspected, initiate the EMS.[73,74]

When exercising at high ambient temperatures (greater than 82 °F/28 °C), persons are at increased risk of heat illness. Factors that increase the risk of heat illness when ambient temperatures are high include exercising at high intensity, exercising for a long duration, and/or poor acclimatization to the higher temperature. Recent illness, dehydration and the use of antidepressants, alcohol or drug abuse, obesity, low fitness levels, sleep deprivation, infection, and sunburn can each increase the risk of developing heat-related illness.

Immediate recognition of heat illness is critical (see Chapter 23). Early signs and symptoms include muscle cramping, disorientation, dizziness, headache, loss of balance, profound fatigue, and hyperventilation. If untreated, these can lead to delirium, seizures, coma, and potentially death. Gradual training in warmer temperatures will promote heat acclimatization. To minimize the risk of heat-related injury, avoid exercising in high temperatures (if not adequately acclimatized to the temperature) and maintain adequate hydration with electrolyte-laden fluids. If heat exhaustion is suspected, terminating the activity, rehydration (with sodium/electrolyte fluids), and cooling the individual are required. Initiate EMS immediately if more severe symptoms are present (eg, falls, collapse, loss of consciousness) because rapid cooling is required for survival. Long-term heat intolerance is possible after surviving an episode of heat illness; patients with a history of heat-related illness will require additional monitoring and modifications to minimize future risks of heat-related illness.[73,74]

In high-altitude environments, expect lower exercise tolerance. Because the air is thinner (less oxygen is available) at high altitudes, the body needs to produce more red blood cells, so additional time needs to be allotted for acclimatization.

## *Additional Medical Considerations When Developing an Aerobic Exercise Program*

### Anemia

Monitoring laboratory values for hemoglobin levels before exercise is essential for these patients. If hemoglobin is less than 10 g/dL, exercise intensity should be decreased. Hold therapy if hemoglobin is less than 8 pending a discussion with the physical therapist, nursing, and/or physician. Expect a significant increase in HR at lower workloads and decreased exercise tolerance with lower hemoglobin levels.[47,48]

### Angina

Aerobic exercise is not appropriate for persons with unstable angina. For persons with stable angina, physician clearance and regular vital sign monitoring is indicated before initiating exercise. Clinicians should be aware of the patient's angina threshold, and exercise intensity is determined by a GXT or at a preanginal intensity level. The patient should have nitroglycerin (NTG) available at each session. If the patient experiences chest pain, stop exercise, assist the patient to a seated position, take vital signs, and have the patient take NTG. If the patient's vital signs are abnormal, symptoms increase, or if NTG is ineffective (after prescribed doses are taken), the clinician should initiate the EMS.[47,48,75]

### Asthma

Always ensure patients have their emergency inhaler at all therapy sessions. Patients should monitor respiratory status using a peak flow meter. For persons diagnosed with exercise-induced bronchospasms, treatment often includes a gradual, prolonged warm-up and taking a short-acting beta-agonist 5 minutes before exercise if prescribed by a physician. Persons taking long-term inhaled corticosteroids are at an increased risk of osteopenia and osteoarthritis, so weight-bearing exercise may be preferred with fall risk protocols implemented. Avoid exercising when environmental triggers are present (cold, pollution, etc).[48,75]

### Chronic Fatigue Syndrome

Patients with chronic fatigue syndrome may benefit from initiating an exercise program with postural exercises, diaphragmatic breathing, and a gentle strengthening program before initiating aerobic exercise. Low-intensity and low-duration exercise with a gradual progression is indicated for these patients to keep symptoms controlled. The patient may have difficulty recognizing internal signals to stop exercise, so it is beneficial to monitor the RPE and the patient's self-rating of fatigue during exercise.[48,75]

### Chronic Obstructive Pulmonary Disease

Baseline testing using the 2-Minute or the 6-Minute Walk Test is beneficial for persons with chronic obstructive pulmonary disease (COPD). Patient education regarding the benefit of regular activity, postural exercises, and pursed lip breathing techniques is important. Aerobic exercise (graded and monitored) and strength training exercises can improve functional tolerance. These patients may benefit in the short and long term from HIIT training.[76] Careful monitoring of oxygen saturation levels is important for patients with COPD.

### Fibromyalgia

Patients with fibromyalgia may benefit from an aerobic exercise program. An aquatic exercise class may be a good environment for these patients because group classes provide additional benefits of social support.[48,75] Initially begin exercises at a low intensity and low duration with a gradual progression that does not increase patient symptoms.

Instruct the patient to use RPE along with vital sign monitoring to maintain the appropriate exercise intensity.

## Insulin-Dependent Diabetes Mellitus

A pre-exercise EKG stress test and physician approval may be indicated for patients with insulin-dependent diabetes mellitus before participating in an aerobic exercise program. Aerobic exercise may be contraindicated if the patient has autonomic neuropathy. Clinicians should educate the patient to avoid injecting short-acting insulin into muscles that are going to be involved in the exercises. The patient should also be instructed not to exercise alone.[48] Exercise should be held if blood sugar is less than 100 mg/dL or greater than 250 mg/dL.[48] If blood sugar is less than 100 mg/dL, give a carbohydrate snack and recheck values before exercising. Have juice/honey available in case the patient becomes hypoglycemic. The patient should not exercise during peak insulin times and should avoid exercising at night (because there is a risk for a delayed hypoglycemic reaction). Encourage the patient to eat about an hour before exercise and to participate in a regular and consistent exercise time/pattern. Patients should hydrate regularly and monitor blood glucose every 30 minutes during prolonged exercise and 15 minutes after exercise (especially if the patient does not exercise regularly). The patient may need to reduce insulin or increase caloric intake for 12 to 24 hours after exercise (depending on intensity/duration and patient response). Exercise in a warm environment or warm water may result in increased insulin uptake and a drop in blood sugar; awareness and additional monitoring are indicated. Exercise-induced hypoglycemia can result if the patient is also taking a beta blocker, diuretic, estrogen, phenytoin, or alcohol.[47,48,75]

## Medication Use

Physical therapist assistants should be aware of the indications for use, the therapeutic effects, and the potential adverse effects that can occur with the use of different medications. Patients who are using specific medications may require additional monitoring or program modification to maintain patient safety. Appendix E provides a summary of the medications typically seen in physical therapy settings, but it is outside the scope of this text to provide a fully comprehensive list of medications and recommended monitoring. Ongoing patient monitoring is vital to safe patient care; staying current with new and existing medications and their side effects is an important responsibility.

## Musculoskeletal Pain and/or Back Pain

The evaluating physical therapist should rule out pathology (ie, cancer, stenosis, nerve impingement, infection, or fracture). Physical therapy interventions typically focus on a focused program to address and treat the causes of pain. If aerobic conditioning is indicated, aquatics or cycling may allow unweighting of painful joints. For patients with cervical or lumbar pain, activities that result in peripheralization of pain should be avoided.[47,48]

## Osteoarthritis

When creating an aerobic training program for patients with osteoarthritis, avoid exercising joints that are acutely inflamed. These patients may better tolerate a cardiorespiratory training program that allows unweighting of the affected extremity. Consider aquatics (water temperature of 83 °F to 88 °F/28 °C to 31 °C), cycling, and an upper body ergometer.[47,48]

## Osteoporosis

Weight-bearing exercises can be beneficial in preventing further decreases in bone density. Avoid exercises/activities that promote trunk flexion and rotation and high-impact activities (ie, the rowing machine, high-impact aerobics, tennis, and bowling).[47,48]

## Peripheral Arterial Disease

PAD is correlated with an increased likelihood of coronary artery disease; the clinician will monitor as appropriate if the patient presents with that comorbidity. PAD presents with symptoms of intermittent claudication. Intermittent claudication is caused by a decrease in blood flow to distal muscles resulting from atherosclerotic deposits in distal arteries. Patients experience muscle pain on mild exertion (described as an ache, cramp, numbness, or sense of fatigue). The symptoms occur in the calf muscle during exercise/walking and are typically relieved by a short period of rest. If the patient is experiencing pain at rest, the physical therapist assistant must notify the physical therapist. For a patient who presents with symptoms during ambulation, a graded exercise program at a duration/intensity below the threshold for intermittent claudication can be initiated. This exercise program typically includes walking (at an intensity that is just below symptom onset) followed by a short rest period, a repeated bout of walking, and rest for 3 to 4 sets based on the patient's tolerance. As the patient's tolerance increases, gradually increase exercise intensity or duration but do not increase both simultaneously. For many patients, increasing walking distance is more functional, so it is advised to increase exercise duration first.[47,48]

## Rhabdomyolysis

Patients who present with rhabdomyolysis secondary to heat exertion–related illness should limit strenuous activity for at least a week and have physician clearance to restart activity. Expect postillness exercise tolerance to be decreased, so initiate retraining at a lower intensity and for a shorter duration than preinjury levels. Avoid training in extreme heat conditions and allow for a gradual reacclimatization to training temperatures before allowing a full return to activity. Carefully monitor for any return of symptoms. Some patients develop long-term intolerance to training in high-heat conditions.[48]

## Common Barriers to Participation in Aerobic Exercise

Clinicians hear many reasons why patients do not participate in exercise including "I can't find time to exercise." "I'm too tired," "I don't have money to ... join a gym/buy a bike/treadmill/purchase free weights," "There is nowhere to exercise in my house," "I'm too ... heavy, clumsy, awkward, uncoordinated," "I'm sick," and "I don't know what to do/how to do the exercises/where to start." The clinicians who recognize that these excuses are more than just excuses can begin to look at ways to help the patient move forward and improve their health. These reasons/excuses are real to patients, and they represent common barriers to improve health, overall fitness, and QOL. Patients are usually more compliant when they participate in group exercise programs.

In life and in health, a person can have excuses or results. Part of the job as a physical therapy clinician is to coach patients, guiding them to remove the excuses to make room for the results. For that to happen, the clinician needs to be able to recognize the reasons, the excuses, and the barriers. The clinician does this to create room to empathize with the patient. Once this occurs, the goal is to guide, coach, and assist the patient to move beyond the barriers.

Changing lifestyle habits is not easy, and the clinician cannot force a patient to take a step they are not ready to take. The clinician should consider the real barriers the patient reports. The clinician must practice listening and thinking about what the patient says without creating judgments. The following are some examples: (1) a 24-year-old with no history of regular exercise who works 2 part-time jobs and whose friends are primarily sedentary; (2) a 40-year-old who has built in a weekly exercise routine who is married, fully employed, and caring for a home and a family of 4; (3) a 32-year-old who is obese with non–insulin-dependent diabetes mellitus and prehypertension with 3 children and 2 jobs and working 60 hours a week; (4) a 63-year-old obese man who presents with non–insulin-dependent diabetes mellitus and congestive heart failure who lives with his son and daughter-in-law working as a driver full time who says that his exercise is "getting in and out of my car" and "helping the people I drive out of the bus"; and (5) a 73-year-old man with coronary artery disease post–coronary artery bypass graft surgery who is afraid of having a heart attack and is afraid to restart an exercise program. What challenges exist to make fitness difficult in these situations? How do clinicians help them create and facilitate lifestyle changes? What are the best coaching strategies in each situation?

Clinicians must first consider the barriers and possible solutions. Then, they problem solve solutions by discussing options with each patient because every situation must be individualized.

Clinicians should encourage task self-efficacy (ie, a person's belief that they can actually complete the task in question [ie, exercising for 20 minutes]), and they guide the patient to improve their barriers to self-efficacy (ie, the ability to believe a person will exercise regularly when faced with common barriers such as lack of time or fatigue). The clinician's focus is first on building task self-efficacy because a patient will not worry about barriers if they do not believe they can first complete the task.[21]

Clinicians need to meet patients where they are, physically, mentally, and emotionally. A patient who is in the early stages of considering exercise but really has no plan to begin exercise benefits most from education about the benefits of exercise based on their personal goals. A patient who is ready to start an exercise program will need guidance about the specific program as well as tips to create exercise as a new habit. Once the patient begins to see the benefits/results, it creates positive reinforcement of the new habit, leading to increased self-efficacy.

## Tips to Increase Compliance With Exercise

Struggling to "stick with" a new exercise program is very common. Let the patient know that they are not alone. Some tips that physical therapist assistants can include to promote patient compliance include the following:

- Review ways to create a new habit/behavior (implement "baby" steps and begin routine performance; complete the new activity for at least 14 to 21 days).
- Demonstrate all exercises and monitor patient performance to ensure proper form.
- Provide short, specific, simple instructions for the HEP.
- Ask patients to provide input on goals and preferred exercises.
- Ask patients to list barriers and discuss them; problem solve for options.
- Use exercise logs and support groups.
- Provide positive feedback and encouragement.
- Encourage/suggest using exercise "buddies" or exercise groups; ensure persons with similar characteristics/goals show up and participate.
- Check up and check in with patients regularly; ask what is working and what is not working and provide education/suggestions as needed.

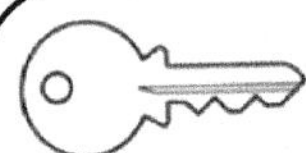

**Key Safety Consideration**

Remember to:

- Monitor for critical vital sign changes.
- Monitor for signs/symptoms to terminate exercise.

## Conclusion

A physical therapist assistant's understanding of the parameters of aerobic exercise and how the presence of varied comorbidities can impact a patient's cardiopulmonary status allows the clinician to create, monitor, and progress aerobic conditioning programs. The ability to educate, coach, and encourage patients through the continuum of care enhances a clinician's ability to promote improved cardiopulmonary conditioning, increased fitness levels, and physical activity in patients. An individual's fitness level directly affects overall health status and their QOL.

## Review Questions

1. Define FITT-VP relative to an aerobic exercise program.
2. List the recommended parameters for components of aerobic exercise (FITT-VP).
3. Discuss the relevance and parameters of a warm-up and cooldown program.
4. What monitoring is indicated for a patient completing aerobic exercise?
5. Describe the typical vital sign response to aerobic exercise.
6. Describe the typical phases and monitoring needed during cardiac rehabilitation.
7. List the reasons to terminate an aerobic exercise or cardiac rehabilitation program.
8. Discuss the indications and contraindications related to aerobic exercise for a patient.
9. Differentiate the expected response to aerobic exercise for a patient with anemia, COPD, and insulin-dependent diabetes mellitus.
10. What additional monitoring is indicated to include when a person taking a beta blocker is completing aerobic exercise? Why?

## Case Study 1

A 45-year-old patient presents with a new diagnosis of atherosclerotic cardiovascular disease with a prescription for an aerobic conditioning program. During the physical therapy evaluation, the patient described a sedentary lifestyle with the only regular exercise being a one-block walk twice a day with the patient's dog. The patient reports "feeling winded" after climbing 3 flights of stairs, and the patient is concerned about "finding time" to exercise. The resting vital signs are blood pressure of 128/68 mm Hg, HR of 84 beats/minute, and RR of 14 beats/minute.

1. Create an appropriate initial conditioning program for this patient. Describe all components and parameters.
2. What is an appropriate initial target HR range? How did you determine this?
3. What patient responses indicate that the patient is ready for progression?
4. List 2 possible progressions that could be used to advance the patient's program.
5. What signs/symptoms indicate the need to terminate the program?
6. What cuing/education could the physical therapist assistant include to address the patient's concern about not having time to exercise?

## Case Study 2

A 64-year-old is admitted to the hospital and diagnosed with a small non–ST-elevation MI. The patient's troponin levels have decreased back to baseline, and the patient is referred for inpatient physical therapy in preparation for discharge to a cardiac rehabilitation outpatient program. The physical therapy evaluation included ambulation and active range of motion. The physician orders state the following: physical therapy: evaluate and treat, activity at MET level 2, and HR and SBP not to increase more than 20 over resting values.

1. What do elevated troponin levels indicate? What values are considered normal?
2. Which interventions are appropriate for the physical therapist assistant to include during the inpatient stay?
3. Which progressions will be appropriate in the outpatient cardiac rehabilitation setting?
4. What patient monitoring is indicated in each level of care?
5. Which changes indicate that the patient is ready for progression?
6. What signs/symptoms indicate the need to terminate the program?

## Suggested Resource

PAR-Q+ Collaboration. The Physical Activity Readiness Questionnaire for Everyone. 2021. Accessed April 18, 2023. https://eparmedx.com/?page_id=75

## References


1. Caspersen CJ, Powell KE, Christenson GM. Physical activity, exercise, and physical fitness: definitions and distinctions for health-related research. *Public Health Rep.* 1985;100(2):126-131.
2. US Department of Health and Human Services. Physical Activity Guidelines Advisory Committee Report, 2008. ODPHP Publication No. U0049. Accessed January 27, 2023. https://health.gov/paguidelines/guidelines/report.aspx
3. US Department of Health and Human Services. *Physical Activity Guidelines for Americans.* 2nd ed. 2018. Accessed January 27, 2023. https://health.gov/paguidelines/second-edition/pdf/Physical_Activity_Guidelines_2nd_edition.pdf
4. Moore G, Durstine J, Painter P. *ACSM EX Management for Persons with Chronic Diseases and Disabilities.* 4th ed. Human Kinetics; 2016.
5. Centers for Disease Control and Prevention. *Healthy People 2030.* Accessed January 27, 2023. https://health.gov/healthypeople
6. National Center for Health Statistics. *Health, United States, 2018.* 2019. Accessed January 27, 2023. https://www.cdc.gov/nchs/data/hus/hus18.pdf
7. Centers for Disease Control. Trends in meeting the 2008 physical activity guidelines, 2008—2018. Accessed January 27, 2023. https://www.cdc.gov/physicalactivity/downloads/trends-in-the-prevalence-of-physical-activity-508.pdf
8. Kenney W, Wilmore J, Costill DL. *Physiology of Sport and Exercise.* 6th ed. Human Kinetics; 2015.
9. Moini J. *Anatomy and Physiology for Health Professionals.* 2nd ed. Jones & Bartlett Learning; 2015.
10. Coglianese D. *Clinical Exercise Pathophysiology for Physical Therapy.* SLACK Incorporated; 2015.
11. McArdle WD, Katch FI, Katch VI. *Essentials of Exercise Physiology.* 5th ed. Lippincott, Williams & Wilkins; 2016.
12. Thomas DT, Erdman KA, Burke LM. American College of Sports Medicine joint position statement. Nutrition and athletic performance [published correction appears in Med Sci Sports Exerc. 2017 Jan;49(1):222]. *Med Sci Sports Exerc.* 2016;48(3):543-568. doi:10.1249/MSS.0000000000000852
13. Ainsworth B, Haskell W, Herrmann S, et al. 2011 Compendium of physical activities: a second update of codes and MET values. *Med Sci Sports Exerc.* 2011;43(8):1575-1581. doi:10.1249/MSS.0b013e31821ece12
14. US Department of Health and Human Services, Public Health Service, Centers for Disease Control and Prevention, National Center for Chronic Disease Prevention and Health Promotion, Division of Nutrition and Physical Activity. *Promoting Physical Activity: A Guide for Community Action.* Human Kinetics; 1999.
15. Borg G. *Borg's Rating of Perceived Exertion and Pain Scales.* Human Kinetics; 1998.
16. Centers for Disease Control and Prevention. Physical activity. Perceived exertion (Borg Rating of Perceived Exertion Scale). Accessed January 27, 2023. http://www.cdc.gov/physicalactivity/basics/measuring/exertion.htm
17. Chen M, Fan X, Moe S. Criterion-related validity of the Borg ratings of perceived exertion scale in healthy individuals: a meta-analysis. *J Sports Sci.* 2002:20(11):873-899.
18. Centers for Disease Control and Prevention. Measuring intensity of physical activity. July 2, 2019. Accessed January 27, 2023. http://www.cdc.gov/physicalactivity/basics/measuring/index.html
19. Fletcher GF, Balady GJ, Amsterdam EA, et al. Exercise standards for testing and training: a statement for healthcare professionals from the American Heart Association. *Circulation.* 2001;104(14):1694-1740.
20. Britannica. Cardiac output. September 6, 2013. Accessed January 27, 2023. https://www.britannica.com/science/cardiac-output
21. American College of Sports Medicine. *ACSM's Guidelines for Ex Testing and Prescription.* 9th ed. Wolters Kluwer/Lippincott Williams &Wilkins; 2014.
22. Higginbotham MB, Morris KG, Williams RS, McHale PA, Coleman RE, Cobb FR. Regulation of stroke volume during submaximal and maximal upright exercise in normal man. *Circ Res.* 1986;58(2):281-291.
23. Hopkins SR. Exercise induced arterial hypoxemia: the role of ventilation-perfusion inequality and pulmonary diffusion limitation. *Adv Exp Med Biol.* 2006;588:17-30.
24. Lauer M, Froelicher E, Williams M, Kligfield P. Exercise testing in asymptomatic adults: a statement for professionals from the American Heart Association Council on Clinical Cardiology, Subcommittee on Exercise, Cardiac Rehabilitation, and Prevention. *Circulation.* 2005;112(5):771-776. doi:10.1161/CIRCULATIONAHA.105.166543
25. Cole C, Blackstone E, Pashkow F, Snader C, Lauer M. Heart-rate recovery immediately after exercise as a predictor of mortality. *N Engl J Med.* 1999;341:1351-1357. doi:10.1056/NEJM199910283411804
26. Gupta MP, Polena S, Coplan N, et al. Prognostic significance of systolic blood pressure increases in men during exercise stress testing. *Am J Cardiol.* 2007;100(11):1609-1613.
27. Kjeldsen SE, Mundal R, Sandvik L, Erikssen G, Thaulow E, Erikssen J. Supine and exercise systolic blood pressure predict cardiovascular death in middle-aged men. *J Hypertens.* 2001;19(8):1343-1348.
28. Taylor A, Beller G. Postexercise systolic blood pressure response: clinical application to the assessment of ischemic heart disease. *Am Fam Physician.* 1998;58(5):1126-1130.
29. Sieira M, Ricart A, Estrany R. Review: blood pressure response to exercise testing. *Apunts Med Esport.* 2010;45(167):191-200.
30. Blackie S, Fairbarn M, McElvaney N, Wilcox P, Morrison N, Pardy R. Normal values and ranges for ventilation and breathing pattern at maximal exercise. *Chest.* 1991;100(1):136-142.
31. Klabunde R. *Cardiovascular Physiology Concepts.* Lippincott Williams & Wilkins; 2012.
32. Lehman L, Saeed M, Talmor D, Mark R, Malhotra A. Critical care medicine: methods of blood pressure measurement in the ICU. *Crit Care Med.* 2013:41(1):33-40.
33. Hillegass E. *Essentials of Cardiopulmonary Physical Therapy.* 3rd ed. Saunders Elsevier; 2011.

34. American College of Sports Medicine; Chodzko-Zajko WJ, Proctor DN, et al. American College of Sports Medicine position stand. Exercise and physical activity for older adults. *Med Sci Sports Exerc.* 2009;41(7):1510-1530. doi:10.1249/MSS.0b013e3181a0c95c
35. Matelot D, Schnell F, Kervio G, et al. Cardiovascular benefits of endurance training in seniors: 40 is not too late to start. *Int J Sports Med.* 2016:37(8):625-632. doi:10.1055/s-0035-1565237
36. Huang G, Wang R, Chen P, Huang S, Donnelly J, Mehlferber J. Dose-response relationship of cardiorespiratory fitness adaptation to controlled endurance training in sedentary older adults. *Eur J Prev Cardiol.* 2016:23(5):518-529. doi:10.1177/2047487315582322
37. Nelson ME, Rejeski J, Blair SN, Duncan PW, et al. Physical activity and public health in older adults: recommendation from the American College of Sports Medicine and the American Heart Association. *Circulation.* 2007:116(9):1094-1105. doi:10.1161/CIRCULATIONAHA.107.185650
38. Haskell W, Lee M, Pate R, et al. Physical activity and public health: updated recommendation for adults from the American College of Sports Medicine and the American Heart Association. *Med Sci Sports Exerc.* 2007:39:1423-1434.
39. Ekelund U, Steene-Johannessen J, Brown W, et al. Does physical activity attenuate, or even eliminate, the detrimental association of sitting time with mortality? A harmonised meta-analysis of data from more than 1 million men and women. *Lancet.* 2016:388(10051):1302-1310. doi:10.1016/S0140-6736(16)30370-1
40. Matthews C, Moore S, Sampson J, et al. Mortality benefits for replacing sitting time with different physical activities. *Med Sci Sports Exerc.* 2015:47(9):1833-1840. doi:10.1249/MSS.0000000000000621
41. Després J. Physical activity, sedentary behaviours, and cardiovascular health: when will cardiorespiratory fitness become a vital sign? *Can J Cardiol.* 2016:32(4):505-513. doi:10.1016/j.cjca.2015.12.006
42. Cowan R. The Exercise is Medicine initiative: physical activity as a vital sign and prescription in adult rehabilitation practice. *Arch Phys Med Rehabil.* 2016;97(9):S232-S237. doi:10.1016/j.apmr.2016.01.040
43. Arena R, Myers J, Guazzi M. Review. The future of aerobic exercise testing in clinical practice: is it the ultimate vital sign? *Future Cardiol.* 2010:6(3):325-342. doi:10.2217/fca.10.21
44. Crookham J. A guide to exercise prescription. *Prim Care.* 2013:40(4):801-820, vii. doi:10.1016/j.pop.2013.08.002
45. Coleman K, Ngor E, Reynolds K, et al. Initial validation of an exercise "vital sign" in electronic medical records. *Med Sci Sports Exerc.* 2012:44(11):2071-2076.
46. Grant R, Schmittdiel J, Neugebauer R, Uratsu C, Sternfeld B. Exercise as a vital sign: a quasi-experimental analysis of a health system intervention to collect patient-reported exercise levels. *J Gen Intern Med.* 2014:29(2):341-348. doi:10.1007/s11606-013-2693-9
47. Goodman C, Helgeson K. *Exercise Prescription for Medical Conditions Handbook for Physical Therapists.* FA Davis; 2011.
48. Goodman C, Fuller K. *Pathology: Implications for the Physical Therapist.* 4th ed. FA Davis; 2015.
49. Gibbons R, Baladt G, Bricker J, et al. ACC/AHA 2002 guideline update for exercise testing: summary article: a report of the American College of Cardiology/American Heart Association Task Force on Practice Guidelines. *J Am Coll Cardiol.* 2002:40(8):1531-1540.
50. American Association of Cardiovascular and Pulmonary Rehabilitation. *Guidelines for Cardiac Rehabilitation and Secondary Prevention Programs.* 5th ed. Human Kinetics; 2013.
51. Canadian Society for Exercise Physiology. Physical Activity Readiness Questionnaire - PAR-Q. Revised 2002. Accessed January 27, 2023. https://exerciseismedicine.org/assets/page_documents/Par-Q.pdf
52. Shephard R. Qualified fitness and exercise as professionals and exercise prescription: evolution of the PAR-Q and Canadian Aerobic Fitness Test. *J Phys Act Health.* 2015:12(4):454-61. doi:10.1123/jpah.2013-0473
53. Rodriguez-Larrad A, Lascurain-Aguirrebena I, Abecia-Inchaurregui L, Seco J. Perioperative physiotherapy in patients undergoing lung cancer resection. *Interact Cardiovasc Thorac Surg.* 2014:19(2):269-281. doi:10.1093/icvts/ivu126
54. Neviere R, Edme J, Montaigne D, Boleslawski E, Pruvot F, Dharancy S. Prognostic implications of preoperative aerobic capacity and exercise oscillatory ventilation after liver transplantation. *Am J Transplant.* 2014:14(1):88-95. doi:10.1111/ajt.12502
55. Smith J, Verrill T, Boura J, Sakwa M, Shannon F, Franklin B. Effect of cardiorespiratory fitness on short-term morbidity and mortality after coronary artery bypass grafting. *Am J Cardiol.* 2013:112(8):1104-1109. doi:10.1016/j.amjcard.2013.05.057
56. Feeney C, Reynolds J, Hussey J. Preoperative physical activity levels and postoperative pulmonary complications post-esophagectomy. *Dis Esophagus.* 2011:24(7):489-494. doi:10.1111/j.1442-2050.2010.01171.x
57. Garber C, Blissmer B, Deschenes M, et al. ACSM position stand: quantity and quality of exercise for developing and maintaining cardiorespiratory, musculoskeletal, and neuromotor fitness in apparently healthy adults: guidance for prescribing exercise. *Med Sci Sports Exerc.* 2011;43(7):1334-1359. doi:10.1249/MSS.0b013e318213fefb
58. Tanaka H, Monahan K, Seals D. Age-predicted maximal HR revisted. *J Am Coll Cardiol.* 2001:37(1):153-156.
59. Gellish RL, Goslin BR, Olson RE, McDonald A, Russi GD, Moudgil VK. Longitudinal modeling of the relationship between age and maximal heart rate. *Med Sci Sports Exerc.* 2007;39(5):822-829.
60. O'Sullivan S, Schmitz T, Fulk G. *Physical Rehabilitation.* 7th ed. FA Davis; 2019.
61. Berne RM, Levy MN. *Cardiovascular Physiology.* 7th ed. Mosby; 2001.
62. Kisner C, Colby LA, Borstad J, eds. *Therapeutic Exercise Foundations and Techniques.* FA Davis; 2018:166-245.
63. Ramos J, Dalleck L, Tjonna A, Beetham K, Coombes J. The impact of high-intensity interval training versus moderate-intensity continuous training on vascular function: a systematic review and meta-analysis. *Sports Med.* 2015:45(5):679-692. doi:10.1007/s40279-015-0321-z
64. Reichert T, Kanitz A, Delevatti R, Bagatini N, Barroso B, Kruel L. Continuous and interval training programs using deep water running improves functional fitness and blood pressure in the older adults. *Age (Dordr).* 2016:38(1):20. doi:10.1007/s11357-016-9882-5

65. Sawyer B, Tucker W, Bhammar D, Ryder J, Sweazea K, Gaesser G. Effects of high-intensity interval training and moderate-intensity continuous training on endothelial function and cardiometabolic risk markers in obese adults. *J Appl Physiol.* 2016;121(1):279-288. doi:10.1152/japplphysiol.00024.2016
66. Ahlborg G, Jensen-Urstad M. Metabolism in exercising arm vs. leg muscle. *Clin Physiol.* 1991:11(5):459-468.
67. Kang J, Chaloupka E, Mastrangelo M, Angelucci J. Physiological responses to upper body exercise on an arm and a modified leg ergometer. *Med Sci Sports Exerc.* 1999:31(10):1453-1459.
68. Pollack R, Brown S, Rea T, et al. Impact of bystander automated external defibrillator use on survival and functional outcomes in shockable observed public cardiac arrests. *Circulation.* 2018:137(20):2104-2113. doi:10.1161/CIRCULATIONAHA.117.030700
69. Thompson PD, Buchner D, Pina IL, et al. Exercise and physical activity in the prevention and treatment of atherosclerotic cardiovascular disease: a statement from the Council on Clinical Cardiology (Subcommittee on Exercise, Rehabilitation, and Prevention) and the Council on Nutrition, Physical Activity, and Metabolism (Subcommittee on Physical Activity). *Circulation.* 2003;107(24):3109-3116. doi:10.1161/01.CIR.0000075572.40158.77
70. El-Ansary D, LaPier TK, Adams J, et al. An evidence-based perspective on movement and activity following median sternotomy. *Phys Ther.* 2019:99(12):1587-1601. doi:10.1093/ptj/pzz126
71. Adams J, Lotshaw A, Exum E, et al. An alternative approach to prescribing sternal precautions after median sternotomy, "Keep Your Move in the Tube." *Proc (Bayl Univ Med Cent).* 2016;29(1):97-100. doi:10.1080/08998280.2016.11929379
72. Bauman A, Merom D, Bull FC, Buchner DM, Fiatarone Singh MA. Updating the evidence for physical activity: summative reviews of the epidemiological evidence, prevalence, and interventions to promote "active aging." *Gerontologist.* 2016;56(suppl 2):S268-S280. doi:10.1093/geront/gnw031
73. Armstrong L, Casa D, Millard-Stafford M, Moran D, Pyne S, Roberts W. American College of Sports Medicine position stand. Exertional heat illness during training and competition. *Med Sci Sports Exerc.* 2007:39(3):556-572. doi:10.1249/MSS.0b013e31802fa199
74. Castellani J, Young A, Ducharme M, Giesbrecht G, Glickman E, Sallis R. American College of Sports Medicine position stand: prevention of cold injuries during exercise. *Med Sci Sports Exerc.* 2006;38(11):2012-2029. doi:10.1249/01.mss.0000241641.75101.64
75. American College of Sports Medicine; Durstine JL, Moore G, Painter P, Roberts S. *ACSM's Exercise Management for Persons With Chronic Diseases and Disabilities.* 4th ed. Human Kinetics; 2016.
76. Guadalupe-Grau A, Aznar-Laín S, Mañas A, et al. Short and long term effects of concurrent strength and HIIT training in octogenarian COPDs. *J Aging Phys Act.* 2017;25(1):105-115. doi:10.1123/japa.2015-0307

# Chapter 10
# Aquatic Therapy

*Jacki Klaczak Kopack, PT, DPT*

**KEY TERMS** Buoyancy | Density | Dive reflex | Drag force | Hydrostatic pressure | Viscosity

## Chapter Objectives

1. Describe the physical principles of water.
2. Explain how the physical principles of water impact the development of an exercise program in water.
3. Discuss the indications and contraindications for aquatic therapy.
4. Compare and contrast the advantages and disadvantages of a land-based vs aquatic exercise program.
5. Describe the effective ways to transition from an aquatic therapy environment to a land-based exercise program.

Aquatic therapy is effective for managing several conditions, such as musculoskeletal, neurologic, and/or cardiopulmonary problems or pathologies.[1-6] Aquatic therapy is also referred to as *hydrotherapy, aqua therapy, pool therapy, aquatic rehabilitation*, or *therapeutic aquatic exercise*. Water has been used for centuries to promote healing and for the medical management of diseases. The ancient Romans and Greeks bathed in hot springs for relaxation. In 1911, hydrotherapy was used to treat patients with cerebral palsy and other patients with spasticity by Charles LeRoy Lowman, the founder of what is now known as Rancho Los Amigos in Los Angeles. The Hubbard tank, which was developed by Leroy Hubbard, was used in 1924 to treat Franklin Delano Roosevelt's polio-related paralysis in Warm Springs, Georgia. Dr. Lowman was the first to use water exercises that had specific parameters and dosing to restore function in 1937.[7] The reported use of therapeutic tubs, pools, and exercise regimens is found in the research as early as the 1930s.

Aquatic exercise treatment interventions that incorporate the properties of water are a safe and effective tool to improve patient outcomes. The physical properties of water provide the clinician with ways to modify exercises to make them easier or more difficult to perform. Patients who have limited weight-bearing status or are unable to perform exercises/activities against gravity because of pain or acuity can perform exercises/activities in an environment that is less stressful on joints than land-based activities. Immersion in water has biological effects that can provide a therapeutic benefit.

During the initial evaluation, the physical therapist considers the advantages and barriers of initiating an aquatic therapy program. The physical therapist needs to determine if an aquatic exercise program is the most appropriate tool to meet the patient's needs given their presentation and



Kopack JK, Cascardi KA. *Principles of Therapeutic Exercise for the Physical Therapist Assistant* (pp 223-240).

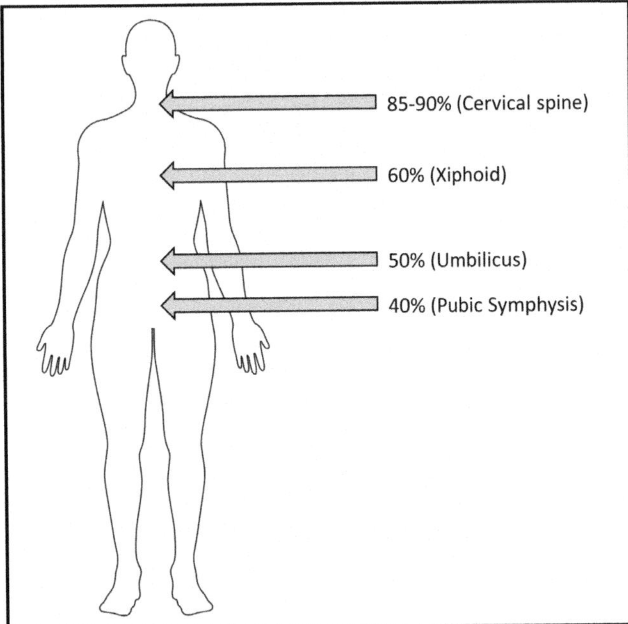


**Figure 10-1.** Buoyancy immersion weight off-loading percentages.[7]

goals and the potential for the aquatic exercises to decrease pain and increase range of motion (ROM), strength, balance, gait, overall function, and quality of life (QOL). A plan must be in place to progress the exercise program from an aquatic environment to a land-based program to ensure the patient's functional goals are being addressed.

## Physical Properties of Water

The properties of water allow clinicians to modify treatments in ways that are not possible in most land-based programs. For example, an athlete who is non–weight bearing may be able to practice underwater running while suspended using flotation devices in deep water. Patients with diminished strength receive gentle challenges to increase strength when moving against the resistance of the water. The risk for injury from falls is also removed when exercising in the water. A clear understanding of the properties of water enables the clinician to create appropriate treatment plans while taking advantage of the unique opportunities offered by exercising in this environment. The properties of water that need to be considered when developing an aquatic exercise program include buoyancy, density, hydrostatic pressure, surface tension, viscosity, thermodynamics, and hydrodynamics.[7,8]

### *Buoyancy and Density*

**Buoyancy** is defined as the power of a fluid to exert an upward force on a body placed in it.[9] A body (or body part) that is immersed in the water will experience this upward force, which decreases the impact of gravity on the body and/or its body parts. Buoyancy acts in the opposite direction of gravity and causes an object to become lighter; it unweights the immersed body or body part. The deeper the body is submerged, the more it is affected by buoyancy. The percentage of body weight that is unweighted is dependent on the depth of submersion (Figure 10-1).[7,10]

The force of buoyancy can assist a body part to move toward the water's surface, creating a sense of weightlessness (eg, having an arm move or float from midline into shoulder abduction). If the surface area of the limb is increased (ie, a fully extended limb or a limb with a mitt on the hand), the forces of buoyancy will work on the larger surface area; this results in a greater/stronger buoying force assisting the limb toward the surface. Buoyancy can serve to unweight the lower limbs. This allows a patient with a restricted weight-bearing status to practice weight bearing, weight shifting, and gait in an environment that allows for compliance with their weight-bearing restrictions. Conversely, when a patient moves a limb downward through the water, the limb moves against the resistance of buoyancy forces. This uses the force of buoyancy to facilitate strengthening. Having a patient pull their arm down from a floating position into shoulder adduction is an example of overcoming buoyancy. If the limb is moving down in the water and the patient is wearing a mitt on the hand, the patient will need to overcome a greater force because of the larger surface area. Similarly, moving the hand through the water with the fingers adducted creates a larger surface area and more resistance than movement with the fingers separated.

An understanding of **density** and center of buoyancy (COB) is important when determining the positions, exercises, and selection of flotation devices. Whether an object will float or sink is dependent on the object's density. Objects that are denser than water will sink, and objects that are less dense will float. Relative densities can be compared using the specific gravity of an object. Specific gravity is the ratio of the object's density to water's density (at 4 °C/39.2 °F). The lower extremities and pelvis have a heavier mass (they are denser) than the thorax, arms, and head. The lungs are filled with air, which contributes to less mass and density (and lower specific gravity) in the upper part of the body. A person with fully inflated lungs displaces a greater volume of water and is more buoyant than a person with deflated lungs. Because air is less dense than water, its presence increases buoyancy. The average specific gravity of a human with lungs inflated is less than water's specific gravity, allowing the person to float.

The ability to float varies from person to person. Floating occurs when the forces created by the person's body are less than the water's buoyant force. The amount of water displaced by an object needs to weigh more than the weight of the actual object for the object to float. Bone structure, bone weight, and body fat are factors that have an effect on buoyancy. A person with a greater percentage of body fat tends to be more buoyant, whereas a person with a lean body mass tends to have a specific gravity that is greater than water's; the lean person is more likely to sink. A person who is denser will need to expend greater energy to stay afloat than a person who is more buoyant.

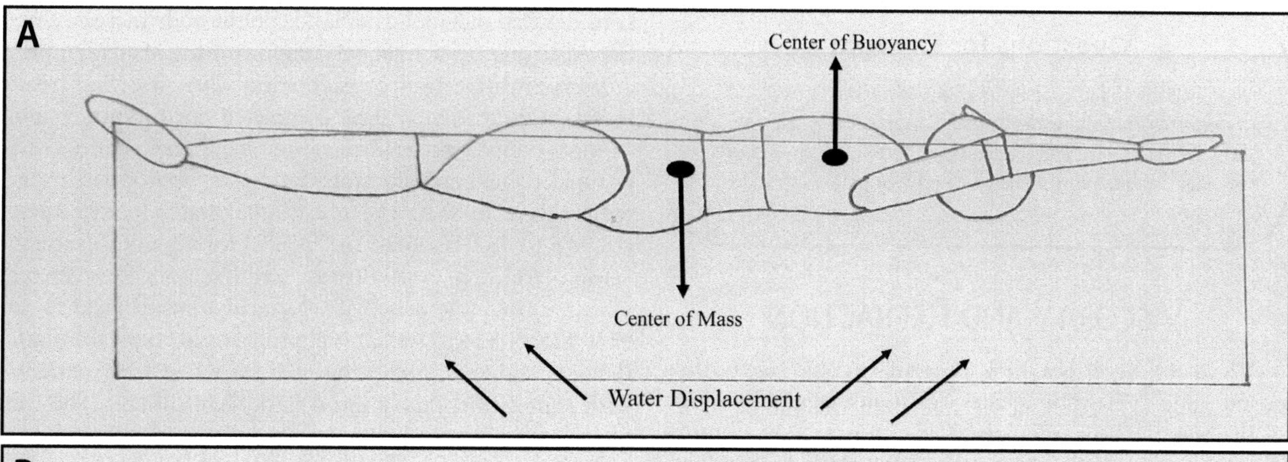


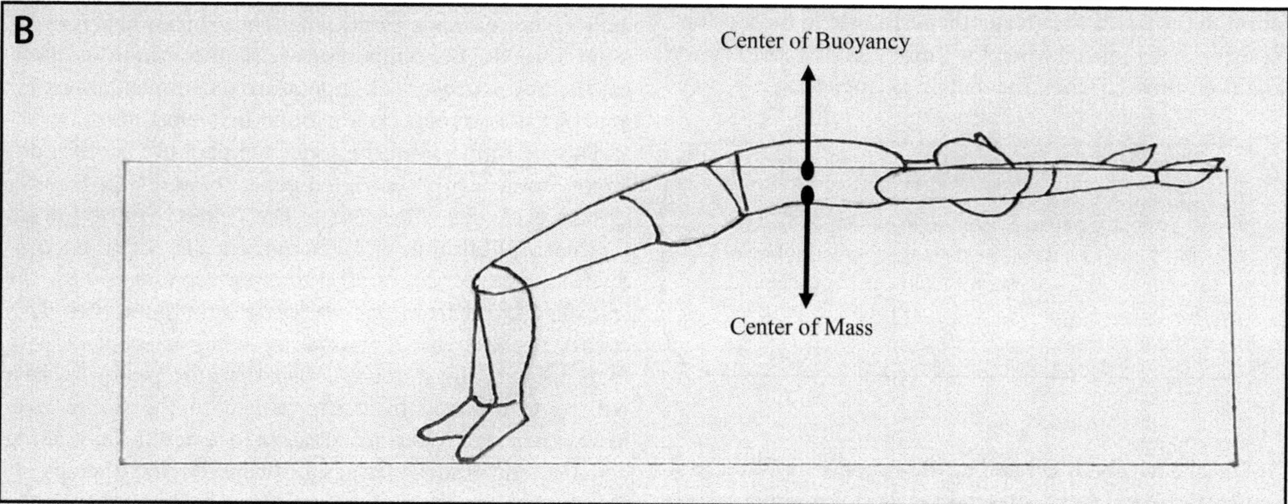


**Figure 10-2.** (A) COB and water displacement. (B) COB aligned with the center of mass. (Graphic created by Buzzy August.)

Every object that floats has a center of gravity (COG) and COB. COG is the point at which weight is equal and balanced in all directions. COB is the reference point where all buoyancy forces are balanced; it is based on the COG of the fluid displaced by the floating object as shown in Figure 10-2A. In humans, the COB tends to be located near the upper torso (due to the lungs filled with air), and the COG or center of mass is located within the pelvis. This is the reason why the lower extremities tend to sink, and the upper trunk tends to move toward the surface when a patient attempts to float on their back. This rotation continues until the COB and COG are vertically aligned (Figure 10-2B). The center of mass will vary slightly in individuals.

> **Questions for Thought**
>
> If a patient is cleared for toe touch weight bearing, what is the appropriate depth of immersion to allow safe ambulation in the pool? If a patient has upper extremity strength of 2/5, which direction is most appropriate to have the patient move the limb in the water?

## Hydrostatic Pressure

**Hydrostatic pressure** is the pressure exerted on the body by the water surrounding it. The pressure increases proportional to the density of the liquid (more density results in greater pressure) and to immersion depth (more pressure is exerted with deeper immersion). Hydrostatic pressure facilitates edema reduction in an injured body part, which can decrease pain and improve ROM. Water exerts pressure equivalent to 1 mm Hg/1.36 cm of water depth, so a body immersed to a depth of 4 feet (121.92 cm) is subjected to a hydrostatic pressure force of 88.9 mm Hg (greater than normal diastolic blood pressure). This pressure facilitates distal blood flow centrally resulting in increased right atrial and pleural surface pressure as well as chest wall compression and upward displacement of the diaphragm. Hydrostatic pressure increases pressure on all areas of the body that are immersed. The increased pressure has a greater impact in patients in whom pathology or organ function compromise already exists. Patients with respiratory muscle weakness may benefit from aquatic therapy because the constant pressure on the chest wall during inspiration and expiration provides a training effect and helps improve the patient's lung capacity.[11] Research indicates that although aquatic therapy is beneficial for persons with pulmonary pathology, it does not clearly indicate that aquatic exercise improves exercise capacity or QOL.[12]

### Questions for Thought

What impact will immersion to neck level have on postinjury edema from an ankle sprain? Consider the ramifications of hydrostatic pressure in a patient with acute congestive heart failure; would exercise in the aquatic setting be appropriate?

## Viscosity and Refraction

**Viscosity** describes how resistant a fluid is to flow or motion.[7] Viscosity creates resistance against motion in the water. The harder or faster a person tries to move through the water, the greater the resistance to the motion.[7] Resistance is reduced when the limb or body moves slower and is eliminated when the motion is stopped.

### Clinical Tip

When a patient is performing an exercise in the water, viscosity creates resistance; if the patient complains of pain, the physical therapist assistant should cue the patient to slow down the movement. Continuing at a slower speed lowers the resistance.

Surface tension is created by the cohesion of water molecules. Cohesion is the attraction of each water molecule to other water molecules. Surface tension creates a mild resistance to motion through the surface of the water (ie, lifting an arm out of the water into the air or lowering it back into the water). This minor increase in resistance typically does not factor into program development, except in cases in which the patient has significant weakness.

Refraction is the bending of light rays as they move from one medium to another. Refraction occurs when light rays pass from the air into the water, causing the light rays to bend downward. Refraction distorts the view of what is seen in the water from the pool deck, making the pool bottom appear closer or shallower than it actually is.[13]

### Considerations for the Physical Therapist Assistant

It is typically more beneficial to be in the pool with the patient. The view from the pool deck is distorted when looking at the patient's body parts that are moving underwater.

### *Thermodynamics*

Water temperature affects physiological responses during aquatic therapy. The effect is determined by the water temperature, the percentage of body immersion, and whether the patient is moving or at rest. Clinicians must consider that metabolic demands on the body increase during exercise in a warm aquatic environment. Water temperature is an important consideration when selecting treatment activities that will be completed during immersion. In most pools, temperature cannot be altered significantly or rapidly. General recommendations for appropriate water temperature indicate the use of cool water temperatures (78.8 °F to 85.1 °F/26 °C to 29.5 °C) for vigorous exercise, aerobic training, and fitness training and for patients with multiple sclerosis (MS). Neutral warmth (92.3 °F to 95.9 °F/33.5 °C to 35.5 °C) is appropriate for typical aquatic therapy exercises and programs geared to treat patients with spinal cord injuries and Parkinson disease. The use of warmer water temperatures (96.8 °F to 101.3 °F/36 °C to 38.5 °C) is most appropriate when the primary goal is relaxation; these higher temperatures are uncommon in physical therapy settings.[7,8] Temperature recommendations for aquatic fitness programs are found in Table 10-1.

During immersion, the water temperature is often different from normal body temperature, and heat transfer or heat exchange will occur as the 2 objects move toward thermal equilibrium.[7,14] Heat transfer can occur via conduction, convection, and radiation. Conduction is the transfer of heat from one object directly to another. This occurs because the 2 objects are in direct contact with each other; if the water is cooler than the person is, heat will be transferred from the patient to the water. Heat loss occurs about 30 times quicker in water vs air, making aquatic temperature very significant during therapy.[7,14] Conduction is the primary means of heat transfer in the water when the patient/water is not moving. Convection occurs when heat is transferred from an object because the air or liquid crosses over it. (If the water moving around a person is cooler than the person, then the person will lose heat to the water.) A patient will experience greater transfer of heat from convection when the patient is moving or the water is turbulent.[7,54] Heat is also lost from the body via radiation (the body radiates heat in all directions to the objects around it); if the ambient air temperature is higher, the body experiences an increase in temperature as the surrounding objects radiate heat onto the body. During land-based exercise, the body relies on evaporation for heat dissipation. Evaporation occurs as sweat is converted from a liquid to a vapor, creating perspiration. Sweat evaporation causes a cooling effect, but in water sweat is washed away and provides little to no cooling effect. Radiation and evaporation are the primary means of heat transfer during land-based exercise, whereas conduction is the primary means of heat transfer during water immersion.[7,14]

Because of all of the combined aspects of heat transfer that occur during immersion, the body experiences heat transfer 40 times quicker in water than it does in air at the same temperature. Heat transfer begins immediately upon immersion, and the body will equilibrate (bringing the body's temperature closer to the water's temperature) more rapidly than the surrounding water temperature will change. The body will work to maintain a stable core temperature by altering blood vessel dilation/constriction,

**Table 10-1**

Temperature Recommendations for Aquatic Fitness Programs[24]

| Activity or Target Population | Temperature Range (°F/°C) |
|---|---|
| Resistance training | 83 to 86/28.3 to 30 |
| Pregnancy | 83 to 85/28.3 to 29.4 |
| MS | 80 to 84/26.7 to 28.9 |
| Parkinson disease | 90 to 92/32.2 to 33.3 |
| Arthritis: Aquatic fitness program | 83 to 90/28.3 to 32.2 |
| Arthritis: ROM; low intensity with no endurance component | 91 to 94/32.8 to 34.4 |
| Older adults (moderate to high intensity) | 83 to 86/28.3 to 30 |
| Older adults (low intensity) | 86 to 88/30 to 31.1 |
| Children | 83 to 86/28.3 to 30 |
| Obese | 80 to 86/26.5 to 30 |
| Note: These reflect recommendations for water temperature for aquatic fitness programs. | |

generating muscle contractions (shivering), and using evaporation. Heat transfer is also impacted by ambient air temperature and humidity.[15]

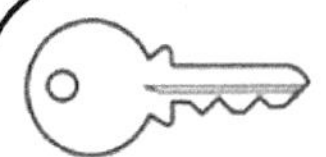

**Key Safety Consideration**

Aerobic activities are more suited to lower aquatic temperatures, and flexibility exercises are more suited to warmer water temperatures.

Recognizing that the temperature of an immersed body will adjust in the direction of the water temperature is an important consideration because this drives the decision regarding the type and intensity of activity. Exercise performed in water temperatures other than the recommended ranges requires modification of the program and additional patient monitoring.

## *Mechanical Properties of Water/Hydrodynamics*

Fluid dynamics (flow, drag, and turbulence) are additional properties of the aquatic environment that clinicians can modify to adjust program intensity.[8,14] Flow describes the motion of water. Streamlined or laminar flow occurs when water molecules are moving in a smooth path. A patient moving in the direction of flow will find the motion assisted. Attempting to move in the opposite direction of flow will result in increased resistance to the motion. **Drag force** is the resistance to motion in the water that is speed dependent. This force occurs parallel to the direction of the movement but in the opposite direction. The faster a person tries to move in the water, the greater the drag force. Additionally, if a patient is attempting to move through water that is against the flow, drag is increased. If equipment is used to increase a body part's surface area (eg, a glove/mitt), drag and resistance to the motion will both be increased. Turbulence occurs when the water molecules move erratically. Motion in turbulent water is more difficult for patients to navigate.

# Effects of Immersion on the Body Systems

The aquatic environment affects multiple body systems because of the various properties of water.[7] Each property should be considered when developing an aquatic therapy program.

## *Musculoskeletal Systems*

Muscle flexibility, strength, and endurance can improve in an aquatic environment. During immersion, blood flow to muscles is significantly increased. Dependent edema is reduced, and venous return increases, resulting in decreased blood pooling in the extremities. There is also improved oxygen delivery and waste removal from the muscles. Pain/muscle spasm may be reduced by warm water temperatures, sensory stimulation from water turbulence, and the patient's generalized relaxation. Aquatic therapy has been shown to be an effective treatment for patients with osteoarthritis (OA).[16]

## Nervous System

Hydrotherapy is useful for treating patients with spasticity.[17] Water temperature has a positive effect on muscle tone. Clinicians must consider the treatment goals and intervention activities when selecting a water temperature. Warm water (neutral warmth and water pressure) may decrease spasticity and allow relaxation of muscles in preparation for strengthening and functional activities. Using cold water has also been shown to be beneficial to decrease tone.[18] The use of cold water, although effective in decreasing tone, may also result in a decrease in functional ability in patients with spasticity (potentially negating the benefit of tone reduction).[19]

## Cardiovascular and Pulmonary Systems

The body responds to the hydrostatic pressure of water by displacing blood from the lower extremities proximally. As blood centralizes in the thoracic cavity (ie, heart vessels and lungs), there is an increase in central venous pressure, cardiac filling, and cardiac output via increased stroke volume. Heart rate during immersion tends to be lower than land-based values, except when the patient is immersed in very warm water (when heart rate generally rises). The increase in cardiac output tends to be age dependent (a greater increase in younger patients) and temperature dependent (a greater increase at higher water temperatures). Peripheral vascular resistance and diastolic blood pressure decrease during immersion, and these decreases can last hours after immersion.

During immersion, hydrostatic pressure results in compression on the thoracic cage, limiting thoracic expansion, and increases the effort of breathing. The increase in central (and pulmonary) blood volume also results in an increased effort of breathing.[7,8] There is a 60% increase in the total work of breathing with immersion to neck level.[7] The increased demand and workload can create training opportunities for many clients/patients. This increased breathing effort increases the demand on the inspiratory muscles, which may be impaired for patients with many pathologies (eg, congestive heart failure and chronic obstructive pulmonary disease). Patients with compromised respiratory status or pulmonary pathology may have difficulty breathing during exercise with immersion or in some cases at rest during immersion. Patients with pulmonary restrictions should begin at waist depth and increase immersion (and activity levels) in a carefully graded pattern. Research studies have reported that water-based exercise has beneficial effects on respiratory muscle and skeletal muscle function compared with land-based exercise for patients with chronic obstructive pulmonary disease.[20] However, the research does not clearly indicate that aquatic exercise improves exercise capacity or QOL for persons with pulmonary pathology.[12] For this reason, before initiating an aquatic program with any patient who has a pulmonary pathology, careful consideration of the individual's presentation and discussion of the risks/benefits of the intervention with the medical team should occur. If initiated, immersion and aquatic exercise for patients with pulmonary disease should be carefully monitored and advanced slowly. Athletes can also benefit from immersion training because it increases pulmonary demands and results in improved physiological training performance.

### Water Immersion Versus Land-Based Heart Rate Calculations

Vital sign monitoring is an important component of any treatment intervention for all patient populations. To maximize patient safety when exercising in water, clinicians must modify the target vital sign to reflect the body's adjusted response when immersed. The clinician should monitor the patient's rate of perceived exertion (RPE) and carefully observe the patient for skin color changes and respiratory rate.

Exercise in an aquatic environment affects heart rate, which tends to be lower during immersion compared with land-based resting values. Generally, a person's RPE is also lower in the water than during land-based exercises. There is a correlation between exercise heart rate and RPE in the aquatic environment in a healthy population.[21] It is believed that this is a result of the **"dive reflex"** decreasing demands on the circulatory system.[22] The dive reflex is defined as decreased cardiac workload when time is spent in a horizontal position supported by buoyancy combined with the cooling effect of the water. Traditionally, conversion to account for this lowering was to reduce the target heart rate by 13% of the tabulated land value. Alternate research suggested subtracting 17 beats/minute (bpm) from the final number tabulated in the heart rate reserve formula.[23] However, using either of these conversions can lead to an over- or underestimation of the target heart rate because of a number of individual factors and the patient's overall fitness level. For that reason, the Aquatic Exercise Association recommends using the Kruel aquatic heart rate deduction formula. A patient's aquatic (heart rate) deduction is calculated by taking a patient's resting heart rate (RHR) for 1 minute while standing in the water at the level of immersion at armpit height and subtracting it from the heart rate taken while standing on land for 1 minute.[23,24] The patient needs to wait 3 minutes before taking the standing heart rates both on land and in the water to adapt to the respective environments. The clinician also needs to know the patient's age and then determine the desired intensity before calculating the patient's target heart rate in the water.

The following equation provides an example for calculating the target heart rate for a 65-year-old patient with an RHR of 70 who will be working at a 60% desired intensity in the pool. The patient's aquatic deduction was 6.

**Application: Using Kruel Aquatic Heart Rate Deduction With the Heart Rate Reserve (Karvonen) Formula**

([220 – age – RHR – aquatic deduction) × desired intensity percentage] + RHR[23,24]

Aquatic deduction = RHR on land – RHR (immersed to armpit level)

(220 – 65 [age] – 70 [RHR] – 6 [aquatic deduction]) × 60% + 70 (RHR) = ______ bpm

(220 – 65 [age] – 70 [RHR] – 6 [aquatic deduction]) = 79

79 × 0.60 (% intensity) + 70 (RHR) = 117.4 bpm

## *Lymphatic and Renal Systems*

In addition to the displacement of blood and fluid from the lower extremities proximally from hydrostatic pressure, lymph flow moves centrally as well. During immersion, there is increased blood flow to the kidneys, resulting in improved (increased) urinary outflow. This causes an increase in sodium and potassium excretion that can increase the risk of dehydration. Regular hydration is important, especially when exercising in warmer water temperatures.

# Indications, Contraindications, and Precautions for Aquatic Therapy

The initial evaluation performed by the physical therapist on land determines if the patient should be treated with water- or land-based interventions. The therapist assesses the patient's level of safety in a pool environment, the patient's comfort level of being in the water, and contraindications or precautions that might inhibit the patient from participating in an aquatic therapy program. If the patient and treatment goals are deemed appropriate for aquatic therapy, the program can be initiated. The plan should include progression to a land-based program as soon as the patient's overall progress, short-term goals, and/or the needed weight-bearing progressions are met. The aquatic environment allows for joint protection, unweighting/unloading the spine and extremities, and compliance with weight-bearing status. Warmer water tends to be a relaxing environment, which can cause positive secondary effects during therapy.

Indications, contraindications, and precautions for aquatic exercise are listed in Table 10-2. Patients who exhibit any precautions need to be closely monitored at all times for safety concerns. When treating patients in the pool, clinicians should err on the side of caution and obtain clinical guidance from the supervising physical therapist.

# The Aquatic Environment and Pool Safety

The clinician will assess the following items when considering safety in the aquatic environment: the pool type, size, and depth; water temperature; chemicals used; pool accessibility; deck conditions; and the types of equipment available for patient transfers and treatment. There are different schools of thought regarding optimal instruction in a pool environment. For generalized fitness classes, the Aquatic Exercise Association recommends deck-based instruction for classes because of a larger number of participants; this allows better exercise demonstrations, more effective observation, and a more rapid safety response (if indicated) by the instructor.[25] Skilled aquatic therapy interventions are best accomplished on a one-to-one patient–clinician interaction in the water. The clinician must ensure their own safety and consider daily immersion time, water temperature, and activity level and should allow for appropriate rest time out of the water as well as maintaining adequate hydration.

The clinician may have access to a number of aquatic options, including traditional pools or small (individual) or self-contained pools. Generally, in the individual pools, the patient enters through a side door or down a few steps, while the therapist instructs the patient from outside the pool. These pools are often used in the outpatient orthopedic environment as a way to build up a patient's tolerance for land-based progressions. Pools may have built-in underwater treadmills or exercise bikes (Figure 10-3) and/or adjustable jets to modify water current or resistance during the treatment.[10] Larger pools usually have ramps or walk-in access, and some may have chair lift access (Figure 10-4). Lifts used for access into/out of the pool should be inspected regularly for safety, and the clinicians should receive safety training for all pool equipment. All steps/ladders should be slip resistant and fully secured. Deck surfaces and all access routes to the locker rooms/changing areas should be nonslip, accessible, and barrier free. Safety rules should be posted and reviewed regularly with all persons involved. Jumping into a pool with flotation equipment on and/or diving into shallow areas (less than 5 feet) should be prohibited. All clinicians should be familiar with emergency evacuations from the pool. Laws require all personnel to be certified in cardiopulmonary resuscitation and to know the location of life preservers and other rescue equipment.

Pool maintenance must follow guidelines set forth by county/state/local health departments. The water quality should be checked at least twice daily, and additional weekly testing and cleaning are required based on a state's pool codes. Any pool condition changes should be reported to appropriate personnel including chemical fumes, cloudy or discolored water, or patient complaints regarding new rashes or throat or eye irritation.[25]

**Table 10-2**

**Indications, Contraindications, and Precautions for Aquatic Therapy Exercise[7,8]**

| Indications | Contraindications | Precautions |
|---|---|---|
| • Edema or swelling<br>• Pain<br>• Decreased ROM<br>• Decreased strength<br>• Decreased muscle endurance<br>• Decreased aerobic endurance<br>• Balance/coordination deficits<br>• Gait deviations<br>• Increased fall risk<br>• Impaired quality of movement<br>• Increased tone or muscle guarding | • Acute myocardial infarction, severe congestive heart failure, or unstable angina<br>• Severe peripheral vascular disease<br>• Open wounds, danger of hemorrhage, or acute burns<br>• Recent postoperative incisions (unless occlusive dressing is secured)<br>• Active infections (ie, influenza, tuberculosis, or gastrointestinal infection)<br>• Contagious skin disease or rash (ie, impetigo, ringworm, or methicillin-resistant *Staphylococcus aureus*)<br>• Severe respiratory dysfunction<br>• Uncontrolled bowel, bladder dysfunction, or urinary tract infection<br>• Uncontrolled seizure disorders<br>• Menstruation without internal protection (ie, tampons)<br>• Client behavior that compromises patient/staff safety<br>• Severe fear or phobia of water<br>• Allergic reactions to pool chemicals | • Controlled seizures<br>• Neurologic disorders (ie, MS [water temperature and fatigue])<br>• Cardiac conditions (ie, angina and abnormal blood pressure)<br>• Severe/chronic ear infections<br>• Tracheotomies<br>• Small wounds, if covered with waterproof dressings<br>• Patients with low body fat and decreased ability to generate heat with movement<br>• Controlled diabetes<br>• Fear of water |

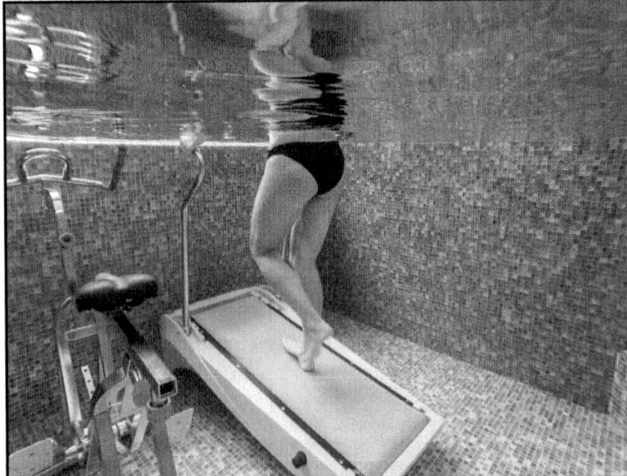

**Figure 10-3.** Underwater treadmill and bike (Elizaveta Galitckaia/Shutterstock.com).

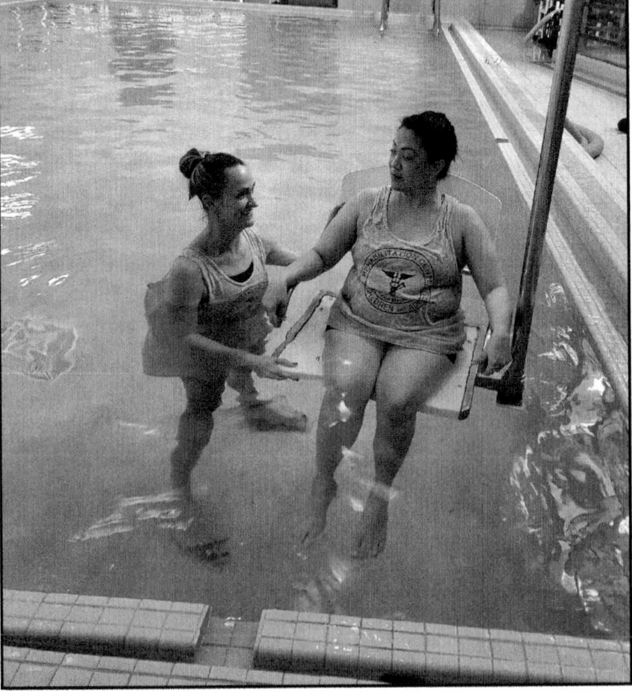

**Figure 10-4.** Chair lift for pool access.

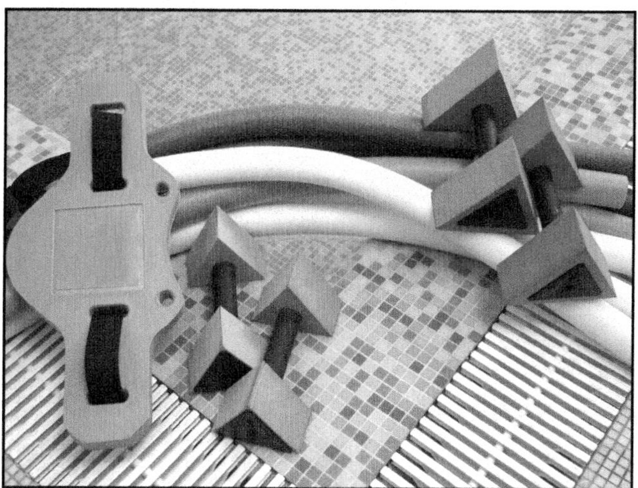

Figure 10-5. Aquatic noodles, flotation vest, and barbells (Pashin Georgiy/Shutterstock.com).

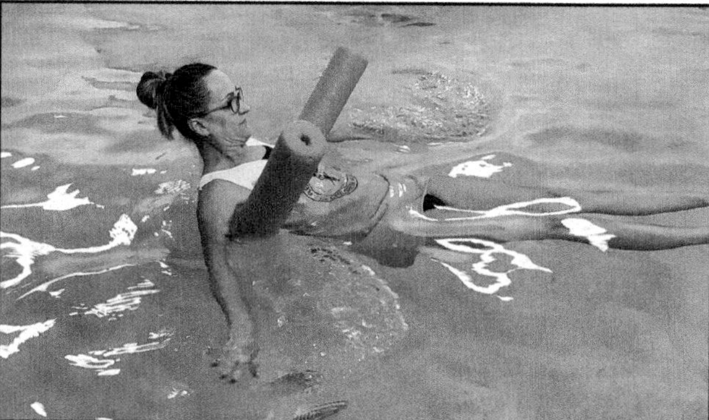

Figure 10-6. A pool noodle used for flotation.

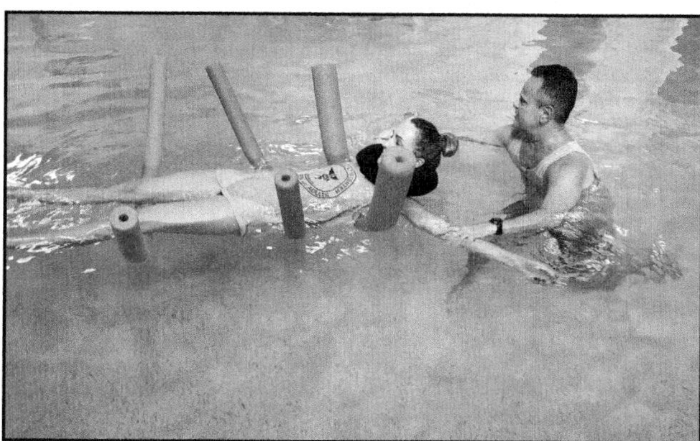

Figure 10-7. Using noodles and a cervical collar for support and buoyancy.

## Types of Equipment

Aquatic equipment can be used to assist with buoyancy/flotation or for resistance, balance, aerobic training, and/or gait training (Figure 10-5). Flotation vests, noodles, belts, or rings are used to add buoyancy (Figure 10-6). Rings are used to support the extremities, and vests or belts are often used during deep water activities to maintain flotation in supine or in the vertical position for exercise (Figure 10-7). Kickboards are used for buoyancy but can also provide resistance (if held vertically; Figure 10-8). The patient can practice sitting or stepping on a kickboard that is immersed to challenge balance (Figure 10-9). Buoyant barbells (or swim bars) can be used to assist with supporting the patient in an upright position and for maintaining balance (Figure 10-10). There are a variety of barbells that can also be used for resistance training (Figure 10-11). Webbed gloves or hand paddles are used to increase resistance during upper extremity exercise (Figure 10-12). Fins or boots can be added to increase lower extremity resistance to motion.[8,26]

## Exercise Guidelines and Clinical Applications

After reviewing the patient's goals and plan of care, the patient's ability to enter/exit the pool, precautions/contraindications, and vital signs, clinicians must consider the properties of water, water depth, types of equipment, thermodynamics, and hydrodynamics to select the appropriate exercise type and activity intensity for the patient.

Warm-up exercises should include large body motions to elevate core temperature, and exercise interventions must occur at an adequate intensity to maintain body temperature. ROM, flexibility, controlled strengthening, gait and balance training, modified functional activities, and cardiovascular endurance training can be safely performed in the pool. Cooldown after exercise may need to be adjusted to ensure that body temperature does not drop too much.[8]

Water temperature above the recommended range will warrant program modification, and the intensity and length of the exercise interventions may need to be lowered to prevent overheating. An extended cooldown with emphasis on stretching and relaxation is beneficial.

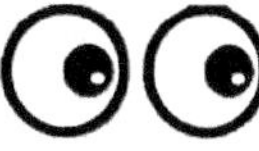

### Eye on the Research

Frohman et al[27] reported that aquatic exercise can be an ideal environment for patients with MS. Sweating is reduced in many patients with MS, and aquatic exercise improves heat conduction away from the core, essentially assisting to overcome their impaired thermoregulatory regulation. Additionally, buoyancy reduces the risk of falls and fracture during exercise. Hydrostatic pressure promotes venous return, which can assist in minimizing orthostasis (common in patients with MS). Many community pools control temperatures between 80 °F (26.7 °C) and 88 °F (31.1 °C), which is ideal for heat transfer during aquatic exercise in patients with MS; however, each individual patient with MS must be carefully monitored to determine their own particular comfort zone (based on individual response) with respect to water temperature.[27]

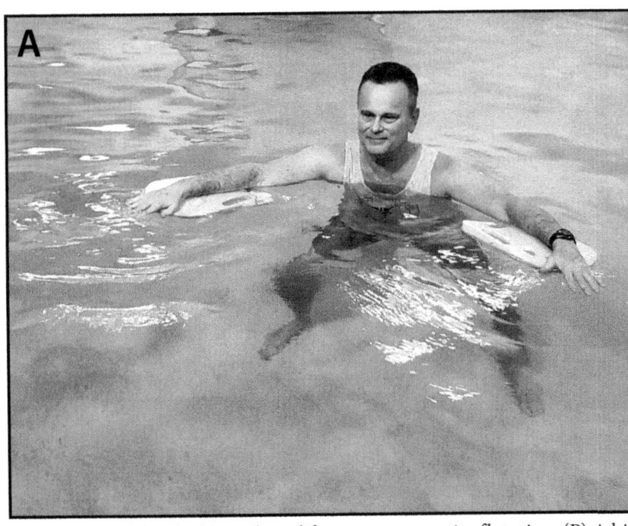



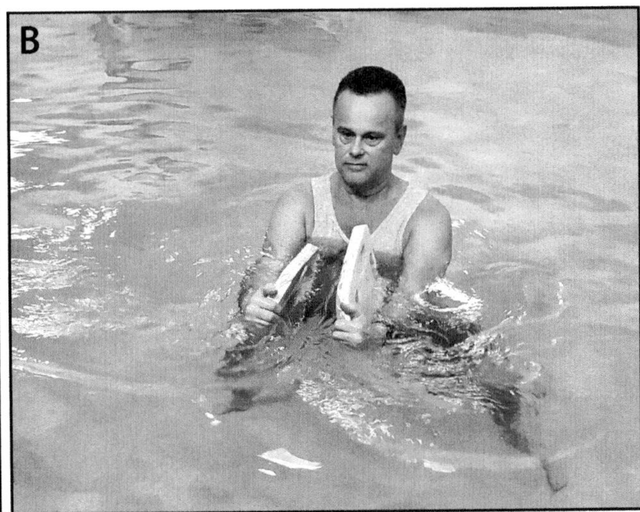



**Figure 10-8.** (A) A kickboard used for upper extremity flotation. (B) A kickboard used for upper extremity resistance and core stabilization training.

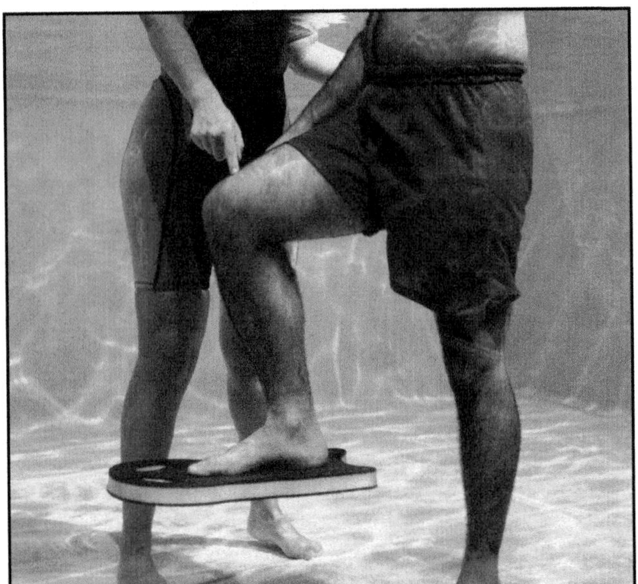

**Figure 10-9.** Stepping on a kickboard: A balance challenge.

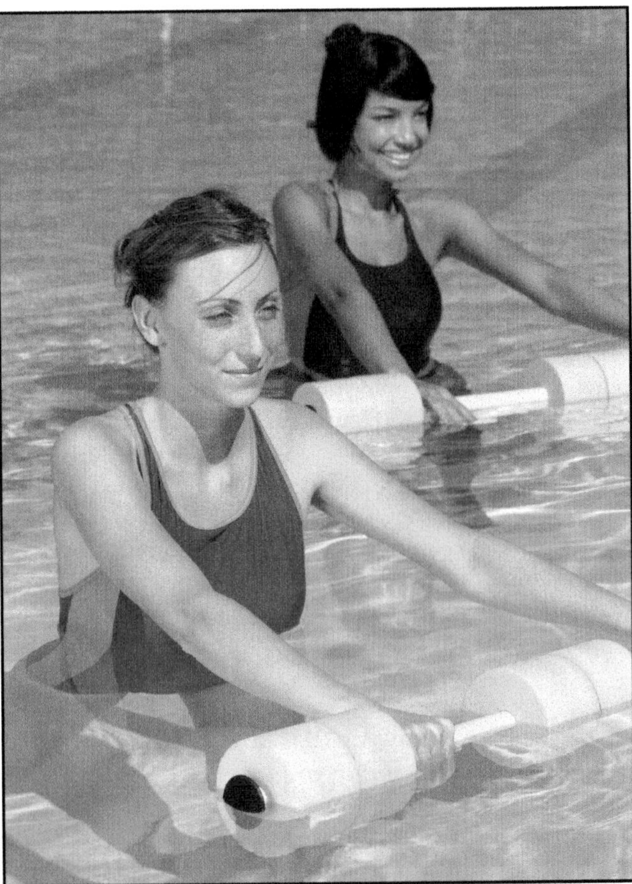

**Figure 10-10.** Buoyant barbells (or swim bars) used to assist with maintaining balance (Ground Picture/Shutterstock.com).

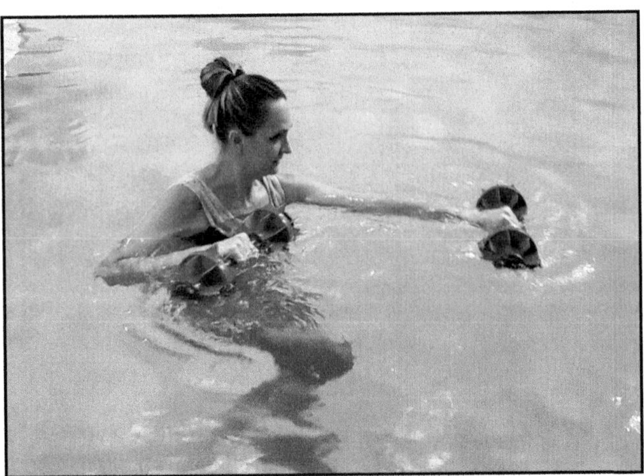

**Figure 10-11.** Water barbells for resistance training.

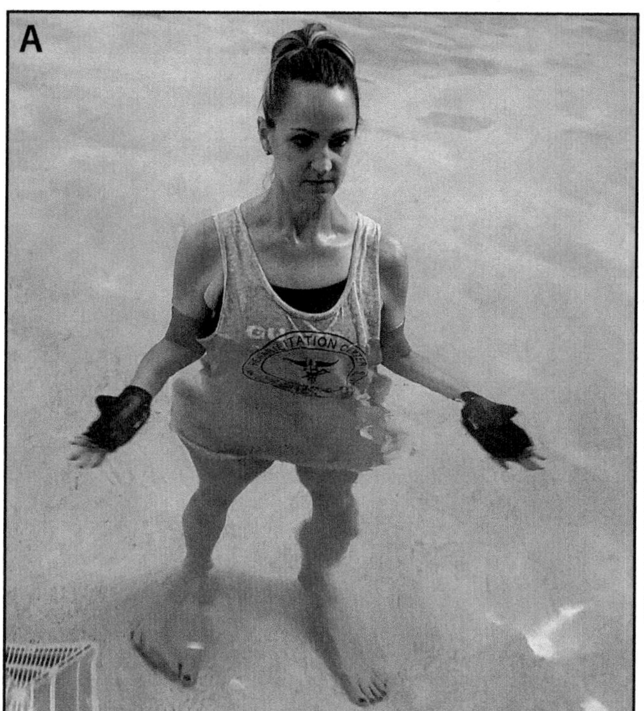


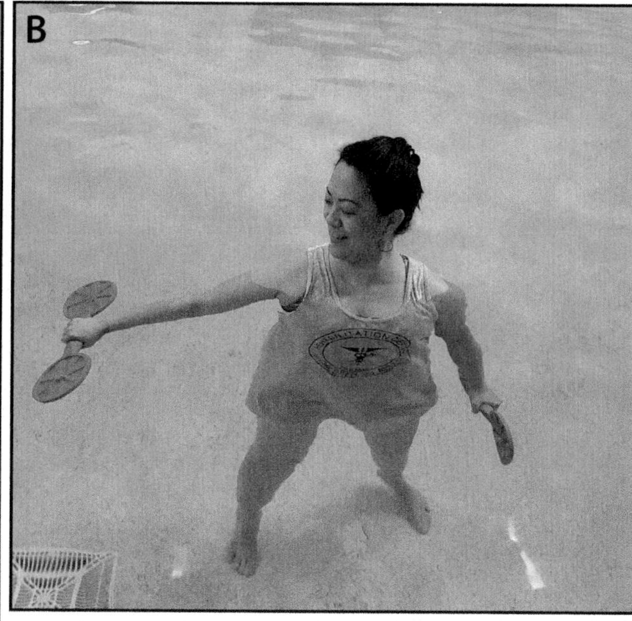


**Figure 10-12.** (A) Webbed aqua gloves (or hydrogloves) used for resisted shoulder internal/external rotation. (B) Aqua paddles used for resisted shoulder abduction/adduction.

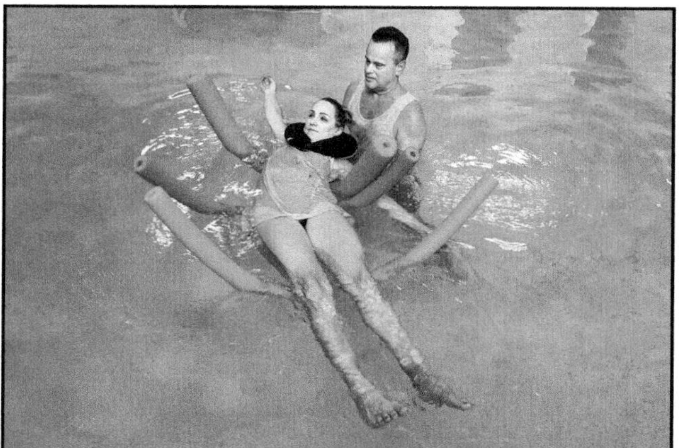

**Figure 10-13.** Passive lateral trunk flexion.

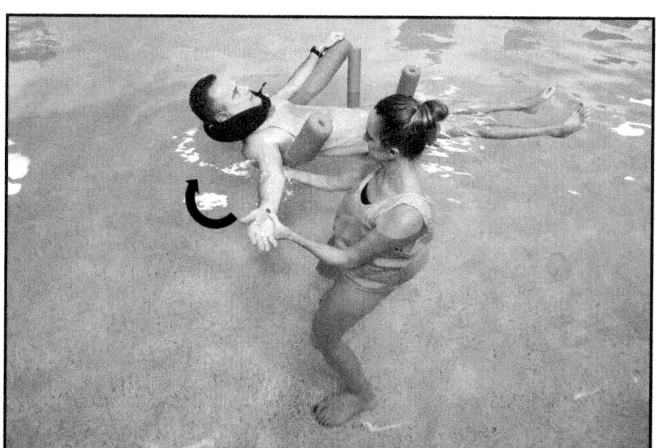

**Figure 10-14.** Passive shoulder abduction.

## *Range of Motion and Stretching*

The properties of water can facilitate the effectiveness of ROM and stretching programs. Exercise in the water may decrease a patient's pain and allow a more effective ROM. Passive and self-stretching interventions for the spine and upper and lower extremities can be performed with the patient supported in supine with a vest and flotation rings. Stretching techniques with the patient supported supine in the water allow the therapist better control and patient access when performing the techniques compared with a land-based program. The therapist can apply passive stretching to most joints in this position. Figures 10-13 through 10-15 illustrate passive ROM exercises.

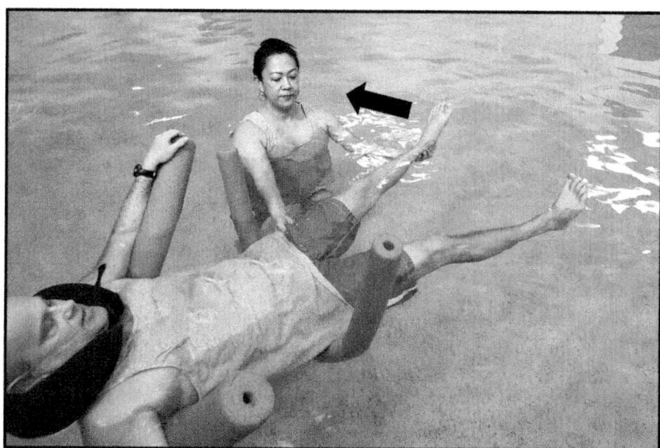

**Figure 10-15.** Passive hip abduction.

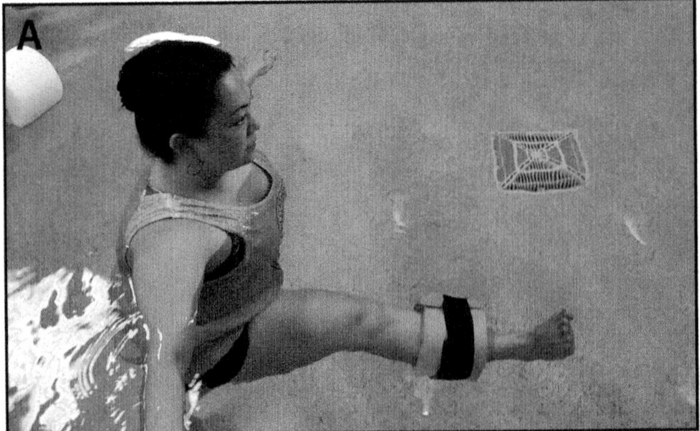


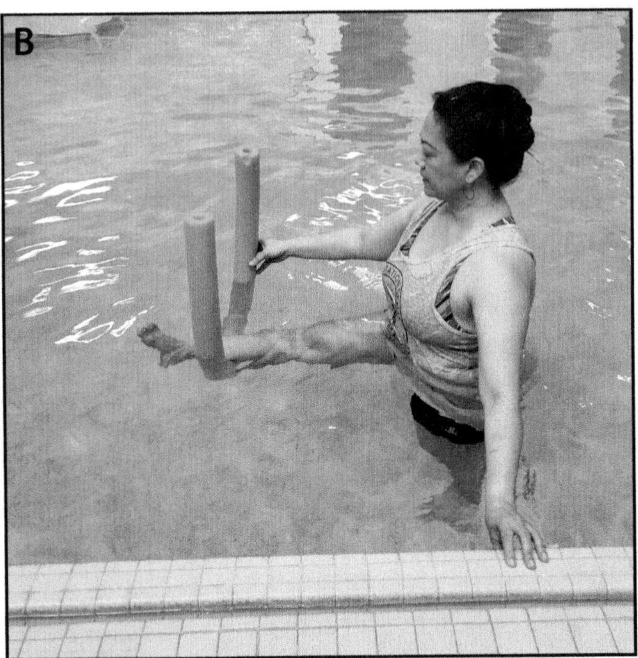


**Figure 10-16.** Hamstring self-stretch using (A) a flotation ring and (B) a noodle. For purposes of demonstration/ease of viewing, the patient is standing with upper extremity support. Optimal positioning would include the patient positioned in stance with the back resting on the pool wall.

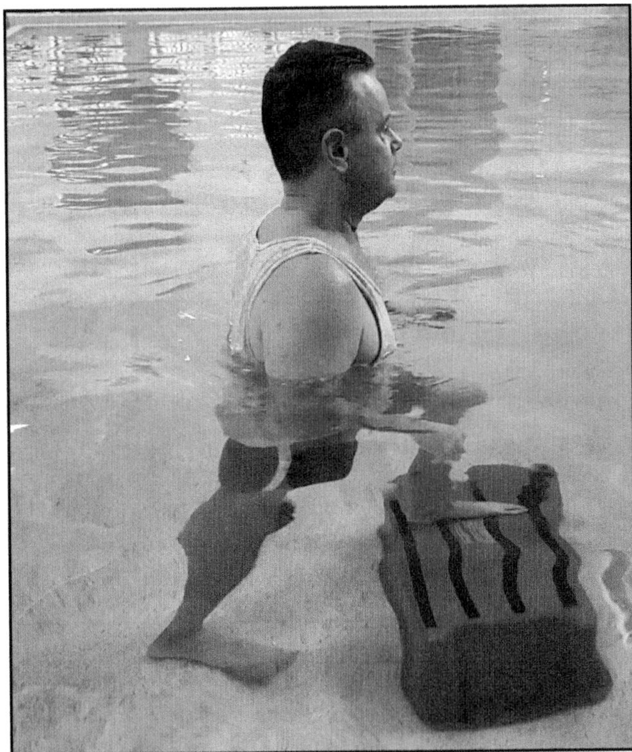

**Figure 10-17.** Step-ups.

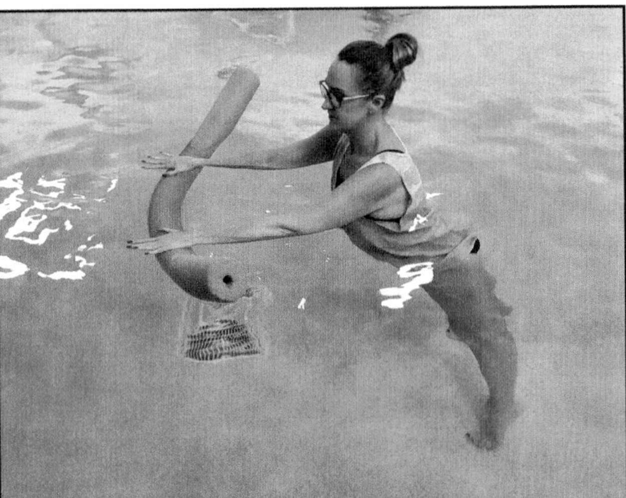

**Figure 10-18.** Core exercises; a noodle is used for promoting core and upper extremity stabilization.

The property of buoyancy can also be used to assist with self-stretching (Figure 10-16). Patients must have adequate muscle control to ensure that overstretching and injury do not occur. If the patient cannot overcome the forces of buoyancy, passive stretching by the clinician is initially safer. Buoyancy rings can be used to increase the stretch, but they are not required because the forces of buoyancy work on any submerged limb. Stretching positions are similar to those used for land-based programs. As with a land-based program, clinicians should provide instruction, demonstration, and verbal/tactile cues to ensure that the stretches are performed correctly and that overstretching is avoided.

## *Strengthening*

Strength training can be initiated as a part of many postoperative protocols in the aquatic environment once incisions are closed and the physician clears the patient. Patients often find that they can initially perform water-based exercises with less pain compared with a land-based program. Open and/or closed kinetic chain (Figure 10-17) exercises can be modified using the properties of water. Motion in the water can occur in any direction using diagonal planes (proprioceptive neuromuscular facilitation patterns) of motion to replicate functional activities. Postural and trunk stabilization exercises (Figure 10-18)

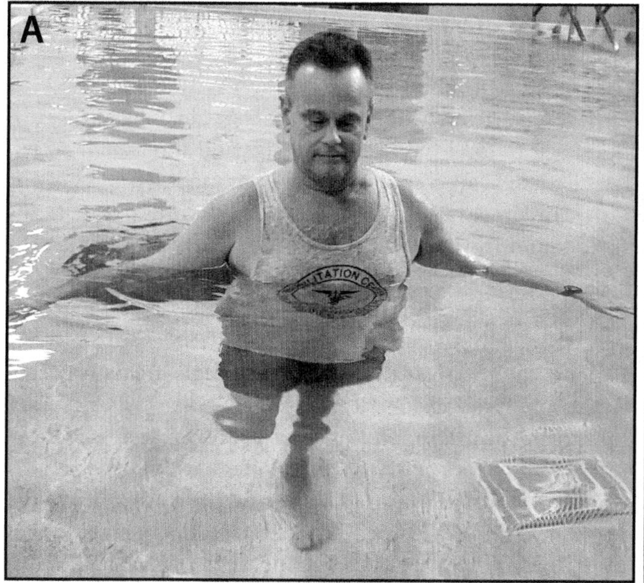
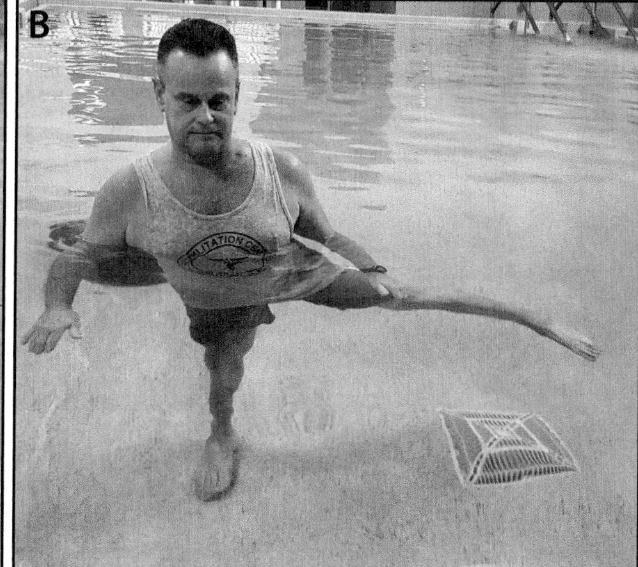

**Figure 10-19.** (A and B) Balance exercises: Single-leg standing variations.

can be performed in the water with the potential benefit of increasing strength with decreased pain due to the unloading of spinal compression forces.

Progressions for strengthening include transitioning an exercise from a buoyancy-assisted to a buoyancy-supported to a buoyancy-resisted direction. Increasing the speed of the motion in water increases the resistance. Adding hydrogloves or other types of equipment can further increase exercise. Other ways to increase the resistance of an exercise include the following: (1) increasing the length of the lever arm (ie, transitioning from shoulder abduction with the elbow flexed to an elbow-extended position), (2) moving in the opposite direction of flow or turbulence, and (3) increasing the size of buoyancy devices while having the patient create motion down/toward the pool bottom.

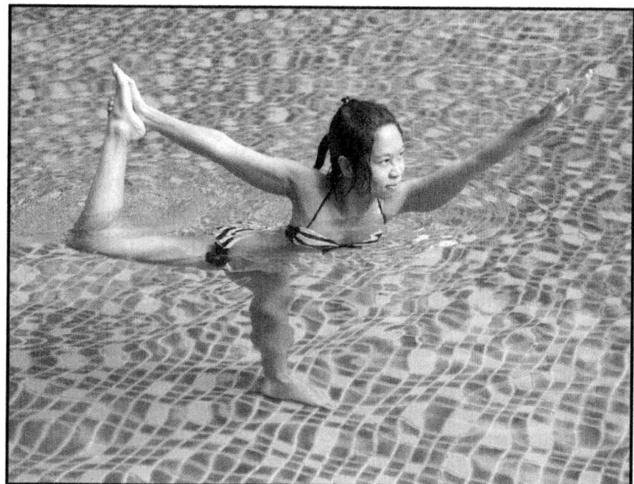

**Figure 10-20.** Balance progression using a yoga pose (Benjavisa Ruangvaree Art/Shutterstock.com).

## Balance and Coordination

The aquatic environment provides a safe environment with a reduced risk of injury from falls when initiating balance progressions. Typical seated and standing balance progressions can be performed in the aquatic environment. Clinicians can progress balance activities by starting a patient in a double-limb stance, transitioning to tandem standing, adding arm movements, and finally progressing to a single-limb stance without (Figure 10-19) and then with arm movements. Adding upper extremity motion creates drag and turbulence, challenging the patient to overcome the disturbances to maintain upright. Advanced balance activities, including yoga poses, are appropriate, especially for athletes preparing for the rigor of land-based single-limb activities and plyometrics (Figure 10-20).

## Gait Training

Initiating ambulation in the aquatic environment is beneficial because buoyancy reduces compressive forces through the joints and decreases the mechanical stresses of ambulation, and hydrostatic pressure enhances venous return. Walking in the water promotes some weight bearing, and an aquatic walking program can improve strength and overall endurance. However, walking in water is different from normal gait biomechanics on land (ie, step lengths are shorter, cadence is decreased, and ground forces are reduced); patients generate forces more slowly during ambulation in this environment. Although initiating gait training in water is beneficial, gait training for full, normalized functional return must progress to a land-based program.[8]

Vertical non–weight-bearing ambulation can be initiated with a patient wearing a buoyancy vest and simulating "ambulation" in deep water. During deep water walking activities, clinicians must instruct and carefully monitor the patient's form. Initially, ambulation can be progressed from chin-deep water ambulation for maximal limb unloading to a more tolerable weight-bearing status as water depth is

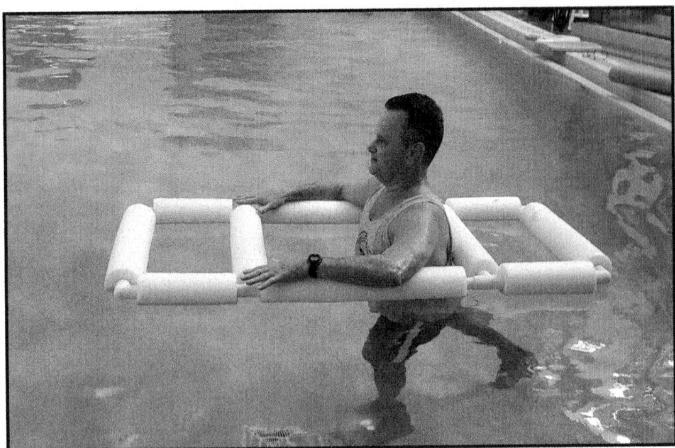

**Figure 10-21.** Supported ambulation.

decreased (Figure 10-21). Flotation devices can be used in the initial phases for additional support/balance, and they can be removed as the patient improves. Underwater stairs and treadmills can be used during aquatic gait training.

## Endurance/Aerobic Conditioning

Aerobic conditioning activities that can occur in the aquatic environment include ambulation, deep water jogging or running, deep water cross-country skiing, underwater treadmill use, immersed cycling, and swimming. Deep water jogging and running typically occur with patients suspended in deep water so that the feet are unable to touch the pool floor.

Careful attention to proper body mechanics and running form is important to minimize the risk of injury. The patient should be instructed to maintain a neutral cervical spine position with the trunk slightly forward of vertical, also maintaining a neutral spine position. A patient is typically suspended with a waist buoyancy belt. Patients can run against the resistance of water (jets) or may run in place while tethered to the side of the pool if the pool area is small.[8]

Swimming (using a preferred stroke) is another option for patients who enjoy this activity, have the required ROM and strength, and are able to tolerate being in the supine/prone position as required for proper stroke execution. Swimming may provide a bigger challenge to the cardiac and respiratory systems than other aquatic aerobic activities because both upper and lower extremity movement is needed to perform swimming strokes.

## Progressions: Functional Training and Plyometrics

The aquatic environment can be an ideal way to transition back to land-based plyometrics and functional activities. Patients can complete functional mobility tasks in the water in preparation for land-based training. Practicing sit to stand in the water allows the patient to practice the task with buoyancy acting to assist with the transfer and decrease the eccentric demands on the lower extremities when going from standing to sitting (Figure 10-22). Patients can progress through low- to high-intensity activities in preparation for return to land-based, work-related, or sports-specific activities. For example, if a patient is required to perform lifting techniques at work, this activity can be performed initially in the water to lower the chance of injury (Figure 10-23). The clinician can make corrections to faulty mechanics during these water-based lifts that can later be transitioned to land-based lifting using improved lifting mechanics.

Water-based high-intensity aerobic training is an option to reduce injury risk and improve the patient's overall level of conditioning. Equipment such as aquatic step benches and/or balls of different sizes and shapes can be used to build an appropriate exercise program to target the patient's goals. Plyometric exercises that can be adapted for use in the pool include (but are not limited to) jumping in place, hopping, box jumps, and directional jumps. Integrating aquatic training tasks before land progressions is an effective way to prepare the patient to return to their prior level of function or sport participation.

## Other Specialized Aquatic Interventions

There are several specialty interventions that can be used in the aquatic setting, including Watsu (water shiatsu), Bad Ragaz Ring, ai chi, and Poolates (a water-based version of Pilates).[8] Buoyancy devices are often used during these treatments. Determining the most appropriate intervention for a patient is made based on their presentation, goals, and how to best harness the benefits of the properties of water to achieve patient treatment goals.

Watsu is a form of passive aquatic therapy. This intervention is hands-on, and therapist certification in the technique is required. Bad Ragaz Ring is a method that incorporates manually guiding the patient through specific

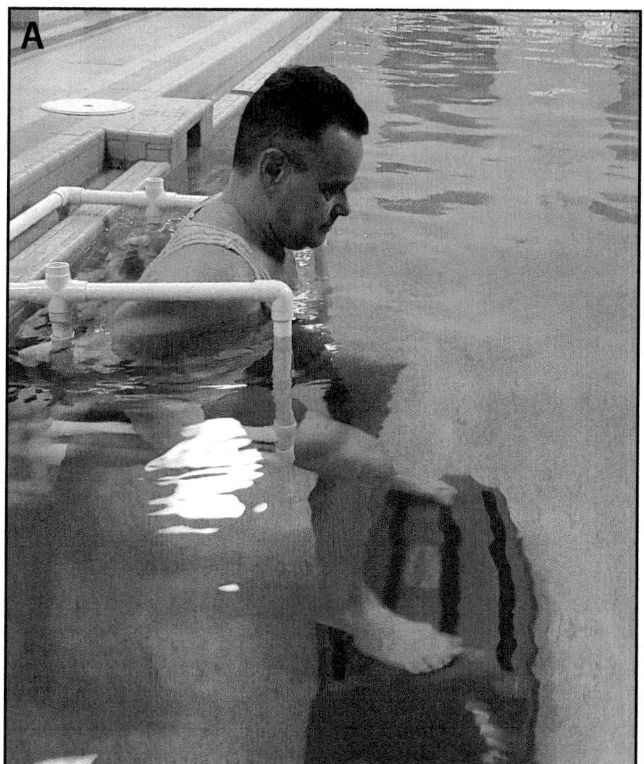


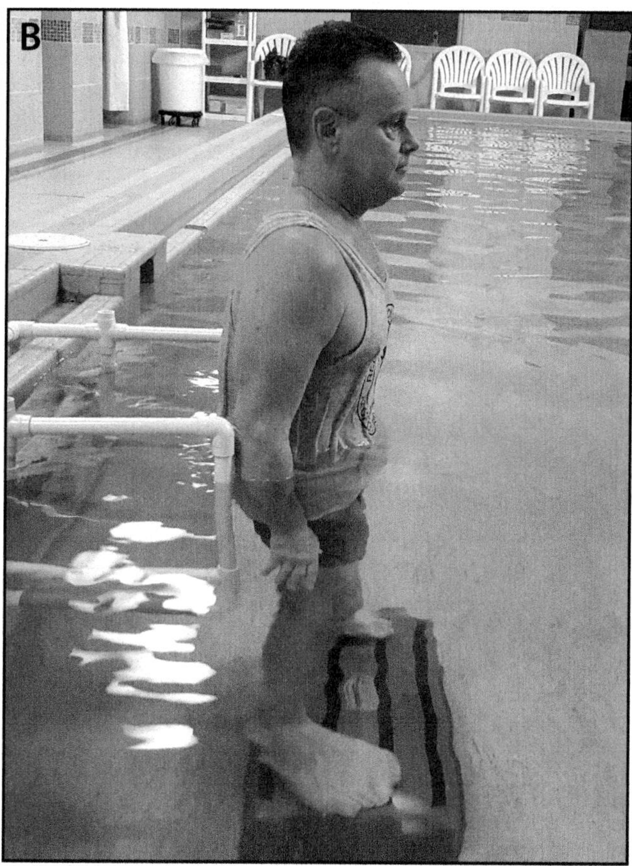


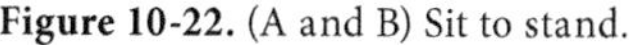
**Figure 10-22.** (A and B) Sit to stand.

motions, facilitating muscle elongation and relaxation (for pain modulation), with the goal of improving proprioception and neuromuscular function. This technique uses the properties of water for relaxation, muscle re-education, and strengthening.[26] Ai chi is an aquatic version of tai chi focusing on balance and movement control. Poolates pairs the use of equipment with motions that are geared to increase core stability, balance, and flexibility.

## Aquatic Exercise Effectiveness for Varied Diagnoses

Researchers have investigated the effectiveness of aquatic therapy for different patient populations, but these studies are often limited by patient population sizes and other constraints, making the results difficult to generalize. Although larger studies are often suggested, the results of the existing research indicate that exercise completed in an aquatic environment can be beneficial for a variety of patient populations.

Aquatic exercise has beneficial effects on persons with different chronic diseases. In a small research study completed by Ayán et al,[28] their results suggest that both water- and land-based exercise programs can improve gait impairments in patients with Parkinson disease. Patients with mild to moderate Parkinson disease demonstrated improved function, pain perception, balance, and functional capacity after ai chi treatment.[29]

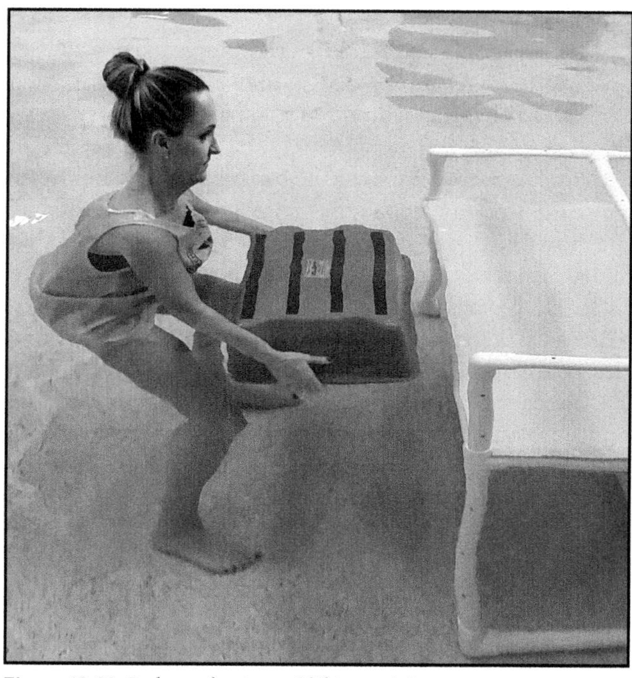
**Figure 10-23.** Body mechanics and lifting activity.

Aquatic exercise may be a safe option to improve activity levels and for persons with non–insulin-dependent diabetes mellitus. Researchers noted improvement with the patient's cardiovascular function (maximum oxygen consumption and blood pressure) and basic metabolic profile in men with non–insulin-dependent diabetes mellitus.[30]

Aquatic exercise for persons with mild deficits after stroke resulted in significantly more improvement (vs the control group) in the 2-Minute Walk Test, the Functional Reach Test, the Timed Up and Go Test, and the Berg Balance Test.[31] A larger systematic review determined that at least fair evidence exists to support the ability of an aquatic program to increase dynamic balance and gait speed in persons with cerebrovascular accident and MS.[4] Kim et al[32] demonstrated the benefit of aquatic dual-task training for balance and gait in patients with stroke.

Neville et al[33] completed a small study incorporating aquatic exercise targeting strength, agility, flexibility, balance, and relaxation for patients with dementia. The results indicated that a dementia-specific, aquatic exercise intervention reduced behavioral symptoms and improved psychological well-being in people with moderate to severe dementia.

Patients with sickle cell disease reported that aquatic therapy interventions resulted in significant improvement in pain, trunk ROM and strength, and hip extension and abduction muscle strength in comparison to a land-based exercise program.[34] Pechter et al[35] completed a 10-year study that examined the impact of aquatic exercise on persons with chronic kidney disease who were not yet on dialysis. None of the members in the aquatic exercise group reached dialysis or died during the 10-year study, but 55% in the sedentary control group started dialysis or died. In this particular study, regular supervised aquatic exercise was correlated to slowing chronic kidney disease progression.[35]

When patients with spinal cord injuries participated in an aquatic exercise program, pulmonary function results improved compared with those who participated in a land-based program.[36]

Dundar et al[3] compared the benefit of a home exercise program with an aquatic exercise program for patients diagnosed with ankylosing spondylitis and concluded that aquatic exercises produced better improvement in pain and QOL. Deep water running included along with a multimodal physical therapy exercise program has also been shown to decrease cancer-related fatigue in breast cancer patients.[37]

Kanitz et al[38] compared deep water endurance training and deep water strength training combined with endurance training (concurrent training). The study found that 2 training programs were effective at producing a significant increased improvement in cardiorespiratory and muscular strength responses in older adult men associated with deep water endurance training. Aquatic exercise can result in improved performance (using the 6-Minute Walk Test) for patients with stable congestive heart failure (vs land-based programs), which can lead to improvements (similar to those seen in land-based programs) in muscle strength and QOL. This may be an effective alternative exercise option for persons with congestive heart failure.[39]

A large systematic review concluded that aquatic exercise can have beneficial effects on pain, physical function, and QOL in adults with musculoskeletal conditions, similar to outcomes achieved with land-based exercise.[1] There is evidence of short-term benefits of aquatic exercise compared with land-based exercising and nonexercising patients with knee OA.[6] Bressel et al[40] determined that patients with knee OA had decreased joint pain and improved balance, sit-to-stand function, and ambulation speed after participating in high-intensity interval training and underwater treadmill training. They noted that patient adherence was exceptional, indicating that aquatic treadmill exercise and aquatic high-intensity interval training may be useful in managing symptoms of OA.[40]

Patients with chronic back pain experienced decreased levels of back pain and disability, increased QOL, improved body composition, and improved health-related fitness after intensive aquatic therapy.[41] Both aerobic training and aquatic exercise resulted in moderate to large increases in cardiorespiratory endurance and improvement in activities of daily living in persons with fibromyalgia.[42] Another systematic review reported statistically significant improvements on Fibromyalgia Impact Questionnaire scores, stiffness, and 6-Minute Walk Test results in patients with fibromyalgia after participating in aquatic physical therapy.[5]

Older adults also benefit from participating in aquatic therapy because it provides a safe environment when performing balance training. It can improve postural control, balance, and motor and cognitive skills as well as improve attitudes toward exercise and overall physiological wellness.[43]

There is at least one patient population for whom land-based exercise programs may be more effective than an aquatic program. Murtezani et al[44] determined that significant improvements in physical function and bone mass density occurred with a land-based exercise program but not with aquatic exercise for postmenopausal women with osteoporosis.

### Considerations for the Physical Therapist Assistant

Clinicians can use the following questions to confirm that aquatic therapy is appropriate for a patient:

- Do patient presentations and goals support an aquatic environment as the best treatment environment?
- Is the patient comfortable in the aquatic environment?
- Are there any patient contraindications to aquatic therapy?
- Can the patient safely enter and exit the pool?
- Has the target heart rate been determined using the aquatic heart rate deduction formula?
- When and/or how quickly will the patient transition to land-based exercise?
- Do aquatic interventions specifically address patient goals?

## Conclusion

Aquatic therapy interventions can be used to improve ROM, cardiopulmonary function, strength, flexibility, gait training, and overall relaxation. These improvements can lead to improved functional mobility and gains when transitioned to land-based activities. Aquatic exercise is considered a specialty area in rehabilitation. Practitioners who are interested in working in this setting will benefit from continuing education courses and/or certifications.

## Review Questions

1. Describe the primary impact each principle of water can have on a patient who is exercising in the water.
2. What effect does wearing hydrogloves during immersed shoulder horizontal abduction exercises have?
3. A patient is supported in deep water with a buoyancy vest. What effect will the addition of a buoyancy ring on the ankle have? Will the buoyancy ring increase or decrease resistance if the patient is completing hip extension in supine?
4. A patient is holding on to the edge of the pool while supine with a buoyancy ring attached to one ankle. What position will the lower extremity move into? What structure will be stretched in this position?
5. Which of the properties of water creates a force that assists a patient with performing shoulder flexion from 0 to 90 degrees when immersed in a standing position?
6. A patient's partial weight-bearing status is 40%. When standing in the water, how far should the patient be immersed?
7. Which property of water is most effective for controlling edema?
8. List the indications and contraindications for aquatic therapy.
9. Provide 3 advantages of an aquatic exercise program compared with a land-based exercise program.
10. What are 3 ways to transition from an aquatic therapy environment to a land-based exercise program?

## Case Study

A 64-year-old patient had a right total knee replacement 4 weeks ago and is referred for aquatic therapy. The patient walks with an antalgic gait with a decreased step length on the right partially because of limited knee extension and quadriceps muscle weakness. The patient reports a fear of falling when standing and walking. The treatment goals include improved ROM and strength on the right lower extremity, improved static and dynamic balance from fair to good, and improved gait mechanics.

1. List 3 aquatic exercises the patient can perform, and create 2 progressions to address each of the goals.
2. List any equipment that is needed. Identify the properties of water that are affecting each of the activities that you selected.

## Suggested Resources

American Physical Therapy Association. Academy of Aquatic Physical Therapy. 2023. Accessed January 30, 2023. http://www.aquaticpt.org/

Aquatic Exercise Association. 2022. Accessed January 30, 2023. https://www.aeawave.org

## References


1. Barker AL, Talevski J, Morello RT, Brand CA, Rahmann AE, Urquhart DM. Effectiveness of aquatic exercise for musculoskeletal conditions: a meta-analysis. *Arch Phys Med Rehabil.* 2014;95(9):1776-1786. doi:10.1016/j.apmr.2014.04.005
2. Heywood S, McClelland J, Metaplays B, Geigle P, Rahmann A, Clark R. The effectiveness of aquatic exercise in improving lower limb strength in musculoskeletal conditions: a systematic review and meta-analysis. *Arch Phys Med Rehabil.* 2017;98(1):173-186. doi:10.1016/j.apmr.2016.08.472
3. Dundar U, Solak O, Toktas H, et al. Effect of aquatic exercise on ankylosing spondylitis: a randomized controlled trial. *Rheumatol Int.* 2014;34(11):1505-1511. doi:10.1007/s00296-014-2980-8
4. Marinho-Buzelli AR, Bonnyman AM, Verrier MC. The effects of aquatic therapy on mobility of individuals with neurological diseases: a systematic review. *Clin Rehabil.* 2015;29(8):741-751. doi:10.1177/0269215514556297
5. Lima TB, Dias JM, Mazuquin BF, et al. The effectiveness of aquatic physical therapy in the treatment of fibromyalgia: a systematic review with meta-analysis. *Clin Rehabil.* 2013;27(10):892-908. doi:10.1177/0269215513484772
6. Lu M, Su Y, Zhang Y, et al. Effectiveness of aquatic exercise for treatment of knee osteoarthritis: systematic review and meta-analysis. *Z Rheumatol.* 2015;74(6):543-552. doi:10.1007/s00393-014-1559-9
7. Becker BE. Aquatic therapy: scientific foundations and clinical rehabilitation applications. *PM R.* 2009;1(9):859-872.
8. Becker B, Cole A. *Comprehensive Aquatic Therapy.* 3rd ed. Washington State University Publishing; 2010.
9. Merriam-Webster. Buoyancy. *Merriam-Webster Dictionary.* Accessed January 30, 2023. http://www.merriam-webster.com/dictionary/buoyancy
10. Bukowski EL. Aquatic exercise. In: Kisner C, Colby LA, Borstad J, eds. *Therapeutic Exercise Foundations and Techniques.* 7th ed. FA Davis; 2018.
11. Kawadler J. More on hydrostatic pressure and its benefits for hydrotherapy. 2022. Accessed January 30, 2023. https://www.swimex.com/professional/blog/hydrostatic-pressure-benefits2/
12. McNamara RJ, McKeough ZJ, McKenzie DK, Alison JA. Water-based exercise training for chronic obstructive pulmonary disease. *Cochrane Database Syst Rev.* 2013;12:CD008290.
13. Nave CR. HyperPhysics. Georgia State University. Accessed January 30, 2023. http://hyperphysics.phy-astr.gsu.edu/Hbase/geoopt/refr2.html
14. Low J, Reed A, Boston MA. *Physics Principles Explained.* Butterworth-Heinemann; 1994.
15. Torres-Ronda L, Del Alcázar XS. The properties of water and their applications for training. *J Hum Kinet.* 2014;44:237-248. doi:10.2478/hukin-2014-0129

16. De Mattos F, Leite N, Pitta A, Bento PCB. Effects of aquatic exercise on muscle strength and functional performance of individuals with osteoarthritis: a systematic review. *Rev Bras Reumatol Engl Ed.* 2016;56(6):530-542. doi:10.1016/j.rbre.2016.09.003
17. Kesiktas N. The use of hydrotherapy for the management of spasticity. *Neurorehabil Neural Repair.* 2004;18(4):268-273.
18. Bellew J, Michlovitz S, Nolan T. *Michlovitz's Modalities for Therapeutic Intervention.* 6th ed. FA Davis; 2016.
19. Denton A. Superficial warming and cooling of the leg affects walking speed and neuromuscular impairments in people with spastic paraparesis. *Ann Phys Rehabil Med.* 2016;59(5-6):326-332. doi:10.1016/j.rehab.2016.04.006
20. Wu W, Lui X, Lui J, Li P, Wang Z. Effectiveness of water-based Liuzijue exercise on respiratory muscle strength and peripheral skeletal muscle function in patients with COPD. *Int J Chron Obstruct Pulmon Dis.* 2018;13:1713-1726. doi:10.2147/COPD.S165593
21. Pinto SS, Alberton CL, Zaffari P, et al. Rating of perceived exertion and physiological responses in water-based exercise. *J Hum Kinet.* 2015;49:99-108. doi:10.1515/hukin-2015-0112
22. Panneton M. The mammalian diving response: an enigmatic reflex to preserve life? *Physiology (Bethesda).* 2013;28(5):284-297. doi:10.1152/physiol.00020.2013
23. Chewning, JM, Krist PS, Poli de Figueiredo PA. Monitoring Your aquatic heart rate: increasing accuracy with the Kruel Aquatic Adaptation. Aquatic Exercise Association Research Committee Project, May 2008-July 2009. Aquatic Exercise Association. Accessed January 30, 2023. https://aeawave.org/Portals/0/Monitoring%20Your%20Aquatic%20Heart%20Rate%20Increasing%20Accuracy%20with%20the%20Kruel%20Aquatic%20Adaptation.pdf
24. Kruel LF, Peyré-Tartaruga LA, Coertjens M, Dias AB, Da Silva RC, Rangel AC. Using heart rate to prescribe physical exercise during head-out water immersion. *J Strength Cond Res.* 2014;28(1):281-289. doi:10.1519/JSC.0b013e318295d534
25. Aquatic Exercise Association. AEA standards and guidelines. Aquatic Fitness. February 2014. Accessed January 30, 2023. https://aeawave.org/Portals/0/AEA_Cert_Docs/AEA_Standards_Guidlines_2020.pdf?ver=2019-12-18-131623-417%C3%97tamp=1576696862726
26. Hoogenboom BJ, Lomax NE. Aquatic therapy in rehabilitation. In: Prentice WE. *Rehabilitation Techniques for Sports Medicine and Athletic Training.* 6th ed. SLACK Incorporated; 2015.
27. Frohman AN, Okuda DT, Beh S, et al. Aquatic training in MS: neurotherapeutic impact upon quality of life. *Ann Clin Transl Neurol.* 2015;2(8):864-872. doi:10.1002/acn3.220
28. Ayán C, Cancela JM, Gutiérrez-Santiago A, Prieto I. Effects of two different exercise programs on gait parameters in individuals with Parkinson's disease: a pilot study. *Gait Posture.* 2014;39(1):648-651.
29. Pérez-de la Cruz S, García Luengo AV, Lambeck J. Effects of an Ai Chi fall prevention programme for patients with Parkinson's disease. *Neurologia.* 2016;31(3):176-182. doi:10.1016/j.nrl.2015.05.009
30. Cugusi L, Cadeddu C, Nocco S, et al. Effects of an aquatic-based exercise program to improve cardiometabolic profile, quality of life, and physical activity levels in men with type 2 diabetes mellitus. *PM R.* 2015;7(2):141-148; quiz 148. doi:10.1016/j.pmrj.2014.09.004
31. Zhu Z, Cui L, Yin M, et al. Hydrotherapy vs. conventional land-based exercise for improving walking and balance after stroke: a randomized controlled trial. *Clin Rehabil.* 2016;30(6):587-593. doi:10.1177/0269215515593392
32. Kim K, Lee DK, Kim EK. Effect of aquatic dual-task training on balance and gait in stroke patients. *J Phys Ther Sci.* 2016;28(7):2044-2047. doi:10.1589/jpts.28.2044
33. Neville C, Henwood T, Beattie E, Fielding E. Exploring the effect of aquatic exercise on behaviour and psychological well-being in people with moderate to severe dementia: a pilot study of the Watermemories Swimming Club. *Australas J Ageing.* 2014;33(2):124-127. doi:10.1111/ajag.12076
34. Zanoni CT, Galvão F, Cliquet Junior A, Saad ST. Pilot randomized controlled trial to evaluate the effect of aquatic and land physical therapy on musculoskeletal dysfunction of sickle cell disease patients. *Rev Bras Hematol Hemoter.* 2015;37(2):82-89. doi:10.1016/j.bjhh.2014.11.010
35. Pechter Ü, Raag M, Ots-Rosenberg M. Regular aquatic exercise for chronic kidney disease patients: a 10-year follow-up study. *Int J Rehabil Res.* 2014;37(3):251-255. doi:10.1097/MRR.0000000000000063
36. Jung J, Chung EJ, Kim K, Lee B-H, Lee JY. The effects of aquatic exercise on pulmonary function in patients with spinal cord injury. *J Phys Ther Sci.* 2014;26(5):707-709. doi:10.1589/jpts.26.707
37. Cuesta-Vargas AI, Buchan J, Arroyo-Morales M. A multimodal physiotherapy programme plus deep water running for improving cancer-related fatigue and quality of life in breast cancer survivors. *Eur J Cancer Care (Engl).* 2014;23(1):15-21. doi:10.1111/ecc.12114
38. Kanitz AC, Delevatti RS, Reichert T, et al. Effects of two deep water training programs on cardiorespiratory and muscular strength responses in older adults. *Exp Gerontol.* 2015;64:55-61. doi:10.1016/j.exger.2015.02.013
39. Adsett JA, Mudge AM, Morris N, Kuys S, Paratz JD. Aquatic exercise training and stable heart failure: a systematic review and meta-analysis. *Int J Cardiol.* 2015;186:22-28. doi:10.1016/j.ijcard.2015.03.095
40. Bressel E, Wing JE, Miller AI, Dolny DG. High-intensity interval training on an aquatic treadmill in adults with osteoarthritis: effect on pain, balance, function, and mobility. *J Strength Cond Res.* 2014;28(8):2088-2096. doi:10.1519/JSC.0000000000000258
41. Baena-Beato PÁ, Artero EG, Arroyo-Morales M, Robles-Fuentes A, Gatto-Cardia MC, Delgado-Fernández M. Aquatic therapy improves pain, disability, quality of life, body composition and fitness in sedentary adults with chronic low back pain. A controlled clinical trial. *Clin Rehabil.* 2014;28(4):350-360. doi:10.1177/0269215513504943
42. García-Hermoso A, Saavedra JM, Escalante Y. Effects of exercise on functional aerobic capacity in adults with fibromyalgia syndrome: a systematic review of randomized controlled trials. *J Back Musculoskelet Rehabil.* 2015;28(4):609-619. doi:10.3233/BMR-140562
43. Turner AJ, Chander H, Knight AC. Falls in geriatric populations and hydrotherapy as an intervention: a brief review. *Geriatrics (Basel).* 2018;3(4):71. doi:10.3390/geriatrics3040071
44. Murtezani A, Nevzati A, Ibraimi Z, Sllamniku S, Meka VS, Abazi N. The effect of land versus aquatic exercise program on bone mineral density and physical function in postmenopausal women with osteoporosis: a randomized controlled trial. *Ortop Traumatol Rehabil.* 2014;16(3):319-325. doi:10.5604/15093492.1112533

Section II

# Therapeutic Exercise Interventions for Orthopedic Conditions

# Chapter 11
# Orthopedic Considerations

*Jacki Klaczak Kopack, PT, DPT*

**KEY TERMS** Human movement system | Mechanical Diagnosis and Therapy | Movement system–based approach | Pain neuroscience education | Pathoanatomical approach | Psychologically informed care | Regional interdependence model | Rehabilitation management approach | Treatment-based classification | Yellow flags

## Chapter Objectives

1. Compare and contrast the classification of treatment diagnoses based on a pathoanatomical diagnosis vs a treatment-based classification system, mechanical diagnosis, or movement system impairment.
2. Define the term *human movement system* and briefly describe the American Physical Therapy Association's (APTA's) vision statement.
3. Define the regional interdependence model.
4. Define what the acronym SINSS (Severity, Irritability, Nature of complaint, Stage, Stability) represents and its relevance to patient monitoring.
5. Summarize the importance of clinical reasoning when working with persons with orthopedic diagnoses.
6. Define differential diagnosis as it relates to physical therapy.
7. Summarize the signs and symptoms that serve as red flags when working with patients who present with an orthopedic diagnosis.
8. Define and briefly describe pain neuroscience education.
9. List the manual interventions that may be included in the management of orthopedic patients.
10. Describe how common research terms are relevant to physical therapy practice (sensitivity, specificity, and reliability).

## Understanding the Movement System and Treatment Approaches

Physical therapist assistants treat patients who present with varied orthopedic diagnoses. The physical therapy profession is shifting away from assigning diagnoses related to specific body tissue or structure and toward the use of mechanical, movement system, and treatment-based classification systems to guide the diagnosis of patients. The APTA adopted a vision statement in 2013 that stated that the role of physical therapy is "transforming society by optimizing movement to improve the human experience."[1] This vision statement links the identity of physical therapists and physical therapist assistants to the movement system. "The movement system is the integration of body systems



Kopack JK, Cascardi KA.
*Principles of Therapeutic Exercise for the Physical Therapist Assistant* (pp 243-260).

that generate and maintain movement at all levels of bodily function. Human movement is a complex behavior within a specific context, and is influenced by social, environmental, and personal factors."[2] The **human movement system** is the "collection of systems (cardiovascular, pulmonary, endocrine, integumentary, nervous, and musculoskeletal) that interact to move the body or its component parts."[3] Physical therapists are educated to examine, evaluate, and diagnose movement system disorders and to create individualized treatment plans to address deficits.[3] The use of a movement system approach can ensure that the therapy team is considering all aspects of the patient and developing a plan that is focused on returning the patient to their highest level of function.

The physical therapist completes the physical examination and evaluation, generates a treatment diagnosis, and creates a treatment plan of care (POC) to address the patient's goals. The 2010 APTA House of Delegates position stated the following:

> A diagnosis is a label encompassing a cluster of signs and symptoms commonly associated with a disorder or syndrome or category of impairments in body structures and function, activity limitations, or participation restrictions ... When the patient/client is referred with a previously established diagnosis, the physical therapist should determine that the clinical findings are consistent with that diagnosis. If the diagnostic process reveals findings that are outside the scope of the physical therapist's knowledge, experience, or expertise, the physical therapist should then refer the patient/client to an appropriate practitioner.[4]

During the evaluation, the physical therapist will complete a screening to rule out other potential medical (non-orthopedic) causes for a patient's symptoms. Differential diagnosis is the process of reviewing a patient's presentation and comparing patient-specific information with known diagnostic criteria (inclusionary and exclusionary). Knowledge of each body system and the typical presentation of orthopedic and medical pathologies is required to create an accurate diagnosis and to effectively rule out other possible diagnoses; the physical therapist is responsible for creating the physical therapy diagnosis. The physical therapist assistant will monitor each patient to verify that the patient's presentation remains consistent with the diagnosis; any changes are reported to the supervising therapist. The assistant monitors the patient's response to treatment interventions, completes data collection, observes and corrects patient exercise/activity performance, and modifies progression during treatment (as indicated by patient presentation and response). The assistant must be aware of typical/expected patient progress, factors that may indicate a patient is not progressing as expected, and the signs/symptoms that warrant immediate communication to the therapist including but not limited to new presentation of red flags. The ability to recognize and apply this knowledge allows the physical therapist assistant to function effectively as part of the physical therapy team, promoting optimal patient outcomes.

### Considerations for the Physical Therapist Assistant

- Review the medical record and be aware of treatment indications, precautions, and contraindications.
- Establish professional rapport with patients.
- Collect relevant subjective and objective patient data, including vital signs.
- Safely apply appropriate interventions as per the physical therapy POC.
- Provide appropriate oversight of treatment activities and interventions.
- Carefully observe the patient during each session and report the following to the supervising therapist:
  - Any significant new findings or red flags
  - Changes in patient status
  - Patient progress (or lack thereof)
- Provide clear and concise instructions when educating patients.

The APTA's vision statement creates a shift away from a strictly pathoanatomical focus on diagnosis. Diagnoses that use the **pathoanatomical approach** focus on identifying a pathoanatomical tissue as the cause of a patient's symptoms. The pathoanatomical approach has been a foundation for assessment and intervention when treating patients with musculoskeletal diagnoses. A limitation to the pathoanatomical approach is that a patient's signs or symptoms may not all clearly arise from one tissue or structure. Additionally, the determination of a single physiological cause of symptoms is not always possible because a patient's symptoms may be impacted by impairments in surrounding tissues. A comprehensive physical therapy examination of a patient includes screening areas above and below the primary area of the musculoskeletal complaint; the results of that screening are not always easy to incorporate into a single pathoanatomical diagnosis.[4] A pathoanatomical diagnosis is often made by a physician (based on medical testing or imaging). The physical therapist reviews the medical diagnosis, the results of diagnostic testing, and the patient's presentation during the evaluation and then synthesizes this information to determine the physical therapy diagnosis. Physical therapy treatment is based on the diagnosis and stage of healing. Goals may address improving deficits in range of motion (ROM) or strength based on the assumption that these improvements will lead to an increase in function. The APTA's vision statement prioritizes the integration of the therapist's knowledge of the anatomy and biomechanics of each joint with the assessment of the patient's movement patterns, coordination, and skill activity. This shifts the focus of evaluation away from extremely detailed examination tests (some of which are not well supported by evidence) and toward the use of a biopsychosocial model that considers the whole person (including physical impairments and psychosocial variables). This model creates a shift from a detailed, localized assessment to a broader assessment of the local and the surrounding regions. This approach supports treatment-based classifications as part of the physical therapy diagnosis.[4] When the physical therapist focuses on optimizing each person's movement, the physical therapy diagnosis will address the components of the movement system that appear to be causing deficits in the patient's functional abilities. The POC will then include interventions focused on improving each area of impaired mobility, and the physical therapist assistant will implement and monitor the outcomes of each intervention. The movement system approach encourages the development of a treatment plan that focuses on the whole patient; most therapists already assess the impact of all body systems on a person's abilities, so this vision reflects the profession's effort to highlight the importance of this approach.

## *Movement System Approach*

The **movement system–based approach** recognizes the importance of observing the patient's motor control, coordination, and movement quality (including distal and proximal control) as well as their strength, ROM, medical diagnosis, and the results of special tests. A person may present with good strength in a muscle but decreased muscular endurance or coordination, which can present as pain or dysfunction. These issues might be overlooked if medical diagnosis, strength, or joint special tests were assessed in isolation. Assessing joint-specific and global movement patterns enables the clinician to define deficits and target treatment interventions to improve patient outcomes.

What makes the movement system approach an effective approach? Consider that an impairment-based diagnosis (ie, decreased hamstring length) may direct the clinician to look at and address the muscle length impairment but not the impact that the resultant posterior pelvic tilt may have on the patient's posture and trunk mobility. A medical diagnosis (eg, trochanteric bursitis) may encourage interventions that address inflammation, resulting in a short-term treatment that effectively reduces symptoms but does not address the underlying cause (ie, faulty running biomechanics). This approach can result in the same patient returning to physical therapy requiring additional treatments (after being discharged) for the same pathology. Approaching patient care from a single treatment approach may result in treatments focused on improving a single component of the person's limitations. A movement-based diagnosis describes the motions that are impaired and provides direct insight into which intervention strategies will be most appropriate/effective. This approach encourages a more comprehensive assessment of the patient and a more thorough framework for developing the treatment plan.

The physical therapist's examination and evaluation result in a treatment diagnosis, and the physical therapist assistant will follow the therapist's POC. A typical treatment progression often focuses on decreasing a patient's symptoms; then promoting movement control (stability); and, finally, guiding the patient to produce optimal movement patterns. During the initial evaluation, the physical therapist assesses the patient's ROM (of primary, proximal, and distal joints), muscle strength, and gross movement patterns. The therapist assesses the patient's ability to move, the quality of the movement, and the ability to transition from one posture to another (eg, sit to stand). The ability to analyze movement patterns allows physical therapy professionals to effectively diagnose and treat patients; this analysis is key to optimizing a patient's functional ability and independence. The therapy team can also play an effective role in preventing pathologies and future movement system dysfunction. Physical therapy interventions focus on improving patient function while incorporating education about pain control (potentially reducing the need for pain medications). Encouraging patients to move and actively participate in physical therapy may have an added benefit in addressing the opioid epidemic.

## *Regional Interdependence Model*

The **regional interdependence model** indicates "that seemingly unrelated impairments in a remote anatomical region may contribute to, or be associated with, the patient's primary complaint."[5] There are numerous examples in the literature of regional impairments that impact a patient's primary complaint.[6] Research that fully supports this model is limited; however, the evolution toward a biopsychosocial model supports interdependence. Knowledge of the interactions between body systems (musculoskeletal, neuromuscular, and somatic/visceral) continues to evolve. The model of regional interdependence will benefit from continued research to better define and describe the complex relationships between body systems. Given the current knowledge of these interactions, it is likely that clinicians will be integrating concepts of regional interdependence into patient care as further research becomes available.[6]

## *Treatment-Based Classification System*

The profession's focus on shifting to a movement system–based approach supports research encouraging physical therapists to classify patients into treatment categories. Treatment-based classification is a clinical approach that categorizes a patient into a specific treatment category based on their clinical presentations and impairments.[7] Research indicates that this treatment model can result in better care and outcomes.[7-10] Treatment-based classification models for the lumbar spine are reliable and valid.[9,11,12] A cervical spine treatment-based classification[12,13] has been proposed as well as shoulder and hip classification systems,[14-16] although these systems have not

## Box 11-1

### Treatment-Based Classification

Step 1: Initial triage

- Medical management: Appropriate medical screening, testing, and follow-up.
- Self-care management: Patient education, medication, work/activity modification, and progressions.
- Rehabilitation management (physical therapy interventions).

Step 2: If assigned to rehabilitation management

- Symptom modulation approach.
- Movement control approach.
- Functional optimization approach.

been fully tested for reliability. The treatment-based classification system for the lumbar spine is presented in greater detail in Chapter 15.

The classification system creates a general pathway/framework for treatment reflective of the patient's clinical presentation while allowing for individualized treatment interventions that address the patient's goals. Just as the movement system approach creates a shift away from the pathoanatomical focus of treatment so does the treatment-based classification system. Within the pathoanatomical model, some of the diagnostic labels may not be consistently reliable in accurately diagnosing or guiding treatment[7,14,15] and may not provide the best clinical guidance considering that the majority of physical therapy interventions focus on the treatment of pain and/or movement impairments. The treatment-based classification models provide a structure for grouping patients based on clinical presentation and movement patterns while also considering tissue irritability/symptoms.

The primary goal of this approach is to categorize a patient based on their clinical presentation into a classification where the patient is most likely to respond favorably. A patient may fit into more than one category, but the evaluating therapist will prioritize the most significant impairment to create the basis for treatment. Each treatment-based classification is intentionally broad to allow for flexible treatment interventions. The consistent use of treatment-based classification categories can create greater uniformity in treatment selections.[11,12,17] The use of this classification system relies on a thorough screening for possible underlying medical issues, comorbidities, and the patient's psychological status, in addition to the actual presentation of the impairment that led the patient to seek treatment. A careful review of these factors by the therapist ensures that the patient is classified correctly and treated appropriately.[17,18]

The 2 key steps in using a treatment-based classification approach to patient care are described in Box 11-1. The first step determines the overall management approach to the patient's care. This step is a triage approach, which is completed by a health care practitioner competent in treating the affected area (eg, primary care physician, orthopedic surgeon, physical therapist). The purpose of this step is to determine if the patient is appropriate for rehabilitation management, if a medical workup is indicated (medical management), or if self-care management appears to be adequate. The evaluating practitioner will screen the patient and assign them to 1 of the 3 approaches.[17] Medical management (physician referral) is indicated for patients who present with red flags for serious pathologies (eg, cancer, ligament tear, fracture) or comorbidities that require medical management before rehabilitation interventions (eg, poorly managed thyroid disease, rheumatoid arthritis, depression).

If a patient passes the medical screening with no apparent red flags, they are selected for either rehabilitation or self-care management. A small percentage of patients may benefit from a self-care management approach. The criteria for placement into this category are limited—low levels of distress, no (or well-controlled) comorbidities, normal neurologic presentation, and a low likelihood that the pain will increase to disabling levels. Screening for fear avoidance beliefs and pain catastrophizing is important. The Fear Avoidance Beliefs Questionnaire (FABQ) is a useful screening tool for identifying patients with high fear avoidance beliefs who are at risk for prolonged disability (see the Suggested Resource section at the end of this chapter). The FABQ considers how a patient's fear avoidance beliefs about work and activity may impact their pain and the resultant level of function or disability.[18,19] Recognition of these traits can guide clinicians to tailor interventions to meet patient needs (including a multidisciplinary approach, such as cognitive behavioral therapy, patient education, and graded exposure to physical activity).[20] Patients who score low in these areas are more appropriate for placement in the self-care management group. These patients will receive patient education focused on the general prognosis for the impairment (eg, chronic low back pain [LBP]), medication, work, and activity modifications and progressions.

Most patients who present with pain and impairments are appropriate for the **rehabilitation management approach.** When this approach is indicated, the physical therapist will select the most appropriate approach based on the patient's presentation, the patient's perception of pain and disability, and the clinician's assessment. This approach is not typically based on the time elapsed from the onset of injury. The patient may then be classified into a symptom modulation approach, movement control approach, or functional optimization approach.[17] Symptom/pain modulation is recommended for patients with significant symptoms, a recent (acute) or recurrent history of impairment, and very high disability and visual analog scale scores. The movement control approach is assigned to patients presenting with moderate pain/disability. The functional optimization approach is recommended for patients with low pain and disability. As a patient's impairments progress and/or change as a result of treatment, the clinician reassesses the classification if/when appropriate.[17] These approaches are described later using a patient who presents with LBP.

## Symptom Modulation Approach

The symptom modulation approach is most appropriate when the initial examination reveals a patient with a history of recent (or recurrent) neck/back pain with active symptoms and significant pain. These patients tend to avoid certain postures and have limited and/or painful ROM. They may also present with positive responses during a neurologic examination (reproducing peripheralization or centralization of symptoms). Optimal treatment interventions are individualized, focusing on decreasing the patient's symptoms; they typically include manual therapy, traction, and directional preference exercises (ie, exercises that centralize the symptoms). Directional preference exercises are typically consistent with the **Mechanical Diagnosis and Therapy (MDT)** or McKenzie approach for spinal and/or joint conditions. This approach is discussed in Chapter 15. Optimal results when using MDT are more likely observed in persons presenting with chronic LBP vs acute LBP.[21,22] However, in some acute cases, positional traction or immobilization techniques are indicated.

## Movement Control Approach

The movement control approach is indicated for patients who demonstrate one or more of the following presentations: moderate to low pain, gradual onset of pain, pain that increases with certain activities but dissipates after the aggravating activity is terminated, or recurrent episodes of pain triggered by certain movements (but are typically asymptomatic between episodes). The physical therapist may reclassify patients who initially presented in the symptom modulation category who now have decreased pain but continued symptoms with certain activities/motions. These patients report impairments caused by their inability to complete distinct tasks without increased pain.

The physical therapy examination assesses localized mobility and stability. Using a patient with LBP as an example, the therapist will assess posture, joint mobility (ie, spine and hip active ROM/passive ROM), and the quality of spinal movement during spine and lower extremity motion as well as soft tissue mobility. The therapist records observations related to motor control (specifically postural control and spine motion during hip active ROM, spinal active ROM, activities of daily living (ADLs), and functional mobility tasks) and notes areas of decreased mobility and stability. Muscle strength, muscle activation patterns during isometric contractions, and active ROM are also examined (refer to Chapter 15 for abdominal hollowing/bracing, multifidi contractions, and breathing activities at rest/activity).[23] The therapist also assesses the patient's neural mobility. Neural dynamic assessments include a straight leg raise test (sciatic nerve), femoral nerve tension test (femoral nerve), and slump test (general). The clinician assesses the patient's performance in those activities that correspond to complaints of increasing symptoms. Higher-level tasks (eg, lifting, reaching, and reciprocal motions) may also be included in the assessment.

Once impairments are determined, the therapist creates a POC so the physical therapist assistant can determine/select appropriate interventions to meet the treatment goals. Treatment progressions often address neural mobility impairments first and then joint mobility and soft tissue limitations followed by motor control training interventions and endurance training.[24]

## Functional Optimization

A functional optimization approach is indicated for those patients who are relatively asymptomatic. These patients are generally independent and pain free with ADLs, but they need to return to higher levels of physical function to return to a job or sport. Their symptoms are often only reproduced when they are fatigued with endurance or repetitive activities/tasks. These patients benefit from interventions that focus on task-specific performance. Endurance training or plyometric activities should focus on movement quality and maintaining good form throughout the activity.

### Considerations for the Physical Therapist Assistant

- If the patient's symptoms cannot be reproduced, do not initiate treatment. (This often indicates that the source of the symptoms may not be musculoskeletal.)
- If medical red flags are present, report the findings to the supervising therapist to refer out.
- If a patient presents with traits consistent with more than one classification, the therapist will prioritize presentations and select the most appropriate classification for initial treatments.
- A patient's presentation can change as treatment progresses; this will warrant a reassessment by the therapist and a potential change in treatment classification.
- Extensive patient education (simplified and issued in small, frequent information chunks) can improve outcomes. For patients presenting with significant psychosocial factors, education regarding pain theories, the importance of good sleep habits, coping skills, relaxation techniques, mindfulness, and avoiding catastrophizing about pain will be a beneficial inclusion to the treatment plan.[24]

### Mechanical Diagnosis and Therapy

MDT "is a specific classification-based musculoskeletal examination and intervention system that uses repeated end range and/or sustained movement to classify patients into mechanical syndromes."[25] The MDT system is commonly accepted and used for patients with spinal pathologies (ie, the McKenzie approach) but less widely used as a basis for treatment with peripheral joint diagnoses. The McKenzie approach classifies patients using 1 of 3 mechanical diagnostic categories: postural syndrome, dysfunction syndrome, or derangement syndrome. Postural syndrome is reflective of a patient's presentation that includes symptoms that are related to posture, postural fault, or symptoms that correlate to sustained positions/postures. Dysfunction syndrome reflects the presence of symptoms associated with motion (typically presenting as difficulty or inability to complete full ROM). Derangement syndrome includes 7 categories that are classified by the location of a patient's symptoms and are typically treated with repeated end range motions. These motions are completed in the opposite direction of the motion that creates the patient's symptoms. In the spine, derangement treatment theory is based on the physiological motion of the nucleus pulposus. For example, a posterolateral herniated nucleus pulposus typically produces symptoms with neck or trunk flexion (especially repeated flexion) and would be treated with extension bias exercises for the trunk (ie, prone on elbows or hands, repeated standing trunk extension, and cervical retraction with extension). An anterior derangement produces symptoms with extension, warranting flexion bias exercises (ie, knee to chest and trunk flexion). Depending on patient presentation, a lateral shift (motion in the transverse or frontal plane) may also be required to reduce the derangement in the lumbar spine.[26] As stated earlier, the McKenzie approach is described in Chapter 15. Cervical retraction and extension exercises are commonly used for the neck (refer to Chapter 14).

The MDT system has been proposed as a viable option for the treatment of some peripheral joint disorders, but preliminary research suggests that outcomes using this approach are most consistent when MDT-trained and -certified clinicians provide the treatment. Further research is indicated before selecting this as the first line of treatment for peripheral joints.[25,27]

The **treatment-based classification** system can capture and guide treatment for both pathoanatomical diagnoses as well as movement system impairments, perhaps making it the easiest model to apply. There is no clear and definitive research to state that one approach is preferred. Sound clinical judgment and integrating evidence-based research are important for physical therapist assistants to apply throughout their careers.

## Clinical Reasoning and the Physical Therapist Assistant

The physical therapist assistant will review patient indications, precautions, and contraindications before selecting and implementing interventions as per the POC. The assistant applies clinical reasoning within each patient interaction because each patient will progress at a different rate. Patient status and progression are impacted by what the clinician does during treatment and what the patient does between sessions with "normal life" activities. Because a patient's status can change during the treatment session, the assistant should perform at least one of the following tasks every session based on patient presentation and response:

- Continue treatment as per the POC.
- Modify the treatment as per the POC.
- Report changes to the physical therapist or physician depending on the severity/medical acuity of observations.
    - In this situation, the assistant may decide to "hold therapy" (delay/reschedule a session because of patient status change) pending communication with the therapist.

Physical therapist assistants need to use clinical decision-making skills when monitoring patients and assessing SINSS.[28] The assistant should collect SINSS data from the patient each session to help guide the clinician in determining if continuation or modification of the treatment is indicated (Table 11-1).

### *Red Flags and Yellow Flags*

Physical therapist assistants must be able to recognize significant changes in a patient's presentation that probably indicate a change in their medical status, a need for medical follow-up, or a pending or evolving medical emergency. These changes are referred to as *red flags*, and they warrant immediate communication with the physical therapist or initiation of the emergency medical services depending on individuals' presentations and their urgency. Red flag items and appropriate actions are provided in Table 11-2.[29]

**Yellow flags** are psychological, social, or environmental risk factors that (if present) may prolong disability or result in pain becoming more chronic in nature. Some examples of yellow flags include a person's attitude or beliefs about their pain, behavior, withdrawal from typical activities, patient-reported concerns about their diagnosis or treatment as well as their emotions, and family or work expectations. Determining the presence of yellow flags may help determine psychosocial risk that can assist the clinician in recognizing which patients may benefit from cognitive or behavioral management. In cases in which yellow flags are present, the physical therapist should determine if the physical therapy interventions should proceed with a modified approach or if a referral to a more appropriate medical provider is indicated.[30]

**Table 11-1**

## Monitoring the Orthopedic Patient Using SINSS

Any significant change in the patient's presentation may warrant reassessment by the supervising therapist.

| Element | Definition | Monitoring Guidelines |
|---|---|---|
| S: Severity | The intensity of symptoms reflects the degree to which symptoms limit activity | Assess patient's symptom intensity: Pain scale (VAS), ADL limitations, amount of medication taken to control pain, and presence or absence of resting and/or night pain<br>High = elevated pain levels and severe ADL restrictions<br>Low = little resting pain, low pain with activity |
| I: Irritability | Relationship between amount of activity-producing symptoms, magnitude of symptoms, and the time it takes symptoms to subside<br>Note: Condition may be highly irritable but not severe; therefore, symptoms are tolerable | Determine: Are symptoms easily provoked? How persistent are the symptoms?<br>High = pain lasts longer than 24 hours<br>Moderate = pain occurs midway through ROM, subsides in a few minutes<br>Mild = pain with full ROM or end ROM; pain stops immediately after activity is terminated |
| N: Nature of the complaint | Physical therapy diagnosis and any special considerations accompanying the diagnosis and prognosis | Include: Therapist's diagnosis of tissue/structures involved and/or pathology that produces signs/symptoms, any examination results or PMH that is a precaution, presence of red flags, personality traits of the patient (eg, FABQ, reported perception of pain) |
| S: Stage | Clinician's assessment of the stage in which the disorder is presenting | What is the stage of healing (based on time)?<br>Acute (typically < 3 weeks)<br>Subacute (> 3 weeks but < 6 weeks)<br>Chronic (> 6 weeks)<br>Acute on chronic (new onset of acute injury in an area with a history of injury/pain) |
| S: Stability | Progression of patient's symptoms over time | Stability is often judged by asking patient how the problem has changed since onset: Better? Worse? Unchanged? Stable? Unstable? |

PMH = past medical history; VAS = visual analog scale.

**Table 11-2**

Red Flags[29]

In all scenarios, the first step should be to stop activity, assist the patient to seated/supine, and assess vital signs. In all situations, if the actions state "intervene by (whatever action stated)" or "contact physical therapist," but patient's status continues to decline, the assistant should contact the physician and/or initiate EMS as indicated by patient status

| Signs/Symptoms | Concern/Cause | Indicated Follow-Up Actions |
|---|---|---|
| Inappropriate vital sign response to exercise | Cardiac or pulmonary compromise | Stop activity; assess vital signs. Contact the physical therapist, nurse, or physician. Monitor patient. Initiate EMS if patient status declines (vital signs remain unstable or patient becomes unresponsive). Start CPR if indicated. |
| New-onset cardiac signs/symptoms: Chest pain, left arm or jaw pain, excessive sweating, pallor, and fainting | MI | Stop activity, and assess vital signs. Initiate EMS. Monitor patient; start CPR if indicated. |
| Sweating, unsteadiness, weakness, clumsiness, confusion, and shakiness | Hypoglycemia | Administer sugar. Notify physical therapist. Have the patient check blood sugar. |
| Severe fatigue, lethargy, dry/flushed skin, extreme thirst/urination, and dizziness | Hyperglycemia | Call for medical assistance/administer insulin. Notify therapist. |
| Unexplained weight loss, fever, constant pain, night pain, fatigue, and changes in bowel and bladder | Cancer | Notify therapist and/or refer for medical screening. |
| Lower extremity swelling, tenderness/cramping in calf, and localized warmth | DVT | Complete Well's criteria (Suggested Resources in Chapter 3). Notify therapist and physician based on Well's criteria scoring. |
| Swollen limb, severe pain in local area, sensory deficits in the area and distal, motor loss in area/distal, and decreased/absent peripheral pulse | Compartment syndrome | Notify therapist and refer to physician or emergency room immediately. |
| Local edema, erythema, and heat; cellulitis; evidence of pus/purulent exudate; discoloration; and abnormal smell | Infection | Notify therapist and refer to physician. |
| Bowel and bladder changes/new incontinence, diminished reflexes, and motor/sensory loss | Cauda equina syndrome (spine related) | Notify therapist and refer to physician or emergency room immediately. |
| Signs/symptoms inconsistent with diagnosis or expected stage of healing and new neurologic or vascular changes | Change in patient status | Notify therapist for reassessment. |

Caution flags: These are signs/symptoms that warrant follow-up with a physical therapist; the assistant should modify treatment interventions and proceed with caution. Signs/symptoms of excessive stress/strain from exercise are soreness after exercise that lasts more than 2 hours or is still present after 24 hours, increased pain with activity (compared with prior tolerance), increased stiffness or loss of ROM, and decrease/loss of strength in the affected region.

CPR = cardiopulmonary resuscitation; DVT = deep vein thrombosis; EMS = emergency medical services; MI = myocardial infarction.

## Understanding Pain and Patient Education

A primary reason patients seek out physical therapy treatment is often because of pain, and they typically ask the doctor/physical therapy team "What is causing my pain?" or "What is wrong with me?" Routine patient education after an acute injury or surgical procedure typically informs the patient about highlights of the healing process and includes education regarding pain management but may not necessarily focus on pain itself. Pain is associated with injury and is often present during the rehabilitation process. The perception of pain is influenced by many factors. Historically, therapists and assistants spent a lot of time educating patients about their injured body part but not as much time talking about the aspects of pain typically associated with recovery and healing. This focus on anatomy is consistent with a biomedical approach, but a shift to a biopsychosocial model appears to improve patient outcomes. With acute, short-term injuries, the historical approach to pain education may not present an issue. However, when a patient presents with a chronic illness or history of repeated injury to a body part, patients are often familiar with having pain and, in many cases, are fearful of the experience of pain. Patients who are fearful of pain many times associate pain with "hurting myself more." Research indicates that anxiety, anticipation of pain, fear avoidance behaviors, and pain catastrophizing negatively effect musculoskeletal function and pain perception, resulting in poorer long-term outcomes.[31-33] Patient education often focuses on home exercises and explanations of the mechanism of injury and/or pathology. It must also prioritize education about the biopsychosocial elements of pain; clinicians should inform patients that discomfort/pain does not necessarily equate to harm. This education is especially important for patients who demonstrate fear avoidance traits, anxiety, and catastrophizing because patients' beliefs about pain can hinder their progression.

The biopsychosocial model demonstrates the relationship between the physiological pathology, psychology (ie, emotions, fear avoidance, stress), and social factors (ie, economic, culture, and work/family situations). Research indicates that changing fear avoidance beliefs/behaviors in patients with chronic LBP results in a more positive outcome.[34,35] Additional time spent on education, building trust, and reinforcing the clinician–patient alliance can make a difference between successful outcomes or less than optimal results. The physical therapist assistant should consider the patient's FABQ results when selecting the best educational information to provide; addressing the patient's physical activity avoidance is important, especially if avoidance occurs because of fear.[36]

Incorporating **pain neuroscience education (PNE)** during treatment can improve patient outcomes. PNE is a patient-centered educational approach that focuses on teaching patients about their pain, including education about the neurobiological and neurophysiological processes. Research supports that patients who understand the biology/physiology of pain better understand their pain and become less fearful. The inclusion of PNE has been shown to improve pain ratings, fear avoidance behaviors, movement limitations, and dysfunction.[37] **Psychologically informed care** acknowledges contextual factors about the patient and their pain while considering both the pain and the musculoskeletal diagnosis.[30] Contextual factors include, but are not limited to, the patient's expectations, the patient's medical and social history, the patient's personality, the clinician's behaviors/suggestions and use of therapeutic touch, the patient's perception of their therapeutic encounters, the use of a patient-centered approach, and the patient's perceptions of the health care system/office/clinician.

PNE is based on the pain neuromatrix model, which proposes that the brain processes inputs from varied areas (sensory, vision, limbic system/emotion, and stress regulation systems) to produce outgoing neural messages that produce the sensation of pain.[38] Providing patient education that describes the pain may help these patients to be less fearful of their pain. Consider an example in which a patient is told they have torn a ligament in their knee. For the patient, this is a fear-inducing diagnosis ("Oh no, something is torn!") that can lead to increasing their focus on the pain; anxiety regarding healing; and escalated fear about the return to their prior level of function, return to work, and/or ability to pay their bills. This can increase the threat perceived by their brain, increasing the pain response and creating fears about the effect that activities/exercises might have on healing. This is also true when a patient experiences pain associated with a chronic diagnosis. Patient "self-talk" providing negative reinforcement can inhibit participation and progress (ie, "This is making my pain worse," "Moving hurts," "I don't think anyone else feels like this," and "I'm never going to get better"). Education to alleviate this perception can be beneficial, but is education alone enough? Research indicates that the best clinical approach pairs PNE with graded movement/exercise.[37,39] The clinician should inform the patient that after an acute injury (or surgery) the initial pain is associated with the inflammatory response and healing process. Patients need to understand and accept that the pain they are experiencing is solely associated with the injured tissues and should diminish as healing progresses.

Patients with chronic-type pain continue to have pain generated from the neuromatrix/nervous system after the localized tissues have healed. This pain is often associated with an increase in the perceived threat of reinjury with movement, negative self-talk, and fear of the pain itself. This creates a negative cycle whereby patients experience pain and begin to self-limit activity. Pairing graded exercise with PNE can help condition patients to increase levels of activity while experiencing less pain. Graded exercise exposure is recommended for patients with chronic LBP who display clear signs of fear of pain or reinjury and are experiencing activity avoidance.[30] Desensitizing a patient to fear while gradually increasing physical activity can

## Box 11-2

### Sample Pathway for a Graded Exercise Intervention[30,40]

This progression can be used with exercises, treatment activities, and/or work-related activity simulations.

- Session 1: Complete FABQ, determine appropriate activities/interventions, and initiate interventions at a duration/intensity/frequency that does not increase symptoms or fear.
- Session 2: Reassess patient's fear and symptoms, complete fear-inducing exercises/activity with close monitoring by the therapist or assistant, and complete postactivity assessment of fear and symptoms.

Are fear ratings for activity decreasing?

If yes:

- Offer encouragement and positive reinforcement (feedback targets completion of the task and the ability to confront symptoms).
- Complete exercises/activities again. Do not increase any parameter by more than 10% at a time. As with any progression, increase duration, frequency, or intensity (but typically increase only one parameter at a time).
- Reassess fear ratings for activity; if decreased, repeat this process.

If no:

- Provide education highlighting the importance of completing the activity and confronting the present symptoms.
- Repeat exercise at initial exercise parameters.
- Reassess fear ratings for activity; repeat process at session 2.

facilitate patient progress. Box 11-2 provides a template for patient progression when implementing graded exercise interventions with patients who report a fear of activity performance.[40] Individual progression is based on the patient's response to each activity/session.[30,40]

Using modalities (to decrease localized pain or inflammation), therapeutic exercise, and/or manual interventions are useful adjuncts to this education. Treating patients with pain requires a comprehensive approach and a willingness to use all available treatment tools at a clinician's disposal. Appropriate selection of interventions, the use of psychologically informed care, patient education, judicious use of modalities, and manual interventions addressing the patient's individualized presentation can optimize outcomes.

## Implementing Orthopedic Interventions

The physical therapist assistant should approach treatment intervention plans systematically to ensure that interventions are effective, safe, and appropriate to achieve the patient's functional goals as outlined in the initial evaluation. Table 11-3 provides a sequential list of steps for assistants treating orthopedic patients. Physical therapist assistants should use active listening, foundational knowledge, clinical skills, and clinical decision making to help patients achieve their goals. If a patient is not showing significant improvement, the assistant should collect objective data and review it with the supervising therapist to determine if treatment modification is indicated or if other treatment methods should be implemented. Patient-centered interventions require collaboration between the therapist and the assistant.

## Manual Interventions: Ischemic Compression, Nerve Glides, and Mobilizations for Orthopedic Conditions

The initial evaluation includes the therapist's assessment of orthopedic diagnoses, trigger points, nerve compression or adhesions, and/or spinal malalignment. These presentations can benefit from using manual therapy interventions to improve function and decrease symptoms. Manual treatment interventions that can be delegated to the physical therapist assistant are defined within the individual state practice act. Using manual therapy techniques is based on the scope of practice regulations in each state, and the delegation of these techniques is at the discretion of the physical therapist. When manual techniques must be provided by therapists only, assistants may initiate treatment interventions before these mobilizations to prepare the patient and continue treatment after mobilization techniques have been performed by the therapist.

Vertebral malalignment is often addressed with spinal mobilizations using high-velocity thrust manipulations. Spinal mobilization techniques are not entry-level skills and should not be performed by an assistant. Some state practice acts even prohibit physical therapists from performing high-velocity manipulative thrusts on the spine.

## Table 11-3

## A Guide to Orthopedic Intervention Sequencing

Steps that guide clinical decision making and problem-solving processes for physical therapist assistants.

1. Select interventions based on the initial physical therapy evaluation and POC that address goals.
   a. Review the medical record for contraindications and precautions; obtain additional medical clearance if indicated/appropriate.
2. Verify changes in status, medications, or new subjective complaints since the last visit.
   a. Inquire: Any new orthopedic restrictions (ie, recent fracture/tendon/ligament tear, infections, or cancer).
   b. Obtain pain level: At rest, what makes it worse and/or better.
   c. Determine how the patient perceives their pain as it relates to specific position/movement avoidance.
3. Obtain consent to treat and vital signs pretreatment.
4. Determine which muscle groups to stretch, strengthen, and/or stabilize.
   a. Review treatment-based classification, movement system impairment, or mechanical diagnosis.
   b. Check passive ROM/active ROM to determine a starting point for exercises; consider results of movement testing from evaluation.
5. Select the most appropriate exercises:
   a. Based on diagnostic classification and stage of healing.
   b. Select exercises that target the treatment-based classification, diagnosis, and movement preference. Encourage gradual movement into fear-based positions while monitoring pain.
6. Select the most appropriate exercise parameters based on patient presentation and data collection; be specific (FITT [frequency, intensity, time, type]).
   a. Consider patient positioning: Can the patient comfortably attain the desired position? Does the selected position allow for optimal stabilization?
   b. Select the parameters to address the treatment goals.
7. Once an exercise and parameters are selected, demonstrate the exercise to the patient.
   a. Have the patient return, demonstrate the exercise, and monitor for correct form.
      i. Ensure appropriate body mechanics, proper breathing (no Valsalva), and no substitution/compensation.
      ii. Verify exercise does not increase patient symptoms.
8. Complete task-specific training as indicated.
9. Record posttreatment patient: Vital signs, status, and subjective report. Document signs of discomfort/pain and difficulty/progress performing any part of the intervention.
10. Issue home exercise program (HEP):
    a. Only if the patient can demonstrate exercises safely independently.
    b. Provide written/electronic HEP and/or educational materials (video clips and web links). (See Appendices C and D for HEP development resources).

Assessment and modification:

- Assess patient functional activity/exercise performance and modify FITT appropriately during each treatment session to meet short- and long-term goals.
- *Important:* Follow up with physical therapist during treatment session if the patient reports new pain, pain in a new location, or severe/increased pain; increased swelling; any new cardiac or neurologic signs/symptoms; or lack of progression within the expected time frame.
- If no significant improvement, collect objective data and review it with supervising therapist; treatment modification may be indicated.

## Box 11-3

### Nerve Flossing and Neural Glides

*Important:* Neural mobilization is not appropriate if unstable neurologic signs are present; these incidents, as well as localized infection or local neoplasm, warrant immediate medical referral.

Nerve slide/flossing: Place the patient in the position that produces the onset of symptoms, and then the 2 joints are moved simultaneously; the clinician creates tension in one end of the nerve while simultaneously releasing tension on the other end.

- The motion at one joint counterbalances the strain created by the second joint motion.

Nerve tension/glides: Place the patient in the position that produces the onset of symptoms, and move one joint.

- Gently and slowly move the limb in and out of the point of tissue resistance or symptoms.

Key: A positive test will reproduce patient symptoms with the glide movement sequence and should decrease symptoms with motion out of the sequence pattern. Progressive practice will desensitize the patient and decrease symptoms.

If a patient's symptoms are related to the presence of a trigger point, the primary goal of treatment is to relieve pain and then improve ROM and strength that address the factors contributing to trigger point irritation. Interventions include ischemic compression massage to the trigger point and ice (or vapocoolant spray applied as part of a "spray and stretch" intervention). Ischemic compression massage is typically achieved using the thumb or therapeutic tool to apply deep pressure directly onto the trigger point. The clinician begins gently and then gradually increases downward pressure with sustained deep pressure over the trigger point for 20 to 30 seconds; the process can be repeated 3 to 4 times. This intervention is followed by gentle stretching and then postural exercise/retraining. The clinician reassesses the tissues to see if there is less localized muscle tension and decreased trigger point sensitivity after the intervention.

Most initial physical therapy examinations include an examination of the nervous system (assessed by checking reflexes, sensation, myotome muscle strength, and neural tension). When the evaluation indicates a presence of neural adhesions, the POC often includes neural mobilization techniques.

When a nerve is injured or compressed, it sometimes loses its ability to glide normally through the surrounding sheath and tissues, resulting in pain or paresthesia. Nerves can be stretched carefully to reduce this inflammation/compression, ultimately allowing the nerves to glide normally. Typical muscular stretching parameters could irritate the nerve and possibly exacerbate symptoms. For this reason, neurodynamic tension treatments (nerve glides or flossing) are used. Neurodynamic tension tests and treatments apply controlled gradual increasing stress to the neural tissues/structures. Increases in symptoms during testing indicate that a patient's pain may be caused by tension in the spinal nerve root or the peripheral nerve. This may indicate that techniques to mobilize nerve tissue are appropriate. Neural mobilization techniques are used to both assess and treat neural adhesions; 2 common techniques include nerve tension (neural glide) techniques and nerve slide (flossing) techniques. Nerve glides work to separate the nerve from the surrounding structures by gently sliding the nerve, using joint movements to gently lengthen a nerve. Sliding, or flossing, is an intervention used to improve the extensibility of a nerve by providing a mild stretch and release repeatedly. Box 11-3 briefly describes neural glides and flossing. The following basic management rules should be followed when using nerve glides or flossing:

- Always modify the intensity of the technique based on the irritability of symptoms (more irritable = more gentle treatment/slower progression).
- Do not apply nerve glides or flossing at an intensity that increases the patient's symptoms.
- Monitor for signs or symptoms that indicate vascular compromise or a rapidly worsening condition; these warrant reassessment by the physical therapist.

Neural mobilization is effective for treating neck and LBP.[41] Nerve glides are generally accepted and used to treat several peripheral nerve injuries (including carpal tunnel syndrome), but there remains a need for high-quality research to support the use for treating peripheral neural diagnoses.[41,42] Table 11-4 describes the appropriate testing position for the peripheral nerves and possible conditions.[43] Figures 11-1 through 11-6 illustrate positions for nerve tension tests. Progression is based on the patient's response. Passive limb motion should be stopped when the patient describes the provoking symptoms that lead to pain or paresthesia distally in the related dermatome or when the clinician feels tension in the tissue. Once the end position is reached, the clinician should passively move one joint in and then out of the end position slowly. When performing upper limb tension tests, the addition of cervical lateral flexion promotes full elongation of the neural structures. Once the appropriate end position is found and the patient's response is appropriate (no severe pain and mild symptoms stop immediately with movement out of the end position), the clinician can initiate nerve flossing techniques. Flossing creates tension at one end of the nerve while simultaneously releasing tension on the other end. This repetitive motion glides the nerve back and forth through its path, which releases adhesions that have

**Table 11-4**

Common Neurodynamic Tests/Treatment Technique Positions[43]

| | |
|---|---|
| ULTT 1 or ULTT A (median nerve bias; see Figure 11-1) | • Position the patient supine.<br>• Passively move the upper extremity into abduction to 110 degrees; elbow flexion to 90 degrees; wrist, finger, and thumb extension; and supinate the forearm.<br>• Then externally rotate the shoulder.<br>• Then slowly extend the elbow.<br>Assess the patient's response with cervical spine lateral flexion away from the test side and then toward the test side. Do symptoms increase, decrease, or remain unchanged?<br>Common indications: Carpal tunnel syndrome and median nerve symptoms. |
| ULTT 2 (radial nerve bias; see Figure 11-2) | • Position the patient in supine.<br>• Passively move the shoulder girdle into depression and abduct the shoulder to 10 degrees.<br>• Internally rotate the upper extremity and pronate the forearm; extend the elbow; add wrist, finger, and thumb flexion; and then add ulnar deviation.<br>• Slowly abduct the shoulder.<br>Assess the patient's response with cervical spine lateral flexion away from the test side and then toward the test side. Do symptoms increase, decrease, or remain unchanged?<br>Common indications: Radial nerve symptoms, lateral epicondylitis, de Quervain tenosynovitis, and radial tunnel syndrome |
| ULTT 3 (ulnar nerve bias; see Figure 11-3) | • Position the patient in supine.<br>• Passively extend the wrist and fingers, pronate the forearm, and flex the elbow.<br>• Then laterally rotate the shoulder and depress the shoulder girdle.<br>• Then slowly abduct the shoulder up to 110 degrees.<br>Assess the patient's response with cervical spine lateral flexion away from the test side and then toward the test side. Do symptoms increase, decrease, or remain unchanged?<br>Common indications: Lower brachial plexus or radial nerve symptoms, medial epicondylitis, and pronator syndrome |
| SLR (sciatic nerve; see Figure 11-4) | • Position the patient in supine.<br>• Passively move the patient into SLR position (hip flexion with knee extension), and add ankle dorsiflexion.<br>• Once the end point is determined, the technique can be modified to better target varied nerve tracts.<br>  ○ Dorsiflexion with eversion stresses tibial nerve.<br>  ○ Dorsiflexion with inversion stresses the sural nerve.<br>  ○ Plantar flexion with inversion stresses the common peroneal nerve.<br>  ○ Dorsiflexion with great toe extension stresses the plantar nerves.<br>One must distinguish between increased symptoms due to hamstring tightness.<br>Assess patient response with motion from hip/knee flexion into hip/knee extension. Do symptoms increase, decrease, or remain unchanged?<br>Common indications: Sciatic nerve symptoms and tarsal tunnel syndrome<br>*(continued)* |

**Table 11-4 (continued)**

## Common Neurodynamic Tests/Treatment Technique Positions[43]

| | |
|---|---|
| Slump/sitting (sciatic nerve; see Figure 11-5) | This position stresses the sciatic nerve, increasing overall neural tension.<br>• Position the patient in a sitting position.<br>• Ask the patient to slump into trunk/neck flexion; apply gentle overpressure into cervical flexion.<br>• Dorsiflex the ankle and then have the patient actively extend the knee.<br>• Release the overpressure.<br>Assess patient response with cervical extension and flexion. Do symptoms increase, decrease, or remain unchanged?<br>Common indications: Sciatic nerve symptoms |
| Prone knee bend (femoral nerve; see Figure 11-6) | This position stresses the femoral nerve.<br>• Position the patient in prone, spine neutral, and hips extended to 0 degrees.<br>• Flex the knee and slightly extend the hip.<br>One must distinguish between increased symptoms due to rectus femoris or psoas major tightness or facet pain. Ensure that the spine is in a neutral position.<br>Assess patient response with motion from knee flexion into extension. Do symptoms increase, decrease, or remain unchanged?<br>Common indications: Femoral nerve symptoms at high lumbar levels (L2-L4) |
| SLR=straight leg raise; ULTT=upper limb tension test. | |

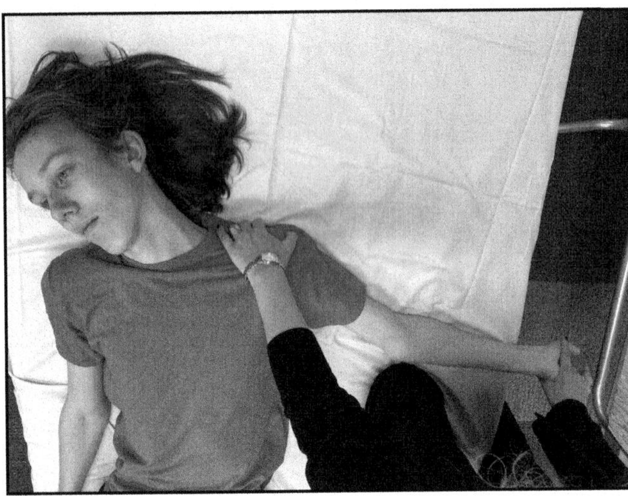

**Figure 11-1.** ULTT 1/A (median nerve bias).

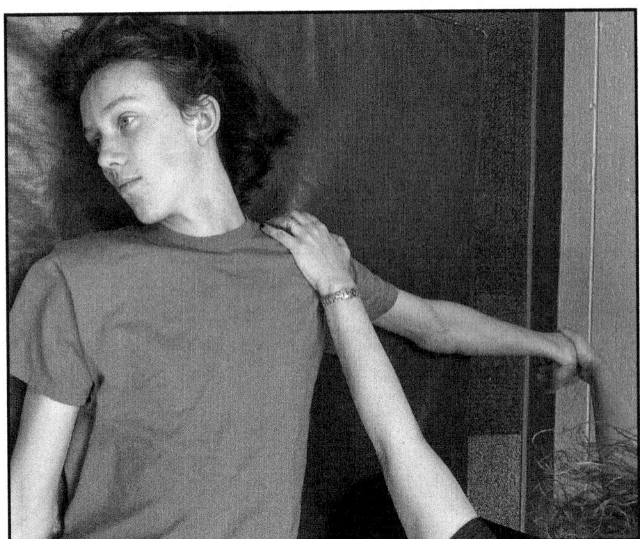

**Figure 11-2.** ULTT 2 (radial nerve bias).

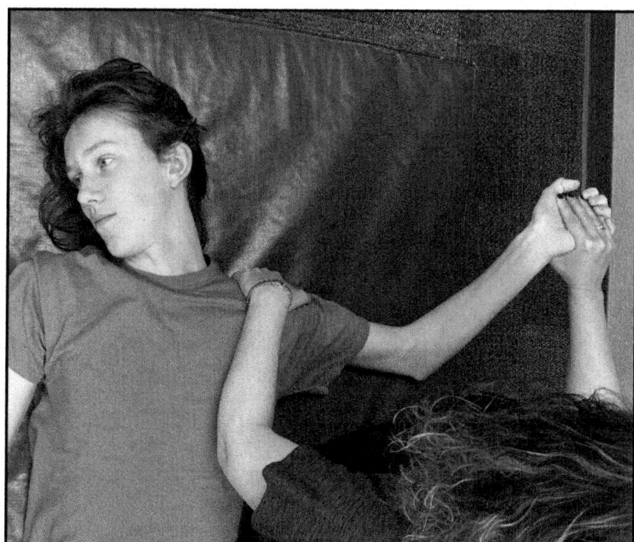

Figure 11-3. ULTT 3 (ulnar nerve bias).

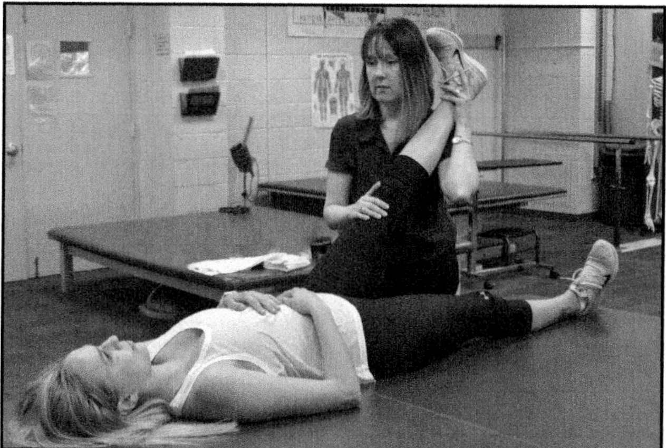

Figure 11-4. SLR test (sciatic nerve).

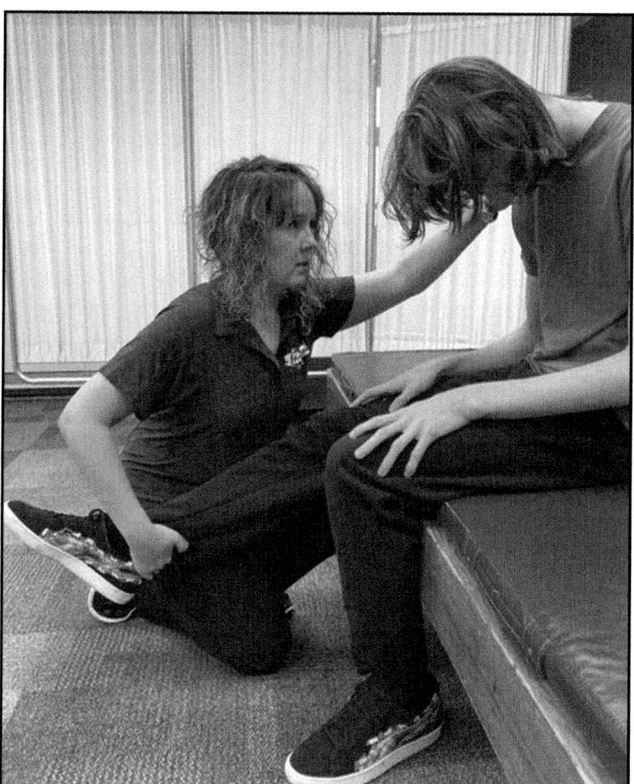

Figure 11-5. Slump test/nerve tension test (sciatic nerve).

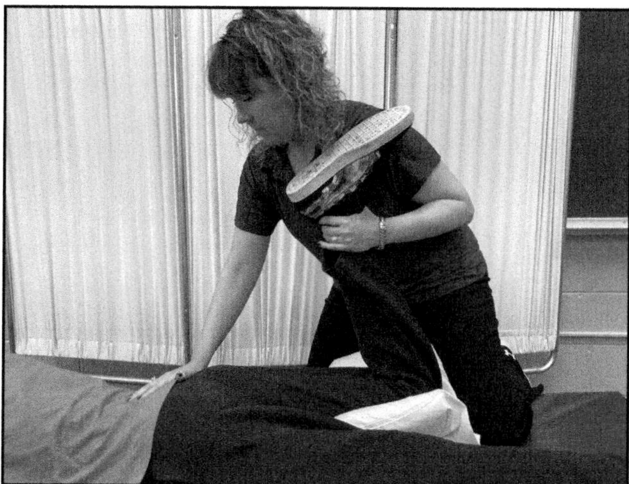

Figure 11-6. Femoral nerve tension test: Prone knee bend.

developed in the path. The patient can also be instructed in self-mobilization techniques once the patient's response is positive and consistent.

Contraindications for neural mobilization interventions include unstable or acute neurologic signs (eg, partial or complete paralysis or sensation loss of a limb), spinal cord injury, cauda equina syndrome, cancer, and infection.

## Understanding Basic Research Terminology

When practicing physical therapy, physical therapist assistants will read medical research articles that include research terms. Becoming familiar with commonly used research terms helps the assistant interpret research articles and understand the effectiveness of special tests that are used in a clinical diagnosis of patients. Commonly used research terms used to describe special tests include reliability, validity, sensitivity, and specificity (Table 11-5). Clinical diagnostic tests with high (close to 100%) specificity are effective at ruling in a pathology/condition if the patient has a positive result, and tests with a high sensitivity are effective at ruling out a condition/pathology if the patient has a negative result.

**Table 11-5**

Commonly Used Research Terms[44]

| Term | Definition | Relevance | Clinical Application |
|---|---|---|---|
| Reliability | The consistency of a measurement | The extent to which the results can be reproduced when the research is repeated under the same conditions. | If the same results are consistently achieved by using the same methods, the measurement is considered reliable. |
| Validity | The accuracy of a measure | The extent to which the results measure what they are supposed to measure. | If a tool has high validity, it means that it produces results that correspond to real characteristics. |
| Sensitivity | The ability of a test to identify patients who have a particular disorder. It represents a positive result on a diagnostic test (true positives). Tests are useful for ruling out a disorder. People who test negative are more likely not to have the target disorder. | "SnNout" is an acronym that can be used to remember a highly sensitive test with a negative result is good at ruling out the disorder/diagnosis in question. | For example, if a test has a sensitivity rating of 0.95 for detecting a disorder and a patient has a negative result on the test, the clinician can be confident that the patient does not have the disorder. |
| Specificity | The ability of a test to identify those who do not have a particular disorder. It represents a negative result on a test for a disorder (true negatives). Highly specific tests are useful for ruling in a disorder. | "SpPin" is an acronym that is used to remember a test with high specificity and a positive result is good for ruling in a disorder. | For example, if a test has a specificity of 98% and a patient has a positive test result, the patient likely has the disorder. |

## Conclusion

Knowledge of pathoanatomical and mechanical diagnoses, movement system, and treatment-based classification systems helps guide the physical therapist assistant when developing treatment plans. Effective treatment development and provision rely on the application of clinical reasoning and appropriate data collection (subjective and objective) from the patient. A firm grasp on the red and yellow flags and understanding of the importance of monitoring SINSS when paired with effective communication skills and regular communication of pertinent data to the supervising therapist will promote patient safety. The application of this knowledge allows the assistant to function as an effective rehabilitation team member.

## Review Questions

1. Compare and contrast the pathoanatomical approach and the treatment-based classification system.
2. What is the significance of the term *human movement system* to physical therapy practice?
3. What is regional interdependence? Provide an example of how a patient's pain/symptoms in one area of the body could be impacted by another body region.
4. List at least 4 responsibilities of a physical therapist assistant when treating an orthopedic patient.
5. What does the acronym SINSS represent?
6. What is the most appropriate action for a physical therapist assistant to take if a patient presents with a significant increase in both the severity and irritability of their symptoms?

7. Are clinical reasoning skills important to a physical therapist assistant? Why/why not? Describe a scenario in which the assistant would need to apply clinical reasoning when working with an orthopedic patient.
8. What is the differential diagnosis? Which team member has the primary responsibility to create a differential diagnosis for a physical therapy patient? When should the process of differential diagnosis occur?
9. List at least 5 possible red flags that an assistant would be expected to recognize and define what action is most appropriate for the assistant to take once that red flag is noted.
10. Define specificity and sensitivity. A clinical special test had a sensitivity of 94%. What is the clinical relevance of that information?

## Suggested Resource

Waddell G, Newton M, Henderson I, Somerville D, Main CJ. A Fear-Avoidance Beliefs Questionnaire (FABQ) and the role of fear-avoidance beliefs in chronic low back pain and disability, *Pain*. 1993;52(2): 157-168.

## References

1. American Physical Therapy Association. Vision statement for the physical therapy profession. Accessed January 30, 2023. http://www.apta.org/Vision/
2. American Physical Therapy Association. Movement system management. Accessed January 30, 2023. http://www.apta.org/MovementSystem/
3. American Physical Therapy Association. Physical therapist practice and the movement system. August 2015. Accessed January 30, 2023. https://www.apta.org/patient-care/interventions/movement-system-management/movement-system-white-paper
4. American Physical Therapy Association. Diagnosis by physical therapists. HOD P06-12-10-09. Accessed January 30, 2023. http://www.apta.org/uploadedFiles/APTAorg/About_Us/Policies/Practice/Diagnosis.pdf
5. Wainner RS, Whitman JM, Cleland JA, Flynn TW. Regional interdependence: a musculoskeletal examination model whose time has come. *J Orthop Sports Phys Ther.* 2007;37(11):658-660.
6. Sueki DG, Cleland JA, Wainner RS. A regional interdependence model of musculoskeletal dysfunction: research, mechanisms, and clinical implications. *J Man Manip Ther.* 2013;21(2):90-102. doi:10.1179/2042618612Y.0000000027
7. Delitto A, Erhard RE, Bowling RW. A treatment-based classification approach to low back syndrome: identifying and staging patients for conservative treatment. *Phys Ther.* 1995;75(6):470-485; discussion 485-489.
8. Hebert JJ, Koppenhaver SL, Walker BF. Subgrouping patients with low back pain: a treatment-based approach to classification. *Sports Health.* 2011;3(6):534-542.
9. Brennan G, Fritz J, Hunter S, et al. Identifying subgroups of patients with acute/subacute nonspecific low back pain. *Spine (Phila Pa 1976).* 2006;31:623-631.
10. Fritz J, Brennan G, Clifford S, et al. An examination of the reliability of a classification algorithm for subgrouping patients with low back pain. *Spine (Phila Pa 1976).* 2006;31:77-82.
11. Fritz J, Delitto A, Erhard R. Comparison of classification-based physical therapy with therapy based on clinical practice guidelines for patients with acute low back pain. *Spine (Phila Pa 1976).* 2003;28:1363-1372.
12. Fritz JM, Brennan GP. Preliminary examination of a proposed treatment-based classification system for patients receiving physical therapy interventions for neck pain. *Phys Ther.* 2007;87(5):513-524.
13. Childs JD, Fritz JM, Piva SR, Whitman JM. Proposal of a classification system for patients with neck pain. *J Orthop Sports Phys Ther.* 2004;34(11):686-696; discussion 697-700.
14. McClure PW, Michener LA. Staged approach for rehabilitation classification: shoulder disorders (STAR-shoulder). *Phys Ther.* 2015;95(5):791-800. doi:10.2522/ptj.20140156
15. Ludewig PM, Kamonseki DH, Staker JL, Lawrence RL, Camargo PR, Braman JP. Changing our diagnostic paradigm: movement system diagnostic. *Int J Sports Phys Ther.* 2017;12(6):884-893.
16. Martin R, Kivlan B. Classification-based treatment of hip pathology in older adults. *Top Geriatr Rehabil.* 2013;29(4):218-226. doi:10.1097/TGR.0b013e3182940bb4
17. Alrwaily M, Timko M, Schneider M, et al. Treatment-based classification system for low back pain: revision and update. *Phys Ther.* 2016;96(7):1057-1066.
18. Westman AE, Boersma K, Leppert J, Linton SJ. Fear-avoidance beliefs, catastrophizing, and distress: a longitudinal subgroup analysis on patients with musculoskeletal pain. *Clin J Pain.* 2011;27(7):567-577. doi:10.1097/AJP.0b013e318219ab6c
19. Waddell C, Newton M, Henderson I, et al. A Fear-Avoidance Beliefs Questionnaire (FABQ) and the role of fear-avoidance beliefs in chronic low back pain and disability. *Pain.* 1993;52:157-168.
20. Fritz JM, George S. Identifying psychosocial variables in patients with acute work-related low back pain: the importance of fear-avoidance beliefs. *Phys Ther.* 2002;82(10):973-983.
21. Garcia AN, Costa LDCM, de Souza FS, et al. Reliability of mechanical diagnosis and therapy system in patients with spinal pain: a systematic review. *J Orthop Sports Phys Ther.* 2018;48(12):923-933. doi:10.2519/jospt.2018.7876
22. Lam OT, Strenger DM, Chan-Fee M, Pham PT, Preuss RA, Robbins SM. Effectiveness of the McKenzie method of mechanical diagnosis and therapy for treating low back pain: literature review with meta-analysis. *J Orthop Sports Phys Ther.* 2018;48(6):476-490. doi:10.2519/jospt.2018.7562
23. Luca B, Bussard L, Kimmons K. Exercises for lumbar instability. Physiopedia. June 9, 2017. Accessed January 30, 2023. https://www.physio-pedia.com/index.php?title=Exercises_for_Lumbar_Instability&oldid=175115
24. Alrwaily M, Timko M, Schneider M, et al. Treatment-based classification system for patients with low back pain: the movement control approach. *Phys Ther.* 2017;97(12):1147-1157. doi:10.1093/ptj/pzx087
25. Maccio JR, Carlton L, Levesque K, Maccio JG, Egan L. Directional preference of the extremity: a preliminary investigation. *J Man Manip Ther.* 2018;26(5):272-280. doi:10.1080/10669817.2018.1505022

26. McKenzie R, May S. *The Lumbar Spine: Mechanical Diagnosis and Therapy.* 2nd ed. Spinal Publications New Zealand Ltd; 2003.
27. May SJ, Rosedale R. A survey of the McKenzie classification system in the extremities: prevalence of mechanical syndromes and preferred loading strategies. *Phys Ther.* 2012;92(9):1175-1186. doi:10.2522/ptj.20110371
28. Baker SE, Painter EE, Morgan BC, et al. Systematic clinical reasoning in physical therapy (SCRIPT): tool for the purposeful practice of clinical reasoning in orthopedic manual physical therapy. *Phys Ther.* 2017;97(1):61-70.
29. Goodman C, Fuller K. *Pathology: Implications for the Physical Therapist.* 4th ed. Saunders; 2015.
30. Nicholas MK, George SZ. Psychologically informed interventions for low back pain: an update for physical therapists. *Phys Ther.* 2011;91(5):765-776. doi:10.2522/ptj.20100278
31. Bialosky JE, Bishop MD, Cleland JA. Individual expectation: an overlooked, but pertinent, factor in the treatment of individuals experiencing musculoskeletal pain. *Phys Ther.* 2010;90(9):1345-1355. doi:10.2522/ptj.20090306
32. Wertli MM, Rasmussen-Barr E, Weiser S, Bachmann LM, Brunner F. The role of fear avoidance beliefs as a prognostic factor for outcome in patients with nonspecific low back pain: a systematic review [erratum in Spine J. 2014;14[8]:a18]. *Spine J.* 2014;14(5):816-836.e4. doi:10.1016/j.spinee.2013.09.036
33. Wertli MM, Burgstaller JM, Weiser S, Steurer J, Kofmehl R, Held U. Influence of catastrophizing on treatment outcome in patients with nonspecific low back pain: a systematic review. *Spine (Phila Pa 1976).* 2014;39(3):263-273. doi:10.1097/BRS.0000000000000110
34. Burton AK, Waddell G, Tillotson KM, Summerton N. Information and advice to patients with back pain can have a positive effect. A randomized controlled trial of a novel educational booklet in primary care. *Spine (Phila Pa 1976).* 1999;24(23):2484-2491.
35. Henrotin YE, Cedraschi C, Duplan B, Bazin T, Duquesnoy B. Information and low back pain management: a systematic review. *Spine (Phila Pa 1976).* 2006;31(11):E326-E334.
36. Gibson G, Werrick K. Fear Avoidance Belief Questionnaire. Accessed January 30, 2023. https://www.physio-pedia.com/Fear%E2%80%90Avoidance_Belief_Questionnaire
37. Louw A, Zimney K, Puentedura EJ, Diener I. The efficacy of pain neuroscience education on musculoskeletal pain: a systematic review of the literature. *Physiother Theory Pract.* 2016;32(5):332-355. doi:10.1080/09593985.2016.1194646
38. Melzack R. From the gate to the neuromatrix. *Pain.* 1999;Aug(suppl 6):S121-S126.
39. Moseley GL. A pain neuromatrix approach to patients with chronic pain. *Man Ther.* 2003;8(3):130-140.
40. George SZ, Stryker SE. Fear-avoidance beliefs and clinical outcomes for patients seeking outpatient physical therapy for musculoskeletal pain conditions. *J Orthop Sports Phys Ther.* 2011;41(4):249-259. doi:10.2519/jospt.2011.3488
41. Basson A, Olivier B, Ellis R, Coppieters M, Stewart A, Mudzi W. The effectiveness of neural mobilization for neuromusculoskeletal conditions: a systematic review and meta-analysis. *J Orthop Sports Phys Ther.* 2017;47(9):593-615. doi:10.2519/jospt.2017.7117
42. Ballestero-Pérez R, Plaza-Manzano G, Urraca-Gesto A, et al. Effectiveness of nerve gliding exercises on carpal tunnel syndrome: a systematic review. *J Manipulative Physiol Ther.* 2017;40(1):50-59. doi:10.1016/j.jmpt.2016.10.004
43. Kisner C, Armstrong CJ. Peripheral nerve disorders and management. In: Kisner C, Colby LA, Borstad J, eds. *Therapeutic Exercise Foundations and Techniques.* 7th ed. FA Davis Company; 2018:382-401.
44. Sackett DL, Straws SE, Richardson WS, et al. *Evidence-Based Medicine: How to Practice and Teach EBM.* 2nd ed. Harcourt Publishers Limited; 2000.

Chapter 12

# Therapeutic Exercise for the Upper Extremity

*John Morris, PT, MBA, OCS, Cert MDT and Karen A. Cascardi, PhD, MS, ATC, PTA*

**KEY TERMS** Adhesive capsulitis | Bankart lesion | Carpal tunnel syndrome | Cluster tests | FOOSH (falling on an outstretched hand) | Hill-Sachs lesion | Lateral epicondylalgia | Medial epicondylalgia | SLAP (superior labrum anterior to posterior) lesion | Subacromial impingement | Volkmann ischemic contracture

## Chapter Objectives

1. Recall the basic anatomical structures of the upper extremity (UE; shoulder girdle, glenohumeral [GH] joint, elbow, wrist, and hand).
2. Identify and describe the common injuries and pathologies involving the UE.
3. Describe the impact of structural or muscle weakness or tightness on range of motion (ROM), strength, pain, and function.
4. Identify the common special tests used in a physical therapy evaluation of the shoulder, elbow, wrist, and hand.
5. Discuss and select the common treatment exercise interventions and progressions used to address various diagnoses of the UE.
6. Recognize the contraindications and precautions related to UE diagnoses.
7. Demonstrate median nerve glides and tendon glides for wrist and hand diagnoses.
8. Given a patient diagnosis and physical therapy plan of care (POC), design and progress a basic exercise and intervention program for a patient with a UE injury.

Normal joint motions for all segments of the upper quarter allow for the functional movement needed to perform activities of daily living (ADLs) and occupational or recreational activities efficiently. Trauma, congenital factors, tissue degeneration, and/or repetitive activity can disrupt normal biomechanics of the UE and lead to pain, mobility restrictions, and functional loss. When treating the UE, effective screening is important to rule out the cervical spine as the origin of symptoms. It is critical to remember that referred pain patterns, paresthesia, and/or muscle weakness in the UE can be due to cervical spine nerve root involvement, injury, or other pathologies. The physical therapist will evaluate the patient to determine the most likely source of the patient's symptoms, and the physical therapist assistant should continue to monitor the patient during treatment. It is important to report any signs or symptoms that may indicate a change in the pain pattern or presentation to the therapist.



Kopack JK, Cascardi KA.
*Principles of Therapeutic Exercise for the Physical Therapist Assistant* (pp 261-349).

**Table 12-1**

Shoulder Range of Motion[2]

| Shoulder Motion | Degrees |
|---|---|
| Flexion | 180 |
| Extension | 60 |
| Abduction | 180 |
| External (lateral) rotation | 70 |
| Internal (medial) rotation | 90 |

Note: There is variation in normative values based on sex and age. Values are based on the American Academy of Orthopedic Surgeons.

## Upper Extremity Anatomy

This section briefly reviews the anatomy of the shoulder girdle, GH joint, elbow, wrist, and hand. There are 30 bones in the UE.[1] It is suggested that readers refer to kinesiology textbooks for more details on the UE anatomy and function.

### *Shoulder Anatomy and Function*

The bony anatomy of the UE begins proximally with the shoulder girdle. The shoulder girdle joints include the sternoclavicular (SC), acromioclavicular (AC), scapulothoracic (ST), and GH joints.

The SC joint, which is composed of the proximal sternum and the medial clavicle, is the only bony attachment of the UE to the axial skeleton. It is stable with strong support provided by the costoclavicular, anterior and posterior SC, and infraclavicular ligaments. The AC joint consists of the distal end of the clavicle, which attaches to the acromion process. The AC joint is stabilized by the coracoclavicular ligament, the superior AC ligament, and the inferior AC ligament. There are 3 degrees of freedom that occur at the AC and SC joints during shoulder movement, including elevation/depression, protraction/retraction, and passive rotation of the clavicle. These motions contribute to normal shoulder biomechanics.

The ST joint motions include elevation/depression, abduction/adduction (or protraction/retraction), and upward/downward rotation. These motions occur in combination with the clavicle at the AC and SC joints. An injury to the clavicle or AC/SC joints will affect scapular and GH joint motion. Tipping and winging are accessory motions occurring at the ST joint. Tipping occurs when the inferior angle moves posterior to the thorax (lifting the inferior angle away from the trunk), and winging occurs when the vertebral border of the scapula moves posteriorly in relation to the thorax (lifting the vertebral border away from the trunk).

The GH joint has 3 degrees of freedom, including flexion/extension, abduction/adduction, and internal/external rotation. The GH joint is composed of the glenoid fossa (concave surface) of the scapula and the proximal head of the humerus (convex surface). The humeral head is much larger than the fossa, but the glenoid labrum increases joint stability; it deepens the socket. The labrum creates a seal around the head of the humerus, which also enhances the stability of the joint. The superior, middle, and inferior GH ligaments and the coracohumeral ligament provide additional stability.

Normative values for ROM at the shoulder are listed in Table 12-1. The closed-pack position of the GH joint is 90 degrees of abduction and 90 degrees of external (lateral) rotation. The open-packed position is 50 to 55 degrees of abduction and 30 degrees of flexion. The shoulder joint capsular pattern includes limitations that are greatest in external (lateral) rotation, abduction, and internal (medial) rotation, respectively. Shoulder motions have a firm end feel.

#### Shoulder Muscles and Nerve Innervations

The scapula stabilizers (Table 12-2) provide primary musculature support of the shoulder girdle together with the rotator cuff (RC) muscles (Table 12-3).[1,3] The RC muscles are a group of 4 muscles: the supraspinatus, infraspinatus, teres minor, and subscapularis (referred to as *SITS muscles*). The RC muscles originate on the scapula and insert on the proximal humerus. The supraspinatus initiates humeral abduction (providing the original approximately 0 to 5 degrees of motion). The infraspinatus is a larger triangular-shaped muscle that primarily performs shoulder external rotation. The teres minor (the smallest RC muscle) assists in shoulder external rotation. The subscapularis (the strongest RC muscle) is located on the anterior surface of the scapula and performs GH internal rotation. The RC muscles create a force couple with the deltoid muscles, which allows for normal, pain-free shoulder flexion and abduction. As a group, the RC muscles act to compress and depress the humeral head, preventing any superior migration of the humerus, whereas the deltoid muscle group acts to distract and elevate the humerus.

**Table 12-2**

Scapulothoracic Muscles

| Scapulothoracic Muscle | Actions | Origin | Insertion | Nerve Innervations |
|---|---|---|---|---|
| Trapezius | Upper fibers: Upper trapezius<br>Bilaterally: Extends the head/neck<br>Unilaterally: Lateral flexion of head/neck to same side, rotates head/neck to the opposite side, elevates the scapula, and upward rotation of the scapula<br>Middle fibers: Middle trapezius, adducts the scapula, and stabilizes the scapula<br>Lower fibers: Lower trapezius, depresses the scapula, and upward rotation of the scapula | External occipital protuberance, medial portion of superior nuchal line of the occiput, ligamentum nuchae, and spinous processes of C7 through T12 | Lateral one-third of clavicle, acromion, and spine of the scapula | Spinal portion of cranial nerve XI (accessory) and ventral ramus (C2, C3, C4) |
| Levator scapula | Unilaterally: Elevates the scapula, downwardly rotates the scapula, laterally flexes the head/neck, and rotates the head/neck to the same side<br>Bilaterally: Extends the head/neck | Transverse processes of 1 through 4 cervical vertebrae | Medial border of scapula, between superior angle and superior portion of spine of scapula | C3 and C4 and dorsal scapular (C4, C5) |
| Serratus anterior | With the origin fixed: Abducts the scapula, upwardly rotates the scapula, depresses the scapula, and holds the medial border of the scapula against the rib cage<br>If scapula is fixed, elevate the thorax during forced inhalation | External surfaces of upper 8 or 9 ribs | Anterior surface of medial border of the scapula | Long thoracic (C5, C6, C7, C8) |

(continued)

**Table 12-2 (continued)**

Scapulothoracic Muscles

| Scapulothoracic Muscle | Actions | Origin | Insertion | Nerve Innervations |
|---|---|---|---|---|
| Pectoralis minor | Depresses the scapula<br>Abducts the scapula<br>Downwardly rotates the scapula<br>If scapula is fixed, assists to elevate the thorax during forced inhalation | 3 to 5 ribs | Medial surface of coracoid process of the scapula | Medial pectoral, with fibers from a communicating branch of the lateral pectoral (C6, C7, C8, T1) |
| Rhomboid major and minor | Adducts the scapula<br>Elevates the scapula<br>Downwardly rotates the scapula | Major: Spinous processes T2 to T5<br>Minor: Spinous processes C7 and T1 | Major: Medial border of the scapula between the spine of the scapula and inferior angle<br>Minor: Upper portion of medial border of the scapula, across from spine of the scapula | Dorsal scapular (C4, C5) |

**Table 12-3**

**Shoulder: Glenohumeral Joint Muscles and Rotator Cuff Muscles**

| | Actions | Origin | Insertion | Nerve Innervations |
|---|---|---|---|---|
| ***Glenohumeral Muscles*** | | | | |
| Latissimus dorsi | Extends the shoulder<br>Adducts the shoulder<br>Medial (internal) rotation of the shoulder | Inferior angle of scapula, spinous processes of last 6 thoracic vertebrae, last 3 to 4 ribs, thoracolumbar aponeurosis, and posterior iliac crest | Intertubercular groove of the humerus | Thoracodorsal (C6, C7, C8) |
| Pectoralis major | All fibers: Adduct the shoulder, medially rotate the shoulder, and assist to elevate the thorax during forced inhalation (with arm fixed)<br>Upper fibers: Flex the shoulder and horizontally adduct the shoulder<br>Lower fibers: Extend the shoulder | Medial half of clavicle, sternum, and cartilage of 1 to 6 ribs | Crest of greater tubercle of humerus | Upper fibers: Lateral pectoral (C5, C6, C7)<br>Lower fibers: Lateral and medial pectoral (C6, C7, C8, T1) |
| Teres major | Extends the shoulder<br>Adducts the shoulder<br>Medial (internal) rotation of the shoulder | Inferior angle and lower one-third of lateral border of the scapula | Crest of the lesser tubercle of the humerus | Lower subscapular (C5, C6, C7) |
| Coracobrachialis | Flexes the shoulder<br>Adducts the shoulder | Coracoid process of the scapula | Medial surface of midhumeral shaft | Musculocutaneous (C6, C7) |
| Deltoid | All fibers: Abduct the shoulder<br>Anterior fibers: Flex the shoulder, medial (internal) rotation of the shoulder, and horizontally adduct the shoulder<br>Posterior fibers: Extend the shoulder, lateral (external) rotation of the shoulder, and horizontally abduct shoulder | Lateral one-third of clavicle, acromion, and spine of scapula | Deltoid tuberosity | Axillary (C5, C6) |

*(continued)*

**Table 12-3 (continued)**

Shoulder: Glenohumeral Joint Muscles and Rotator Cuff Muscles

| | Actions | Origin | Insertion | Nerve Innervations |
|---|---|---|---|---|
| ***Rotator Cuff Muscles*** | | | | |
| Supraspinatus | Abducts shoulder and is prime agonist 0 to 15 degrees and then assists deltoid muscle to 90 degrees<br>Stabilizes humeral head in glenoid fossa | Supraspinous fossa of the scapula | Greater tubercle of the humerus | Suprascapular (C4, C5, C6) |
| Infraspinatus | Lateral (external) rotation of the shoulder<br>Adducts the shoulder<br>Stabilizes humeral head in glenoid fossa | Infraspinous fossa of the scapula | Greater tubercle of the humerus | Suprascapular (C4, C5, C6) |
| Teres minor | Lateral (external) rotation of the shoulder<br>Adducts the shoulder<br>Stabilizes humeral head in glenoid fossa | Upper two-thirds of lateral border of the scapula | Greater tubercle of the humerus | Axillary (C5, C6) |
| Subscapularis | Medial (internal) rotation of the shoulder<br>Stabilizes humeral head in glenoid fossa | Subscapular fossa of the scapula | Lesser tubercle of the humerus | Upper and lower subscapular (C5, C6, C7) |

A total of 17 muscles attach to the scapula, some of which work together to create force couple actions. These muscles pull on the scapula in different directions simultaneously, creating synchronized ST and GH movement. The serratus anterior and upper and lower trapezius muscles upwardly rotate the scapula during shoulder flexion and abduction, whereas the levator scapulae, rhomboids, and pectoralis minor work together to downwardly rotate the scapula.

The brachial plexus provides neural innervation to the muscles of the UE. It emerges from 5 levels of the spinal cord and is formed by the anterior (ventral) rami of the spinal nerve roots of C5-T1. The plexus has 3 primary trunks: the superior, middle, and inferior. Each trunk splits into an anterior and posterior division, which give rise to the lateral, posterior, and medial cords. The 5 peripheral nerves that arise from the cords include the axillary, musculocutaneous, radial, median, and ulnar nerves.

## *Elbow and Forearm Anatomy and Function*

The humeroulnar joint and the humeroradial joint are the articulations that form the elbow joint. The trochlea on the distal humerus is convex, and the trochlear notch of the ulna is concave. The head of the radius (concave) articulates with the capitulum (convex) of the humerus. The elbow is a hinge joint with one degree of freedom and flexion/extension (0 to 145 degrees). The normal end feel during flexion is soft, and extension is hard or bony.

Pronation and supination (0 to 80 degrees) of the forearm occur at the proximal and distal radioulnar joints as the radius moves around the ulna. The radius and ulna are parallel when the forearm is supinated and crossed when the forearm is pronated. The side of the head of the proximal radius is convex; it articulates with the concave radial notch on the ulna. Distally, the concave radius moves on the convex ulna. During forearm motions at the proximal joint, there is joint surface gliding and rolling in opposite directions, and at the distal joint there is gliding and rolling in the same direction.

The medial and lateral collateral ligaments provide elbow stability. The annular ligament surrounds the radial head and stabilizes the proximal radioulnar joint.

### Elbow and Forearm Muscles and Nerve Innervations

The major muscles of the elbow are the flexors and extensors (Table 12-4).[4] Elbow flexors are located on the anterior surface of the arm, crossing in the front of the elbow. The brachialis is the strongest flexor, and brachialis action is not affected by the forearm position. The biceps brachii is strongest in the midrange. The prime mover for elbow extension is the triceps brachii assisted by the anconeus. Nerve innervations for the muscles of the elbow and forearm are located in Table 12-4.

## *Wrist and Hand Anatomy and Function*

The wrist provides the control and stability needed for functional hand positions. The wrist is composed of the distal ends of the radius and ulna, 8 carpal bones (4 in each row), and the proximal ends of the 5 metacarpals. The articulation between the proximal row of carpals and the radius is called the *radiocarpal joint*, and the joint between the metacarpals and the distal row of carpals is the carpometacarpal (CMC) joint.

Proceeding distally, the metacarpal heads (convex) attach to the base (concave) of the proximal phalanges, forming the metacarpophalangeal (MCP) joints. The joint between the proximal phalange and the middle phalange is the proximal interphalangeal (PIP) joint, and the distal interphalangeal (DIP) joint is the articulation between the middle and distal phalanges. There are 14 phalanges (3 in each finger and 2 in the thumb).[4]

The radiocarpal motions include flexion (0 to 80 degrees), extension (0 to 70 degrees), radial deviation (0 to 20 degrees), and ulnar deviation (0 to 30 degrees). Radial deviation is also called *wrist abduction*, and ulnar deviation is called *wrist adduction*.[2] A neutral wrist position with slight ulnar deviation is the open-packed position; this is the position where joint play is at its greatest. The carpal bones in the proximal row are convex, and the radius is concave, so carpal motion occurs opposite to that of hand motion. For example, during wrist flexion, the proximal carpal bones roll anteriorly and glide posteriorly, and with extension, they roll posteriorly and glide anteriorly. The wrist capsular pattern includes limitations that are equal for flexion and extension.

Thumb motions (the first CMC joint) include flexion, extension, abduction, adduction, and opposition. Flexion and extension occur at the PIP and DIP joints of the fingers and the interphalangeal (IP) joint of the thumb.

### Wrist and Hand Muscles and Nerve Innervations

The muscles that control the wrist originate proximally at the elbow and forearm and insert onto the carpals, metacarpals, and/or phalanges (Table 12-5). Several muscles create motion solely at the wrist, and others move both the wrist and the thumb or fingers (Table 12-6). The wrist and finger flexors are located on the palmar or anterior surface of the forearm, and the extensors are on the dorsal side.

The wrist extensors are innervated by the radial nerve. The wrist flexors are innervated by the median or ulnar nerves. Sensory nerve patterns for the hand are found in Figure 12-1. Nerve innervation for the wrist and hand muscles are found in Tables 12-5 and 12-6.

**Table 12-4**

Elbow and Forearm Muscles

| Muscle | Actions | Origin | Insertion | Nerve Innervations |
|---|---|---|---|---|
| Biceps brachii | Flexes the elbow<br>Supinates the forearm<br>Flexes the shoulder | Short head: Coracoid process of scapula<br>Long head: Supraglenoid tubercle of scapula | Tuberosity of the radius and aponeurosis of the biceps brachii | Musculocutaneous (C5, C6) |
| Brachialis | Flexes the elbow | Distal half of anterior surface of humerus | Tuberosity and coronoid process of ulna | Musculocutaneous, small branch from radial (C5, C6) |
| Brachioradialis | Flexes the elbow<br>Assists pronation/supination of the forearm when these movements are resisted | Proximal two-thirds of the lateral supracondylar ridge of humerus | Styloid process of radius | Radial (C5, C6) |
| Triceps brachii | All heads: Extend the elbow<br>Long head: Extends the shoulder and adducts the shoulder | Long head: Infraglenoid tubercle of the scapula<br>Lateral head: Posterior surface of proximal half of the humerus<br>Medial head: Posterior surface of distal half of the humerus | Olecranon process of the ulna | Radial (C6, C7, C8, T1) |
| Anconeus | Extends the elbow | Lateral epicondyle of the humerus | Olecranon process and posterior, proximal surface of ulna | Radial (C7, C8) |
| Pronator teres | Pronates the forearm<br>Assists flexion of the elbow | Common flexor tendon from medial epicondyle of humerus and coronoid process of the ulna | Middle of lateral surface of the radius | Median (C6, C7) |
| Pronator quadratus | Pronates the forearm | Distal one-quarter ulna | Distal one-quarter radius | Median (C8, T1) |
| Supinator | Supinates the forearm | Lateral epicondyle of humerus, proximal ulna | Anterior surface of proximal radius | Radial (C6) |

**Table 12-5**

Wrist and Hand Muscles

| Wrist/Finger Extensor Muscle | Actions | Origin | Insertion | Nerve Innervations |
|---|---|---|---|---|
| Extensor carpi radialis longus | Extends the wrist<br>Abducts (radial deviation) the wrist<br>Assists to flex the elbow | Distal one-third of the lateral supracondylar ridge of humerus | Base of second metacarpal | Radial (C5, C6, C7, C8) |
| Extensor carpi radialis brevis | Extends the wrist<br>Abducts (radial deviation) the wrist | Common extensor tendon from the lateral epicondyle of humerus | Base of third metacarpal | Radial (C6, C7, C8) |
| Extensor carpi ulnaris | Extends the wrist<br>Adducts (ulnar deviation) the wrist | Common extensor tendon from the lateral epicondyle of humerus | Base of fifth metacarpal | Radial (C6, C7, C8) |
| Extensor digitorum | Extends second through fifth fingers at MCP and PIP joints<br>Assists to extend the wrist | Common extensor tendon from the lateral epicondyle of humerus | Bases of middle and distal phalanges of second through fifth fingers | Radial (C6, C7, C8) |

*(continued)*

**Table 12-5 (continued)**

Wrist and Hand Muscles

| Wrist/Finger Extensor Muscle | Actions | Origin | Insertion | Nerve Innervations |
|---|---|---|---|---|
| Flexor carpi radialis | Flexes the wrist<br>Abducts the wrist | Common flexor tendon from medial epicondyle of humerus | Bases of second and third metacarpals | Median (C6, C7, C8) |
| Flexor carpi ulnaris | Flexes the wrist<br>Adducts (ulnar deviation) the wrist<br>Assists to flex the elbow | Humeral head: Common flexor tendon from medial epicondyle of humerus<br>Ulnar head: Posterior surface of proximal two-thirds of ulna | Pisiform, hook of the hamate and base of fifth metacarpal | Ulnar (C7, C8, T1) |
| Palmaris longus | Tenses the palmar fascia<br>Flexes the wrist | Common flexor tendon from medial epicondyle of humerus | Flexor retinaculum and palmar aponeurosis | Median (C6, C7, C8) |
| Flexor digitorum superficialis | Flexes the second through fifth fingers at MCP and PIP joints<br>Flexes the wrist | Common flexor tendon from medial epicondyle of humerus, ulnar collateral ligament (UCL), coronoid process of ulna, interosseous membrane, and proximal shaft of radius | Sides of middle phalanges of second through fifth fingers | Median (C7, C8, T1) |
| Flexor digitorum profundus | Flexes the second through fifth fingers at MCP and PIP joints<br>Assists to flex the wrist | Anterior and medial surfaces of proximal three-quarters of ulna | Bases of distal phalanges, palmar surface of second through fifth fingers | First and second: Median (C7, C8, T1)<br>Third and fourth: Ulnar (C7, C8, T1) |

**Table 12-6**

Thumb and Intrinsic Muscles of the Hand

| Muscle | Actions | Origin | Insertion | Nerve Innervations |
|---|---|---|---|---|
| Abductor pollicis longus | Abducts the thumb<br>Extends the thumb<br>Abducts (radial deviation) the wrist | Posterior surface of radius and ulna and interosseous membrane | Base of first metacarpal | Radial (C6, C7, C8) |
| Abductor pollicis brevis | Abducts the thumb at CMC and MCP<br>Assists in opposition of the thumb | Flexor retinaculum, trapezium, and scaphoid tubercles | Base of proximal phalanx of thumb | Median (C6, C7, C8, T1) |
| Extensor pollicis longus | Extends the thumb at IP joint<br>Extends the thumb at CMC and MCP joints<br>Assists to abduct (radial deviation) the wrist | Posterior surface of ulna and interosseous membrane | Base of distal phalanx of thumb | Radial (C6, C7) |
| Extensor pollicis brevis | Extends the thumb<br>Extends the thumb at CMC and MCP joints<br>Assists to abduct (radial deviation) the wrist | Posterior surface of radius and interosseous membrane | Base of proximal phalanx of thumb | Radial (C6, C7, C8) |
| Flexor pollicis longus | Flexes the thumb (IP)<br>Flexes the thumb (CMC and MCP)<br>Assists to flex the wrist | Anterior surface of radius and interosseous membrane | Base of distal phalanx of thumb | Median (C6, C7, C8, T1) |
| Flexor pollicis brevis | Flexes the thumb at CMC and MCP joints<br>Assists in opposition of the thumb | Superficial head: Flexor retinaculum<br>Deep head: Trapezium, trapezoid, and capitate | Base of proximal phalanx of thumb | Superficial head: Median (C6, C7, C8, T1)<br>Deep head: Ulnar (C8, T1) |
| Opponens pollicis | Opposition of the thumb at CMC joint (bringing the pads of the thumb and fifth finger together) | Flexor retinaculum and tubercle of the trapezium | Entire length of first metacarpal bone, radial surface | Median (C6, C7, C8, T1) |

*(continued)*

**Table 12-6 (continued)**

Thumb and Intrinsic Muscles of the Hand

| Muscle | Actions | Origin | Insertion | Nerve Innervations |
|---|---|---|---|---|
| Adductor pollicis | Adducts the thumb at CMC and MCP joints<br>Assists to flex the thumb | Capitate, second and third metacarpals | Base of proximal phalanx of thumb | Ulnar (C8, T1) |
| Lumbricals of the hand | Extends second through fifth at PIP and DIP joints<br>Flexes second through fifth fingers at MCP joints | Surfaces of the flexor digitorum profundus tendons | Extensor aponeurosis on dorsal surface of phalanges | Second and third fingers: Median (C6, C7, C8, T1)<br>Fourth and fifth fingers: Ulnar (C7, C8, T1) |
| Palmar interossei | Adducts the thumb, second, fourth, and fifth fingers toward the third finger<br>Assists to flex the thumb, second, third, and fourth fingers at MCP<br>Assists to extend the thumb, second, fourth, and fifth fingers at IP joints | Base of first, second, fourth, and fifth metacarpals | Base of the proximal phalanx of the related finger and the extensor aponeurosis | Ulnar (C8, T1) |
| Dorsal interossei | Abducts second, third, and fourth fingers at MCP<br>Assists to flex second, third, and fourth fingers at MCP<br>Assists to extend second, third, and fourth at IP joints | Adjacent to sides of all metacarpals | Base of the proximal phalanx of the second, third, and fourth fingers and the extensor aponeurosis | Ulnar (C8, T1) |
| Abductor digiti minimi | Abducts the fifth finger at MCP<br>Assists in opposition of the fifth finger toward the thumb at MCP joint | Pisiform and tendon of flexor carpi ulnaris | Base of proximal fifth phalanx, ulnar surface | Ulnar (C7, C8, T1) |
| Flexor digiti minimi brevis | Flexes the fifth MCP joint<br>Assists in opposition of fifth finger toward the thumb | Hook of hamate and flexor retinaculum | Base of proximal phalanx of fifth finger, palmar surface | Ulnar (C7, C8, T1) |
| Opponens digiti minimi | Opposition of the fifth finger at the CMC joint | Hook of hamate and flexor retinaculum | Shaft of fifth metacarpal, ulnar surface | Ulnar (C7, C8, T1) |

## Tools to Assess Shoulder, Elbow, Wrist, and Hand Progress

ROM, manual muscle testing (MMT), special tests, subjective questionnaires, and functional performance tests are used during the initial physical therapy evaluation to assess a patient's current status and performance as well as during the course of treatment to track progress. Special tests used to assess each joint of the UE are discussed later in the chapter. The reader is referred to test and measurement textbooks for full descriptions of the special tests listed throughout this chapter.

There are subjective tests or questionnaires that describe a patient's functional status from their perspective. Two of the more commonly used tools are the Disability of the Arm Shoulder and Hand (DASH) and the Upper Extremity Functional Index. The Western Ontario Rotator Cuff is a tool that is useful for patients with RC pathology. Each of these tests has good reliability and validity, and the Western Ontario Rotator Cuff correlates well with the DASH.[5-7]

It is recommended that athletes (high school, college, and older recreational) who participate in overhead sports (eg, tennis, baseball, volleyball) complete functional physical performance tests before returning to their sport. Commonly used performance tests to assess UE functional status include the Y Balance Test-Upper Quarter, the Closed Kinetic Chain Upper Extremity Stability Test, and the Seated Medicine Ball Throw.[8] A link (Rehabilitation Database Measures) to descriptions of these tests can be found in the Suggested Resources section at the end of this chapter.

## Management and Treatment of Shoulder Pathologies

The shoulder is the most dynamically mobile joint in the body, and it allows for large amounts of motion in all 3 planes. Recovery from a shoulder pathology is often slow and has a recurrence rate of 25%. The most common causes of shoulder pain include RC, GH joint, and AC joint pathologies.[9]

Examination of the shoulder by the physical therapist includes a thorough history to determine the onset, location, nature, and behavior of the patient's primary complaints, symptoms, and functional restrictions. The patient's prior level of function and the effect of the injury on current function are assessed. If a specific event or injury occurred, the mechanism of injury (MOI) may assist in determining the primary diagnosis and secondary structure involvement. The therapist also reviews subjective questionnaires completed by the patient, normal ADLs, and occupational and/or sports-related activities. The therapist's clinical examination commonly includes the following:

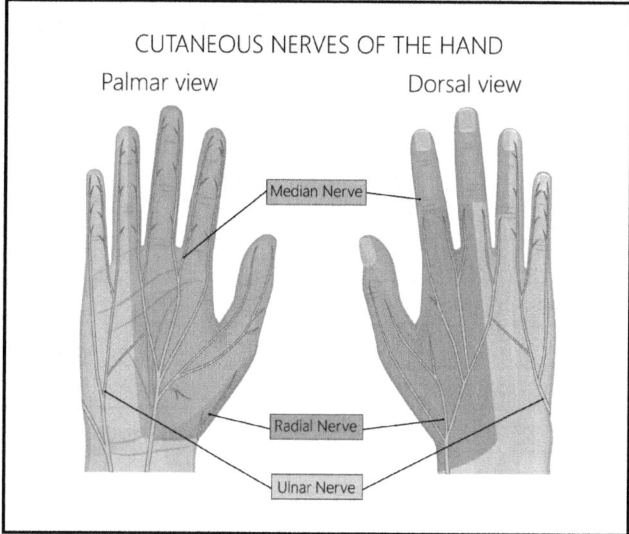


**Figure 12-1.** Sensory innervation patterns of the hands (Aksanaku/Shutterstock.com).

- Postural assessment for symmetry and deviations
- A cervical spine screen (rule in/out referred pain into the shoulder) and general systems screening
- Passive range of motion (PROM)/active range of motion (AROM), MMT, and special tests

During a cervical spine screening, the physical therapist will ensure that the patient's complaints of pain are originating from the shoulder vs the neck. The therapist assesses the scapula position on the thorax and GH/ST rhythm during active motions as well as special tests to rule in/out musculoskeletal diagnoses. Current research supports the use of certain tests in combination vs using a single test for a more reliable joint pathology diagnosis. A specific group of tests (usually greater than 3) that are used to better identify the specific diagnosis causing shoulder pain are called **cluster tests.** The cluster of tests for RC tears include the drop arm, infraspinatus muscle, and painful arc tests; these tests are referred to as the *DIP cluster* (named for the first letter of each test). The cluster of tests to determine shoulder impingement include the Hawkins-Kennedy, infraspinatus muscle, and painful arc tests (known as the *HIP cluster*). If all 3 tests are positive for the DIP or HIP clusters, the probability of having a full-thickness RC tear is 91% and 95% for shoulder impingement, respectively.[10]

### Considerations for the Physical Therapist Assistant: Nonmusculoskeletal Referred Pain Patterns

Right shoulder blade referred pain is commonly associated with gallbladder conditions; left arm pain could be a sign of cardiovascular problems (ie, a heart attack). Kehr's sign is a classic symptom of a ruptured spleen (referred pain into the left shoulder). An acute ulcer or diverticulitis can also present as referred pain into the left shoulder.[11] Refer to Appendix G for a list of all referred pain patterns.

**Table 12-7**

Special Tests for Various Shoulder Pathologies

| Special Test | Possible Shoulder Pathology if Positive |
|---|---|
| Drop arm | RC tear |
| Infraspinatus[a,b] | RC tear, impingement |
| Painful arc[a,b] | RC tear, impingement |
| Hawkins-Kennedy impingement | Impingement (usually of the supraspinatus muscle) |
| Liftoff | Subscapularis tear |
| Empty can (supraspinatus test) | Supraspinatus tear |
| Yergason's test | Biceps tendonitis and SLAP lesion |
| Compression rotation (grind test) | SLAP lesion |
| Surprise (active release) | Instability |
| Sulcus sign (with inferior distraction) | Instability |
| Apprehension | Instability |

Note: It is suggested that a cluster of tests (vs a single test) should be performed to confirm suspected diagnosis.
[a]DIP cluster for RC tears.
[b]HIP cluster for impingement.
SLAP = superior labrum anterior to posterior.

Patients present with varied shoulder pathoanatomical diagnoses, and treatment for most of these diagnoses is often based on the patient's presentation rather than a specific medical diagnosis. Although there are certain diagnoses that have specific precautions and restrictions based on the postinjury/surgery timeline and bone and soft tissue healing times, most interventions should be based on the patient's severity of symptoms, level of irritability, identified impairments, and long-term goals.

After the initial examination, the patient's shoulder injury/dysfunction can be categorized into one or more of the following classifications: instability, joint degeneration, mobility, and/or overuse. Once the condition is categorized, the initial treatment and long-term management can be determined.

Physical therapist assistants treat patients with a variety of shoulder pathologies during different phases of the healing/rehabilitation process. The assistant performs ROM measurements and MMTs and should be familiar with the common special tests (Table 12-7). Physical therapist assistants implement various treatment interventions (ie, modalities and soft tissue/joint mobilizations) and exercise/protocol progressions, recognize contraindications/precautions, and provide appropriate patient education to improve patient outcomes. The assistant should monitor patients throughout each treatment session and be alert to any significant changes in signs/symptoms. Those findings should immediately be discussed with the therapist before continuing treatment.

## *Shoulder Joint Mobilization Techniques*

As discussed in Chapter 4, joint mobilization techniques are used to reduce pain and muscle guarding (grades I and II), increase joint play, and increase ROM (grades III and IV). Joint mobilizations described in this section are suggestions; the physical therapist will determine the most appropriate mobilizations based on the patient's presentation. The type of mobilization (sustained or oscillation) and the amount of force or grade are determined by the therapist. A sustained distraction is usually held for 10 seconds for several repetitions, and oscillations are usually performed for about 60 seconds but no longer than 2 minutes.

The physical therapist assistant must abide by state regulations regarding joint mobilization and always gain consent from the supervising physical therapist before performing these techniques. The therapist must feel comfortable and confident in the skill level of the assistant in providing any intervention before delegating a task.

Before mobilizing a joint, it is best to warm up the tissues surrounding the involved joint.[12,13] The patient should be relaxed in a comfortable position, and the clinician should use good body mechanics. The clinician needs to pay close attention to hand placement and the direction of pull and/or size of oscillations and use the minimal amount of force to achieve the selected grade desired. Constant and repetitive communication with the patient during the technique is essential. It is important that the clinician asks the patient for feedback about pain level and/or discomfort

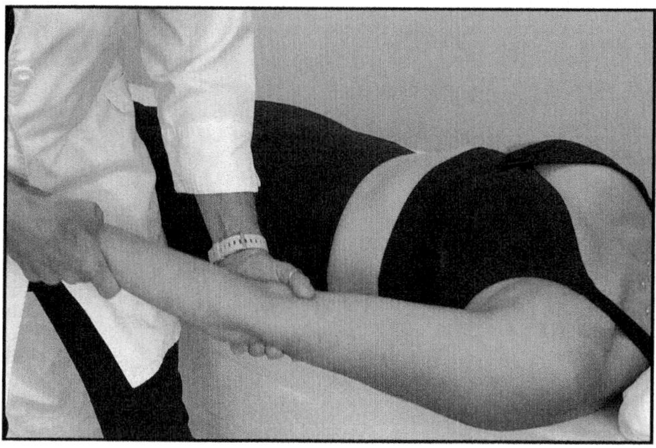

**Figure 12-2.** The patient's arm in the resting position of 55 degrees of abduction and 30 degrees of horizontal adduction.

("Does this feel better or worse?") throughout the intervention. Safe and effective performance of joint mobilization techniques requires good tactile sensation, attention to detail, and a significant amount of practice.

Before performing any joint mobilization technique, the clinician must know which joint surface is convex and which is concave and which bone is to be stabilized and mobilized. The resting position (Figure 12-2) for the shoulder is about 55 degrees of abduction and 30 degrees of horizontal adduction (anterior to the frontal plane) with the forearm in neutral (thumb up). The clinician must ensure the scapula is stabilized before performing GH joint mobilization. Many of the shoulder joint mobilization techniques are performed with the patient's arm in the resting position, but they can be performed at any point in the range where a restriction is experienced.

## Lateral Distraction of the Glenohumeral Joint

Lateral distraction of the GH joint is commonly used for pain control (grades I and II) and to promote generalized mobility (when a grade III force is applied). Grade I or II oscillations reduce muscle guarding and can be performed before any grade III mobilization. To perform lateral distraction, the patient is placed in a supine position with the scapula stabilized and the arm in the resting position. The clinician should face forward toward the patient's head on the side to be treated. The clinician supports the patient's involved extremity (the patient's forearm is supported between the clinician's trunk and humerus). The clinician's hand stabilizes the humerus by grasping the distal end around the epicondyles. The other hand should be firmly situated in the axilla with the palm facing outward just below the joint. The clinician's proximal hand should apply the lateral force distracting the head of the humerus while the other hand stabilizes the distal end of the humerus (Figure 12-3).

## Posterior Glide of the Glenohumeral Joint

A posterior glide of the humeral head increases shoulder flexion, internal (medial) rotation, and external (lateral) rotation.[13] The patient is positioned supine with the shoulder in the resting position. The clinician should face the patient's head and stabilize the patient's arm between the clinician's forearm and trunk. Before beginning the technique, the clinician should palpate the humeral head (Figure 12-4A) to locate its position and then place the hand over the anterior surface of the humeral head as shown in Figure 12-4B and apply the appropriate amount of posterior force (sustained or oscillations) depending on the goal of the treatment.

## Increasing External (Lateral) Rotation of the Glenohumeral Joint

External rotation can be increased when a grade III force is applied while the patient's arm is in the resting position. This is the preferred position when attempting to increase external rotation because there is a reduced risk of dislocating or subluxing the shoulder.

To perform this technique (Figure 12-5), the clinician should face forward toward the patient's head and position the clinician's hand that is closer to the patient's feet in the axilla in preparation to apply a lateral distraction. The clinician's other hand should grasp the most distal aspect of the humerus and apply an external (lateral) rotation force to the end of the patient's available range. Once the arm is rotated to that point, the clinician should then apply a grade III lateral distraction. Current research suggests using a grade III posterior glide may be more effective in increasing shoulder external rotation (compared with other directional glides) for patients with adhesive capsulitis.[12,13]

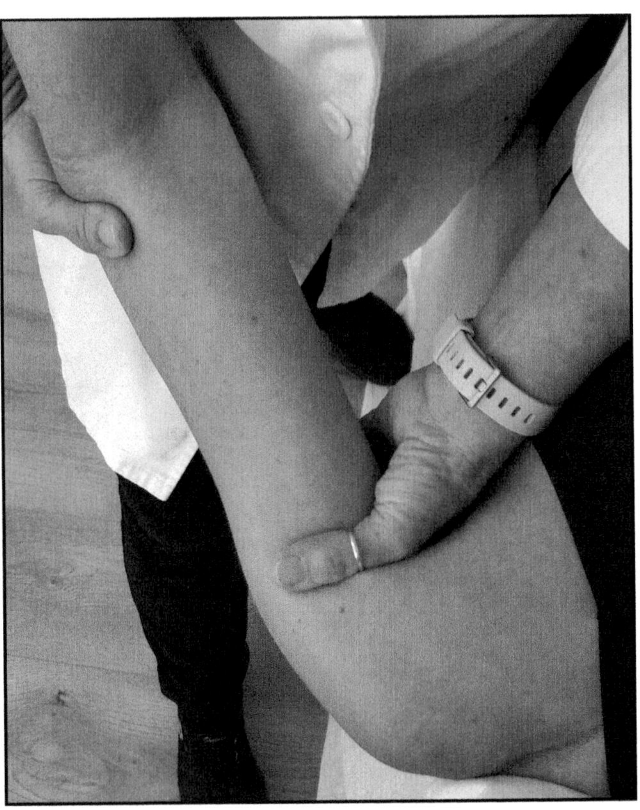

**Figure 12-3.** Shoulder distraction with lateral force applied to the proximal humerus.

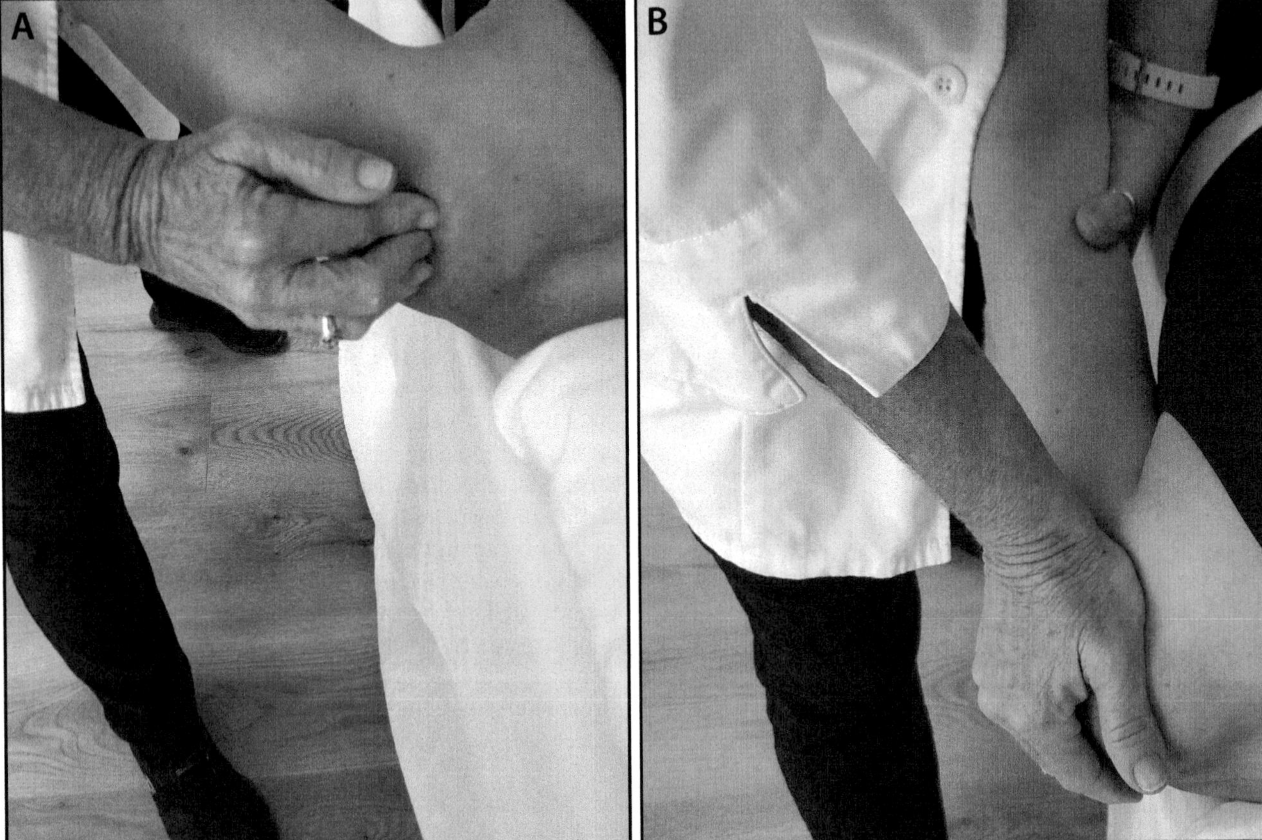

**Figure 12-4.** (A) Palpate the humeral head just inferiorly to the acromion and then slide the hand anteriorly. (B) A posterior glide with the hand placed on the anterior surface of the humeral head increases shoulder flexion and internal or external rotation.

### Inferior or Caudal Glide of the Glenohumeral Joint

There are 2 primary reasons for using this technique: (1) to lower the position of the humeral head in the glenoid if it sits superiorly in the socket (possibly causing an impingement during movement) and (2) to increase shoulder abduction.

This technique can be performed with the arm in the resting position (Figure 12-6A) or abducted at the end of the patient's available range or where the humeral head migrates superiorly during abduction (Figure 12-6B). Regardless of the patient's arm position, the clinician should face the patient's side. The web space of the hand closest to the patient's head is positioned just lateral to the acromion on the superior aspect of the humeral head. The clinician's other hand grasps the humerus and applies a grade I distraction before gliding the head inferiorly. The clinician should first use a grade II caudal force to take up the slack in the capsule and then slowly apply a sustained grade III pressure to increase abduction.

Long-axis distraction in the resting position can be used to create an inferior (caudal) glide using a grade III mobilization to reposition the head of the humerus or grades I or II (sustained or oscillations) for pain control or to reduce muscle guarding. The clinician faces the patient's head and grasps the distal shaft of the humerus with one hand and the distal forearm with the other. To apply a grade III mobilization force, the clinician should lean back (Figure 12-6C) to create the force. For a grade II joint mobilization, the clinician grasps the distal forearm with both hands and slightly leans back to take up the slack in the joint for a sustained distraction or while performing rhythmic vertical oscillations.

### Scapulothoracic Joint and Soft Tissue Mobilization

There are several muscles that attach to the scapula and are responsible for its movement. If muscle guarding is present, the scapula cannot glide or rotate efficiently, which limits scapula mobility and impacts GH joint arthrokinematics, resulting in decreased or compensated shoulder motions.

Scapular mobilization is used to increase and restore scapula mobility. Position the patient in the side-lying position on the unaffected side close to the edge of the table. It is advised to place a pillow between the clinician and the patient to avoid direct body contact with the patient's chest (especially when they are of different sexes). The clinician places one hand on the acromion and the other gently grasping the inferior angle of the scapula (Figure 12-7A). This hand position allows the clinician to control scapula elevation by sliding the scapula upward using the hand on the inferior angle and depression by using the hand positioned superiorly on the acromion. To rotate the scapula (upward or downward), the hand on the inferior angle guides the motion, and the hand on the acromion assists.

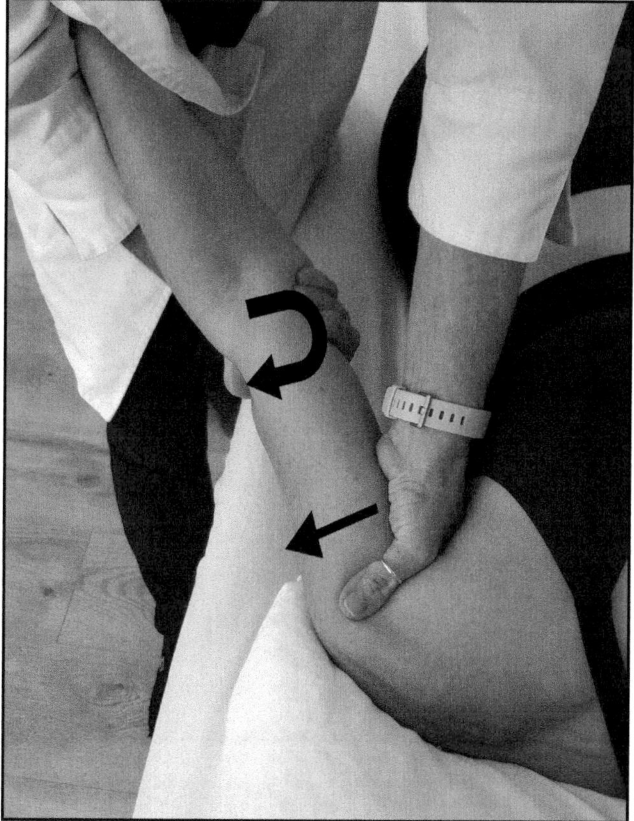

**Figure 12-5.** The clinician's left hand applies a grade I lateral distraction, and the right hand externally rotates the humerus to increase the motion.

To improve protraction and retraction, one hand should be positioned on the acromion and the other on the vertebral border of the scapula with the fingers gently grasping the anterior surface (Figure 12-7B). The easiest way to achieve this is to slide the scapula into retraction first with the hand positioned on the acromion. Once the hand is positioned on the vertebral border of the scapula, gently lift it off the rib cage and slide it laterally.

These techniques can be repeated several times in each direction. Once scapula mobility is restored, scapula proprioceptive neuromuscular facilitation (PNF) should be progressed from PROM to AROM to resisted motion.

## Shoulder Instability

Shoulder instability can occur when surrounding joint structures become stretched or torn, creating GH hypermobility. Instability can range from mild unobservable subluxations caused by congenital joint laxity or microtraumatic injury (due to repetitive activities) to severe, resulting from a dislocation (major instability) from a single traumatic event.[14] A traumatic instability occurs when a significant force disrupts the supporting structures (ie, the labrum or ligaments) of the shoulder, resulting in partial separation of the humeral head from the glenoid fossa (subluxation) or a complete separation (dislocation). The shoulder is the most commonly dislocated joint in the body (accounting for about 50% of the dislocations seen in emergency departments).[15]

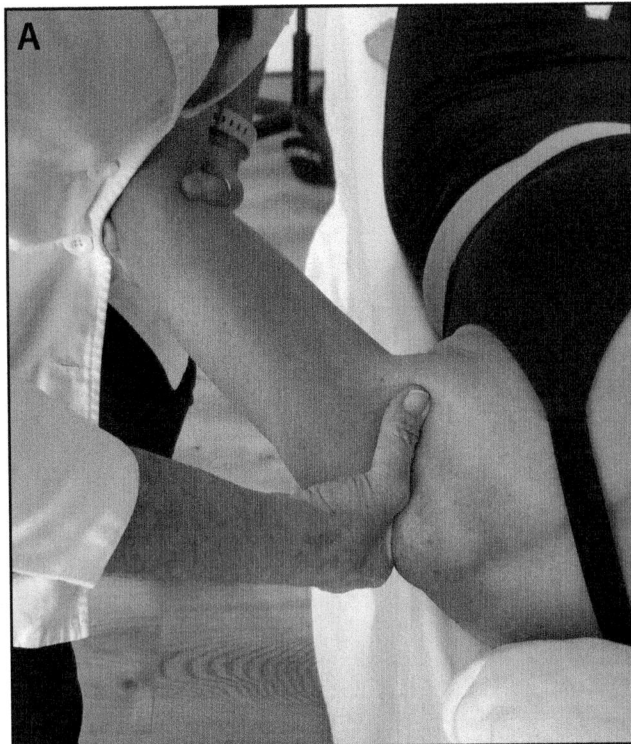


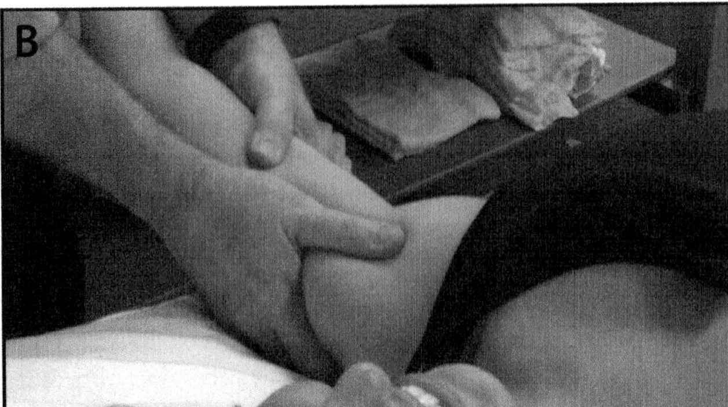


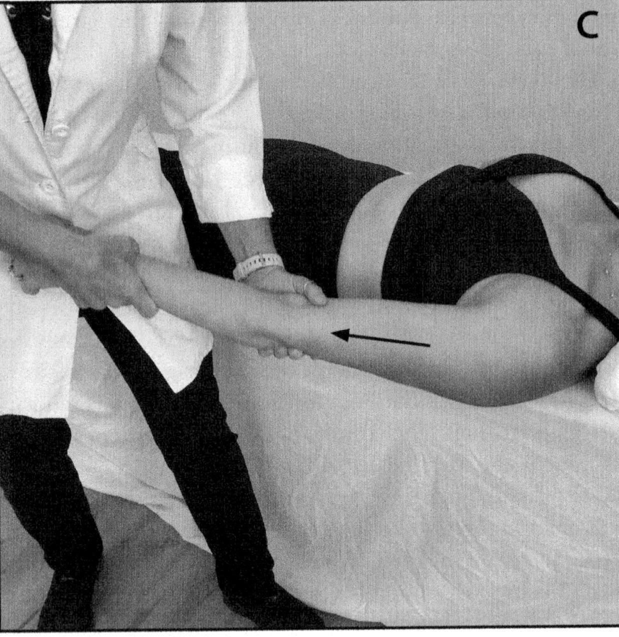


**Figure 12-6.** (A) The resting position with an inferior or caudal guide to increase shoulder abduction. (B) Bring the arm to the end of the available range then apply a grade I distraction with a caudal glide to reposition the humerus and increase ROM past 90 degrees. (C) Long-axis caudal traction can be used for increasing joint mobility or reducing muscle guarding depending on the grade.

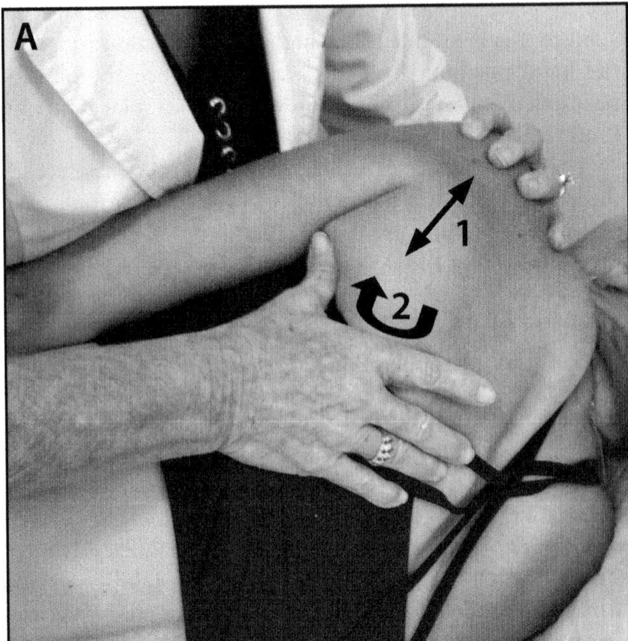


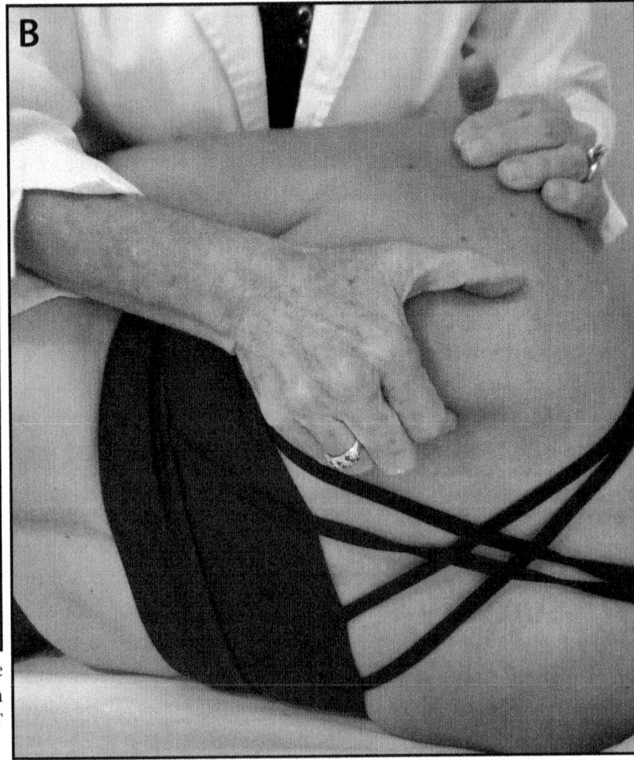


**Figure 12-7.** (A) The clinician's hand on the inferior angle moves the scapula in the directions of elevation, depression (arrow 1), and rotation (arrow 2) while the hand on the acromion assists and stabilizes. (B) ST mobilization: Grasp the vertebral border and gently lift it off the thorax.

Immediate medical management after a dislocation involves a reduction of the joint by a physician. Once reduced, the arm is immobilized in a sling to allow for rest and tissue healing. Immobilization time varies depending on the severity of the injury, prior occurrences, or other concerns related to further injury to the surrounding structures. The most common concern associated with dislocations or repeated subluxations is damage to the glenoid labrum. This can occur when the humeral head is forcefully compressed or sheared against the labrum. A mild (grade I), first-time subluxation requires a short period of rest before resuming activities, whereas patients experiencing a traumatic or recurring dislocation usually present with muscle weakness and/or loss of mobility requiring longer healing times.

### Unidirectional Instability and Dislocations

Unidirectional instability occurs in one direction (anterior, posterior, or inferior), with the majority occurring anteriorly. A patient's clinical presentation varies based on the MOI, degree of instability, prior occurrences, and medical management after the injury. Understanding the MOI can help the clinician predict the extent of damage sustained to the joint and surrounding soft tissues and nerves. Shoulder dislocations should be medically or surgically reduced as soon as possible.

The most common dislocation is in the anterior direction (accounting for about 95% of shoulder dislocations).[15,16] The incidence rate of anterior dislocations is between 8.2 and 23.9 per 100,000 people, with a prevalence of 1.7%.[17,18] A large percentage of dislocations occur in the younger population, with the highest rate of incidence occurring in men 16 to 20 years of age. There is an increased risk of recurrences in this age group, with studies reporting a 60% to 75% recurrence rate in 11- to 18-year-old patients.[19,20] Anterior dislocations most commonly occur when an excessive force is applied as the arm is externally rotated and abducted (90/90 closed-pack position), forcing the humeral head anteriorly. An anteriorly directed blow to the posterior or posterolateral aspect of the shoulder can also result in an anterior dislocation.

A posterior dislocation, although less frequent (2% to 4% occurrence), can occur when the shoulder is internally rotated as one **falling on an outstretched hand (FOOSH)**. The impact to the shoulder from the fall forcefully translates the humeral head posteriorly, which can be associated with lesser tubercle fractures, posterior labrum injury, and/or subscapularis tear/avulsion.[15]

Less than 1% of shoulder dislocations occur inferiorly. Inferior dislocations occur when the shoulder is hyperabducted (eg, when grasping for an object overhead to prevent a fall), forcing the humeral head inferiorly. Disruption of the inferior capsule is often associated with axillary nerve and artery injury as well as RC injury.[15]

### Multidirectional Instability

There are 2 causes of multidirectional instability (MDI). First, the shoulder joint itself has generalized laxity and may slide in and out of the glenoid fossa in more than one direction. Patients who present with MDI may have this clinical presentation in both shoulders (indicating a congenital problem) and may also present with general laxity in other joints (eg, the hips). MDI in one or both shoulders can also be due to repetitive overhead activities that are commonly associated with swimmers, gymnasts, and/or throwing athletes. These patients may complain of pain with pushing, pulling, lifting, and/or overhead movements. Patients may also report numbness and/or weakness in the arms/hands. Depending on the severity of the patient's injury, the clinical examination may reveal painful or empty end ranges with PROM or AROM that is impaired due to weakness of the RC and/or scapular stabilizing musculature. The patient may have a positive apprehension or active release test and/or a sulcus sign and will typically describe specific movements/activities that provoke symptoms.

## *Conservative Treatment for Shoulder Instability*

Once the patient is referred to therapy, the physical therapist will complete a clinical examination and identify the primary impairments. It is common for the patient's shoulder to be stiff and to have limited motion after immobilization.

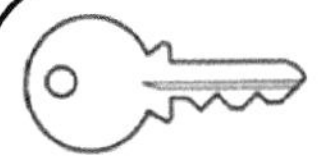

**Key Safety Consideration: Treating Patients With Shoulder Instability**

Patients should avoid the combined positions/motions or MOI that caused the dislocation/subluxation, especially during the early phases of rehabilitation.

- Anterior dislocation: Avoid abduction and external rotation (especially at 90/90 degrees)
- Posterior dislocation: Avoid flexion, horizontal adduction, and internal rotation
- Inferior dislocation: Avoid end-range flexion or abduction
- MDI: Avoid those directions where there is increased laxity as determined by the physical therapist (eg, anterior inferior).

To restore normal, pain-free shoulder mobility while minimizing the risk to the healing tissues, working in safe ranges below the level of the shoulder is recommended

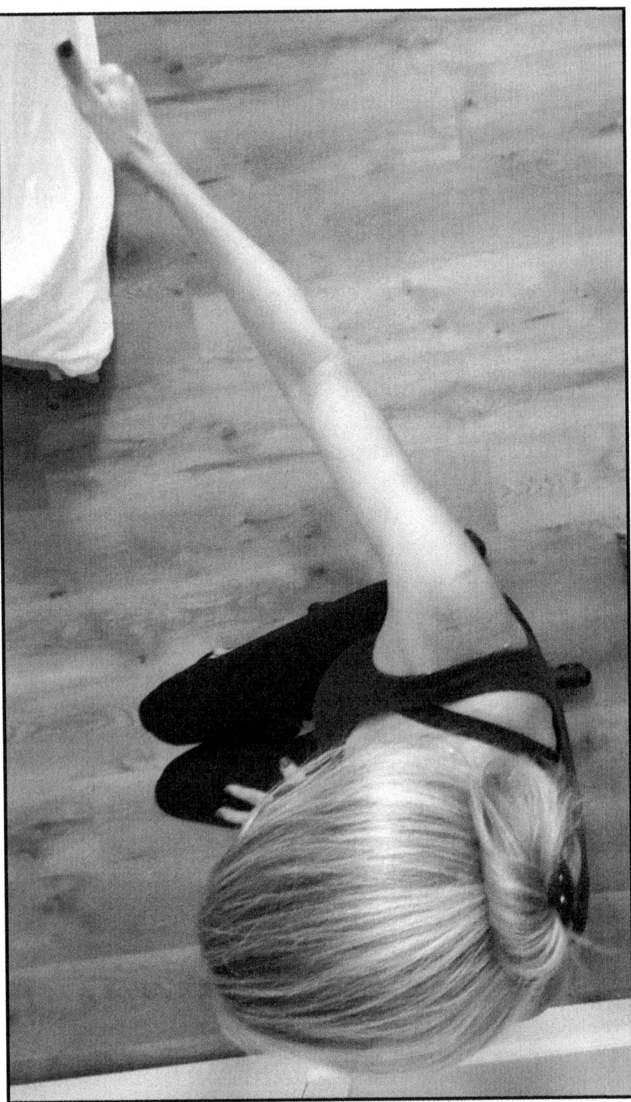

**Figure 12-8.** The plane of the scapula.

(for the first 1 to 2 weeks). ROM and strengthening exercises are often performed with the arm in neutral or in the plane of the scapula or scaption, which is 30 to 40 degrees anterior from the frontal plane (Figure 12-8). For example, when performing external (lateral) rotation ROM, placing the arm in this position avoids stressing the healing joint capsule (especially after an anterior dislocation) and reduces the chance of impinging the supraspinatus and other structures under the acromion. Instruct the patient to limit the time their involved arm hangs down unsupported and avoid full adduction because these positions stress the GH ligaments and the weakened RC muscles (especially the supraspinatus muscle).

### Clinical Tips

After the physician clears the patient to discontinue the use of the sling, the shoulder joint may still need to be supported when the arm hangs down. Initially, the RC muscles fatigue easily due to weakness. The assistant can educate the patient on ways to reduce stress on the soft tissue structures as follows:

- Instruct the patient to place a small, rolled towel in the axilla on the involved side.
- Have the patient support the arm by placing the thumb on the involved side in a side pocket or through a belt loop.

Physical therapy management includes appropriate stretches and progressive strengthening of both RC and scapular stabilizing musculature while monitoring the patient to ensure that proper arthrokinematics and osteokinematic movements are occurring at the ST and GH joints in order to prevent secondary injury. The patient in Figure 12-9 is demonstrating poor shoulder joint mechanics; the normally expected downward gliding of the humeral head is not occurring, and the humeral head remains positioned on the superior portion in the glenoid fossa. This deviation from normal biomechanics not only limits the patient's ROM, but it can also create an impingement of the structures that lie superior to the humeral head and inferior to the acromion. Forward head posture and rounded shoulders can also contribute to impingement and/or ROM loss.

Open kinetic chain (OKC) strengthening and stretching exercises isolate specific weakened (or tightened) muscles, whereas closed kinetic chain (CKC) exercises promote cocontractions of several muscles (Table 12-8). If the patient's symptoms are highly irritable, it is appropriate to start with isometric strengthening exercises because these allow patients to control the level of muscle activity while minimizing pain. Patients can perform isometric exercises using a graded scale (ie, 25%, 50%, and 75% amount of effort) and gradually increase the intensity of the contractions until a pain-free maximal isometric contraction can be achieved. Initially, the isometrics should be performed with the elbow flexed to 90 degrees with the arm in the neutral position. Isometrics can be self-resisted (Figure 12-10) or completed against a stable surface (Figure 12-11). As the patient progresses, the isometrics can be performed with the elbow straight (Figure 12-12).

Pain-free CKC exercises can be initiated to facilitate the RC muscles to act as a group, encouraging joint approximation.

As pain resolves and mobility improves, patients can progress to resistance bands or hand weights, initially starting with exercises below shoulder level and in single-plane movements and then motions above shoulder height and multiplanar activities as tolerated. Eventually, higher-level dynamic and plyometric exercises should be used during the minimal protection/return-to-function phase.

Exercise progressions for conservative management of shoulder instability and dislocations are located in Table 12-9. The physical therapist assistant must understand that the severity of the injury and the patient's response to exercise vary from patient to patient; therefore, the rate of exercise progression will also vary. Neuromuscular control is a key component for safe return to the patient's prior level of function, so exercises to improve neuromuscular control should be initiated early in the rehabilitation process.

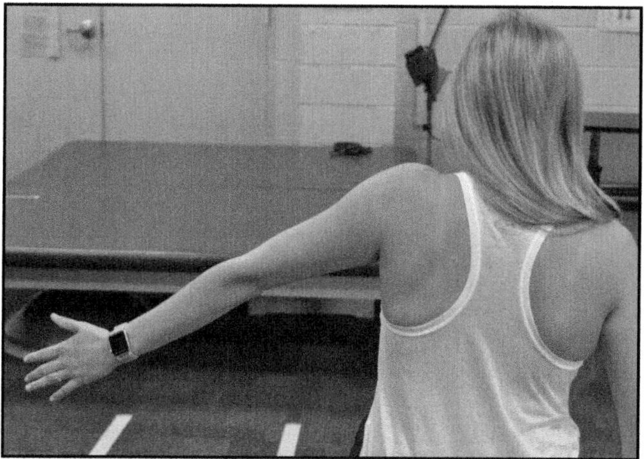

**Figure 12-9.** Faulty shoulder joint biomechanics during shoulder abduction can create an impingement.

## *Shoulder Instability Surgical Procedures and Postoperative Rehabilitation Management*

When conservative management is unsuccessful in stabilizing shoulder joint instability, surgical intervention is common. Evidence indicates that earlier surgical management may produce better outcomes. A systematic review (14 studies) reported surgical interventions after a first-time traumatic shoulder anterior instability (especially in younger athletes) reduced the rate of recurrent instability. A 2-year follow-up found that surgical intervention "produced significantly lower rates of recurrent instability (7%) compared with non-surgical treatment (46%)."[21]

### Shoulder Instability Complications and Surgical Interventions

Several complications are associated with an anterior shoulder dislocation. Two studies found the prevalence of injuries most commonly associated with anterior shoulder instability (for one-time and recurrent dislocations) include Bankart (100% and 97%, respectively) and Hill-Sachs (71% and 93%, respectively) lesions.[22,23] A **Bankart lesion** is an avulsion of the anterior-inferior labrum that may also include a tear of the inferior GH ligament and/or bony damage to the inferior aspect of the glenoid fossa. A **Hill-Sachs lesion** is a compression fracture or indentation defect of the posterolateral humeral head that can occur when it contacts the anterior glenoid during anterior dislocation. Small or medium defects are usually treated conservatively, whereas large defects require surgical intervention. Other lesions associated with instability include tears of the **SLAP** (prevalence of 20.19%) and RC muscles (prevalence of 11.53%).[23] The long head of the biceps brachii tendon (which attaches in the superior glenoid) may also be injured with SLAP lesions. Supraspinatus tendon tears can be associated with anterior dislocations, but this is not as common.

Surgical (open or arthroscopic) procedures can restore dynamic stability of the shoulder, allowing patients to resume their prior level of function and return to work/sport activities. A capsular shift (capsulorrhaphy) is performed to tighten the lax area(s) of the capsule. The 2 arthroscopic techniques that can be performed include a "pinch-tuck" method to gather and tighten the capsule using sutures or a thermal method that shrinks the stretched part of the capsule.[24] During an arthroscopic Bankart repair, the surgeon reattaches the torn area of the labrum to the anterior-inferior rim of the glenoid and repairs the involved ligaments using sutures and anchors/tacks. A capsulorrhaphy may also be performed to improve joint stability. To repair a SLAP lesion, the surgeon debrides the torn portion of the labrum and smooths the surface of the glenoid before reattaching the labrum back in place. The long head of the biceps brachii may also be reattached, but this is at the discretion of the surgeon.

## *Postoperative Rehabilitation Management*

All postoperative management is dictated by the surgeon's protocol. These protocols include prescriptive immobilization time and staged progressions of ROM, strengthening, and functional activities. The physical therapist assistant must follow the physician's postoperative precautions because they are developed to protect healing structures and to minimize the risk of damaging the surgical repair. Patients are usually immobilized anywhere from a few days to 6 weeks depending on the extent of the surgical repair and the physician's protocol. During the immobilization phase, the patient is usually instructed to wear the sling or brace 24 hours a day; however, the physician may allow sling removal only to perform prescribed exercises, but the UE must be fully supported during that time. An example of a shoulder immobilizer is shown in Figure 12-13; the surgeon selects the type of immobilizer.

**Table 12-8**

Shoulder Exercises

| ROM Exercises and Stretches | OKC and CKC Strengthening | Neuromuscular Exercises |
|---|---|---|
| • PROM: Pendulums: Abduction/adduction, flexion/extension, circles<br>• AAROM: Pulleys flexion, abduction, internal rotation<br>• AAROM: Tabletop slides to increase flexion, horizontal abduction/adduction, abduction, external rotation<br>• AAROM: Wall waking to increase abduction and flexion<br>• AAROM/stretching using a cane: Supine with cane[a]: Flexion, abduction, internal/external rotation in neutral or 90/90<br>• Side-lying sleeper stretch targets external rotation muscles and posterior capsule<br>• Cross-chest stretch: Posterior capsule stretch<br>• Anterior capsule, pectoralis major and internal rotation stretch with arm straight<br>• Towel stretch: Targets external rotation muscles<br>• Inferior capsule self-stretch and adductor | Isometrics<br>• Scapula muscle setting/isometrics all directions: Retraction—targets rhomboids; elbows in back pocket—targets lower traps<br>• GH muscle setting⇨isometrics: Submaximal⇨maximal self-resisted or against a wall: With elbow flexed to 90 degrees for flexion, extension, abduction, internal/external rotation⇨ arm straight; multiangle isometrics can be performed<br>• Sustained large ball punches with 30- to 60-second hold to facilitate RC muscles<br>• Dynamic isometric exercises using resistance band for various directions<br>OKC Exercises[b]<br>• Manual resistance for all scapula motions<br>• Manual resistance for UE D1 and D2 PNF<br>• Supine protraction for serratus anterior with weights or standing with resistance band<br>• Resisted band or free weight exercises varied positions for maximal resistance against gravity flexion, extension, abduction, adduction, internal/external rotation, and in plane of scapula thumbs up and PNF<br>• Standing rows with resistance band with thumbs up targets middle trapezius<br>• Standing military press targets upper trapezius, levator scapulae, and middle deltoid | • Upper body weight shifting seated⇨wall⇨quadruped then add perturbations to shoulders/trunk<br>• Quadruped single extremity lifts and then opposite arm and leg lifts<br>• Supine scapula stabilization against clinician resistance in all directions at various speeds<br>• Supine PNF with manual resistance<br>• Standing PNF with resistance bands<br>• Large ball punches with isometric holds progress to multidirectional perturbations<br>• Smaller ball circles against wall for scapula stabilization<br>• Body blade: With arm by the side, then shoulder at 90 degrees elbow straight: Blade held horizontally and vertically<br>• Ball toss/catch supine to self, against a wall or mini trampoline (1 or 2 hands)<br>• Stair stepper with UEs<br>• Spider-Man wall walking with resistance band<br>• All other advanced exercises<br>• Note: Push-up and plank progressions considered as neuromuscular control exercises. More advanced exercises can include UE step-ups (on a step) and plyometric push-ups. |

*(continued)*

**Table 12-8 (continued)**

Shoulder Exercises

| ROM Exercises and Stretches | OKC and CKC Strengthening | Neuromuscular Exercises |
|---|---|---|
| • Upper trapezius stretch<br>• Levator scapulae stretch<br>• Pectoralis major muscle stretches | • Prone "I" and "Y" for lower trapezius serratus anterior and "T" palms down: Rhomboids, thumbs up: Middle trapezius (progression prone on large ball)<br>• Prone shoulder extension targets latissimus dorsi, teres major, and posterior deltoid<br>• Supine chest press for pectoralis major and anterior deltoid strengthening<br>• Pull downs target latissimus dorsi and teres major<br>• Combined scapula retraction, horizontal abduction, and external rotation in prone 90/90 (or standing) targets middle trapezius, rhomboids, posterior deltoid, infraspinatus, and teres minor<br>CKC Exercises<br>• Large ball pushes with perturbations<br>• Ball against wall circles<br>• Seated shoulder depression<br>• Push-up progression: Against wall⇨table⇨floor on knees then with legs straight, then with feet on a ball or hands on a balance disc or wobble board. Push-up plus for any of the above push-ups targets serratus anterior<br>• Plank progression (refer to Chapter 15) | |

[a]These can also be used as stretches targeting the antagonist muscle group (ie, a stretch into shoulder flexion stretches the shoulder extensors).
[b]Resistance bands or weights can be added to any of these exercises as a progression.
AAROM = active assisted range of motion.

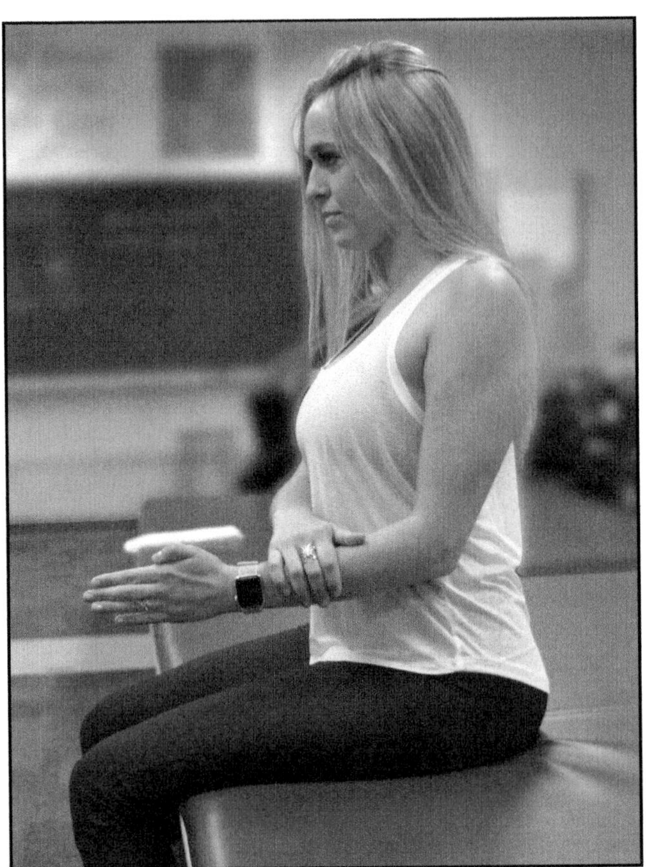

**Figure 12-10.** Self-resisted isometric external rotation.

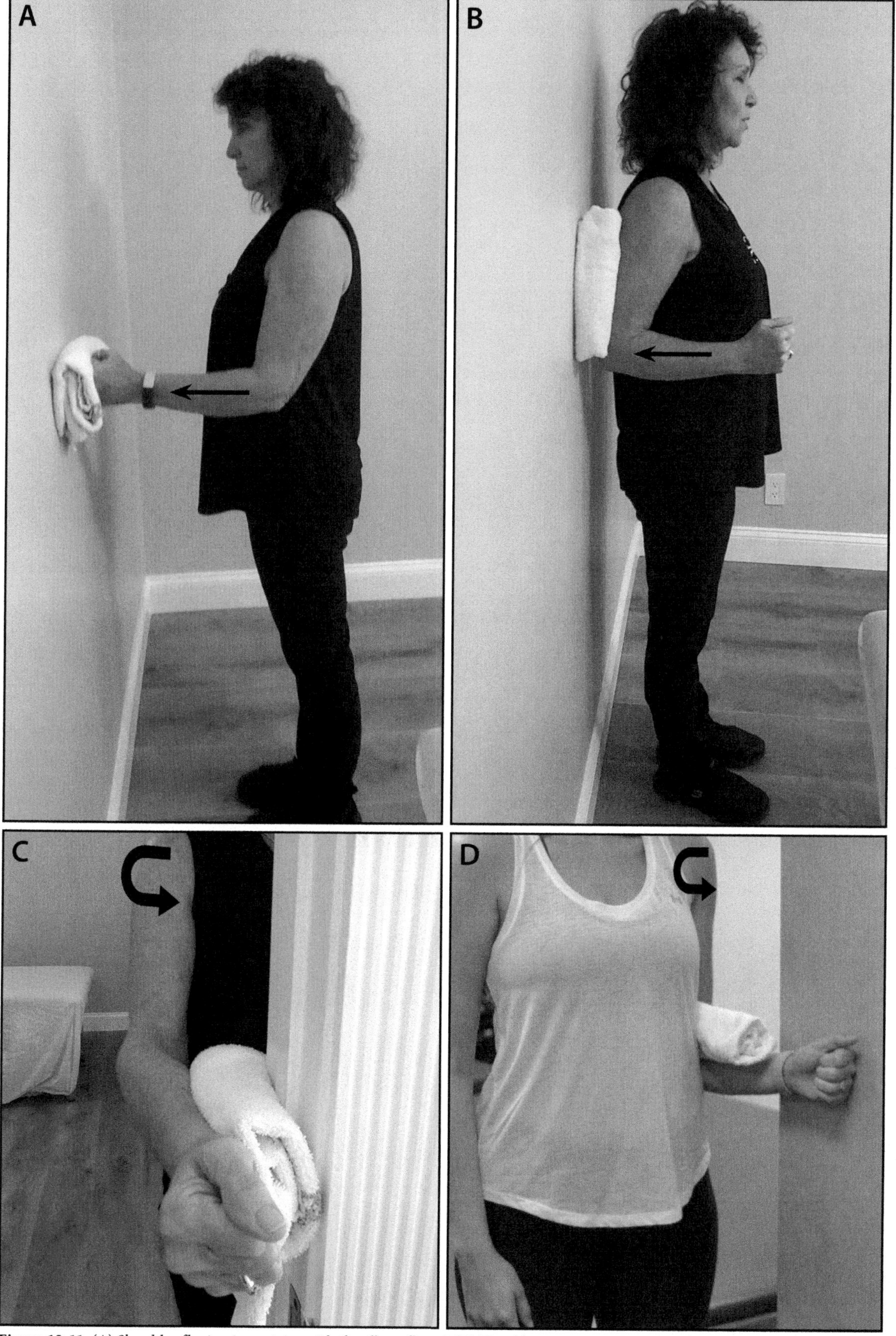


**Figure 12-11.** (A) Shoulder flexion isometrics with the elbow flexed. (B) Shoulder extension isometrics. (C) Shoulder internal rotation isometric contraction. (D) Shoulder external rotation isometrics.

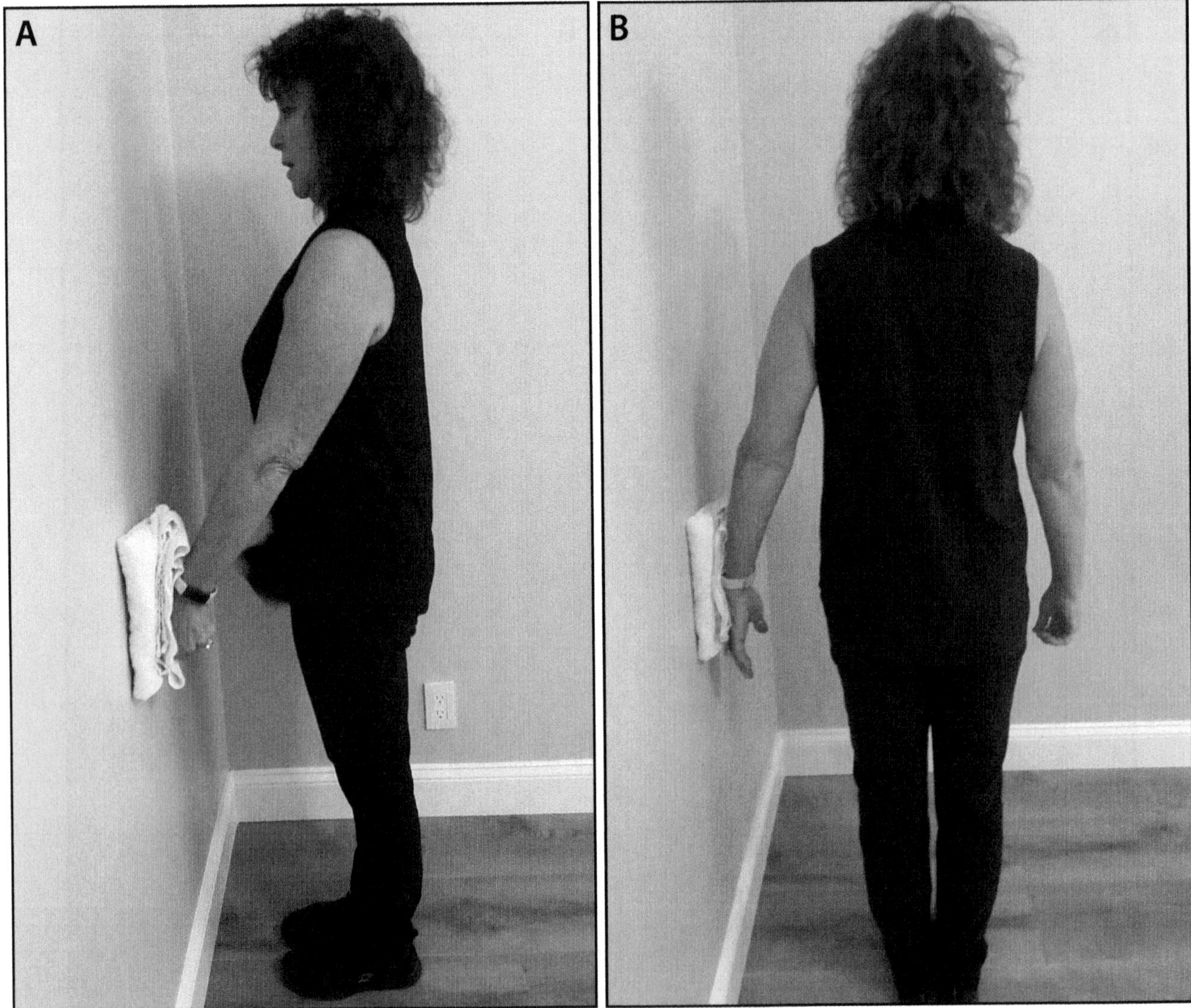


**Figure 12-12.** (A) Shoulder flexion with the elbow extended. (B) Shoulder abduction isometrics.

**Table 12-9**

General Exercise Progressions for Shoulder Dislocations and Shoulder Instability

| Dislocation/Instability | Phase 1: Maximal Protection Phase (Day 1 to Week 4-6) | Phase 2: Moderate Protection Phase (Week 4-6 to 10-12) | Phase 3: Minimal Protection Phase (12+ Weeks) |
|---|---|---|---|
| Dislocations:<br>• Common MOI for an anterior dislocation = abduction, external rotation at 90/90 degrees<br>• Common MOI for posterior dislocation = FOOSH flexion, internal rotation<br><br>Instabilities:<br>• Unidirectional instability: Avoid exercises in direction of the positions/motions that created the instability | Goals<br>• Reduce pain, inflammation, and muscle guarding<br>• Protect healing tissues; wear sling/brace<br>• Avoid positions that created the dislocation/instability especially during ADLs<br>Note: Immobilized 1 to 3 weeks in a sling/brace following injury (nonsurgical); 3 days to 6 weeks postoperative depending on type of repair. Surgical precautions found in Table 12-10.<br>Exercises<br>• Nonsurgical ROM: Follow precautions; pendulum exercises (no weight), PROM/AAROM in safe, pain-free ranges only in plane of scapula week 1 to 2; progress from AAROM with wall walking, cane, or pulleys to full AROM by week 6 to 7<br>• Postoperative ROM: Follow precautions in Table 12-10 for ROM if no protocol was provided. Pendulums (no weight) week 4, PROM flexion to 90 degrees may be permitted by week 4. | Goals<br>• Discontinue brace (postoperative)<br>• Continue with joint protection and pain control<br>• Restore full AROM; stretch tight structures<br>• Normalize ST and GH rhythm<br>• Increase muscle strength and endurance<br>• Increase neuromuscular control<br>Exercises<br>• Nonsurgical ROM: Gain full AROM early-midphase<br>• Postoperative ROM: Follow precautions in Table 12-10. Begin with AAROM with cane, pulleys, and wall walking; progress from AAROM⇨AROM with good GH/ST mechanics; flexion 135 degrees PROM, about 115 degrees AROM; rotation 50 degrees PROM in plane of scapula by week 7 to 8; by week 12 full PROM, AROM WNL<br>• Nonsurgical stretching/strengthening: Stretching upper trapezius, levator scapulae, pectoralis major posterior capsule, cane/towel for internal/external rotation progress to 90 degrees abduction week 8 to 9. Begin CKC push-up progression; OKC exercises using weights and resistance band for ST and GH muscles (see Table 12-8) early in the phase; progress to 90/90 internal/external rotation with resistance band week 8 | Goals<br>• Increase dynamic strengthening and motor control<br>• Enhance endurance with functional use of UE<br>• Good ST/GH mechanics (negative scapula dyskinesis) during abduction and flexion for 5 repetitions with 5 pounds (lb)<br>• Gradual return-to-sport activities: Nonsurgical patients ⇨12 weeks; ⇨16 weeks for postoperative patients<br>Exercises<br>• Postoperative ROM: Full pain-free AROM early in the phase<br>• Nonsurgical stretching/strengthening: Continue internal/external rotation strengthening at 90 degrees of abduction; begin plyometrics and eccentric strengthening<br>• Postoperative stretching/strengthening: Use more aggressive internal/external rotation stretching if necessary, with 90 degrees of abduction; progress with ST/GH muscle strengthening as per Table 12-8 |

*(continued)*

**Table 12-9 (continued)**

General Exercise Progressions for Shoulder Dislocations and Shoulder Instability

| Dislocation/ Instability | Phase 1: Maximal Protection Phase (Day 1 to Week 4-6) | Phase 2: Moderate Protection Phase (Week 4-6 to 10-12) | Phase 3: Minimal Protection Phase (12+ Weeks) |
|---|---|---|---|
| • MDI: Exercises strengthening anterior and posterior structures; avoid end-range flexion and abduction due to hypermobile inferior capsule | • Nonsurgical strengthening: Elbow and forearm AROM: Wrist flexion/extension/adduction/abduction AROM; light isometrics with arm supported; ball squeezes early in this phase; ST AROM, muscle setting, and isometrics all directions; submaximal GH isometrics with arm in neutral elbow flexed to 90 degrees week 1 to 2, progress to maximal isometrics (elbow flexed or straight) week 3 to 4; light resistance in safe ranges and nonprovocative positions if pain free. Begin CKC push-up progression week 4 to 5.<br>• Postoperative strengthening: Seated (forearm supported): Elbow/forearm AROM; wrist flexion/extension/adduction/abduction AROM; ball squeezes early in this phase; ST AROM with clinician, muscle setting for retraction, and elbows in back pocket for retraction and depression<br>Neuromuscular control<br>• Nonsurgical only: Weight shifting into forearms or hands progression week 2; initiate rhythmic stabilization supine and isometric large ball pushes, progress with ball in plane of scapula against wall week 3<br>• Postoperative: No weight bearing into surgical arm; clinician-assisted rhythmic stabilization OKC in small circles | • Postoperative stretching/strengthening: Stretching upper trapezius, levator scapulae, pectoralis major, posterior capsule, cane exercises for internal/external rotators in plane of scapula and neutral. Progress to maximal isometrics; begin dynamic isometrics in neutral for internal/external rotation with light resistance band, begin light weight resistance straight planes and plane of scapula in midphase; OKC serratus anterior strengthening week 4 to 5; begin CKC progression week 7 to 8 if permitted<br>Neuromuscular control<br>• Nonsurgical: Rhythmic stabilizations against wall with ball in plane of scapula, flexion and abduction (progress by increasing time); progress to quadruped activities, push-ups and planks midphase; progress to plyometrics, body blade mid-late phase<br>• Postoperative: OKC rhythmic stabilization supine with perturbations; begin weight shifting and gentle large ball push isometrics when weight bearing is permitted and as early as possible and progress with ball in plane of scapula against wall; begin AROM PNF and progress to light resistance week 8 to 9 | • Postoperative stretching/strengthening: Use more aggressive internal/external rotation stretching if necessary, with 90 degrees of abduction; progress with ST/GH muscle strengthening as per Table 12-8<br>Neuromuscular control<br>• Nonsurgical: Progress to more dynamic overhead plyometric exercises and PNF; progress to sports-related activities and return to sport<br>• Postoperative: Continue PNF strengthening and more dynamic exercises; begin plyometrics with arm below shoulder level week 12 and progress to overhead activities after week 12 |

*(continued)*

**Table 12-9 (continued)**

General Exercise Progressions for Shoulder Dislocations and Shoulder Instability

| Dislocation/ Instability | Phase 1: Maximal Protection Phase (Day 1 to Week 4-6) | Phase 2: Moderate Protection Phase (Week 4-6 to 10-12) | Phase 3: Minimal Protection Phase (12+ Weeks) |
|---|---|---|---|
| | Aerobics<br>• Nonsurgical: Bike without sling and initiate upper body ergometer midphase forward/backward<br>• Postoperative: Recumbent or stationary bike with arm in sling/brace<br>• Additional exercises (with arm supported): Lower extremity exercises seated or standing holding on with uninvolved UE<br>Notes<br>• Also avoid shoulder extension and horizontal abduction after anterior dislocation.<br>• Cross-chest stretch for posterior capsule can be performed with an anterior instability diagnosis if indicated (nonsurgical). | Aerobics<br>• Nonsurgical: Recumbent or stationary bike; progress upper body ergometer forward/backward for endurance as tolerated; light jogging week 8<br>• Postoperative: Recumbent or stationary bike; begin upper body ergometer forward/backward to tolerance progress to increase endurance | Aerobics<br>• Nonsurgical and postoperative: Continue with upper body ergometer for endurance; running or jogging |

WNL=within normal limits.

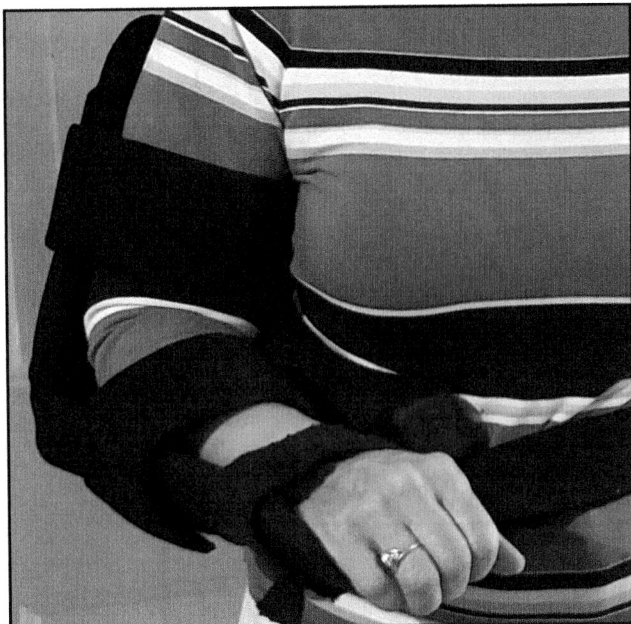

**Figure 12-13.** A shoulder immobilizer is often used for a variety of shoulder diagnoses. The arm is slightly abducted.

Finger and wrist AROM exercises can be performed while in the immobilizer or sling. Elbow flexion/extension and forearm pronation/supination AROM exercises can also be performed but only if the biceps tendon is not involved/repaired and if the humerus is fully supported during those exercises. Suggested postoperative precautions for the common surgical procedures discussed in the prior section are listed in Table 12-10 and are based on evidence-based research.[24-27] Sample exercise progressions for postoperative patients are included in Table 12-9 and are illustrated at the end of the chapter. These exercises do not supersede a surgeon's protocol and are provided only as a general guide. The physical therapist assistant should always follow the protocol and POC.

## Shoulder Pain: Rotator Cuff Injuries and Subacromial Pain

Shoulder pain is the third most common orthopedic complaint,[28] and the most common injuries causing shoulder pain and affecting RC muscles include acute tendinitis, tendinopathy, and impingement. Injury to the RC can affect general and athletic populations. These muscles maintain joint stability during all shoulder movements but can be susceptible to injury with repetitive overuse. By definition, soft tissues that are in an active inflammatory state are referred to as acute tendinitis or bursitis depending on the structures identified as the source of the pain. Patients with shoulder tendinitis or bursitis diagnosis usually report pain with overhead activities. Generally, tendinopathy is considered a chronic problem with prolonged pain, vascular changes, tendon tissue breakdown (or degradation), and fibrosis affecting function.[29] At the GH joint, this condition is usually due to wear and tear of the RC tendons, leading to progressive tissue weakness and resulting in the tearing of one or more RC muscles. Injuring any of these structures can lead to loss of motion, muscle weakness, and compensatory muscle substitution due to poor joint arthrokinematics, especially during activities at or above shoulder height.

**Subacromial impingement** refers to shoulder pain that arises due to compression (impingement) of the structures situated below the acromion process in the subacromial space (Figure 12-14). Some clinicians refer to this as *subacromial pain syndrome*. The 3 structures that pass through this narrow space include the supraspinatus tendon, the subacromial bursa, and the long head of the biceps brachii tendon. These structures can be compressed or entrapped in the space between the superior humeral head and the undersurface of the acromion and coracoacromial ligament (coracoacromial arch). The space is the smallest when the arm is in 90 degrees of abduction and internally rotated and the supraspinatus is closest to the coracoacromial arch. The supraspinatus tendon is most commonly impinged during overhead activities.[30]

Structural (anatomic) or functional mechanical causes can also create an impingement of the soft tissues in the subacromial space. Structurally, the shape of the acromion (ie, curved or hooked), joint/capsule laxity (due to recurrent dislocation or instability), and/or faulty posture (ie, forward head, rounded shoulders, or increased kyphosis) can alter normal GH/ST position and joint mechanics. An inadequate muscle response or fatigue during repetitive overhead activities can affect shoulder joint mechanics. A muscle imbalance between the internal (medial) and external (lateral) rotators and decreased ability of the RC muscles to dynamically stabilize the humeral head and/or inability of the ST muscles to work with the RC muscles can affect the efficiency of ST rhythm, altering joint arthrokinematics. A patient's clinical presentation can vary depending on symptom acuity and irritability levels. The most common complaints associated with an impingement include anterior and lateral shoulder pain with active movements or lifting and night pain when sleeping (especially on the involved shoulder). Excessive loading of the RC muscles can lead to degeneration of the tendons, eventually leading to tears.[31] The hallmark signs of an RC tear are pain with active movement, an inability to raise the arm, and significant muscle weakness during MMT.

Neer[32] first described the following staging of RC impingement in 1983:

- Stage I is associated with acute inflammation and edema of the RC tendon and most commonly affects younger patients (less than 25 years old). The patient usually reports pain that is the worst with shoulder abduction greater than 90 degrees. This stage can be treated successfully with conservative physical therapy interventions.

**Table 12-10**

Postoperative Precaution Suggestions[a]

| Arthroscopic Capsular Shift ("Pinch-Tuck" or Thermal Techniques)[24] | Bankart Lesion Repairs (With/Without Subscapularis Repair) | SLAP Lesion Repairs[b] (With/Without Labral or Biceps Repair) |
|---|---|---|
| • Thermal technique: Patients wear immobilizer 2 to 3 weeks; allowed to perform pendulums and PROM/AAROM in safe ranges depending on the direction of instability[24]<br>• "Pinch-tuck" technique: Immobilizer worn for 4 weeks; PROM, AAROM, and isometric exercises; AROM at 6 weeks[24,26]<br>• Prescribed ROM limitations depend on the part of the capsule repaired; ROM should be performed passively within safe ranges (refer to Key Safety Considerations)<br>• Avoid stressing the specific part of the capsule that was repaired.<br>• Avoid overhead activities and 90 degrees flexion/90 degrees abduction/external rotation until week 12[24] | • Patient wears immobilizer 2 to 6 weeks depending on amount of repair[25,26]<br>• Avoid stressing anterior capsule for at least 6 weeks (ie, avoid shoulder external rotation, extension, or horizontal abduction)<br>• PROM flexion and abduction to < 90 degrees; external rotation in plane of scapula to only 20 degrees by week 3 to 4[25,26]<br>• No PROM into external rotation past 0 degrees for 6 weeks following subscapularis reattachment[25,26]<br>• No internal rotation AROM after subscapularis reattachment after week 4 to 6[25,26]<br>• Avoid aggressive external rotation stretching until after week 10[25,26] | • Patient wears sling 3 to 4 days with simple debridement/no labrum reattachment or 4 to 6 weeks with reattached labrum and/or if there is biceps tendon involvement[27]<br>• PROM/AAROM started postoperatively within pain-free range for flexion and internal/external rotation in plane of the scapula (if only debridement, can work to full ROM by 2 weeks).[27] Otherwise, with labral reattachment:<br>  ○ PROM flexion: 60 degrees by week 2; 90 degrees by week 3 to 4<br>  ○ PROM rotation: External to 0 to 15 degrees; internal 45 degrees by week 2[26,27]<br>• Avoid stressing the biceps' attachment to the glenoid:<br>  ○ No combined shoulder and elbow extension with supination[26]<br>  ○ No shoulder abduction with external rotation<br>• With biceps reattached, include AROM by 4 to 6 weeks and avoid eccentrics until 10 to 12 weeks[27] |

[a]Progressions are guidelines; follow the surgeon's protocol and the physical therapist's POC.
[b]Discussion of the various types of SLAP lesions is beyond the scope of this book. Specific progressions vary depending on the type of lesion.[27]

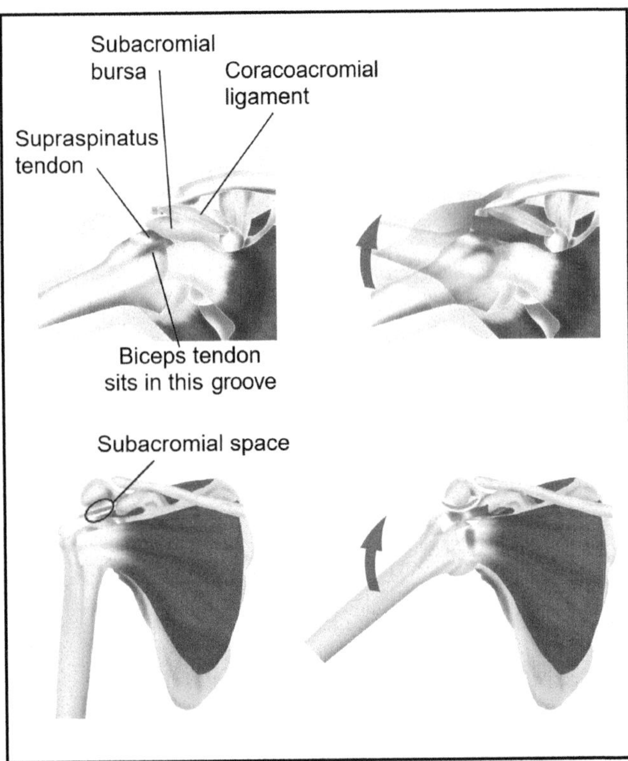


**Figure 12-14.** The subacromial space and impingement (Chu KyungMin/Shutterstock.com).

- Stage II affects patients 25 to 40 years old and is a continuation of the previous stage, but the subacromial structures (the bursa, supraspinatus, and biceps tendons) become more inflamed and develop fibrotic characteristics to the point where the condition is irreversible because of the ongoing friction of the tendons. The patient commonly describes pain with ADLs and during sleep.
- Stage III usually affects patients older than 40 years in whom further degeneration of the tendons occurs, resulting in either a partial or complete tear. These patients usually have a long history of shoulder pain, muscle weakness/atrophy, and poor joint mechanics, resulting in degenerative changes to the coracoacromial arch (ie, osteophyte formation).[30,32]

## *Conservative Rehabilitation Management After Rotator Cuff Injury and Impingement*

When designing and implementing an exercise program after an RC injury, it is important to consider those impairments identified by the physical therapist in the medical record. During the initial evaluation, the therapist will determine where in the range the patient's greatest pain is reported. Most patients with RC pathology report pain during AROM between 60 and 120 degrees of shoulder abduction or in the plane of scapula with or without internal/external rotation.[28] These points in the range are referred to as a *painful arc*, and the physical therapist assistant should have the patient avoid working in this area. The assistant should have the patient work above and below the painful arc when initiating strengthening early in the rehabilitation process. The ultimate goal is for the patient to perform resisted exercises through the full ROM without pain.

When a patient has decreased passive joint mobility, a primary focus of physical therapy is to restore full/functional, pain-free ROM. In addition to manual stretching and joint and soft tissue mobilization techniques, the clinician should teach the patient self-stretching joint mobilization or stretching to help regain mobility (Figures 12-15 and 12-16). Active assisted exercises minimize muscle activity and are appropriate interventions to restore shoulder mobility during the early phase and can also be given to the patient as part of their home exercise program (HEP). All selected exercise interventions should respect the stage of healing and the patient's level of symptoms/tissue irritability.

The physical therapist assistant should continually monitor and educate patients to ensure good-quality GH/ST movements during all ROM and strengthening exercises to avoid impingement, pain, or reinjury. Controlled progressive static to dynamic loading (isometric to concentric and then eccentric) of the RC muscles is important for tissue remodeling.[28] It is acceptable to have mild amounts of pain during the first few repetitions of a strengthening exercise, but it should either disappear or decrease during the exercise set; it should totally dissipate once the exercise is completed.

### Considerations for the Physical Therapist Assistant

It is important to continuously monitor patients in real time to ensure proper joint arthrokinematics/osteokinematics and muscle sequencing during all exercises. The assistant should recognize when the targeted muscles being strengthened become fatigued and make appropriate exercise corrections and/or modifications. This is necessary to reduce the risk of further tissue irritation or injury to the joint structures and to improve patient outcomes.

Scapula stabilization and submaximal isometric strengthening can be initiated early in the acute phase and progressed as long as pain is controlled and good joint mechanics are maintained (Table 12-11). Initiate strengthening of the RC muscles in straight planes below shoulder height and progress to above shoulder and overhead multiplane activities during the later phases. Progressive dynamic CKC stabilization and plyometric exercises can be initiated and then progressed to work/sports/recreational-specific activities unique to the patient's goals during the final phase. Photographs of various exercises are found at the end of the chapter.

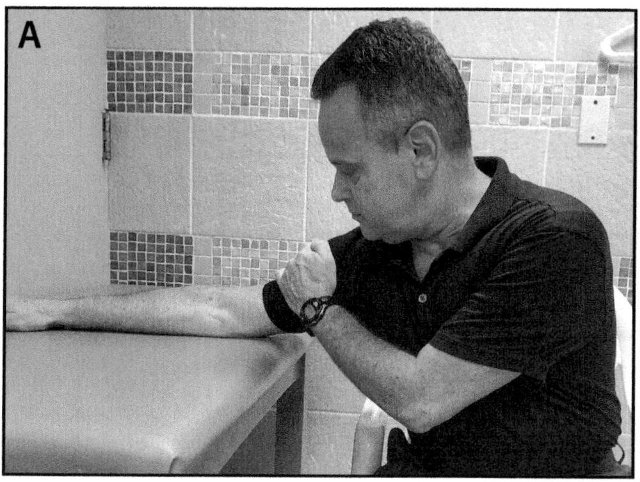


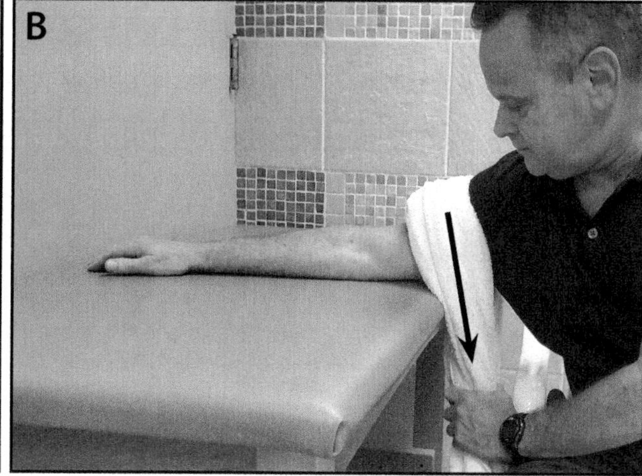


**Figure 12-15.** (A) Self-joint mobilization or stretching to increase shoulder abduction using an inferior glide. (B) Self-joint mobilization or stretching using a towel to achieve the same goal. Ensure the patient's hand or towel is positioned over the humeral head prior to applying pressure.

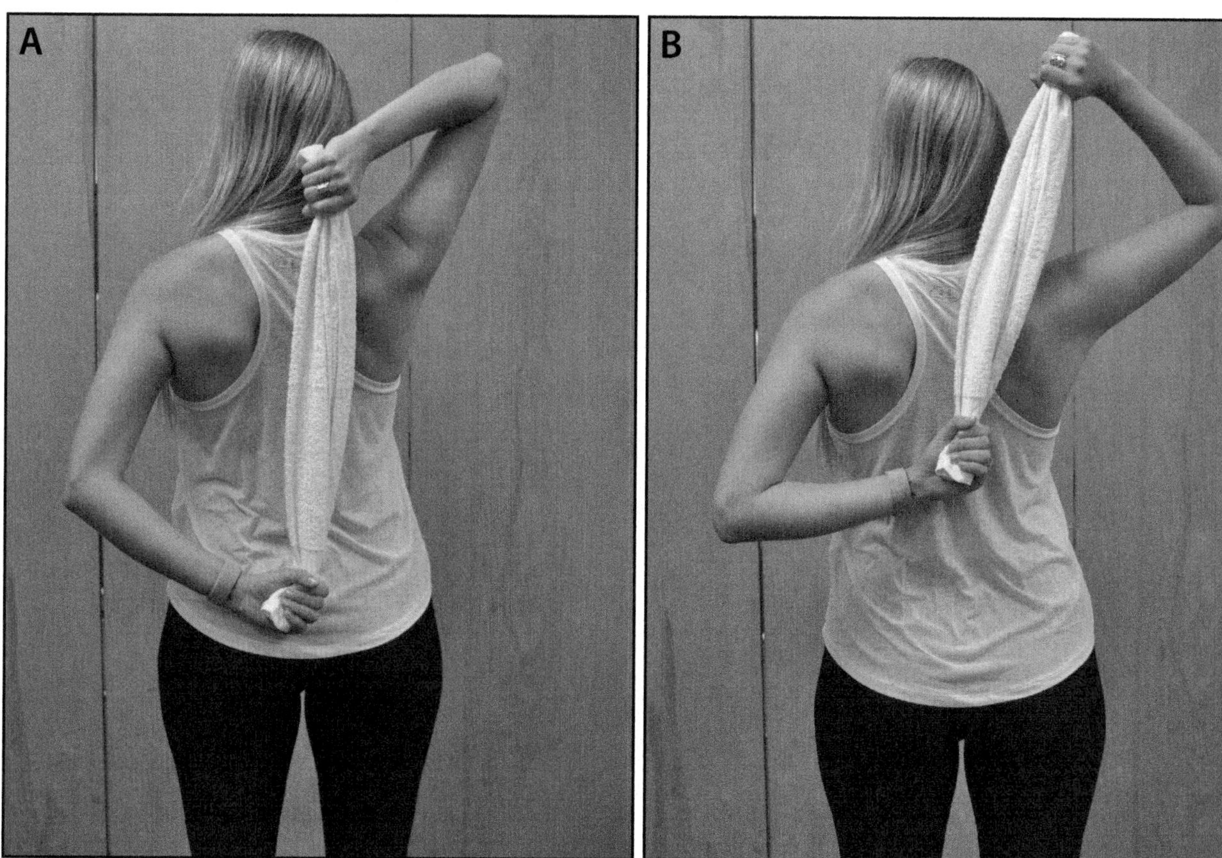


**Figure 12-16.** (A) A self-stretch using a towel to increase shoulder internal rotation; the starting position. (B) A self-stretch using a towel to increase shoulder internal rotation moving the right hand upward to increase motion on the left.

## Rotator Cuff Repair and Subacromial Decompression

When conservative management is unsuccessful in alleviating pain and improving function, patients may decide that surgery is the best option. Arthroscopic repair is the most common surgical intervention for patients with RC tears. For a patient without an RC tear who continues to have prolonged pain and limited mobility, the surgeon may recommend joint debridement and subacromial decompression. The procedure involves removing part of the acromion (acromioplasty), which creates more space in the subacromial space so structures can move unimpeded. It also reduces the chance of impingement and provides pain relief. The healing time is quicker because no tendon repair is performed. A subacromial decompression procedure is often used in conjunction with an RC repair, especially if the acromion is curved or hooked.

**Table 12-11**

**Suggested Exercise Progression for Nonsurgical Rotator Cuff Injury, Impingement, and Adhesive Capsulitis**

| | |
|---|---|
| RC injury with subacromial impingement | Phase 1: Modalities for pain control/inflammation, all exercise < 80 degrees, no overhead activity, and avoid horizontal abduction. Pendulums, slow/gentle pain-free posterior capsule stretch. Pain-free AAROM with wall walking, pulleys, and/or wand supine; sitting or standing all directions < 90 degrees (progress as tolerated near end of the phase); supine external rotation in plane of scapula or neutral only; and wall walking in plane of scapula < 90 degrees. Muscle setting and submaximal isometrics with GH joint in neutral all directions. Scapular AROM, pain-free isometrics for scapular retraction and depression, and supine serratus punches. CKC: Large ball pushes pain free and then progress to perturbations and wall push-ups. Wrist and forearm strengthening with the arm supported.<br>Phase 2: Progress to AROM all planes and plane of scapula in pain-free ranges first to 90 degrees and then progress to full ROM with good joint arthrokinematics. Shoulder, upper trapezius, levator scapulae, and pectoralis major stretches. Seated shoulder depression, prone shoulder extension to hip level only, prone "I" and "Y" AROM, "T" palms down and thumbs up with light weights, resistance band exercises, dynamic isometrics all directions and then AROM in all directions against resistance bands, rows, adduction, and latissimus dorsi pull downs. Light weight and/or ball against a wall in the plane of scapula and PNF. CKC: Quadruped exercises, initiate push-ups, and plank progression. *Check for good ST/GH mechanics and that there is no scapula dyskinesis.*<br>Phase 3: Add prone "T," "I," and "Y" 90/90 with lightweight progress dynamic strengthening and neuromuscular control exercises; advanced push-up and plank progression and plyometrics. *Monitor good ST/GH mechanics with advanced exercises ensuring no scapula dyskinesis.* |
| Adhesive capsulitis | Phase 1: Modalities for pain control/inflammation, grade I and II joint mobilizations decrease pain/reduce guarding. PROM; progress to AAROM/AROM as pain decreases. Pendulums (no weight). Wand/cane exercises, all directions, pulleys, tabletop slides, and/or wall walking. Upper trapezius, levator scapulae, pectoralis major, and wrist stretches. Muscle setting and pain-free submaximal isometrics for GH/ST joints. Scapular AROM; progress to isometric/resisted retraction and depression. Maintain normal elbow, wrist and hand mobility. Maintain or improve cervical ROM.<br>Phase 2: Progress to full AAROM, AROM single planes. Initiate AAROM PNF. Progress to pain-free multiangle isometrics to resistance bands/free weights with good arthrokinematics and begin CKC weight shifting progression table to wall to quadruped.<br>Phase 3: Progress to full AROM with good arthrokinematics as tolerated. Progress with CKC perturbations, balance board, and/or therapy ball. Progress to increasing strength at shoulder height in single planes and progress to PNF with resistance bands.<br>Note: Patient may need vigorous stretching/mobilization if joint ROM is restricted. Joint manipulation by surgeon may need to be performed and physical therapy initiated day of or day after procedure. Patients should be re-evaluated by the therapist after procedure. |

## *Rotator Cuff Tears*

RC tears can result from a traumatic injury, repetitive overhead activities, or degenerative changes. As stated earlier, the supraspinatus tendon is most commonly affected, but any other of the RC muscles may also be involved. RC tears are described as partial (incomplete) or full thickness (complete) and are defined by the size of the tear (small to massive). Partial-thickness tears involve part of the tendon from either the top (acromial side) or the bottom (humeral side). Full-thickness tears can run perpendicular or parallel to fiber alignment, creating a hole or cut in the tendon. RC full-thickness tear sizes are categorized as small (less than 1 cm), medium (1 to 3 cm), large (greater than 3 cm but less than 5 cm of the supraspinatus and infraspinatus), or massive (greater than 5 cm involving the supraspinatus, infraspinatus, and subscapularis). Small- and medium-sized tears involve the supraspinatus only.[33]

Research suggests that younger, active, symptomatic, and healthy patients should have surgery sooner rather than later, whereas older inactive patients with low functional demands should be treated with conservative management first and assessed to determine if surgery is a good option.[34] A patient should not be considered a surgical candidate, even if diagnosed with an RC tear (based on magnetic resonance imaging results), if they report little to no pain or limitation.

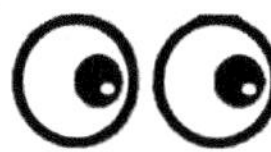

### Eye on the Research

As age increases (greater than 60 years), the prevalence of RC tears increases. According to several literature reviews, the RC tear rates include 15% to 20% of 60-year-olds, 26% to 30% of 70-year-olds, and 36% to 50% of 80-year-olds. The incidence rate of RC repairs in the United States is 15 per 103.[33,34] Younger patients appear to heal better than older patients; patients older than 70 years have about a 50% healing rate. These studies found that small and medium tears heal better than large or massive tears, with an average time of 12 months for healing after a repair. Twelve weeks after RC repair, 71% to 87% of small and medium tears healed compared with 56% to 62% for large and massive tears.[33,34]

Shoulder immobilization (4 to 8 weeks) after RC repair may cause some initial joint stiffness but did not affect ROM compared with early implementation of ROM 1 year after surgery. Although statistically insignificant, early and aggressive therapy using passive mobilization increased retears in medium to larger repairs. Another study reported that poor patient physical therapy compliance after RC surgery could increase the risk of tendon failure or retear.[33-35]

## *Postoperative Rehabilitation Management After Rotator Cuff Repair*

Physical therapy management after RC repair can vary based on the type of repair, the size of the tear, age, medical history, and the functional demands of the patient. After the repair, rehabilitation management is typically divided into phases of recovery. Treatment progression usually follows the surgeon's protocol. The general phases include the following[35-37]:

- Immediate postoperative/maximum protection phase (day 1 to 6 weeks)
- Moderate protection/AAROM and AROM phase (6 to 12 weeks)
- Early strengthening/minimum protection phase (10 to 16 weeks)
- Advanced strengthening phase (16 to 22 weeks)

Physical therapist assistants should understand the extent of the injury and surgical repair, the tissue healing timeline (inflammatory, proliferation, and maturation periods), and the precautions to be followed throughout the rehabilitation process. The criteria to progress from one phase to another differ and are dependent on the surgeon's protocol.[26,35-37] There is no high-level evidence in the research supporting one evidence-based RC postoperative rehabilitation program.[34] However, activity restrictions or precautions after RC repairs do appear to be relatively consistent in the literature (Table 12-12).[35-37] The assistant should educate patients on the physician's postoperative restrictions and reinforce the importance of being compliant with all restrictions.

### Considerations for the Physical Therapist Assistant

The assistant should continue to reinforce all precautions and restrictions based on the surgeon's protocol. All lifting, pushing, pulling, or reaching using the operative arm is contraindicated for at least 6 weeks. Weight bearing into the surgical arm is typically prohibited during this time. Continued lifting restrictions of less than 10 lb for up to 10 to 12 weeks after surgery are dependent on the extent of the repair and the structures repaired.

Although shoulder immobilization is common practice to protect healing tissues, the duration of immobilization varies due to the size of the tear, the patient's age, and the surgeon's preference. Smaller tears are usually immobilized for about 2 weeks, medium to large tears 3 to 6 weeks, and massive tears 4 to 8 weeks.[26] Joint stiffness due to immobilization is a common complaint, but one large randomized study found it did not lead to joint stiffness and it did not affect overall ROM in the long term.[38] Gentle grade I and II joint mobilizations (with the limb fully supported in the resting position) can reduce stiffness, pain, and muscle guarding.[35] The physical therapist assistant should not perform these techniques without the consent of the supervising physical therapist (and in accordance with state practice act/laws).

PROM is often initiated early during the rehabilitation process, but initiation depends on the size of the tear/extent of the repair and the surgeon's protocol. Before performing PROM, position the patient in supine with a folded towel placed under the humerus so the arm is positioned slightly anterior to neutral to prevent shoulder extension and provide support. The clinician should support the humerus with one hand and the forearm with the other and then slowly move the arm in safe and pain-free ranges (and according to the physician's protocol), avoiding stress on healing structures. PROM does not have a negative effect on healing tissues and usually is started while the patient is still immobilized.[34,38] Patients often require frequent verbal cues to relax the arm as the clinician moves it. The patient should achieve passive shoulder flexion to about 90 degrees between 6 and 8 weeks after surgery. Supine passive shoulder external (lateral) rotation should be limited to less than 35 degrees with the arm in the plane of the scapula as long as there is no repair to the subscapularis. If

**Table 12-12**

**Activity Restrictions or Precautions After Rotator Cuff Repair**

| Small- or Medium-Sized Tears | Large to Massive Size Tears |
|---|---|
| No shoulder AAROM until week 3 to 5; no AROM until week 5 to 6 | No (painful) PROM before week 4 to 5 |
| No pushing off or supporting body weight through the hands until week 6 | No using surgical UE for eating, dressing, or showering until week 5 to 6 |
| No reaching behind the back until week 7 to 8 | No driving until out of immobilizer (about 6 weeks) |
| No lifting (0 to 6 weeks); lifting objects < 10 lb; starting week 8: 10 lb or greater after week 12 | No pushing off or supporting body weight through the hands until week 7 to 8 |
| Avoid abrupt or sudden jerky movements until week 12 | No AAROM until week 7; no AROM until week 8 |
| No excessive end-range stretches until after week 12 | No shoulder extension past anterior trunk until week 6 to 7 (when supine avoid humerus passing the anterior aspect of the trunk) |
| | No lifting (0 to 6 weeks); lifting ≤ 5 lb week 6; 10 lb week 12 |
| | No reaching overhead until week 10 |
| | No pulling or pushing of objects with involved UE until week 10 to 12 |
| | No reaching behind back until week 10 |
| | Avoid lifting overhead with weight until week 14+ |
| | Avoid abrupt or sudden jerky movements until week 16+ |

the subscapularis is repaired, the external rotation should not occur past neutral for up to 6 weeks.[39] Internal rotation should be limited to no more than 30 degrees, and it should also be performed in the plane of the scapula.[35-37]

Pendulum exercises (Figure 12-17) are considered PROM, but physical therapist assistants must emphasize that the patient's shoulder muscles should not contract during the activity. The arm must hang freely, and the gentle rocking of the body (ie, forward/back/side to side or circles) creates the momentum of the arm movement in small amplitudes (about 7 inches/20 cm in any direction). Larger pendulums or performing the exercise incorrectly increases muscle contraction activity in the RC muscles and should be avoided early in the rehabilitation process. These exercises could be delayed until 3 to 5 weeks after RC repair.[35,40]

Elbow, wrist, and hand/finger AROM can be performed, but the UE must be supported so as not to stress the repair. Active biceps brachii exercises should not be performed if it was repaired or reattached for 6 to 8 weeks after surgery or until cleared by the surgeon. ST AROM and postural corrections can be initiated during this initial phase of rehabilitation. CKC exercises for the surgical UE should not begin until indicated by the protocol; they are typically permitted about 6 weeks postoperatively.[26,35-37] This exercise facilitates the scapula and RC muscles.

As healing progresses, patients can begin AAROM (using a cane and/or pulleys) and progress to full AROM by week 12 (depending on the size of the tear). The physical therapist assistant needs to focus on ST/GH motions during exercises to ensure joint arthrokinematics are normalized. No strengthening activities above 90 degrees should be performed until those joint mechanics are normal. It is important to avoid superior migration of the humeral head, which can cause irritation or reinjury to healing tendons (Figure 12-18). AROM in the plane of the scapula can be difficult for patients to initially perform, so doing it with the elbow flexed is a good way to initiate supraspinatus muscle activity. This is called the *salute exercise*.[35]

Muscle setting and submaximal isometrics for scapula retraction and depression can begin during the initial phase (week 2 to 4).[35-37] Once the patient can perform supine AAROM shoulder flexion to 90 degrees or a simulated bench press exercise without weight, small active oscillations in various directions or circles can improve scapular neuromuscular control in the OKC (Figure 12-19). This exercise can be progressed by having the clinician provide rapid random directional perturbations (see Figure 12-18) once the patient is cleared to initiate resisted exercises. Normal scapular muscle firing capability, sequencing, and timing are vital for good shoulder girdle arthrokinematics and avoiding impingement or injury to the healing tendons. Physical therapist assistants should have patients focus on strengthening the lower trapezius and rhomboid muscles and stretching the upper trapezius (Figure 12-20) and levator scapulae (Figure 12-21). These exercises help reduce overactivation of these muscles during GH movements, which is a common occurrence in patients with shoulder pathologies. Active scapular protraction can be performed during the initial rehabilitation phase, progressed to using

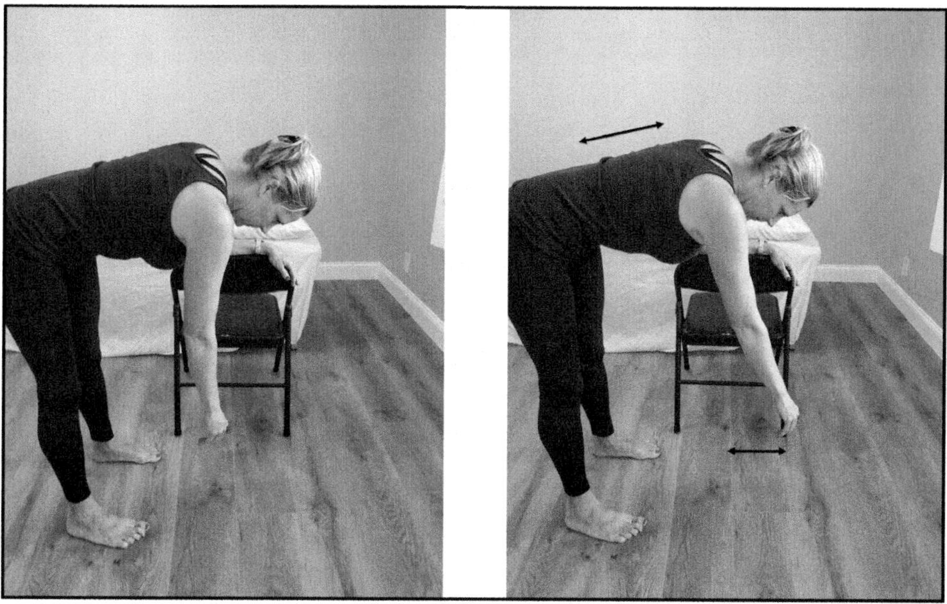

**Figure 12-17.** The pendulum exercise. The direction of body motion creates the shoulder motion. Shoulder muscles should not contract.

OKC weights (Figure 12-22), and in later phases progressed to CKC push-up progressions with added protraction (called a *push-up plus*). Push-up progressions are included in figures at the end of the chapter.

End-range stretching into internal/external rotation should be avoided at least until week 12 to allow for tendon healing. Excessive end-range internal rotation stretching stresses the infraspinatus, and external rotation stretching stresses the subscapularis; therefore, both should be avoided until week 16 after the repair of a large or massive tear (because these structures were repaired along with the supraspinatus tendon).[36,37,39]

It is important for physical therapist assistants to remember that it takes a minimum of 12 to 16 weeks for maximal tendon tensile strength to occur, which must be taken into account as patients are progressed.[35-37]

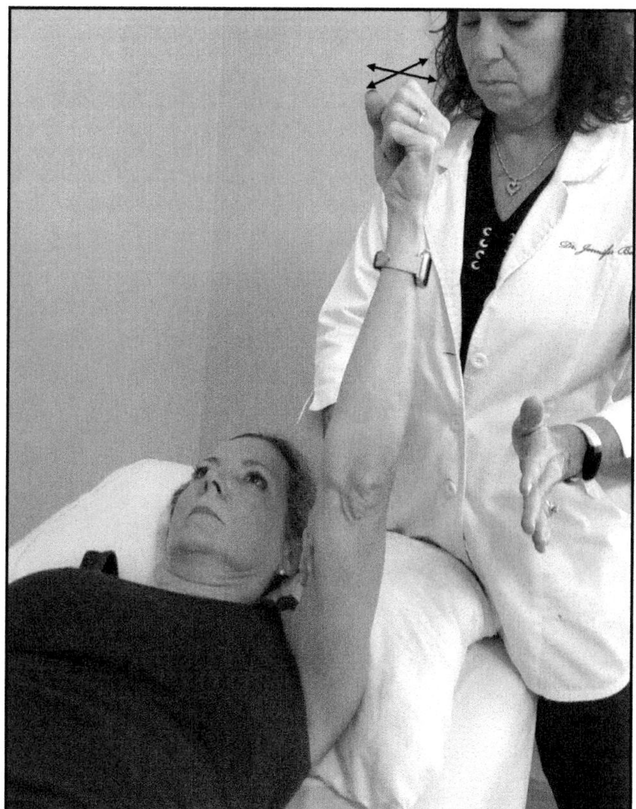

**Figure 12-18.** The patient performs small multidirection oscillations for neuromuscular control for shoulder girdle muscles as the clinician guards the patient.

## Osteoarthritis of the Shoulder

Although osteoarthritis is more commonly seen in weight-bearing joints in older patients, the GH joint can also become arthritic over time. Osteoarthritis of the shoulder most commonly affects adults over the age of 60 years. Patients usually complain of pain, limited movement, and/or weakness because of friction created between the joint surfaces leading to the breakdown of the articular surfaces and thickening of the joint capsule. RC muscles can also degenerate over time, and when it occurs in combination with GH arthritis, it is called *shoulder arthropathy.* Risk factors for shoulder osteoarthritis include advanced age, genetics, sex, weight, joint infection, systemic/metabolic disorders, a history of shoulder dislocation/instability, and/or previous injury. Heavy construction work, prolonged overhead work activities, or participation in overhead sports are also risk factors.[41-43]

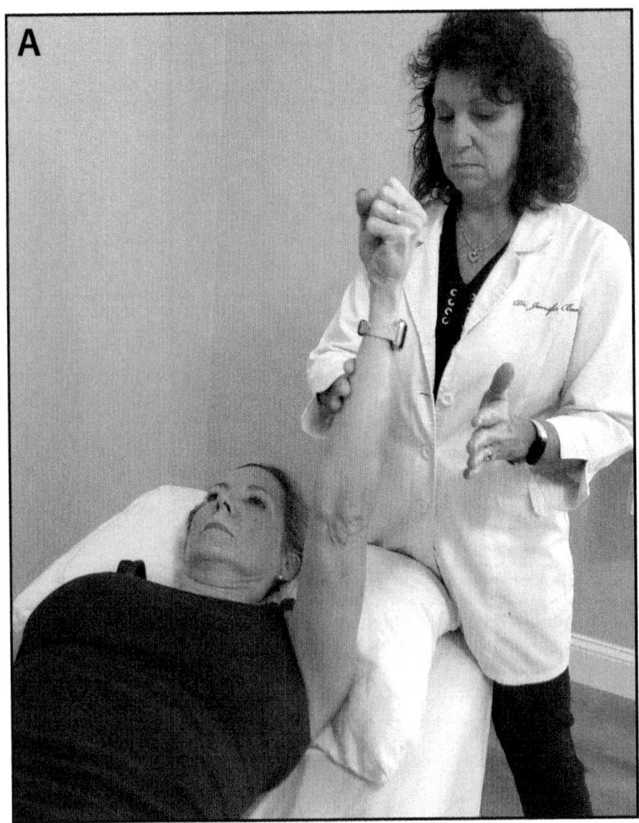

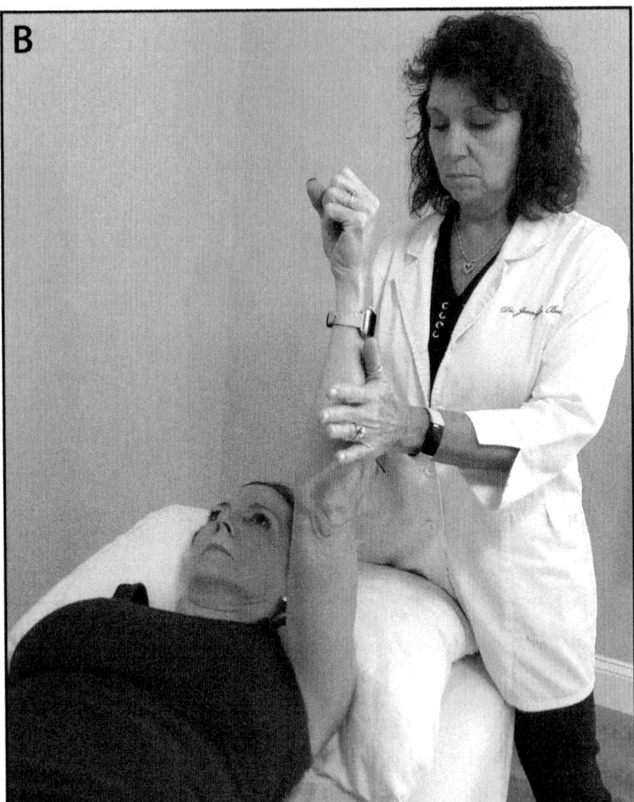

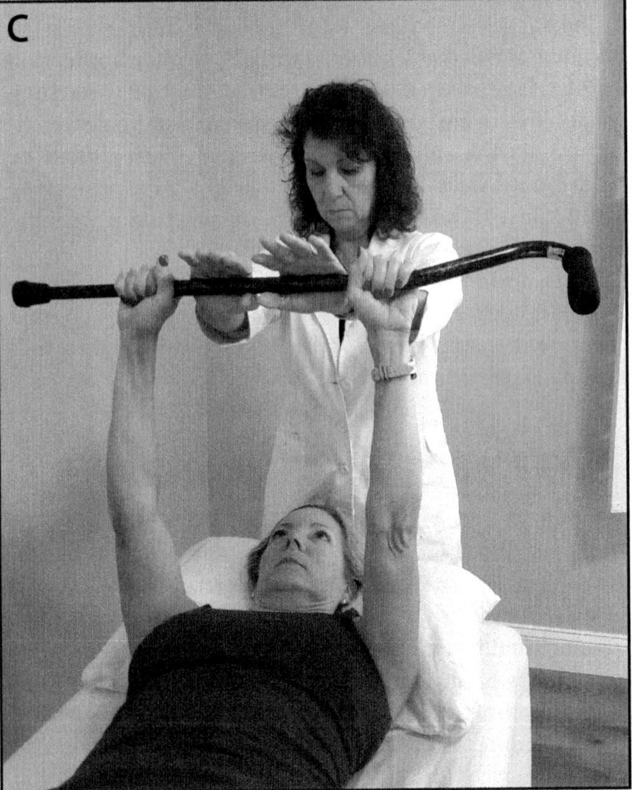

**Figure 12-19.** (A) The clinician provides rapid perturbations as a neuromuscular control progression. (B) The clinician also provides random directional perturbations. (C) Using the cane gives the clinician the ability to add a rotational component to the perturbations.

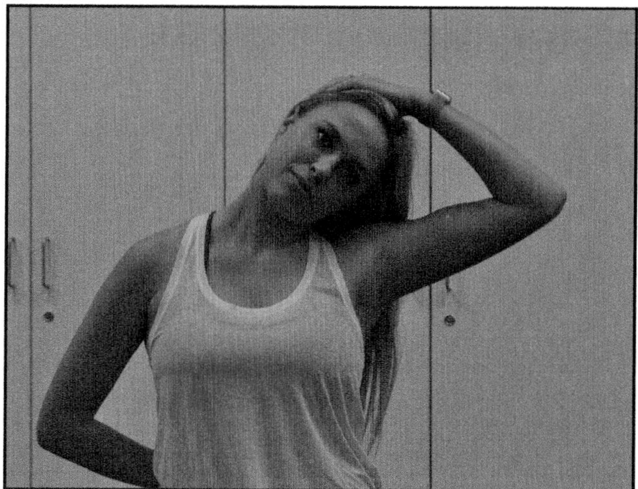

**Figure 12-20.** An upper trapezius stretch.

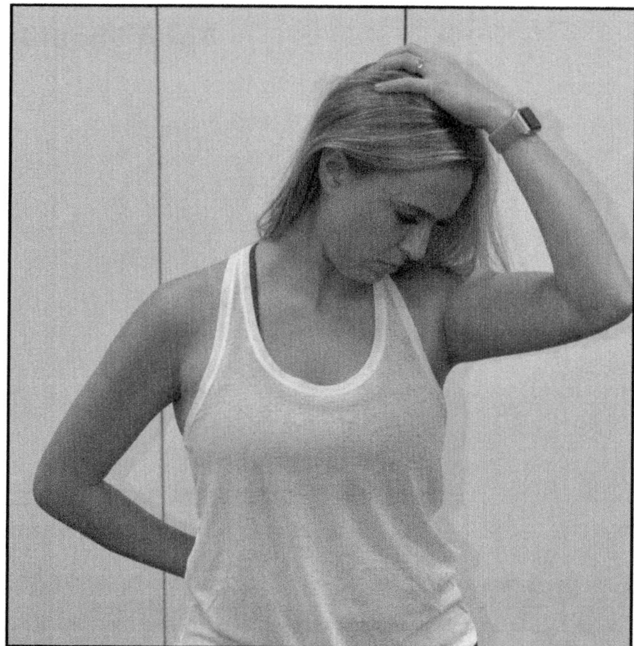

**Figure 12-21.** A levator scapulae stretch.

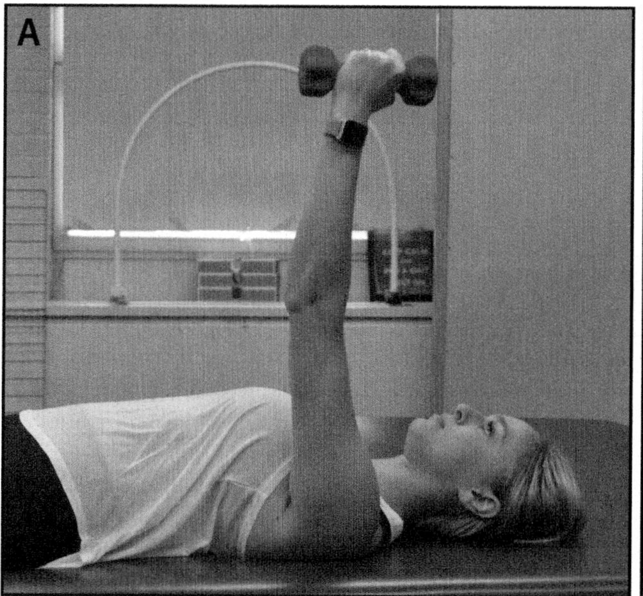

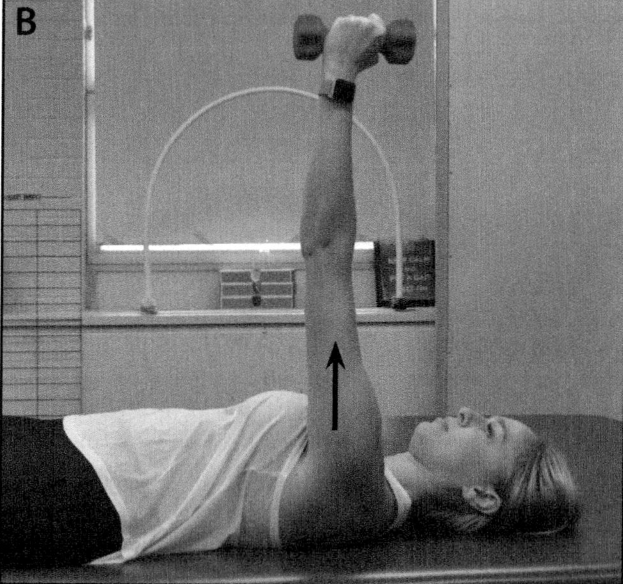

**Figure 12-22.** (A) The scapular protraction OKC-resisted exercise starting position. (B) The scapular protraction end position.

## *Conservative Rehabilitation Management*

Mild to moderate cases of shoulder arthritis are usually managed with physical therapy, targeting the primary goals of reducing pain and regaining functional mobility and strength. When starting an exercise program, the physical therapist assistant should focus on both mobility and strengthening exercises that minimize the patient's pain while considering the impairments identified and the current ROM and MMT documented by the evaluating physical therapist. Forward head posture, shoulder internal rotation or excessive scapular protraction, and thoracic kyphosis may be contributing factors to the patient's increased pain and/or decreased ROM. Postural deviations need to be corrected with the appropriate stretching and strengthening exercises (refer to Chapter 7) before working on increasing shoulder AROM because faulty posture can create shoulder impingement.

These patients can follow the phase 1 and 2 exercise sequences shown in Table 12-11 as long as posture has been addressed and pain is controlled. Exercise progressions can vary from patient to patient depending on the patient's level of irritability and/or residual pain after the exercises; exercise programs should be modified based on the patient's response (for soreness guidelines, see Chapter 6). Clinicians should avoid giving patients multiple new exercises during a treatment session; if too many exercises are added,

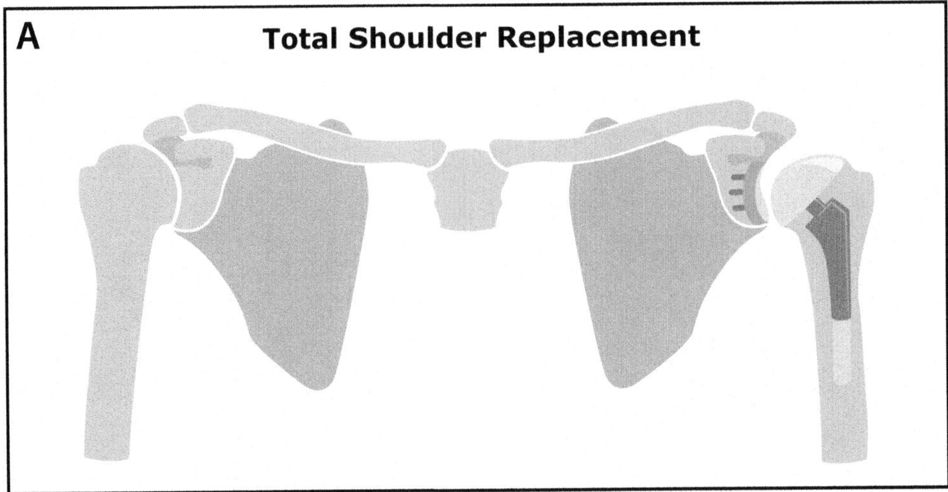


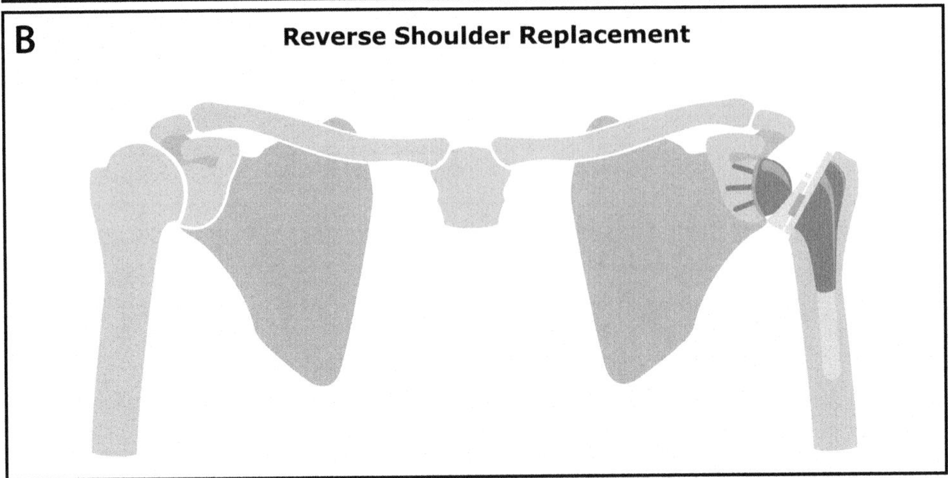


**Figure 12-23.** (A) TSA (juliawhite/Shutterstock.com). (B) RTSA (juliawhite/Shutterstock.com).

it is difficult to determine which ones may have increased or created symptoms. Continually monitoring patients for proper form, joint mechanics, and pain level during exercise performance is important because weak muscles fatigue rapidly. Muscle fatigue affects arthrokinematics, which can lead to injury and pain.

Conservative management does not stop the progression of osteoarthritis, but it can be effective at reducing pain, restoring ROM, and improving strength and ST mechanics, which may delay or eliminate the need for surgical intervention. Physical therapy is advised before surgery and is beneficial to correct faulty posture, improve ROM, strengthen the surrounding muscles, and reduce the chance of developing contractures.

## Types of Shoulder Arthroplasties and Postoperative Rehabilitation Management

Patients who fail to conservatively manage shoulder degenerative joint disease may elect to undergo surgery. The most common surgical interventions include arthroscopic debridement for younger patients (55 to 60 years old) who present with moderate pain and shoulder arthroplasty for more severe cases. Arthroscopic debridement involves resurfacing of the joint surfaces, providing significant pain relief for those with less severe/debilitating conditions. This procedure can improve function for a while but does not stop the degenerative joint disease process; it may delay the need for a shoulder replacement.[41,42]

Shoulder arthroplasty is indicated when patients experience a significant reduction in ROM and strength, increased persistent pain (especially night pain), and RC arthropathy due to severe osteoarthritic changes, joint instability, and/or muscle insufficiency.[43] Three types of shoulder arthroplasties that are commonly performed include hemiarthroplasty (only the humeral head is replaced), total shoulder arthroplasty (TSA), and reverse total shoulder arthroplasty (RTSA). TSA (Figure 12-23A) includes replacing both the humeral head and the glenoid fossa (using a cuplike prosthesis). However, when the RC muscles are damaged, RTSA is indicated. During RTSA, the convex surface of the prosthesis is inserted into the glenoid, and the concave surface is fixed onto the proximal end of the humerus (Figure 12-23B).[41-43] An open procedure is used for all 3 of these surgical interventions, and the subscapularis is detached and reattached during surgery.

## *Postoperative Rehabilitation*

The physical therapist assistant needs to adhere to postoperative precautions and exercise guidelines for both TSA and RTSA because some of them are different. However, in both cases, it is imperative that the subscapularis muscle specifically be protected for several weeks after surgery.[26,42-46] Compliance with precautions is critical to healing. Several ROM precautions should be maintained well beyond the initial phase. Specific precautions typically included postoperatively are listed in Table 12-13. In addition to procedure-based precautions, patients who undergo either procedure also typically have the following restrictions:

- Wear a sling/shoulder immobilizer as directed by a physician; this usually includes during sleep for 3 to 6 weeks.
- No reaching behind the back (eg, dressing, toileting)
- No stretching (PROM is not stretching)
- No PROM beyond safe ranges determined by the physician or as listed in Table 12-13
- No driving (determined by the physician and usually restricted until at least week 5 or 6 postoperatively)
- Keep all activities at waist height (computer work, writing, and eating with the surgical arm may be prohibited based on the surgeon's protocol)

After surgery, TSA and RTSA patients are usually immobilized for 4 to 6 weeks, respectively, to allow for appropriate healing and protection.[42-46] A common type of shoulder immobilization includes an abduction pillow with the shoulder positioned anywhere between 15 and 20 degrees of abduction after RTSA.[45] After TSA, a sling or other type of shoulder immobilizer is used depending on the surgeon's preference.[44-46]

A 2019 systematic review of 16 studies provided a general consensus for rehabilitation guidelines for TSA and RTSA.[46] Physical therapy will typically be initiated by the surgeon sometime between weeks 2 and 4 to allow gentle PROM of the shoulder and AROM for joints above and below the shoulder (cervical spine, elbow, wrist, and hand).[26,44-46] Physical therapy interventions and precautions are most commonly dictated by the surgeon's protocol. The suggested rehabilitation guidelines for TSA and RTSA are listed in Table 12-13; these suggestions summarize several sources and research reports.[26,44-46] The assistant should defer to the physician's specific rehabilitation protocol.

During the course of care, the physical therapist assistant should not only monitor the patient during treatment but also check with the patient for any increases in resting or night pain and notify the supervising physical therapist of changes.

# Adhesive Capsulitis: A Mobility Classification

The most common diagnosis under the mobility classification is **adhesive capsulitis** (also referred to as *frozen shoulder*). Patients in this classification are identified by the primary need to regain ROM of the shoulder. Adhesive capsulitis is characterized by a progressive loss of both active and passive shoulder mobility that can last for 1 to 3 years.[47-49]

The etiology of adhesive capsulitis is unknown but has been linked to diabetes and other metabolic conditions, such as hypothyroidism. There is a significantly higher prevalence of adhesive capsulitis in both men (38%) and women (23%) with diabetes compared with their age-matched counterparts (6.5% in men and 4.7% in women) without diabetes.[47] However, it is most prevalent in women 40 to 65 years old, and it tends to resolve over time.[47] When an arm injury or medical event such as a stroke occurs, immobilization or disuse can also lead to adhesive capsulitis. Active external rotation is usually the first motion lost followed by progressive loss of ROM in all planes. Patients commonly report pain before motion loss.[26,47-49]

There are 4 stages of progression for adhesive capsulitis. During the first stage, patients usually experience sharp pain at end range and often describe feeling "achy" at rest and sleep. This stage may last up to 3 months. The second stage lasts between 3 to 9 months and is referred to as the *freezing* or *painful stage*. During this stage, pain becomes more persistent and intense, with all ranges limited after the shoulder capsular pattern. Stage 3 is known as the *frozen stage* because capsular adhesions and fibrotic tissue have developed, severely limiting the patient's motion in all directions and resulting in shoulder musculature atrophy. This stage can last for 9 to 15 months. The thawing stage is the final stage; in this stage, pain tends to lessen, and there is a gradual reduction in ROM limitations. Symptoms do not always fully resolve, and some patients may not regain full ROM.[26,47,49]

Physical therapy interventions can help reduce pain and muscle guarding and restore shoulder motion, strength, and neuromuscular control. As shoulder mobility improves, strengthening of the RC and ST muscles is indicated to regain normal force couple sequencing, promoting functional return and preventing long-term disability (see Table 12-11).

**Table 12-13**

Suggested Rehabilitation Guidelines for Total Shoulder Arthroplasty and Reverse Total Shoulder Arthroplasty

| Maximal Protection<br>0 to 4 Weeks (TSA)<br>0 to 6 Weeks (RTSA) | Moderate Protection<br>4 to 12 Weeks (TSA)<br>6 to 12/16 Weeks (RTSA) | Minimal Protection<br>12+ Weeks (TSA)<br>12+/16+ Weeks (RTSA) |
|---|---|---|
| PRICE: Immobilize 4 to 6 weeks, cryotherapy for pain and edema control, and grade I and II joint mobilizations<br>TSA: Sling for 3 to 4 weeks can be removed as per protocol (ie, during the day, bathing) and to provide support.[26,44,46]<br>RTSA: Abduction splint, 24 hours per day for 4 to 6 weeks but can be removed for pendulums several times a day[26,44,45]<br>Non–weight bearing: No leaning on surgical UE<br>Supine positioning: Immobilizer/sling or arm supported, elbow flexed 90 degrees, shoulder slight abduction, flexion 10 to 20 degrees, head of bed 30 degrees<br>TSA PROM restrictions: PROM 90 to 130 degrees flexion or in plane of scapula, 15 to 30 degrees of external rotation. No extension past neutral (anterior aspect of the trunk); horizontal abduction past neutral[26,46]<br>RTSA PROM restrictions: 60 to 90 degrees of flexion or in plane of scapula, external rotation to neutral. No extension past neutral or anterior aspect of the trunk; no horizontal abduction past neutral[45,46] | TSA ROM restrictions: PROM 135 to 150 degrees flexion or in plane of scapula, 33 to 45 degrees external rotation, and AROM as tolerated with good arthrokinematics.[26,45,46] Begin AROM for internal rotation after week 6 to 7. No extension past neutral (or beyond anterior aspect of the trunk).[26]<br>RTSA ROM restrictions: 90 to 120 degrees of flexion in plane of scapula, external rotation 20 to 30 degrees. Progress to AAROM (various positions); initiate AROM as tolerated with elbow flexed.[26,44-46] No extension past neutral (anterior aspect of the trunk). No horizontal abduction past neutral.[26]<br>Note: Delay internal and external rotation isometrics until after week 8 for TSA and after week 12 for RTSA to protect RC[44,45] | TSA AROM: Full shoulder AROM as tolerated[2,44,46]<br>RTSA limited 12 weeks or more: AAROM⇨AROM pain free as tolerated. No extension or internal rotation past neutral.[26,46] No combined extension, adduction, or internal rotation. Weight bearing initiated week 12.[26,46]<br>TSA lifting: Limited 10 to 15 lb; gradual return to function[26,46]<br>RTSA lifting: Limited to unilateral 6 lb, bilateral 10 to 15 lb, gradual return to functional activities[26,44,45]<br>*(continued)* |

**Table 12-13 (continued)**

## Suggested Rehabilitation Guidelines for Total Shoulder Arthroplasty and Reverse Total Shoulder Arthroplasty

| Maximal Protection<br>0 to 4 Weeks (TSA)<br>0 to 6 Weeks (RTSA) | Moderate Protection<br>4 to 12 Weeks (TSA)<br>6 to 12/16 Weeks (RTSA) | Minimal Protection<br>12+ Weeks (TSA)<br>12+/16+ Weeks (RTSA) |
|---|---|---|
| TSA exercises:<br>PROM as per restrictions<br>Pendulums<br>Scapula muscle setting progress to submaximal isometrics<br>AROM: Cervical spine, hand, wrist, elbow<br>Week 2 (end): scapular motion, stabilization activities<br>Self AAROM: Wand, pulley week 3 to 4<br>AAROM supine 2 to 3 weeks progress to sitting<br>Shoulder rolls to move the scapulae<br>OKC submaximal isometrics of deltoids in scapular plane[26,46]<br>Gentle muscle setting excluding internal rotation; elbow flexed, shoulder in plane of scapula or neutral[25,46]<br>RTSA exercises:<br>AROM scapula and distal joints only<br>PROM as per restrictions, pendulums<br>Scapula isometrics retraction, depression | TSA exercises:<br>Light resisted isometric strengthening<br>Resisted scapular stabilization<br>Begin light CKC stabilization exercises (low resistance)<br>Dynamic strengthening elbow/wrist<br>Begin upper bike ergometer: Light resistance for muscle endurance<br>RTSA exercises:<br>Progress to submaximal isometrics (no internal rotation until week 12); dynamic strengthening elbow/wrist.<br>Note: Non–weight bearing positions through week 12[26,45] | TSA exercises:<br>Progress progressive resistive exercise in functional patterns (low load, high reps); PNF<br>CKC and progress as tolerated<br>RTSA exercises:<br>Begin CKC gradual progression[45]<br>Progress isometric to isotonic with light progressive resistive exercises single planes then in functional patterns[26,44,45]<br>Begin upper bike ergometer light resistance for muscle endurance |

PRICE = protection, rest, ice, compression, elevation.

When treating these patients, the physical therapist assistant should consider the patient's level of tissue irritability. Any exercise that increases tissue irritability is counterproductive and is likely to increase pain, muscle guarding, and a greater reduction in ROM. The goal of rehabilitation should be to control pain and muscle guarding while attempting to increase ROM. Patient progression should be gradual, keeping the patient's level of tissue irritability to a minimum. One high-quality study reported that gentle ROM in pain-free ranges and pendulum exercises were more effective than aggressive therapy. Another study indicated that ROM exercises in ranges with no or minimal pain combined with pain-free ST strengthening were more effective at increasing range than programs that did not include ST strengthening.[47,48]

Patients should understand their diagnosis and be instructed on activity modifications, methods of pain control (ie, heat and ice), and the performance of exercises that do not increase pain.[47] Exercises performed in the clinic should be included as part of the HEP. The clinician should teach patients pain-free supported arm positions during sitting, standing, walking, and sleeping. Faulty postural positions should be avoided, and using the involved UE as normally as possible in the pain-free ranges is encouraged. UE activities should initially be kept below shoulder height to avoid painful arcs. As the patient regains full AROM, strengthening can be progressed to above shoulder height first in single planes and then progressing to multiplanar and functional movements consistent with daily demands.

### Other Mobility Classification Conditions

There are other injuries/pathologies that fall under this classification. Fractures to the proximal humerus, clavicle, and scapula all require different immobilization periods and are based on the type of fracture, site of fracture, age, sex, and past medical history.

Proximal humeral fractures are the third most common fracture observed in older adults (prevalence of 250/100,000) in the United States and most commonly occur from falling. Because a good percentage of these fractures are minimally displaced (50% to 65%), nonsurgical management is a common course of treatment for older patients. However, there are humeral fractures that may require surgical intervention to stabilize the humeral fragments. There is no consensus regarding which criteria determine the use of surgical vs nonsurgical intervention. Physical therapy is usually initiated 3 to 6 weeks after injury, and the timeline is dependent on whether the intervention was nonsurgical or surgical. Physical therapy typically starts once the fracture demonstrates radiologic healing or once surgically stabilized.[50] As with all shoulder protocols discussed in this chapter, restoring normal shoulder mobility and strength so patients can return to their prior level of function is the goal, but the progression is dependent on the patient's levels of irritability and good ST/GH rhythm.

AC joint separations account for more than 40% of all shoulder injuries and are more commonly observed in the younger population and athletes.[51] The joint can separate due to direct trauma to the joint or a FOOSH. Other causes include falling on the lateral aspect of the shoulder with the arm adducted, sport-related collisions, or motor vehicle accidents. Technically, there are 6 grades of separation, but grades I through III are the most common. Grade I (AC ligament sprain with no clavicular displacement) and grade II separations (AC ligament torn and coracoclavicular ligament sprained with some displacement of the clavicle) are treated nonsurgically, and patients are placed in a sling to avoid stressing the ligaments. A grade III separation (AC and coracoclavicular ligaments are torn) may require surgery but is sometimes treated nonsurgically. This is often determined based on the percentage of clavicular displacement.[51]

A grade I separation requires rest, and patients usually return to normal activities in about 2 weeks. Physical therapy interventions for grades II and III are initially the same; patients are in a sling for 1 to 4 weeks, and modalities are used for pain control. Interventions are progressed more cautiously/slowly for patients with grade III separations. Gentle PROM can be initiated early in the rehabilitation process for nonoperative patients or approximately 4 weeks after injury/surgical repair. As with all shoulder rehabilitation programs, the physical therapist assistants should monitor patients during all exercises to limit the risk of shoulder impingement as ROM is restored. Patients with a grade III separation can usually return to normal activities between 6 and 12 weeks after the initial injury.[51] If patients return to sports, the joint should be protected with a brace and/or padding.

## Introduction to the Management and Treatment of Elbow and Forearm Pathologies

Elbow injuries can affect individuals at any age and occur due to a traumatic event or overuse. Falls can cause elbow dislocations and fractures, especially a FOOSH. Overuse injuries are commonly seen in those who participate in throwing activities, racket sports, or golf, but painters, plumbers, and carpenters can also experience pain because of the repetitive nature of these occupations.

The elbow is a very stable joint, with less motion available compared with the shoulder. Elbow and forearm motions are important for performing activities such as carrying objects, opening doors, turning keys, eating, reaching, and using hand tools. Limited elbow motion or arm strength can make these functional activities difficult. Restrictions in forearm motion have an impact on shoulder joint mobility. For example, a limitation in forearm supination increases the need for shoulder adduction and external (lateral) rotation as a compensatory motion (or

**Table 12-14**

Elbow, Forearm, and Wrist Range of Motion[4]

| Elbow, Forearm, and Wrist Motion | Degrees |
|---|---|
| Elbow flexion | 150 |
| Elbow extension | 0 |
| Forearm pronation | 80 |
| Forearm supination | 80 |
| Wrist flexion | 80 |
| Wrist extension | 70 |
| Wrist abduction (radial deviation) | 20 |
| Wrist adduction (ulnar deviation) | 30 |
| Note: There is variation in normative values based on sex and age. Values are based on the American Academy of Orthopedic Surgeons. | |

substitution patterns) to having your palm face upward. The opposite shoulder actions occur when there are limitations in pronation.

**Quick Class Activity**

Hold your forearm in neutral so your thumb is pointing upward. Without pronating your forearm, try to get the palm of your hand to face the floor. What actions occurred at the shoulder to achieve this task?

## *Clinical Assessment of the Elbow and Forearm*

Part of the physical therapist's initial evaluation includes the patient's MOI; primary complaints; functional limitations; and a thorough history to determine the prior level of function and the onset, location, nature, and behavior of the symptoms. The MOI may help determine the primary diagnosis as well as the secondary structures that may also be involved. The therapist's initial examination typically includes the following:

- Assessment of the elbow resting position in standing, looking for any obvious deformities (eg, excessive varus/valgus)
- A cervical/shoulder screen: the cervical spine and shoulder can refer pain into the elbow, making it essential to clear the joints above the elbow
- Palpation of the common points of tenderness (medial/lateral epicondyles, distal biceps, and triceps tendons)
- ROM testing (AROM and PROM) of the elbow and wrist (Table 12-14)
- MMT for elbow and wrist and grip strength with a dynamometer (Figure 12-24; refer to https://www.sralab.org/rehabilitation-measures for normative values)

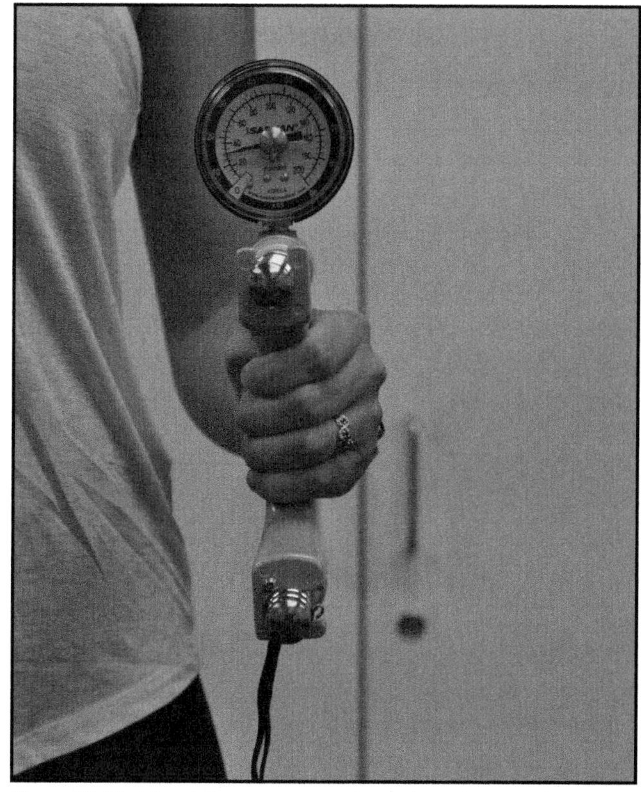

**Figure 12-24.** A hand dynamometer to determine grip strength.

- Special tests to help determine joint stability, tendinopathy, or neuropathy
- Neurodynamic testing of the median, radial, and ulnar nerves
- Notation regarding hand dominance (right or left hand)

The physical therapist assistant should be able to recognize the tests reported in the evaluation. ROM normative values are provided in Table 12-14, and a list of special tests is presented in Table 12-15. Neurodynamic testing related to specific nerves is described in Chapter 11; these techniques may also be used as interventions.

**Table 12-15**

Special Tests for Various Elbow Pathologies

| Special Test | Possible Pathology if Positive |
|---|---|
| Chair push-up test and push-up test[52]* | Posterior lateral rotary instability |
| Valgus stress or moving valgus stress test[52] | Medial collateral ligament (MCL) stability |
| Varus stress test | Lateral collateral ligament stability |
| Golfer's elbow test | Medial epicondylalgia or tendinopathy |
| Resisted tennis elbow test (Cozen's test) | Lateral epicondylalgia or tendinopathy |
| Elbow flexion test | Median nerve distribution involvement |
| Tinel's sign (at the elbow) | Ulnar nerve distribution involvement |
| Resisted wrist extension | Radial nerve distribution involvement |

*It is suggested that these tests be performed together for best results.

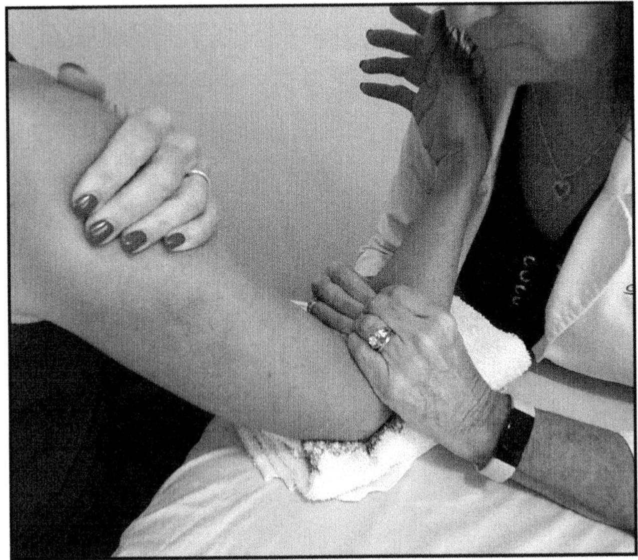

**Figure 12-25.** Elbow joint distraction.

Some special tests have good sensitivity and specificity to determine elbow instability. The moving valgus test is performed with the patient sitting, the shoulder abducted to 90 degrees and maximally externally rotated, and the elbow maximally flexed. The clinician applies a constant valgus force as the elbow is extended to 30 degrees of flexion. A positive test produces pain over the medial aspect of the elbow between 70 and 120 degrees of elbow flexion. To reconfirm the positive test, the same valgus pressure should be applied as the elbow is moved back into flexion. This test has 100% sensitivity and 75% specificity for determining MCL injury.[52] The chair push-up and push-up test have 87.5% sensitivity when using one test and 100% sensitivity when both are performed. A chair push-up test is performed starting with the patient sitting in a chair with the elbows abducted or turned outward and flexed to 90 degrees and their hands on the armrests with the forearms supinated. The patient should use the arms to push off, creating elbow joint loading and valgus stress. To perform the push-up test, the patient assumes a push-up position with the hands turned and the fingers pointing laterally. These tests determine if posterior lateral rotary instability causes pain and apprehension. If the radial head is unstable, it may dislocate.[52]

## *Elbow and Forearm Joint Mobilization Techniques*

Hypomobile humeroulnar, humeroradial, and proximal and distal radioulnar joints often result from elbow immobilization and can limit ROM. The physical therapist determines the type of joint mobilization technique or neurodynamic stretching most beneficial to improve motion. If neurodynamic nerve glides are indicated, they should target the specific nerve distribution causing the patient's symptoms. Specific wrist and hand nerve glides (discussed later in this chapter and illustrated in Figures 12-50 and 12-52) can improve mobility.

Some basic elbow and forearm mobilization techniques are discussed here, but the physical therapist assistant should not perform any of these techniques without the direct consent of the physical therapist before treatment (if permitted by state practice act/laws/statutes).

### Elbow Joint Distraction

Elbow joint distraction is used for general elbow mobility. The resting position for the elbow is 70 degrees of flexion and 10 degrees of forearm supination. The patient is usually positioned in a supine position, but the technique can be performed in a sitting position. Place a towel under the distal humerus just proximal to the olecranon process. Stabilize the humerus and support the forearm against the clinician's shoulder (Figure 12-25). Distract both the ulna and radius on a slight downward angle to take up the slack.

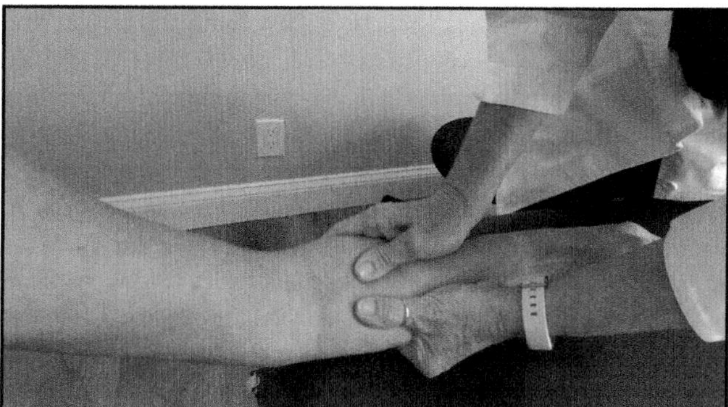

**Figure 12-26.** Humeroradial glides. Dorsal glides of the radius increase elbow extension, and proximal glides increase flexion.

### Humeroradial Glides

The purpose of humeroradial glides is to increase elbow flexion and/or extension. The concave radius glides on the convex surface of the capitulum on the humerus. Extend the elbow and supinate the forearm to the patient's end range. The patient should stabilize the humerus with their other hand, and the clinician can stabilize the ulna with their left hand (Figure 12-26). The clinician pushes downward (performing a dorsal glide) with the right hand at the point indicated by the clinician's right thumb on the radial head. Dorsal glides increase elbow extension. To increase elbow flexion, the clinician maintains the same hand placements but pulls upward on the radius with the fingers (of the right hand) to perform a volar glide.

### Proximal and Distal Radioulnar Glides

Proximal and distal radioulnar glides are used to increase forearm pronation and supination. Proximally, the convex head of the radius sits in the concave radial notch on the ulna. Distally, the concave ulnar notch of the radius articulates with the convex ulna head. The resting position for the proximal radioulnar joint is 70 degrees of elbow flexion and 30 degrees of forearm supination.

The patient's ulna is supported on the table with the thumb side facing upward. The clinician stabilizes the ulna with the left hand and uses the right hand to create a volar glide to increase supination and a dorsal glide to increase pronation as illustrated in Figure 12-27. For distal radioulnar glides, the patient's forearm is supinated 10 degrees. The clinician stabilizes the distal ulna with the left hand and uses the right hand to create a volar glide to increase pronation or a dorsal glide to increase supination (Figure 12-28).

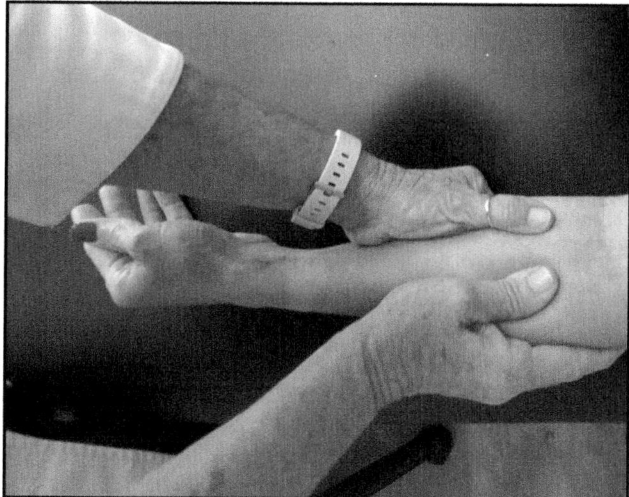

**Figure 12-27.** Proximal radioulnar glides. Volar glides increase supination, and dorsal glides increases pronation.

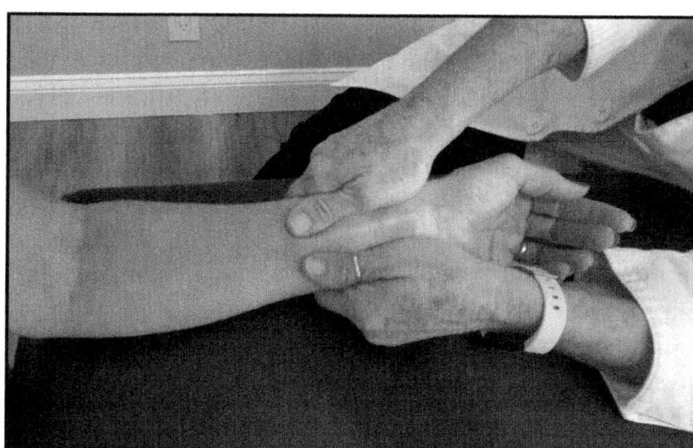

**Figure 12-28.** Distal radioulnar joint glides.

## *Treatment and Rehabilitation for Elbow and Forearm Diagnoses*

### Treatment and Rehabilitation Management of Elbow Dislocations

Because elbow dislocations occur from direct trauma (ie, FOOSH), they can sometimes result in an elbow fracture. The most common position of the outstretched arm during a fall includes elbow extension and forearm pronation with the shoulder abducted and flexed. The combination of these positions significantly increases elbow valgus stress and joint compression (axial loading), causing injury to the MCL/UCL.[53]

As with shoulder dislocations, the severity, direction of dislocation, associated soft tissue damage, and/or fracture must be considered when treating patients with elbow dislocations. Simple dislocations are reduced nonoperatively, and the patient's arm is placed in a sling for 7 to 10 days. If the joint is stable, patients can usually start AROM exercises immediately. More severe dislocations reduced nonoperatively may present with a more unstable joint; these patients are placed in a sling or brace for 3 to 4 weeks to rest. In either case, wrist and gripping/squeezing exercises are encouraged while immobilized. Scapula isometrics and shoulder AROM in all planes can be performed if cleared by the physician.

Once mobility exercises are permitted, physical therapist assistants should work on regaining elbow/forearm full PROM. Gaining full elbow extension is of primary importance to prevent flexion contractures. If this is not achieved after several weeks, more aggressive static stretching (ie, using light cuff weights around the wrist for a prolonged time) or using a static extension brace may be indicated.

## Considerations for the Physical Therapist Assistant: After Elbow Dislocations

- Monitor the patient for evidence of neurovascular signs or symptoms.
- All activities that increase valgus stress on the elbow should be avoided for at least 6 weeks.
- Lifting, pushing, and pulling activities are contraindicated for several weeks.
- Shoulder isometric strengthening exercises are safe to perform, except for internal and external rotation because of the increased stress on the elbow. Avoid these motions for at least 6 weeks.

After about 6 weeks, patients can start strengthening with light weights and begin using the upper bike ergometer. Elbow, forearm, and wrist strengthening can be progressed as tolerated using weights and/or resistance bands (Table 12-16). Placing the hand (gloved) in a bucket of rice (just proximal to the wrist) and moving the fingers, wrist, and forearm in all directions (for 2- to 3-minute bouts) is a good way to strengthen the muscles and increase muscular endurance (Figure 12-29).

Shoulder and scapular muscle strengthening for all motions should be progressed without stressing the elbow. Internal and external rotation exercises are typically permitted by week 6 or 8 if AROM is tolerated. Gentle strengthening can be initiated using light weights as per the physician. CKC activities can be introduced and progressed gradually based on the patient's pain tolerance. Patients can usually return to normal functional activities by week 12 and more demanding sports or work activities between 4 and 6 months.

Patients requiring surgical repair after an elbow joint dislocation are typically splinted for 4 to 6 weeks. The splint may be removed (per the physician) for AROM of the wrist and forearm. Shoulder pendulum exercises, scapular exercises, and wrist/grip AROM are usually permitted in the early days postoperatively while in the brace/splint. Exercise progressions outlined in the physician's protocol are based on the joint stability attained with the repair.

### Treatment and Rehabilitation Management for Elbow Fractures

There are different types of elbow fractures. A supracondylar fracture is a transverse disruption of the distal third of the humerus and is the most common elbow fracture often seen in young children (ages 5 to 7 years).[54] These fractures are commonly treated with a nonoperative closed reduction and immobilized for 4 to 6 weeks. A fracture of both humeral condyles (called an *intercondylar fracture*) and radial head fractures involving the radius are other examples of elbow fractures. Elbow fracture medical management and physical therapy progression are highly dependent on several factors, including the site and type of fracture, the associated dislocation, soft tissue and nerve injury, and the patient's age and past medical history. A simple, nondisplaced fracture will benefit from early mobilization, whereas more complex fractures that may require open reduction and internal fixation surgery will need a longer period of immobilization to rest/heal.

Once cleared for physical therapy, the physical therapist assistant should follow the physician's protocol and POC, which usually begins with ROM exercises to regain lost motion due to injury and/or immobilization. Mobility and strengthening exercises for joints proximal and distal to the elbow are also initiated based on the patient's current status, which is found in the physical therapist's initial evaluation.

The physical therapist assistant should be aware of complications that can occur after any fracture including a nonunion or malunion, joint contracture, and vascular compromise. Vascular injury can lead to compartment syndrome due to bleeding and swelling, which increases pressure in the area. If this complication is not treated in a timely manner, it can lead to ischemia called **Volkmann ischemic contracture.** Volkmann contracture is characterized by a flexed elbow, pronated forearm, wrist flexion, and MCP joint extension.[54] The assistant needs to be alert to the signs and symptoms (refer to Key Safety Considerations: Recognizing Signs of Vascular and Nerve Compromise) and report to the physical therapist immediately for urgent follow-up with the physician. This problem can occur during any phase of the rehabilitation process.

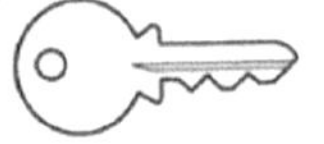

## Key Safety Consideration: Recognizing Signs of Vascular and Nerve Compromise[54]

- Loss of radial pulse
- Severe forearm pain
- Severe finger pain and decreased mobility
- Discoloration of the hand (purplish color)
- Paresthesia followed by loss of sensation

The malunion of a supracondylar fracture affecting the child's growth plate can result in a cubitus varus deformity called *gunstock deformity*. This deformity used to be a common occurrence (58% of cases), but the incidence has significantly decreased because of newer minimally invasive pinning techniques when surgically fixing the fracture.[54]

**Table 12-16**

Elbow, Forearm, and Wrist/Hand Exercises

| ROM Exercises and Stretches | OKC and CKC Strengthening | Neuromuscular/Plyometric Exercises |
|---|---|---|
| Supine passive biceps stretch to gain elbow extension<br>Biceps stretch in doorway but with the forearm pronated<br>Triceps stretch<br>Wrist extensor stretch<br>Wrist flexor stretch | Isometrics/multiangle isometrics<br>• Elbow: Flexion (forearm supinated, pronated, neutral)/extension<br>• Forearm: Pronation/supination<br>• Wrist/hand: Flexion/extension<br>OKC exercises (using resistance bands or weights)<br>• Three-way elbow flexion: Palm up, down, and in neutral<br>• Elbow extension for triceps brachii: Prone, supine, sitting/standing<br>• Rice bucket: For forearm, wrist, and finger strengthening<br>• Wrist strengthening: Flexion/extension<br>• Forearm pronation/supination<br>• Ball squeezes or gripper<br>• Finger extensor strengthening using rubber bands<br>CKC exercises<br>• Push-up progression<br>• Pull-ups with forearms pronated and supinated | PNF exercises: Manual resistance, using resistance bands or weights<br>Ball tosses: Use weighted balls self-toss supine, against a wall, against mini-trampoline (1 to 2 hands), passes to a partner<br>Body blade for entire upper quarter using 1 or both hands: Holding blade vertically/horizontally<br>Stair stepper with UEs<br>Step-ups/downs on a step while in push-up position |

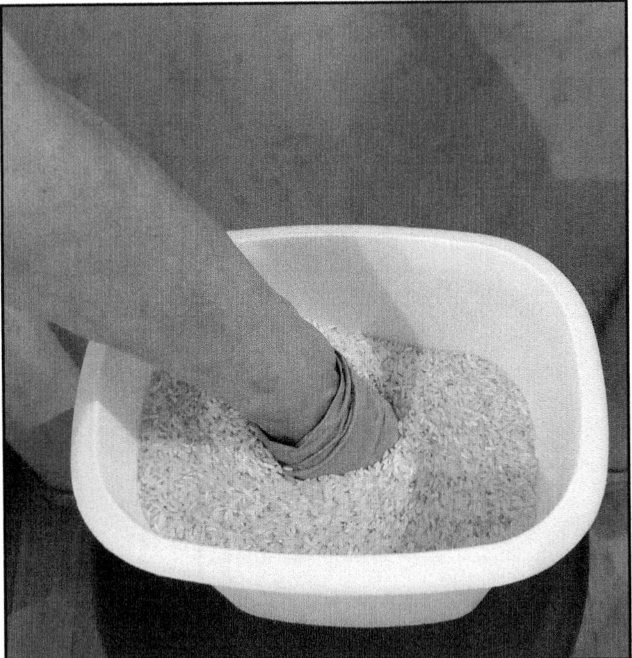

**Figure 12-29.** Finger, wrist, and forearm muscle strengthening using a rice bucket.

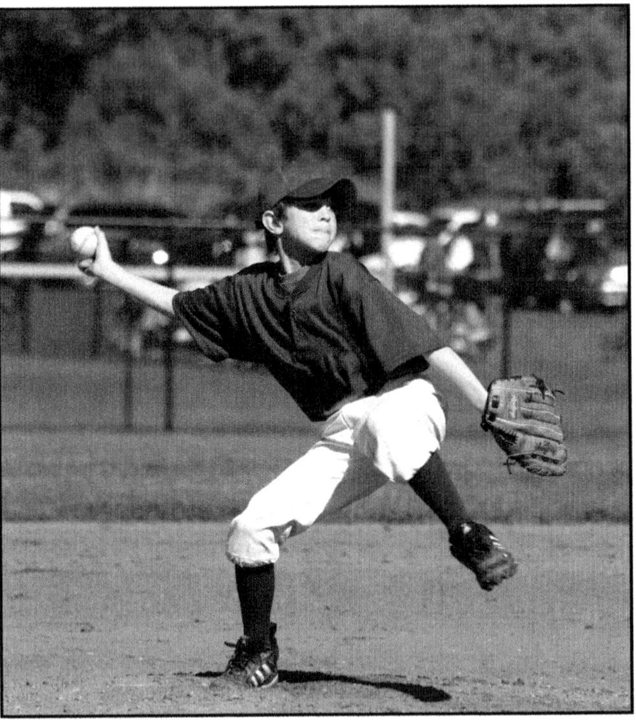

**Figure 12-30.** Little League elbow (sonya etchison/Shutterstock.com).

## Conservative Treatment and Rehabilitation Management of Ulnar Collateral Ligament Injuries

Injury to the UCL usually occurs due to an excessive valgus force to the medial side of the elbow. A traumatic event (ie, a FOOSH causing elbow dislocation or fracture) and repetitive microtrauma commonly seen in overhead throwing athletes (eg, baseball) are the most common causes of UCL injuries. The repetitive nature of throwing in baseball places significant valgus stress on the medial aspect of the elbow with each throw during the acceleration phase.[55] Sports such as tennis and golf also place significant valgus stress on the elbow.[55] Approximately 3 million children play baseball in the United States, and a significant number continue on to play high school and college ball.[56] Medial elbow pain associated with overloading the medial aspect of the growing elbow in children/adolescents is referred to as *Little League elbow* (Figure 12-30). This condition can lead to UCL tissue breakdown, which is occasionally (but not commonly) linked to avulsion fractures of the medial epicondyle.[57] Improper training and overuse usually cause Little League elbow in young athletes; surgical intervention is rare in children. A 4- to 6-week rest from activity and the use of cryotherapy to reduce pain and inflammation combined with gentle pain-free wrist and elbow ROM allows injured tissues to heal during the initial course of treatment.[55,57] Pain-free submaximal isometrics for all wrist and forearm motions can also be started during this time.[55]

The physical therapist will identify movement restrictions and/or muscular weakness throughout the upper quarter; these should be addressed first. Full pain-free ROM for the elbow, wrist, and forearm should be achieved by week 6. Strengthening the elbow, wrist (see Table 12-16), shoulder, and scapular muscles can be initiated at this time. Resistance exercises should be progressed to simulate the throwing motion using PNF. Neuromuscular control exercises are also important for the UE because muscle fatigue has been associated with poor neuromuscular control leading to reinjury.[55,58] Lower extremity strengthening (eg, lunges, squats) and core stabilization exercises are extremely beneficial and should begin early in the rehabilitation process because these do not stress the injured elbow. These strengthening exercises are important to reduce excessive strain on the injured elbow and will improve muscle efficiency once throwing resumes. Once cleared by the physician, the young athlete can slowly return to throwing but should follow age-specific throwing guidelines (ie, pitch count limits per game, per week, and per season).[58] Participating in the Thrower's Ten exercise program (refer to the Suggested Resources section at the end of the chapter) and practicing good throwing mechanics[59] are key to decreasing the risk of reinjury. Specific pitching progression programs for teens from 13 to 14 years old are also available in recent research.[55]

Professional baseball pitchers usually have about 7 degrees less elbow extension and 5.5 degrees less flexion on their throwing arm compared with their nondominant arm, which is consistent with elbow muscle contractures.[55] After a UCL injury, these patients are typically immobilized with a brace, but pain-free motion and submaximal isometrics for the elbow and wrist are encouraged early in the rehabilitation process. Nonoperative management for a UCL injury is similar to Little League elbow rehabilitation, and the rate of progression through the intervention program depends on the severity of the injury to the ligament. There is limited evidence regarding nonoperative management for UCL injuries; however, the general consensus in the literature finds that addressing strength and neuromuscular control for the upper quarter, core, and lower extremities in throwers is advised to reduce the forces through the elbow for several months, even before considering surgery as an option.[55,58,60]

## Ulnar Collateral Ligament Repair and Postoperative Rehabilitation Management

Patients who fail conservative management for a UCL injury and who are unable to regain preinjury functional abilities are usually candidates for surgery to either repair or reconstruct the ligament. The anterior portion (bundle) of the UCL is the structure that is most commonly involved (Figure 12-31). The UCL is a static stabilizer along with the flexor carpi ulnaris and the flexor digitorum superficialis (dynamic stabilizers). It resists most of the valgus stresses that occur during the throwing motion between 30 degrees and 90 degrees of elbow flexion.[60]

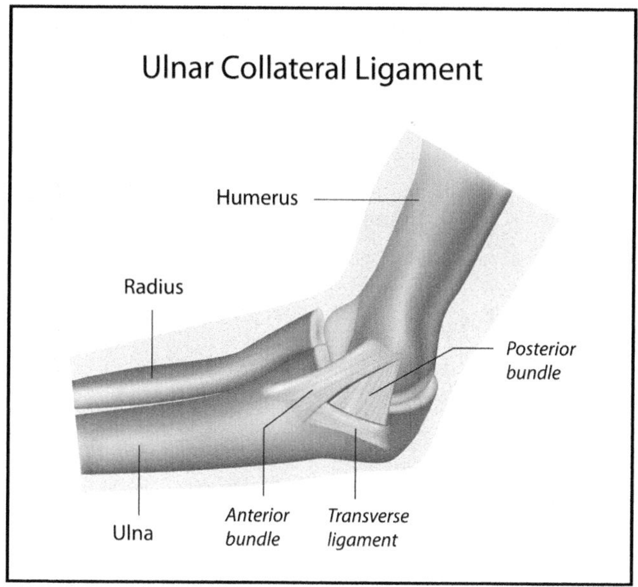


**Figure 12-31.** UCLs. The anterior bundle is most commonly stressed during overhead throwing activities, and graft replacement is placed in this location (Alila Medical Media/Shutterstock.com).

A UCL reconstruction is called *Tommy John surgery.* The basic procedure includes drilling holes in the ulna and medial epicondyle and securing a tendon graft (from the palmaris longus, gracilis, or other autograft tissues) to the bones. In many instances, the ulnar nerve is moved to protect it.[55,60]

The surgeon's protocol dictates the rehabilitative process after reconstruction. Patients are usually put in a hinged brace locked in elbow flexion at 90 degrees for the first week, and then PROM is progressed to full motion in the brace over the next 4 to 6 weeks.[55,60] Because a pitcher's ROM on their throwing arm is less than their nondominant arm before surgery, the primary goal is to reach (at least) equal preoperative measurements after UCL repair in order for the pitcher to return to play.[55]

During the first week, wrist ROM can be initiated, and then submaximal wrist isometrics and gripping exercises can begin in week 2. Between weeks 4 and 8, wrist isometrics can progress to lightweight isotonic exercises, whereas shoulder and scapular stabilization exercises can also be started early in the rehabilitation process. The Thrower's Ten exercise program[59] can be implemented around week 6, and more progressive and dynamic stabilization exercises for the elbow joint can begin at week 9. Eccentric and plyometric exercises can begin around week 12 and an interval throwing program at week 16, assuming that there is appropriate healing and that this is consistent with the physician's protocol. Players do not usually return to competitive baseball until about 9 months after surgery.[55,60] Elbow, forearm, wrist, and hand exercise progressions are listed in Table 12-16. Pictures for wrist stretches, tendon glides, and nerve glides are shown in Figures 12-33, 12-37, and 12-39, respectively. Elbow, wrist, and hand muscle strengthening exercises are found in Figures 12-60 through 12-62.

## Neuropathic Pain: Cubital Tunnel Syndrome and Conservative Treatment

The groove between the medial epicondyle and the olecranon process or cubital tunnel is the most common site of ulnar nerve impingement or stretching (Figure 12-32A), and irritation to the ulnar nerve at this location is called *cubital tunnel syndrome.* This injury is also common in throwers. The nerve can become stretched during valgus stress at the elbow or entrapped where it enters the forearm between the 2 heads of the flexor carpi ulnaris (see Figure 12-32A).[61] Patients usually complain of tenderness at the medial elbow, paresthesia down to the fourth and fifth digits (Figure 12-32B), and pain with elbow flexion in the acute stage. Patients may report waking at night due to pain because the elbow is commonly flexed when sleeping, which increases nerve compression. If not treated, increased muscle weakness can progress to muscle atrophy of the flexor carpi ulnaris, flexor digitorum profundus, adductor pollicis, third and fourth lumbricals, and interossei, with visual intrinsic hand muscle wasting of the hypothenar eminence. If left untreated, permanent damage to the ulnar nerve can occur.[61]

Conservative rehabilitation management can be effective for patients with minor signs and symptoms. A physical therapist assistant should address cubital tunnel syndrome by first reviewing the impairments identified by the evaluating physical therapist as the underlying cause. Patients should avoid end-range elbow flexion and compression to the medial aspect of the elbow in order to prevent further tissue irritation. Some physicians may prescribe a resting night splint. Passive elbow mobility exercises can help prevent or reduce elbow stiffness. As symptoms subside, neurodynamic ulnar nerve stretches or glides (refer to Chapter 11) can restore normal, pain-free motions. An exercise progression should include elbow and forearm AROM, progressing to resisted motions; putty, stress ball, or gripper squeezes; and resisted finger/wrist/forearm motions in the rice bucket. Cervical and shoulder ROM and strengthening should also be addressed.

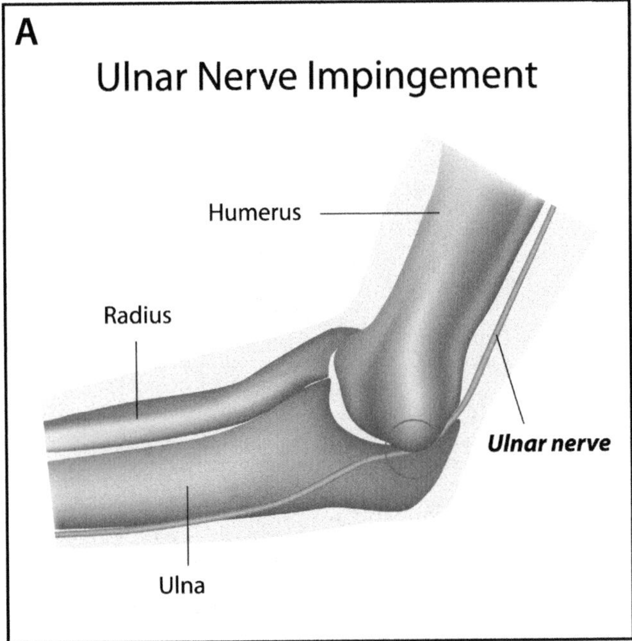


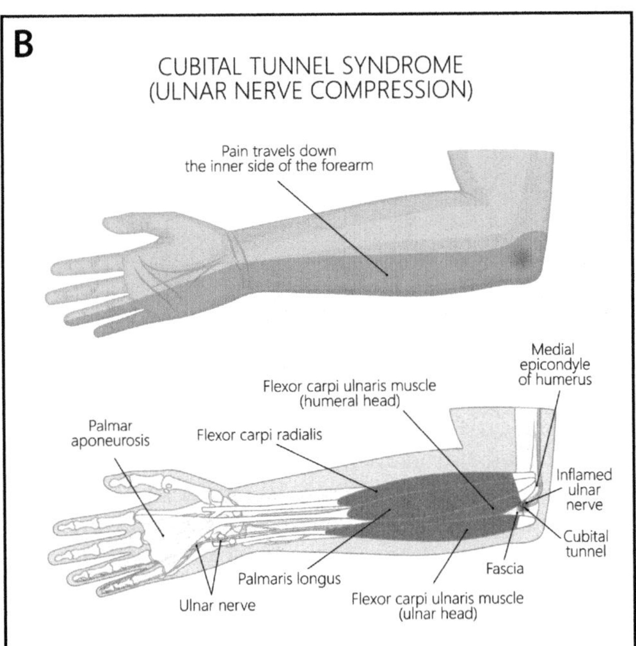


**Figure 12-32.** Cubital compartment syndrome. (A) Nerve impingement (Alila Medical Media/Shutterstock.com). (B) Paresthesia pattern (Aksanaku/Shutterstock.com).

## Medial and Lateral Epicondylalgia/Tendinopathy Rehabilitation Management

The most common forms of tendinopathy occur at both the medial and lateral epicondyles of the distal humerus. These conditions are commonly called *golfer's elbow* and *tennis elbow*, respectively, due to patients reporting symptoms during participation in those recreational activities. Medical professionals refer to these diagnoses as **medial and lateral epicondylalgia** (or tendinopathy). Special tests for these conditions are presented in Table 12-15.

Lateral epicondylalgia refers to pain (especially during gripping activities and resisted wrist extension) in the lateral elbow where the common wrist extensor tendons attach. Lateral epicondylalgia is seen in both men and women (between the ages of 35 and 54 years), most commonly on the dominant UE. It has been reported that 75% to 80% of elbow pain complaints are contributed to lateral epicondylalgia, and 50% of all tennis players experience elbow pain at some point.[62] This can also be a work-related injury in workers (17%) who perform a high rate of repetitive hand tasks (eg, factory poultry/meat cutters, deli meat slicers).[62] Common clinical findings are palpable tenderness on the lateral epicondyle, pain with active elbow/wrist motion, and painful and weak grip strength and finger extension.

Medial epicondylalgia refers to pain on the medial aspect of the elbow at the common wrist flexor tendon attachment. This condition affects men and women equally, with the highest incidence between the ages of 40 and 60 years. Although medial epicondylitis is more commonly associated with overhead throwing, tennis, and golf, the literature reveals other sports such as bowling, football, and heavy weight lifting can also cause this condition. Work-related injuries associated with medial epicondylalgia are due to the exposure of constant vibratory forces (eg, jackhammering) and jobs that include repetitive forceful gripping and continually handing/moving heavy loads (greater than 44 lb).[63] Common findings for medial elbow tendinopathy include point tenderness on the medial epicondyle, pain with active motion at the elbow and wrist, and/or weakness with resisted wrist and finger flexion as well as painful, weakened grip strength testing.

A physical therapist usually screens the cervical and thoracic spine during the initial evaluation to assess for any spinal contribution to the patient's source of pain. Other causes of medial elbow pain that should be ruled out include UCL injury, ulnar nerve pain, or pronator syndrome (compression of the median nerve by the pronator teres muscle).

Therapeutic exercises for both elbow tendinopathies should target regaining full, pain-free mobility at the elbow, wrist, and hand. Stretching the wrist extensors and flexors (Figure 12-33) and OKC strengthening of the elbow, wrist, forearm, and hand muscles should be addressed.[62-64] However, it is common practice to combine these exercises with modalities (eg, ice, heat, ultrasound/phonophoresis, iontophoresis, friction massage) and neurodynamic nerve glides to reduce inflammation and pain and promote improved function.

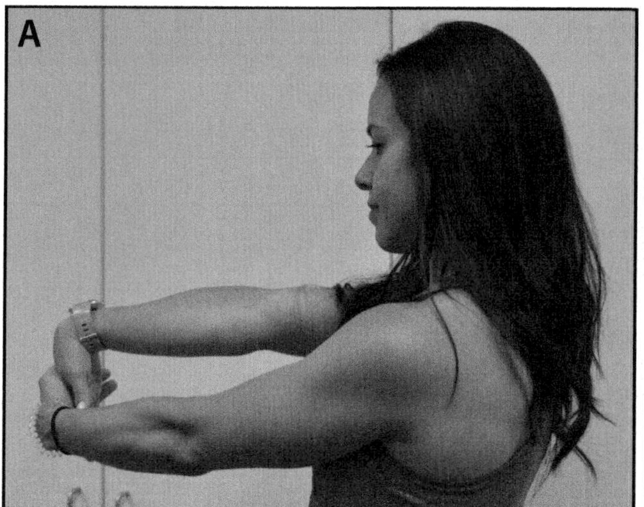


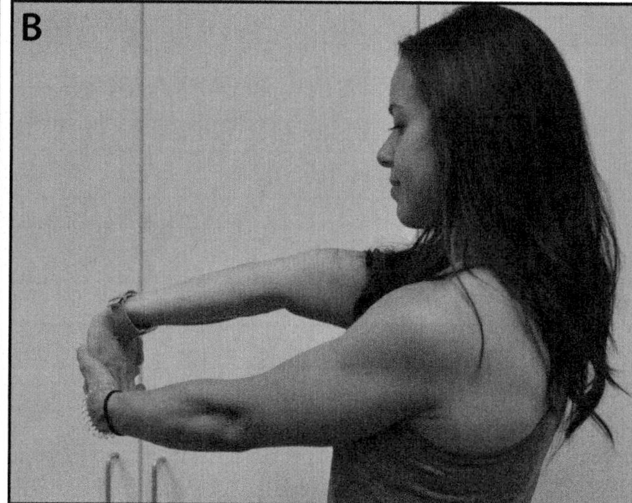


**Figure 12-33.** (A) Wrist extensor muscle stretch. (B) Wrist flexor muscle stretch.

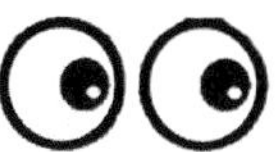

### Eye on the Research: Eccentric Strengthening and Elbow Epicondylalgia

For patients presenting with lateral epicondylalgia, eccentric strength training of the wrist extensors can be effective in both reducing pain and regaining strength.[62,65] A number of randomized controlled studies found that patients who completed eccentric exercises had significantly better pain relief compared with friction massage or ultrasound.[62]

There is a small amount of evidence supporting eccentric strength training for medial elbow pain as well, with patients demonstrating reduced pain and increased grip strength after a 12-week strength training program.[64]

It is important to include ST and GH exercises (to ensure good joint arthrokinematics) and core and lower extremity exercises (to improve overall fitness) for patients after an elbow injury before returning to throwing, other overhead sports, or work-related activities. Proper body mechanics and equipment use should be reviewed before returning to these activities.

## Introduction to the Management and Treatment for Wrist and Hand Pathologies

Fractures, sprains, and overuse injuries can occur in the wrist, thumb, and fingers. ADLs, various occupations, recreational activities (eg, hobbies, art), and sports activities require precise and often repetitive use of these joints. Wrist and hand injuries are common in sports, with an injury rate between 3% and 9%.[66] The incidence of distal radial fractures varies between 100 and 300 per 100,000 when adjusted for age. Eighty-five percent of sports-related hand fractures occur in contact sports such as football, hockey, and lacrosse. A FOOSH is a common MOI for distal radial and scaphoid fractures. Distal radial fractures can also be associated with extensor pollicis longus injury or ruptures. Overuse wrist injuries account for 25% to 50% of all wrist/hand injuries.[66]

### *Clinical Assessment of the Wrist and Hand*

The wrist-hand complex region has more than 25 joints and is made up of 29 bones, including the distal radius and ulna. When examining the wrist or hand, the physical therapist must assess gross movements of multiple joints and how each joint moves in isolation. A detailed history can assist in identifying the onset (trauma/overuse) and location of pain, the MOI, and the types of symptoms to determine the diagnosis. Components of the physical therapist's initial examination typically include the following:

- Observation and palpation: assess for wrist/hand deformities, pain (ie, anatomical snuffbox), and joint motions
- A cervical and proximal screen: assess other contributing factors (ie, spinal involvement, thoracic outlet syndrome, and shoulder or elbow pathology)
- Neurodynamic assessment: ulnar, radial, and median nerves
- Gross movements: open/close hand, hook fist, straight fist, cylinder grip, and thumb opposition
- Wrist (see Table 12-14), thumb, and finger ROM (Table 12-17)
- MMT: wrist flexion/extension/abduction (radial deviation)/adduction (ulnar deviation) and individual finger flexors/extensors/abductors/adductors
- Grip strength testing using a dynamometer
- Pinch grip testing: pad to side (holding a key), tip to tip, and 3-point pinch

**Table 12-17**

**First Carpometacarpal, Metacarpophalangeal, and Interphalangeal Joints Range of Motions[4]**

| Joint/Motion | Degrees |
|---|---|
| ***First Carpometacarpal Joint (Thumb)*** | |
| Flexion | 15 |
| Extension | 20 |
| ***Metacarpophalangeal Joints*** | |
| Flexion/extension (thumb) | 50/0 |
| Flexion/extension (fingers) | 90/45 |
| ***Interphalangeal Joints*** | |
| IP flexion/extension (thumb) | 80/20 |
| PIP flexion/extension (fingers) | 100/0 |
| DIP flexion/extension (fingers) | 90/0 |
| Note: These normative values are based on the American Academy of Orthopedic Surgeons. | |

- Special tests (Table 12-18)
- Notation of right- or left-hand dominant

Cluster testing is common for **carpal tunnel syndrome (CTS),** scaphoid fractures, and de Quervain tenosynovitis diagnoses. Rather than relying on single tests for these diagnoses (ie, Phalen's or Tinel's test), physical therapists use multiple tests (cluster testing) to improve the accuracy of the diagnosis. Confirmation of a diagnosis is based on the clinical evidence and patient's presentation; the number of positive tests is a predictor for each of these diagnoses (see Table 12-18).

The components of the carpal tunnel test cluster include wrist ratio greater than .67, symptom severity scale greater than 1.9, age greater than 45 years, diminished sensation in median sensory field 1 (thumb), and the shaking of the hands to relieve symptoms.[67] A wrist ratio index is the measurement (in centimeters) using a caliper of anteroposterior and mediolateral wrist width at the distal wrist crease. It is calculated by dividing the anteroposterior by mediolateral wrist widths. The median nerve sensory test compares the level of sensation at the thumb pad to the level of sensation at the proximal thenar eminence using the point of a paper clip. The Symptom Severity Scale is a questionnaire (11 items) targeting signs/symptoms for CTS (pain, paresthesia, numbness, weakness, nocturnal symptoms, and overall functional status). The patient reports symptoms on a scale of 1 (mild) to 5 (severe). A score less than 1.9 is indicative of CTS, but the higher the score, the more severe the case.[67]

Scaphoid cluster testing is used to rule out a scaphoid fracture.[68,69] The de Quervain Screening Tool was developed to better determine the presence of this condition. The presence of 5 of the 7 criteria included in Table 12-18 indicate the presence of de Quervain tenosynovitis with 100% specificity and sensitivity.[70]

## *Wrist Joint Mobilization Techniques*

Clinicians need to understand wrist joint arthrokinematics and how various joints move in relation to each other before performing joint mobilizations. The radiocarpal joint includes the distal radius (concave) and scaphoid, lunate, and triquetrum (convex surfaces). The proximal row and distal row of the carpal bones (trapezius, triquetrum, capitate, and hamate) make up the midcarpal joint. The distal row of the carpal bones (convex) articulating with the bases of the metacarpals (concave) form the CMC joints.

When the wrist moves from full wrist flexion to extension, the distal row of the carpal bones moves on the proximal row to neutral, and then the proximal row moves on the radius until full extension is achieved. When moving from full extension to flexion, the reverse joint actions occur; the proximal row moves on the radius to neutral, and then the distal row moves on the proximal row to complete full flexion. The open-packed position for the wrist is in a neutral position, and the closed-pack position is full extension.

**Table 12-18**

**Cluster (Special) Testing for Various Wrist and Thumb Pathologies**

| Cluster Testing | Possible Pathology if Positive |
|---|---|
| Clinical prediction rule (5 components): 45 years and older, hand shaking produces pain relief, wrist ratio index > .67, median nerve sensory test, and Symptom Severity Scale[67] | CTS diagnosis based on the number of positive tests:<br>• ≥3 positive tests: .98 sensitivity and .54 specificity<br>• ≥4 positive tests: .77 sensitivity and .83 specificity<br>• All 5 positive tests: .18 sensitivity and .99 specificity[67] |
| Scaphoid cluster testing (3 items): Tenderness over the anatomical snuffbox, scaphoid tubercle tenderness, and pain with long compression of the thumb[68,69] | Scaphoid fracture diagnosis: If all 3 are positive, 100% sensitivity and specificity of 74%[68,69] |
| The de Quervain Screening Tool (7 criteria): Positive Finkelstein test, pain, swelling over the radial styloid, pain in the first dorsal (extensor) compartment with wrist movement, pain with resisted thumb abduction, and thickening of the tendon sheath[70] | De Quervain tenosynovitis diagnosis if 5+/7 criteria (100% sensitivity and specificity)[70] |

### General Distraction of the Radiocarpal Joint

Radiocarpal long-axis distraction is an effective technique that is used to reduce pain and increase general wrist mobility. The patient can be seated or supine with the forearm supported on a folded towel and the wrist placed in neutral with the forearm pronated. The clinician's hand closest to the patient grasps the distal radius and ulna to stabilize the proximal joint, and the other hand grasps the proximal row of the carpal bones (Figure 12-34), distracting it from the stabilizing hand.

### Radiocarpal Glides to Increase Wrist Flexion and Extension

The clinician can apply a volar glide by gliding the proximal row of carpals downward to increase wrist extension. As stated previously, when the wrist is moved into extension from a neutral position, the proximal carpal row moves on the radius so there is gliding (down) and rolling (up) in opposite directions. To increase wrist flexion, the gliding force of the carpals is applied in the dorsal direction or upward.

The patient is seated or supine, and the clinician's hand positions are the same as for distraction. Depending on the ROM to be targeted, the clinician should apply the gliding force in the volar direction to increase wrist extension or in the dorsal direction to increase flexion (Figure 12-35).

## *Treatment and Rehabilitation for Wrist, Hand, and Thumb Diagnoses*

### Treatment and Rehabilitation Management for Scaphoid and Colles Fractures

The most common MOI for wrist fractures is a FOOSH. A Colles fracture occurs when the distal radius is displaced dorsally and is commonly seen in young male athletes and older female adults. Most of these fractures can be reduced and casted, but unstable fractures may require open reduction and internal fixation surgical intervention.

A scaphoid fracture (Figure 12-36) is the most common carpal bone fracture (82% to 89%). These fractures commonly occur in younger active men, and the typical MOI is a FOOSH with the wrist abducted.[69] These fractures present similarly to wrist sprains and are commonly missed on early radiographs. During treatment, the physical therapist assistant should note if a patient continues to present with nondiminishing symptoms and continued pain with pinch/grasp activities during the initial weeks of treatment. The assistant should contact the physical therapist requesting a re-evaluation as soon as possible. The therapist can complete scaphoid cluster testing (see Table 12-18) to identify a potential scaphoid fracture.[68,69] If positive tests are found, the patient should be referred to an orthopedist for further assessment.

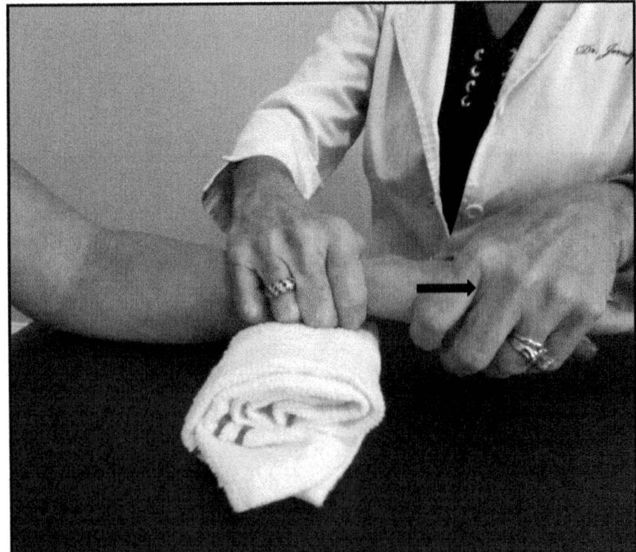

Figure 12-34. The direction for general distraction of the radiocarpal joint is indicated by the black arrow.

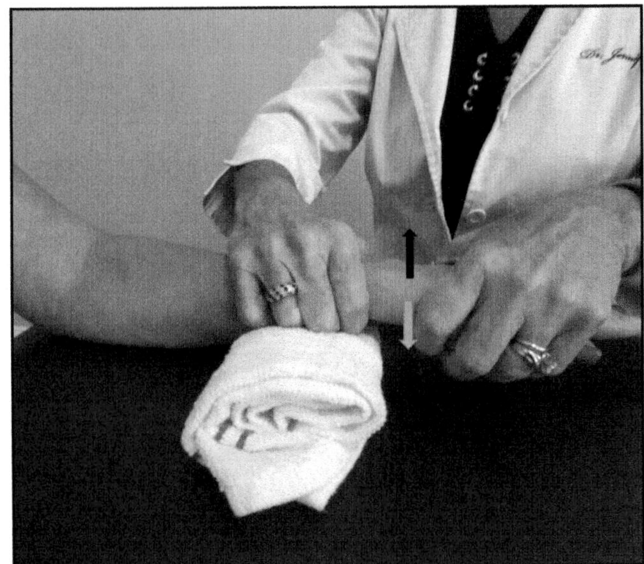

Figure 12-35. The black arrow illustrates dorsal glides to increase flexion. The gray arrow illustrates volar glides to increase extension.

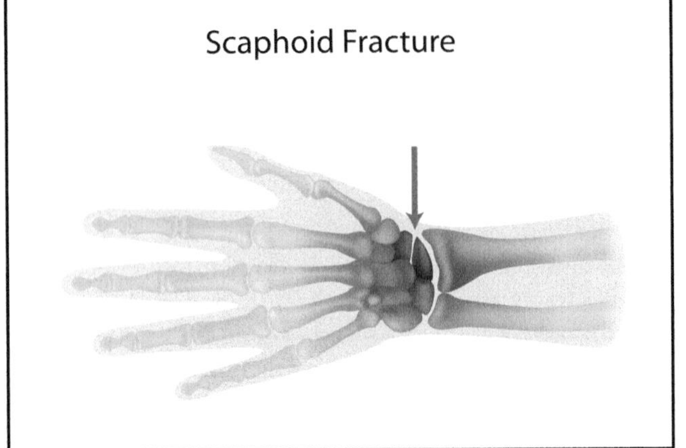


Figure 12-36. A scaphoid fracture (Alila Medical Media/Shutterstock.com).

Once these fractures are stabilized, early active finger movements and gentle pain-free forearm motions in the cast are encouraged, but wrist extension should be avoided.[71] There are 6 finger/hand exercises (referred to as *6-pack active hand exercises*) patients should perform several times a day in order to maintain normal metacarpal and IP joint motion. The first 4 exercises (Figure 12-37) allow for smooth flexor tendon gliding (targeting the flexor digitorum profundus and superficialis) as the tendons pass over the wrist, hand, and fingers. The 6-pack active hand exercises can be given as a HEP (refer to the Suggested Resources section at the end of this chapter). Exercises for the core, lower extremities, and uninvolved UE are initiated if included in the POC.

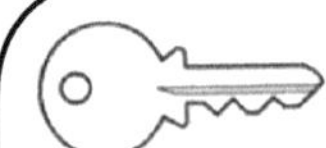

### Key Safety Consideration: Appropriate Monitoring of Patients Who Are Casted

If the patient is in a cast and complains of severe pain, numbness, or tingling in the fingers or if the fingers appear discolored, that is a red flag indicating the cast is too tight. Immediate medical attention is needed.[71]

Once the cast is removed, AAROM and AROM elbow, wrist, and hand exercises should be performed in all directions. Gripping, pinching exercises, and using the rice bucket for strengthening and muscle endurance can be initiated as tolerated. Patients begin with multiangle submaximal isometrics. Four to 5 weeks after cast removal, exercises are progressed to include pain-free dynamic strengthening. CKC exercises can be initiated around this time.[72] Upper body ergometer, stretches, and strengthening exercises for the shoulder on the involved side should be initiated as long as they do not create pain at the fracture site. The physical therapist assistant can use cuff weights around the patient's wrist (proximal to the fracture site) instead of using dumbbell weights for shoulder and elbow strengthening.

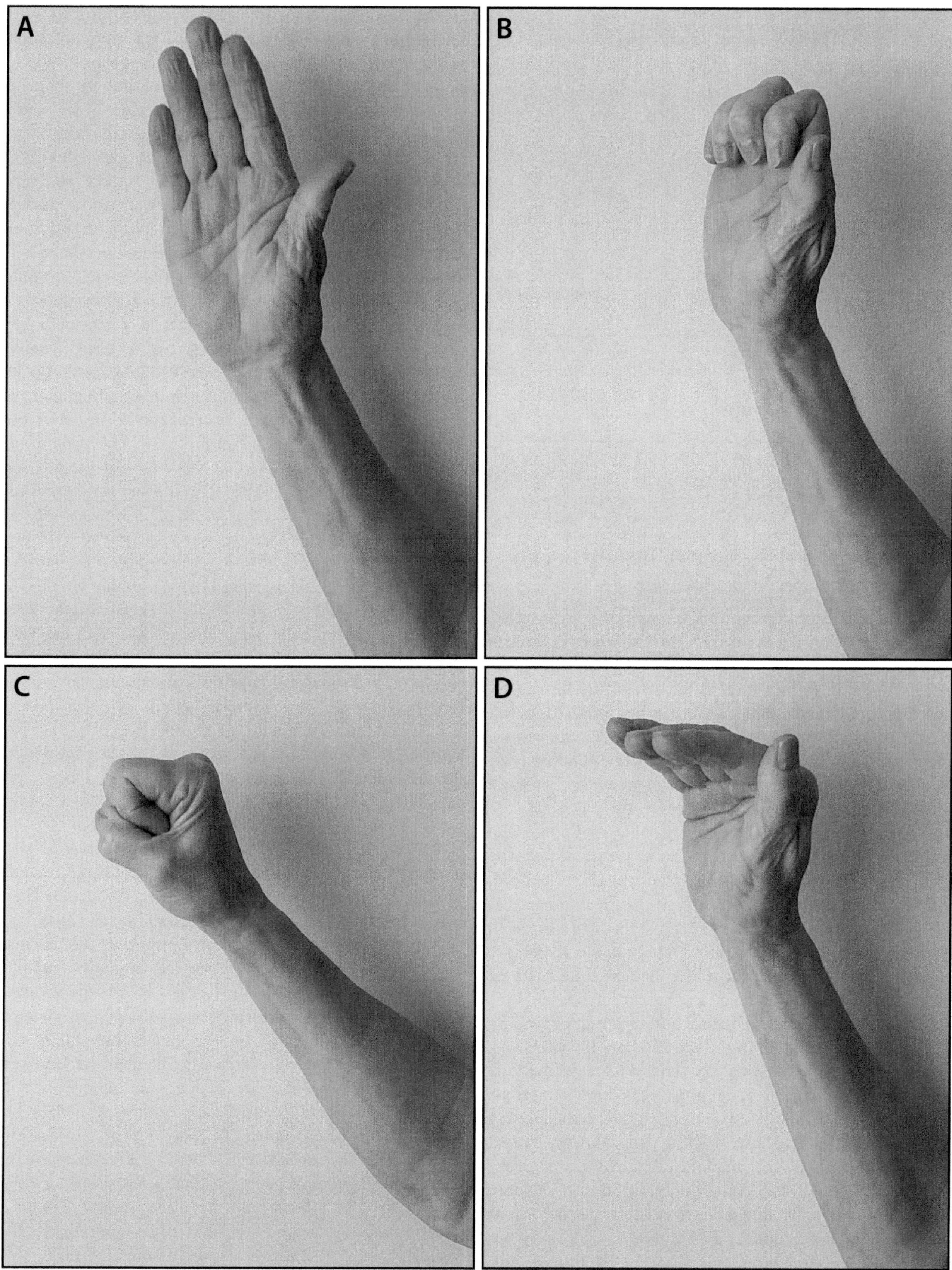


**Figure 12-37.** (A) Flexor tendon glide position 1: Straight hand. (B) Flexor tendon glide position 2: Flexion of the PIP and DIP joints. (C) Flexor tendon glide position 3: Full fisted. (D) Flexor tendon glide position 4: MCP flexion IP extension (lumbricals).

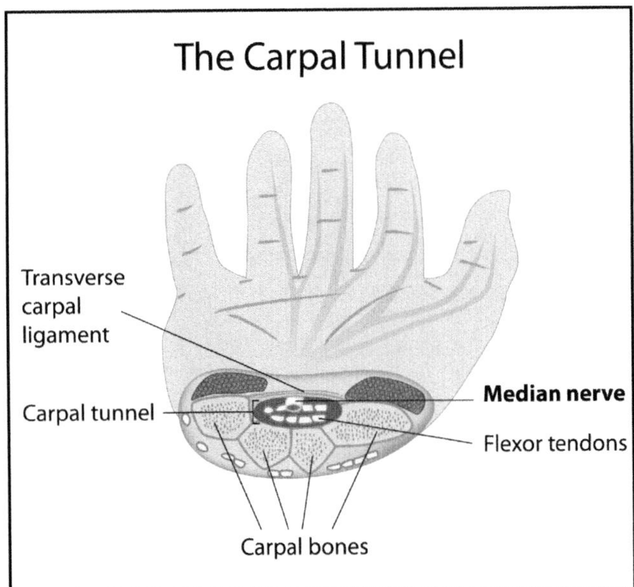


**Figure 12-38.** CTS: a palmar view of the median nerve compression between the transverse carpal ligament (or flexor retinaculum) and carpal bones (Alila Medical Media/Shutterstock.com).

## Carpal Tunnel Syndrome: Treatment and Rehabilitation Management

CTS is the most common of all compressive neuropathies, with a prevalence of 3.8% in the general population, and it is more prevalent in adults between 40 and 60 years old and in women more than men.[73] Risk factors for developing CTS include being female, work-related highly repetitive hand/wrist motions or the use of vibratory tools, increased body mass index (obesity), previous wrist fracture, rheumatoid arthritis, diabetes, pregnancy, high wrist ratio index, and hypothyroidism.[73,74]

The carpal tunnel is composed of the carpal bones, the transverse carpal ligament (the flexor retinaculum), the median nerve, and all finger flexor tendons (Figure 12-38). CTS results from the compression of the median nerve at the wrist, where it passes through a narrow space between the carpal bones on the palmar side and the transverse carpal ligament. Repetitive wrist flexion and extreme extension decrease the space in the carpal tunnel, thus increasing compartment pressure and resulting in median nerve compression and diminished capillary blood flow.[73]

Patients with CTS experience sensory changes (or loss) and muscle weakness. Common signs and symptoms include pain, numbness, and/or tingling along the median nerve distribution and hand swelling that wakes the patient at night. Patients often complain of clumsiness or dropping of objects. If the condition progresses to median nerve palsy, atrophy and muscle wasting of the thenar eminence and hand muscles are commonly seen (ape hand deformity). The clinician should be aware that other conditions may present with similar symptoms to CTS, such as cervical radiculopathy (commonly C6-C7), pronator syndrome, diabetes mellitus, Raynaud syndrome, and other polyneuropathies.[73]

The physician usually prescribes nonsteroidal anti-inflammatory drugs and/or steroidal injections to reduce pain and inflammation and a wrist splint to avoid further nerve irritation. Conservative physical therapy management prioritizes educating the patient about their condition, modification, or avoidance of activities that exacerbate symptoms and recommendations regarding changes in the work environment or workstation. To reduce pain and regain mobility and strength, modalities, tendon glides (see Figure 12-37) and median nerve glides, joint and soft tissue mobilization, pain-free ROM, and a gradual progression of wrist/hand strengthening exercises (isometrics, isotonic, and putty and ball squeezes) are common interventions.

All glides and exercises should be performed gently to minimize swelling and improve mobility. Median nerve glides should be started early but progressed gradually based on symptom irritability and symptom changes. There are 6 nerve glide exercises that should be performed in the order presented in Figure 12-39. The patient can progress on to the next exercise and continue the progression until a tingling sensation in the nerve distribution pattern is experienced. At that point, the patient should halt the progression at that exercise, go back to perform the previous exercise (that did not cause the symptoms), and then attempt the exercise that caused the symptoms once again. The patient should go back and forth alternating between the 2 exercises until the symptoms subside with the more advanced exercise. Once the more advanced exercise can be performed symptom free, the patient can move on to the next exercise. These exercises should be performed for 3 to 5 repetitions each with a 5-second hold 3 times a day. If the exercises make the symptoms worse, then the patient should reduce the number of repetitions and times per day. The physical therapist assistant should check on the patient's progression and symptoms each session.

Recent research indicates low-quality evidence supporting that various exercises and mobilization techniques provide significant benefits for improving CTS; researchers conclude that future high-quality research is needed.[75]

Surgical intervention is another option for CTS that may be considered instead of conservative management or if conservative treatment was unsuccessful. A surgical carpal tunnel release can be performed using an open, mini-open, or endoscopic (minimally invasive) approach. During this procedure, the transverse carpal ligament is cut, and scar tissue is removed to increase the space and relieve pressure on the median nerve.[76] Patients are usually splinted for 1 to 2 weeks after the procedure. To control/minimize swelling after surgery, the surgical arm should be elevated above the heart, and finger movement is initiated. Recovery time may take weeks to months depending on the amount of damage to the median nerve and how long it was compressed. The initial physical therapy goals are to manage postoperative pain and swelling and to initiate mobility exercises to the distal UE. Tendon and nerve glides and wrist/fingers and thumb AROM can be performed as long as pain or symptoms are not increased. Massage to reduce scarring

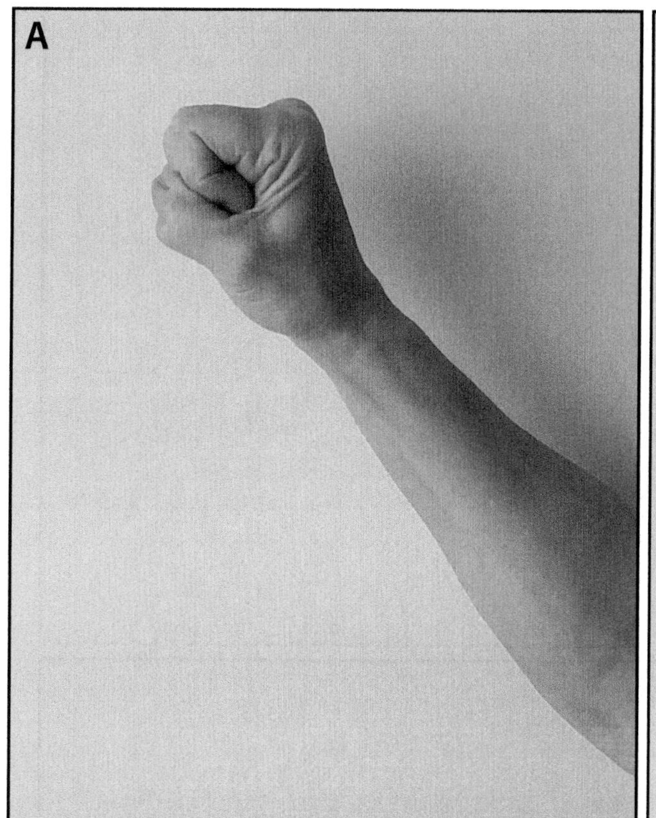


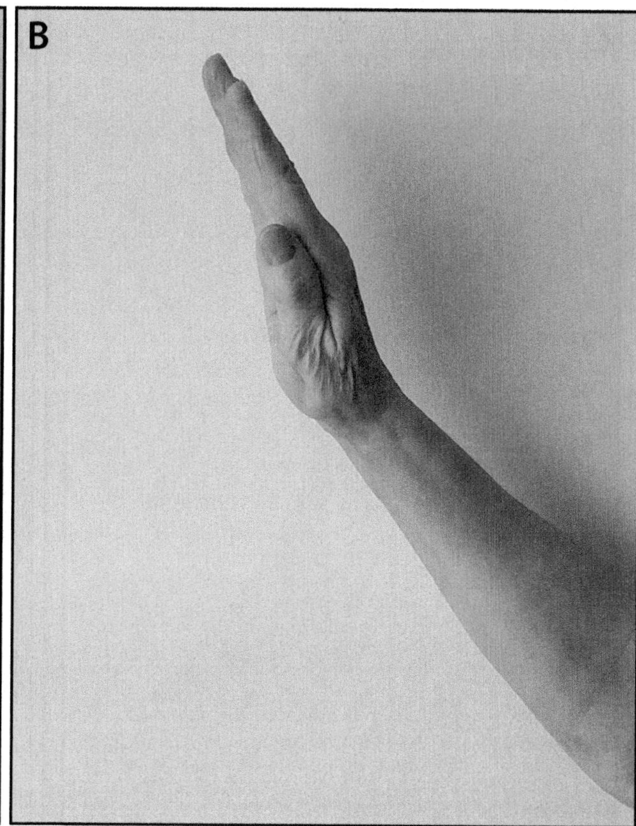


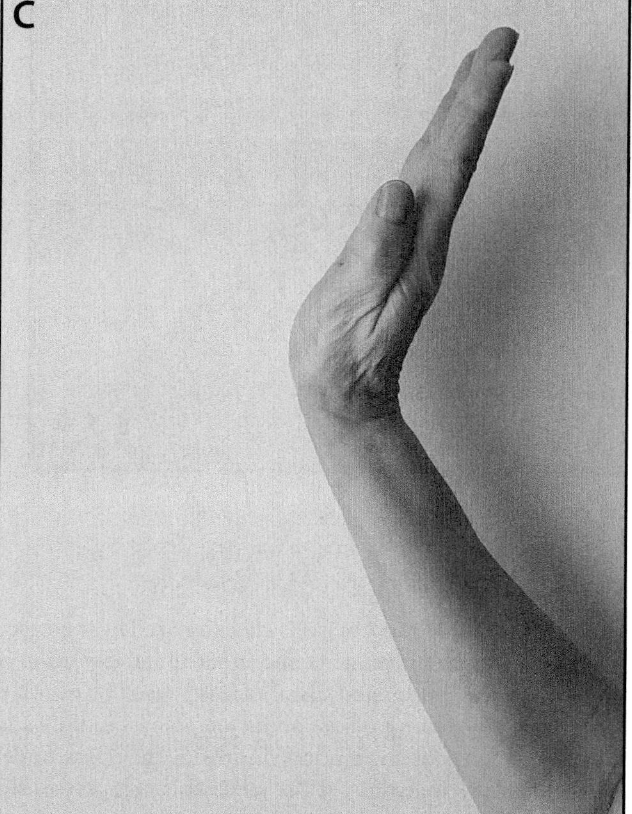


**Figure 12-39.** (A) Nerve glide position 1: Full fisted. (B) Nerve glide position 2: Straight hand. (C) Nerve glide position 3: Wrist extension. *(continued)*

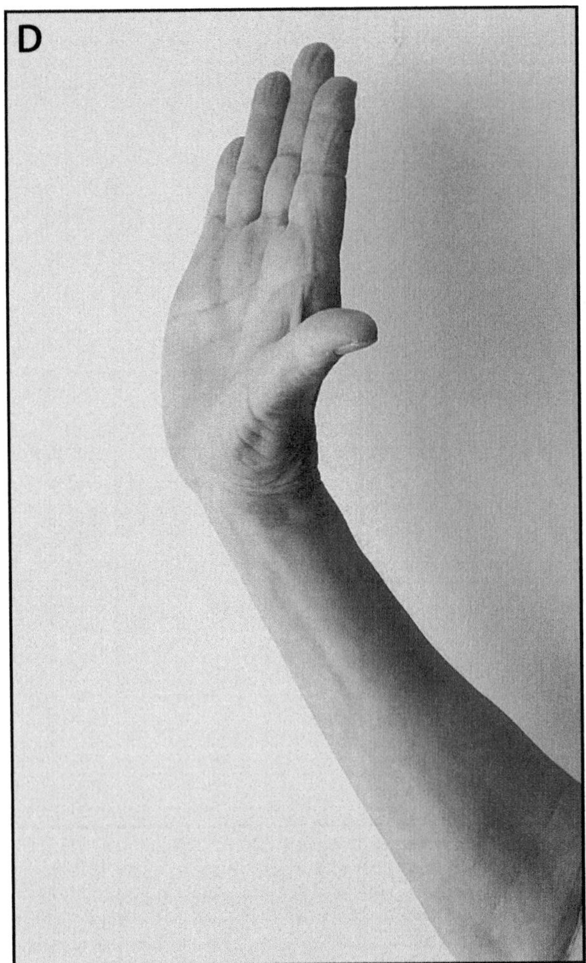


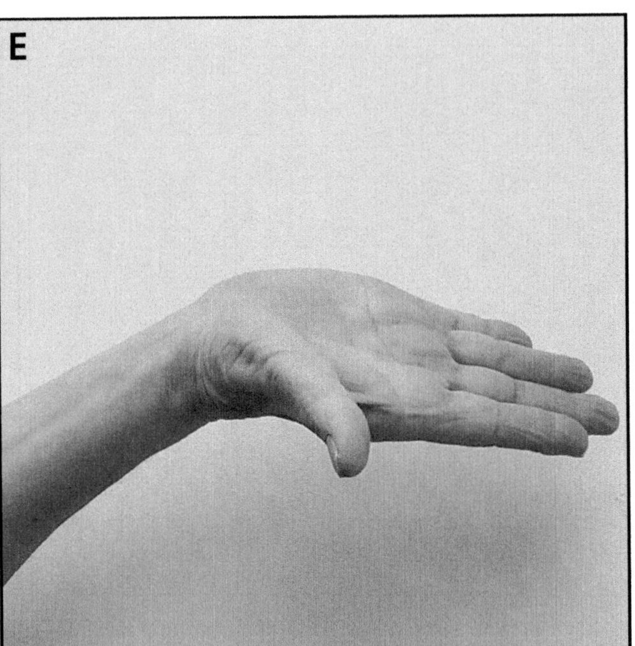


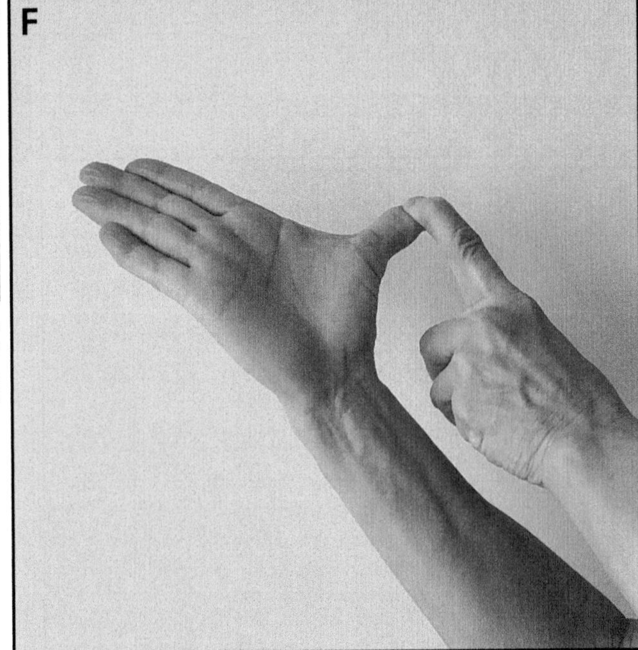


**Figure 12-39 (continued).** (D) Nerve glide position 4: The wrist, fingers, and thumb are extended. (E) Nerve glide position 5: The forearm supinated with the wrist, fingers, and thumb extended. (F) Nerve glide position 6: The forearm supinated and the wrist and fingers extended with the thumb stretched into extension.

can be started once the incision is healed. Desensitization exercises to reduce symptoms may be indicated. Repetitive gripping or lifting should be avoided until cleared by the physician.

An extensive mapping research study summarized that there is an abundance of evidence available in support of exercise, orthotic, and educational interventions for commonly treated wrist and hand diagnoses. Researchers suggested that further evidence is needed "for activity-based, behavioral, and quality-of-care outcomes."[77]

## De Quervain Tenosynovitis: Treatment and Rehabilitation Management

De Quervain tenosynovitis is characterized by increased pain with thumb movements and ulnar/radial deviation at the base of the thumb and distal radius caused by overuse. There is a thickening of the abductor pollicis longus and extensor pollicis brevis tendon sheaths as they pass under the extensor retinaculum at the wrist; this compresses the tendons and affects the normal tendon gliding, resulting in pain (Figure 12-40).[78,79] Patients typically complain of a gradual onset of pain at the radial styloid process while the forearm is in neutral and the ulnar side of the wrist is deviated with the thumb in MCP flexion (simulating the

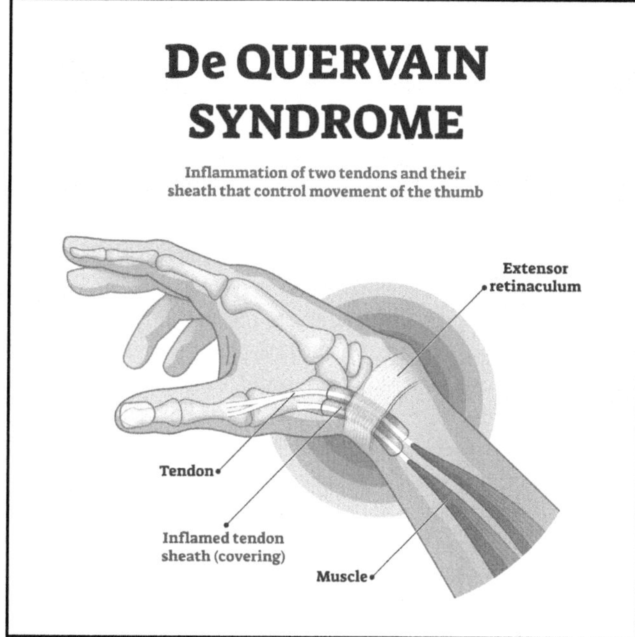


**Figure 12-40.** De Quervain tenosynovitis occurs because of the thickening of the abductor pollicis longus extensor and pollicis brevis tendon sheaths and the extensor retinaculum (VectorMine/Shutterstock.com).

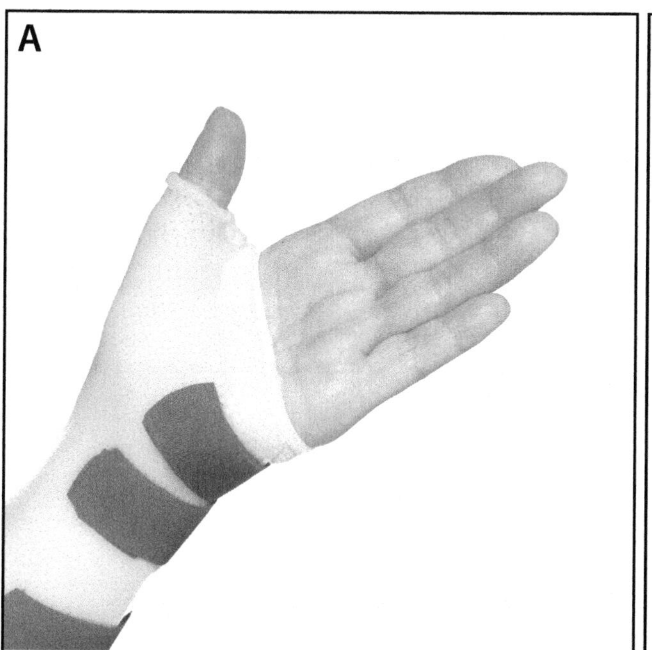


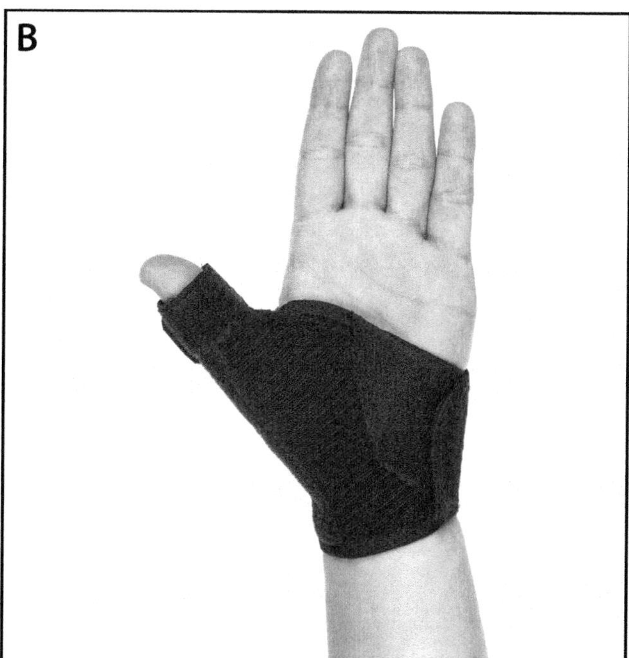


**Figure 12-41.** Thumb spica splints. (A) This is a hard splint limiting thumb and wrist movements (TasfotoNL/Shutterstock.com). (B) This soft splint allows for some wrist motions but still limits thumb movements (gcafotografia/Shutterstock.com).

Finkelstein Test position). Pain is most commonly reported when performing activities such as grasping objects, picking up a child, wringing out a washcloth, or using a hammer.[79] Radial styloid and scaphoid fractures, first CMC arthritis, and radial sensory nerve pain can mimic signs/symptoms of de Quervain tenosynovitis.[79,80]

Current evidence supports the use of a thumb spica splint (Figure 12-41), nonsteroidal anti-inflammatory drugs, steroidal injections, and patient education for activity modification and avoidance that increases pain.[78-80] Pain-free wrist and thumb PROM can be initiated, gradually progressing to AROM and then resistance exercises. These patients are commonly treated by occupational therapists or certified hand specialists as opposed to physical therapy practitioners. Current clinical practice guidelines indicate that therapeutic modalities such as ultrasound, exercise, and Kinesiotaping can be included in management.[80]

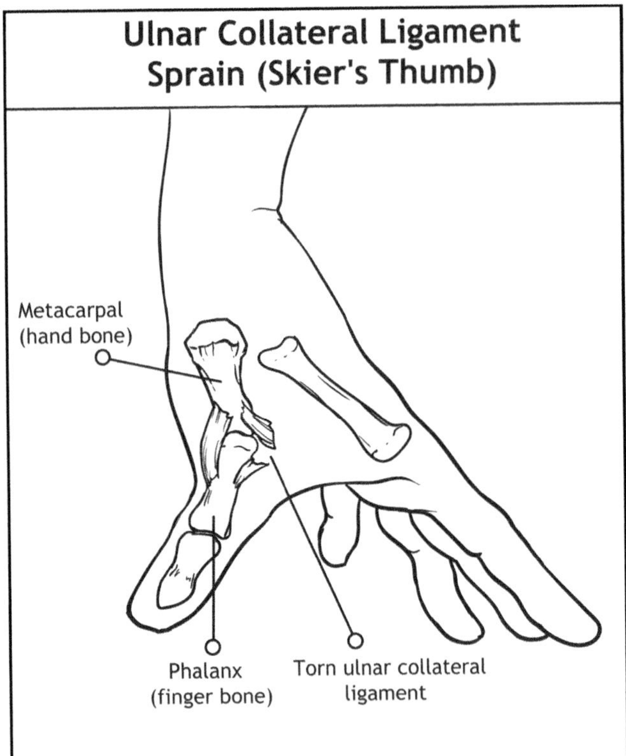


**Figure 12-42.** A UCL sprain also known as *gamekeeper's thumb* or *skier's thumb* (Drp8/Shutterstock.com).

## Gamekeeper's or Skier's Thumb and Other Tendon Injures in the Hand

Gamekeeper's or skier's thumb is an injury to the UCL from trauma or repetitive valgus stress to the first MCP joint. It commonly occurs when a skier falls on an abducted thumb while holding a ski pole (Figure 12-42) and may also occur during soccer, basketball, and volleyball injuries. There are about 200,000 occurrences a year in the United States. If the ligament is ruptured or lacerated, surgery is required. Certified hand therapists see these patients post-operatively for splinting to protect the healing tendon while promoting movement at other hand/finger joints (called *protected mobilization*).[81] Because of the severity of these injuries and the complexity of surgical tendon repairs, treatment of these patients is not considered to be entry level for the assistant.

## Shoulder Exercises

This section presents various ROM, stretching, strengthening, and neuromuscular control exercises that can be used to treat various shoulder diagnoses. Table 12-8 provides a list of various exercises and general exercise progression for each diagnosis. The physical therapist assistant should also include elbow, wrist, and hand stretching and strengthening in order to improve overall function.

### *Range of Motion and Stretching*

Figures 12-43 through 12-49 illustrate ROM and stretching.

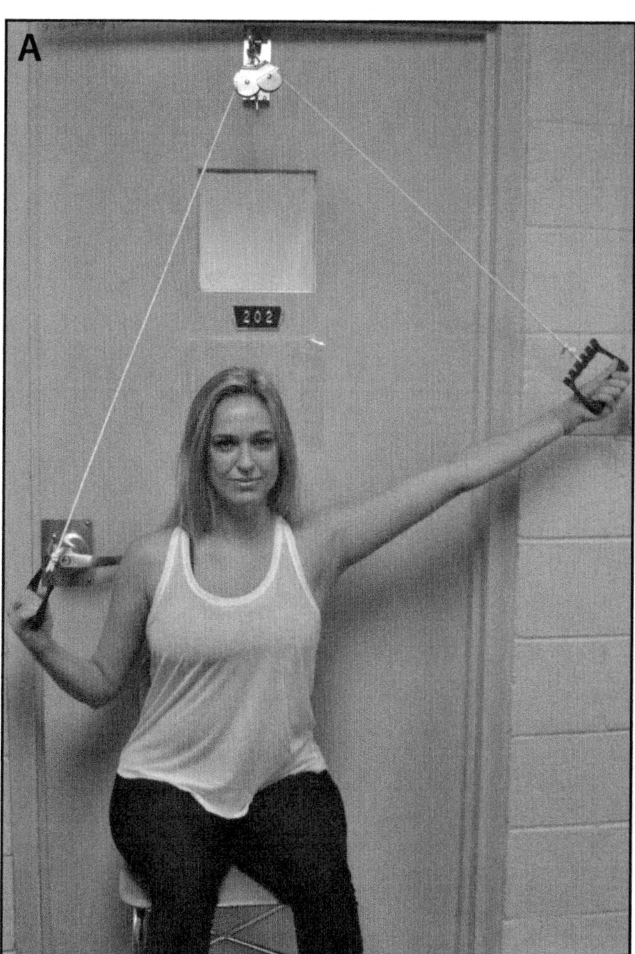


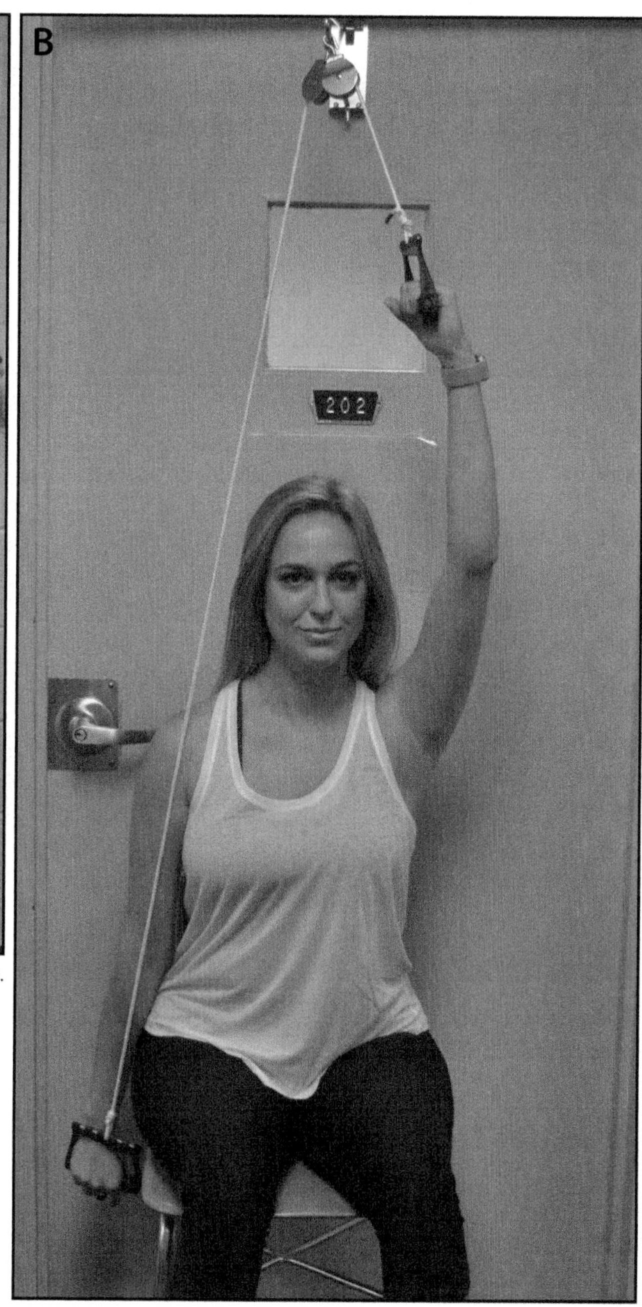


**Figure 12-43.** (A) AAROM for shoulder abduction using pulleys. (B) AAROM for shoulder flexion using pulleys.

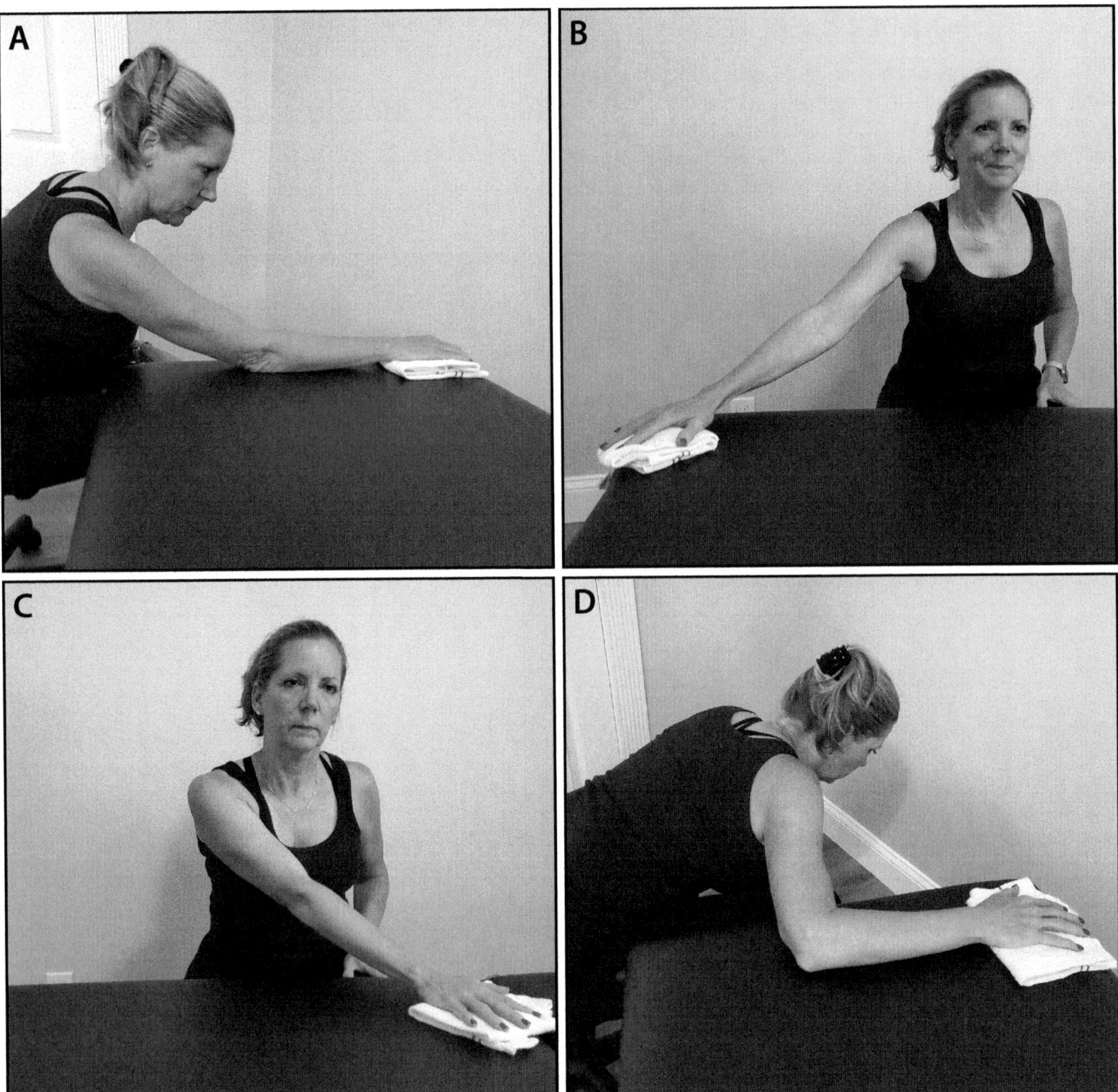


**Figure 12-44.** (A) Tabletop AAROM slides for shoulder flexion ROM and stretching. (B) Tabletop arm slides for AAROM horizontal abduction. (C) Tabletop AAROM for horizontal adduction ROM. (D) Seated PROM external rotation in 90/90. The patient flexes the trunk forward with the arm stabilized on the treatment table to increase external rotation.

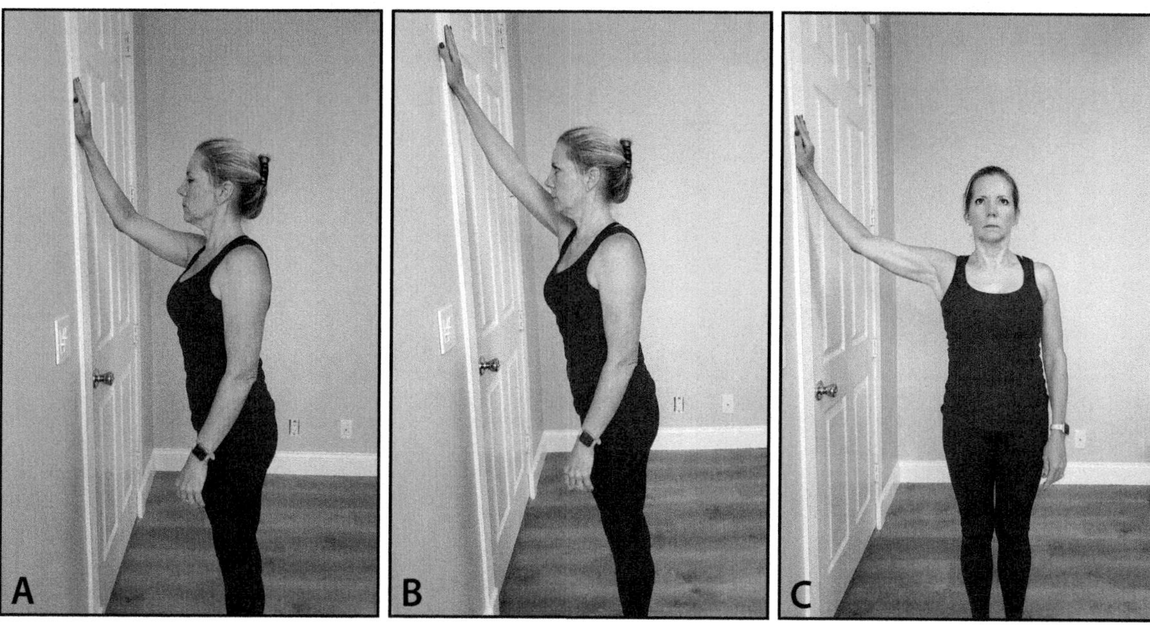

**Figure 12-45.** (A) Wall walking AAROM shoulder flexion. (B) The patient should reach as high as possible, and the assistant should monitor for proper joint mechanics during the activity. (C) Wall walking for abduction.

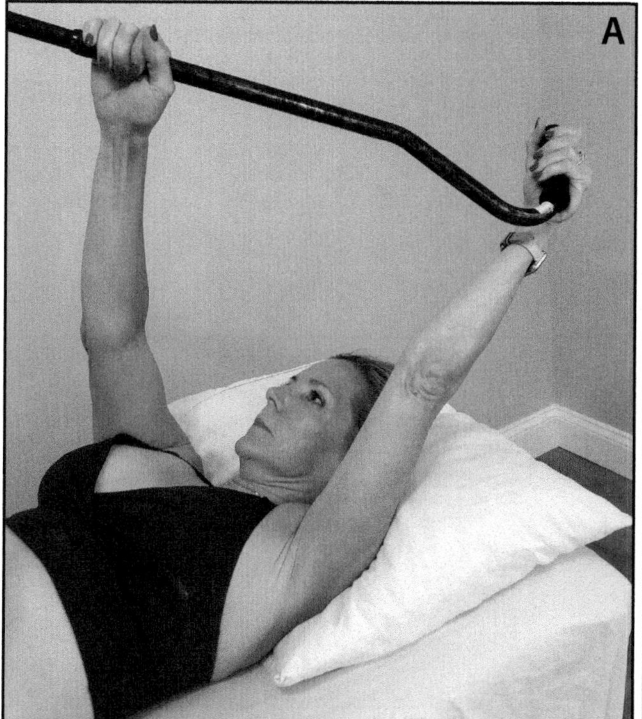

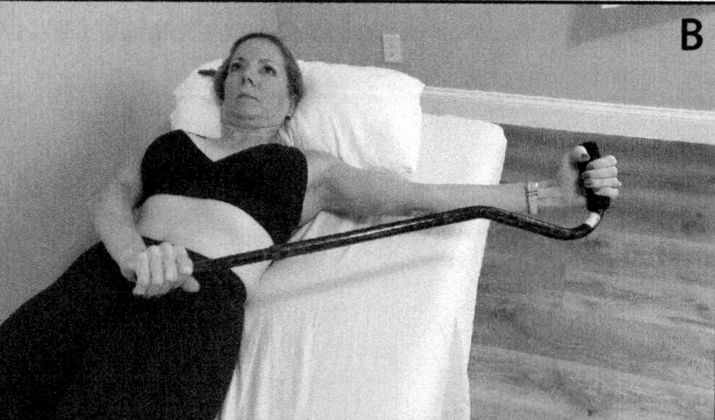

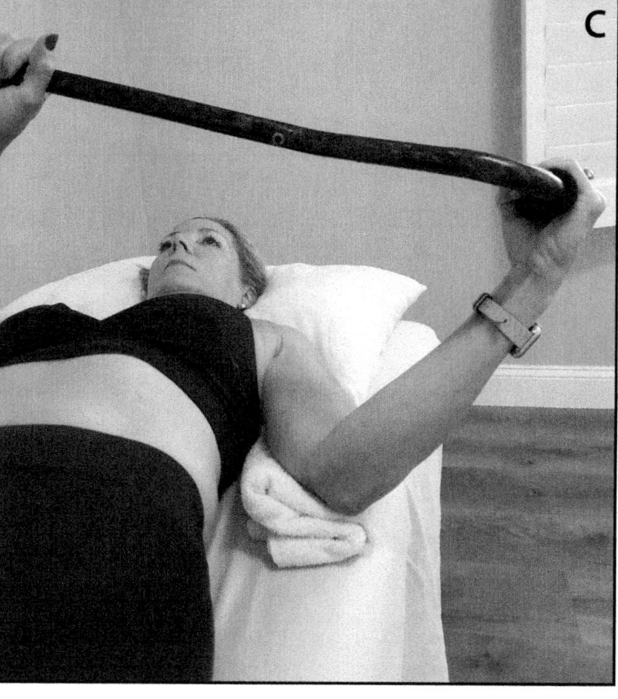

**Figure 12-46.** (A) Shoulder flexion AAROM on the left using a cane. (B) Shoulder abduction AAROM. (C) Shoulder external rotation AAROM or stretching in the plane of the scapula. *(continued)*

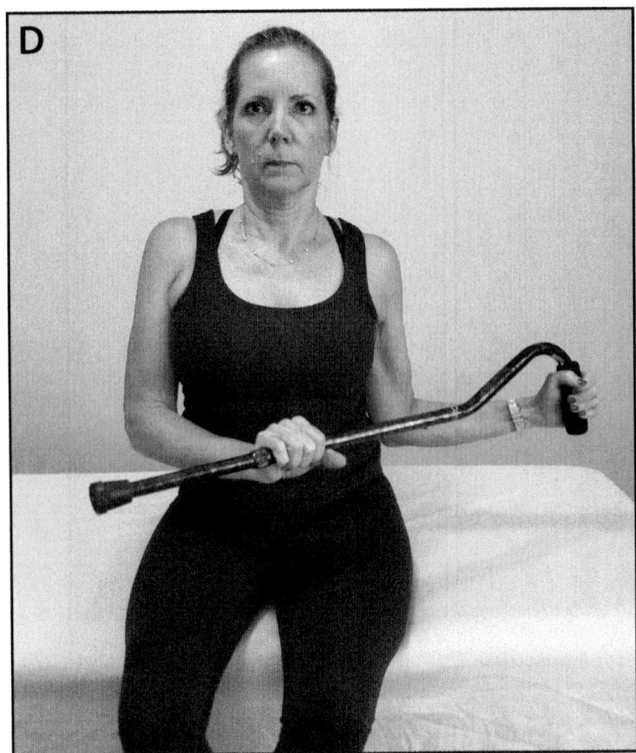


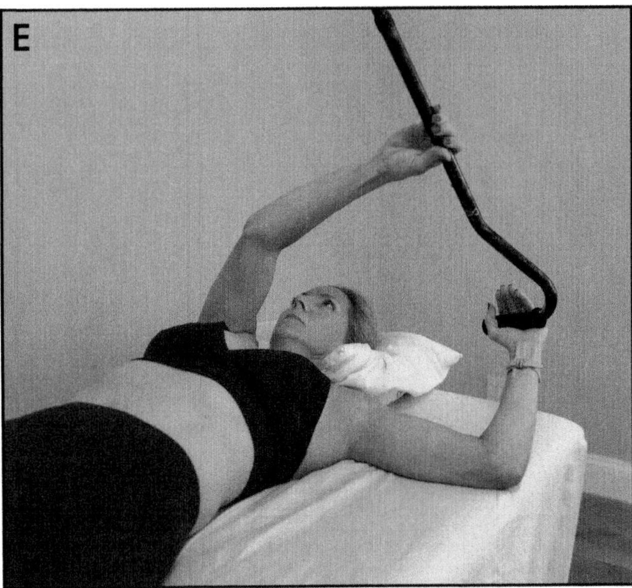


**Figure 12-46 (continued).** (D) Seated AAROM or stretch for the left internal rotator muscles using a cane with the arm in neutral. (E) Shoulder external rotation stretch with 90 degrees of abduction and 90 degrees of elbow flexion.

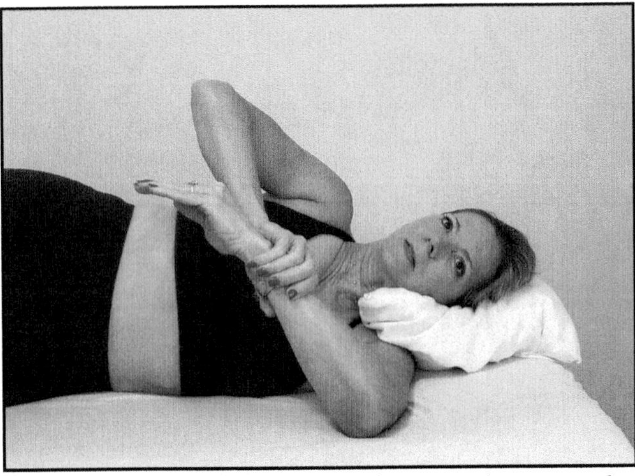

**Figure 12-47.** The sleeper stretch for stretching external rotator muscles.

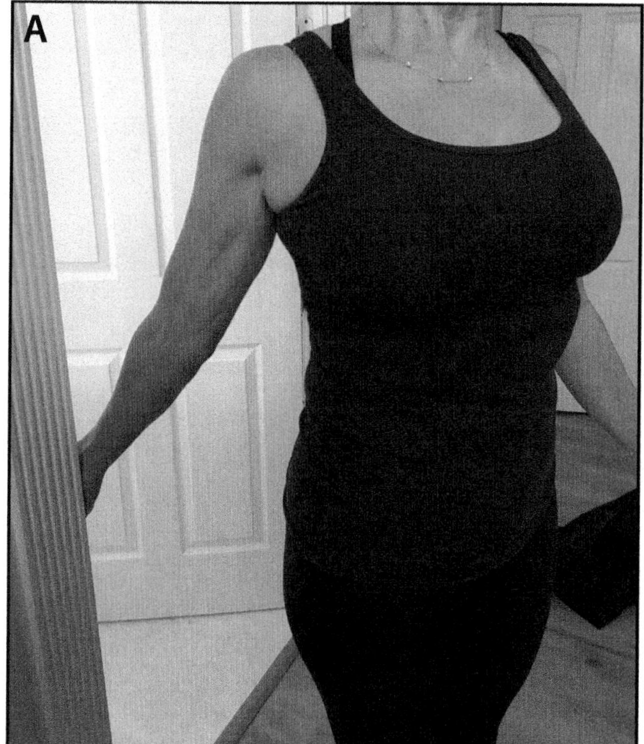

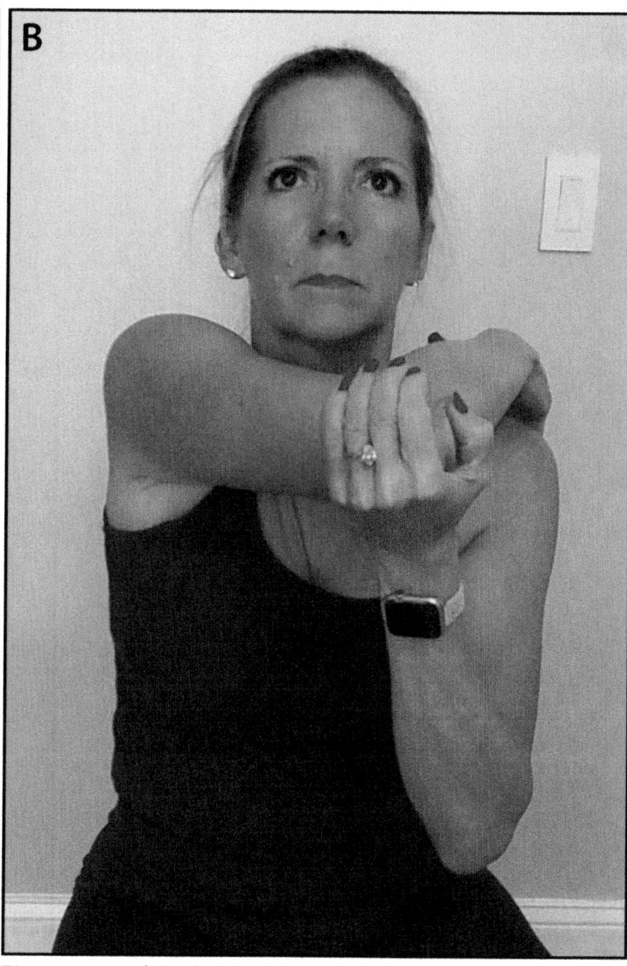

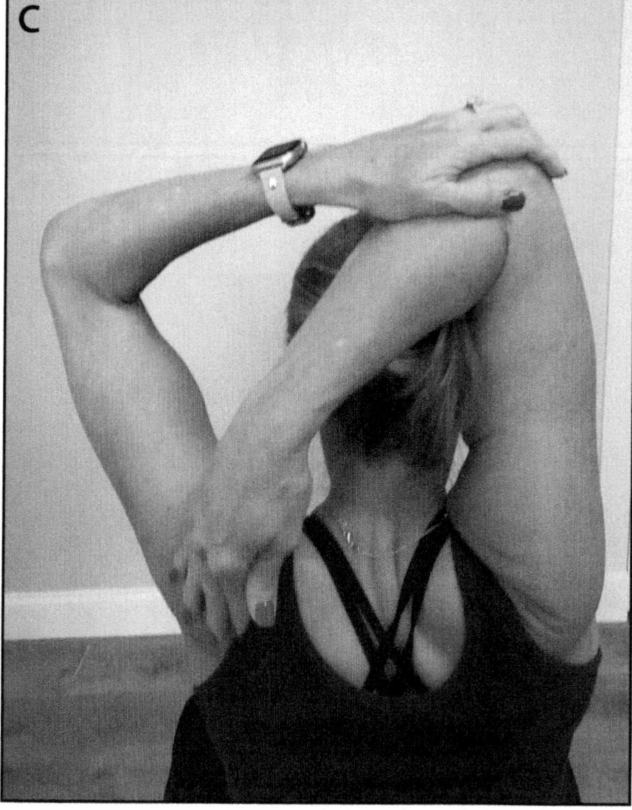

**Figure 12-48.** (A) The anterior capsule stretch and biceps stretch. (B) The cross-chest posterior capsule stretch. (C) The inferior capsule and shoulder adductor muscle stretch also stretches the triceps brachii (posterior view).

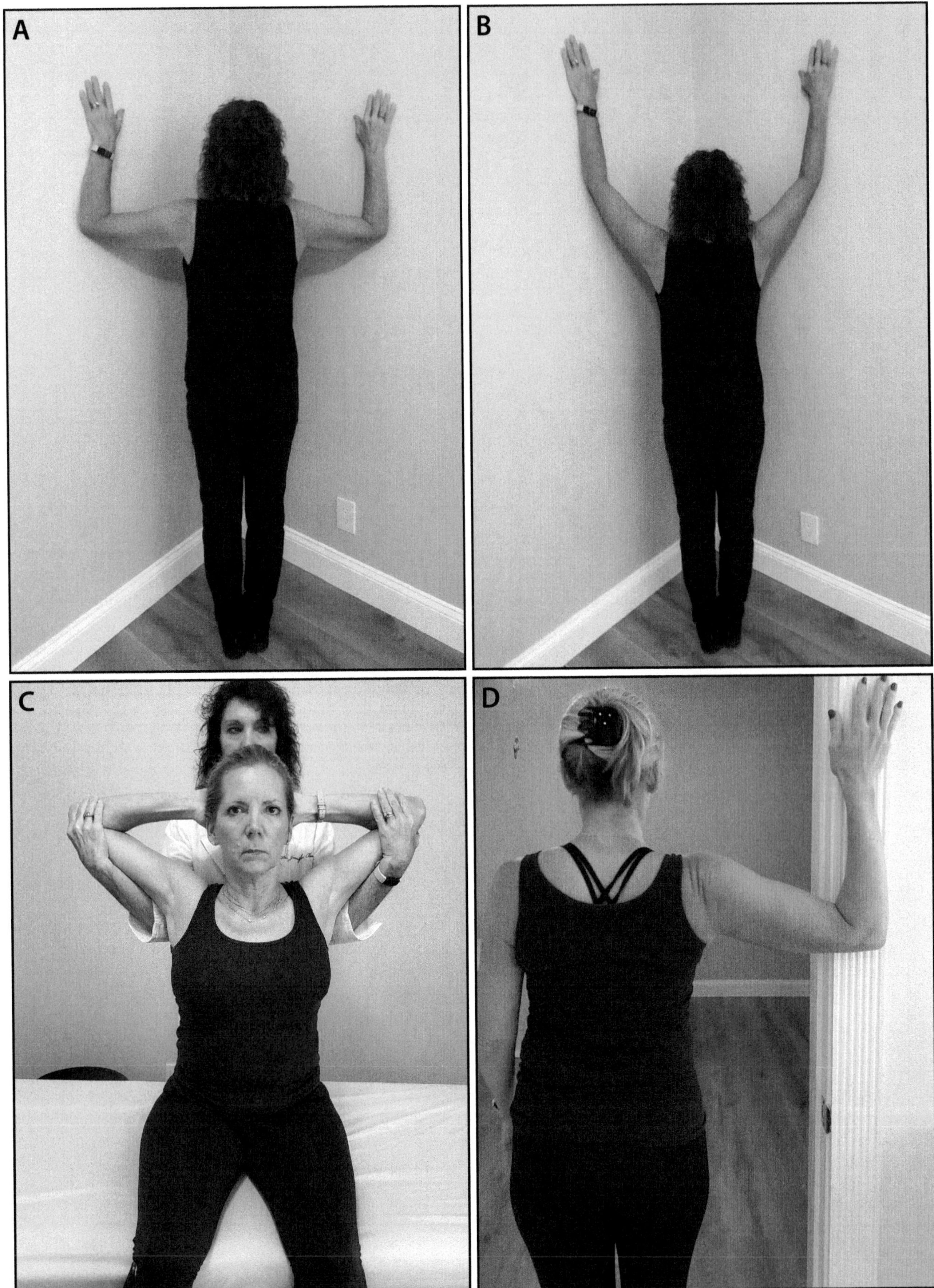

**Figure 12-49.** (A) The corner pectoralis muscle stretch for the clavicular portion of the muscle. (B) The corner stretch for sternal portion of the pectoralis major muscle with the elbows straight and the arms in a V shape. (C) A manually assisted pectoralis major stretch. (D) The doorway unilateral pectoralis stretch and anterior capsule stretch.

## *Strengthening Exercises*

### Isometric and Open Kinetic Chain Exercises

Isometric and OKC exercises are illustrated in Figures 12-11, 12-12, 12-50, 12-51, 12-52, and 12-53.

### Closed Kinetic Chain Exercises and Push-Up Progression

CKC exercises are shown in Figure 12-54, and Figure 12-55 illustrates push-up progression.

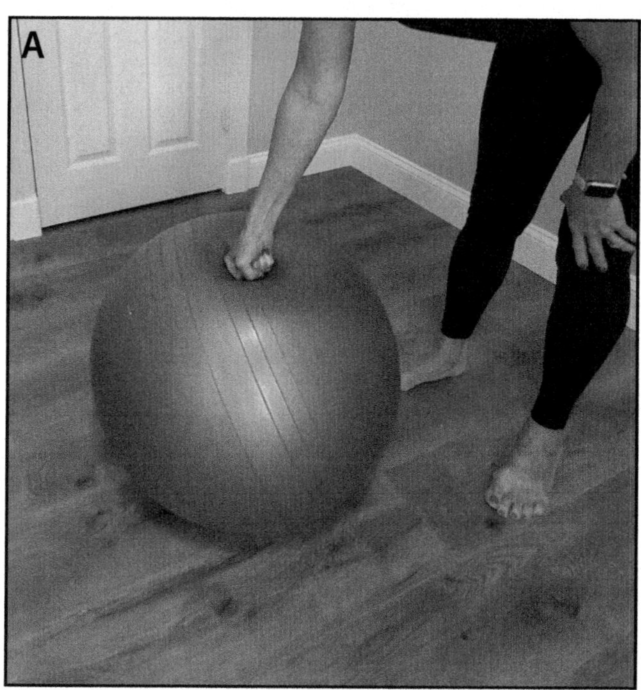


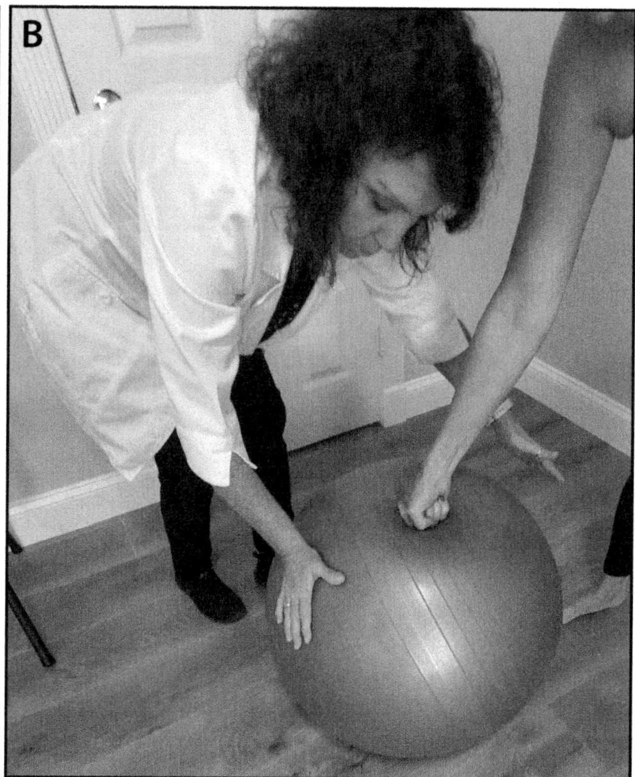


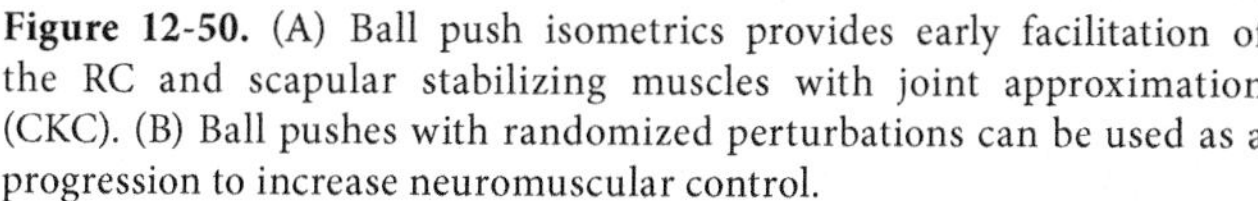

**Figure 12-50.** (A) Ball push isometrics provides early facilitation of the RC and scapular stabilizing muscles with joint approximation (CKC). (B) Ball pushes with randomized perturbations can be used as a progression to increase neuromuscular control.

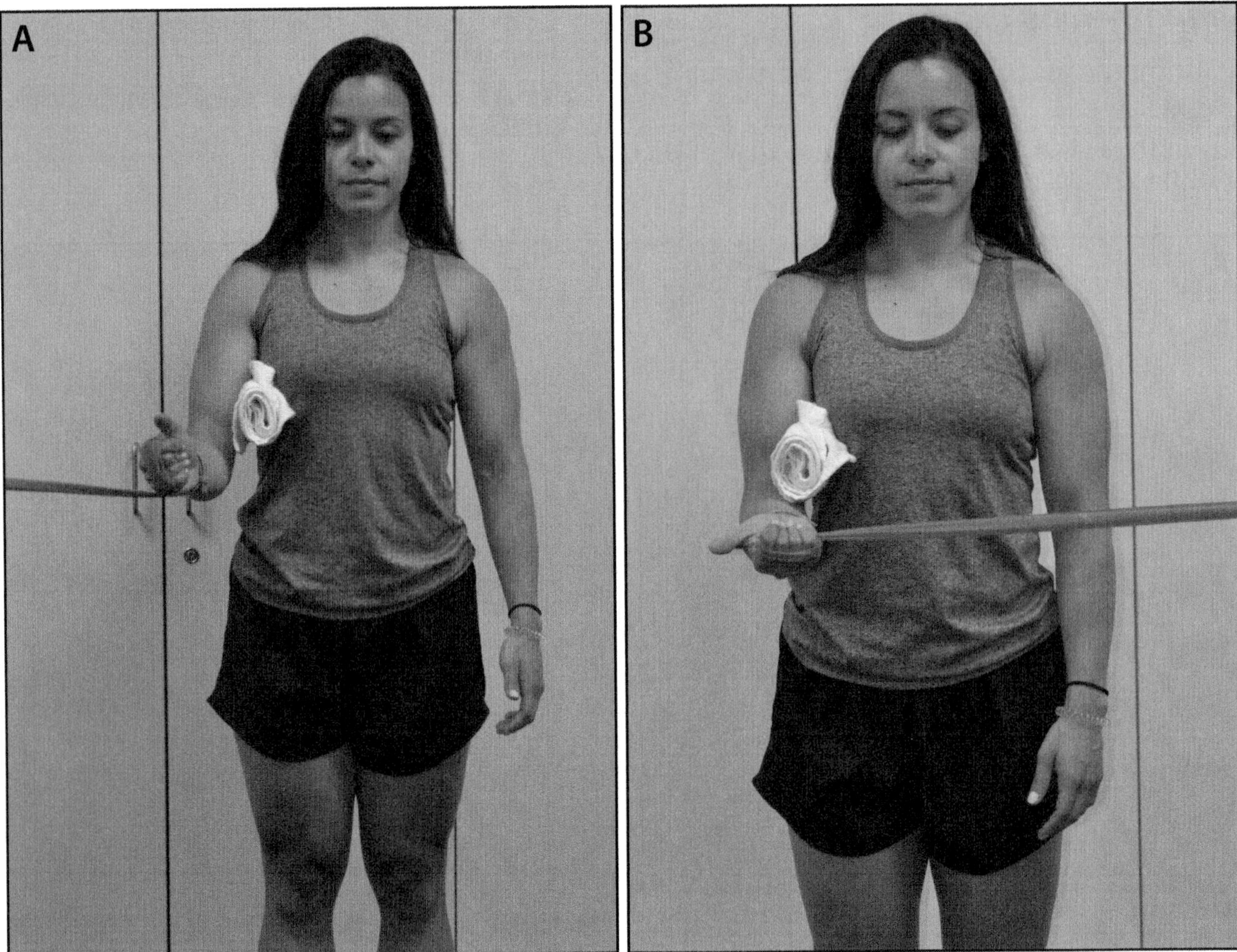


**Figure 12-51.** (A) Dynamic isometrics for internal rotators. The patient keeps the arm in neutral; have the patient side step to the left and back to the right to the starting position. (B) Dynamic isometrics for the external rotators. The patient side steps to the right to increase resistance while maintaining the arm in neutral.

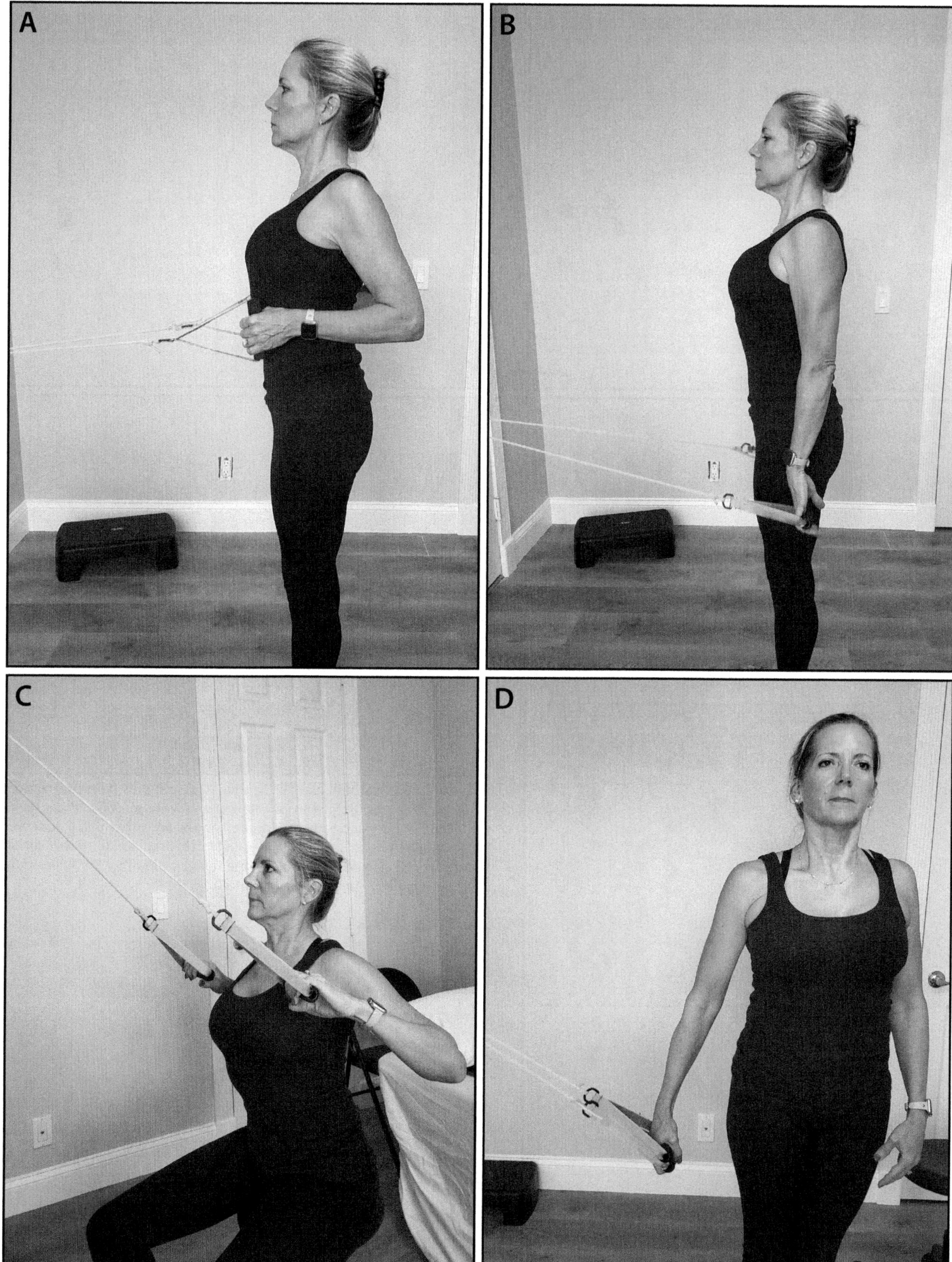


**Figure 12-52.** (A) Rows for rhomboid and middle trapezius strengthening. Shoulder rowing end position. (B) Shoulder extension posterior deltoid strengthening. (C) Pull downs for latissimus dorsi and teres major strengthening. (D) Shoulder adductor strengthening for the pectoralis major and latissimus dorsi. *(continued)*

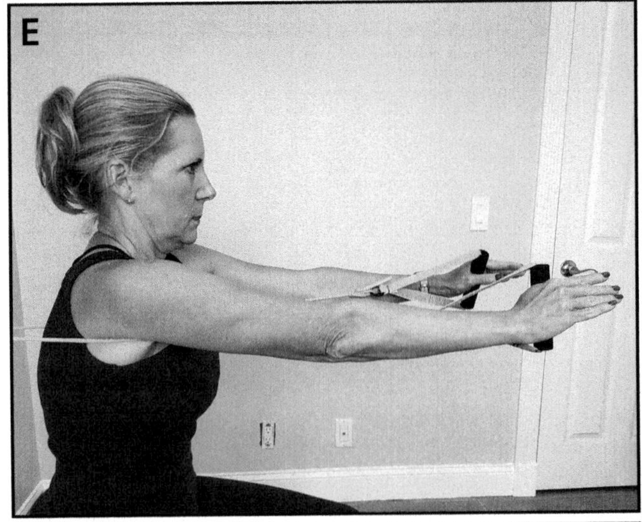


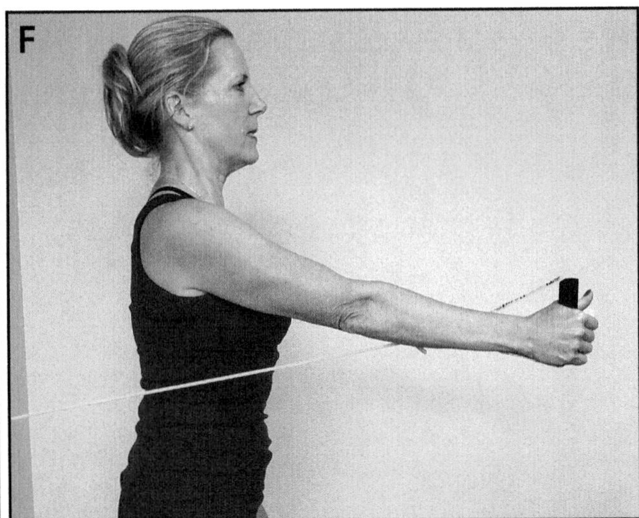


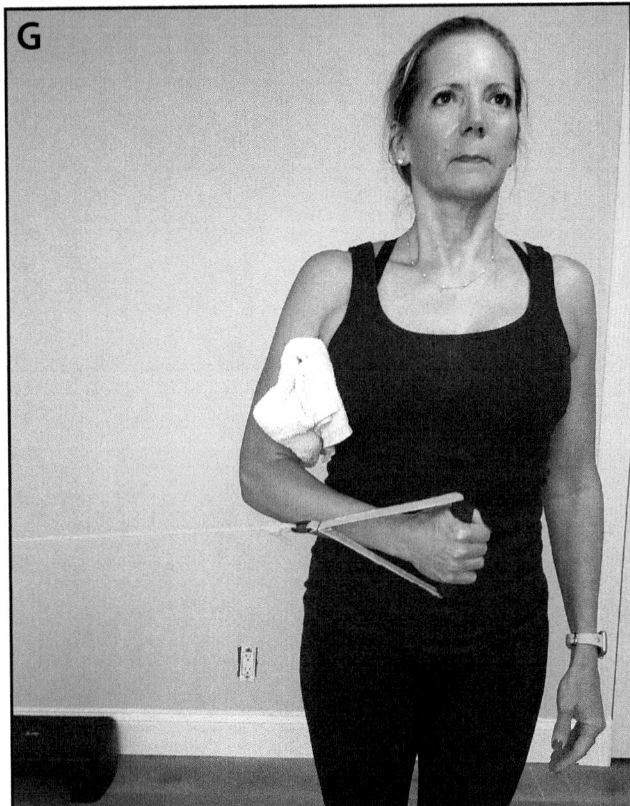


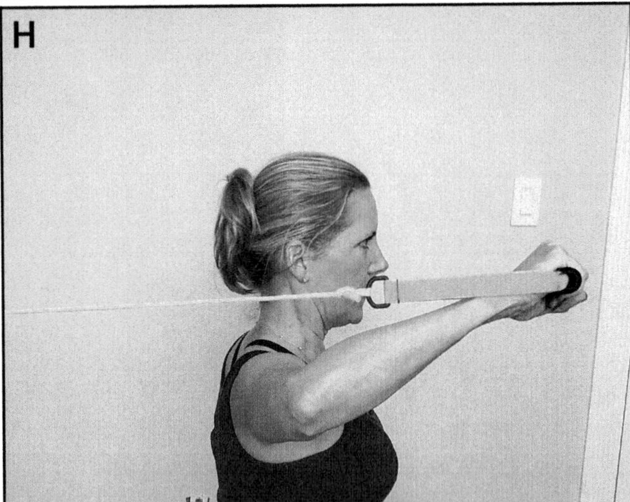


**Figure 12-52 (continued).** (E) The shoulder chest press plus protraction end position for the serratus anterior and anterior deltoid muscles. (F) The shoulder chest press to strengthen the pectoralis major, anterior deltoid, and triceps muscles. (G) Shoulder internal rotation in neutral position. (H) Shoulder internal rotation progression in a 90/90 position for subscapularis strengthening. *(continued)*

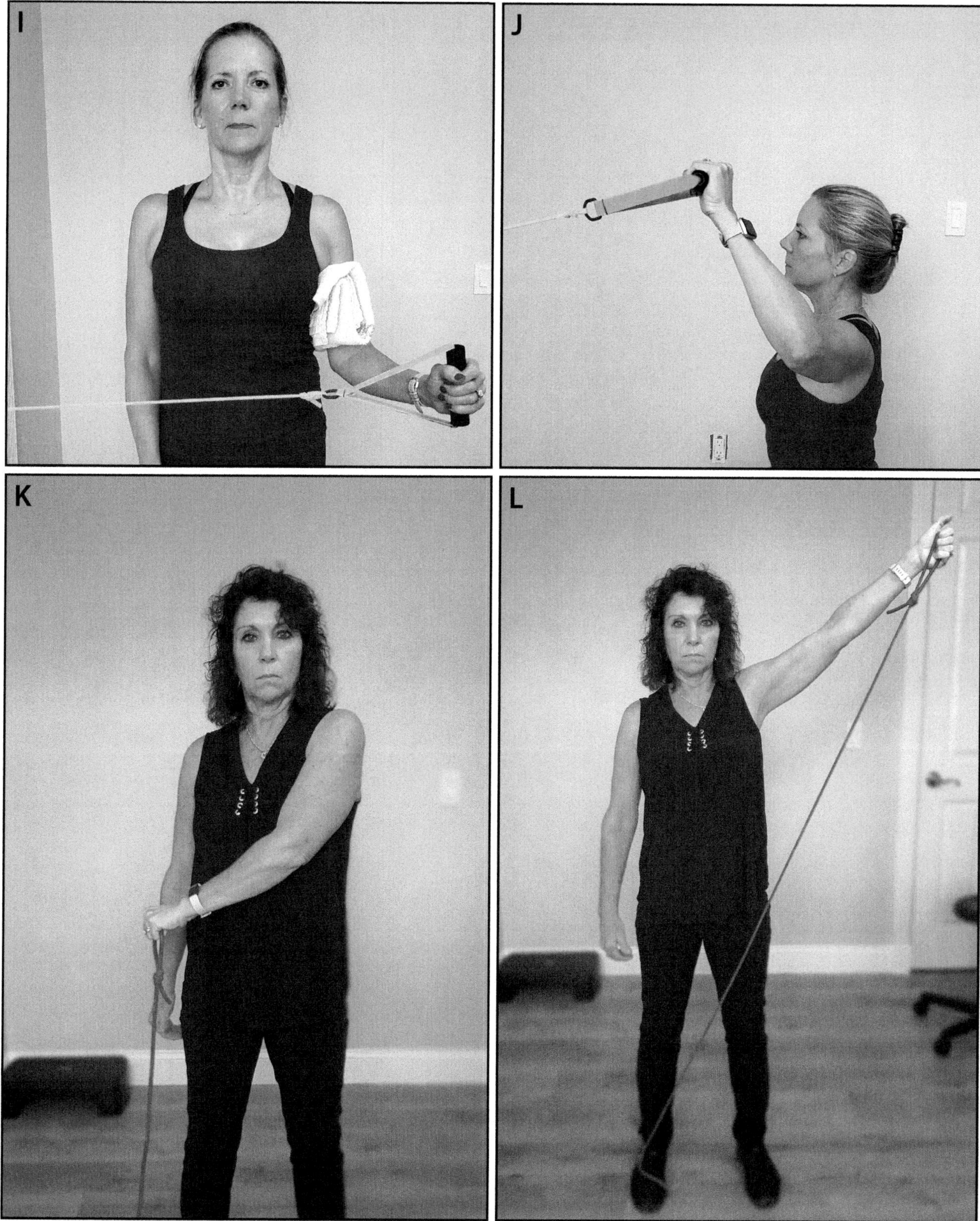


**Figure 12-52 (continued).** (I) Shoulder external rotation for infraspinatus and teres minor strengthening. (J) Shoulder external rotation progression to a 90/90 position. (K) Flexion for UE strengthening. Starting position. (L) The end position for PNF flexion. Notice the band is safely secured around patient's foot. For D2 extension, the band must be secured overhead.

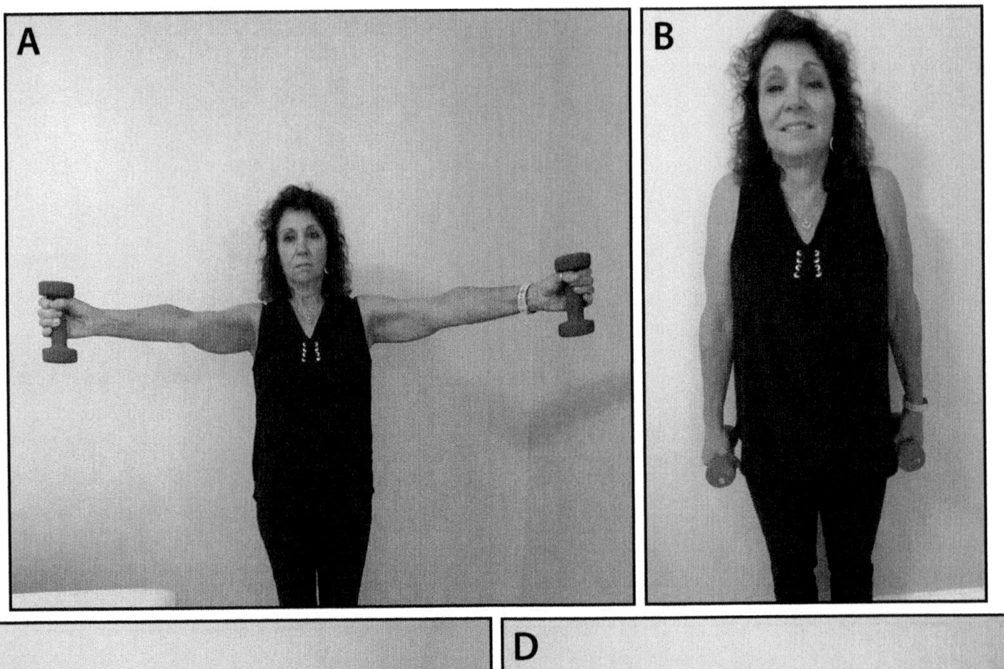

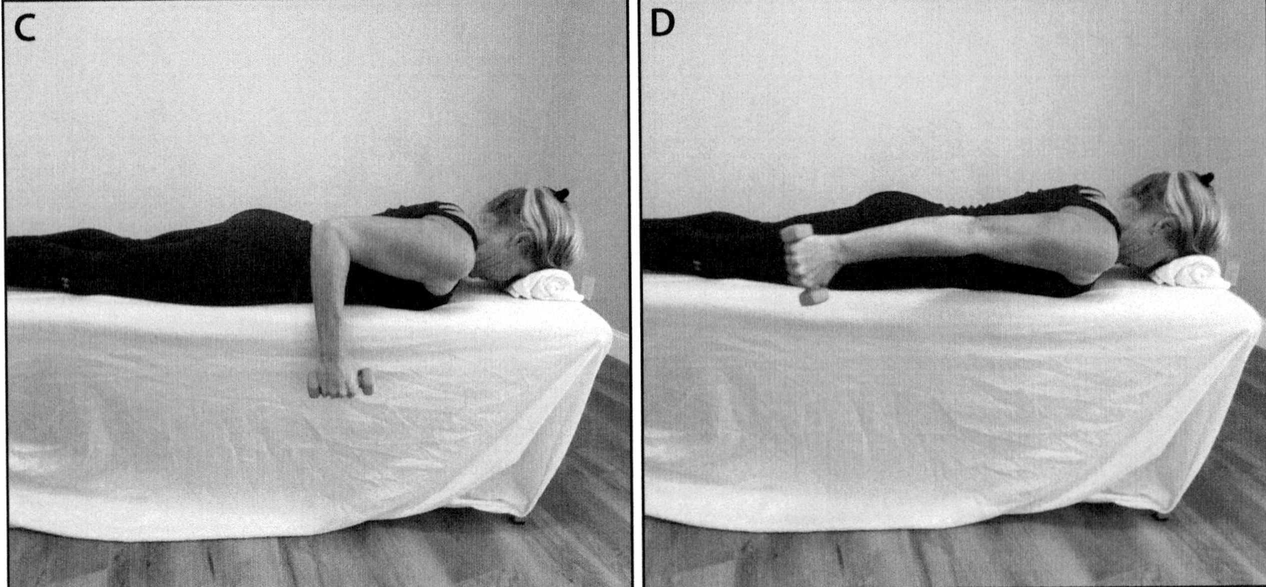

**Figure 12-53.** (A) The plane of the scapula bilaterally targets the supraspinatus muscle. This can be performed with one arm. (B) Shoulder shrugs to strengthen the upper trapezius and levator scapulae muscles. (C) Shoulder extension targets the posterior deltoid and rhomboid muscles. (D) Prone shoulder extension progression with the elbow extended. *(continued)*

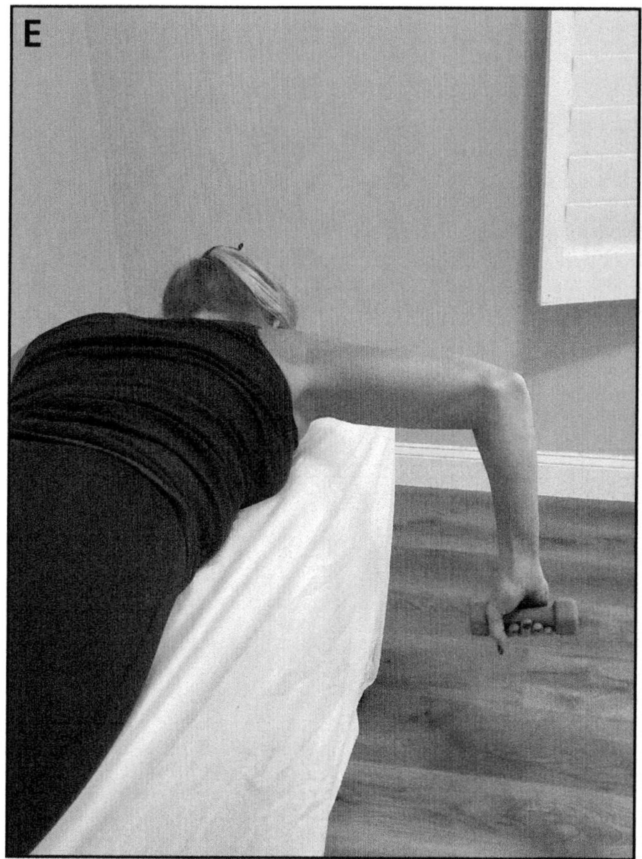


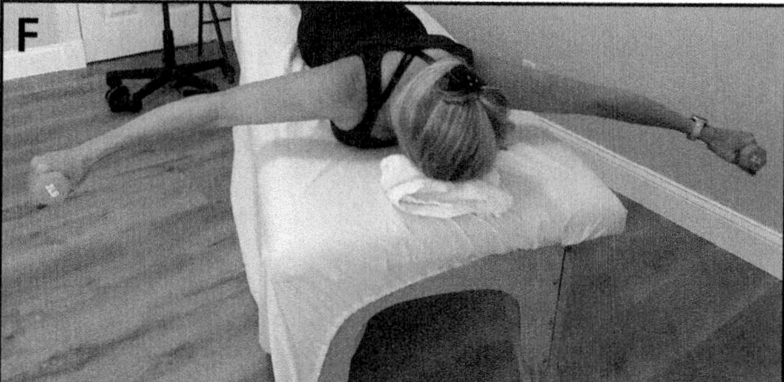


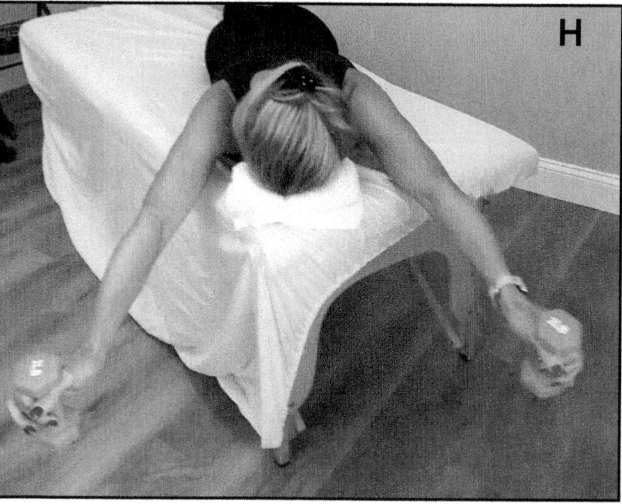


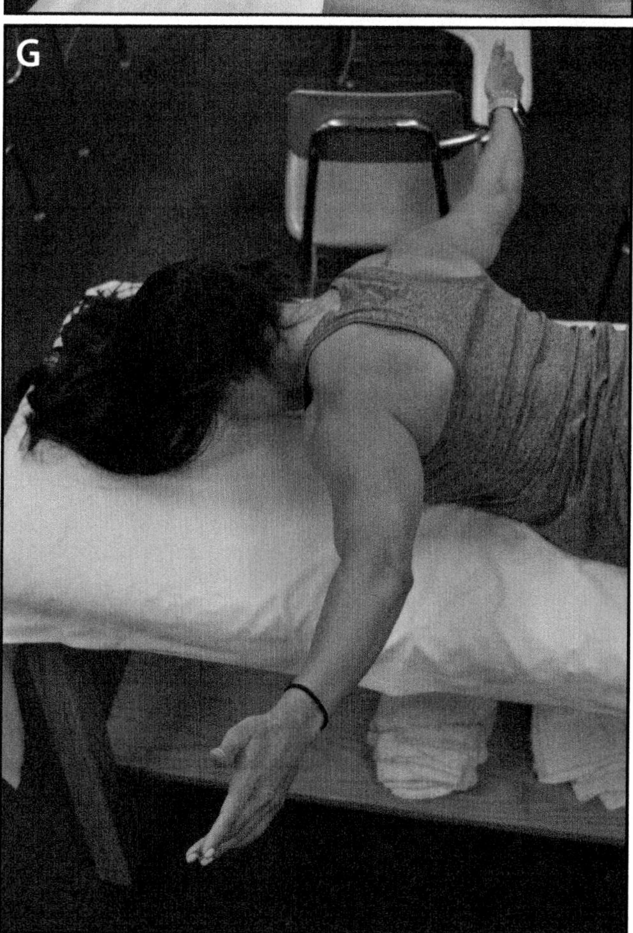


**Figure 12-53 (continued).** (E) Targets the middle trapezius and rhomboid muscles. (F) The prone T exercise palm down targets the rhomboid muscles. (G) Prone T thumb up targets middle trapezius muscles. (H) Prone Y exercise thumb up targets the lower trapezius, supraspinatus, and latissimus dorsi muscles. *(continued)*

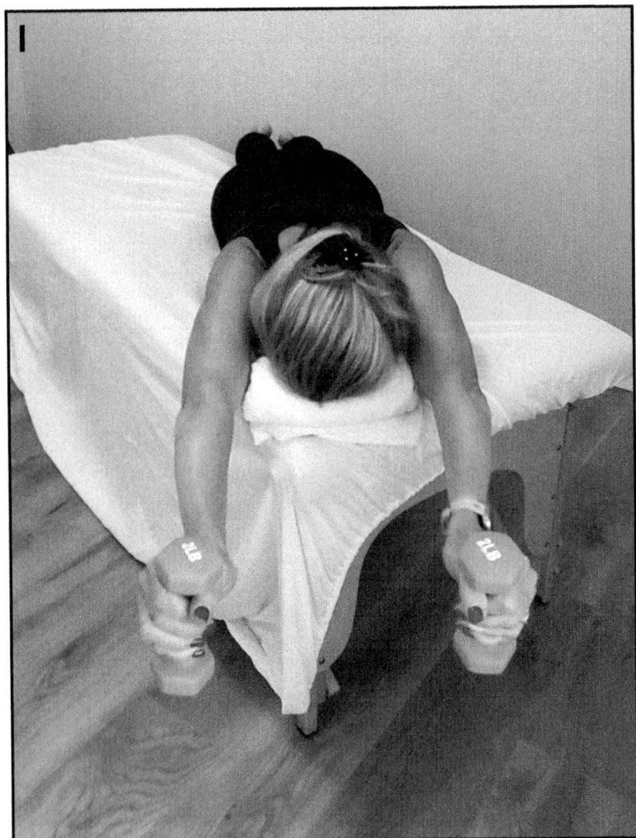

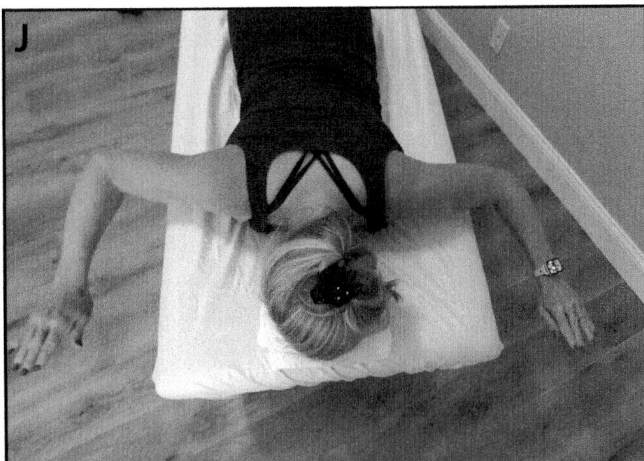

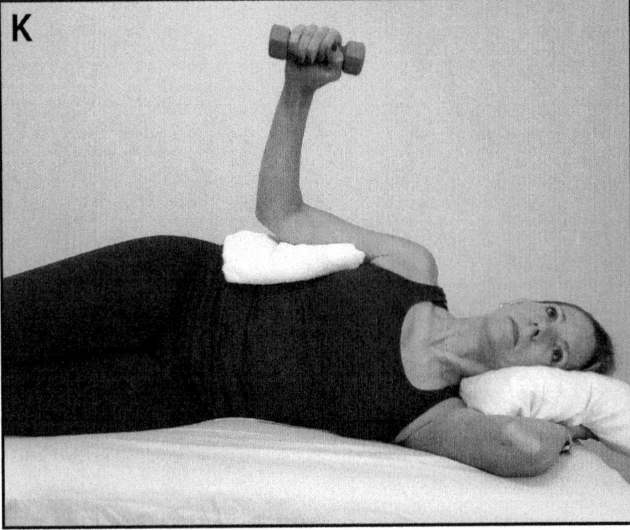

**Figure 12-53 (continued).** (I) Prone I exercise targets upper and lower trapezius, infraspinatus, and teres major. (J) Prone 90-90-90 shoulder retraction and horizontal abduction targets a large group of muscles. (K) Shoulder external rotation side lying.

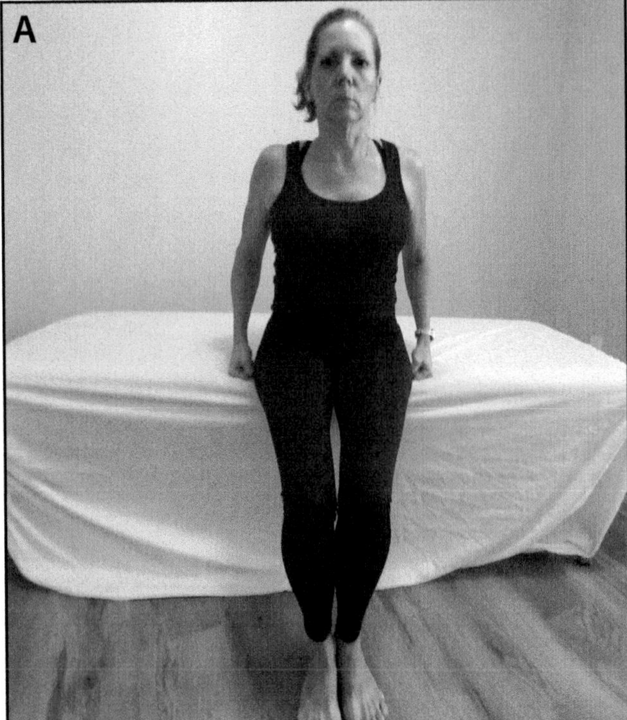

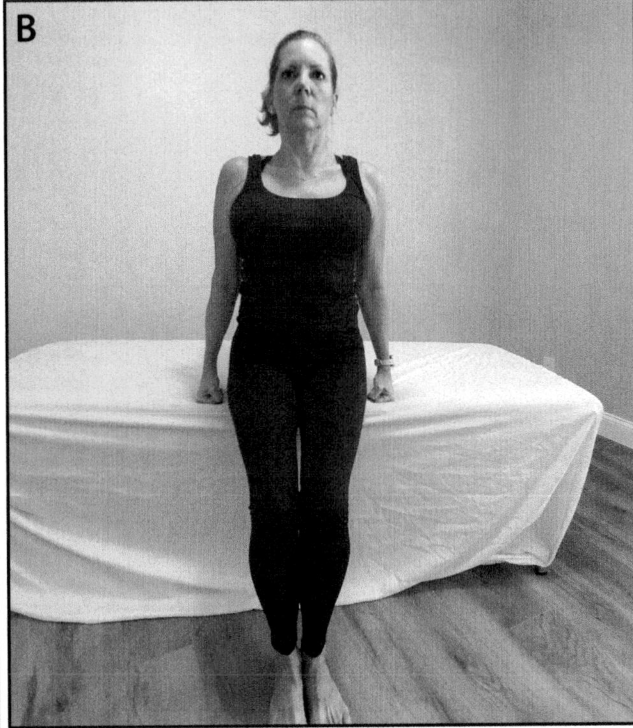

**Figure 12-54.** (A) The shoulder depression starting position. (B) The shoulder depression end position. The patient pushes their fists down into the treatment table, which can be assisted by using feet on the floor.

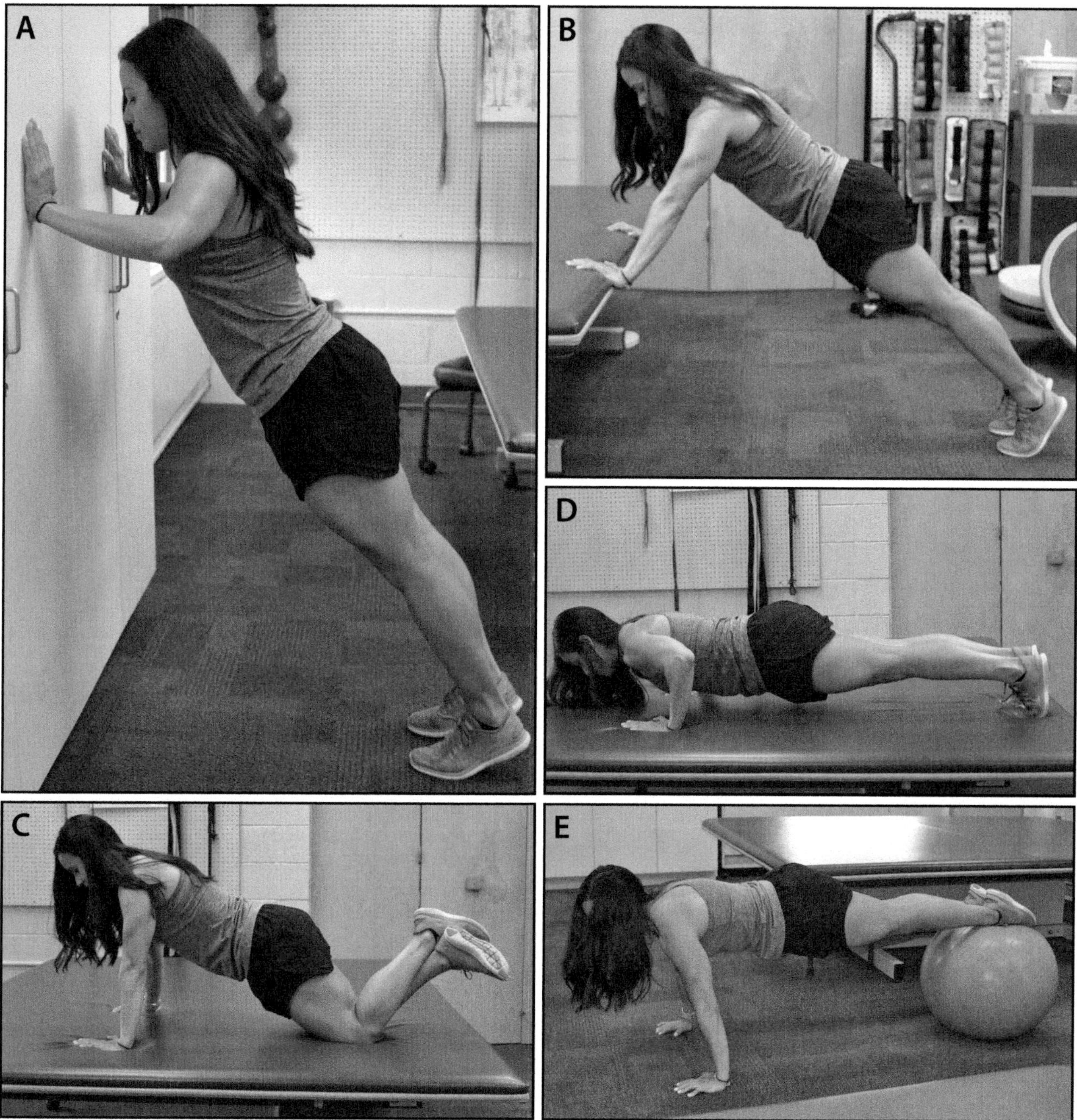


**Figure 12-55.** (A) Push-up progression 1: Against the wall. (B) Push-up progression 2: Increasing the angle makes the exercise more difficult. (C) Push-up progression 3: On knees. (D) Push-up progression 4: Knees straight. To make it more difficult, the hands can be placed on a less stable surface such as foam or balance discs. (E) Push-up progression 5: On a ball. To make it more difficult, hands can be placed on balance discs.

## *Neuromuscular Exercises and Advanced Exercises*

Figure 12-56 illustrates various neuromuscular exercises, with Figures 12-57 through 12-59 showing advanced exercises.

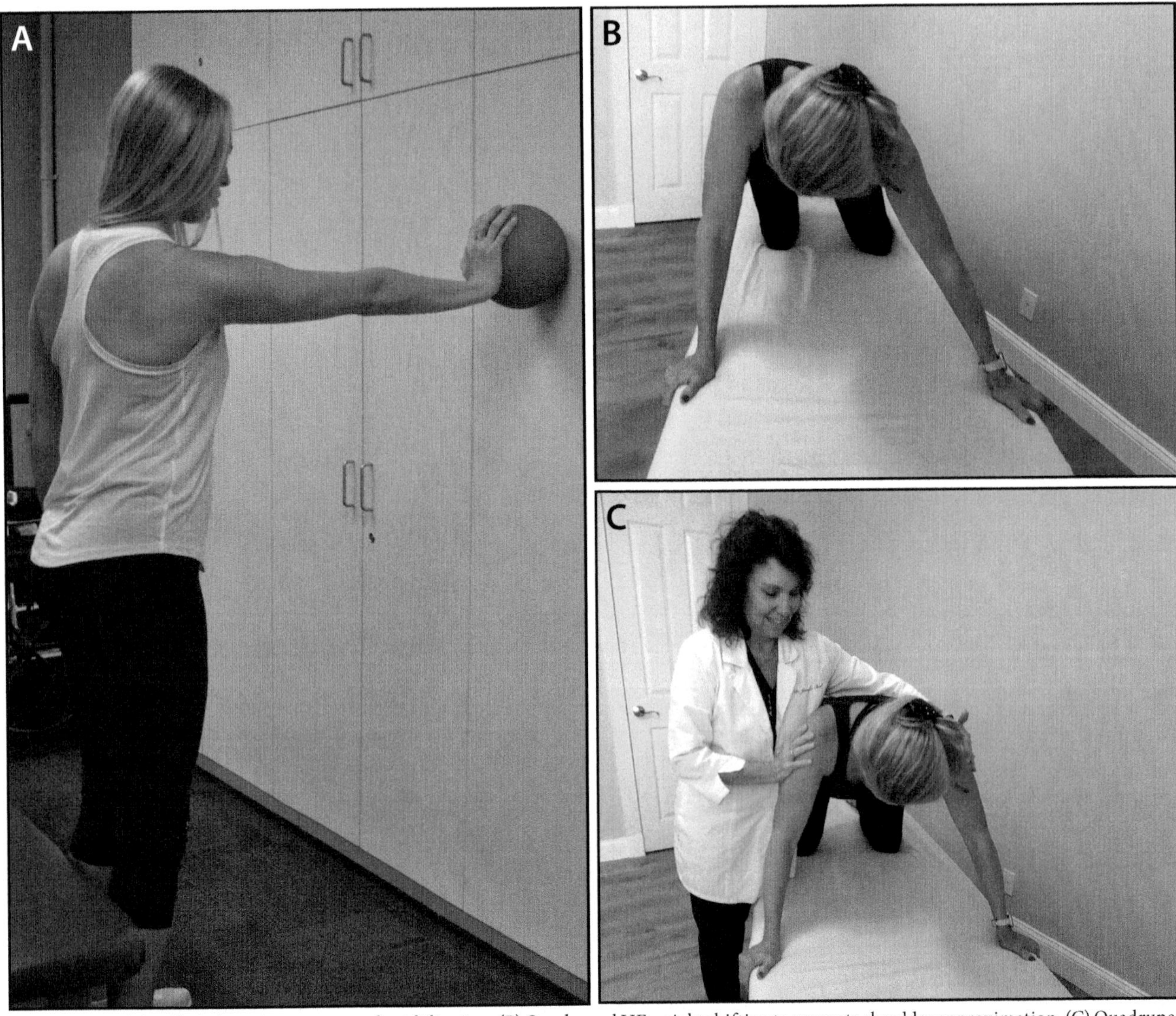

**Figure 12-56.** (A) Ball circles to improve scapula stabilization. (B) Quadruped UE weight shifting to promote shoulder approximation. (C) Quadruped shoulder stabilization with perturbations in all directions to improve neuromuscular control.

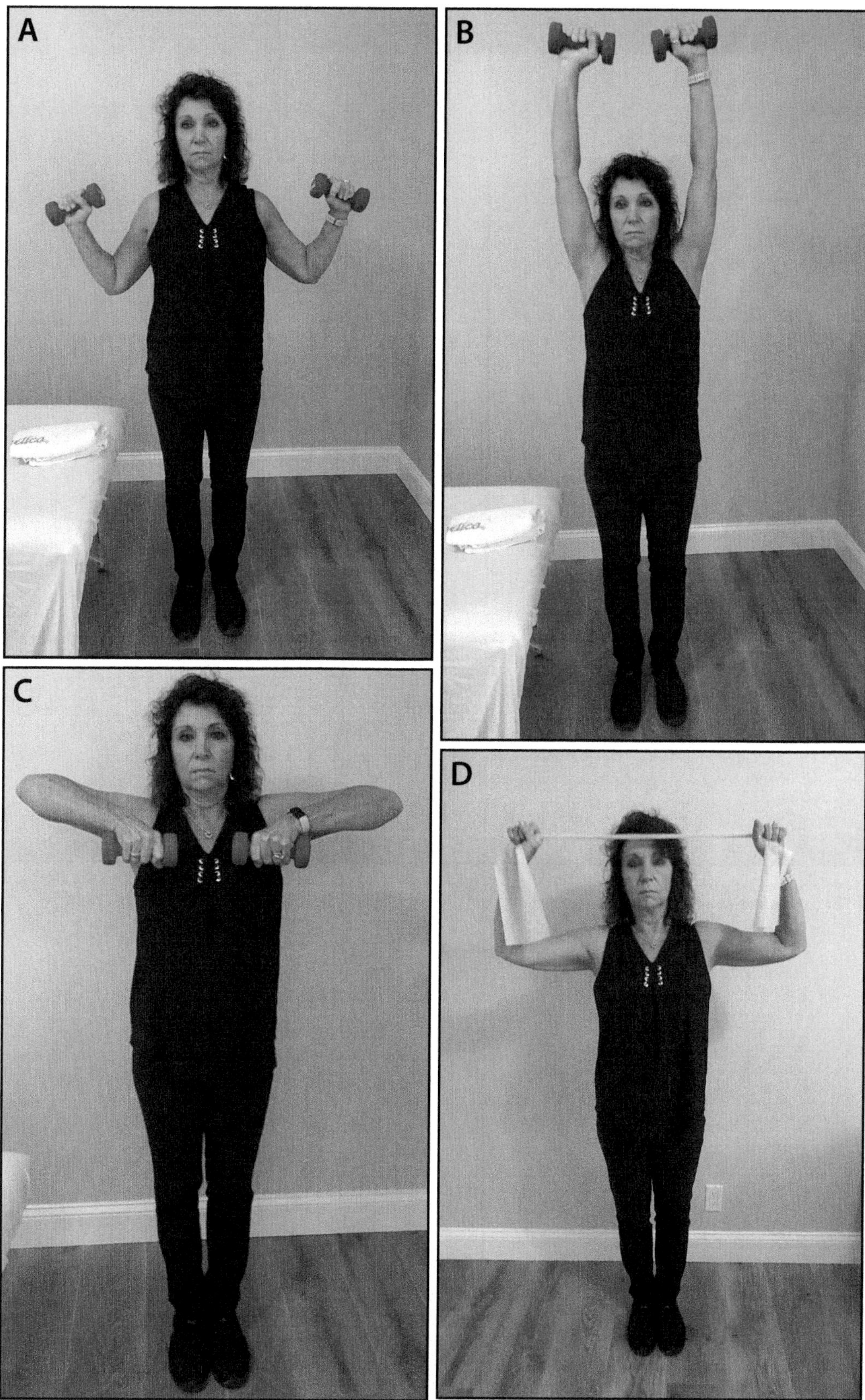


**Figure 12-57.** (A) The military press starting position. (B) The military press end position. (C) Lateral raises target the serratus anterior and anterior and lateral deltoid muscles. (D) Advanced exercises for shoulder stabilizers. The patient starts by creating tension by pulling the hands away from each other.

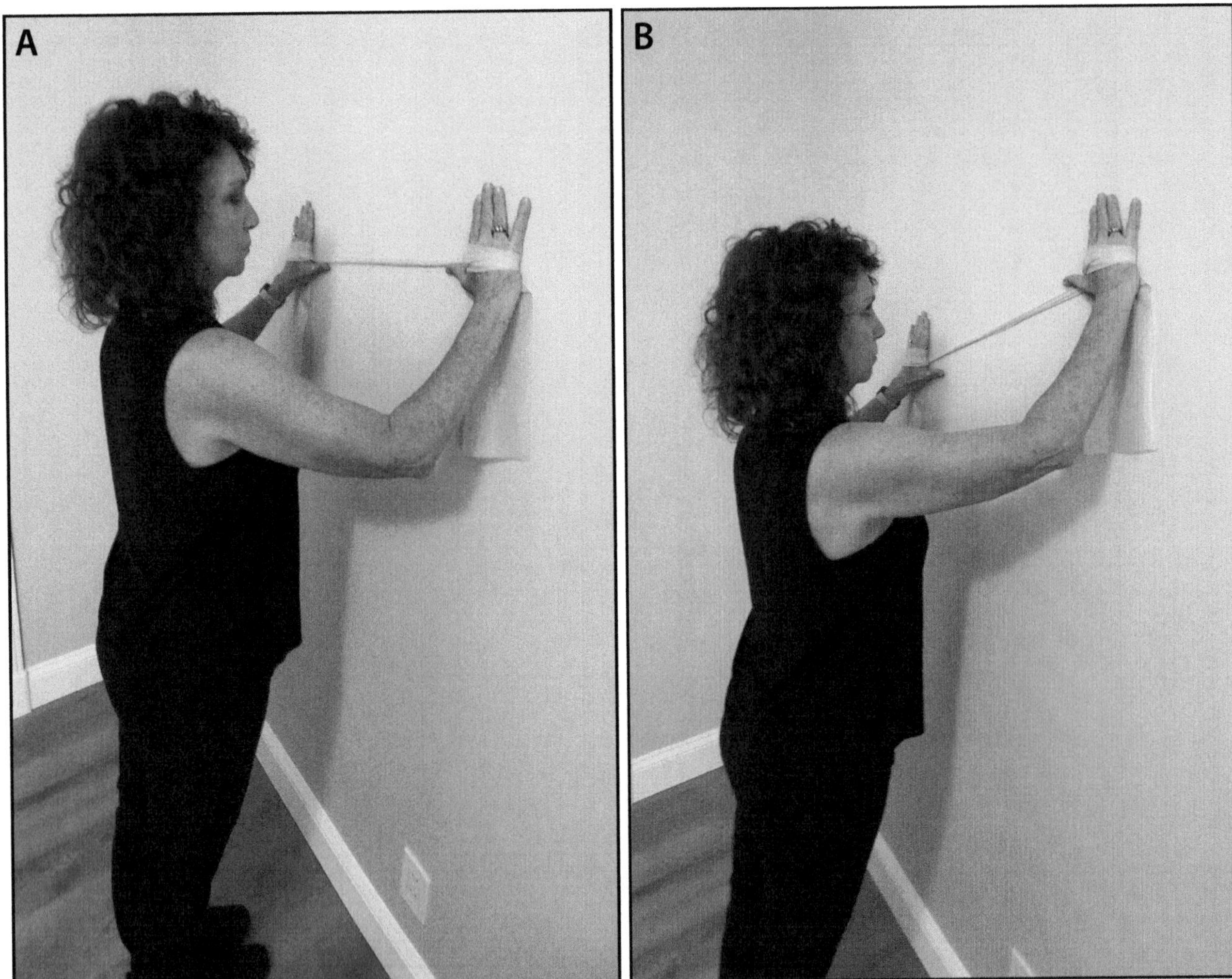


**Figure 12-58.** (A) Advanced exercises. Spiderman wall walking using a resistance band. The hands are positioned with the arms apart and tension on the band. (B) The patient moves one arm at a time to climb up and down the wall while maintaining tension on the band.

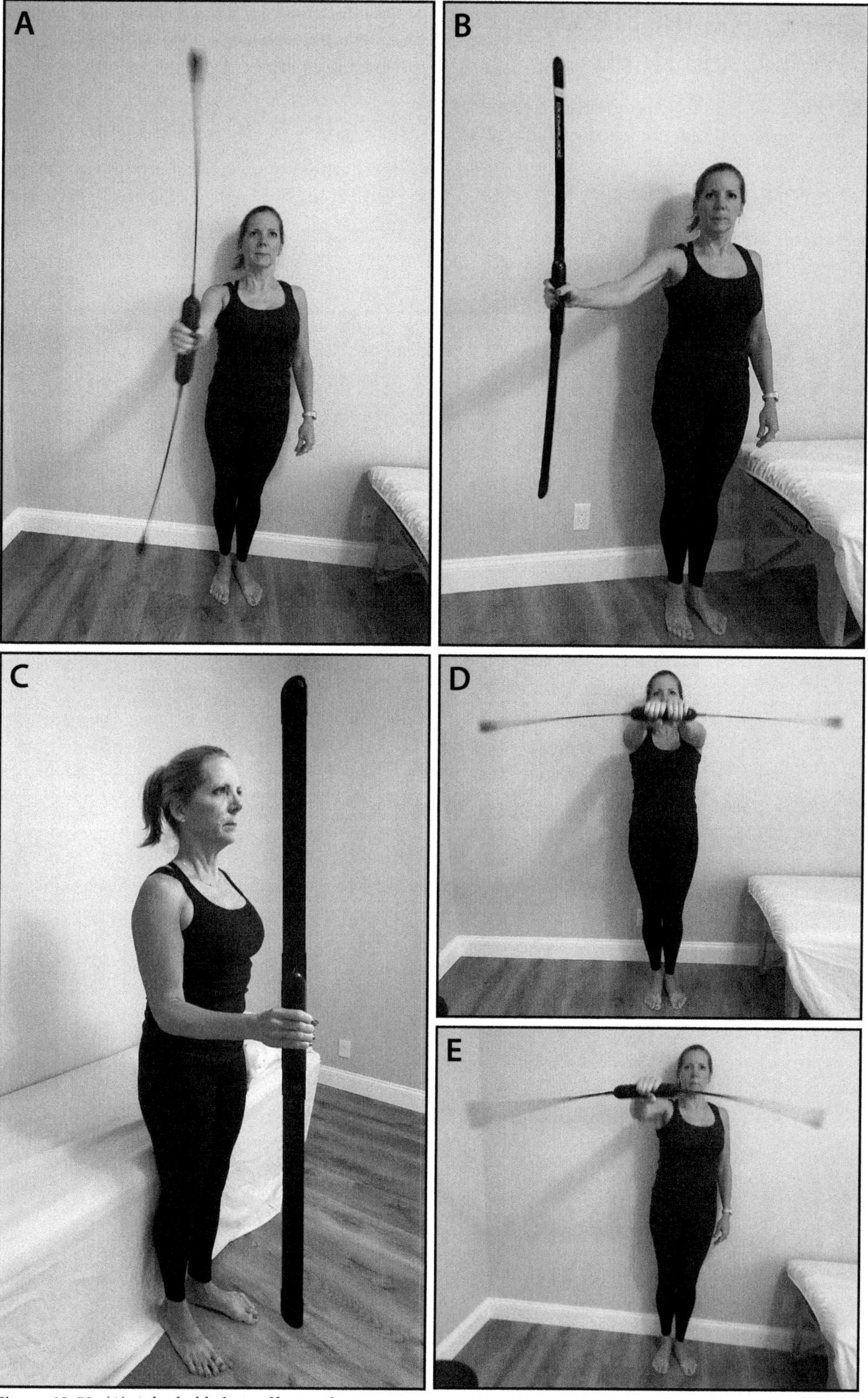


**Figure 12-59.** (A) A body blade is effective for increasing muscle endurance for shoulder stabilization. (B) A body blade exercise in the plane of the scapula. (C) A body blade exercise for shoulder internal and external rotation can be performed with the elbow flexed using small oscillations. (D) A body blade exercise can initially be performed bilaterally and then progressed to using one arm. (E) Body blade exercises can be performed with the elbow straight and on various angles.

# Exercises for the Elbow, Wrist, and Hand

This section presents various strengthening exercises for the elbow, wrist, and hand that are listed in Table 12-16.

## Stretching Exercises

Stretching exercises are illustrated in Figures 12-33 and 12-48A and 12-48C. The physical therapist assistant should understand that shoulder exercises are also important to include; strengthening and stretching above and below the involved joint are necessary to resume normal function.

## Strengthening Exercises

Strengthening exercises are shown for the elbow in Figure 12-60, the wrist in Figure 12-61, and the hand in Figure 12-62.

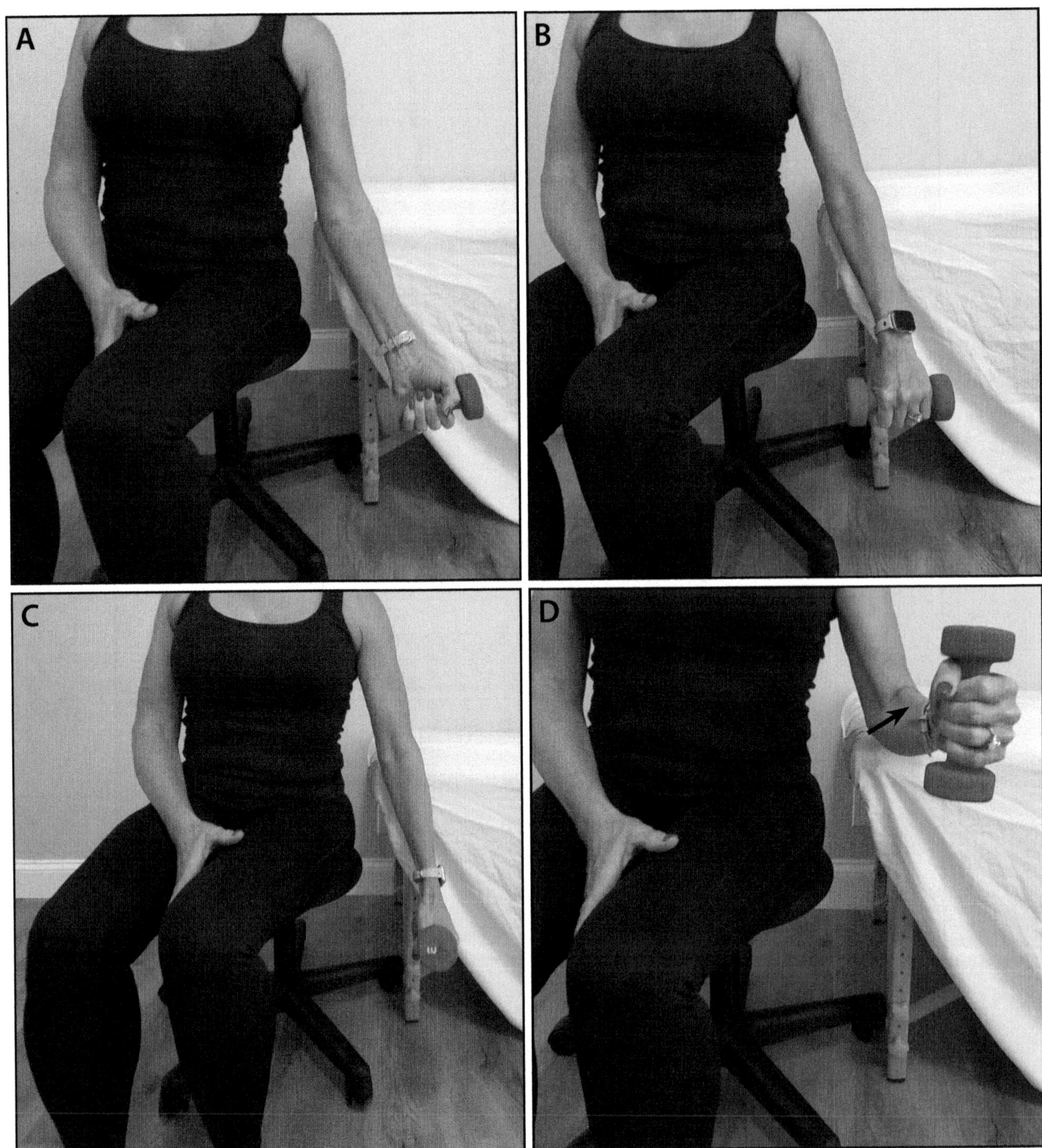


**Figure 12-60.** Three-way elbow strengthening exercise. (A) For the biceps brachii with the palm up. (B) For the brachialis with the palm down. (C) For the brachioradialis forearm in the neutral starting position. (D) Elbow flexion with the forearm in neutral. Notice the observable brachioradialis muscle. *(continued)*

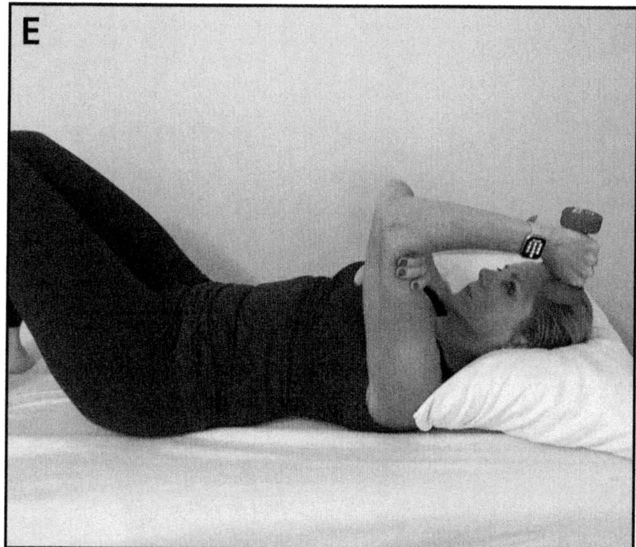


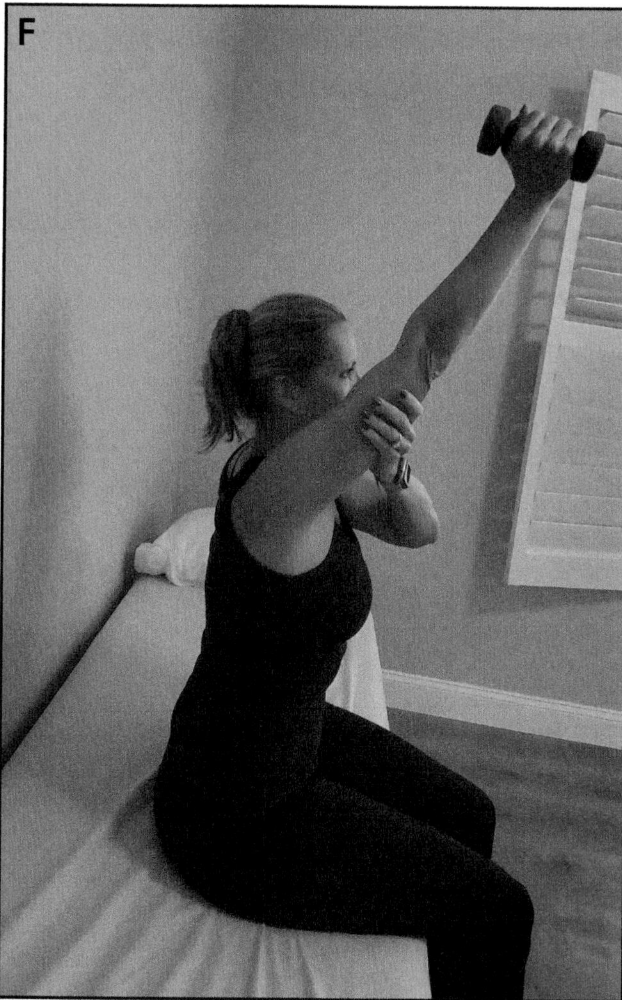


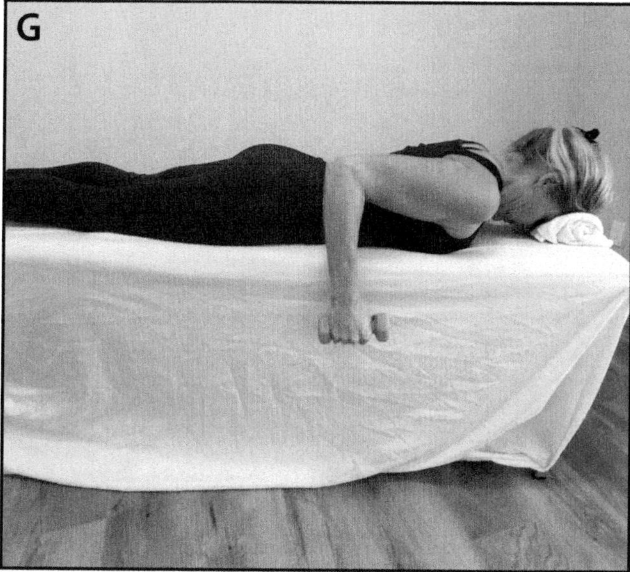


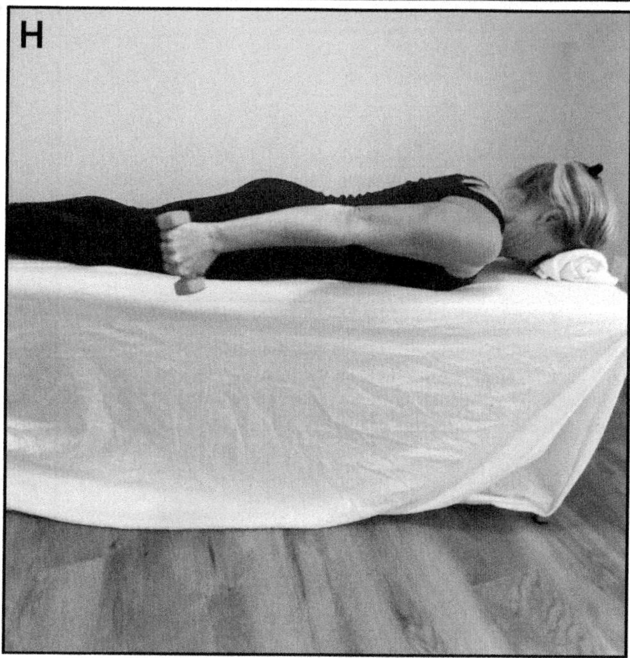


**Figure 12-60 (continued).** (E) Supine elbow extension for triceps brachii muscle strengthening. The patient to straighten the elbow up to the ceiling. (F) The seated triceps muscle strengthening end position. (G) The prone elbow extension starting position. (H) The prone elbow extension end position.

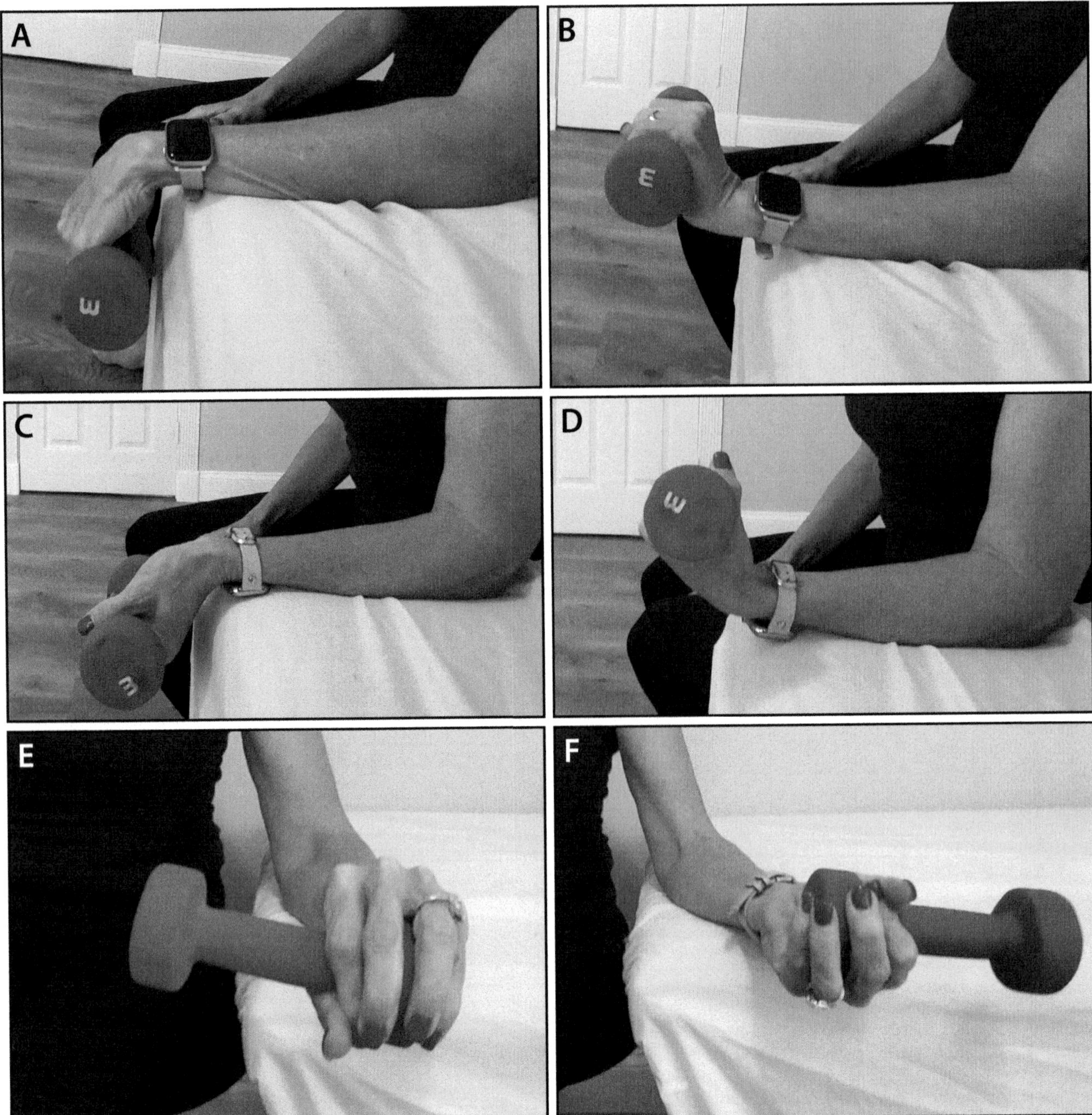


**Figure 12-61.** (A) The wrist extension starting position with the forearm supported. (B) The wrist extension end position for extensor carpi radialis and carpi ulnaris muscle strengthening. (C) The wrist flexion starting position for strengthening the flexor carpi radialis and carpi ulnaris muscles. (D) The wrist flexion muscle strengthening exercise end position. (E) Moving from a pronated position to a supinated position targets the supinator and biceps brachii. Holding the weight at the end increases the resistance. (F) Moving from a supinated position to a pronated position targets the pronator teres and pronator quadratus.

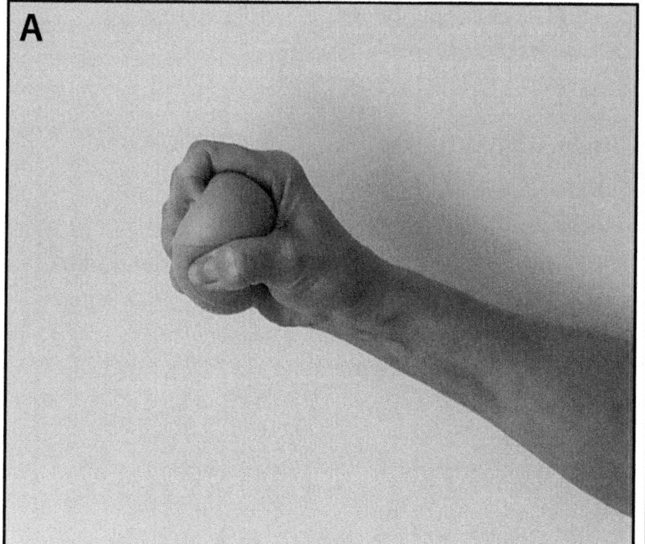


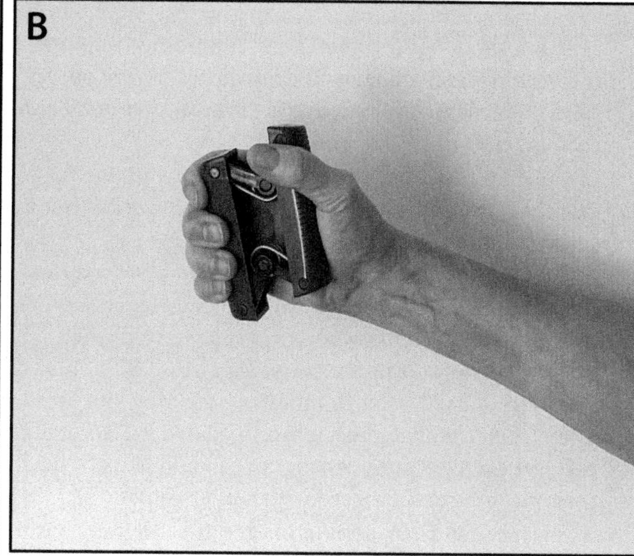


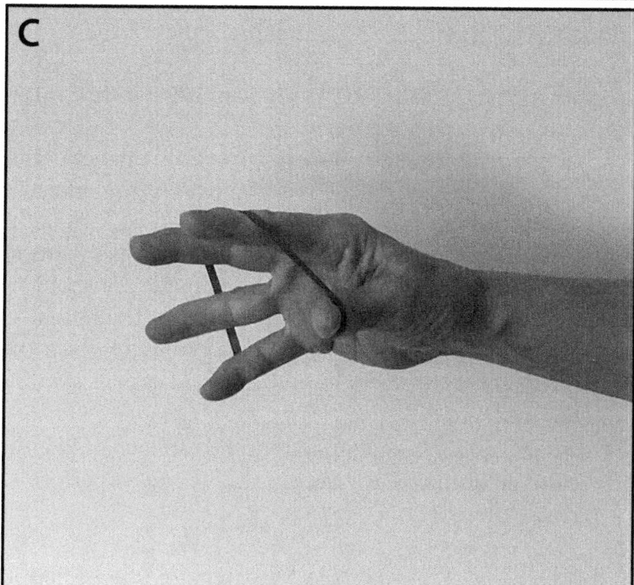


**Figure 12-62.** (A) Stress ball squeezes for finger and wrist flexor muscle strengthening. (B) A hand gripper to increase finger and hand grip strength. Grippers come in various resistances. (C) Finger extension strengthening using resistance or rubber bands.

## Conclusion

Physical therapy is an effective way to promote return to function for patients with a UE pathology. UE trauma, overuse, and tissue degeneration can all disrupt normal and efficient joint movements, creating pain for a patient and limiting participation in ADLs. A physical therapist assistant who understands both functional anatomy and the common MOI should be able to create effective treatment plans that reduce pain, increase ROM and strength, and improve function for the patient. The information in the physical therapy evaluation paired with the assistant's ability to monitor a patient's presentation and response to treatment guides the selection of the most appropriate exercises. The assistant must be able to recognize when and how to progress the patient or modify exercises.

## Review Questions

1. Describe the importance of normal scapular muscle function and strength to shoulder motion.
2. Compare and contrast the clinical presentation of medial and lateral epicondylalgia. Select one stretching and one strengthening exercise that is most appropriate for each condition.
3. What is the impact that forward head and rounded shoulder posture can have on shoulder biomechanics and risk for GH pathology?
4. Differentiate the function/role of the following special tests: empty can, Yergason, elbow varus stress test, and Phalen's test.
5. Describe a clinical presentation (after a Colles fracture with closed reduction and casting) that would indicate the need to follow up immediately with the supervising physical therapist.

6. What is an appropriate exercise to give to a patient with a diagnosis of subacromial pain syndrome (impingement syndrome) who has 75 degrees of active shoulder flexion, 90 degrees of passive flexion, and reports 8/10 pain at rest?
7. List one exercise that is *most* appropriate and one exercise that is *contraindicated* for a patient 2 weeks after a carpal tunnel release.
8. A 32-year-old man receiving therapy after a right shoulder labral tear is 14 weeks postoperative. He reports no resting pain but reports soreness that started when he warmed up on an upper body ergometer. He reports the pain started after 2 minutes of riding but went away after another minute or so. Based on soreness rules of exercise progression, how should the physical therapist assistant proceed with the treatment?
9. A 44-year-old man arrives for his first therapy visit after an initial examination for a left elbow fracture. The patient did not need surgery but was casted for 4 weeks. The patient is right-hand dominant. The primary therapist's clinical examination revealed the following:
   - Elbow ROM: Flexion: 110 degrees AROM, 120 degrees PROM
     - Extension: –25 degrees AROM, –18 degrees PROM
     - Pronation: 75 degrees AROM
     - Supination: 75 degrees AROM
   - Grip strength on Jamar level 2: right 110 foot-pounds and left 90 foot-pounds

   Based on the examination findings, list 3 appropriate exercises for this patient.
10. A 43-year-old man with a primary diagnosis of lateral epicondylalgia has been examined by the physical therapist who has determined that the patient has reduced handgrip strength, pain with gripping objects, and pain with elbow and wrist movements. The patient has had these symptoms for 2 months now and says it is limiting his ability to work as a truck driver. Based on current evidence, what exercises are most appropriate for this patient?

## Case Study 1

A 37-year-old woman presents to physical therapy with a diagnosis of right shoulder pain. She reports the pain first began 4 to 5 weeks ago while reaching in the back seat of her car to pick up a bag. She reports less pain since the initial injury but that it still hurts when reaching overhead or out to the side. She denies any history of shoulder problems. She is right handed and works full time as a mail carrier. She reports being out of work since her injury.

Clinical examination: QuickDASH score of 50
Cervical screen: negative
Shoulder ROM:

| Right: AROM/PROM | Left: AROM/PROM |
|---|---|
| Flexion 132/180 | Flexion WNL |
| Abduction 115/180 | Abduction 180 |
| Internal rotation 53/55 | Internal rotation 75/80 |
| External rotation 60/75 | External rotation 90/90 |

Shoulder strength right:

| Right | Left |
|---|---|
| Flexion 3–/5 (painful) | Flexion 5/5 |
| Abduction 3–/5 (painful) | Abduction 5/5 |
| Internal rotation 5/5 | Internal rotation 5/5 |
| External rotation 4/5 | External rotation 5/5 |

Special tests: positive Hawkins Kennedy, positive infraspinatus muscle test, + painful arc

The physical therapist has diagnosed this patient with right shoulder impingement syndrome. The POC includes patient education, ROM exercises, stretching, and strengthening exercises for 6 weeks. The long-term goals are to reduce the QuickDASH score to less than 30, 5/5 shoulder strength, and return to work without pain or limitation.

1. What ROM exercises are most appropriate given the physical therapist's POC and expected progression for the first week?
2. What signs or complaints from the patient would indicate the need to have the physical therapist perform a reassessment?
3. Four weeks after starting therapy, the patient's ROM and strength are both WNL, and she is expected to start work again next week. Please provide 3 functional-based exercises that she would benefit from performing in preparation for return to work.
4. What does a QuickDASH score of 50 indicate? What does a QuickDASH score of 30 indicate?

## Case Study 2

A 55-year-old woman presents to physical therapy with a primary diagnosis of CTS. She complains of right-handed numbness and weakness, reporting she feels very clumsy holding objects and admits to dropping things quite often. Her orthopedic physician diagnosed her with CTS after an electromyographic study. She continues to work as an administrative assistant but admits to reduced tolerance with computer work. She also reports having trouble sleeping at night because of her hand symptoms. The patient is right-hand dominant. Past medical history is negative for congestive heart failure, sarcoidosis, hypothyroidism, and rheumatoid arthritis.

Clinical examination: Cervical mobility: full and pain free

Elbow mobility: full and pain free

Wrist ROM:

| Right: AROM/PROM | Left: AROM/PROM |
|---|---|
| Flexion 80/85 | Flexion 80/85 |
| Extension 70/75 | Extension 70/75 |
| Radial deviation 18/20 | Radial deviation 20/20 |
| Ulnar deviation 38/40 | Ulnar deviation 40/40 |

Jamar grip strength at L2: right 43 foot-pounds and left 55 foot-pounds

Neurodynamic testing: median nerve tension test (upper limb tension test 1) positive on right for restriction and increase in symptoms

1. What exercises are most likely to be appropriate for initial management assuming a typical course of CTS?
2. List the 2 exercises that would be most beneficial for the patient initially.

After 2 months of therapy and continued symptoms, the patient decides to have surgery and undergoes an endoscopic carpal tunnel release procedure. She arrives 2 weeks postoperatively to initiate therapy.

3. What are appropriate exercises to initiate with the patient on the first visit?
4. What signs or complaints would indicate that the primary therapist should re-examine the patient?

## Suggested Resources

Avery Arora, MD: Surgery of the Hand, Wrist, & Elbow. Six pack active hand exercises. Accessed April 19, 2023. https://arorahandsurgery.com/wp-content/uploads/2017/03/6-pack-Hand_Exercises.pdf

Brigham and Women's Hospital. Physical therapy standards and care of protocol. Accessed April 19, 2023. https://www.brighamandwomens.org/patients-and-families/rehabilitation-services/physical-therapy-protocols

Shirley Ryan AbilityLab. Rehabilitation database measures. 2023. Accessed April 19, 2023. https://www.sralab.org/rehabilitation-measures

University of Florida Department of Orthopedic Surgery and Sports Medicine. Thrower's Ten. Updated October 27, 2021. Accessed April 19, 2023. https://www.ortho.ufl.edu/outreach/handouts

## References

1. Javed O, Maldonado KA, Ashmyan R. *Anatomy, Shoulder and Upper Limb, Muscles*. StatPearls Publishing; 2020. https://www.ncbi.nlm.nih.gov/books/NBK482410/
2. Berryman Reese N, Bandy WD. *Joint Range of Motion and Muscle Length Testing*. 3rd ed. Elsevier; 2017:535.
3. Biel A. Shoulder & arm. In: Biel A, ed. *Trail Guide to the Body: A Hands-on Guide to Locating Muscles, Bones and More*. 4th ed. Books of Discovery; 2010:67-99.
4. Biel A. Forearm & hand. In: Beil A, ed. *Trail Guide to the Body: A Hands-on Guide to Locating Muscles, Bones and More*. 4th ed. Books of Discovery; 2010:132-148, 150-159.
5. Gummesson C, Atroshi I, Ekdahl C. The disabilities of the arm, shoulder and hand (DASH) outcome questionnaire: longitudinal construct validity and measuring self-rated health change after surgery. *BMC Musculoskelet Disord*. 2003;4:11. doi:10.1186/1471-2474-4-11
6. Chesworth BM, Hamilton CB, Walton DM, et al. Reliability and validity of two versions of the upper extremity functional index. *Physiother Can*. 2014;66(3):243-253.
7. St-Pierre C, Dionne CE, Desmeules F, Roy JS. Reliability, validity, and responsiveness of a Canadian French adaptation of the Western Ontario Rotator Cuff (WORC) index. *J Hand Ther*. 2015;28(3):292-299. doi:10.1016/j.jht.2015.02.00
8. Borms D, Cools A. Upper-extremity functional performance tests: reference values for overhead athletes. *Int J Sports Med*. 2018:39(6):433-441. doi:10.1055/a-0573-1388
9. Cadogan A, Laslett M, Hing WA, McNair PJ, Coates MH. A prospective study of shoulder pain in primary care: prevalence of imaged pathology and response to guided diagnostic blocks. *BMC Musculoskelet Disord*. 2011:12:119. doi:10.1186/1471-2474-12-119
10. Park HB, Yokota A, Gill HS, El Rassi G, McFarland EG. Diagnostic accuracy of clinical tests for the different degrees of subacromial impingement syndrome. *J Bone Joint Surg Am*. 2005;87(7):1446-1455. doi:10.2106/JBJS.D.02335
11. Peterson C, Goodman CC. The gastrointestinal system. In: Goodman CC, Fuller KS, eds. *Pathology Implications for the Physical Therapist*. 4th ed. Elsevier; 2015:865-866.
12. Agarwal S, Raza S, Moiz JA, Anwer S, Alghadir AH. Effects of two different mobilization techniques on pain, range of motion and functional disability in patients with adhesive capsulitis: a comparative study. *J Phys Ther Sci*. 2016;28(12):3342-3349. doi:10.1589/jpts.28.3342
13. Johnson AJ, Godges JJ, Zimmerman GJ, Ounanian LL. The effect of anterior versus posterior glide joint mobilization on external rotation range of motion in patients with shoulder adhesive capsulitis. *J Orthop Sports Phys Ther*. 2007;37(3):88-99. doi:10.2519/jospt.2007.2307
14. Wilk KE, Macrina LC, Reinold MM. Non-operative rehabilitation for traumatic and atraumatic glenohumeral instability. *N Am J Sports Phys Ther*. 2006;1(1):16-31.
15. Abrams R, Akbarnia H. *Shoulder Dislocations Overview*. StatPearls Publishing; 2020. https://www.ncbi.nlm.nih.gov/books/NBK459125/
16. Cutts S, Prempeh M, Drew S. Anterior shoulder dislocation. *Ann R Coll Surg Engl*. 2009;91(1):2-7.

17. Milewski MD, Nissen CW. Pediatric and adolescent shoulder instability. *Clin Sports Med.* 2013;32(4):761-779.
18. Zacchilli MA, Owens BD. Epidemiology of shoulder dislocations presenting to emergency departments in the United States. *J Bone Joint Surg Am.* 2010;92(3):542-549.
19. Hovelius L, Olofsson A, Sandström B, et al. Nonoperative treatment of primary anterior shoulder dislocation in patients forty years of age and younger. A prospective twenty-five-year follow-up. *J Bone Joint Surg Am.* 2008;90(5):945-952.
20. Deitch J, Mehlman CT, Foad SL, Obbehat A, Mallory M. Traumatic anterior shoulder dislocation in adolescents. *Am J Sports Med.* 2003;31(5):758-763.
21. Brophy RH, Marx RG. The treatment of traumatic anterior instability of the shoulder: nonoperative and surgical treatment. *Arthroscopy.* 2009;25(3):298-304.
22. Carrazzone OL, Tamaoki MJ, Ambra LF, Neto NA, Matsumoto MH, Belloti JC. Prevalence of lesions associated with traumatic recurrent shoulder dislocation. *Rev Bras Ortop.* 2015;46(3):281-287. doi:10.1016/S2255-4971(15)30196-8
23. Yiannakopoulos CK, Mataragas E, Antonogiannakis E. A comparison of the spectrum of intra-articular lesions in acute and chronic anterior shoulder instability. *Arthroscopy.* 2007;23(9):985-990.
24. Rolfes K. Arthroscopic treatment of shoulder instability: a systematic review of capsular plication versus thermal capsulorrhaphy. *J Athl Train.* 2015;50(1):105-109. doi:10.4085/1062-6050-49.3.63
25. DeFroda SF, Mehta N, Owens BD. Physical therapy protocols for arthroscopic Bankart repair. *Sports Health.* 2018;10(3):250-258. doi:10.1177/1941738117750553
26. Kisner C, Colby L, Borstad J. The shoulder and shoulder girdle. In: Kisner C, Colby L, Borstad J, eds. *Therapeutic Exercise Foundations and Techniques.* 7th ed. FA Davis; 2018:552-593.
27. Wilk KE, Macrina LC, Cain EL, Dugas JR, Andrews JR. The recognition and treatment of superior labral (slap) lesions in the overhead athlete. *Int J Sports Phys Ther.* 2013;8(5):579-600.
28. Spargoli G. Treatment of rotator cuff tendinopathy as a contractile dysfunction. A clinical commentary. *Int J Sports Phys Ther.* 2019;14(1):148-158.
29. The Free Dictionary. Tendinopathy. n.d. Accessed January 31, 2023. https://medical-dictionary.thefreedictionary.com/tendinopathy
30. Khan Y, Nagy MT, Malal J, Waseem M. The painful shoulder: shoulder impingement syndrome. *Open Orthop J.* 2013;7:347-351. doi:10.2174/1874325001307010347
31. Papadonikolakis A, McKenna M, Warme W, Martin BI, Matsen FA. Published evidence relevant to the diagnosis of impingement syndrome of the shoulder. *J Bone Joint Surg Am.* 2011;93(19):1827-1832. doi:10.2106/JBJS.J.01748
32. Neer CS II. Impingement lesions. *Clin Orthop Relat Res.* 1983;173:70-77.
33. Rashid MS, Cooper C, Cook J, et al. Increasing age and tear size reduce rotator cuff repair healing rate at 1 year. *Acta Orthop.* 2017;88(6):606-611. doi:10.1080/17453674.2017.1370844
34. Sambandam SN, Khanna V, Gul A, Mounasamy V. Rotator cuff tears: an evidence based approach. *World J Orthop.* 2015;6(11):902-918. doi:10.5312/wjo.v6.i11.902
35. van der Meijden OA, Westgard P, Chandler Z, Gaskill TR, Kokmeyer D, Millett PJ. Rehabilitation after arthroscopic rotator cuff repair: current concepts review and evidence-based guidelines. *Int J Sports Phys Ther.* 2012;7(2):197-218.
36. Sgroi TA, Cilenti M. Rotator cuff repair: post-operative rehabilitation concepts. *Curr Rev Musculoskelet Med.* 2018;11(1):86-91. doi:10.1007/s12178-018-9462-7
37. Millett PJ, Wilcox RB, O'Holleran JD, Warner JJP. Rehabilitation of the rotator cuff: an evaluation-based approach. *J Am Acad Orthop Surg.* 2006;14(11):599-609.
38. Keener JD, Galatz LM, Stobbs-Cucchi G, Patton R, Yamaguchi K. Rehabilitation following arthroscopic rotator cuff repair: a prospective randomized trial of immobilization compared with early motion. *J Bone Joint Surg Am.* 2014;96(1):11-19. doi:10.2106/JBJS.M.00034
39. Long JL, Ruberte Thiele RA, Skendzel JG, et al. Activation of the shoulder musculature during pendulum exercises and light activities. *J Orthop Sports Phys Ther.* 2010;40(4):230-237. doi:10.2519/jospt.2010.3095
40. Knesek M, Brunfeldt A, Korenczuk C, et al. Patterns of strain and the determination of the safe arc of motion after subscapularis repair--a biomechanical study. *J Orthop Res.* 2016;34(3):518-524. doi:10.1002/jor.23045
41. Millett PJ, Gobezie R, Boykin RE. Shoulder osteoarthritis: diagnosis and management. *Am Fam Physician.* 2008;78(5):605-611.
42. Chillemi C, Franceschini V. Shoulder osteoarthritis. *Arthritis.* 2013;2013:370231. doi:10.1155/2013/370231
43. Mattei L, Mortera S, Arrigoni C, Castoldi F. Anatomic shoulder arthroplasty: an update on indications, technique, results and complication rates. *Joints.* 2015;3(2):72-77. doi:10.11138/jts/2015.3.2.072
44. Boudreau S, Boudreau ED, Higgins LD, Wilcox RB III. Rehabilitation following reverse total shoulder arthroplasty. *J Orthop Sports Phys Ther.* 2007;37(12):734-743. doi:10.2519/jospt.2007.2562
45. Buchmann S, Schoch C, Grim C, et al. Rehabilitation following reverse shoulder arthroplasty. *Obere Extrem.* 2019;14:269-283. doi:10.1007/s11678-019-0513-5
46. Bullock GS, Garrigues GE, Ledbetter L, Kennedy J. A systematic review of proposed rehabilitation guidelines following anatomic and reverse shoulder arthroplasty. *J Orthop Sports Phys Ther.* 2019;49(5):337-346. doi:10.2519/jospt.2019.8616
47. Kelley MJ, Shaffer MA, Kuhn JE, et al. Shoulder pain and mobility deficits: adhesive capsulitis: clinical practice guidelines linked to the International Classification of Functioning, Disability, and Health from the orthopaedic section of the American Physical Therapy Association. *J Orthop Sports Phys Ther.* 2013;43(5):A1-A31.
48. Le HV, Lee SJ, Nazarian A, Rodriguez EK. Adhesive capsulitis of the shoulder: review of pathophysiology and current clinical treatments. *Shoulder Elbow.* 2017;9(2):75-84. doi:10.1177/1758573216676786
49. Manske RC, Prohaska D. Diagnosis and management of adhesive capsulitis. *Curr Rev Musculoskelet Med.* 2008;1(3-4):180-189. doi:10.1007/s12178-008-9031-6
50. Khoriati AA, Antonios T, Bakti N, Mohanlal P, Singh B. Outcomes following non operative management for proximal humerus fractures. *J Clin Orthop Trauma.* 2019;10(3):462-467. doi:10.1016/j.jcot.2019.02.017

51. Kiel J, Kaiser K. *Acromioclavicular Joint Injury*. StatPearls Publishing; 2020. https://www.ncbi.nlm.nih.gov/books/NBK493188/
52. Karbach LE, Elfar J. Elbow instability: anatomy, biomechanics, diagnostic maneuvers, and testing. *J Hand Surg Am*. 2017;42(2):118-126. doi:10.1016/j.jhsa.2016.11.025
53. Schreiber JJ, Warren RF, Hotchkiss RN, Daluiski A. An online video investigation into the mechanism of elbow dislocation. *J Hand Surg*. 2013;38(3):488-494.
54. Kumar V, Singh A. Fracture supracondylar humerus: a review. *J Clin Diagn Res*. 2016;10(12):RE01-RE06. doi:10.7860/JCDR/2016/21647.8942
55. Wilk KE, Macrina LC, Cain EL, Dugas JR, Andrews JR. Rehabilitation of the overhead athlete's elbow. *Sports Health*. 2012;4(5):404-414. doi:10.1177/1941738112455006
56. Melugin HP, Leafblad ND, Camp CL, Conte S. Injury prevention in baseball: from youth to the pros. *Curr Rev Musculoskelet Med*. 2018;11(1):26-34. doi:10.1007/s12178-018-9456-5
57. Benjamin HJ, Briner WW Jr. Little league elbow. *Clin J Sport Med*. 2005;15(1):37-40.
58. Axe M, Hurd W, Snyder-Mackler L. Data-based interval throwing programs for baseball players. *Sports Health*. 2009;1(2):145-153. doi:10.1177/1941738108331198
59. Fleisig GS, Andrews JR. Prevention of elbow injuries in youth baseball pitchers. *Sports Health*. 2012;4(5):419-424. doi:10.1177/1941738112454828
60. Erickson BJ, Harris JD, Chalmers PN, et al. Ulnar collateral ligament reconstruction: anatomy, indications, techniques, and outcomes. *Sports Health*. 2015;7(6):511-517. doi:10.1177/1941738115607208
61. Andrews K, Rowland A, Pranjal A, Ebraheim N. Cubital tunnel syndrome: anatomy, clinical presentation, and management. *J Orthop*. 2018;15(3):832-836. doi:10.1016/j.jor.2018.08.010
62. Bisset LM, Vicenzino B. Physiotherapy management of lateral epicondylalgia. *J Physiother*. 2015;61(4):174-181. doi:10.1016/j.jphys.2015.07.015
63. Amin NH, Kumar NS, Schickendantz MS. Medial epicondylitis evaluation and management. *J Am Acad Orthop Surg*. 2015;23(6):348-355. doi:10.5435/JAAOS-D-14-00145
64. Svernlöv B, Hultgren E, Adolfsson L. Medial epicondylalgia (golfer's elbow) treated by eccentric exercise. *Shoulder Elbow*. 2012;(4)1:50-55. doi:10.1111/j.1758-5740.2011.00152.x
65. Peterson M, Butler S, Eriksson M, Svärdsudd K. A randomized controlled trial of eccentric vs. concentric graded exercise in chronic tennis elbow (lateral elbow tendinopathy). *Clin Rehabil*. 2014;28(9):862-872.
66. Toedebusch B, Washburn B, Marin K. Sports and occupational injuries to the wrist and hand. PM&R Knowledge Now. Updated July 3, 2018. Accessed January 31, 2023. https://now.aapmr.org/sports-and-occupational-injuries-to-the-wrist-and-hand/
67. Wainner RS, Fritz JM, Irrgang JJ, Delitto A, Allison S, Boninger ML. Development of a clinical prediction rule for the diagnosis of carpal tunnel syndrome. *Arch Phys Med Rehabil*. 2005;86(4):609-618. doi:10.1016/j.apmr.2004.11.008
68. Parvizi J, Wayman J, Kelly P, Moran CG. Combining the clinical signs improves diagnosis of scaphoid fractures. A prospective study with follow-up. *J Hand Surg Br*. 1998;23(3):324-327. doi:10.1016/s0266-7681(98)80050-8
69. Rhemrev SJ, Ootes D, Beeres FJ, Meylaerts SA, Schipper IB. Current methods of diagnosis and treatment of scaphoid fractures. *Int J Emerg Med*. 2011;4:4. doi:10.1186/1865-1380-4-4
70. Batteson R, Hammond A, Burke F, Sinha S. The de Quervain's screening tool: validity and reliability of a measure to support clinical diagnosis and management. *Musculoskeletal Care*. 2008;6(3):168-180. doi:10.1002/msc.129
71. Blakeney WG. Stabilization and treatment of Colles' fractures in elderly patients. *Clin Interv Aging*. 2010;5:337-344. doi:10.2147/CIA.S10042
72. Valdes K. A retrospective pilot study comparing the number of therapy visits required to regain functional wrist and forearm range of motion following volar plating of a distal radius fracture. *J Hand Ther*. 2009;22(4):312-319.
73. Genova A, Dix O, Saefan A, Thakur M, Hassan A. Carpal tunnel syndrome: a review of literature. *Cureus*. 2020;12(3):e7333. doi:10.7759/cureus.7333
74. Geoghegan JM, Clark DI, Bainbridge LC, Smith C, Hubbard R. Risk factors in carpal tunnel syndrome. *J Hand Surg Br*. 2004;29(4):315-320. doi:10.1016/j.jhsb.2004.02.009
75. Page MJ, O'Connor D, Pitt V, Massy-Westropp N. Exercise and mobilisation interventions for carpal tunnel syndrome. *Cochrane Database Syst Rev*. 2012;6:CD009899. doi:10.1002/14651858.CD009899
76. Amadio PC. Carpal tunnel syndrome: surgeon's management. In: Skirven TM, Osterman AL, Fedorczyk JM, Amadio PC, eds. *Rehabilitation of the Hand and Upper Extremity*. 6th ed. Mosby Elsevier; 2011:666-677.
77. Takata SC, Wade ET, Roll SC. Hand therapy interventions, outcomes, and diagnoses evaluated over the last 10 years: a mapping review linking research to practice. *J Hand Ther*. 2019;32(1):1-9. doi:10.1016/j.jht.2017.05.018
78. Ilyas AM, Ast M, Schaffer AA, Thoder J. De Quervain tenosynovitis of the wrist. *J Am Acad Orthop Surg*. 2007;15(12):757-764. doi:10.5435/00124635-200712000-00009
79. Goel R, Abzug JM. de Quervain's tenosynovitis: a review of the rehabilitative options. *Hand (N Y)*. 2015;10(1):1-5. doi:10.1007/s11552-014-9649-3
80. Huisstede BM, Coert JH, Fridén J, Hoogvliet P; European HANDGUIDE Group. Consensus on a multidisciplinary treatment guideline for de Quervain disease: results from the European HANDGUIDE study. *Phys Ther*. 2014;94(8):1095-1110. doi:10.2522/ptj.20130069
81. Hung CY, Varacallo M, Chang KV. *Gamekeepers Thumb*. StatPearls Publishing; 2020. https://www.ncbi.nlm.nih.gov/books/NBK499971/

Chapter 13

# Management of Lower Extremity Orthopedic Conditions

*Karen A. Cascardi, PhD, MS, ATC, PTA and Jacki Klaczak Kopack, PT, DPT*

**KEY TERMS** Chondromalacia patella | Lumbopelvic rhythm | Patellofemoral pain syndrome | Screw-home mechanism | Unhappy/terrible triad | Windlass mechanism

## Chapter Objectives

1. Recall the basic anatomical structures of the lower extremity.
2. Describe the common lower quarter sprains, strains, surgical procedures, and injuries.
3. Describe the impact of structural or muscle weakness or tightness on range of motion (ROM), strength, pain, and function.
4. Identify the common tests and measures specific to lower extremity diagnoses.
5. Select exercise interventions and progressions to address lower extremity diagnoses.
6. Given a specific lower quarter diagnosis and plan of care (POC), design and progress a patient through a therapeutic exercise program for each phase of the rehabilitation process.
7. List the contraindications and precautions for the treatment for common lower extremity diagnoses and the surgical procedure.

## Introduction to Lower Extremity Orthopedic Conditions

Physical therapist assistants treat a variety of lower extremity orthopedic conditions. The lower extremity plays an important role in everyday function and mobility, especially during closed kinetic chain (CKC) activities such as walking and sit-to-stand transitions. The ability of the lower extremity to bear weight and transmit forces from the head, arms, and trunk is critical to normal upright mobility and functional movement transitions.

Impairments in any structure during a lower extremity CKC activity can alter the normal biomechanics at other proximal and/or distal joints. Motion in the joints in a weight-bearing limb creates a chain reaction. A change in joint biomechanics related to muscle tightness, ligament laxity, or poor neuromuscular control in one structure will affect the other joints and tissues up and down the chain. For example, iliopsoas tightness can create an increase in hip flexion and an anterior pelvic tilt, resulting in a compensatory lumbar extension when standing. When walking, iliopsoas tightness may limit hip extension, creating



Kopack JK, Cascardi KA. *Principles of Therapeutic Exercise for the Physical Therapist Assistant* (pp 351-461).

subtle shifts in knee and ankle positions and resulting in a decrease in step length and limited use of the hip extensors and plantar flexors. This illustrates that a limitation at one joint can result in a significant change from the normal resting position (or alignment) in other joints and can alter the function and the biomechanics of the surrounding structures. This increases the potential for pathology and pain.

### Considerations for the Physical Therapist Assistant

During unilateral stance, gravity creates an adductor moment in the weight-bearing (CKC) hip; this force is counteracted by contraction of the gluteus medius, preventing a pelvic drop on the (open kinetic chain [OKC]) contralateral side. If the gluteus medius is weak, the adductor moment is not controlled, resulting in pelvic drop on the non–weight-bearing (NWB) side, as well as adduction of the femur and increased valgus at the knee on the CKC leg. Increased valgus at the knee increases stress on the medial knee structures.

A thorough physical therapy examination and evaluation will determine the primary source of a patient's symptoms. The physical therapist assistant must monitor patient performance and observe for signs/symptoms that may indicate additional injury/disease or changes in the inflammatory process. The assistant will select, modify, and determine the appropriate exercise interventions to progress the patient safely to achieve the desired outcomes. Many postoperative rehabilitation progressions will strictly follow a surgeon's postoperative protocol. Suggested guidelines and therapy progressions are included throughout this chapter to aid the assistant in problem-solving exercise progressions, but the assistant should always defer to the surgeon's protocol and the physical therapy POC.

Any new injuries, comorbidities, or changes in the patient's medical status should be brought to the physical therapist's attention immediately. The assistant's observations regarding changes in symptoms or presentation (refer to Chapter 11 [see Table 11-1]) enable the supervising therapist to determine if the structure considered to be the source of symptoms is the actual source or if the treatment diagnosis and POC should be altered. The assistant must consider the entire patient when making observations. Observing the patient's gait pattern, transitional movements, sitting and standing posture, and trends in and location of symptoms up and down the kinetic chain are all part of the ongoing screening and assessment that are critical to maximizing patient outcomes.

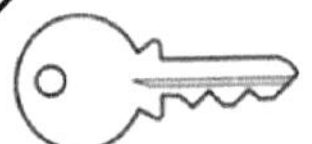

### Key Safety Consideration

- Know the patient's stage of healing (acute, subacute, or chronic) and associated treatment constraints.
- Be alert to the contraindications and precautions relative to the patient's diagnosis or postoperative procedures/protocols.
- Be aware of new or changing signs/symptoms that may indicate a medical vs a musculoskeletal reason for a patient's change in symptoms.

## *Referred Pain Patterns and Red Flag Items*

Referred pain is the patient's perception of pain that originates from somewhere other than the area where the patient is feeling the pain. Radicular pain is perceived in the dermatome of a compressed spinal nerve. Referred pain in the lower extremity can arise from an organ, nerve root, or other musculoskeletal structures. Careful ongoing observation can reveal patterns of symptoms or referred pain patterns (Table 13-1).[1-3] Treatment should be directed to the source of the pain vs the site of the referred pain.

### Clinical Tip

Patients who present with back pain as well as with a limp and groin pain and/or with limitations in hip internal rotation are more likely to have the hip as the source of pain rather than the lumbar spine.[1]

There are medical diagnoses that can also cause lower extremity pain. The physical therapy examination should rule out any red flags before initiating treatment. Because each patient's status evolves, the physical therapist assistant must observe for any new or changing signs or symptoms that may indicate a medical cause vs a musculoskeletal reason for a patient's change in symptoms. Some primary medical diagnoses that may present with lower leg pain or symptoms include deep vein thrombosis (DVT), compartment syndrome, cellulitis, fracture, and septic arthritis (Table 13-2).[4-10] These can be medical emergencies, so the assistant should immediately bring these findings to the supervising physical therapist before continuing treatment. The assistant's ability to observe and perform clinical decision making is crucial to maintaining the patient's health and safety (Box 13-1).

**Table 13-1**

Referred Pain Patterns for the Lower Quarter[1-3]

| Source of Pain | Possible Referred Pain Pattern |
|---|---|
| Hip joint | Posterior pelvic region/buttock, groin, thigh, knee, groin and knee together, foot (<8%) |
| Lumbar disk herniation, lumbar facet disease, sciatica, spinal stenosis | Hip, thigh |
| Sacroiliac dysfunction | Hip/groin |
| Inguinal or femoral hernia | Hip |
| Hip | Knee |
| Iliotibial band (ITB) syndrome | Knee |
| L3 spinal nerve root | Anterior knee |
| S1, S2 spinal nerve root | Posterior knee |
| L4, L5, S1 nerve roots | Foot |

**Table 13-2**

Medical Diagnoses and Typical Presentations

| Medical Diagnosis | Typical Presentation: Signs and Symptoms |
|---|---|
| DVT | Calf pain, redness, warmth, and edema; a recent history of surgery, malignancy, pregnancy, or immobilization; verify using Well's criteria[4,5] |
| Compartment syndrome | Severe, persistent leg pain, swelling, paresthesia, decreased or absent peripheral pulse, exquisite pain; a history of trauma, crush injury, or participation in rigorous training/exercise activity[6] |
| Cellulitis | An area of expanding erythema, warmth, tenderness, or swelling; a history of diabetes mellitus or recent abrasion/wound; may see fever and malaise[7] |
| Fracture | Unwillingness to bear weight on the affected limb, bruising, swelling, hemarthrosis, and point tenderness[8,9]<br>The Ottawa Knee Decision Rules and the Ottawa Ankle Decision Rules provide guidelines for screening after injury[8] |
| Septic arthritis | Swelling, hemarthrosis, warmth, and pain; a history of recent infection, surgery, or injection[10] |

Box 13-1

**Clinical Reasoning for the Physical Therapist Assistant**

- Apply knowledge of treatment indications, precautions, and contraindications.
- Appropriately apply interventions per the POC.
- When treating specific lower extremity conditions, consider the entire lower quarter and the spine.
- Use the data collected and patient observations to continue or modify the treatment (based on SINSS [Severity, Irritability, Nature, Stage, Stability]).
- Based on observations of the patient and any change in status or in the severity/medical acuity, the assistant will need to determine if it is appropriate to "hold therapy." The assistant should also report the findings to the physical therapist or physician.
- The assistant can use the templates in Appendices A and B to guide in the development of a treatment plan.

**Considerations for the Physical Therapist Assistant**

Every patient is different and will progress at their own pace. Patient status and progression are impacted by what we do in the clinic and by what the patient does during their normal activities. For this reason, it is important to ask open-ended questions when a patient reports increased pain. Open-ended questions help the assistant to gather relevant information.

# Lower Extremity Anatomy

The lower extremity is divided into 3 regions. The thigh is the proximal portion of the limb (between the hip joint and knee joint). The lower leg/calf is the region between the knee joint and the ankle joint. The foot is distal to the ankle joint.

## *Hip Anatomy and Function*

The hip joint plays a vital role in locomotion by transmitting the load of the head, arms, and trunk into the lower extremities via the pelvis when standing, walking, and performing activities of daily living (ADLs). The hip joint provides mobility and stability, both of which are critical to its ability to function normally during transfers, gait, and other lower extremity movements.[11] The hip joint is a ball-and-socket synovial joint with the ability to move in 3 planes of motion. Hip motions include flexion/extension, abduction/adduction, and internal (medial)/external (lateral) rotation. Refer to Table 13-3 for normative ROM values, muscle actions, and end feel for the hip motions.[12,13] Normal ROM requires accessory lumbar and/or pelvic motion. To achieve end-range hip flexion, an anterior rotation of the ilium occurs.[12,13] For end-range hip extension, a posterior rotation of the ilium occurs; with hip abduction/adduction, a lateral tilting of the pelvis occurs.[12,13]

The resting position for the hip joint (open pack) is 30 degrees of flexion, 30 degrees of abduction, and slight external rotation. The closed-pack position for the hip joint is full extension, internal rotation, and abduction. The capsular pattern for the hip joint is a restriction in flexion, abduction, and internal rotation in that order.

The head of the femur (convex surface) articulates with the acetabulum (concave surface) of the pelvis forming the hip joint. The femur is the longest and strongest bone in the body. The femur articulates distally with the tibia, forming the knee joint. The acetabulum of the pelvis is the fusion point of the ilium, ischium, and pubic bones of the pelvis. The acetabular labrum (fibrocartilage) deepens the socket, which increases stability of the joint. There is a dense, fibrous, strong joint capsule that surrounds the hip joint, and the capsule blends with the iliofemoral, pubofemoral, and ischiofemoral ligaments (Table 13-4). The labrum, capsule, ligaments, and ligamentum teres provide joint stability. The muscles that contribute to hip mobility (Table 13-5) also assist in stabilizing the joint.

**Considerations for the Physical Therapist Assistant**

The muscle actions listed in Table 13-5 describe the actions that occur during an OKC activity, when the insertion moves toward the origin when the muscle contracts. In CKC activities, many of the muscles will perform a reversal of muscle action when they contract (the origin will move toward the insertion with muscle contraction; ie, when the pelvis moves on a fixed femur). It is useful to understand how the muscles work in both the OKC and CKC.

The femoral shaft has adequate vascularity via branches of the femoral artery. The blood supply to the head of the femur (supplied via branches of the circumflex femoral arteries) travels via the neck of the femur, creating a risk for decreased blood supply with femoral neck fractures.[11] Disruption in the blood supply to the head of the femur can result in avascular necrosis.

Hip pain often presents as a nonspecific complaint, so the physical therapist must carefully assess the patient to determine the actual source of pain. Because the source of pain or inflammation is not always apparent, the assistant should be alert to additional clues that may arise during treatment. Overuse, improper biomechanics, trauma, and muscle or postural imbalances can contribute to hip pain. Any injury that causes inflammation can result in increased fluid in the joint space, which can stretch the joint capsule and result in pain.

**Table 13-3**

Hip Normative Values for Range of Motion, Muscle Actions, and End Feel[12,13]

| Hip Motion | Degrees | Muscle Actions | Normal End Feel |
|---|---|---|---|
| Flexion | 120 | Psoas major, iliacus, and pectineus (sartorius, rectus femoris, tensor fasciae latae, and gluteus minimus) | Soft (tissue approximation) |
| Extension | 20 to 30 | Gluteus maximus, biceps femoris long head, semitendinosus, and semimembranosus (adductor magnus–posterior head) | Firm (tissue stretch) |
| Abduction | 40 | Gluteus medius, gluteus minimus, and tensor fasciae latae (sartorius) | Firm (tissue stretch) |
| Adduction | 20 | Adductor magnus, longus and brevis, gracilis, and pectineus (gluteus maximus—lower fibers) | Firm (tissue stretch) |
| Internal rotation | 45 | Gluteus medius and minimus, pectineus, tensor fasciae latae, (adductor magnus—anterior head), and gracilis—internal rotation (with a flexed knee) | Firm (capsular stretch) |
| External rotation | 45 | Piriformis, gemellus superior and inferior, obturator internus and externus, quadratus femoris, and gluteus maximus (sartorius) | Firm (capsular stretch) |

Note: There are variations in normative values, including variations based on sex and age. Refer to goniometry textbooks for specific age- and sex-specific variations. Muscles in parentheses are muscles that assist with that action.

**Table 13-4**

Primary Ligaments of the Hip

| Ligament | Attachment | Function |
|---|---|---|
| Iliofemoral–Y ligament of Bigelow | Anterior inferior iliac spine of pelvis to intertrochanteric line of femur | Strongest hip ligament; limits hip extension and external rotation. The superior portion tightens with hip adduction. |
| Ischiofemoral | Ischium to greater trochanter | Limits internal rotation (and anterior displacement of head of femur) |
| Pubofemoral | Superior pubic rami to intertrochanteric line of femur | Limits hip extension and abduction |
| Ligamentum teres | Acetabular notch to fovea on the head of femur | Provides blood supply to the head of the femur |
| Transverse acetabular ligament | Covers acetabular arch; creates foramen | Supports joint capsule; prevents inferior displacement of head of the femur |

**Table 13-5**

Muscles of the Hip, Pelvis, and Knee Joints

| Muscle | Actions | Origin | Insertion | Nerve Innervation |
|---|---|---|---|---|
| Gluteus maximus | All fibers: Hip extension, external rotation, abduction<br>Lower fibers: Adduct the hip | Coccyx, edge of sacrum, posterior iliac crest, sacrotuberous and sacroiliac ligaments | Iliotibial tract (upper fibers) and gluteal tuberosity (lower fibers) | Inferior gluteal |
| Gluteus medius | Hip abduction<br>Anterior fibers: Hip flexion, internal rotation<br>Posterior fibers: Hip extension, external rotation | Gluteal surface of ilium, below the iliac crest | Lateral aspect of greater trochanter | Superior gluteal |
| Gluteus minimus | Hip abduction, internal rotation, flexion | Gluteal surface of the ilium between the anterior and inferior gluteal lines | Anterior greater trochanter of femur | Superior gluteal |
| Piriformis | Hip external rotation, hip abduction when hip is flexed | Anterior surface of sacrum | Superior greater trochanter of femur | Sacral plexus |
| Quadratus femoris | Hip external rotation | Lateral border of ischial tuberosity | Intertrochanteric crest, between greater and lesser trochanters | Sacral plexus |
| Obturator internus | Hip external rotation | Obturator membrane, inferior obturator foramen | Medial greater trochanter | Sacral plexus |
| Obturator externus | Hip external rotation | Rami of pubis and ischium, obturator membrane | Trochanteric fossa of femur | Obturator |
| Gemellus superior | Hip external rotation | Ischial spine | Medial greater trochanter | Sacral plexus |
| Gemellus inferior | Hip external rotation | Ischial tuberosity | Medial greater trochanter | Sacral plexus |
| Adductor magnus | Hip adduction, internal rotation; assists to flex the hip<br>Posterior fibers: Extend the hip | Inferior ramus of the pubis, ramus of ischium and ischial tuberosity | Medial linea aspera and adductor tubercle of femur | Obturator and sciatic |
| Adductor longus | Hip adduction, internal rotation; assists to flex the hip | Pubic tubercle | Medial linea aspera and adductor tubercle | Obturator and sciatic |

(continued)

**Table 13-5 (continued)**

Muscles of the Hip, Pelvis, and Knee Joints

| Muscle | Actions | Origin | Insertion | Nerve Innervation |
|---|---|---|---|---|
| Adductor brevis | Hip adduction, internal rotation; assists to flex the hip | Inferior ramus of pubis | Pectineal line and medial lip of linea aspera of femur | Obturator |
| Pectineus | Hip adduction, internal rotation, flexion | Superior ramus of pubis | Pectineal line of femur | Femoral and obturator |
| Psoas major | Origin fixed: Hip flexion, external rotation<br>Insertion fixed: Trunk flexion; tilts pelvis anteriorly<br>Unilaterally: Assists to laterally flex lumbar spine | Bodies and transverse processes of lumbar vertebrae | Lesser trochanter of femur | Lumbar plexus L1, L2, L3, L4 |
| Iliacus | Proximal end fixed: Hip flexion, external rotation<br>Distal end fixed: Trunk flexion; tilts pelvis anteriorly | Iliac fossa | Lesser trochanter of femur | Femoral |
| Tensor fasciae latae | Hip flexion, internal rotation, abduction (with leg slightly anterior to the frontal plane) | Iliac crest, posterior to the anterior superior iliac spine (ASIS) | Iliotibial tract, which runs down lateral thigh, finally attaches to lateral tibial condyle | Superior gluteal |
| Sartorius | Hip: Flexion, external rotation, hip abduction<br>Knee: Flexion, medial rotation of the knee (part of the pes anserine) | ASIS | Proximal, medial shaft of tibia | Femoral |
| Gracilis | Hip: Adduction, internal rotation; assists to flex the hip<br>Knee: Flexes and medially rotates tibia (part of the pes anserine) | Inferior ramus of pubis | Proximal, medial shaft of tibia | Obturator |
| Hamstrings: Semitendinosus | Hip: Extension, assists external rotation, tilts the pelvis posteriorly<br>Knee: Flexion and medially rotates tibia (part of the pes anserine) | Ischial tuberosity | Proximal, medial shaft tibia at pes anserine tendon | Sciatic (tibial branch) |

*(continued)*

**Table 13-5 (continued)**

Muscles of the Hip, Pelvis, and Knee Joints

| Muscle | Actions | Origin | Insertion | Nerve Innervation |
|---|---|---|---|---|
| Hamstrings: Semimembranosus | Extends the hip, tilts the pelvis posteriorly<br>Knee flexion and medially rotates tibia | Ischial tuberosity | Posterior medial condyle of tibia | Sciatic (tibial branch) |
| Hamstrings: Biceps femoris | Long head extends the hip, tilts the pelvis posteriorly<br>Knee flexion, laterally rotates tibia | Long head: Ischial tuberosity<br>Short head: Lateral lip of linea aspera | Head of the fibula | Long head: Sciatic (tibial branch)<br>Short head: Sciatic (peroneal branch) |
| Quadriceps: Rectus femoris | Hip flexion, knee extension | Anterior inferior iliac spine | Tibial tuberosity (patellar ligament) | Femoral |
| Quadriceps: Vastus lateralis | Knee extension | Lateral linea aspera, gluteal tuberosity, greater trochanter | Tibial tuberosity (patellar ligament) | Femoral |
| Quadriceps: Vastus medialis | Knee extension | Medial linea aspera | Tibial tuberosity (patellar ligament) | Femoral |
| Quadriceps: Vastus intermedius | Knee extension | Anterior and lateral shaft of the femur | Tibial tuberosity (patellar ligament) | Femoral |
| Popliteus | Medially rotates to initiate knee flexion in OKC; laterally rotates femur in CKC on a fixed tibia | Lateral condyle of the femur | Proximal, posterior aspect of tibia | Tibial |
| Gastrocnemius | Flexes the knee in OKC and acts as a knee extensor in the CKC<br>Ankle plantar flexion | Condyles of the femur, posterior surfaces | Calcaneus via calcaneal tendon | Tibial |

### Hip Biomechanical Considerations

Pelvic tilting (in the sagittal and frontal planes), lumbopelvic rhythm, and pelvic rotation are biomechanical considerations that influence the amount and quality of motion available at the hip joint (Table 13-6). Soft tissue/muscle length can also affect the motions between the femur, pelvis, and lumbar spine. Limited pelvic motion (in any direction) and poor pelvic muscle control can also affect hip mobility. The direction of the pelvic tilt can be anterior or posterior in the sagittal plane and is named based on the direction of ASIS movement. Pelvic tilting in the sagittal plane can be performed in a CKC or OKC. In the CKC, the head remains stationary, and the pelvis moves, resulting in compensatory movements at the hips and lumbar spine (Figure 13-1). During static standing, the hip and trunk muscles work together to maintain a level pelvis, preventing excessive anterior or posterior pelvic tilting.

**Lumbopelvic rhythm** is the coordinated activity of the lumbar spine and pelvis in the sagittal plane during OKC motions (Figure 13-2). When one bends forward, the head and upper trunk lead, and then flexion at the lumbar spine occurs until the vertebral segments have attained their full range. At that point, the pelvis begins to rotate anteriorly to increase the available range of forward flexion. When returning to a vertical position, the pelvis rotates posteriorly first and then lumbar spine extension occurs followed by upper trunk and cervical extension. Pelvic tilting in the frontal plane and rotation in the transverse plane are described in Table 13-6 and illustrated in Figures 13-3 and 13-4.

The angle of inclination, femoral anteversion, and retroversion are bony biomechanical considerations that impact compressive or shear forces at the hip. Abnormal angles can impact the quality of a person's motion and gait. The angle of inclination is the angle formed between the shaft of the femur in relation to the neck and head of the femur in the frontal plane. A normal angle is approximately 125 degrees (Figure 13-5). Coxa varus describes an angle of inclination greater than 125 degrees, and an angle less than 125 degrees is called *coxa valgus*. Femoral torsion is the angle formed between a line that bisects the femoral condyles and a line that bisects the femoral neck in the transverse plane (Figure 13-6). In adults, the normal angle of anteversion is approximately 15 degrees. An angle greater than 15 degrees is excessive anteversion, and an angle less than 15 degrees is called *retroversion*. Table 13-6 provides a brief summary of these biomechanical factors; more in-depth descriptions of these conditions can be found in kinesiology textbooks. Understanding the biomechanics and likely compensations for faulty biomechanics is useful when selecting treatment interventions.

## *Knee Anatomy and Function*

The knee joint is a complex modified hinge joint composed of the distal femur, proximal tibia (called the *tibiofemoral joint*), and patella. The patella articulates with the trochlear groove of the distal femur (called the *patellofemoral joint*). Flexion and extension are the primary actions occurring at the knee joint, but small amounts of tibial internal and external rotation occur to allow for normal joint biomechanics.

The resting position (open-packed position) of the knee joint is 25 degrees of knee flexion. The closed-pack position is full knee extension and tibial external rotation. The capsular pattern of restriction for the knee joint is a limitation of flexion greater than extension.

### Tibiofemoral Joint Mechanics

Normal knee ROM includes flexion to approximately 130 degrees with a soft end feel and 0 degrees of extension with a firm/capsular end feel.[13] The femoral condyles are convex, and the proximal surface of the tibia is concave. In the OKC, during knee extension, the concave tibia glides and rolls anteriorly on the convex femur (Figure 13-7), and the tibia externally rotates about 10 degrees during the last 20 to 30 degrees of extension.[14] During CKC knee extension, the femur rolls anteriorly but glides posteriorly on the tibia (Figure 13-8), and the femur internally rotates 10 degrees on the tibia during the last 20 to 30 degrees of extension.[14] This rotational component at the end of knee extension is called the **screw-home mechanism.** The screw-home mechanism must occur to "lock" the knee, which increases joint stability.

During knee flexion, the opposite actions occur at the tibia and femur. To initiate knee flexion from full extension, the popliteus contracts and internally rotates the tibia (in an OKC) or externally rotates the femur (in a CKC position). This action "unlocks" the knee, and the hamstrings contract to complete knee flexion.

### Patellofemoral Joint Mechanics

The patella is the largest sesamoid in the body. It sits in the trochlear groove and is embedded in the quadriceps tendon. The patella moves superiorly during knee extension and inferiorly during flexion within the groove. The patella increases the effectiveness of the quadriceps muscles by increasing the mechanical advantage during knee extension. It also decreases friction between the quadriceps and femoral condyles. The patella is stabilized statically by the medial and lateral patellofemoral ligaments and the lateral edge trochlear groove and dynamically by the quadriceps muscle.

When the knee is relaxed and fully extended, the patella sits halfway between the femoral condyles and is very mobile because there are minimal compressive forces. Restrictions in patella mobility can affect ROM and the ability of the quadriceps muscle to fully extend the knee, resulting in an extensor lag.

**Table 13-6**

## Biomechanical Considerations Related to Pelvic and Hip Mobility

| | | | |
|---|---|---|---|
| Pelvic motions in the sagittal plane (CKC) | Anterior pelvic tilt | • Actions: The lumbar extensors (erector spinae) pull upward posteriorly and hip flexors pull downward anteriorly, creating lumbar extension and hip flexion.<br>• Stabilization: The abdominals must contract to prevent an anterior pelvic tilt and stabilize the trunk, which allows for isolated OKC hip flexion.<br>• Pelvic stability in standing: The abdominals and hip extensors contract to counteract excessive anterior pelvic tilting. | |
| | Posterior pelvic tilt | • Actions: The abdominals pull upward anteriorly and gluteus maximus and hamstrings pull downward posteriorly, creating lumbar flexion and hip extension.<br>• Stabilization: To prevent a posterior pelvic tilt, the lumbar extensors must contract and stabilize the trunk, which will allow for isolated hip flexion motion.<br>• Pelvic stability in standing: The iliofemoral ligament and active contraction of lumbar extensors and hip flexors counteract posterior pelvic tilting. | |
| Pelvic motions in the frontal plane | Lateral pelvic tilt (pelvic drop on the OKC side with SLS) | • Actions: A pelvic drop on the OKC side (unweighted limb) results in lateral spinal flexion and hip adduction on the CKC side due to gluteus medius weakness on the CKC side. | • Stabilization: For isolated hip abduction to occur on the OKC side, the internal and external obliques must contract to stabilize the pelvis, preventing rotation and lateral flexion in supine or side lying.<br>• Stability in standing: Gluteus medius on the CKC side needs to effectively contract to counteract a pelvic drop on the OKC (non–weight-bearing) side and keep the pelvis level. |
| | Lateral pelvic tilt (hip hike on the OKC side with SLS) | • Actions: A contraction of the quadratus lumborum on the OKC side (unweighted limb) and reverse muscle action of gluteus medius on the CKC side creates lateral spinal flexion on the OKC side and hip abduction on the CKC side. | |
| Pelvic motions in the frontal plane | Pelvic rotation forward on the OKC side during SLS on the CKC side | • Actions: Hip internal rotators, obliques, and multifidi create hip internal rotation on the CKC side and trunk rotation to the OKC side. | • Stabilization: For isolated hip rotation to occur in the OKC, the transverse abdominis, multifidi, and obliques must contract to stabilize the trunk.<br>• Stability in standing: Gluteus medius on the CKC side needs to effectively contract to keep the pelvis level, and the multifidus and transverse abdominis contract to stabilize the trunk as hip rotation occurs on the CKC side. |
| | Pelvic rotation backward on the OKC side during SLS on the CKC side | • Actions: Hip external rotators create hip external rotation on the CKC side and trunk rotation to the OKC side. | |

(continued)

**Table 13-6 (continued)**

Biomechanical Considerations Related to Pelvic and Hip Mobility

| | | |
|---|---|---|
| Lumbopelvic rhythm (OKC) | Forward bending of the trunk results in: | • A posterior shifting of the pelvis to keep the center of gravity over the BOS<br>• Trunk flexion controlled eccentrically by the trunk extensors<br>• Posterior ligaments of vertebral ligaments becoming taut at the end of lumbar flexion<br>• Superior facet joints shifting superiorly creating passive tension in the capsules<br>• Pelvic rotation forward (anterior pelvic tilt) eccentrically controlled by hamstrings and gluteus maximus<br>Note: Overall forward flexion ROM can be limited if back extensors, fascia, gluteus maximus, and/or hamstrings are restricted. Returning to vertical position occurs via posterior pelvic tilt followed by lumbar and then trunk extension. |
| Angle of inclination | Coxa valga (increased angle of inclination) results in: | • A superior shift of the femoral head in the acetabulum, which decreases joint stability and increases the risk of hip dislocation<br>• A decrease in femoral neck shear and an increase in the compression forces at the head of the femur and superior acetabulum<br>• Hip abductors being placed at a mechanical disadvantage and having to work harder because the lever arm is shortened due to the increased angle. This results in increased joint reaction forces.<br>• The length of the femur is increased, resulting in genu varus at the knee joint. |
| | Coxa vara (decreased angle of inclination) results in: | • A more horizontal orientation of the femoral neck, increasing joint compressive forces and increasing the risk of femoral neck fractures.<br>• Hip abductors are at a mechanical disadvantage because the lever arm is lengthened due to the decreased angle.<br>• The length of the femur is decreased, resulting in genu valgus at the knee joint. |

*(continued)*

**Table 13-6 (continued)**

Biomechanical Considerations Related to Pelvic and Hip Mobility

| | | |
|---|---|---|
| Femoral Torsion | Excessive femoral anteversion (> 15 degrees) results in: | • Femoral head positioned more anterior in the acetabulum<br>• A toe-in (foot inversion/adduction) gait pattern<br>• A relatively shorter leg<br>• Greater hip internal rotation than external rotation<br>• Increased comfort in a W-sitting posture<br>• An increased likelihood of genu valgus |
| | Femoral retroversion (< 15 degrees) results in: | • Femoral head positioned more posterior in the acetabulum<br>• A toe-out (foot eversion/abduction) gait pattern<br>• A relatively longer leg<br>• Greater hip external rotation than internal rotation |

BOS = base of support; SLS = single-leg stance.

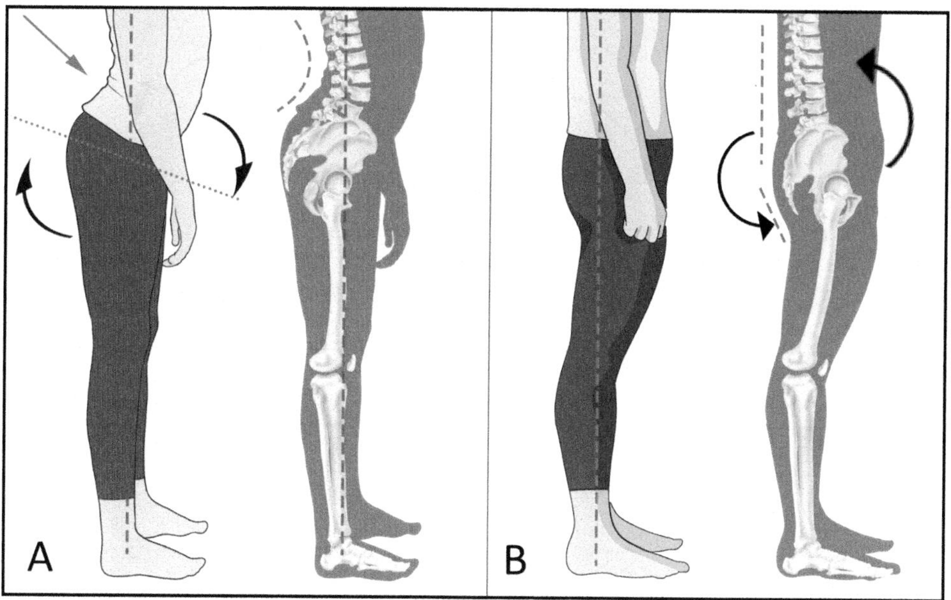


**Figure 13-1.** CKC (A) anterior and (B) posterior pelvic tilts in the sagittal plane (Chu KyungMin/Shutterstock.com).

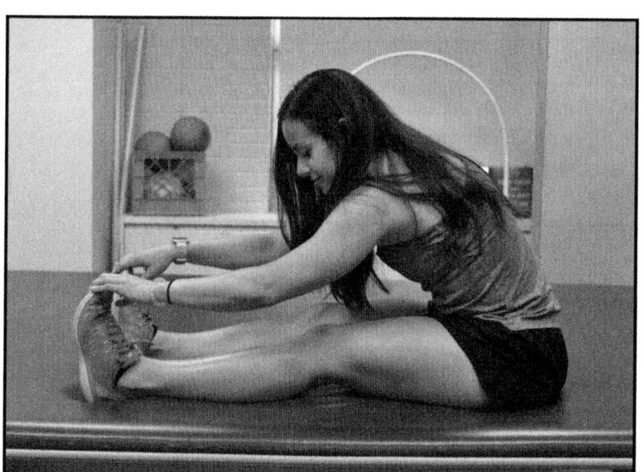

**Figure 13-2.** When lumbopelvic rhythm occurs in the OKC (upper body moves on lower body), there is more available motion because the motion occurs over several joints. The vertebrae of the spine and pelvis contribute to the increased motion, and all move in the same direction.

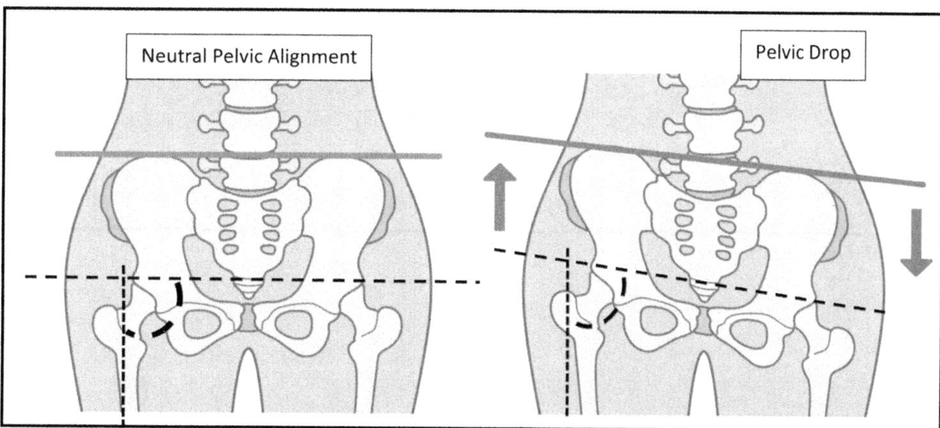


**Figure 13-3.** Pelvic tilting in the frontal plane. Note the changes in the angle between the femur and the pelvis in each position. With a pelvic drop on the left side, the femur on the right side (the weight-bearing/CKC side) is in relative adduction, and the angle between the pelvis and the femur on the right is decreased (matsukiyo8379/Shutterstock.com).

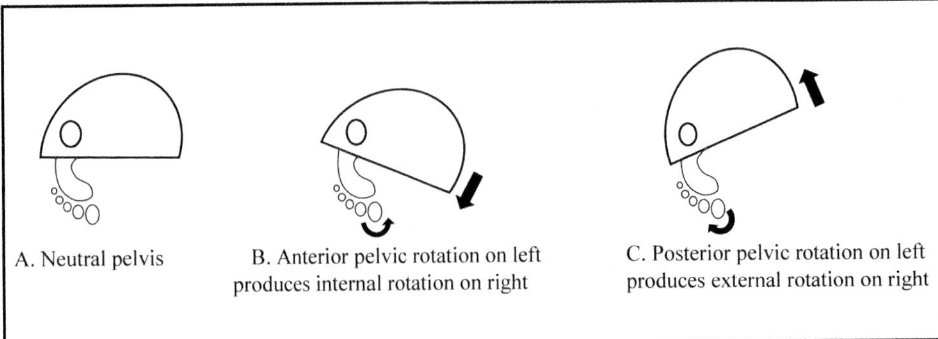


**Figure 13-4.** Pelvic rotation on a CKC leg (looking down on the pelvis).

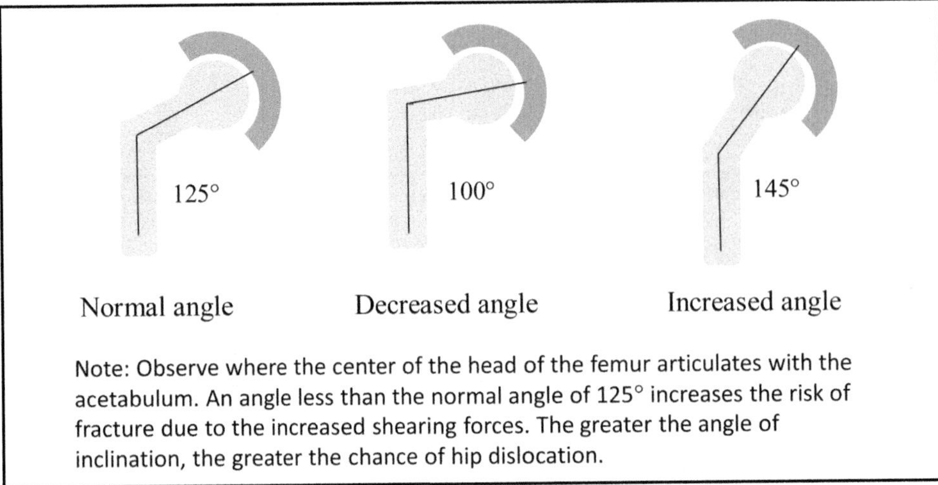


**Figure 13-5.** Angle of inclination of the hip.

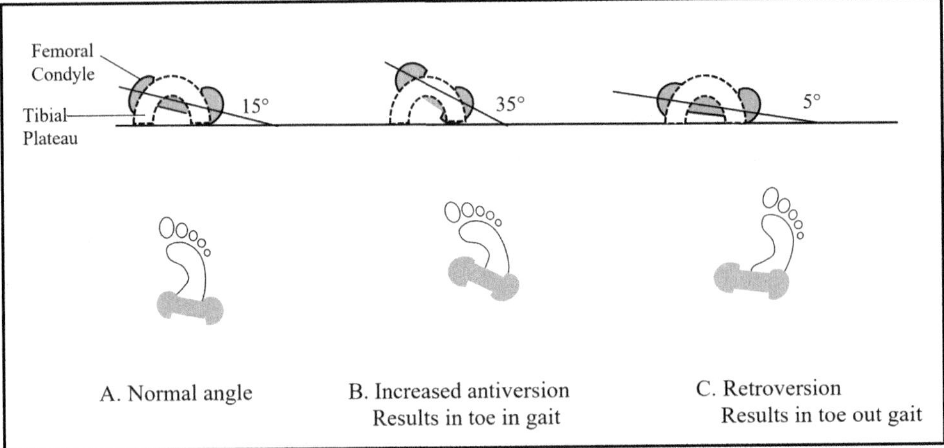


**Figure 13-6.** Angle of torsion.

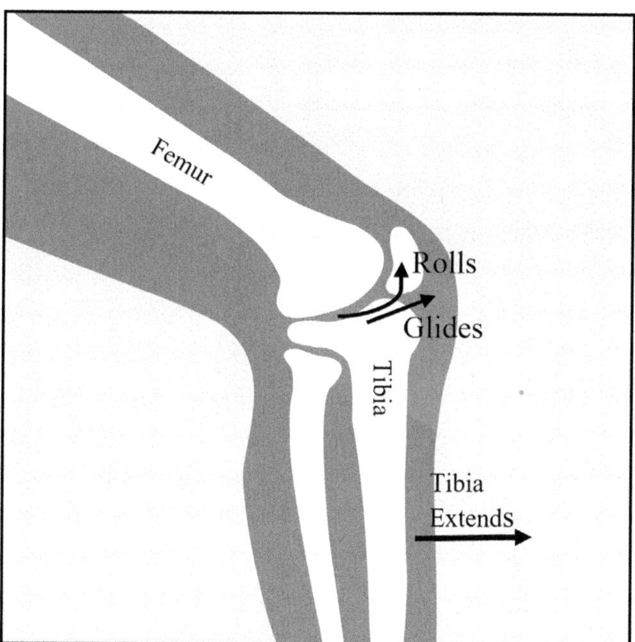


Figure 13-7. OKC arthrokinematic knee extension; the tibia moves on the femur (Oleksandr Malysh/Shutterstock.com).

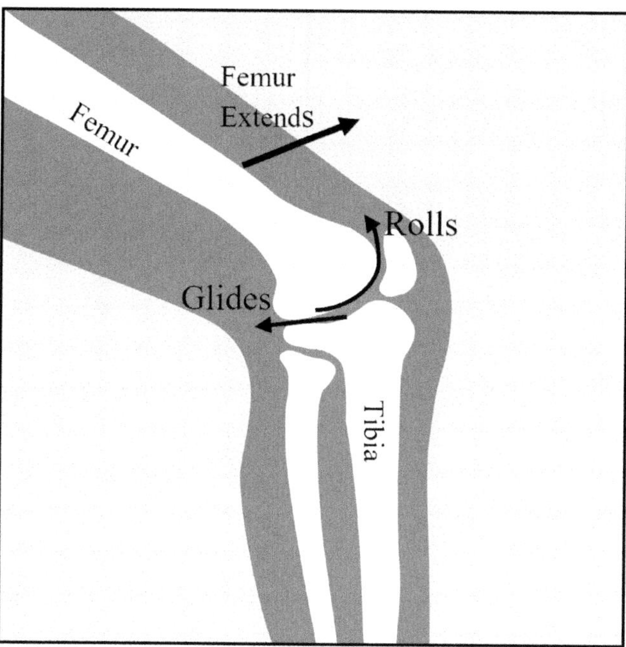


Figure 13-8. CKC arthrokinematic knee extension; the femur moves on the tibia (Oleksandr Malysh/Shutterstock.com).

The amount of joint compression (or reaction) force is directly related to the amount of patella surface area that is in contact with the femur as well as the joint position and amount of muscle tension.[15] A larger contact area between the patellar surface and the femur decreases stress on the articular tissue. A high patellofemoral joint reaction force (PFJRF) combined with a small contact area increases patellofemoral joint stress. This increased stress on the joint may damage joint articular cartilage.[15]

As the knee moves from 0 to 90 degrees of flexion in an OKC, there is an increase in the patellofemoral contact area. This increased contact area results in less compression because the forces are distributed across a greater area of joint surface. The greatest compressive force of the quadriceps muscle occurs when the knee nears full extension and the contact area of the patellofemoral joint is the smallest. For this reason, it is recommended that OKC exercises be performed from 90 to no more than 30 degrees of knee flexion to reduce patellofemoral joint stress. During CKC motion, PFJRF is highest when exercises are performed from 90 to 45 degrees of knee flexion, but the forces are significantly decreased during terminal knee extension (TKE; ie, 20 to 0 degrees).[15,16] These concepts are applied when designing an exercise program for patients with patellofemoral conditions. Activities such as running or deep squats can increase PFJRF by 5 to 8 times the patient's body weight; introducing these activities too early can be detrimental to a patient's recovery.[15]

Poor patella positioning or tracking issues can make the PFJRF worse. Patella malalignment or lateral patella tracking can be due to an increased Q angle, dynamic knee valgus, tight ITB, tight lateral retinaculum, tight plantar flexors (increased pronation), weak hip abductors or external rotators, and weak vastus medialis oblique (VMO).

The Q angle determines the line of pull of the quadriceps muscles and can be measured as shown in Figure 13-9A. The Q angle is the angle formed between a line drawn from the midpatella to the tibial tuberosity and a second line drawn from the ASIS to the center of the patella.

An angle on the lateral aspect of the knee is formed where the femur and tibia articulate. This angle is influenced by the angle of inclination as shown in Figure 13-9B. When the angle of inclination at the hip is 125 degrees, the femur and tibia are closely aligned in the vertical plane. An angle of inclination at the hip less than 125 degrees (coxa valga) results in genu varus (bowed legs). Genu valgus ("knock" knees) results when the angle of inclination is greater than 125 (coxa vara). Table 13-7 lists factors that can affect the patella's ability to move efficiently.

## Clinical Tip

Consider strengthening the VMO, hip abductors, and hip external rotators and stretching the ITB for persons with patellofemoral pain syndrome (PFPS).

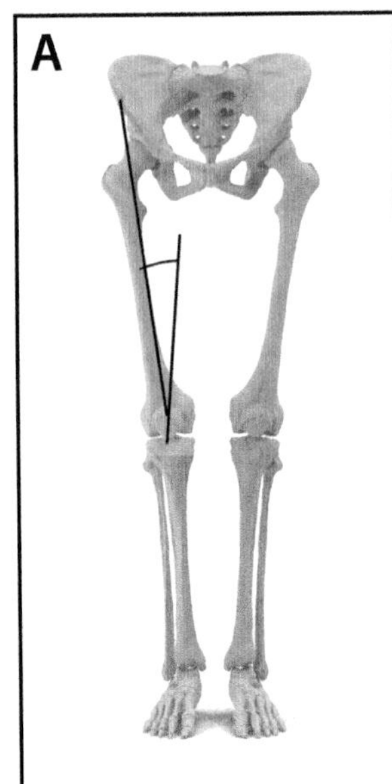


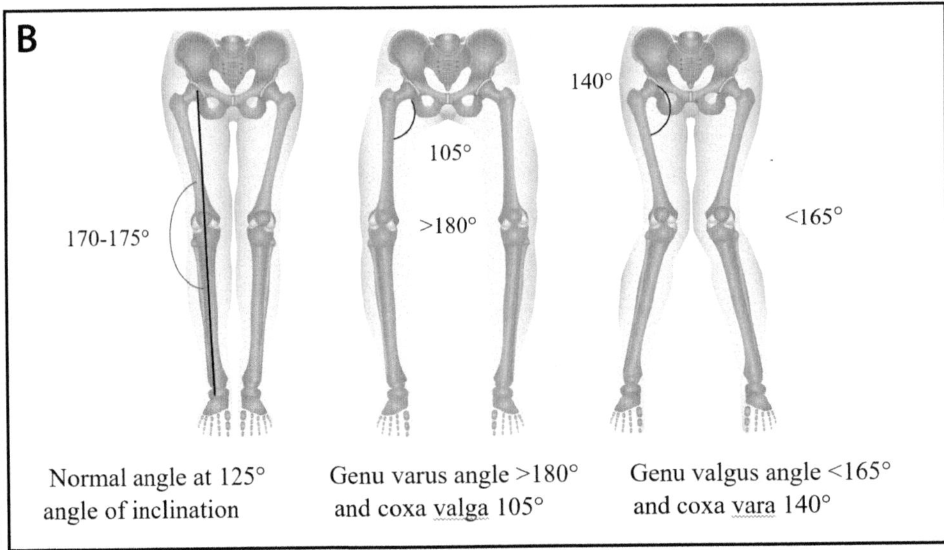


**Figure 13-9.** Knee alignments. (A) Q angle normal 10 to 15 degrees (3DMI/Shutterstock.com). (B) Femur/tibia alignment (lotan/Shutterstock.com).

**Table 13-7**

**Contributing Factors Affecting Proper Patella Alignment and Biomechanics**

| Factor | Description | Possible Consequences |
|---|---|---|
| Quadriceps angle (Q angle) | The Q angle represents the line of pull of the quadriceps muscle. | • A normal Q angle is between 10 and 15 degrees. Women tend to have a larger Q angle because they have a wider pelvis.<br>• Increased Q angle (> 15 degrees) may increase the risk of lateral tracking of the patella and PFPS. An increased Q angle increases the risk for patellar dislocation/subluxation.<br>  ○ Using orthotics to prevent foot pronation may reduce PFPS.<br>  ○ Increased Q angle is associated with genu valgum (knock-knees), coxa vara, femoral anteversion, external femoral torsion, and tibial internal rotation. |
| Patellar positioning | The position of the patella relative to the femur is tabulated as a ratio of patellar tendon length to the greatest length of the patella. | • Normal: The patella is approximately equal in length to the patellar tendon length (ratio range = 0.6 to 1.3 using the Caton-Deschamps Index).<br>• Patella alta: Ratio > 1.3, indicating patella location is elevated. This increases the risk of patellar dislocation.<br>• Patella baja: Ratio < 0.6, indicating patella location is more distal. This is often associated with hypotonia of the quadriceps or knee trauma. |
| Lateral patella tracking | An observable abrupt lateral movement at or near terminal/full knee extension (20 to 0 degrees) | These causes usually are found in combination:<br>• Increased Q angle (see earlier), patella alta, shallow trochlear groove, genu valgum, coxa vara, and foot pronation<br>• Tight lateral structures (ie, ITB and patella retinaculum) and tight hip internal rotators and adductors<br>• Joint hypermobility or stretched medial structures (ie, patella retinaculum, patellofemoral ligament, and MCL)<br>• Muscle weakness (ie, hip abductors and external rotators, VMO, and tibialis posterior [to control for pronation]) |

Clinical implications: If a patient's movement pattern occurs differently than the typical/expected pattern, the clinical team should discern why and whether this variation warrants treatment. Imbalances in one area can alter biomechanics up and down the chain and may present as pain in another area of the kinetic chain.

Consideration of patellar tracking patterns, strength of the stabilizing muscles (especially the hip muscles and VMO), and patellar compressive forces should drive the exercise prescription.

MCL = medial collateral ligament.

### Knee Ligaments, Muscles, Menisci, and Bursae

The knee is frequently injured because of the reliance on soft tissue support and the lack of bony support. The ligaments that support the joint play a significant role in maintaining joint stability and integrity. The major ligamentous support (Table 13-8) for the knee includes the joint capsule, the MCL, the lateral collateral ligament (LCL), the anterior cruciate ligament (ACL), and the posterior cruciate ligament (PCL). The ACL contributes to 85% of knee stabilization and is considered the prime stabilizer.[17]

Specific muscles act as dynamic stabilizers, assisting the ligaments in providing stability during knee movement. Exercises can target specific muscles to improve support to their associated ligament. This is key to achieving improved motor control and joint proprioception and reducing the risk of reinjury.[16,17] Several knee muscles are 2-joint muscles, so the concepts of active and passive insufficiency (refer to Chapter 4) should be considered when developing an exercise program. Table 13-5 provides a list of the knee muscles, attachments, and actions.

The knee menisci assist in increasing stability at the knee joint by deepening the joint surfaces and increasing congruence between the femoral and tibial surfaces. They are thicker peripherally, and they assist in cushioning and lubricating the joint and distributing the weight-bearing forces through the joint. The transverse ligament blends in with the anterior fibers of the ACL and connects the menisci anteriorly. The posterior meniscofemoral ligament runs from the posterior aspect of the lateral meniscus behind the PCL to the medial femoral condyle.[15]

The "C"-shaped medial meniscus is less mobile because it attaches to the capsule and MCL and indirectly to the semimembranosus. The lateral meniscus is more "O" shaped and is attached to the popliteus tendon. The menisci move anteriorly on the tibia during extension and posteriorly during flexion. The medial meniscus moves about half the distance that the lateral meniscus moves because of the limiting structural attachments.[14]

**Clinical Tip**

The outer one-third of the meniscus has a good blood supply, but the inner two-thirds are avascular, limiting the healing ability after a meniscal tear.

The bursae and fat pads reduce friction between the muscles/tendons and the underlying bony prominences. The suprapatellar bursa is posterior to the patellar tendon. Distally, the deep infrapatellar bursa is located anterior to the tibial tuberosity and posterior to the patellar ligament. Overuse, improper biomechanics, trauma, and muscle or postural imbalances can lead to inflammation of these structures, creating pain.

## *Ankle/Foot Anatomy and Function*

The foot and ankle are a complex series of bones and joints that work together to allow the foot to propel the body during walking, adjust and adapt to different terrains, and absorb various mechanical stresses. Ninety percent of the body weight is transmitted through the tibia and 10% through the fibula to the foot. The fibula does not directly contribute to motion at the ankle; however, the fibula does provide critical support and accessory motion that allow normal biomechanics at the ankle joint.

The foot–ankle complex must be both stable and flexible. Stability allows for the transmission of the weight-bearing forces associated with gait, and the foot must be rigid to facilitate push off during gait. Flexibility is required to absorb ground reaction forces and to allow the foot to adjust to uneven terrain during gait. Shock absorption and forward propulsion are primarily accommodated by changes in plantar flexion and dorsiflexion, and adaptation to the terrain is primarily accommodated by pronation/supination.

The foot is divided into 3 sections. The rear foot (hindfoot) includes the talus and calcaneus, and the midfoot is formed by the navicular, cuboid, and cuneiform bones. The forefoot includes the 5 metatarsal bones and 14 phalanges.

### Joints and Motions at the Ankle and Foot

The joints of the hindfoot (or rear foot) include the tibiofibular, the talocrural (ankle), and the subtalar joints. The joint of the midfoot is the midtarsal joint, and the forefoot includes the tarsometatarsal, metatarsophalangeal (MTP), and interphalangeal joints. Table 13-9 provides ROM values, open/closed-pack positions, and the capsular patterns of these joints.

Proximally, the fibula and tibia create the superior tibiofemoral joint, which allows superior/inferior gliding and rotation of the fibula. The inferior tibiofibular joint is a syndesmosis (ie, a fibrous union) in which the tibia and fibula are separated by fibrocartilaginous tissue and supported by the tibiofibular interosseous membrane. The anterior and posterior tibiofibular ligaments and the interosseous membrane form a strong mortise at the proximal end of the ankle joint.[11,12,18] This creates the stability required for normal biomechanics.

**Clinical Tip**

The tibiofibular interosseous membrane is so strong that a distracting force is more likely to result in a distal fibula fracture rather than a ligament rupture.

**Table 13-8**

Primary Ligament Support of the Knee

| Ligament | Attachments | Function | Muscles/Dynamic Support to Assist Ligament Stability |
|---|---|---|---|
| ACL | Anterior intercondylar region of the tibia to posterior femur on the medial aspect of the lateral condyle | • When the femur is fixed, the ACL resists anterior translation of the tibia<br>• When the tibia is fixed, the ACL resists posterior translation of the tibia<br>• Prevents hyperextension<br>• Resists varus/valgus deformations and tibial rotation | Hamstrings also pull the tibia posterior during CKC activities and assist in preventing hyperextension. |
| PCL | Posterior intercondylar region of the tibia to posterior femur on the lateral aspect of the medial condyle | • When the femur is fixed, the PCL resists posterior translation of the tibia<br>• When the tibia is fixed, the PCL resists anterior translation of the femur on the tibia<br>• Resists extreme knee flexion<br>• Resists varus and valgus deformations and tibial external rotation | Quadriceps |
| MCL | Attaches from the medial epicondyle of the femur to the medial proximal tibia. It is part of the capsule and attaches to the medial meniscus. It is wide and flat in shape. | • Resists valgus stresses to the knee | Gracilis, sartorius, and semitendinosus |
| LCL | Attaches from the lateral epicondyle of the femur to the head of the fibula. Lies outside the capsule and is cylindrical in shape. | • Resists varus stresses to the knee | ITB (tensor fasciae latae)<br>Biceps femoris |

**Table 13-9**

**Ankle/Foot Joints, Range of Motion, Open- and Closed-Pack Positions, and Capsular Patterns**

| Joints and Motions | Normal ROM | Open-Packed Position | Closed-Pack Position | Capsular Pattern | End Feel |
|---|---|---|---|---|---|
| Tibiofibular | NA | Plantar flexion | Dorsiflexion (maximal) | Pain with stress | NA |
| Talocrural | Dorsiflexion: 0 to 20 degrees<br>Plantar flexion: 0 to 50 degrees | 10 degrees plantar flexion, halfway between inversion and eversion | Dorsiflexion (maximal) | Plantar flexion, dorsiflexion | Firm |
| Subtalar | Inversion (hindfoot): 0 to 20 degrees<br>Eversion (hindfoot): 0 to 10 degrees | Halfway between maximum end ROM | Supination | Varus, valgus | Firm |
| Midtarsal | NA | Halfway between maximum end ROM | Supination | Dorsiflexion, plantar flexion, adduction, inversion | NA |
| Tarsometatarsal | Supination (plantar flexion, inversion, forefoot adduction): 0 to 35 degrees<br>Pronation (dorsiflexion, eversion, forefoot abduction): 0 to 15 degrees | Halfway between maximum end ROM | Supination | None | Firm |
| MTP | First MTP<br>• Flexion: 0 to 45 degrees<br>• Hyperextension: 0 to 90 degrees<br>Second through fifth MTPs<br>• Flexion: 0 to 40 degrees<br>• Hyperextension: 0 to 45 degrees | Slight extension | Extension (maximal) | Great toe extension, flexion of toes 2 through 5 | Firm |
| Interphalangeal | NA | Slight flexion | Extension (maximal) | Flexion, extension | Firm |

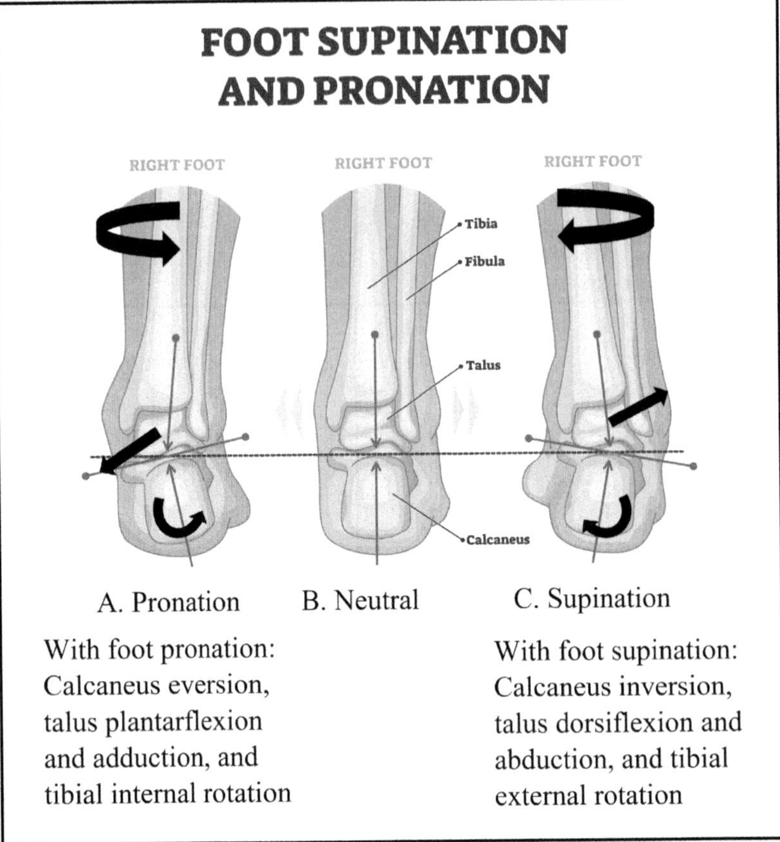


**Figure 13-10.** Right foot pronation and supination in CKC (VectorMine/Shutterstock.com).

The talocrural joint includes the articulation between the tibia, fibula, and talus. The ankle joint is a hinge joint, but the joint axis is at an oblique angle. Dorsiflexion and plantar flexion are the primary motions that occur at the talocrural joint, but the oblique joint axis angle allows for triplanar motion. The talus adducts and slightly inverts (supination) during ankle plantar flexion; the talus abducts and slightly everts (pronation) during dorsiflexion in the OKC. In the CKC, the talus plantar flexes and adducts with pronation and dorsiflexes and abducts with supination. Motions in the horizontal plane include tibia external rotation during supination and internal rotation during pronation (Figure 13-10).[11,12,19] During OKC plantar flexion, the talus glides anteriorly and rolls posteriorly; with dorsiflexion, the talus glides posteriorly and rolls anteriorly.

The subtalar joint (talocalcaneal joint) is composed of the inferior talus and 3 articulations with the superior aspect of the calcaneus. Motions at the subtalar joint are also triplanar because of its oblique joint axis, but the primary actions are ankle inversion and eversion. Inversion and eversion do not occur in isolation; the other components of pronation and supination also occur.

## Clinical Tip

There is approximately a 2:1 ratio of available inversion to eversion at the subtalar joint. In the OKC, the calcaneus moves on the talus, but in the CKC, the talus moves on the calcaneus.

Foot pronation occurs at the subtalar and transverse tarsal joints to absorb shock as the arch of the foot flattens during the loading response of the gait cycle. The foot is more flexible when pronated (the open-packed position). When supination occurs during normal walking, the subtalar joint "locks" the mid- and forefoot, allowing the tibia to translate forward and shift the body weight anteriorly.[20]

The midtarsal or transverse tarsal joint (talonavicular and calcaneocuboid articulations) connects the forefoot to the hindfoot. It assists with force distribution and in raising and lowering the arch of the foot by working with the subtalar joint during pronation and supination. Motions at the subtalar and transverse tarsal joints cannot be separated because they are dependent on each other and linked with the talocrural joint.

The tarsometatarsal joints, MTP, and proximal and distal interphalangeal joints contribute to movement at the toes and foot flexibility and stability during gait.

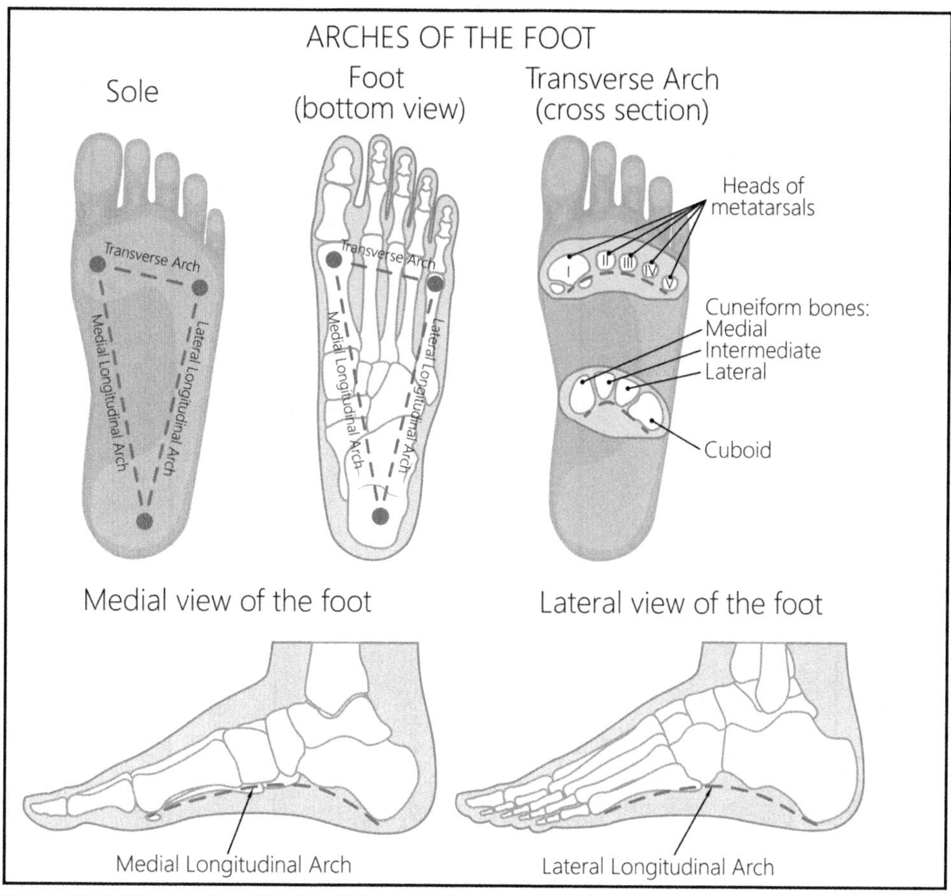


**Figure 13-11.** Three arches of the foot (Aksanaku/Shutterstock.com).

### *Arches of the Foot*

The arches of the foot are critical for normal biomechanics of the lower extremity during weight bearing. The 3 arches stabilize the foot, respond to loads, and adapt to uneven surfaces; they are supported by ligaments and fascia (Figure 13-11). The transverse arch spans across the anterior tarsal bones to the metatarsal heads and is typically more prominent (concave) at the tarsals; the arch flattens as it nears the metatarsal heads at the ball of the foot. There are 2 longitudinal arches that span the foot from the base of the calcaneus to the metatarsal heads, one medially and one laterally. The calcaneus and the fifth and first metatarsal are the 3 bones that bear the most weight when standing; they form a triangle and longitudinally form the medial and lateral arches. The spring ligament (calcaneonavicular ligament) supports the talus and provides the primary support for the medial longitudinal arch, preventing its flattening.

The plantar fascia is the dense fibrous tissue that spans the plantar aspect of the foot, supporting the longitudinal arch. It attaches from the calcaneal tuberosity and plantar aspects of the MTP joints and inserts into the flexor tendons of the toes. The plantar fascia insertion onto the flexor tendons of the toes creates tension in the plantar fascia during weight bearing; this helps to stabilize the arch and create the "forefoot rocker," which contributes to the rigidity needed for normal gait in the terminal stance/preswing phases.[21]

> **Clinical Tip**
>
> An excessive or increased arch is called *pes cavus*. A decreased arch is called *pes planus* and is referred to as *flat feet* in layperson's terms.

### *Ankle Ligaments and Dynamic Muscle Control*

The ligaments of the ankle provide static stability, and the muscles provide dynamic control in order to prevent excessive motion. A list of ligaments is located in Table 13-10, and the muscles are described in Table 13-11.

There are 3 ligaments on the lateral side of the ankle that limit ankle inversion. The anterior talofibular ligament (ATFL) is the weakest of the lateral ligaments; it is stressed when the ankle is plantar flexed and inverted. This ligament is commonly injured with inversion ankle sprains. The calcaneofibular ligament (CFL) resists inversion when the ankle is in neutral or dorsiflexed; it can be injured in more severe lateral inversion ankle sprains. The posterior talofibular ligament (PTFL) is the strongest of the lateral ligaments; it plays a supplementary role in ankle stability when the lateral ligament complex is intact. It is under the greatest strain when the ankle is in dorsiflexion. The peroneus muscles provide dynamic stability to assist these ligaments. These muscles can be strained if the ankle is excessively inverted.

**Table 13-10**

## Ligaments of the Ankle and Foot

| Joint | Ligament | Location/Motion Limited by Intact Ligament |
|---|---|---|
| Tibiofibular | Anterior inferior tibiofibular (AITF) ligament<br>Posterior inferior tibiofibular (PITF) ligament | AITF: Anterior tubercle of the distal tibia and anterior surface of the distal fibula at the lateral malleolus<br>PITF: Posterior tubercle of the distal tibia and posterior surface of the distal fibula at the lateral malleolus<br>• Both stabilize the joint and limit external rotation of the foot on the lower leg and distal fibular motion in relation to the tibia |
| Talocrural | Medial support<br>Deltoid ligament (4 parts): Tibiotalar, tibionavicular (deep and superficial), and tibiocalcaneal ligaments | Medial malleolus to medial talus, calcaneus, and navicular tuberosity<br>Very strong and broad ligament<br>• Limits ankle eversion |
| | LCLs: ATFL, CFL, and PTFL | ATFL: Anterior talus to lateral malleolus; very weak<br>CFL: Lateral calcaneus to lateral malleolus<br>PTFL: Posterior talus to lateral malleolus<br>• Limits ankle inversion |
| Subtalar | Talocalcaneal ligaments | Stabilize the subtalar joint; the medial talocalcaneal and interosseous limit eversion, and the posterior talocalcaneal and lateral talocalcaneal limit inversion |
| | Spring | Calcaneus to navicular (plantar aspect): Limits eversion<br>This ligament also supports/stabilizes the transverse tarsal joint |
| Transverse tarsal | Long and short plantar ligaments, dorsal calcaneocuboid, and bifurcate | Stabilize transverse tarsal joint |

**Table 13-11**

Muscles of the Ankle/Foot

| Muscle | Primary Actions | Origin | Insertion |
|---|---|---|---|
| Gastrocnemius | Flex the knee, plantar flex the ankle | Condyles of the femur, posterior surfaces | Calcaneus via calcaneal tendon |
| Soleus | Plantar flex the ankle (talocrural joint) | Proximal, posterior surface of tibia; posterior aspect of head of fibula and proximal, posterior surface of tibia | Calcaneus via calcaneal tendon |
| Plantaris | Weak plantar flexion of the ankle, weak knee flexor | Lateral supracondylar line of femur | Calcaneus via calcaneal tendon |
| Peroneus (fibularis) longus | Evert the foot, assist to plantar flex the ankle | Head of fibula and proximal two-thirds of lateral fibula | Base first metatarsal, medial cuneiform |
| Peroneus (fibularis) brevis | Evert the foot, assist to plantar flex the ankle | Distal two-thirds of lateral fibula | Tuberosity on base of fifth metatarsal |
| Tibialis anterior | Invert the foot, dorsiflex the ankle | Lateral condyle of tibia; proximal, lateral tibia, interosseous membrane | Medial cuneiform, first metatarsal |
| Extensor digitorum longus | Extend the second through fifth toes, dorsiflex the ankle, evert the foot | Lateral condyle of tibia; proximal, anterior shaft of fibula, interosseous membrane | Middle and distal phalanges of second through fifth toes |
| Extensor hallucis longus | Extend the first toe, ankle dorsiflexion, inverts the foot | Middle anterior surface of fibula, interosseous membrane | Distal phalanx of first toe |
| Tibialis posterior | Invert the foot, ankle plantar flexion | Proximal posterior shafts of tibia and fibula, interosseous membrane | Five tarsal bones, bases of 2 to 4 metatarsals |
| Flexor digitorum longus | Flex toes 2 through 5, inverts foot, weak ankle plantar flexor | Middle posterior surface of tibia | Distal phalanges of second through fifth toes |
| Flexor hallucis longus | Flex the first toe, inverts the foot, weak ankle plantar flexor | Middle half of posterior fibula | Distal phalanx of first toe |

The deltoid ligament is located on the medial side of the ankle, and it is much stronger than the lateral ligaments. The ligament resists eversion of the hindfoot and stabilizes the ankle against plantar flexion and subtalar pronation. The muscles that assist in resisting these motions include the tibialis anterior and posterior, the flexor hallucis longus, and the flexor digitorum longus.

## Objective Tools to Assess the Hip, Knee, Ankle, and/or Foot

In addition to ROM, manual muscle testing (MMT), and special tests, physical performance measures can be used to assess performance and track patient progress. The 6-Minute Walk Test, self-paced walk speed (self-selected gait speed), stair measure test (stair climb test), and Timed Up and Go Test can determine the patient's activity limitations and participation restrictions.[22] The use of validated functional outcome assessment tools provides objective data regarding improvement in impairments and changes in activity limitations and/or participation restrictions. The Orthopedic Section of the American Physical Therapy Association (APTA) recommends using the Western Ontario and McMaster Universities Osteoarthritis Index (WOMAC), the Lower Extremity Functional Scale, and the Harris Hip Score. These tools are reliable and valid. The WOMAC and Lower Extremity Functional Scale are completed by the patient, and the Harris Hip Score is completed by the physical therapist to determine activity limitations and restrictions.[22]

Commonly used tools for patients with knee pathology include the Knee Injury and Osteoarthritis Outcome Score (KOOS) and the Patient-Specific Functional Scale. The KOOS assesses function and symptoms for patients who have experienced a knee injury or who have osteoarthritis (OA). The questions from the WOMAC are included in the KOOS so comparisons can be made between the 2 questionnaires.[23] The Patient-Specific Functional Scale can be used for any musculoskeletal problem; its use is not limited to patients with knee pain. The Ottawa Knee and Ankle Rules have been validated to help determine the need for radiographic imaging.[24,25]

# Management and Treatment of Hip Pathologies and Conditions

Hip pain is a common complaint from both young and old patients.[26,27] Degenerative OA and hip fractures are common diagnoses in older adults, but muscle strains, sprains, impingements, and contusions are more common in younger patients who are more active and/or participate in sports. Anterior hip and/or groin pain is commonly associated with intra-articular pathology, such as OA and labral tears. Posterior hip pain is associated with piriformis syndrome, sacroiliac joint dysfunction, or lumbar radiculopathy, and lateral hip pain is commonly associated with greater trochanteric bursitis or ITB syndrome.

A patient's past medical history, pain location, type of pain, and the results of special tests provide important information regarding the diagnosis during the physical therapist's evaluation. Clinical examination tests are helpful, but they are not sensitive or specific for all diagnoses. Physicians order radiography if acute fractures, dislocations, or stress fractures are suspected. Magnetic resonance imaging (MRI) is valuable to detect less apparent traumatic fractures, stress fractures, and osteonecrosis of the femoral head. An MRI arthrogram using a contrast medium (or dye) injected directly into the injured joint is the diagnostic test of choice for labral tears.

Physical therapist assistants will treat patients with various hip pathologies in a variety of settings and through different phases of the rehabilitation process. The assistant should be familiar with the special tests (Table 13-12), treatment techniques (eg, modalities, soft tissue/joint mobilizations), exercise/protocol progressions, and patient education to improve patient outcomes.

## Hip Osteoarthritis

Hip OA that is idiopathic is considered primary OA. Factors that can increase the risk of developing hip OA include previous joint injury/trauma, being overweight, and increased age. The articular cartilage breakdown affects the surrounding structures (ie, synovium, subchondral bone, joint capsule, ligaments, and muscles) and leads to joint space narrowing and osteophytes development. Secondary OA results from a previous underlying cause due to injury or pre-existing conditions or deformities.[26] Bilateral hip OA is more common in patients who are overweight or have been diagnosed with rheumatoid arthritis (RA).[26,27] Patients with degenerative hip OA usually complain of a gradual onset of aching pain in the groin that may or may not radiate into the thigh.[26] Some patients may complain of pain that goes from the anterior to the lateral hip area in a "C" shape.[27] Most will report limited ROM, joint stiffness, and pain that is worse with prolonged standing and walking.

**Table 13-12**

Special Tests for Various Hip Pathologies

| Special Tests | Possible Hip Pathologies if Positive |
|---|---|
| Scour or quadrant | Hip OA, labral tear, general hip pathologies (ie, capsule tightness) |
| Craig's | Femoral anteversion/retroversion |
| FABER (flexion, abduction, external rotation) | Hip pathologies, sacroiliac joint dysfunction, iliopsoas |
| FADDIR (flexion, adduction internal rotation) | Labral tear, impingement, iliopsoas |
| Trendelenburg | Gluteus medius weakness |
| Ober | Tensor fascia latae, ITB tightness |
| Piriformis | Piriformis tightness, sciatic nerve impingement with pain also down posterior thigh |
| Thomas | Iliopsoas, rectus femoris, ITB if femur abducts |
| Ely | Rectus femoris tightness |
| 90/90 | Hamstring tightness |

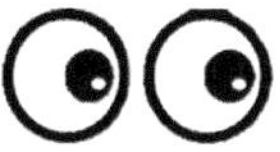

**Eye on the Research: Prediction Rule for Hip Osteoarthritis Diagnosis**

A study was completed to determine how accurate clinical examination items were in predicting hip OA. The 5 items are as follows:

1. Squatting aggravates symptoms (self-reported)
2. Active hip flexion that causes lateral hip pain
3. The scour test with adduction that causes lateral hip or groin pain
4. Active hip extension that causes pain
5. Passive internal rotation is 25 degrees or less

The presence of 3 of the 5 variables indicated the likelihood of having hip OA increased from 29% to 68%, and if 4 of the 5 items were present, the probability increased to 91%.[28]

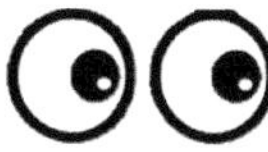

**Eye on the Research: Whole-Body Cryotherapy for Osteoarthritis**

A small study including 31 patients with spondyloarthritis, 10 with knee OA, and 9 with hip OA was completed to assess the effect of whole-body cryotherapy on OA. Whole-body cryotherapy (using a cryochamber) was beneficial for reducing pain, reducing analgesic medication use, and improving physical function after 10 days of treatment. There was improvement or significant improvement in 96% of the patients.[29] Clinicians should remain aware of new research and emerging treatment options.

## *Conservative Treatment for Patients With Hip Osteoarthritis*

Pain control is an important priority. Patients may be prescribed acetaminophen and nonsteroidal anti-inflammatory drugs (NSAIDs) by the physician. The physical therapist assistant should monitor for medication side effects. (See Appendix E for commonly used medications.) A patient can be fitted with a cane to control for pain when walking. It should be used on the contralateral side to reduce forces on the involved leg. If the therapist determines there is a leg length discrepancy due to joint space narrowing, a heel lift can be placed in the patient's shoe to level out the pelvis.

Hip internal rotation and extension motions may be limited because of the narrowing of the joint space. Limited hip motion increases stress on the lumbar spine and may be associated with low back pain. Pain-free active assisted range of motion (AAROM) and active range of motion (AROM) and multiplane isometric strengthening exercises can be initiated in the maximal protection phase. Using pain as a guide, the assistant can progress to dynamic strengthening and stretching exercises and balance training to improve patient function. Hip exercises and progressions are listed in Table 13-13. Pictures of these exercises are included at the end of the chapter.

Patients with hip OA should be instructed to avoid high-impact activities and to use heat or cold to manage pain. These patients are good candidates for aquatic therapy; low-impact aerobic conditioning and lower extremity strengthening are safe options in the water. Recumbent or upright stationary bikes or elliptical machines are other options for low-impact exercise.

**Table 13-13**

Hip Exercises

| Muscle Stretches | OKC/Strengthening[a] | CKC/Strengthening |
|---|---|---|
| Hip flexors<br>• Prone press-up<br>• Thomas test position (psoas) and then passively flex knee (rectus femoris)<br>• Half kneeling rock forward<br>• Stand astride and assume forward lunge position<br>Hip extensors/gluteals<br>• Bilateral knee to chest<br>• Single knee to chest<br>Hip extensors/hamstrings<br>• Sit with leg on table, knee straight; flex forward at hips<br>• Stand foot on stool knee straight; flex forward at hips<br>• Supine straight leg raise (SLR) with towel/strap<br>• Supine towel around thigh at 90 degrees; straighten knee<br>• Short sit and extend knee<br>Hip adductors and internal rotators<br>• Bilateral self-stretch supine (frog, butterfly position)<br>• Supine single-leg hip external rotation with flexed knee<br>• Seated butterfly stretch (soles of feet together, knees flexed and push them all toward floor)<br>• Stand feet shoulder width with hip external rotation, side lunge<br>Hip external rotators<br>• Supine or seated piriformis stretch<br>• Supine or seated knee to opposite shoulder<br>Tensor fascia latae/ITB<br>• Supine, knee straight, bring leg across body<br>• Side lying, knee straight, leg drops posterior/off table (Ober test position)<br>• Stand with involved leg 12 inches (in) from wall, cross other leg in front, and then push level pelvis toward wall and hold | Hip flexion<br>• Supine heel slides<br>• Seated hip flexion isometrics or active<br>• Standing hip/knee flexion<br>• Standing straight leg flexion<br>Hip extensors/gluteals and hamstrings<br>• Gluteal squeezes<br>• Prone hip extension (knees flexed [glutes] or straight [hamstrings])<br>• Quadruped hip extension (leg lifts)<br>• Standing hip extension<br>Hip adductors and internal rotators<br>• Supine or seated isometric pillow squeezes (knees straight or flexed)<br>• Seated hip internal rotation<br>• Side-lying adduction<br>• Standing adduction<br>Hip external rotation<br>• Prone or seated external rotation isometrics<br>• Side-lying external rotation (clamshells)<br>• Quadruped hip external rotation with knee flexed<br>• Sitting external rotation<br>Hip abductors<br>• Supine pelvic drop to hip hike (gluteus medius one side and quadratus lumborum opposite side)<br>• Supine abduction active or isometric<br>• Side-lying abduction<br>• Quadruped hip abduction with straight knee<br>• Standing hip abduction | Dynamic activities<br>• Supine bridging: Double leg, single leg (on table progress to feet on ball)<br>• Wall slides to 90 degrees (double leg progress to single leg)<br>• Partial squats/mini-squats<br>• Step-up/down: Forward, lateral, backward<br>• Standing pelvic drop to hip hike<br>• Partial/full lunges forward, lateral, backward<br>• Single-leg standing progress to partial squat and change to compliant surface<br>Plyometrics<br>• Jumps, skip for height, skip for distance, hopping for height, hopping for distance<br>• Add sport-specific agility drills<br>Note: These are not appropriate for all patients. |

[a]Exercises can be made more difficult by adding weights or using higher-resistance elastic bands.

**Considerations for the Physical Therapist Assistant**

Older patients with hip OA may be deconditioned, so additional monitoring when implementing aerobic exercise programs is indicated (refer to Chapter 9).

# Surgical Interventions for the Hip Joint: Diagnoses, Procedures, and Treatment

Surgical interventions are commonly indicated for patients with severe OA or RA and after hip fractures caused by falls, fragility, or osteoporosis. Arthroscopic procedures are indicated for small articular repairs (eg, chondroplasty, removal of loose bodies), acetabulum labral tears, femoroacetabular impingement (FAI) syndromes, and/or joint laxity. Open procedures are used to repair femoral fractures and for total hip arthroplasties (THAs) and hemiarthroplasties.[30]

## *Arthroscopic Repair of Labrum Tears and Associated Diagnoses*

Acetabular labrum tears and FAI can cause hip pain. These diagnoses are more common in athletes because of high-velocity twisting, ballistic collisions, and violent falls; they often present together.[31,32] Other causes of hip pain include capsular laxity/hip joint hypermobility, hip dysplasia, and degeneration.[31,33]

Anterior hip or groin pain, clicking, locking, and giving way are signs and symptoms of labral tears. Sixty-six percent of patients (39 ± 13 years old) in the general population who present with these symptoms were diagnosed with labrum tears.[32] Damage to articular cartilage (chondral defects) is more severe in patients with tearing (or fraying) of the acetabular labrum, and articular damage often occurs in the same zone/region as the labral tear/lesion.[33] The damaged labrum can be repaired by reattaching it to the acetabulum, or it can be resected and debrided (removed) during an arthroscopic procedure. Hyaline cartilage does not regenerate, so a procedure called *microfracture* (or chondroplasty) is performed to promote fibrocartilage formation at the site of the defect. During this procedure, microfracture picks make small fractures into the subchondral bone in the damaged area to create bleeding so that fibrocartilage can form.

A femoral osteoplasty is performed to correct for FAI. The goal is to restore the normal relationship between the femoral head and acetabulum so that the hip can move through the full ROM without impingement.

### Rehabilitation After Arthroscopic Hip Procedures

Initial rehabilitation interventions after the arthroscopic procedures mentioned previously include patient education, protected weight bearing, and AAROM. Patient education includes avoiding painful positions and ensuring pain does not exceed minimal levels (2 to 3/10) with exercise. Postoperative weight bearing is typically limited to toe-touch weight bearing (TTWB). Hip AAROM is initiated to reduce muscle guarding and scarring. ROM restrictions for the first week include avoiding hip flexion greater than 90 degrees, extension past neutral, and external rotation beyond 20 to 25 degrees.[31,32,34] Some patients may be fitted with a brace to limit hip flexion.

Lumbopelvic and hip muscle control is important for trunk stability and to reduce shearing forces (which can negatively affect tissue healing).[31,34] Regaining motor control and proper sequencing of the lumbopelvic region, hip, and lower extremity are more important than maximizing strength or power, so continual monitoring is required during the rehabilitation process.

**Considerations for the Physical Therapist Assistant**

It is essential for patients to observe postoperative weight-bearing restrictions to allow for proper healing. The assistant should defer to physician protocol. General weight-bearing guidelines include the following:

- Labral repair: TTWB for 3 to 6 weeks postsurgery
- Labral resection/debridement only: Partial weight bearing (PWB) or 50% weight bearing for 10 days to 2 weeks postsurgery
- Osteoplasty for FAI: TTWB for 4 to 6 weeks postsurgery
- Microfracture (chondroplasty): TTWB for 4 to 6 weeks and up to 8 weeks postsurgery[30]

After the recommended timelines, the patient progresses to weight bearing as tolerated (WBAT) and then to full weight bearing (FWB) based on the physician's protocol and the patient's tolerance.

Patient progression is based on tissue healing times and the patient reaching certain criteria determined by the physician's protocol. Intra-articular swelling from the surgical intervention usually takes 4 to 6 weeks to resolve. Exercise guidelines and criteria for the progression for various arthroscopic procedures are summarized in Table 13-14.[30-34]

**Table 13-14**

**Postoperative Rehabilitation Suggested Guidelines After Hip Arthroscopies**

| Phase 1 (Day 1 to Week 3 to 5) Maximal Protection Phase | Phase 2 (Week 3 to 5 to Week 7 to 8) Moderate Protection Phase | Phase 3 (Week 8 to 12)/Phase 4 (Week 12+) Return to Function |
|---|---|---|
| • Ankle pumps, gentle calf stretches, toe crunches<br>• Pain free or ≤3/10 pain with passive and active-assisted hip ROM: Flexion ≤90 degrees; extension to 0 degrees, limit abduction to about 45 degrees all for 2 to 3 weeks, internal rotation with legs extended limited by pain, external rotation to 20 to 25 degrees for first 2 weeks. Progress to full ROM by week 3 to 4; begin pain free or ≤3/10 pain AROM during week 2 to 3.<br>• Prone on elbows is safe initially, but *avoid* passive extension past neutral for 2 to 3 weeks.<br>• Transverse abdominis and gentle pelvic tilts and pelvic clocks. Progress to supine marching with no pelvic motion or pain about week 3.<br>• Isometrics: Gluteal (prone and with knees flexed), hip abduction, quadriceps sets, hip adduction, and internal rotation<br>• Stationary bike with limited hip flexion to 90 degrees no resistance (no recumbent bike).<br>• Observe weight-bearing precautions.<br>• *Avoid* any activity creating "pinching feeling/pain" in the anterior hip region.<br>• *Avoid* any exercise that creates excessive iliopsoas activity for about 2 to 4 weeks. Tendonitis is a side effect. | • Normalize gait pattern, speed, and endurance. Progress weight bearing as per protocol or pain limits. (Microfracture restrictions may be up to week 7 to 8.)<br>• Progress AROM all motions in various positions gravity minimized to against gravity (supine, prone, side-lying, standing)<br>• Progress to treadmill, elliptical, and bike with resistance<br>• Stretching: Gentle hip flexion and single knee to chest stretches, hamstring stretch, adductor stretch<br>• Strengthening OKC: Hip flexion SLR week 4 with minimal pinching or hip pain, add resistance for SLR for abduction, adduction and extension, clams, supine opposite arm/leg for rectus abdominals and obliques progress to core stabilization on/with ball, resisted band standing trunk rotation, quadruped opposite arm/leg, half-kneeling chops/PNF<br>• Strengthening CKC: Bridging, (double more than single leg), forward, lateral backward step-ups/downs, planks, wall slides, mini-squats, side stepping<br>• Balance when FWB: Double-leg wobble board, 2 legs stand on foam/mini-trampoline eyes opened/closed, ball tossing, single-leg stand on firm surface<br>• Precautions: No post activity soreness > 24 hours and no ballistic or forced stretching; limit excessive or repetitive hip flexion activities that cause discomfort | Phase 3 advanced exercises<br>• Increase cardiovascular aerobic endurance<br>• Progress to squats, single-leg squats, multidirectional lunges, lunges with trunk rotation and weighted ball<br>• Single-leg standing on foam/mini-trampoline eyes open/closed, ball tossing, step-ups/downs 4- and 6-in steps control eccentrics<br>• Straight-line slow jogging week 10 or later, resisted side stepping, forward and backward walking<br>• Advanced and dynamic core stabilization exercises and side planks<br>Phase 4 sport-specific training<br>• Begin running, skipping, and jumping; progress to hopping<br>• Straight-line running progressing to starts/stops, cutting drills on command<br>• Plyometric training<br>• Step up and down from 8-in step with control and balance |

PNF = proprioceptive neuromuscular facilitation.

The criteria to proceed to the second phase include healing time, pain less than 3/10, and passive range of motion (PROM) to 90% of normal limits (maintain any ongoing postprocedural protocol restrictions; ie, no hip extension greater than 10 degrees or external rotation greater than 20 to 25 degrees). Hip flexion should be approximately 110 degrees. AROM can be initiated at approximately 2 to 3 weeks postoperatively. The goals of phase 2 include AROM within normal limits and a normalized gait pattern. Patients should work on normalizing their gait pattern while abiding by weight-bearing restrictions. Once the patient is able to tolerate FWB, goals include normalizing gait speed, step length, and walking endurance; increasing static and dynamic lumbopelvic and postural motor control; and increasing strength and muscle endurance for all hip musculature.

The criteria to progress to the third phase include passive hip flexion 120 to 130 degrees without anterior hip pinching, 20 degrees of hip extension, and 45 degrees of external rotation. The patient must demonstrate 75% FABER test performance, a symmetrical squat with 70 degrees of knee flexion, a negative Trendelenburg test, and a normal symmetrical gait pattern.[31] Additionally, the patient must be able to complete single-leg standing on the uninvolved leg while performing active hip flexion to 90 degrees and extension to 20 degrees on the involved leg and 30 repetitions of prone hip extension to 20 degrees.[31] Goals focus on progressing the patient for returning to work or sport.

## *Total Hip Arthroplasty and Hemiarthroplasty*

More than 1 million hip arthroplasties are performed worldwide per year, and this number is expected to double within the next 20 years. THAs or total hip replacements are one of the most common surgical interventions for patients with severe hip OA who have resting pain and severe hip pain during motion and weight bearing. THAs are also indicated for patients with RA, ankylosing spondylitis, avascular necrosis, fractures, or other failed surgical procedures (eg, osteotomy, hemiarthroplasty of the femoral component).[30,35-38] Figure 13-12 shows a radiographic view of a hip implant after a THA procedure.

A hemiarthroplasty is a procedure in which only one component is replaced (most commonly the femoral component), typically due to disease/degeneration or after a femoral fracture. The femoral head replacement can be either unipolar or bipolar. A unipolar prosthesis is a one-piece design in which all hip movement occurs directly between the prosthesis and the acetabulum. A bipolar femoral prosthesis has 2 components (the stem and head) that articulate; this articulation allows for some motion between the stem and head in addition to the motion that occurs between the head of the prosthesis and the patient's own acetabulum. Both the femoral head and acetabulum are replaced in THA.

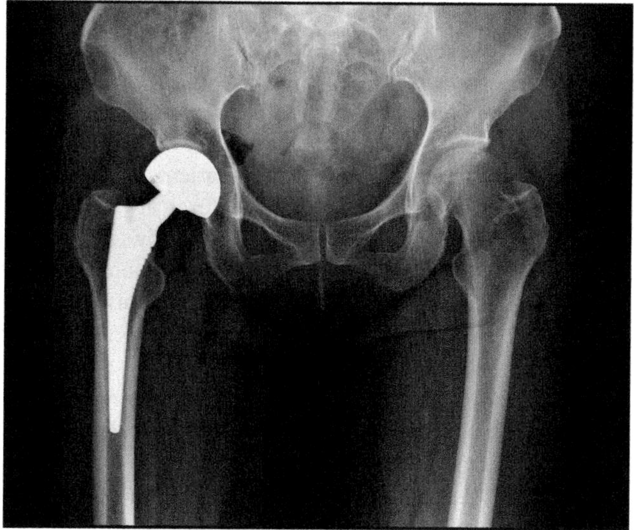

**Figure 13-12.** A radiographic view of the hip after total hip replacement (ChooChin/Shutterstock.com).

### Surgical Procedure Approaches, Hip Precautions, and Possible Complications

There are several surgical approaches that are used to perform a THA. Patient presentation, regional practice patterns, and the surgeon's preference are factors that determine which surgical approach is selected for a patient. The assistant will educate the patient regarding postoperative hip precautions. Knowing the precautions for each approach allows the assistant to select only those exercises that are appropriate and to guide the patient to maintain the hip precautions with functional mobility.

A posterior or posterolateral approach requires the surgeon to cut the tensor fasciae latae where the gluteus maximus attaches (sparing the gluteus medius) and to detach the hip external rotators and the gluteus minimus where they attach to the greater trochanter. Historically, this procedure presents with a higher risk for postoperative dislocations; surgeons work to reduce this risk by increasing the size of the femoral head and reattaching the short hip external rotators and posterior capsule to the greater trochanter.[35,37,38] Hip precautions postoperatively include avoiding hip flexion past 90 degrees, hip adduction across the midline, and hip internal rotation past neutral. These motions should especially be avoided in combination; performing these motions is contraindicated because they can increase the chances of dislocating the surgical hip. Patients should also avoid flexing the trunk forward past 90 degrees (eg, picking something off the floor, tying shoes) or standing on the surgical leg and twisting because these motions create CKC hip flexion and internal rotation, respectively.

During an anterior surgical approach, the surgeon makes an incision just below and lateral to the ASIS and just medial to the tensor fasciae latae.[30,35] The advantages of the anterior approach include less postoperative pain (the muscles are retracted not cut), a decreased risk of dislocation, and increased ROM. These patients can usually tolerate more weight bearing into the surgical hip sooner because they tend to have less pain. One study found that patients with anterior hip replacements were able to walk without an assistive device 6 days earlier than patients who had other types of hip replacements.[35] Hip precautions for the anterior approach include avoiding excessive hip extension, but patients should be able to walk using a near-normal step and stride length. These patients should avoid lying prone, performing bridges, and standing trunk extension because these activities exaggerate hip extension. Hip external rotation in either an OKC or CKC is considered a precaution. The physician determines the length of time the precautions should be observed.

Other approaches include anterolateral, direct lateral, transtrochanteric, and minimally invasive techniques. Clinicians should be aware of the physician's protocols and postoperative precautions, which are typically located in the postoperative physical therapy orders and documented in the initial evaluation.

There are postoperative complications associated with THA procedures. One meta-analysis study compared lateral and posterior approach complications. The researchers reported a significant reduction in the risk of a Trendelenburg gait and stem malposition with posterior approaches. There was no significant difference in heterotopic ossification, and the researchers concluded that neither approach had a functional advantage over the other.[39] Although mortality rates are low, DVT and pulmonary edema are serious complications of THA, and the physical therapist assistant should be familiar with their signs and symptoms. Early mobility out of bed, ambulation, and exercises such as ankle pumps and heel slides reduce the risk of these complications. The risk of infection is also low (1% to 2%) but higher for patients who are overweight or have diabetes, RA, or blood clotting disorders. Warmth, heat, or swelling over the hip area may indicate a possible infection, and the assistant should report these findings to the physical therapist and/or the physician. Additional complications include dislocation, implant component loosening, possible leg length discrepancy, and nerve injury.[26,39-42] Hip dislocations usually occur early in the recovery period, and the chances of dislocation can be reduced through adherence to hip precautions. Dislocation rates are lower after an initial procedure compared with surgical revisions. Within 3 months after THA surgery, one study found that hip dislocation rate was reported in 3.1% of the cases.[41]

Implant component loosening is a complication that can occur months/years after the initial surgery; loosening will require a surgical hip replacement revision. Signs and/or symptoms include thigh pain with walking (often persistent and worsens over time), popping (because of the loosened component) often with pain, and complaints of "something just doesn't feel right." The assistant should notify the therapist immediately if any of these complications are reported.

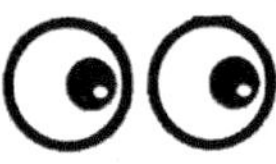

**Eye on the Research: Implant Loosening**

One study found no significant difference in the length of time an implant maintained its function/integrity between cemented and uncemented THA.[40] Another study reported men were at a higher risk of cemented stem component loosening, but older patients were at a lower risk of loosening of the same cemented component. Patients with a body mass index greater than 25 kg/m$^2$ have an increased risk of cemented stem loosening.[42]

## Rehabilitation Management After Total Hip Arthroplasties

Physical therapy interventions usually start the day of or the day after THA as long as the patient is medically stable. Table 13-15 provides suggested exercises and activities for each phase of the rehabilitation program after THA and hemiarthroplasty procedures. These are guidelines; they do not replace a physician's protocol or the physical therapist's POC.

A patient immediately after THA is in the acute stage of healing (maximum protection phase), and emphasis during this phase is to prevent surgical complications and to promote safe mobility. The clinician should follow the specific hip precautions based on the surgical approach used. Patient education and compliance are crucial to achieving safe mobility and minimizing the occurrence of complications.

Weight-bearing considerations depend on the surgeon's decision to use cemented, uncemented, or a hybrid technique. Patients are usually permitted to WBAT immediately after surgery with cemented replacements. Weight-bearing restrictions with uncemented or hybrid prostheses vary from TTWB to PWB for 6 weeks or longer, but the physician determines the weight-bearing status. When weight bearing is restricted, it is done so based on the theory that the weight bearing may cause very small movements of the components, leading to prosthetic loosening. Growing evidence indicates that allowing patients to bear weight as tolerated is safe.[30,41] Early weight bearing after surgery helps to reduce the chances of bone demineralization and allows for easier mobility.[30,35,41] It is the responsibility of the therapy team to follow the weight-bearing guidelines included in the physician's protocol.

During the moderate protection phase, general recommendations include maintaining hip precautions at least through week 12 postoperatively.[30] There is evidence of variability in precaution timelines; the risk of dislocation

**Table 13-15**

Postoperative Rehabilitation Suggested Guidelines for Hemiarthroplasty and Total Hip Arthroplasty

| Maximum Protection Phase (Day 1 to 3 Weeks Postoperatively) | Moderate Protection Phase (3 to 12 Weeks Postoperatively) | Return to Function Minimum Protection Phase (12 to 16 Weeks) |
|---|---|---|
| Goals: Increase ROM (within precautions)<br>• Increase strength<br>• Pain control (cold pack)<br>• Bed mobility/transfer training<br>• Hip precautions education to prevent dislocation, prevent postoperative complications (ie, DVT)<br>• Gait training within weight-bearing restrictions as per physician.<br>Bed mobility/transfers<br>• Adhere to hip precautions with these activities: Supine to long sit to sit (no logrolling or rolling to side)<br>• Weight bearing: WBAT with assistive device; even if FWB, use assistive device. Follow physician-specific weight-bearing restrictions. | Criteria to progress to moderate protection phase<br>• Reduced pain to 3 to 4/10<br>• Quadriceps strength is at least 3/5<br>• Compliance with hip precautions<br>• Independent with bed mobility and transfers<br>Safe and independent with gait with increasing weight-bearing status as tolerated or permitted<br>Note: Patients *must* have adequate hip extension and abduction strength before walking without an assistive device. | Criteria to progress to minimal protection phase<br>• Normalized pain-free gait pattern with least restrictive assistive device or without assistive device<br>• Improve balance, coordination and proprioception, and endurance<br>• Functional ROM and strength in surgical hip<br>• Independent with ADLs<br><br>*(continued)* |

**Table 13-15 (continued)**

Postoperative Rehabilitation Suggested Guidelines for Hemiarthroplasty and Total Hip Arthroplasty

| Maximum Protection Phase (Day 1 to 3 Weeks Postoperatively) | Moderate Protection Phase (3 to 12 Weeks Postoperatively) | Return to Function Minimum Protection Phase (12 to 16 Weeks) |
|---|---|---|
| Exercises<br>• Supine: Ankle pumps/circles, AAROM to AROM heel slides, TKE, hip abduction/adduction to midline (using hip precautions)<br>• Isometrics: Quadriceps and gluteal sets, pillow squeezes (submaximal or setting)<br>• Standing: Hip flexion < 90 degrees, abduction, extension, active knee flexion/extension<br>• Weight shifts limited by weight-bearing status<br>• Additional exercises: Deep breathing exercises, pelvic tilts, OKC/CKC ROM and strengthening on uninvolved lower extremity; strengthen both upper extremities<br>Note: Encourage patient to use as normal gait pattern as possible while abiding by weight-bearing restrictions. | Exercises<br>• Seated/semirecumbent: Knee flexion/extension with resistance<br>• Supine: Bridges hook-lying* resisted hip external rotation<br>• Side lying: Hip external rotation, abduction<br>• Standing: Hip abduction/adduction, flexion/extension,* straight plane with resistance bands (no hip rotation)<br>• CKC: Can begin 3 to 8 weeks postoperatively (delay 2 to 3 weeks for uncemented/hybrid as per protocol). Calf raises, weight-shifting progress to single-leg standing, partial squats. Lunges forward and lateral, mini–step-ups forward/lateral (2-in step) when FWB is permitted. Standing resisted band TKE.<br>• Stretches: Calf stretches, supine hip/knee flexor stretch in Thomas test position only if cleared by physician<br>• Seated hamstring stretches (avoid with posterior/posterior-lateral approach unless able to maintain precautions).<br>Aerobics: Stationary bike (raised seat), upper bike ergometer, aquatic exercises<br>Balance: Ankle and hip strategies progress to balance with one leg on step or wobble board<br>Gait training: Walking treadmill backward and forward<br>*Anterior approach THA: No bridging/limit hip hyperextension | Exercises<br>• Proprioception and coordination<br>• Lunges forward/backward/lateral<br>• Side stepping with resistance bands<br>• Lateral step-ups, 3- to 4-in step<br>Aerobics: Stationary bike, upper bike ergometer, aquatic exercises, treadmill<br>Balance: Single-leg standing (eyes open/closed, foam, mini-trampoline, balance beam). In quiet stance and Romberg rhythmic stabilization/alternating isometrics, balance with self-initiated perturbations.<br>Gait: Walk on uneven surfaces, stair training, walk up and down ramps, gait with head movements.<br>Task-specific training: Stairs, carrying loads with walking<br>Progress to community exercise class, increase walking distance and speed. |

plateaus between 10 and 13 weeks, the rate of infection plateaus between 4 and 6 weeks, and pulmonary edema risk is stabilized by about week 6.[41] Strengthening exercises are progressed to resisted OKC activities targeting hip extensors and hip abductors. When the patient is able to achieve FWB status, double- and single-leg CKC exercises can be initiated. A patient can be progressed from using a cane to no assistive device but only if the patient has adequate hip extension and abduction strength to prevent an antalgic or atypical gait (ie, Trendelenburg or lurch gait pattern). The assistant should check the POC and/or the physician's protocol before progressing the patient to ambulation without an assistive device.

The minimum protection or return-to-function phase ends at about 16 weeks after surgery, but it may take up to 1 year for full recovery. There is controversy regarding the types of sporting activities patients can engage in after THA surgery. Patients can usually return to nonimpact activities such as bicycling, swimming, dancing, golf, and tennis (doubles).[41] Specific questions regarding readiness to return to other types of sports or activities should be directed to the surgeon.

## Fractures and Surgical Repair

Fall risk, fall rates, and the incidence of hip fractures increase with age. In the United States, the rate of hip fracture in women ranges from 0.2% for those 60 to 64 years old to 2.5% for those 85 years or older; the risk for women is double that of men. Hip fractures in older adults can have a negative impact on their quality of life and can result in a loss of independence. Mortality rates among older patients after hip fractures range between 14% and 36% within 1 year after surgery; the rate is higher among men older than 75 years of age.[43,44] Osteoporosis causes more than 8.9 million fractures annually worldwide. About 20% of osteoporotic fractures occur at the proximal femur.[45] Risk factors associated with increased mortality after an osteoporotic hip fracture include being older than 75 years, being male, moderate to severe liver disease, diabetes mellitus, living in a nursing home, chronic obstructive pulmonary disease, myocardial infarction, and dementia.[44]

Fractures to the femoral neck and head are called *intracapsular fractures*. These fractures can disrupt blood flow to the femoral head, resulting in avascular necrosis or nonunion. Trochanteric fractures occur between the greater and lesser trochanter, and subtrochanteric fractures occur just distal to the lesser trochanter; these fractures are extracapsular fractures.

The type of surgical intervention used to secure the fracture site depends on the patient's age, location, severity of fracture, bone quality, prior level of function, presence of additional soft tissue injury, and the goals to return to activity or prior level of function. Open reduction and internal fixation (ORIF) techniques are used to stabilize the fracture. Fractures can be repaired using several internal fixation techniques (ie, plates and screws) or with a hemiarthroplasty.

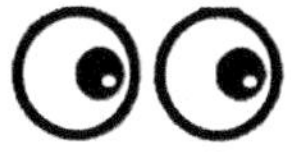

**Eye on the Research: Femoral Neck Fracture Repairs**

Preservation of the femoral head (using multiple screws to fix the fracture) is the treatment of choice for nondisplaced femoral neck fractures for both general orthopedists and orthopedic specialists.[46] In displaced femoral neck fractures, replacing the femoral head is preferred by both groups of orthopedic surgeons, but orthopedic specialists preferred THA, whereas general orthopedists preferred a hemiarthroplasty.[46]

Comparison of cemented vs uncemented procedures indicated a significantly lower occurrence of postoperative infection in the cemented group compared with the uncemented group. There was no significant difference in postoperative ambulation ability. Researchers concluded that the selective use of a cemented stem and bipolar hemiarthroplasty could be a desirable procedure for patients with poor bone quality and a higher risk of infections.[47]

### Rehabilitation Management After Hip Fractures

After hip fracture surgery, physical therapy usually begins the day of or the day after surgery. The patient's weight-bearing status is based on the surgical procedure; it can range from non–weight bearing (NWB) to TTWB to WBAT. Avoiding prolonged bed rest; early mobility and exercise reduce the likelihood of surgical complications (eg, DVTs and pneumonia). Patients may be discharged to a skilled nursing facility (to continue therapy) or home with home health care based on the patient's living situation (ie, living alone or physical barriers at home) and the postoperative need for assistance with ADLs.

Patient education focuses on reducing excessive forces that may be placed on the surgical hip during bed mobility and transfers. Clinicians should have patients practice safe bed mobility and transfer training techniques, stressing the importance of following the physician's protocol and weight-bearing precautions using an assistive device during ambulation. When the patient is in bed, ensure that the knee of the surgical leg is positioned in extension, and avoid placing a pillow under the knee because this increases the risk for developing a knee flexion contracture.

Exercises are initially focused on restoring ROM and regaining muscle control in the surgical leg. Table 13-16 provides rehabilitation treatment suggestions and progressions across the phases of rehabilitation.

**Table 13-16**

**Postoperative Rehabilitation Suggested Guidelines for Hip Fractures**

| Acute Stage/Phase 1<br>Maximum Protection (Day 0 to 3 Weeks) | Subacute Stage/Phase 2<br>Moderate Protection (3 to 6 Weeks) | Return to Function/Phase 3<br>Minimal Protection (6 to 12 Weeks) |
|---|---|---|
| Goals<br>• Prevent postoperative complications; reduce pain/swelling<br>• Protect surgical limb<br>• Increase upper extremity strength<br>• Increase hip ROM, muscular control of hip<br>• Patient education for bed mobility, transfers, and gait with assistive device<br>Weight bearing<br>• As per physician protocol<br>Exercises<br>• Supine: Ankle pumps, heel slides, hip abduction/adduction, and internal/external rotation<br>• Standing: Hip flexion, SLRs, and hip extension and abduction with surgical leg<br>• Submaximal isometrics: Gluteal, quadriceps, hamstring, and abductors/adductors<br>• Additional exercises: Deep breathing exercises, pelvic tilts, OKC/CKC ROM and strengthening on uninvolved lower extremity and both upper extremities | Goals<br>• Improve ROM, strength, and aerobic conditioning<br>• *Avoid* stresses at fracture site for 4 to 6 weeks<br>• By week 6, WBAT is usually permitted to FWB as tolerated.<br>Weight bearing is dictated by rate of bone healing (about 10 to 18 weeks) or as recommended per physician protocol<br>Exercises (Note: Hold supine SLR until week 6 postoperatively)<br>• Standing OKC: 4-way SLR; progress to light resistance; use resistance bands and/or ankle weights<br>• CKC bilateral: Heel/toe raises, mini-squats, partial wall squats, and step-ups. Adjust for weight-bearing restrictions or perform in pool.<br>• Stretches: Calf stretches, and seated hamstring stretches<br>Aerobics: Stationary bike, recumbent stepper, and upper bike ergometer<br>Balance: Quiet stance, Romberg stabilization stance (rhythmic stabilization/alternating isometrics), balance with self-initiated perturbations | Goals<br>• Normal gait using a cane or no assistive device by about week 12 as tolerated<br>• *Avoid* twisting in CKC on surgical leg.<br>• Resume instrumental activities of daily living (IADLs) as age and health status allows<br>Weight bearing: Progress functional activities to FWB either as tolerated or as per physician protocol<br>Exercises<br>• CKC: Partial squats, heel raises with table/walker for support, lunges, and forward/lateral step-ups<br>• OKC: Hip/knee with resistance (up to 5 pounds); emphasize hip extension and abduction for gait carryover<br>• Stretches: Calf stretches, hip flexor stretches (Thomas test position), and hamstring stretches<br>Aerobics: Stationary bike, recumbent stepper, upper bike ergometer, treadmill, and aquatics<br>Balance: When FWB, ankle and hip strategies progress to balance with one leg on step or wobble board. Progress to SLS, tandem standing, and balance activities with eyes open and closed.<br>Task-specific training: Stairs, carrying loads with walking<br>Progress to community activities; increase walking distance and speed |

### Considerations for the Physical Therapist Assistant: Exercise Precautions

- When performing CKC exercises and/or supine bridging, always maintain compliance with weight-bearing restrictions on the surgical leg.
- Patient should avoid performing SLRs on the surgical hip for at least 4 weeks following surgery or if cleared by the surgeon.
- Confer with the physical therapist for guidance before increasing resistance or lengthening the lever arm during exercises.

The long-term goal is to have the patient return to their prior level of function and maintain independence if possible. Because many patients are discharged before meeting this goal, they should be encouraged to participate in a supervised exercise program for several months after being discharged from physical therapy to continue improving functional activities. Several studies reported that extended progressive resistive exercise programs for mild to moderately frail older adults resulted in strength gains on the surgical leg equal to that of the uninvolved leg, reinforcing the value of continued physical therapy for this population.[30]

## Musculotendinous and Bursae Injuries: Nonsurgical Interventions

Soft tissue injuries are common in the hip and thigh areas. Common mechanisms of injury (MOIs) include repetitive overuse, trauma due to explosive muscle contractions, or sudden muscle stretching associated with stopping/deceleration. Muscle strains commonly affect the hamstrings, hip flexors, and hip abductors. Lower extremity strains present similarly. A mild strain typically presents with minimal pain with little to no loss of strength or ROM. A moderate strain results in pain with motion and an antalgic gait; the patient may require short-term use of crutches. Moderate strains present with loss of ROM and weakness in the affected muscle and delayed bruising in that region. A severe strain may present with the patient reporting a popping sound and is associated with a significant loss of ROM and strength. Common bursitis diagnoses include trochanteric, ischial, and iliopectineal (psoas).

Hamstring muscle injury is one of the most common strains noted in athletes. The most common MOI includes explosive forceful contractions during rapid acceleration or deceleration or rapid overstretching of the muscle. The patient presents with weakness during resisted knee flexion and hip extension and delayed bruising on the posterior thigh. Hip adductor (or groin) strains can be caused by kicking (eg, soccer), sudden lateral changes in direction when running, or twisting or overstretching the muscles. More severe strains (grades II and III) cause bruising in the medial aspect of the thigh and result in weak hip adduction. Hip flexor strains commonly affect dancers, gymnasts, cyclists, and those who participate in martial arts and are often a result of repetitive overuse. A sudden trauma may also be a cause of injury to the iliopsoas muscles. Patients complain of pain in the anterior groin/thigh and weakness with stair climbing and hip flexion.

Trochanteric bursitis causes dull or burning pain on the lateral aspect of the hip and thigh. Causes include a direct blow (falling on the lateral hip), excessive walking or stair climbing, or repetitive ITB rubbing. Repetitive ITB rubbing irritates the bursa; this is exacerbated by tight adductors or large Q angles (more common in women) and when running with a slightly adducted leg (eg, when running on a cambered sidewalk/road). Ischial bursitis is often observed in people who sit on hard surfaces for long periods of time, or it can be caused by a direct blow from a fall on the ischial tuberosity. It can also occur due to excessive uphill walking or stair climbing. Pain occurs on or around the ischial tuberosity and increases during sitting. If there is swelling of the bursa, the sciatic nerve can become irritated, resulting in radicular symptoms down the leg. Iliopectineal or psoas bursitis can be caused by repetitive hip flexion activities, causing groin or anterior hip and thigh pain. It can be mistaken for a hip flexor strain.

### *Rehabilitation Management After Musculotendinous Strains and Bursitis*

Treatment of sprains and strains should follow the rehabilitation phases and stages of healing described in Chapter 3. Refer to Table 13-17 for suggested treatment interventions for these diagnoses.

During the acute stage (maximal protection phase), patients should be educated on how to limit or modify their activities, assume proper sleeping positions to reduce symptoms, ways to control swelling and pain (eg, cryotherapy techniques), and to only perform gentle exercises that do not increase symptoms. Gentle ROM exercises and muscle setting or submaximal isometrics are indicated but must be pain free. The assistant can include core stabilization exercises, upper extremity aerobic and strengthening exercises, and exercises for the uninvolved lower extremity.

During the moderate protection phase, the patient can initiate gentle stretching to the injured structures and can begin light strengthening exercises targeting those muscles on the involved lower extremity. Progression is based on the POC.

The ultimate goal is to return the patient to their prior level of function and eventually return to work or sport. Patients may be discharged from therapy before all goals are met. In these cases, the clinician should strongly encourage the patient to participate in a supervised exercise program or to work with an athletic trainer to continue sport-specific progressions.

**Table 13-17**

Suggested Exercise Progression Guidelines for Muscle Strains, Nerve Entrapment, and Bursitis Diagnosis

| Diagnosis | Treatment/Exercise Guidelines |
|---|---|
| ITB | Acute/maximal protection: Modalities for pain control/inflammation reduce irritating stresses and activities. Underlying cause: Adducted gait, weak hip abductors external rotators, leg length discrepancy, genu varus, and Q angle.<br>Subacute/moderate protection: Hip AROM, gentle stretching of tight structures, and submaximal isometrics<br>Return to function/minimal protection: More aggressive stretching of tight structures, cross friction massage/IASTM, dynamic strengthening (typically hip abductors, external rotation), plyometrics in preparation for return to sport. |
| Piriformis tightness (sciatic nerve entrapment) | Acute/maximal protection: Modalities for pain control/inflammation, avoid prolonged hip external rotation positions (ie, prolonged sitting/standing). Underlying cause: Lumbar disk issue, muscle tightness/guarding/nerve entrapment, creating radicular symptoms. Educate on positions that reduce symptoms, initiate use of McKenzie sequence for pain reduction/positioning.<br>Subacute/moderate protection: Submaximal isometrics for hip extensors, abductors, and external rotators; education for correction of faulty movement patterns; gentle piriformis stretching, progress McKenzie sequence as indicated. Nerve glides may be included if sciatic nerve irritation is present.<br>Return to function/minimal protection: Progressive strengthening for hip extensors, abductors, and external rotators; piriformis stretching; plyometric exercise that focuses on gluteal strengthening to correct faulty biomechanics as indicated |
| Hip muscle strains: Hip flexors, hamstrings (sciatic nerve entrapment), hip adductor (obturator nerve entrapment) | Acute/maximal protection: Modalities for pain control/swelling (ie, cryotherapy and compression). Avoid exacerbating activities. Gait: Protected weight bearing with assistive device (grade II and III). Review sleeping posture to ensure no stress on injured structure. Gentle pain-free ROM all directions, muscle setting of the involved muscle.<br>Subacute/moderate protection: Gentle pain-free stretching of the involved muscle group and submaximal isometrics.<br>Hip flexor strain: Quadriceps stretch, Thomas test position stretch.<br>Hamstring strain: Supine knee extension stretch; progress to seated single-leg knee extension stretch. If radicular symptoms are reported, nerve glides to mobilize the sciatic nerve. Progressive strengthening.<br>Hip adductor strain: Hip adductor and flexor muscle stretches (ie, seated butterfly stretch). Submaximal isometrics; progress to resistance through ROM. Nerve glides may be included if obturator nerve irritation is present.<br>Return to function/minimal protection: More aggressive stretch and dynamic strengthening and plyometrics for return to sport. |
| Hip bursitis: Trochanteric, ischial, psoas | Acute/maximal protection: Modalities for pain control/swelling. Pain-free ROM; avoid aggravating activities.<br>Subacute/moderate protection: Stretch what is tight. Stretch lateral thigh (ITB and tensor fasciae latae), external rotators, quadriceps, hip flexors, and adductors. Strengthen support muscles (hip external rotators, gluteus medius, gluteus maximus, psoas, quadriceps, and hamstrings).<br>Exercises: Quadriceps strengthening, hamstring curls, partial squats, and leg press<br>Return to function/minimal protection: Strengthening/stretching activities, balance, and coordination; progress to more difficult activities to return to work or sport. |

IASTM = instrument-assisted soft tissue mobilization.

## Nerve Entrapment Pain in the Hip and Nerve Glides

Nerves can be stretched or compressed around bony, ligamentous, and/or musculotendinous structures. The nerves can be injured as a result of local trauma or entrapped, thus preventing the nerves from gliding normally. Nerve entrapment signs and symptoms may mimic muscle strains or other hip conditions.[48] Treatment suggestions for these conditions are provided in Table 13-17. Nerve glides should be performed carefully and cautiously to avoid additional irritation to the involved structures. They are progressed based on the patient's response. Refer to Chapter 11 for information about nerve glides.

### *Sciatic Nerve Entrapment*

The sciatic nerve can become entrapped where it passes under the piriformis and over the other hip external rotator muscles. The proximal hamstring muscles and ischium can also entrap the sciatic nerve (referred to as *ischial tunnel syndrome*), which may occur associated with a gluteal injury.[49] Patients complain of burning pain and/or paresthesia along the sciatic nerve distribution, but pain in the buttocks area may be a better indicator of the nerve being entrapped. Patients have difficulty sitting for longer than 30 minutes and during the transition from midstance to terminal stance during walking. Posterior thigh radicular symptoms (to the popliteal fossa) increase during running, especially at the heel strike, when the knee is extended and the hip is flexed.[48,49]

Treatment can include sciatic nerve glides using the combined movements of hip flexion, knee extension, and ankle dorsiflexion. The patient can be supine or seated in a slumped position to increase tension along the nerve (refer to Chapter 11 [see Figures 11-4 and 11-5]).[30,48] Other treatments can include modalities, soft tissue mobilization to the piriformis and hamstring muscles, and stretching and strengthening to improve function.

### *Obturator Nerve Entrapment*

The obturator nerve can be entrapped as it exits the obturator foramen, or it may be entrapped more distally by the adductor muscles.[48] Patients with obturator nerve entrapment report exercise-induced medial thigh pain originating near the origin of the adductor muscle group, which can also radiate distally along the medial thigh. These symptoms can be reproduced with hip abduction and slight extension, which stretches the nerve. Resisted hip adduction is painless but may be weak.[48] This differentiates obturator entrapment from an adductor muscle strain.

Nerve glides can be performed to mobilize the obturator nerve. The patient begins in a short sitting and slumped position with the neck flexed, and then the thigh is abducted to place the obturator nerve on stretch. To relieve the tension on the nerve, the patient will sit tall, extend the neck, and adduct the leg back to neutral.

### *Femoral Nerve Entrapment*

The femoral triangle is formed superiorly by the inguinal ligament, medially by the adductor longus muscle, and laterally by the sartorius muscle. The femoral nerve can be entrapped at the spinal level between L2-3 or L3-4 due to disk involvement, at the inguinal ligament level, or at the iliopsoas muscle. Hip extension and knee flexion increase symptoms, which can radiate from the anteromedial knee along the medial aspect of the lower leg and into the foot. In severe cases, the primary sign in patients with femoral nerve entrapment is quadriceps weakness. Pelvic or proximal femoral fractures or trauma to the anterior pelvis (ie, during contact sports) can cause femoral nerve entrapment.[48]

Combined knee flexion and hip extension either in the supine position (eg, Thomas test position) or prone position can mobilize the femoral nerve (refer to Chapter 11 [see Figure 11-6]).[30,48]

## Hip Joint Mobilizations

Hip joint mobilizations may be indicated for patients with hip joint hypomobility, hip OA, or capsular restrictions. There are several ways to perform hip joint mobilizations, but the direction of the force (ie, anterior or posterior) should target the restricted motion(s). For example, long-axis distraction is for pain control and general mobility, whereas a posterior glide is to increase hip flexion and internal rotation, and an anterior glide will increase hip extension and external rotation.

The examples of joint mobilizations in this section are guidelines; it is at the discretion of the physical therapist to select the appropriate technique, type (sustained or oscillation), and amount of force or grade. Grades I and II may be performed in the acute stage to reduce pain and muscle guarding. Grades III and IV are used to increase ROM. Refer to Chapter 4 for general information regarding joint mobilizations, patient preparation, application, monitoring, and progression.

### *Long-Axis Hip Distraction*

Hip long-axis distraction occurs in the caudal direction. To perform long-axis distraction, the patient is comfortably positioned supine with the hip abducted and flexed to 30 degrees with slight external rotation (joint resting position). The patient's body weight or the use of a gait belt around the patient's pelvis can stabilize the patient's trunk. The clinician grasps the distal tibia and fibula and applies traction by leaning back, creating, and holding a gentle pull (Figure 13-13A). The clinician should modify the mobilization for persons with a history of knee pathology, using a modified caudal glide distraction (Figure 13-13B) and grasping the distal femur (around the epicondyles) to perform the distraction.

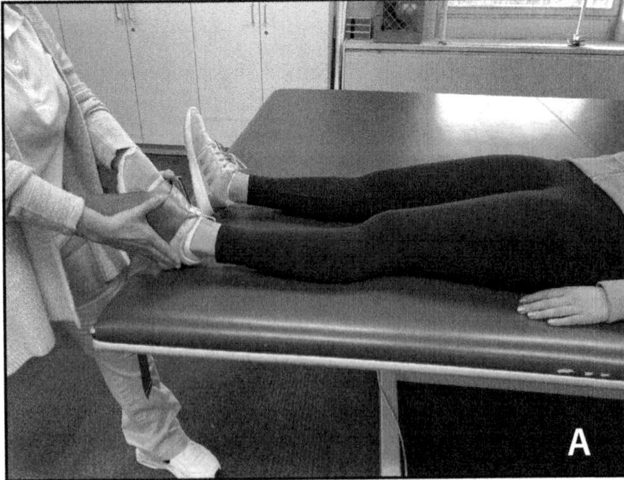


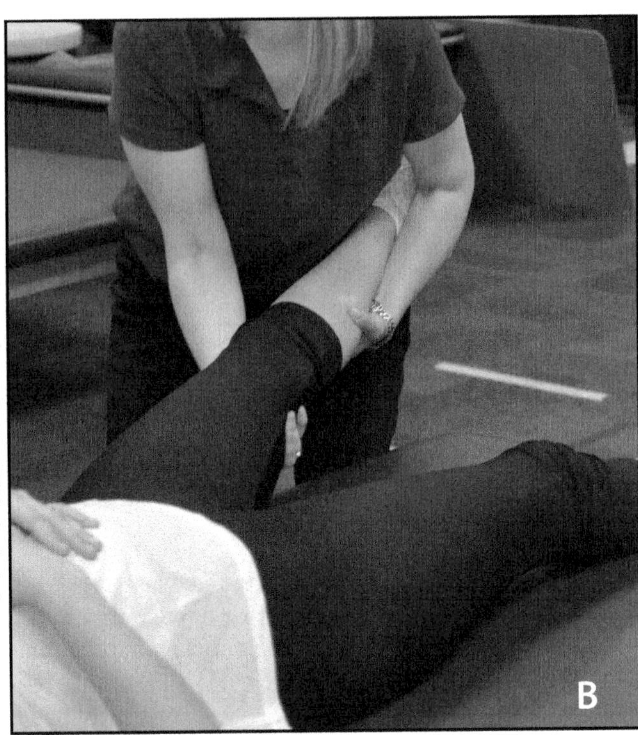


**Figure 13-13.** (A) Long-axis caudal hip distraction. Grasp the distal tibia and fibula or use a strap around the foot as shown; the clinician then leans back to create distraction. (B) Modified long-axis hip distraction. The clinician grasps the distal femur to protect the knee and leans back to create the hip distraction.

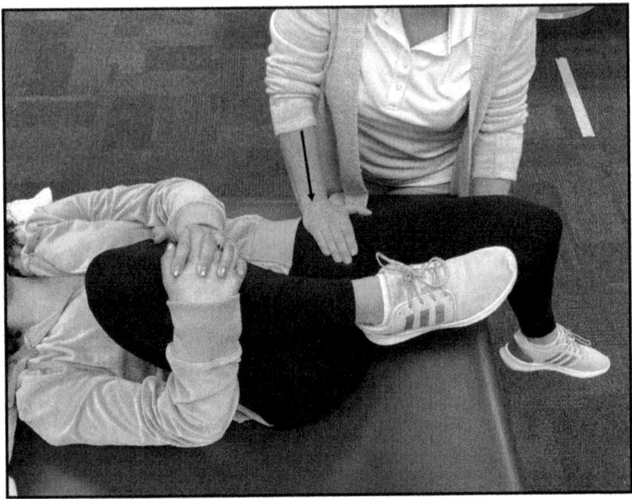

**Figure 13-14.** A posterior glide to increase hip flexion and internal rotation. A downward force, shown by the arrow, is applied to the proximal anterior femur.

## Posterior Glide

A posterior glide increases hip flexion and internal rotation. The patient is positioned supine with the uninvolved leg flexed at the hip and knee. The clinician stands on the same side of the involved hip and places one hand under the femur for support and the other hand proximally at the crease of the hip joint on the anterior aspect. The clinician applies a downward force with the proximal hand (Figure 13-14). Placing a folded towel under the involved pelvis before applying the force can increase pressure on the posterior hip capsule.

## Anterior Glide

An anterior glide increases hip extension and external rotation. The patient is positioned side lying with the involved hip up with a pillow between the knees. The clinician stands behind the patient with an anterior/posterior staggered stance. One hand (the one closer to the patient's head) is placed firmly on the ASIS to stabilize the pelvis. With a fully extended elbow, the other hand is placed on the proximal femur, posterior to the greater trochanter. Keeping the distal arm stiff, the assistant leans forward toward the patient, creating an anterior force on the femur to stress the anterior capsule, and simultaneously pulls posteriorly with the other hand to stabilize the pelvis (Figure 13-15A).

An alternate anterior glide technique can be performed by placing the patient in a prone position with the knee flexed on the involved side and the thigh in neutral or slight extension. The patient's uninvolved leg is on the floor for stability. The clinician stands on the involved side facing the patient's buttocks and supports the flexed limb by using a strap to support the thigh and the distal hand holding the lower leg (Figure 13-15B). The patient must totally relax the involved extremity; the table stabilizes the pelvis. The clinician places the other hand on the most proximal posterior aspect of the femur and places a force in the anterior direction. The amount of passive hip extension can be increased by lifting the distal femur with the strap as the patient's ROM increases.

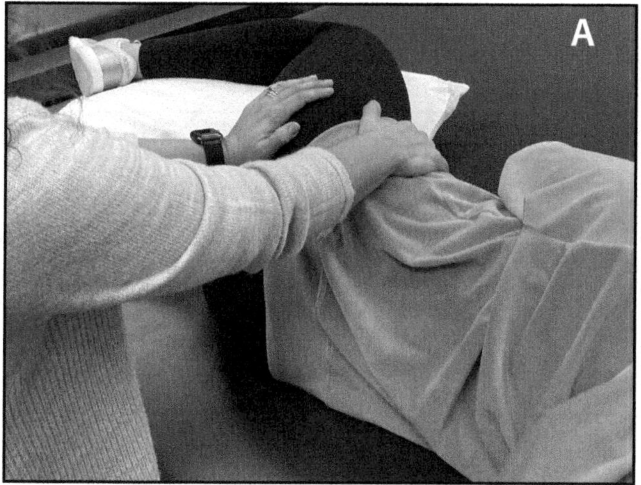


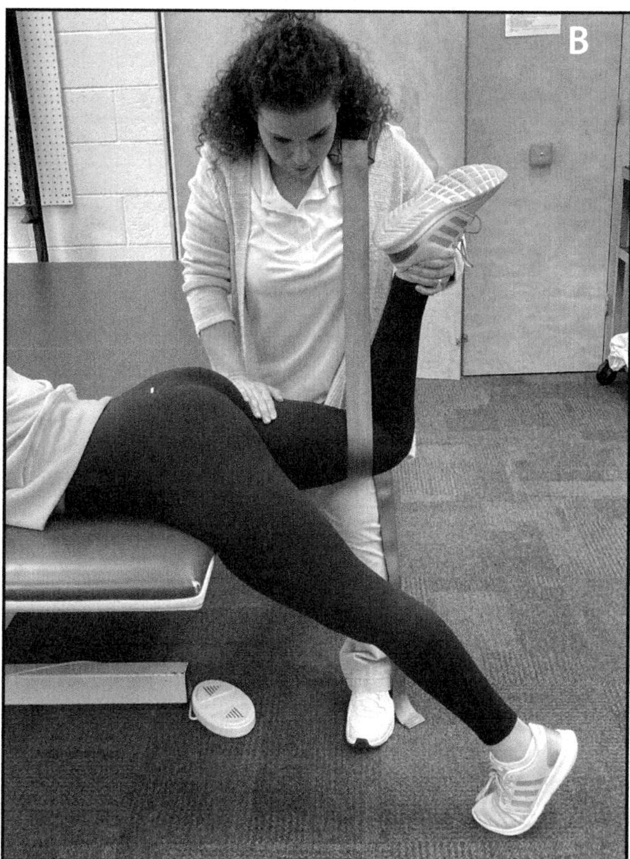


**Figure 13-15.** An anterior glide for the hip. (A) An anterior glide to increase hip extension and external rotation (the side-lying position). (B) An anterior glide to increase hip extension and external rotation (the prone position).

# Management and Treatment of Knee Pathologies and Conditions

The physical therapy team will treat patients of all ages with a variety of knee conditions. The physical therapist assistant should have a working knowledge of tissue healing responses, MOIs, and special tests for specific structures (Table 13-18) performed by the physical therapist during the initial evaluation. Pictures of commonly prescribed knee exercises are included at the end of this chapter (Figures 13-49 through 13-51).

# Knee Osteoarthritis

Knee OA is common in adults 60 years and older. About 13% of women and 10% of men who are older have symptomatic knee OA pain, decreased function, and increased disability (ie, difficulty walking or stair climbing); these are the most common reasons for obtaining a total knee replacement.[50,51] Risk factors for developing knee OA include being older and female, being obese or overweight, prior knee injury (due to sports participation or work-related excessive kneeling/squatting), reduced bone density and joint laxity, and/or muscle weakness. Because the population is aging and living longer, the reports of disability and the prevalence of knee replacements continue to rise.[50-52]

The onset of knee pain caused by OA is gradual. The characteristics of knee OA include persistent pain, decreased function, morning stiffness, joint crepitus, restricted motion, and an enlarged joint.[51,52] Pain is usually more severe with activity and subsides with rest, ice, and NSAIDs. In severe cases, patients may display genu varus (more common) or valgus due to compressive forces and narrowing of the joint space as the joint surfaces continue to break down. It is common for patients with knee OA to walk with an abnormal gait pattern (ie, antalgic gait) due to pain, limited ROM, or deformity.

## *Conservative Treatment for Patients With Knee Osteoarthritis*

Conservative treatment for knee OA is similar to that discussed earlier for hip OA. Treatment options during the maximal protection period include modalities, joint mobilization (grade I and II), NSAIDs for pain control, fitting the patient with a cane or walker (to reduce stresses on the involved knee during gait), and performing pain-free ROM and muscle setting.

Hip weakness is a contributing factor for knee pain and disability. Hip weakness is a contributing factor associated with knee pain and disability. Stretching and strengthening exercises that target the hip abductors, external rotators, and extensors (see Table 13-13) should be included in the patient's rehabilitation program.[51] During the initial phase of knee rehabilitation (regardless of the diagnosis), decreasing knee edema must be prioritized. Even small amounts of swelling/knee joint effusion can "shut down" or inhibit the quadriceps muscle, specifically the VMO.

**Table 13-18**

**Special Tests for Various Knee Pathologies**

| Special Test | Possible Pathologies if Positive |
|---|---|
| Q angle test | Patellofemoral conditions |
| Patella apprehension test | Patellofemoral conditions |
| Patella compression/grind | Patellofemoral conditions |
| Squat test | Patellofemoral conditions |
| Apley's compression | Meniscus tear |
| Bounce home test | Meniscus tear |
| McMurray test | Meniscus tear |
| Lachman test | ACL injury |
| Anterior drawer test | ACL injury |
| Slocum test (with internal/external tibial rotation) | ACL anterolateral instability/ACL anteromedial instability |
| Posterior drawer test | PCL injury |
| Posterior sag test | PCL injury |
| Valgus stress test | MCL injury |
| Varus stress test | LCL injury |

### Considerations for the Physical Therapist Assistant

Quadriceps muscle control is a primary goal during the initial phase of rehabilitation. To regain neuromuscular control of the knee joint, the patella needs to be able to glide superiorly in the groove; this allows effective facilitation of the VMO to occur. After patellar mobility is attained, the clinician should prioritize the patient's ability to perform an SLR without an extension lag before transitioning to walking without an assistive device.

In the moderate protection phase, the patient can progress to knee stretching and strengthening exercises as long as they are pain free (Table 13-19). With progression to light weights for seated knee flexion/extension, the physical therapist assistant should have the patient initially work in ranges from 30 to 90 degrees, where patellofemoral forces are lowest. The patient can progress from 90 degrees to full extension if there are no complaints of patellar pain. CKC TKE (or quadriceps set) can be performed in prone (Figure 13-16) or in standing (Figure 13-17) and can be initiated at 20 degrees of knee flexion to full extension. If there are no complaints of patellar pain, the knee flexion can be increased to no greater than 45 degrees. The clinician should progress the patient's strengthening program slowly and only add 1 or 2 exercises at a time. This reduces the chance of increasing symptoms and allows the clinician to determine which newly added exercise contributed to increased symptoms if the patient experiences a change in status. Soft tissue mobilizations or joint mobilizations can be included for patients with limited ROM. Patient education should include preventive positioning, avoiding high-impact activities, limiting or avoiding stair climbing, suggesting weight loss if indicated, and promoting a healthy lifestyle.[15,16] Preventive positioning includes avoiding prolonged sitting with the knees in a moderately flexed position (sometimes called the *theater sign*; ie, knee pain when standing from a desk or theater seat).

The physician or physical therapist may suggest the use of a knee brace to unload forces from the area of pain or deformity. Intra-articular corticosteroid injections may be used for short-term pain relief, but repetitive injections should be avoided because they may damage joint cartilage.[51,53] Hyaluronic acid injections into the joint act as a joint lubricant and may increase production of the body's normal hyaluronic acid. (Hyaluronic acid production is typically decreased in patients with knee OA.[51])

**Table 13-19**

Knee Exercises

| Stretches | OKC/Strengthening[a] | CKC/Strengthening and Balance |
|---|---|---|
| Knee extension<br>• Prone lower leg hang<br>• Supine heel prop-up<br>• Seated or standing hamstring stretches<br>• Standing or seated calf stretches<br>Knee flexion<br>• Seated self-stretch with uninvolved lower extremity<br>• Supine or seated heel slides (hip/knee flexion/extension)<br>• Thomas test position with knee flexion<br>• Standing knee flexion—quadriceps stretch<br>ITB (see Table 13-13)<br>• Foam roll fascia release: Side lying with involved leg on roll | Knee extension<br>• Quadriceps setting<br>• Multiangle isometrics<br>• TKE<br>• SLRs<br>• Straight leg eccentric lowering<br>• Long-arc quadriceps (LAQ)<br>• PNF D1 extension<br>Knee flexion<br>• Hamstring sets<br>• Multiangle isometrics<br>• PNF D1 flexion<br>• Standing or prone hamstring curls<br>Hip strengthening (see Table 13-13) | Strengthening with or without resistance<br>• TKE prone and progress to standing with resistance bands<br>• Heel digs for hamstrings or for cocontractions<br>• Lateral weight shifts (abiding weight-bearing precautions)<br>• Stool pulls/scoots (these are not appropriate or safe for persons with decreased balance; complete with close guarding only)<br>• Partial/mini-squats and wall slides<br>• Step-up/down: Forward/backward/lateral<br>• Partial and full lunges forward/backward/lateral<br>• Plyometrics: Hopping, skipping, jumping, box jumps/hops<br>• Sport-specific drills<br>Balance<br>• Anterior/posterior sways, ankle strategies<br>• Perturbations all directions for proper strategy selection<br>• Eyes opened/closed vary BOS and SLS on firm/foam surfaces, rocker board, Biomechanical Ankle Platform System (BAPS) board (Spectrum Therapy Products), mini-trampoline |

[a]Add resistance progress.

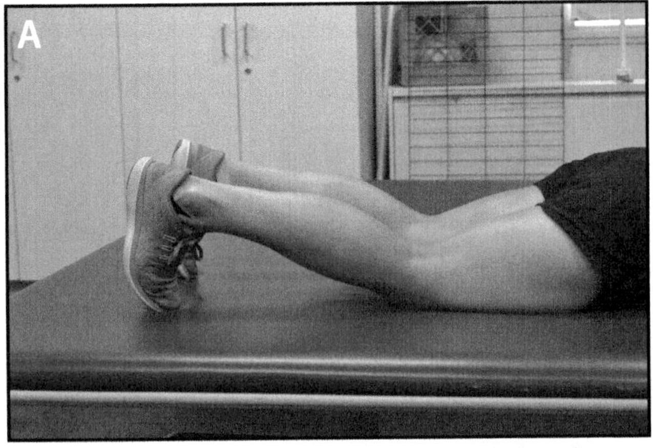


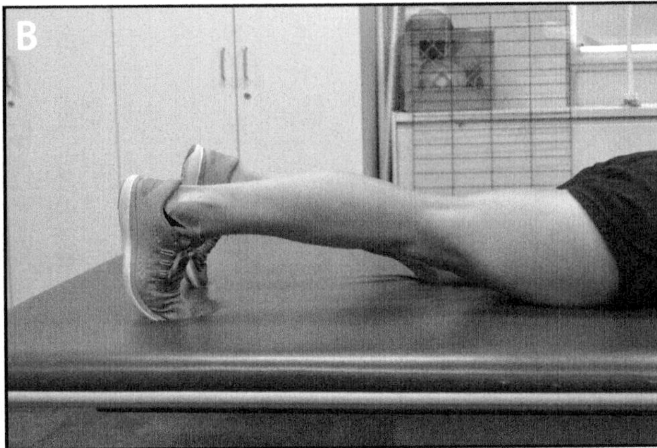


**Figure 13-16.** Prone TKE. (A) The starting position. (B) The end position.

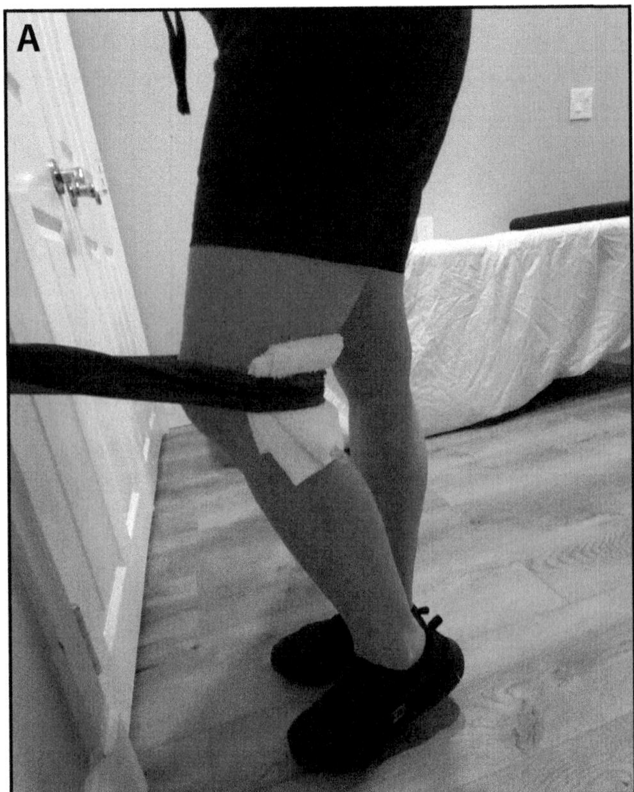


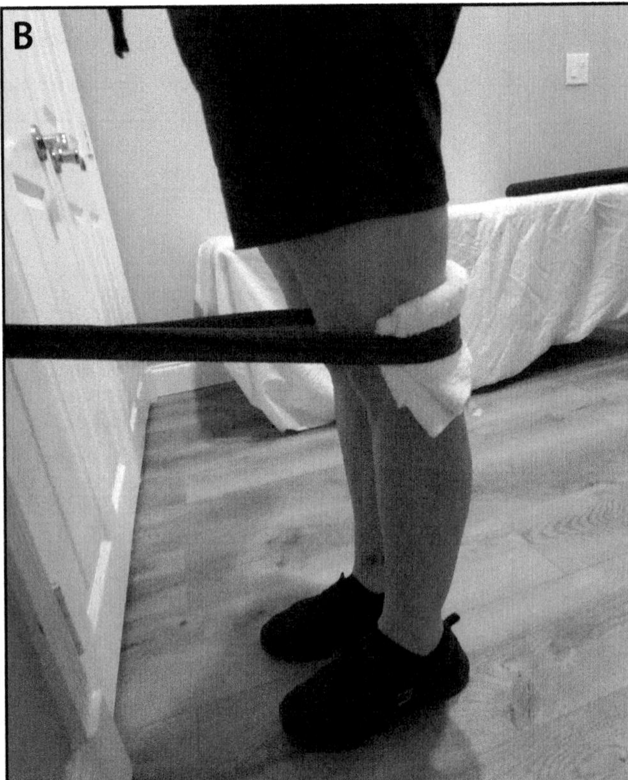


**Figure 13-17.** Standing TKE. (A) The starting position. (B) The end position.

## Surgical Options for Knee Osteoarthritis and Rehabilitation Management

When conservative management has been unsuccessful, surgery is considered. The primary goals of knee surgery for advanced OA include reducing pain, correcting varus deformity, and improving function. The most commonly used surgical options to achieve these goals include high tibial osteotomy (HTO), unicompartmental (or unicondylar) knee arthroplasty (UKA), or total knee arthroplasty (TKA). The orthopedic physician selects the procedure that will best address the patient's individual presentation, symptoms, and goals. The physical therapy team works with the medical team and the patient to promote recovery and return to optimal strength and functional levels postoperatively.

HTO corrects varus alignment of the knee, reducing pressure on the medial arthritic portion of the joint (Figure 13-18). This procedure is most often recommended for patients before the development of advanced stages of knee OA, without ligamentous instability, and with minimal ROM limits and in younger more active persons (60 to 65 years old or younger). In an open wedge osteotomy, a wedge of bone is cut from the proximal aspect of the tibia, and a bone graft is placed to fill the space to realign the knee joint. A closed wedge osteotomy removes the wedge, brings the cut edges together, and stabilizes the site. Surgeons perform ORIF using various types of hardware (ie, plates

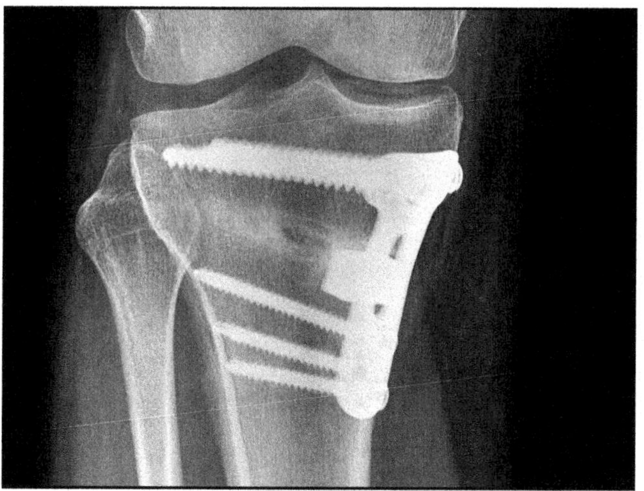

**Figure 13-18.** HTO. The medial wedge of bone is used to correct the varus deformity and then stabilized in position (J. GALIANO/Shutterstock.com).

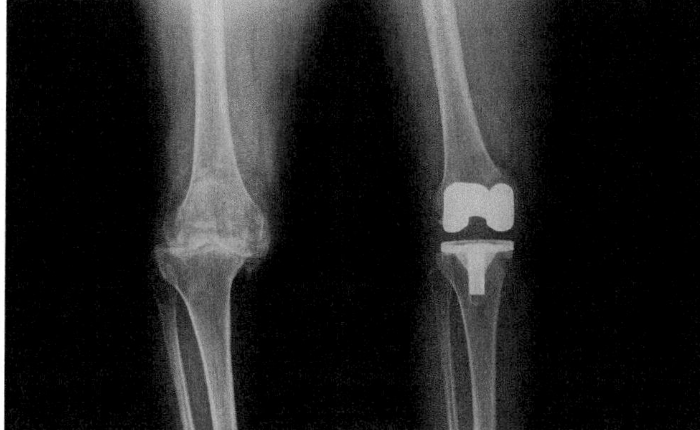

**Figure 13-19.** Severe OA with varus deformity shown in the image on the left. TKA corrects the deformity and is shown in the image on the right (Yok_onepiece/Shutterstock.com).

and screws) to stabilize the site where the bone wedge was removed and to correct the deformity. These procedures reduce the load-bearing forces on the medial compartment and prolong the time (up to 10 years) until a TKA procedure is needed.[51,54] Once the patient has completed their rehabilitation program, these patients can usually return to high-impact activities 6 to 9 months postoperatively after clearance from the physician. The number of HTO procedures has declined because of the advances and improvements associated with TKA procedures.[54,55]

UKA is most appropriate for patients who have advanced arthritic changes in either the medial or lateral compartment of the joint with an intact ACL. These patients are typically older and not overweight but are often less active. This procedure is associated with less pain, shorter hospital stays, and faster recovery than TKA.[51,55,56]

TKA is indicated for patients with advanced stages of OA, greater joint limitations, knee instability, deformity, and/or severe pain that restricts normal activities (Figure 13-19). Two of the most common types of TKA are the bicompartmental and the tricompartmental implants. A bicompartmental prosthesis uses an implant that has a femoral and tibial component with a rotating polyethylene platform inserted between the 2 components to reduce the wear on the tibial component (this is used in younger active patients). A tricompartmental implant is indicated when the patella is severely damaged and a patellar component is implanted, in addition to the femoral and tibial prosthetics.[55,57]

Cemented fixation is more common than uncemented in both UKA and TKA. The surgical procedure selected for knee fixation depends on the patient's age, bone quality, and prior level of function. Long-term viability of the implant is significantly better for cemented implants.

Potential TKA postoperative complications include infection, wound healing issues, DVT, joint instability, component loosening, and patella subluxation/dislocation.[51,58] Limited knee ROM (commonly in flexion) and improper patella tracking can cause pain and affect the patient's functional ability. The medical and therapy team will observe for signs/symptoms of postoperative complications. Following the physician's protocol and the physical therapist's POC ensures the best outcomes for the patient.[58]

## *Knee Osteoarthritis Postoperative Rehabilitation Management*

Exercise guidelines for HTO, UKA, and TKA across the stages of healing and rehabilitative phases are listed in Table 13-20. These are suggestions to guide the rehabilitation process based on current evidence; the physician's protocol and the physical therapist's POC should guide the physical therapist assistant with treatment interventions.

### High Tibial Osteotomy Treatment Interventions

Typically, weight-bearing instructions after HTO include protected weight bearing (crutches) and the use of a hinge brace at all times for up to 6 weeks.[54,59-61] Weight-bearing guidelines are determined by the physician based on the amount of deviation correction that was performed and the type of hardware used for the ORIF. Initial weight-bearing status ranges from NWB to PWB up to 25% for the first 2 to 6 weeks (with the brace locked in extension). Progression to WBAT may be initiated between weeks 2 and 8 (with the brace limited to 90 degrees). Research supports that FWB without crutches should be achieved by week 12 if gait is normalized.[54,59-61]

During the acute phase, exercises are initiated the day after surgery. All exercises focus on increasing the patient's pain-free AROM as quickly and safely as possible, prioritizing full knee extension. Strengthening and stretching should only be performed in NWB positions.

**Table 13-20**

**Postoperative Rehabilitation Suggested Guidelines for High Tibial Osteotomy, Unicompartmental Knee Arthroplasty, and Total Knee Arthroplasty**

| Diagnosis | Acute Stage/Phase 1<br>Maximal protection (0 to 4 Weeks) | Subacute Stage/Phase 2<br>Moderate Protection (4 to 8 Weeks) | Return to Function/Phase 3<br>Minimal Protection (8 to 12 Weeks) |
|---|---|---|---|
| HTO | Goals<br>• Limit weight bearing as per protocol.<br>• AAROM/AROM 0 to 90 degrees full knee extension by week 2 to 4.<br>• Patella joint mobilizations. Modalities for pain/inflammation<br>• Protect incision and joint structures from forces that impede healing.<br>Exercises<br>• Supine: Ankle pumps, gluteal and quadriceps sets, heel slides, hip internal/external rotation. Breathing and core stabilization exercises. In knee brace locked in full extension: SLR 4 ways in standing on uninvolved leg or supine, prone, and side lying.<br>• CKC: Strengthening on uninvolved extremity only.<br>• NWB stretches: Calf, hamstring, and hip flexors if included in physician protocol | Goals<br>• Progress weight-bearing status as per protocol.<br>• Normalize gait abiding by weight-bearing restrictions in brace (brace restricts knee flexion to < 90 degrees).<br>• AAROM/AROM at least 0 to 120 degrees pain free by week 6 (consider the use of a stationary bike for ROM).<br>Exercises: SLR 4 ways—progress to weights/bands, side-lying hip external rotation or supine with resistance band—knees flexed, plantar flexion/dorsiflexion with resistance band. Standing/prone knee flexion.<br>• CKC: As per weight-bearing status: Bridges, weight shifts, mini-squats to 45 degrees, calf raises, resistance band TKE. Pool exercises/water walking.<br>• Stretches: Calf, hamstring, and hip flexors.<br>Aerobics: Upper bike ergometer, stationary bike, deep water exercises (treading or running/cycling actions) | Goals<br>• FWB, advance to no crutches.<br>• Full pain-free ROM.<br>Exercises: Progress/increase OKC resistance exercises from previous phase and move to more functional activities.<br>• CKC: Step-ups (forward, backward, lateral). Single-leg calf raises and squats.<br>• Stretches: Calf, hamstring, and hip flexors.<br>Balance: Anterior/posterior sways—ankle strategies. Eyes opened/closed vary BOS and SLS on firm/foam. BOSU Balance Trainer, rocker board, mini-trampoline.<br>Aerobics: As previous phase and progress to swimming, treadmill running at end of month 3. Progress with dynamic training beginning month 4.<br>Sport-specific training: Typically, not initiated until 6 to 9 months postoperatively. Physician clearance required.<br>*(continued)* |

**Table 13-20 (continued)**

Postoperative Rehabilitation Suggested Guidelines for High Tibial Osteotomy, Unicompartmental Knee Arthroplasty, and Total Knee Arthroplasty

| Diagnosis | Acute Stage/Phase 1<br>Maximal protection (0 to 4 Weeks) | Subacute Stage/Phase 2<br>Moderate Protection (4 to 8 Weeks) | Return to Function/Phase 3<br>Minimal Protection (8 to 12 Weeks) |
|---|---|---|---|
| UKA and TKA | Goals<br>• WBAT during gait with assistive device or as per protocol.<br>• AAROM/AROM 0 to >90 degrees full knee extension by week 2 to 4. Can use stationary bike for ROM.<br>Exercises: PROM/AAROM/AROM seated/supine. Ankle pumps, supine heel slides, TKE, seated knee LAQ flexion/extension, quadriceps sets, hamstring sets, gluteal sets, bridges and hip adductor isometrics in hook lying. SLR 4 ways in standing on uninvolved leg or supine, prone, and side lying.<br>• CKC strengthening on uninvolved extremity.<br>• Stretches: Calf, hamstring, hip flexors if included in physician protocol. | Goals<br>• Progress to FWB.<br>• AAROM/AROM 0 to >110 degrees; use stationary bike for ROM with a lower seat.<br>Exercises: AAROM/AROM/progressive resistance exercise (PRE) seated knee flexion/extension, multiangle isometrics quadriceps, hamstrings, resisted hip flexion, extension, abduction, external rotation.<br>• CKC: Bridges, resistance band TKE, mini-squats to 45 degrees, wall slides, step ups-forward, backward, lateral 2 to 4-in steps, quarter-forward lunges, calf raises.<br>• Stretches: Calf, hamstring, hip adductors and flexors.<br>Balance: Anterior/posterior sways on rocker board. Eyes opened/closed vary BOS, SLS on firm/foam.<br>Aerobics: Swim/water walking, elliptical, stationary bike with raised or normal height seat. | Goals<br>• Progress to FWB without assistive device and normal gait stride and speed.<br>• AROM knee flexion >120 degrees<br>Exercises: Continue to increase lower extremity strength >4/5 using exercises from the previous phase; increase weights/resistance.<br>• Stretches: Calf, hamstring, hip adductors, flexors.<br>Balance: Combine balance and advanced functional activities on various surfaces: BOSU Balance Trainer, mini-trampoline, grass, sand.<br>Aerobics: As previous phase. |

As the patient progresses to the subacute phase, a minimum of 0 to 120 degrees of pain-free ROM should be achieved by week 6 (ideally, 135 degrees is preferred). CKC exercises can be initiated as long as the prescribed weight-bearing status is maintained. Pool exercises and water walking can begin as long as the incision is healed and the activities maintain weight-bearing restrictions/guidelines. If FWB is permitted, retro walking on the treadmill can help normalize the patient's gait pattern. A stationary bike can be used for aerobic conditioning.

During the return-to-function phase, the patient should be able to walk without assistance and with a normal gait pattern at good velocity. Progressions includes resistance training, functional training, and balance activities. The patient can begin a jogging program at the end of this phase if cleared by the physician and/or physical therapist.

## Unicompartmental and Total Knee Arthroplasty Treatment Management

After UKA, patients typically experience a shorter rehabilitation time, and they are usually permitted to be WBAT. They are typically cleared to resume FWB sooner than those patients who had an HTO.[62,63] After TKA, patients are also usually allowed to be WBAT, but weight-bearing restrictions vary based on the fixation of the prosthesis (cemented/uncemented) and/or the physician's protocol. The suggested treatment guidelines for UKA and TKA are similar and are listed in Table 13-20; variation in the physician's protocol or the therapist's POC should be respected. The goals in the acute stage (0 to 4 weeks) include decrease swelling, control pain, increase knee ROM, improve muscle control, and increase hip and knee strength. Patient education includes how to perform safe bed mobility and transfer techniques, to avoid twisting when standing on the surgical leg, and proper gait training with an assistive device while maintaining weight-bearing restrictions on flat surfaces and stairs. The patient should be educated about possible postoperative complications such as signs and symptoms of pulmonary edema, DVT, and infection (incisional/general). Exercises should begin the day of or day after surgery as long as the patient is medically stable. As the incision heals, gentle scar mobilization and patella mobilization should be performed to improve soft tissue mobility and quadriceps function.

### Considerations for the Physical Therapist Assistant: Quadriceps Weakness and Knee Extensor Lag

When a patient performs straight leg exercises in any direction, the knee should always be fully extended (Figure 13-20A) with no evidence of a knee extensor lag. A knee extensor lag occurs when the quadriceps muscle is unable to complete and/or maintain the contraction in full extension when the leg is lifted off the table, resulting in a position of slight knee flexion when the leg is in the air (Figure 13-20B). Knee extensor lag indicates quadriceps weakness or poor neuromuscular control. The ability to hold the knee in full extension is important with any exercise that targets the quadriceps muscle group. If a patient is unable to perform a strong quadriceps contraction, they will not be able to perform an SLR effectively. Techniques that can facilitate a quadriceps muscle contraction so SLRs can be performed correctly are described in the patellofemoral pain syndrome rehabilitation section of this chapter.

The criteria that indicate readiness for progression to the moderate protection phase include decreased pain and joint swelling, greater than 3/5 knee extension muscle strength, and the ability to walk independently with an assistive device with increased weight bearing using a normalized gait pattern. FWB and reduced reliance on the assistive device are based on the physician's protocol, the patient's tolerance, and the quality of the patient's gait. The focus of treatment in this phase is on increasing core stability, knee and hip strength, and muscle endurance and control. Aerobic conditioning should begin during this phase. Patients can usually resume driving approximately 6 weeks after surgery.[51]

Improving balance is an important goal after TKA. Static and dynamic balance training is introduced as early as safely possible. Standing balance is often compromised in older patients with knee OA. Twenty-five percent of TKA recipients fall within 2 years after surgery.[64] Weight-bearing biofeedback (WBB) has emerged as a retraining program to improve balance performance. Nintendo Wii, Wii Fit (Nintendo), and Xbox Kinect each have WBB and balance training exercises. (Although the Wii products are no longer being produced, they are still useful

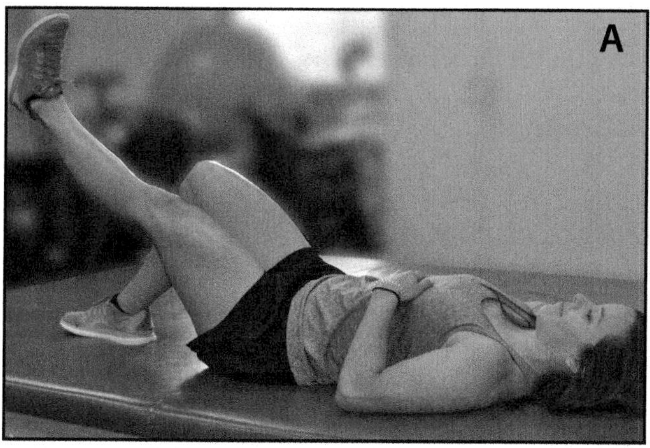


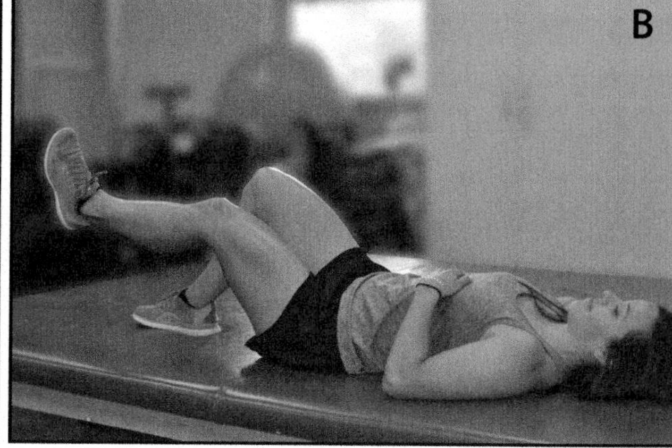


**Figure 13-20.** SLR. (A) A properly performed SLR. (B) Improper completion of SLR with the knee extensor lag evident.

training options; other companies continue to release fitness programs that are compatible with their online gaming platforms). Biodex and LiteGait are 2 of the companies that offer WBB equipment that can be used in the clinic. Compared with control groups, patients who participated in WBB programs had better outcomes in the 5 Times Sit-to-Stand Test 6 weeks after surgery and better knee movement at 26 weeks.[64]

The patient can progress to the return-to-function phase approximately 8 weeks after surgery if little to no pain or swelling is evident, knee flexion is greater than 110 degrees, and lower extremity strength is 4/5 or greater. Soft tissue and patella mobility should be within normal limits. During this phase, the patient should be able to perform ADLs and IADLs with minimal difficulty, and more challenging balance activities can be added based on the patient's goals.

The physician will provide the clearance when medically appropriate for patients to return to sports. The mean time to return to low-impact type sports (golf and walking) is 12 weeks after UKA.[63,65]

# Meniscal Injuries: Conservative and Postoperative Management

## *Meniscal Injuries: Mechanism of Injury, Types of Tears, and Signs and Symptoms*

The menisci distribute forces and provide knee joint lubrication, stability, and shock absorption. Meniscus tears can occur due to an acute injury or as a result of cumulative stresses (resulting in a degenerative tear). One-quarter of all knee injuries involve the meniscus, and there are an estimated 850,000 meniscal tear cases occurring in the United States per year.[66] During sports participation, most meniscal injuries occur during a noncontact event or incident (eg, cutting, decelerating, landing from a jump). When the foot is firmly planted on the ground and the femur rotates on the tibia, a rotational force and increased axial loading at the knee joint create a shearing of the meniscus, which can result in a tear. This MOI is also associated with ligamentous and articular cartilage injuries.[67] When a varus or valgus force is applied to a flexed knee (especially when combined with a twisting motion of the leg), there is the potential for a ligamentous injury also. The type of injury is dependent on the direction and intensity of the force. Deep squatting can impinge the meniscus between the femur and tibia, also resulting in a tear. Meniscal integrity begins to diminish in people over the age of 30 years; these degenerative changes increase susceptibility to meniscal tears during normal activities. About 30% of all meniscal tears occur between the ages of 41 and 50 years for men and 61 and 70 years for women.[67] Men are 4 times more likely than women to sustain a meniscal injury.[67]

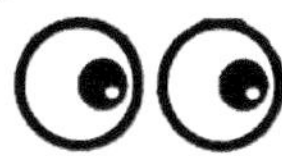

### Eye on the Research: Meniscal Tears

In a study of 392 randomly selected patients, 32.4% of the meniscal tears were sports related, 38.8% were non–sports related, and 28.8% of the patients could not identify a specific incident causing the injury. Older patients had a higher rate of meniscal tears.[66,67] The mean age of meniscal injury in a sporting group was 33 years, 41 years in a nonsporting group, and 43 years in a nonactivity group. Acute meniscal tears have a peak incidence in men 21 to 30 years old and in women 11 to 19 years old.[67]

The medial meniscus is more commonly injured because of its attachment to the MCL and its location within the joint capsule. Meniscal tears are categorized as complete (full-thickness) tears or incomplete (partial-thickness) tears (Figure 13-21). An incomplete tear extends partially through the meniscus, and a complete tear extends through the meniscus to the tibia. Tears are further described based on the direction (vertical, longitudinal, horizontal, or oblique) and location of the tear in relation to the tibia. The type and extent of the tear can be determined with

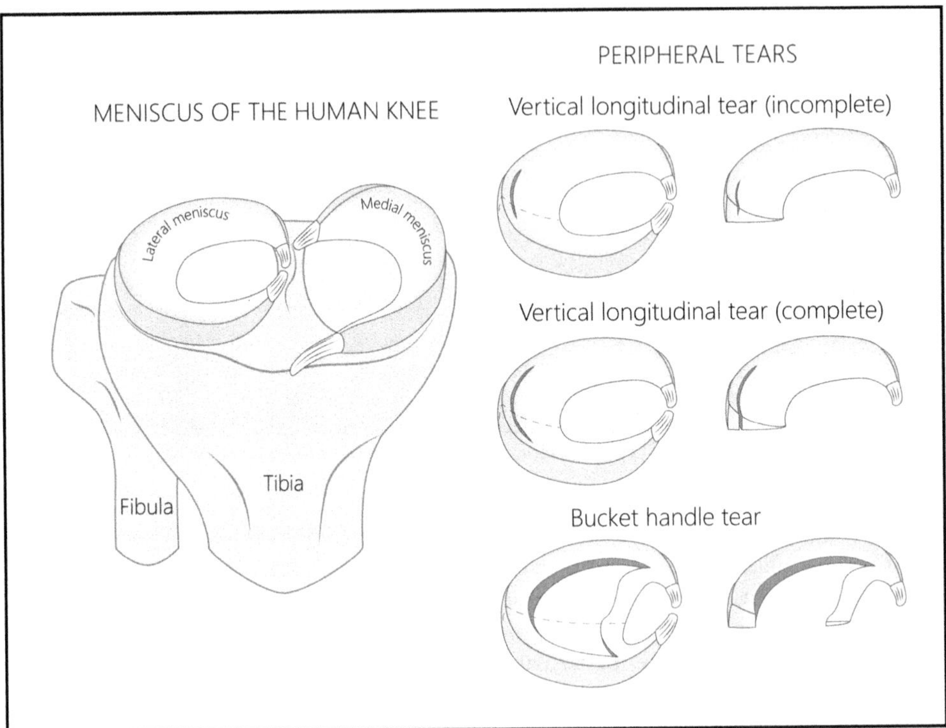


**Figure 13-21.** The types of meniscal tears (Aksanaku/Shutterstock.com).

MRI.[66-68] A vertical-longitudinal or bucket handle tear is the most common type, and it is most often observed in younger patients.[68]

Younger people or athletes often report a "popping or snapping" at the time of the injury during an acute or traumatic incident. Older adults are predisposed to degenerative tears, and they may not associate the tear with a specific incident. A tear may occur during IADLs or leisure activities. Signs and symptoms of meniscal injuries include pain with squatting or weight bearing; a sensation of the knee "catching," locking, or buckling; pain along the joint line; and/or swelling. Full knee extension may be limited due to joint swelling, or it may be associated with catching and locking. Table 13-18 provides a list of the special tests the therapist may use during the evaluation.[66,68]

## Conservative Rehabilitation Management for Meniscal Tears

If a tear occurs along the outer one-third/peripheral edge of the meniscus, it may heal without surgical intervention due to good vascularization in that area. The initial treatment after an acute meniscal tear is to use the PRICE (protection, rest, ice, compression, elevation) protocol to control for swelling and pain. If the tear is degenerative in nature, the physician may prescribe anti-inflammatory and analgesic medications, a knee brace, and physical therapy if surgery is not initially indicated.[69] The guidelines outlined for conservative treatment for knee OA can be followed for patients with a nonsurgical meniscal tear. The focus of treatment is on controlling pain and swelling, incorporating lower extremity OKC and CKC strengthening, stretching, and activity modification to guide the patient back to their prior level of function. Conservative treatment guidelines are typically followed for about 3 months before considering surgical interventions.[68,69]

## Postoperative Rehabilitation Management After Meniscal Repairs and Meniscectomy

Most meniscal surgical procedures are performed arthroscopically, and surgical options include partial or total meniscectomy, meniscal repair, and/or meniscal reconstruction.[68,69] A partial meniscectomy removes the damaged area and preserves the healthy part of the meniscus. A total meniscectomy removes the entire meniscus; this is only performed if the meniscus cannot be salvaged.[55,68,69] Preserving as much of the meniscus as possible can help reduce the occurrence of premature OA. Partial meniscectomies are usually performed when the tear is located in the inner part (avascular area) of the meniscus or when the fibrocartilage is frayed. Meniscal repairs are more commonly performed if the tear is along the peripheral area of the meniscus where there is good blood supply. The edges of the torn meniscus are approximated and sutured together.[68]

Meniscal reconstruction techniques (meniscal scaffolds and meniscal allograft transplantation) are used to fill in the space after a partial meniscus resection or to replace the meniscus after a total meniscectomy.[69] The goal of these procedures is to use an anatomically shaped meniscus to restore knee mechanics to improve joint function, reduce pain, and delay joint degeneration. Meniscal allograft transplantation is used to replace the entire meniscus. Meniscal scaffolding is used to replace the resected portion of the meniscus using either collagen or polyurethane-based material. Whether these procedures meet the goal of preventing or delaying joint degeneration is under debate.[69]

## Partial Meniscectomy Rehabilitation

After a partial meniscectomy, the patient is usually permitted to WBAT. Regaining a normal gait pattern using an assistive device and progression to FWB as quickly as possible is encouraged. The criteria for progression to FWB include having no pain, the ability to achieve full active knee extension (without an extension lag), and the ability to walk without limping.

The PRICE protocol is initiated immediately after the procedure. ROM (to gain full extension and increase flexion) and quadriceps muscle strengthening (ie, quadriceps sets and TKEs) should begin the day of or day after surgery. Oftentimes, the patient will receive the list of exercises before the surgery and will practice them so that there will be no delay in starting them at home after the surgery. Implementing exercises early helps prevent muscle atrophy. Depending on the age and prior level of function, exercises (see Table 13-19) can be progressed quickly as long as quadriceps muscle motor control is regained. Athletes or young adults are usually FWB and performing functional activities 4 to 6 days after surgery, but less active adults may take longer. Pain, swelling, and quadriceps muscle control will determine the pace of patient progression. By week 3 or 4, patients can be progressed to the minimal protection phase. Monitor for any increase in joint swelling and pain because these may indicate that the exercises are being progressed too quickly.

## Meniscal Repair Rehabilitation

Rehabilitation protocols after a meniscal repair are more conservative than the protocols used after a partial meniscectomy. Physical therapy after a meniscal repair typically includes progressive ROM and weight bearing, strengthening of the hip and knee muscles, and neuromuscular training. Early progressive weight bearing in patients after meniscal repairs is determined by the physician, and it depends on several factors (eg, repair location, surgical techniques).[55,66,70,71] Table 13-21 provides rehabilitation guidelines for postoperative meniscus repair.

Some physicians may require that the patient wear a hinged knee brace locked in full extension for the first few weeks postoperatively during all ambulation. If the patient is permitted to walk with a brace that allows for flexion to 90 degrees, the clinician should encourage the patient to ambulate with their assistive device with a heel-toe gait to encourage a normal gait pattern regardless of weight-bearing restrictions. Walking on an underwater treadmill or walking in a pool are also good ways to practice proper gait mechanics when weight bearing is restricted. Refer to Chapter 10 for estimated weight-bearing percentages for in-water activities.

Patient progression to FWB is typically permitted between weeks 4 and 6 (or as per protocol) if the repair was in the peripheral area of the meniscus. The knee brace may be discontinued around week 6, but it may be beneficial to have the patient continue using a cane or one crutch until the patient's confidence and quadriceps control are consistent.[55] Weight-bearing restrictions may be maintained for a longer period of time if the repair or reconstruction was in the avascular area of the meniscus.

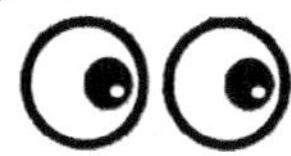

### Eye on the Research: Weight-Bearing Restrictions After Meniscal Repairs

One systematic review compared accelerated and conservative ROM and weight-bearing protocols, reporting that 70% to 94% of patients who followed a conservative protocol and 64% to 96% of those who followed an accelerated protocol had good outcomes. Researchers acknowledged that direct comparison was difficult because of a lack of consistency in both the objective criteria and the surgical techniques.[70]

Another study compared restricted and unrestricted rehabilitation programs. The restricted program required patients to wear a hinged brace and maintain TTWB, with progressive increases in brace ROM (up to 90 degrees) for 6 weeks. The unrestricted ("free") program restricted weight bearing to toe touch without a brace for 2 weeks and then allowed ROM to 90 degrees and unrestricted activity going forward.[66,71] The researchers concluded that an unrestricted rehabilitation program was safe and that there was no significant increase in postoperative failure rates compared with a restricted rehabilitation program.[71]

Aerobic conditioning can be initiated immediately after surgery using an upper bike ergometer, and activity can be progressed a few weeks later by transitioning to a stationary bike with the seat as high as possible (to avoid excessive knee flexion) or deep water jogging with a vest (once the incisions are healed).

Exercises during the maximal and moderate protection phases should focus on hip strengthening (especially abductors and extensors) and ankle strengthening. The patient will progress from initially wearing the brace locked, to an unlocked brace during CKC exercises, and finally to exercises without the brace per the physician's protocol.[55,70]

During the late stage of rehabilitation, a functional progression to sport- or work-specific activities should be introduced. Patients can return to sport activities at about 16 weeks after surgery if the tear was in a vascular area and 24 weeks after surgery if the repair was in the avascular part of the meniscus depending on the sport and physician clearance.[68]

**Table 13-21**

**Postoperative Suggested Rehabilitation Guidelines After Meniscal Repair**

| Acute Stage/Phase 1<br>Maximum Protection (0 to 4 Weeks) | Subacute Stage/Phase 2<br>Moderate Protection (4 to 6 Weeks) | Return to Function/Phase 3<br>Minimal Protection (6 to 16 Weeks) |
|---|---|---|
| Goals<br>• Gradual progressive ROM to 90 degrees brace locked in extension and/or hinged brace set to 0 to 90 degrees<br>• TTWB/WBAT or FWB for 4 to 6 weeks (weight-bearing restrictions per physician protocol)<br>• Pain and edema control<br>• Patella mobilization<br>• Quadriceps muscle control<br>Exercises<br>• OKC: AAROM/AROM to 90 degrees heel slides; TKE, gluteal, quadriceps sets, progress to SLR, seated knee flexion/extension, 4-way hip strengthening, ankle strengthening all directions, core stabilization<br>• CKC: Progress to CKC bilateral calf raises if weight bearing is 50% or greater<br>• NWB stretches: hamstrings, gastrocnemius/soleus<br>Aerobics: Upper bike ergometer | Goals<br>• Discontinue knee brace after about 6 weeks or as per physician's protocol<br>• Good quadriceps control (no extension lag)<br>• Gradually increase ROM to > 110 degrees<br>• FWB by week 6; normalize gait pattern; progress to CKC activities<br>• Minimal pain/swelling after exercise/activity<br>Exercises<br>• OKC: Resisted 4-way hip strengthening, prone gluteal strengthening, resisted TKE and LAQ light resistance<br>• CKC: Mini-squats to 45 to 60 degrees (< 90 degrees), quarter-forward lunges to 45 to 60 degrees, calf raises, step-ups/downs forward 2-in steps, stool pulls to knee flexion 60 degrees<br>• Stretching: Same as previous phase, add CKC ankle stretching, OKC hip flexors, and ITB<br>Balance: Eyes open/closed firm and foam; perturbations, rocker board, begin single-leg activities as per physician's protocol<br>Aerobics: Stationary bike minimal resistance with high seat or if ROM is > 110 degrees; deep water: Treading water or running/cycling | Note: Patient progression is dependent on the location of the repair or reconstruction.<br>Goals<br>• FWB and ROM to 135 degrees; normalize gait pattern<br>• Increase strength, neuromuscular control with CKC activities<br>• Gradually increase power and endurance; begin light plyometrics and running (week 14)[72]<br>• Gradual progression to return to activity/sport after 16 weeks if cleared by physician<br>• *Avoid* deep squats and twisting for at least 14 weeks<br>Exercises<br>• CKC: Step-ups/downs forward, backward, lateral 4-, 6-, and 8-in steps. Week 12 to 14: Begin controlled jumping progress from 2-foot (ft) landings to 1-ft landings then hopping activities all directions.<br>Balance: BOSU Balance Trainer or mini-trampoline add upper extremity activities, advanced functional activities and SLS activities on various surfaces.<br>Aerobics: Same as previous phase, but bike resistance can be increased with normal seat height; treadmill walking, elliptical about week 8 to 9 based on pain and swelling response |

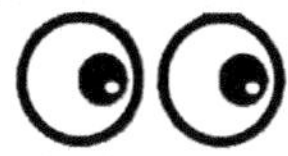

**Eye on the Research: Return to Sports**

According to a 2019 systematic review,[72] return to sports was based on the type of repair. Most athletes returned to sports 7 to 9 weeks after a partial meniscectomy and (on average) 5.6 months after an isolated meniscal repair. Return to sports occurred in a range from 7.6 to 16.5 months after repair using a meniscal allograft transplantation; 81% to 88.9% of athletes were able to return to sports after a meniscal repair, and 67% to 85.7% returned after a meniscal allograft transplantation.[72]

## Ligamentous Injuries: Conservative and Postoperative Management

The knee ligaments are the primary static stabilizers for the joint, and they are commonly sprained during lower leg twisting (rotary) motion, during weight-bearing activities with a sudden change of direction, and/or due to direct contact injuries to the joint.

Conservative treatment interventions are applied when treating grade I and II sprains. Some grade III sprains may also be treated with conservative management initially to reduce pain and inflammation and to strengthen the surrounding musculature. Conservative management may be recommended as part of a prehabilitation program before surgery for persons with grade III injuries. Physicians often postpone surgical interventions for several weeks until swelling is reduced and ROM, muscle control, and strength are restored. Good quadriceps strength before surgery results in quicker postoperative muscle return.[68,73,74]

### *Mechanism of Injury for Various Ligamentous Structures*

It is important to understand the MOI for each ligament because those motions or activities that injured the ligament should be avoided early in the rehabilitation process. Knowing the static function of each ligament allows the clinician to select exercises that target the dynamic (muscle) stabilizers that support the specific ligamentous structure while minimizing stress on the injured ligament. The ACL and MCL are injured more often than the PCL and LCLs. The special tests that assess ligament integrity are provided in Table 13-18.

The ACL can be injured either due to direct or nondirect contact, with the latter mechanism occurring more often. Women are 2 to 8 times more likely to sustain an ACL sprain than men.[73] Female athletes may have an increased risk for ACL sprains due to increased knee valgus, ligamentous laxity due to estrogen, and knee recurvatum (knee hyperextension). The ACL is commonly torn when a person rapidly changes direction, quickly decelerates from running, or when landing from a jump in a flat-footed position. During these scenarios, the knee is near full extension and vertically "loaded" with a valgus stress and tibia internal rotation (about 15 degrees), creating an anterior shear of the tibia in relation to the femur.[73,74] The vertical (axial) loading of the joint with rotational component can also create a meniscal tear, and if the valgus stress is significant, it can also result in an MCL sprain. This combined injury is referred to as the **unhappy triad** or **terrible triad**. An ACL injury can also occur when the foot is firmly planted with the knee slightly abducted (ie, when decelerating or changing directions suddenly) and the leg is hit from the posterolateral direction, creating valgus, internal rotation, and an anterior shear force at the knee.[74] After an ACL injury, the patient may report a "pop or popping" sound, severe pain, immediate swelling, and difficulty walking due to the pain and a feeling of instability or "giving way." A complete ACL tear usually requires surgery, but the decision to proceed with a surgical repair is dependent on the patient's age, prior level of function, and the patient's report of knee instability.[74]

The PCL is almost twice as strong as the ACL and is injured less often. Men experience PCL injuries twice as often as women. Motorcycle accidents and soccer-related injuries are the most common causes for PCL injury.[75] A PCL injury can result due to a blow to the anterior tibia while the knee is flexed (ie, if the shin hits the dashboard during a car crash). In a noncontact situation, a player can land on a hyperflexed knee with either the foot plantar flexed on the ground or sustain an additional downward force on the femur, creating significant posterior displacement of the tibia stressing the PCL.[75] Mild to moderate joint effusion (swelling) can occur immediately or hours after injury; however, the amount of swelling tends to be less than that seen in ACL injuries. The swelling may be so mild that it may go unnoticed. Dull or sharp pain is often reported in the back of the knee, and it can occur immediately or days after the injury. The patient may or may not report popping, but they usually complain of pain and or stiffness with prolonged weight bearing and difficulty walking.[76] The severity of the injury correlates with the intensity of the signs and symptoms the patient experiences.

MCL injuries are extremely common and account for approximately 40% of ligamentous knee injuries and about 7.9% of all knee injuries.[77,78] The most common MOI is a direct blow to the lateral aspect of the knee joint (or the lower leg) when the foot is planted, creating a valgus stress to the ligament (common in football or soccer). If the force is minor, the superficial fibers are usually injured, but if the force is severe, both the superficial and deep fibers of the ligament will be disrupted. Noncontact injury to the MCL is less common and typically results in less severe injury. The MCL is stressed when any valgus stress to the knee is combined with an external rotary force, which occurs during cutting or pivoting activities (eg, skiing and soccer).[78] Patients often report a pop or experience a giving way with sudden pain on the medial side of the knee along the ligament and/or medial joint line. Swelling appears immediately, but ecchymosis may appear 2 to 3 days later depending on the severity of the injury. Patients may have difficulty walking due to pain or instability.[77,78]

Injury to the LCL is rare and the least common of the ligament sprains. The MOI is almost always due to a direct force to the medial aspect of the knee that creates a varus stress.

## *Types of Anterior Cruciate Ligament Reconstruction Surgeries*

The primary reason for knee reconstruction surgery is to restore joint stability. Between 100,000 and 300,000 ACL repair procedures are performed each year in the United States.[79] There are several arthroscopic procedures that are used to repair the ACL. Intra-articular reconstruction places an autograft (patient's tissue) or allograft (synthetic or cadaver graft) within the joint to replace and simulate the function of the ligament. The bone-patellar tendon-bone technique is an example of an intra-articular procedure that uses the middle third of the patient's patellar tendon to replace the ACL by attaching it to the femur and tibia. This technique, commonly used in athletes, tends to be the gold standard of ACL reconstruction.[74,80] The semitendinosus and/or the gracilis tendons can be used as a tendon graft to replace the ligament. The patient often has less pain and can recover faster, but some investigators feel that the hamstring graft is not as strong as the bone-patellar tendon-bone graft.[74,80,81] A graft is at its strongest immediately after surgery but becomes weaker 4 to 6 weeks after surgery as the tissue breaks down and reforms. Autografts need time to vascularize and remodel, which takes about 16 weeks. During this revascularization/healing process, the graft is weak and prone to stretching or tearing, so stress on the graft should be minimized during this time.[73,74,79,81] The tensile strength of the autograft continues to increase to about 56% at 6 months and then increases to about 87% 9 months postoperatively.[80]

Extra-articular reconstruction uses a structure (ie, tendon or ligament) placed outside the joint capsule to provide stability. Extra-articular procedures can be used in conjunction with intra-articular procedures. Extra-articular reconstruction techniques are not performed in isolation because they do not allow for the same joint mechanics as intra-articular procedures.[55,80,82]

## *Anterior Cruciate Ligament Postoperative Rehabilitation*

Surgical interventions are indicated for athletes who wish to return to sport and for people who experience repeated events of instability during ADLs or sports/work-related activities.[74] Patient progression should include an evidence-based functional program dependent on tissue healing, ROM, strength, and neuromuscular control. It is important to include interventions to reduce pain and swelling. Progressing from isolated muscle strengthening to functional strengthening and restoration of neuromuscular function is imperative for the patient to return to sporting, recreational, and work activities safely. Table 13-22 provides rehabilitation guidelines based on current evidence-based research.[83-88]

Weight-bearing status and brace use postoperatively are debated in the literature. Guidelines for weight-bearing status and brace use will reflect the physician's protocol. Protocols often base patient readiness for progression on evidence of adequate quadriceps/hamstring muscle control. One systematic review summarized that FWB using a normalized gait pattern by day 10 after surgery reduced PFP, improved quadriceps motor control, and did not affect joint stability.[83,84,88] There is evidence that indicates bracing the knee after ACL repair may not be required; these studies determined that bracing the knee did not necessarily protect against injury, decrease pain, affect motion, or improve stability after surgery.[84,85,88] However, many physicians still prescribe a brace with either limited motion (0 to 90 degrees) or locked in full extension.[80,83-85] If the brace is locked during weight bearing, it can typically be opened to 90 degrees once the patient can perform an SLR without an extension lag. The criteria for brace removal during gait often includes clearance for FWB (by week 4 to 6) and a normal gait pattern with no evidence of limping.[83] Quadriceps weakness is a common cause for an antalgic gait pattern, so initiating quadriceps strengthening exercises early is important.[83-85,87,88]

During the acute stage, pain and swelling must be controlled. Improving ROM (especially knee extension) and reestablishing quadriceps motor control are primary focuses immediately postoperatively. Patella mobilizations in all directions are initiated to help facilitate knee ROM and quadriceps muscle contraction.[83-85] A home exercise program should be provided to the patient either before or immediately after the procedure. From postoperative day 0 to 2 weeks after surgery, isometrics for quadriceps and hamstrings are completed using CKC exercises in a range of 0 to 30 to 60 degrees. Exercises for OKC knee extension are limited to 90 and 40 degrees; this protected ROM is used to minimize stress on the ACL graft.[83,84,86,88] ROM and quadriceps strengthening exercises include heel slides, seated knee extension from 90 to 40 degrees, quadriceps sets, and SLRs (without extension lag). Although there is some research that indicates that 90 to 0 degrees may not compromise the graft, many clinicians incorporate the protected ROM. The assistant should defer to the physician's protocol.[83]

Weight shifting and mini-squats 0 to 30 degrees can be performed in standing.[84,88] Initiating CKC strengthening early in the rehabilitation program can result in full quadriceps strength sooner and without compromising graft stability.[85,89] Increasing strength and initiating isometric hamstring strengthening very early in the rehabilitation process result in decreased swelling and significant improvements in ADLs 4 weeks after surgery.[86,88] The

**Table 13-22**

Postoperative Suggested Rehabilitation Guidelines After Anterior Cruciate Ligament Reconstruction

| Acute Stage/Phase 1<br>Maximum Protection (0 to 6 Weeks) | Subacute Stage/Phase 2<br>Moderate Protection (6 to 14 Weeks) | Return to Function/Phase 3<br>Minimal Protection (14 to 22 Weeks)<br>Phase 4 (More Than 22 Weeks) |
|---|---|---|
| Goals<br>• Control swelling/pain<br>• Protect graft; good patella mobility<br>• ROM 0 to 90 degrees by week 2; 0 to 120 degrees by week 4 to 6<br>• Quadriceps muscle control; SLR no lag<br>• FWB work on normalized gait<br>Note: Avoid reciprocal descent on steps (avoid eccentric contraction)<br>Exercises<br>• OKC: Heel slides, stationary bike for ROM, quad sets, SLR no lag, 4-way hip strengthening, seated knee extension ROM, and hamstring isometrics 90 to 40 degrees; add light resistance week 3 and core stability<br>• CKC: Mini-squats 0 to 30 to 60 degrees add light band resistance about week 3, backward walking treadmill; week 6 begin 2-in step-ups (no step-downs) if FWB and no pain, calf raises (when weight bearing is > 50%)<br>• Stretches: Gastrocnemius/soleus, gentle hamstrings, hip flexors<br>Balance: Weight shifting (when weight bearing is > 50%) progress to foam/rocker board and gentle multidirectional perturbations<br>Aerobics: UBE, stationary bike (when ROM is > 100 degrees); pool exercises, underwater treadmill | Goals<br>• Full ROM 0 to 135 degrees and FWB with normal gait and speed<br>• Ascend/descend 8-in step with no pain and good control<br>• No patellofemoral pain (PFP) with activities or exercise<br>Exercises<br>• Hip and ankle PRE strengthening; knee resistance training CKC 0 to 60 degrees, OKC 90 to 40 degrees; can progress to OKC PRE when ROM 0 to 130 degrees if no pain at week 12, forward step-ups 4-, 6-, and 8-in progression; then initiate step-down progression (about week 12 to 13); lunges, leg press wall slides to 90 degrees vertical shin week 14.<br>• Stretches: Gastrocnemius/soleus, hamstrings, hip flexors<br>Balance: Rocker board or foam eyes open/closed, progress to SLS on firm to foam/mini-trampoline; add perturbations and upper extremity tasks<br>Aerobics: Stationary bike, elliptical (forward/backward), swimming (no breaststroke), deep water treading and running; backward walking on incline on treadmill | Goals<br>• Pain-free running<br>• 5/5 strength quadriceps/hamstrings<br>• Lower extremity flexibility adequate for sport demands<br>• No PFP with activities<br>• Clearance by physician to return to sport about week 26<br>• Good confidence with plyometrics and agility<br>Exercises<br>• Progress functional strengthening. Begin squat program ≥90 degrees after week 16 progress to SLS squats with control. Eccentric hamstring strengthening.<br>Neuromuscular training: When no pain with 8-in step-down, begin plyometrics: Jumping to box jumps, etc; progress to single hop test = to uninvolved leg. Isokinetic testing ≥90%. Week 18 work on good biomechanics (vertical shin) with various sport agility drills at various speeds.<br>Aerobics: Same as last phase. Begin backward treadmill running before forward treadmill running. Forward running can be initiated if no knee pain and good quadriceps control with 8-in step-downs and > 14 weeks.<br>Note: Make sure there is no evidence of valgus stress and that the shin is vertical (knee not to extend past the toes) with all CKC activities. |

hamstrings are the dynamic stabilizers for the ACL, and they help to prevent anterior translation of the tibia, so progressive hamstrings strengthening is important. After a hamstring tendon graft, the physician may delay hamstring strengthening and stretching for a few weeks because of the harvesting location of the tendons for the graft, but as long as pain is controlled, gentle isometrics and stretching may be permitted.[85] Research indicates that quadriceps muscle weakness, extension lag during SLRs, and the inability to actively attain full knee extension 5 weeks postoperatively increase the risk of ongoing quadriceps weakness 6 months after surgery.[84]

Patients need to understand that the ligament repair is at its weakest point during the second phase of the rehabilitation process, so all exercise and ADL precautions must be followed. Light resistive CKC exercises can be performed staying within the 0 to 60 degree range. If no PFP is reported, the range can be gradually increased to 90 degrees. Gradual progressive resistance OKC exercises from 0 to 90 degrees may be initiated after week 6.[83,89] Eccentric quadriceps strengthening (in the safe/protected range) and isokinetic hamstring strengthening can be added at the beginning of this phase to improve knee strength. Some investigators have reported that this could begin 3 weeks after ACL surgery, but accelerated strengthening should be determined by the physician's protocol or the physical therapist.[88,89] Hip strengthening and core stabilization exercises can be progressed as long as they do not place stress on the healing ligament.

In the minimal protection phase, the focus shifts to more aggressive OKC strengthening and CKC functional activities (ie, step-ups) as long as PFP is controlled.[84,85] Squats may be progressed to 90 degrees and in the fourth phase to greater than 90 degrees with a gradual increase in resistance, but avoid irritating the patellar tendon. Eccentric hamstring strengthening can be initiated early in phase 3 and should continue even after return to sport.[86] Neuromuscular training includes more challenging tasks (ie, hopping), but instruction and monitoring of good knee mechanics (maintaining a vertical shin) during squatting and dynamic activities are vital to limiting stress on the graft. After these mechanics become learned and automatic, the patient can progress to more challenging plyometric and agility drills before returning to sport. Some physicians may prescribe a functional brace in the latter phases of rehabilitation and for use when returning to sports or recreational activities to prevent reinjury.[55]

## *Posterior Cruciate Ligament Rehabilitation*

There is variability and a lack of consensus in recommendations and guidelines for the management of PCL tears.[75,80,90-92] The physical therapist assistant should follow the physical therapist's POC and physician's protocol.

### Conservative Management of a Posterior Cruciate Ligament Sprain

Acute isolated grade I or II PCL injuries are initially treated with conservative management using PRICE interventions. Isolated grade III sprains can be treated with conservative treatment if symptoms are mild and the patient does not participate in moderate- or high-demand activities. PCL surgical reconstruction is indicated when conservative management is unsuccessful in controlling knee pain and instability or when there is damage to additional knee ligaments.[90,91] Conservative and postoperative treatment protocols are similar, but conservative management of milder sprains requires less time to rehabilitate.[80,91,92] There is variability regarding a recommended time for return to work/sport, with a range from 4 to 12 weeks depending on the degree of injury and physician's protocol. The following information reflects general recommendations from peer-reviewed protocols.

Because the quadriceps muscles are the dynamic stabilizers for the PCL, quadriceps sets and SLRs should be initiated as soon as possible, and strengthening these muscles is the primary focus during the rehabilitation process.[75,80,90,91] OKC hamstring strengthening should be avoided until later in the exercise program because it stresses the PCL.

During nonoperative treatment of a PCL tear, in phase 1 (week 1 to 6), the knee may be braced either locked in extension or allowing 0 to 60 degrees of motion for the first 2 to 4 weeks depending on the severity of the sprain (bracing prevents posterior tibial sag). Modalities are used to address pain and inflammation. Patients should be instructed to elevate the limb with the entire lower leg fully supported (preventing posterior tibial translational forces/sag). Weight bearing may be restricted (PWB or WBAT) during the first 2 weeks, but it is recommended that FWB be achieved by week 6. Passive knee flexion and extension ROM should be performed with the patient lying prone to prevent the hamstrings from contracting. Avoid hamstring contraction because it creates a posterior translation of the tibia, placing stress on the PCL. Knee flexion may be limited to 90 degrees for the first 2 weeks and then gradually progressed to full pain-free range. According to biomechanical studies, the least amount of stress placed on the PCL occurs between 40 and 90 degrees of knee flexion.[90,91] Once the patient achieves 115 degrees of knee flexion, the patient can use a stationary bike with no resistance for aerobic conditioning. Hamstring and gastrocnemius/soleus stretches can be included. Hip muscle strengthening exercises can be initiated early as long as they do not create a posterior tibial sag. Quadriceps sets and SLRs (with no extension lag) can be initiated as long as joint swelling is controlled. Implementing these exercises early helps minimize the risk of quadriceps muscle inhibition. Russian stimulation (or neuromuscular electrical stimulation) can be used in conjunction with active quadriceps muscle setting exercises to "jump start" the muscles. Weight shifting,

CKC TKEs, and partial squats (or leg press) are initiated (0 to 45 degrees) and should not exceed 70 degrees of knee flexion. Avoid knee hyperextension because it is contraindicated during all activities. The clinician may need to manually support the lower limb when initiating AROM exercises to ensure that the knee does not hyperextend. The clinician should ensure that the patient has equal weight bearing on both lower extremities and that genu valgus is avoided during squats. Standing on a rocker board or foam can improve proprioception and balance.[90,91]

Patients should achieve full ROM and weight bearing with a normal gait pattern by phase 2 (week 6 to 12). The goals for this phase include increasing lower extremity strength, neuromuscular control, and proprioception and then progressing from double-leg to single-leg activities on various surfaces. Continue to monitor the patient's knee position, avoiding genu valgus and knee hyperextension during exercises. CKC exercises are more appropriate than resisted OKC exercises. Forward and lateral step-ups/downs, resisted squatting, and lunges limited to 70 degrees can be initiated. Cocontractions of the quadriceps during these activities will help control posterior translation of the tibia and reduce patellofemoral irritation.[80,90] Implement more advanced hip strengthening exercises (ie, using a resistance band for all motions) targeting the gluteal and hip rotator muscles (ie, bridges on therapy ball knees straight and clamshells).

Jogging and CKC strengthening beyond 70 degrees of flexion with double- and single-limb activities can be initiated between 12 and 16 weeks. Good-quality lower leg neuromuscular control is important, and it requires good joint proprioceptive and kinesthetic awareness during all exercises to prevent reinjury (ie, step-ups/downs, lunges, and single-leg squats). Targeted hamstring strengthening (ie, double- and single-leg bridges with knees flexed on therapy ball) should be progressed. More advanced trunk and hip strengthening and dynamic stabilization can be progressed as long as there is no evidence of pain or swelling. Beginning week 14 to 16, running, cutting, plyometrics, and agility drills can be introduced and progressed to prepare the patient for return to play (16 to 24 weeks). Return to play can be as early as 2 to 4 weeks; the rate of progress for grade I and II tears is only limited by pain and swelling because there is usually minimal functional limitations.[75,80] The progression presented previously is a relatively conservative timeline. Patient progression varies depending on the degree of the tear and the individual inflammatory response to exercise progression. If grade III PCL tears do not respond well in phase 2, surgical intervention should be revisited.

### Postsurgical Management of a Posterior Cruciate Ligament Sprain

In the initial weeks after a postoperative PCL repair, a brace is typically worn until the patient is cleared for FWB and demonstrates adequate quadriceps muscle control. OKC AROM exercises are avoided, and hip exercises and SLR exercises are completed while braced. PROM for the knee is completed in prone, and quadriceps sets and ankle and hip ROM exercises are included. In phase 2, emphasis continues on CKC exercises; wall slides and mini-squats (to 45 degrees) and leg presses (limited to 60 degrees) are initiated. The physician may delay hamstring strengthening exercises until week 6 to 8. A stationary bike may be used for aerobic training (seat elevated). In phase 3, treadmill training and CKC exercises are progressed.

Most postoperative return-to-sport timelines range from 4 to 12 months, but there are not many studies on PCL postsurgical outcomes. The ability to return to play is often determined using a combination of the postoperative timeline, lower extremity strength, and the results of functional performance testing (ie, single-hop test).[92]

## *Medial Collateral Ligament Rehabilitation*

All degrees of isolated MCL injuries usually heal well with conservative treatment because the ligament has good blood supply. As with all injuries, protecting the joint and PRICE should be initiated immediately after injury. Controlling the swelling and pain as quickly as possible will help reduce inhibition of the quadriceps muscles.[77,80,93]

Grade I MCL sprains are treated symptomatically. Pain-free ROM, quadriceps sets, SLRs (if no extension lag), and WBAT can be initiated the day after injury and can be progressed more aggressively than with more serious MCL injuries. Early pain-free ROM, weight bearing, and (normalized) gait indicate readiness to progress to pain-free OKC and CKC strengthening. Initiating more advanced balance and dynamic/plyometric activities (similar to those for ACL injuries) will help the patient return to sport and high-demand physical jobs. Pain, swelling, neuromuscular control, and strength gains will determine how fast the patient can return to ADLs (usually in 1 to 2 weeks), and many patients return to sport competitively in 3 to 5 weeks.[80] The clinician should also focus on maintaining core and hip strength during the rehabilitation process.

**Considerations for the Physical Therapist Assistant**

Patients who plan to return to sports or work tasks that require them to move laterally and/or pivot on the involved knee at high rates of speed need to be able to perform those movements confidently. This may require a longer rehabilitation episode of care (depending on the severity of injury) compared with patients with lower mobility demands. The ligament and the dynamic stabilizers for the MCL need to be challenged in order to adapt to these higher demands before returning to the job or sport.

Patients with grade II sprains may require a few days for the swelling and pain to decrease, but initiating exercises (ROM and quadriceps neuromuscular control) as soon as possible after injury should be encouraged. Initially using heel slides to gain range and then progressing these patients to a stationary bike (lowering the seat height) to regain pain-free full ROM is indicated. As with most knee injuries, regaining full knee extension and achieving good quadriceps neuromuscular control are priorities because these are necessary for normal walking.

Because grade II MCL injuries present with some ligament instability, WBAT and the use of crutches for 1 to 2 weeks are indicated. The physician may prescribe a knee immobilizer or brace for the same length of time for comfort and to prevent stressing the MCL.[77,78] Once pain and swelling are controlled, standing knee flexion and seated knee extension ROM against gravity should be performed. OKC and CKC strengthening and balance exercises should follow the same progression as for a grade I MCL rehabilitation program. Refer to Table 13-19 and the figures at the end of the chapter. A functional brace reduces valgus and rotational stresses on the ligament and may be worn as the patient returns to sports or high-demanding physical labor–type work (eg, construction worker, plumber, roofer).

Grade III MCL injuries are often associated with injuries to other local structures such as the ACL, PCL, LCL, and/or meniscus.[77,78,80,93,94] There is a 78% likelihood of concurrent injury to another knee ligament/structure when a patient sustains a grade III MCL sprain.[93] However, most isolated grade III MCL sprains and injuries involving other structures are initially treated conservatively. Multistructural injuries can be surgically repaired if conservative treatment is unsuccessful after 3 weeks.[93] Progression depends on the patient's prior level of function, their motivation, the physician's protocol, and the physical therapy POC.

The patient is initially placed in a hinged knee brace for about 6 weeks to prevent valgus stress. Just as with grade II sprains, bracing can be continued until the patient feels confident and stable, and the brace may also be used when the patient is cleared to return to sport if necessary. Early motion after grade III MCL injury improves the alignment of collagen cells, increasing the ability of the healing tissue to resist load and protecting against damage to articular cartilage.[93,94]

During the initial phase of rehabilitation (0 to 4 weeks), the goals are to control pain and swelling using cryotherapy and electric stimulation. ROM and weight bearing can be initiated immediately. OKC knee (pain-free) flexion and extension strengthening/stretching can begin and quadriceps neuromuscular control restored. During this phase, ROM should be restored to at least 0 to 100 degrees and quadriceps and hamstring strength restored to at least 4/5.[93,94] FWB with normal gait pattern is expected by week 4.[93,94] The clinician should include interventions to address hip and trunk strength and stability throughout the rehabilitation program while protecting the knee from valgus stress.

During phase 2 (4 to 6 weeks), full ROM should be achieved and muscle strength increased to within normal limits (5/5). FWB CKC strengthening is included, and single-leg balance can be challenged (varied surfaces) as long as pain and swelling are controlled.[93]

During the third phase (6 to 10 weeks), the patient can return to light jogging on the treadmill and progress to more dynamic balance activities (on a mini-trampoline). Later in this phase, the assistant can introduce controlled lateral movements (eg, Fitter Slide Board [Fitter International]) and light progressive agility drills and plyometrics.[93]

During weeks 8 to 12, the patient can progress by implementing activities such as varying running speeds, starts/stops, cutting, full plyometric training, and sport-specific training. These tasks must be performed without pain or evidence of increased swelling during or after the activities. If the patient plans to return to sports, the following goals should be achieved first: quadriceps strength at 90% and a single-leg hop at 90% of the contralateral leg, no signs or symptoms of knee joint instability, and successful sport-specific skill performance testing without pain or evidence of swelling.

The success of any nonoperative rehabilitation treatment of medial knee injuries is dependent on the presence of an intact ACL. "Protocols that prioritize early weight bearing and include immediate knee ROM exercises and progressive strength training produce good outcomes and are associated with high rates of return to the patient's prior level of activity."[94]

## Patellofemoral Joint Pain: Diagnoses, Mechanism of Injury, and Signs and Symptoms

PFP is a common multifactorial problem most often seen in physically active individuals. The treatment of PFP pain should address the actual diagnosis as well as any underlying causes of the pain. This is important because effective long-term outcomes for PFP require a multimodal approach. The inability to address the underlying causes can result in ongoing symptoms that can negatively affect the patient's quality of life and physical function.

There are a number of conditions and contributing factors (see Table 13-7) that affect the patellofemoral joint and cause anterior knee pain. PFPS, chondromalacia, infrapatellar fat pad syndrome, patella tendinopathy, and patella subluxations/dislocations are some examples.

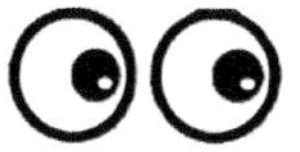

### Eye on the Research: Patellofemoral Pain Prevalence and Outcomes

According to the 2019 clinical practice guidelines, PFPS can affect individuals of all ages and sex.[95] Some studies found that PFPS was most common in individuals between the ages of 12 and 19 years, whereas others reported a higher likelihood in ages 50 to 59 years; this variation may be due to the type of clinical environment where the data were collected. There is variability in the reported incidence rates between men and women, which may be related to the environments where data are collected and the expected level of physical activity of the participants. Although one meta-analysis reported that 55% of people with PFP were women, another study found that women are 2.23 times more likely to develop PFPS. Other studies noted that the lifetime prevalence of PFP in high school runners is 21% in women and 16% in men.[95]

Recurrence rates of PFP are high (70% to 90% of patients report recurrent symptoms). Long-term outcomes for those with PFP are not encouraging. More than 50% of individuals with PFP report unfavorable outcomes 5 to 8 years after a diagnosis, and 50% to 56% of adolescents continue with pain 2 years after their diagnosis.[95]

Patients who experience **PFPS** commonly complain of retropatellar or peripatellar anterior knee pain. The pain tends to be gradual, may be present in both knees, and is often activity related (associated with repetitive knee flexion/extension). It is important to determine if there are underlying factors contributing to the patient's PFPS. Several factors that may contribute to PFPS include an excessive Q angle creating genu valgus, patella location (ie, patella alta or lateral tilting), and muscular imbalance and/or weakness in the hip and knee, all of which can affect patella alignment and biomechanics.[15,16,55,80,95] Although older research reported that subtalar pronation was a contributing factor,[15] current clinical practice guidelines indicate that there is a minimal relationship between subtalar pronation and an increased risk for developing PFP.[95]

**Chondromalacia patella** is a softening and deterioration of the articular cartilage on the posterior surface of the patella. This deterioration may be associated with PFPS, and it can occur as a result of any of the conditions associated with lateral patella tracking.[15,16,55,80,95] Patients who do not have patella tracking issues may also develop chondromalacia because direct impact/injury can damage the back side of the patella, which can also cause chondromalacia.[80] Patients usually complain of pain and a "grinding" feeling, and they may describe an audible grating sound with knee flexion and extension. These patients often have a positive compression/grind test.

Patellar tendinopathy is characterized by chronic anterior knee pain, but the pain usually occurs where the patella tendon attaches to the inferior pole of the patella.[80,96] This condition is also called *jumper's knee* because it occurs in athletes whose sports require repetitive jumping (eg, volleyball, basketball).[80] It is more common in men 15 to 30 years of age. The repetitive "load-related pain" occurs because of the high demands placed on the quadriceps during jumping and landing; with this repetitive motion, the patellar tendon stores and releases energy, and this creates a chronic inflammation.[80,96]

Another potential cause of anterior knee pain is infrapatellar fat pad syndrome. The infrapatellar fat pad sits behind the distal portion of the patella tendon, is fairly mobile, and can be palpated on either side of the tendon. Injury to the infrapatellar fat pad can be due to a direct blow (eg, fall, motor vehicle accident) or related to overuse. This usually results in swelling of the fat pad; it becomes less mobile and can be impinged between the posterior patella tendon and the lateral femoral condyle. Patients who have genu recurvatum (hyperextended knees) or who wear high heels often (which can create knee hyperextension) may also be prone to irritating this structure.[97]

Patients with any of these diagnoses usually have similar complaints. They typically report pain during activities that require repetitive knee flexion/extension such as climbing stairs, running, jumping, or squatting. Patients may have a positive "movie theater" sign (ie, knee pain with the transition to standing after prolonged sitting), and they are likely to report pain with increased activity intensity as well as pain that occurs during ambulation, jogging, or running (especially over changing surfaces; ie, road to sand). Patients report audible popping/cracking in the knee. Pain with palpation and swelling may be evident in the front of the knee as well as along the patella tendon area.

Patients may be predisposed to acute lateral patellar subluxation or dislocation. The incidence of lateral patellar tracking increases if the patient has a shallow trochlear groove, a short lip on the lateral condyle, patella alta, an increased Q angle (genu valgus), and/or genu recurvatum. These mechanical factors can increase the risk of patellar subluxation or dislocation. The most common MOI for an acute subluxation or dislocation is a strong quadriceps contraction that occurs when the foot is planted and the femur rotates internally on the tibia, creating a valgus stress. These actions occur when an individual quickly decelerates and changes directions away from the planted leg. Another mechanism for acute lateral dislocation occurs when the foot is planted and another athlete hits the medial aspect of the patella, pushing it laterally.[98] The majority (70% to 100%) of lateral patella dislocations are associated with concurrent damage to the medial patellar stabilizers (medial retinaculum and medial patellofemoral ligament).[97]

## *Rehabilitation Management and Patellofemoral Pain Syndrome*

It is important for physical therapist assistants to understand joint mechanics related to the patellofemoral joint when working with patients with patellofemoral diagnoses. As discussed in the Patellofemoral Joint Mechanics section earlier in this chapter, the clinician should have the patient perform OKC exercises between 90 and 30 degrees of knee flexion to reduce patellofemoral joint stress. During CKC exercises, forces are significantly decreased during TKE, so these exercises should initially be performed from 20 degrees to full extension; they can be progressed to about 45 degrees if pain free (but should not exceed 60 degrees).[15,55,80,97] Activities such as running or deep squats can increase patellofemoral forces by 5 to 8 times the patient's body weight and should not be introduced until much later in the rehabilitation program (Table 13-23).[15,55,80]

The assistant should monitor and target any of the following when creating an exercise plan for a person with PFPS: weak VMO muscle, tight lateral structures (ie, the lateral retinaculum, ITB, and vastus lateralis), weak hip musculature (especially hip extensors, abductors, and external rotators), tight quadriceps, hamstrings and gastrocnemius, and knee joint mechanics.[15,55,80,95,97,99,100] Most lateral patella tracking occurs between 0 and 30 degrees of knee flexion, and the assistant should carefully monitor patellar tracking during exercise.[97]

During the initial phase of rehabilitation, rest, ice, and avoiding painful ADLs are indicated. Exercises can be performed but only if they do not irritate the patella or create pain. Quadriceps exercises should be used in conjunction with hip external rotation and hip abduction exercises for at least 4 weeks because isolated quadriceps strengthening has been shown to increase patella irritation. PNF stretching for hip flexors and extensors has been shown to be more effective in reducing pain and improving function compared with classic stretching exercises.[95,99]

CKC strengthening exercises that target both hip and knee musculature have been shown to be effective for improving strength and reducing PFP.[15,55,80,95,97,99,100] If the patient experiences pain during FWB activities, modify the status to WBAT during CKC activities and then gradually increase the weight-bearing status. Once the patient can tolerate FWB, progress to bilateral and then unilateral strengthening and balance exercises. The physical therapist assistant should closely monitor the patient and ensure all exercises are performed with good knee positioning (the shin should be vertical and not pass the toes) and joint mechanics to reduce patellofemoral irritation. Table 13-23 provides suggested rehabilitation guidelines for patients with PFPS; progression is determined by the patient's pain level.

Patellar bracing or taping may help reduce pain and forces on the patella. Clinical practice guidelines suggest that clinicians use tailored patellar taping (in combination with exercise) to assist in pain reduction and to enhance short-term outcomes. The guidelines note that taping may not be beneficial in the long term or when used with more intense exercises. Taping is not recommended for goals of enhancing muscle function. Some patients may benefit from shoe inserts or orthotic use combined with exercise during the early weeks of rehabilitation if they exhibit increased pronation.[95] Any consideration to use taping, bracing, or orthotics should first be discussed with the physical therapist. Patients who have a high baseline of pain (severity of pain) and PFP symptoms for a long period of time tend to have poorer outcomes and recovery rates.[95]

**Considerations for the Physical Therapist Assistant**

Strengthening the VMO, hip extensors, abductors, and external rotators and stretching the ITB as part of the treatment plan for persons with PFPS are effective to reduce knee pain and improve function.[15,80,95,97,99]

### Techniques to Facilitate Quadriceps Setting and Straight Leg Raise Progression

The VMO stabilizes the patella both statically and dynamically; abnormal patellar tracking creates undue stress on the joint.[15] A key component for reducing pain and improving alignment is to increase hip muscle and quadriceps strength, especially of the VMO. Gluteus medius and hip external rotation strength are important for preventing femur adduction and internal rotation (which increases valgus stress and alters patellar tracking).

A factor that significantly impacts knee rehabilitation is the relationship between knee edema and quadriceps contractility. Swelling around the knee inhibits the ability of the quadriceps muscle to contract, and it must be addressed immediately. Ice, elevation, compression, and early implementation of quadriceps set exercises are indicated to retain or improve quadriceps contractility, especially during TKE.

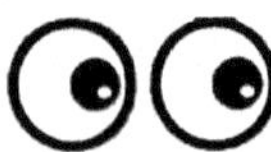

**Eye on the Research**

Muscle balance between the vastus lateralis and VMO is essential to reducing pain and improving patella tracking.[100,101] Several studies have reported that interventions focused on improving VMO force and firing time (facilitating VMO contraction before vastus lateralis contraction during knee extension) are difficult to achieve. Interventions targeted at improving VMO firing time and force do not necessarily lead to better pain outcomes.[99] Electromyography studies found that CKC exercises induce VMO activation.[100,101] The incorporation of CKC activities may assist with achieving muscle balance.

## Table 13-23

### Conservative Management: Suggested Rehabilitation Guidelines for Patellofemoral Pain Syndrome and Patella Dislocation/Subluxation

| Acute Stage/Phase 1<br>Maximum Protection (Day 1 to 4 Weeks) | Subacute Stage/Phase 2<br>Moderate Protection (4 to 8 Weeks) | Return to Function/Phase 3<br>Minimal Protection (More Than 8 Weeks) |
|---|---|---|
| Goals<br>• Joint protection, control pain, and swelling (knee immobilizer for dislocations, 2 to 4 weeks)<br>• Gain full pain-free ROM<br>• Increase hip muscle and quadriceps strength<br>• Soft tissue mobilization to tight lateral structures (ITB and lateral retinaculum)<br>• Stretch tight structures<br>• Avoid painful activities<br>Note: Progression depends on control of swelling and pain. Monitor for genu valgus with CKC exercises; stop performance if improper form.<br>Exercises<br>• OKC: Side-lying hip external rotation (clamshells), hip abduction and prone extension for gluteals and hamstrings (add resistance if pain free), quadriceps sets, multiangle isometrics, and SLR if pain free hamstring curls standing.<br>• CKC: TKEs and mini-squats<br>Additional exercises: Core stabilization and pelvic control (ie, pelvic clocks)<br>Stretches: PNF contract relax stretching for quadriceps/hip flexors and hamstrings, hip external rotators and adductors (ie, independent hip rotation ITB and CKC gastrocnemius/soleus)<br>Balance: Perturbations, rocker board bilaterally, partial step-ups, and progress to controlled SLS<br>Aerobics: UBE, stationary bike no resistance (if pain free and no residual complaints) | Goals<br>• Continue joint protection and pain control<br>• Continue with hip strengthening and neuromuscular control bilaterally and unilaterally<br>• Continue stretching tight structures<br>• Increase strengthening OKC and CKC at progressive ROM pain free (ie, squats between 45 to 60 degrees)<br>Note: Watch for genu valgus and knee passing the toes with CKC exercises; stop performance if improper form.<br>Exercises<br>• OKC: Increase resistance with weights around the ankles for hip and knee strengthening or resistance bands above the knee joint for hip strengthening. Isokinetic machine (higher speeds) in pain-free ROM.<br>• CKC: Mini-squats to 45 to 60 degrees (< 90 degrees), quarter-forward lunges to 45 to 60 degrees, calf raises, step-ups/downs forward and lateral 2-in steps, stool pulls to knee flexion 60 degrees, resistance band side stepping and backward walking.<br>Balance: Rocker board or foam eyes open/closed, progress SLS on firm to foam/mini-trampoline, add perturbations and upper extremity tasks<br>Aerobics: Stationary bike slight resistance, treadmill or elliptical (forward/backward), swimming (no breast stroke), deep water treading and running | Goals<br>• Increase pain-free functional strength in preparation for return to activities/sport<br>• Introduce pain-free dynamic and plyometric activities. Progress as tolerated back to prior level of function.<br>• Begin running program with gradual increases. No hills until running on level surfaces is pain free (probably > 2 weeks).<br>Exercises<br>• OKC: Knee flexion/extension weight machine full ROM (or isokinetic machine all speeds)<br>• CKC: Mini-squats to 90 degrees; forward lunges to 90 degrees; calf raises; step-ups/downs forward and lateral 4-, 6-, and 8-in steps; stool pulls to knee flexion 60 degrees; resisted side stepping; SLS mini-squats<br>Light jumping with controlled landing progress to hopping pain free (about 10 to 12 weeks). Add plyometrics as tolerated (pain free) after 12 weeks.<br>Balance: Rocker board or foam eyes open/closed, progress SLS on firm to foam/mini-trampoline, BAPS board, and add perturbations and upper extremity tasks<br>Aerobics: Stationary bike vary resistance, elliptical with resistance, swimming, begin treadmill jogging, and progress to level ground running. Add specific cutting drills and acceleration and deceleration drills. |

UBE = upper body ergometer.

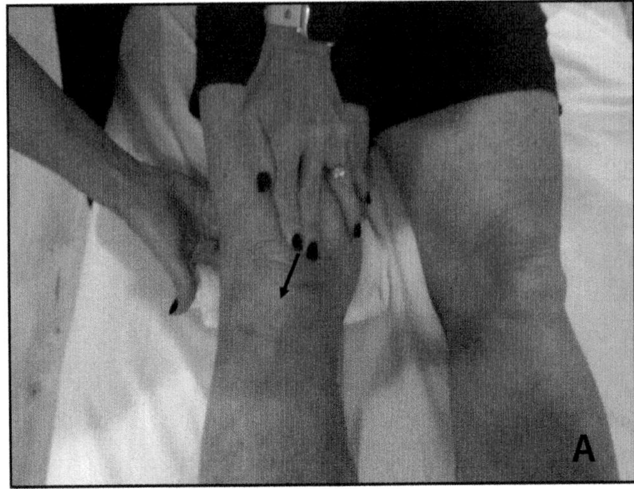


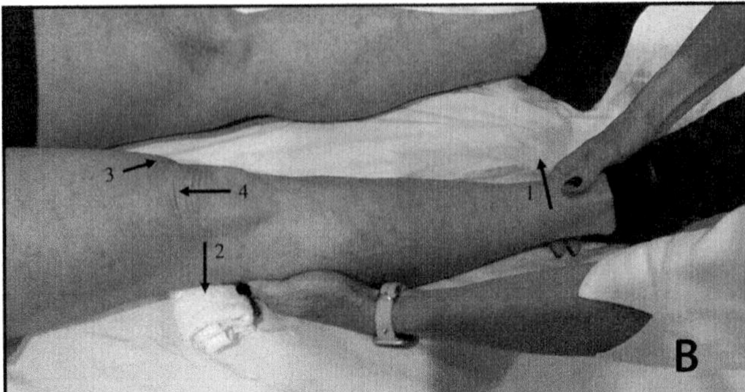


**Figure 13-22.** Facilitation for VMO quadriceps set. (A) Using a patella prestretch. The clinician places one hand under the knee and 2 fingers of the other hand on the medial superior border of the patella. The clinician provides a quick prestretch inferiorly and then instructs the patient to push the back of the knee down into the clinician's hand or towel. Note: The pressure is released once the patient is instructed to push the knee down. The clinician is looking for the patella to move superiorly and the medial quadriceps muscle to contract. (B) Using hip adduction isometric contraction. (1) The patient is instructed to first perform an isometric hip adduction contraction as the clinician resists. (2) The patient is then instructed to push the back of the knee down into the small towel. The clinician is feeling for the knee motion and observing the knee for (3) a muscle contraction and (4) proximal movement of the patella.

There are techniques that can enhance the ability to facilitate a quadriceps contraction while targeting the VMO. Providing an inferior patella prestretch (Figure 13-22A) or resisting hip adduction isometrically (Figure 13-22B) while simultaneously providing instruction to perform a quadriceps set are good techniques to achieve this goal. Once the patient is able to elicit a quadriceps contraction, it is helpful to have the patient perform 3 to 4 very quick quadriceps set contractions followed by one contraction with a 3-second isometric hold. Regardless of the technique used or the hold time parameter, the clinician should give verbal cues to "push the back of the knee down" either into a small towel roll or clinician's hand. It is helpful to cue the patient to watch their patella move superiorly during the contraction. This provides useful reinforcement and acts as a type of biofeedback for the patient. A prone CKC quadriceps set (or TKE) exercise is also a useful technique (see Figure 13-16). Have the patient lie prone, dorsiflex the foot, and place the toes on the treatment table. Instruct the patient to straighten the knee and "push the back of the knee up toward the ceiling." This is a modified CKC TKE.

Once the patient can maintain an isometric quadriceps contraction, they can progress to SLRs. If the patient cannot perform an SLR in a supine position, initiate the SLR in standing or in a lean-back retrograde position. The patient progresses to a supine position when the exercise can be performed without an extension lag in the gravity-minimized positions. The clinician needs to ensure that an extension lag is avoided during SLR performance because this lag often denotes muscle fatigue or weakness. The patient's program can be gradually progressed as long as edema and pain are controlled.

## *Patella Tendinopathy: Conservative Management*

The initial treatment for patients with patella tendinopathy includes education to avoid all activities that increase pain (ie, no running or jumping) and the use of cryotherapy to reduce pain and inflammation. Adequate warm-up exercises are an important component of treatment. Low- to moderate-intensity eccentric quadriceps strengthening exercises are indicated.[80,96] General lower extremity stretching and a gradual increase of eccentric training are beneficial. Before the patient can return to play, good strength, flexibility, neuromuscular control, and proper biomechanical jump landing skills need to be achieved.[80]

## *Patella Dislocation and Subluxation: Conservative Management*

After a patella dislocation, patients are usually immobilized for 2 to 4 weeks and allowed to perform WBAT with crutches. As with any injury, the PRICE treatment regimen should be followed. Swelling control allows for early ROM and VMO activation.[98,102] Gentle pedaling on a stationary bike forward and backward helps increase ROM.

Restoring a normal gait pattern is of particular importance with these patients. They either walk with the leg fully extended or avoid completing full knee extension (ie, lacking the terminal 20 to 30 degrees) during gait; these deviations can increase the chance of dislocating the patella again.[102] Backward walking can help to normalize the gait pattern (the clinician can hold the patient's hands as the patient walks backward). Table 13-23 provides suggested rehabilitation guidelines.

**Clinical Tip**

The clinician needs to remember that lateral step-ups and lunges require a significant amount of VMO muscle activation (85% and 76%, respectively, during electromyography), and these exercises are very effective for increasing strength and muscle endurance.[103]

## Knee Joint Mobilization

A concave tibial plateau and convex femoral condyles are the articulating surfaces of the knee joint. To increase knee flexion, the tibia must glide posteriorly on the femur. To increase knee extension, the tibia needs to glide anteriorly. The patella moves superiorly in the trochlea groove of the femur to achieve full knee extension, and it moves inferiorly to achieve knee flexion.

The quadriceps, hamstrings, ITB, gastrocnemius, and hip adductors should be assessed for muscle length and guarding. Muscle tightness or guarding can result in decreased joint mobility. Soft tissue guarding can limit the muscles' ability to effectively contract.

### *Tibiofemoral Distraction*

There are a few ways to position the patient to perform long-axis tibial distraction (Figure 13-23). Having the patient short sitting is one of the easier ways because the femur is stabilized by the table. The knee is placed in 25 degrees of flexion, and the clinician sits on a stool or squats down facing the patient's lower leg. One hand is placed on the distal femur to stabilize it. The clinician grasps the distal aspect of the tibia and fibula just above the ankle with the other and gently pulls the tibia toward the floor while maintaining the angle. The distraction force will separate the joint space. This position is used for grade I and II mobilizations for pain control.

### *Tibiofemoral Posterior Glide to Increase Flexion*

The patient should be positioned in short sitting at the end of the treatment table. To increase knee flexion, the clinician stands facing the patient and then moves the patient's lower leg to the end of available flexion with one hand placed just above the ankle. The clinician should then gently distract and internally rotate the tibia with one hand and place the other hand on the proximal tibia just lateral to the tibial tuberosity (Figure 13-24). Keeping the elbow straight, the clinician leans into the top hand and applies a posterior glide with medial pressure to the proximal tibia as the distal hand continues to move the lower leg into flexion.

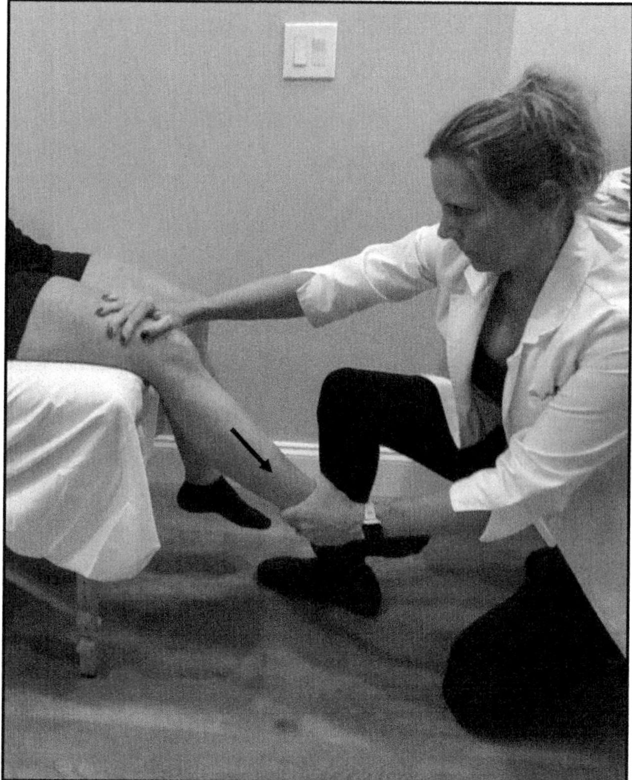

**Figure 13-23.** Tibiofemoral distraction. The clinician gently pulls downward.

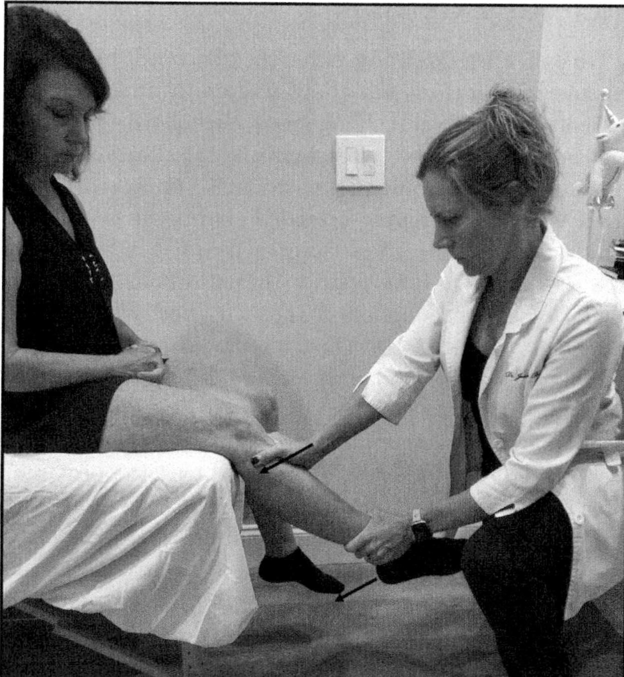

**Figure 13-24.** A tibiofemoral posterior glide to increase knee flexion. The directional force is the same direction as the joint motion (knee flexion) due to the concave tibial surface moving on convex femoral condyles.

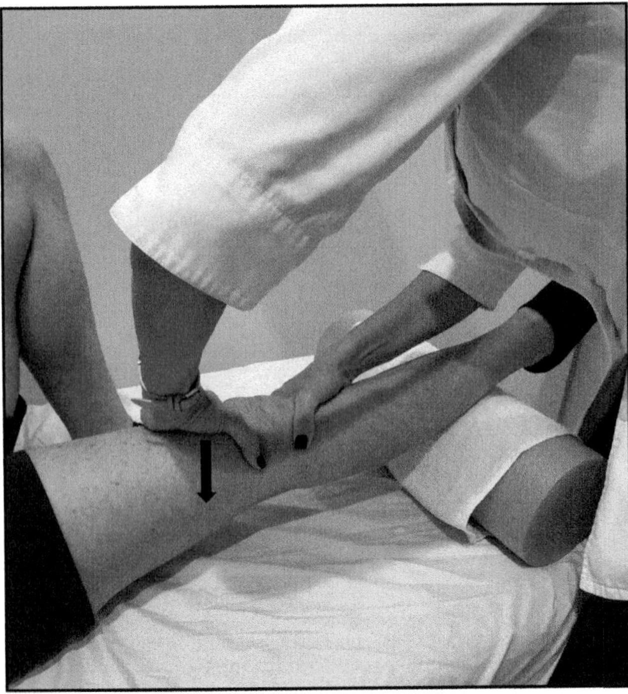

**Figure 13-25.** A posterior femoral glide to increase knee extension. The clinician stabilizes the tibia with the right hand and pushes the femur in the posterior directions with the left hand.

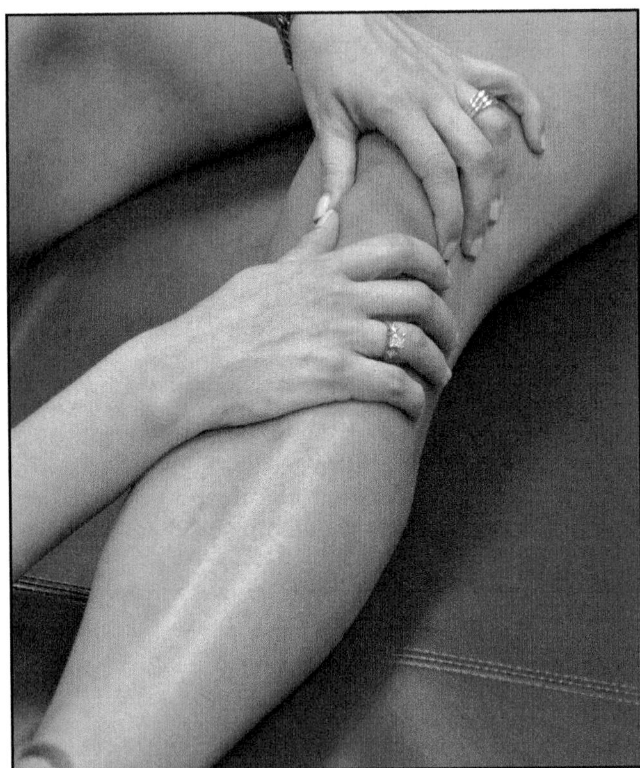

**Figure 13-26.** Patella glides to increase extension and flexion.

## *Femoral Posterior Glide to Increase Extension*

To gain knee extension, either the tibia needs to be glided anteriorly or the femur glided posteriorly. Because some patients cannot tolerate lying prone, the following method may be easiest for both the patient and the clinician.

The patient should be positioned supine with the involved lower extremity extended as straight as possible and a towel roll placed just proximal to the Achilles tendon. The clinician stands next to the patient's leg facing the lateral aspect of the involved knee with both elbows fully extended (Figure 13-25). The table should be lowered to a height to allow for good body mechanics. The web space of one hand is placed proximal to the patella with the palm of the hand on the anterior surface of the distal femur. The web space of the other hand is placed over the proximal tibia (below the joint line) and stabilizes the lower leg. The clinician leans gently into the straight proximal arm, placing a gentle downward force into the femur only. Grade III or IV oscillations are best to use for this technique, so the clinician should gently rock up and down to achieve the mobilization. Ongoing assessment of the patient's symptoms is important; there should not be any report of increased pain.

## *Patella Superior and Inferior Glides*

The patella has to be mobile to obtain normal knee ROM. The patient should be positioned supine with the involved knee as straight as possible; the clinician then assesses the patella to see if it moves freely. The clinician places the fingers of the distal hand around the edges of the patella (Figure 13-26) and gently glides the patella toward the patient's head. The clinician should not push down on the patella because this compresses the patella against the femur, which may cause pain. The patella needs to move superiorly to perform a quadriceps muscle setting contraction.

If the patient has limited patellar motion inferiorly, the patient's knee flexion will be limited. In this case, the patient should sit at the end of the treatment table and flex the involved knee as much as possible. The clinician sits facing the patient's lower leg and places the pads of the fingers on the edge of the superior aspect of the patella. As the knee is passively flexed, a gentle inferior force is applied on the patella as the knee is flexed further. The clinician should avoid compressive pressure into the tibia.

# Management and Treatment for Common Ankle and Foot Pathologies

The therapy team will apply criteria-based therapeutic exercise progressions across the various phases of rehabilitation for common ankle and foot conditions. It is useful for the physical therapist assistant to understand MOI and treatment options for ankle sprains, ankle/foot fractures,

**Table 13-24**

Special Tests for Various Ankle and Foot Pathologies

| Special Test | Possible Pathology if Positive |
|---|---|
| Lower leg compression test (tibia/fibula squeeze test) | Fibula fracture[a] or high ankle sprain |
| Anterior drawer test | ATFL sprain/tear |
| Talar tilt test into inversion | ATFL and/or CFL sprain/tear |
| Talar tilt test into eversion | Deltoid ligament tear |
| Thompson test | Achilles tendon rupture |
| Feiss line test | Various degrees of pes planus or excessive pronation |
| Windlass weight-bearing test | Plantar fasciitis |

[a]Radiography indicated to rule out a possible fracture.

Achilles tendon ruptures, and plantar fasciitis. Special tests targeting structures are initially performed by the physical therapist during the initial evaluation for various ankle and foot pathologies (Table 13-24). Examples of ankle and foot exercises are located at the end of this chapter.

## *Mechanisms of Injury and Signs and Symptoms for Various Ankle Pathologies*

Lateral ankle sprains are a common occurrence in sports. Approximately 2 million ankle sprains occur in the United States each year, and about one-half of those treated in emergency departments are not sports related. The incidence of ankle sprains may be higher than reported because some athletes who participate in organized sports or higher levels of physical activity are not necessarily treated in emergency departments, especially if the injury is not serious. Acute lateral ankle sprains (involving at least the ATFL) account for more than 75% of all ankle sprains, and the remaining 25% are either high/syndesmosis ankle sprains (affecting AITF or PITF ligaments) or medial (affecting the deltoid ligaments) sprains.[104]

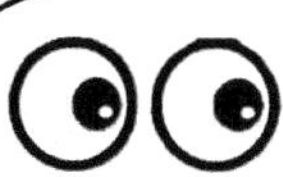

**Eye on the Research: Ankle Sprains**

One meta-analysis of 181 studies found a higher incidence of ankle sprains occurred in women (13.6/1000) compared with men (6.4/1000), with the highest risk activity occurring with indoor court sports. Participants are at a significantly higher risk of sustaining a lateral ankle sprain (vs a syndesmotic or medial ankle sprain).[105]

Another study found that the majority of high ankle sprain injuries in collegiate sports resulted from player contact/collision (most commonly in football, wrestling, and ice hockey) during competition (56.7%). The researchers reviewed 25 different collegiate sports nationwide and found 47.1% of athletes were restricted from sports participation 7 days or more, and 15.8% of injuries resulted in more than 21 days of restricted participation as a result of high ankle sprains. Lateral ankle sprains were more commonly seen in collegiate basketball for both men and women.[106] Both studies noted that lateral ankle sprains were the most common type, and high ankle sprains were associated with longer recovery times.[104-106]

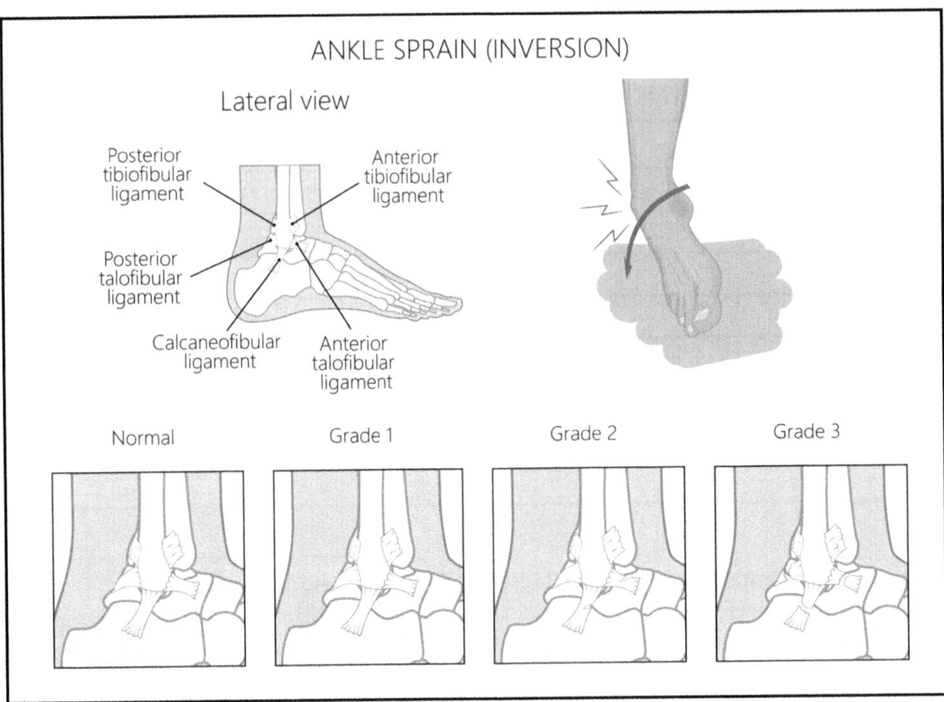


**Figure 13-27.** Inversion ankle sprain grades (Aksanaku/Shutterstock.com).

The most common MOI associated with lateral ankle sprains is a combined motion into ankle inversion and plantar flexion. The ATFL is usually injured first with those motions (Figure 13-27). If the injury is more severe, the peroneal (fibularis) brevis can also be strained because it tries to prevent excessive motion. Inversion ankle sprains commonly occur when an individual steps off a step/curb improperly (especially if wearing high heels), makes sharp changes in direction, turns/pivots, or comes down from a jump or hop. Isolated calcaneal fibular ligament (CFL) sprains are very rare. The CFL can be injured along with the ATFL in more severe sprains (ie, grade II) and when more inversion forces occur during the acute injury. This occurs in approximately 20% of lateral ankle sprains.[107,108] Injury to the PTFL is very rare; this injury only tends to occur when the forces placed on the other ligaments are so extreme that both the ATFL and the CFL tear, which can result in dislocation and/or instability. Disruption of the PTFL rarely occurs because extreme dorsiflexion, not plantar flexion, places the most stress on the ligament.[107,108]

Signs and symptoms are dependent on the severity/grade of the injury (see Figure 13-27). A grade I sprain results in little pain and swelling with minimal to no loss of function or ankle instability. Grade II sprains involve the partial tearing of the ATFL with lateral ankle pain and swelling immediately after the event and ecchymosis presenting 24 to 48 hours later. The patient may report hearing a pop, is often unable to bear weight, has limited movement, and has minimal to moderate joint instability. A grade III sprain involves a complete tear of the ATFL and significant damage (or possibly complete rupture) to the CFL with total loss of function, abnormal joint motion, and ankle instability.[107,108] With grade II or III inversion sprains, the peroneal (fibularis) brevis may be strained and/or the base of the fifth metatarsal partially or totally avulsed due to the extreme amount of inversion force that is placed on the peroneus brevis attachment during injury.

The distal tibiofibular joint (syndesmosis joint) is stabilized by the interosseous membrane and AITF and PITF ligaments (see Figure 13-27 top left). These structures help prevent the separation of the tibia and fibula and act as a shock absorber. Syndesmosis or high ankle sprains account for 11% to 17% of ankle injuries.[109] The most common MOI includes tibial external rotation and/or extreme dorsiflexion,[108] but injury to this joint may also be associated with any other ankle motions. An external rotary force with the foot planted causes injury to the tibiofibular ligaments but typically spares the other structures.[107,109] This mechanism occurs during forward acceleration paired with a quick change of direction. There is also an increased incidence of high ankle sprains associated with player contact during a collision in sports.[106] Regardless of the MOI, high ankle sprains are difficult to manage, and the recovery time and time to return to sport are prolonged. As with any sprain, the severity of the injury is graded, but grade III high ankle sprains are very rare. Signs and symptoms include tenderness with palpation on the anterolateral aspect of the ankle and radiating pain along the syndesmosis reproduced with a compression test of the tibia and fibula. Radiating pain may be experienced when the tibia is stabilized and the foot dorsiflexed and externally rotated forcibly by the clinician. Patients may also report radiating pain upward from the ankle during walking, but swelling and bruising are less common with these sprains. These injuries may be more severe than they appear.[107-109]

Deltoid ligament sprains are extremely rare, but when they do occur, they are often associated with avulsion fractures of the medial malleolus as opposed to ligament tearing because of the strength of this ligament.[110-112] The MOI for deltoid ligament sprains includes ankle dorsiflexion and eversion. Deltoid ligament injuries can result in persistent pain, and the patient may be prone to developing significant foot pronation postinjury.[112]

Ankle fractures are common injuries among people of all ages, but individuals with osteoporosis are more likely to incur a fracture as opposed to a sprain with an ankle injury. Lateral malleolus fractures are the most common type of ankle fracture, accounting for 55% of all ankle fractures. Common causes of fractures include falls (61% of lateral malleolus fractures) followed by sports participation (22%).[112,113] Bimalleolar fractures are the second most common type (Figure 13-28). Complete deltoid ligament tears are associated with lateral malleolar and bimalleolar fractures; approximately 40% of ankle fractures also present with deltoid ligament sprains.[112] Ankle fractures can result from inversion or eversion MOI, and these fractures tend to occur before syndesmosis ligaments rupture.[109] Individuals usually experience immediate swelling, severe pain, and the inability to bear weight.[112]

The Achilles tendon is the strongest tendon in the body; yet, it is one of the most common tendons to rupture. Achilles tendon ruptures are most prevalent in men 20 to 39 years of age, but there has been a significant rise in occurrence in middle-aged men 40 to 59 years old.[114-117] Approximately 82% of all ruptures are sports or exercise related, and the male-to-female ratio is 71.1% to 22.9% for acute ruptures. It is hypothesized that the rise in middle-aged male incidence is likely because of the increase in participation rates in recreational sports. Basketball injuries account for 47% of all acute ruptures in men, and volleyball injuries account for 15% of tendon ruptures. Older adults (in their 60s through 80s) are also prone to Achilles tendon ruptures because of tendon degenerative changes and tendon stiffening.[114-116]

A strong eccentric muscle contraction is the most common MOI for Achilles tendon ruptures. Not all injuries to the Achilles tendon result in a rupture. Total rupture (grade III strain) or varying degrees (grades I or II) of injury are most likely to occur during plyometric activities (eg, jumping) in which a large eccentric loading activity is followed by a ballistic concentric contraction.

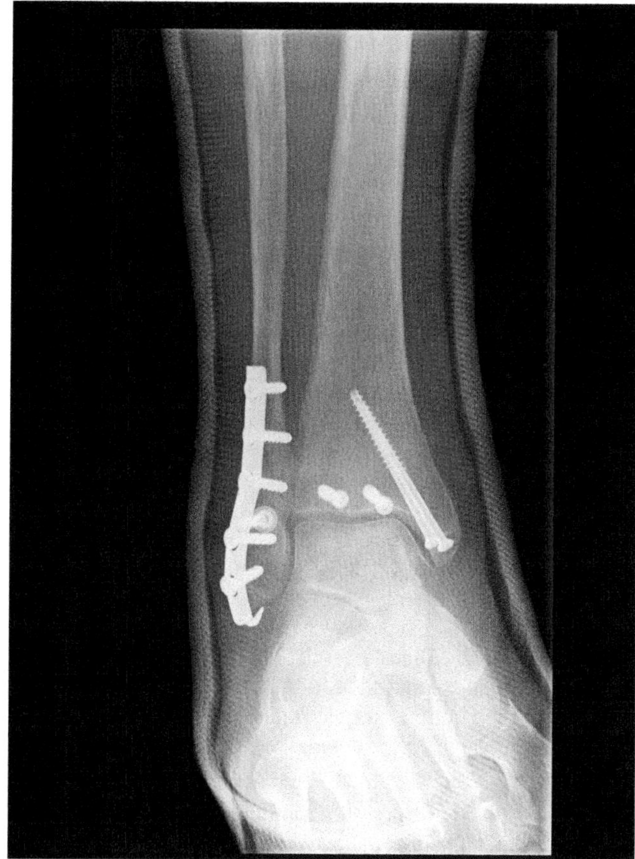

**Figure 13-28.** A bimalleolar fracture (Thomas Schauer/Shutterstock.com).

Achilles tendon pain can be a result of wearing high heels (which increases gastrocnemius/soleus muscle tightness and tendon shortening), running, and/or repetitive jumping/landing during sports-related activities. Mild to moderate symptoms are associated with less severe sprains and include a sudden onset of some degree of pain, swelling and tenderness over the tendon, and pain with heel raises (or resisted plantar flexion). With an acute rupture, the patient may report hearing a popping or snapping sound at the time of the injury and is unable to achieve terminal stance (pushing off) when walking. Other signs and symptoms of a complete rupture may include onset of sharp pain and severe swelling posterior calcaneus, the inability to plantar flex or perform a heel raise, and a positive Thompson test.

**Considerations for the Physical Therapist Assistant: Medication Side Effects and Achilles Tendon Ruptures**

When treating patients with tendon injuries, the physical therapy team should review the patient's medication list for recent or past use (up to 6 months prior) of fluoroquinolones. These antibiotic medications are used to treat illnesses such as respiratory infections, gastrointestinal infections (ie, diverticulitis), and/or urinary tract infections. Some examples are Cipro (ciprofloxacin), Factive (gemifloxacin mesylate), Levaquin (levofloxacin), Avelox (moxifloxacin hydrochloride), and Noroxin (norfloxacin). There is a growing body of evidence indicating that fluoroquinolones can cause pathologic lesions in tendon tissue, in some cases resulting in a complete rupture. Evidence suggests that these adverse effects can occur within hours of beginning treatment and up to months after discontinuing the use of these drugs.[116] An additional medication-based consideration arises for patients who are taking corticosteroids. Low-dose corticosteroids have also been associated with an increased risk of Achilles tendon rupture. Concurrent use of fluoroquinolones appears to increase the risk further. Patients taking both fluoroquinolones and corticosteroids have a significantly higher risk of Achilles tendon rupture than those taking neither medication.[116]

Clinicians should use increased caution when developing a treatment plan for patients with a history of taking these medications. Recovery from tendon injury associated with these medications may be slower and requires a less aggressive approach early during rehabilitation compared with other types of tendinopathy. Eccentric training regimens are commonly used for the treatment of tendinopathy; these exercises result in the tendon being subjected to a sustained physiological load. Although eccentric exercise programs lead to successful outcomes in the majority of active individuals with tendinopathy, more sedentary patients may not respond as well to the increased loads associated with eccentric training. Additionally, loading a tendon with eccentric exercise may not be the best option for treating fluoroquinolone-induced tendon conditions during the early stages. Patients with fluoroquinolone-related tendinopathy may benefit from a 2-phase approach.[116] The initial treatment includes a period of bracing and support to allow the tendon to recover from damage caused by the fluoroquinolone followed by a period of gradual, progressive loading.[116]

## *Ankle Injuries: Conservative and Postoperative Management*

Because ankle injuries are common, knowledge of the anatomy and the static and dynamic stabilizers of the ankle will help the physical therapist assistant select the most appropriate treatment interventions. General guidelines and progressions are outlined in the following sections. The assistant should implement and modify interventions based on the patient's progress and goals, the physician's protocol, and the physical therapist's POC.

### *Conservative Rehabilitation Management for Ankle Sprains*

Conservative rehabilitation is more common than surgical interventions for ankle sprains. Research indicates that when comparing conservative treatments with surgical interventions for ankle instability, there was no significant difference between long-term outcomes.[108] However, conservative treatment resulted in better ROM and allowed the patient to return to work/sport sooner.[108] Studies indicate that early functional mobility and neuromuscular training are significantly more effective than immobilization (ie, casting); patients who received these interventions early returned to work/sport sooner and had a lower incidence of reinjury.[108]

The severity of injury is the leading factor in determining the timeline for return to work/sport. Grade I injuries present with no instability, so these patients can usually return to their normal activities in a few (about 5 to 7) days. Grade II and III ankle sprains do exhibit joint instability, so temporary joint protection is needed (ie, taping, elastic wrap, or bracing) during the early phases of rehabilitation, but it is important to implement ROM early.

Table 13-25 provides suggested guidelines for ankle sprains across the rehabilitation phases. During the acute stage of healing, the focus is on joint protection and controlling pain and swelling for the first 24 to 48 hours. With grade II and III sprains, the patient will use crutches and is usually permitted to perform WBAT; AROM can be initiated early but only within pain-free ranges. Ankle pumps (dorsiflexion/plantar flexion) are best performed several times a day with the involved ankle elevated to help reduce swelling. The patient can be progressed to tracing the alphabet with the foot and ankle with the leg also elevated to increase ROM and continue to control swelling. Ankle inversion tends to be limited by pain early in recovery, and dorsiflexion and eversion should be emphasized. Pain-free submaximal isometrics can be performed with the ankle in a neutral position only to avoid stressing the healing ligaments.

During the moderate protection phase, ankle dorsiflexion and eversion strength and muscle endurance training (through full pain-free ROM) should be prioritized. Because plantar flexion and inversion increase the stress on the ATFL, OKC strengthening in these directions is not initiated until late in the subacute phase so the ligament has time to heal. However, CKC strengthening and balance activities are encouraged because these activities facilitate active pronation and supination. The tibialis posterior helps to maintain the medial arch during supination, and the peroneus (fibularis) brevis and longus play an important role in supporting the transverse arch. Once swelling and pain are controlled, the next goal is to regain full ROM as early as possible to reduce the risk of joint dysfunction. Gaining full dorsiflexion is extremely important to restore normal talocrural joint function. Gastrocnemius and soleus stretching can begin in a NWB position but should be progressed to standing or using a slant board as soon as possible. Limited posterior glide of the talus may occur in

**Table 13-25**

Conservative Management: Suggested Rehabilitation Guidelines for Ankle Sprains[a]

| Acute Stage/Phase 1<br>Maximum Protection Phase (Days 1 to 4 for Grade I, up to 14 Days for Grade II, up to 4 Weeks for Grade III) | Subacute Stage/Phase 2<br>Moderate Protection (Grade I Days 4 to 14, Grade II up to 6 Weeks, Grade III up to 2 Months) | Return to Function/Phase 3<br>Minimal Protection<br>(2 to 6 Weeks for Grade I to II, up to 3 to 4 Months for Grade III) |
|---|---|---|
| Goals<br>• Joint protection, control pain and swelling, PRICE<br>• Progress to full pain-free ROM<br>• Maintain hip, knee, and core strength<br>Exercises<br>• OKC: AROM in pain-free ROM (ie, dorsiflexion, eversion, initiate alphabet if appropriate), toe curls/crunches and ankle eversion with a towel on the floor, submaximal pain-free isometrics in neutral position only for dorsiflexion, plantar flexion, eversion, and inversion<br>• CKC: Mini-squats, seated heel raises (for soleus), walking in the pool<br>• Stretches: OKC gastrocnemius/soleus progress to CKC, plantar fasciitis, and hip/knee stretches<br>• Additional exercises: Core stabilization, OKC hip and knee strengthening, CKC strengthening and balance on uninvolved leg | Goals<br>• Full ROM all directions, pain free (use joint mobilization to aid in the process)<br>• Progress to FWB and normalize gait; reduce brace use to none as tolerated<br>• Restore proprioception and neuromuscular control<br>Exercises<br>• OKC: Increase resistance with weights around the foot, with resistance bands, or isokinetic machine for ankle strengthening dorsiflexion and eversion in pain-free ROM progress speeds as tolerated to resisted full ROM, initiate with plantar flexion if tolerated based on patient presentation; ankle D1/D2 flexion/extension with manual resistance or resistance bands<br>• CKC: BAPS board for ROM seated increasing size of ball for more range (progress to standing), heel raises knee straight and flexed, forefoot raises (progress to SLS eccentric then concentric contractions), and toe and heel walking; hip/knee strengthening: Step-ups/downs forward, lateral, backward 4- to 6-in steps, resistance band side stepping, and backward walking<br>• Stretches: Achilles tendon stretches | Goals<br>• Increase pain-free functional strength in preparation for return to activities/sport<br>• Introduce pain-free dynamic and plyometric activities; progress as tolerated back to prior level of function<br>• Begin running program with gradual increases and varied surfaces; running patterns<br>Exercises<br>• OKC: Resistance bands (various band resistance) for strength and muscle endurance for dorsiflexion, eversion, and PNF D1/D2, isokinetic machine high and low speeds if available.<br>• CKC: Light jumping with controlled landing progress to hopping pain free; add plyometrics as tolerated pain free; progress until running, jumping, and hopping are pain free. |

*(continued)*

**Table 13-25 (continued)**

Conservative Management: Suggested Rehabilitation Guidelines for Ankle Sprains[a]

| Acute Stage/Phase 1<br>Maximum Protection Phase (Days 1 to 4 for Grade I, up to 14 Days for Grade II, up to 4 Weeks for Grade III) | Subacute Stage/Phase 2<br>Moderate Protection (Grade I Days 4 to 14, Grade II up to 6 Weeks, Grade III up to 2 Months) | Return to Function/Phase 3<br>Minimal Protection<br>(2 to 6 Weeks for Grade I to II, up to 3 to 4 Months for Grade III) |
|---|---|---|
| Balance: Weight shifting all directions pain free; progress to partial step-up balance<br>Aerobics: UBE, stationary bike minimal resistance, deep water running (with aqua vest) | Balance: Rocker board (used anterior/posterior and laterally), foam eyes open/closed, progress to SLS on firm to foam/mini-trampoline/BOSU Balance Trainer, maintain calf raises, and add perturbations and upper extremity tasks<br>Aerobics: Stationary bike, treadmill (with no limping) progress to light jogging or elliptical (forward/backward) | Balance: SLS on firm to foam/mini-trampoline, BAPS board, and BOSU Balance Trainer eyes open/closed; add perturbations and upper extremity tasks; hop stabilization all directions<br>Aerobics: Progress to treadmill running and progress to level ground running, progress to sand or uneven surface running; add specific cutting drills and acceleration and deceleration drills.<br>Return-to-sport suggested tests<br>• Star Excursion Balance Test: For dynamic balance<br>• Side hop test: Perform 10 lateral hops as fast as possible, hopping a distance of >30 cm<br>Strength should be >85% of the uninvolved ankle.<br>Note: The patient may continue to need support (taping/bracing) with return to sport; ligament healing can take 6 to 12 months. |

[a]Progression and time frames depend on the severity of injury and how well pain and swelling are controlled. The return-to-function phase should target the patient's prior level of function, but balance exercises should be included for all patient populations.

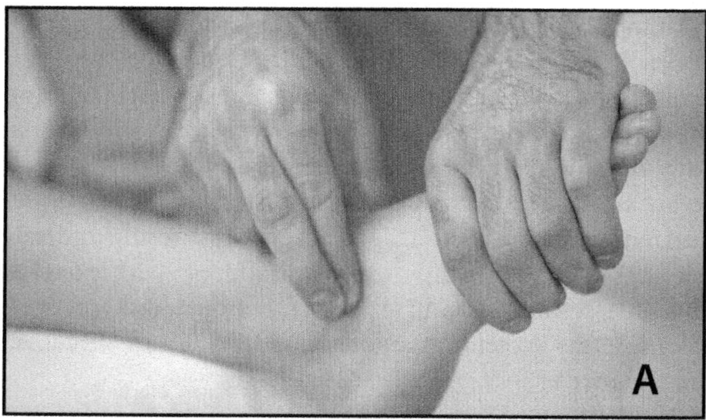


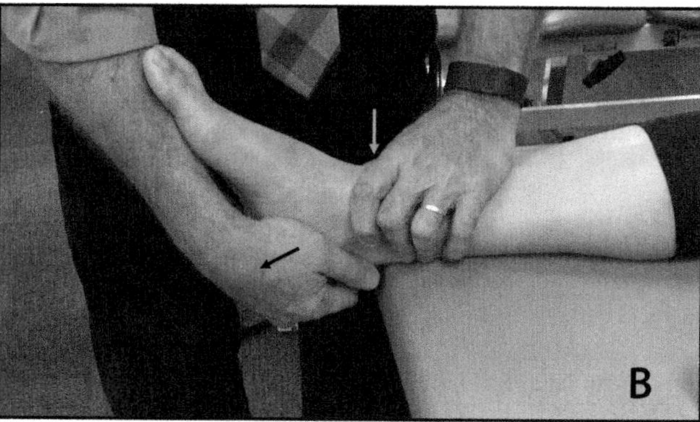


**Figure 13-29.** Posterior glide of the talus to increase ankle dorsiflexion. (A) Locating the talus. The talus can be palpated just anteriorly to the tibia and fibula. The talus can be palpated when inverting and everting the ankle to reconfirm its location (wavebreakmedia/Shutterstock.com). (B) Performing an anterior-to-posterior glide of the talus. The clinician supports the foot and dorsiflexes the patient's foot until slight resistance is felt and then applies a gentle caudal glide on the calcaneus (black arrow). The clinician then glides the anterior aspect of the talus posteriorly with the web space of the proximal hand (gray arrow).

## Box 13-2

### Proprioceptive Neuromuscular Facilitation Ankle Strengthening

- D1 flexion: Start in plantar flexion and eversion with toes flexed and end in dorsiflexion and inversion with toes extended.
- D1 extension: Start in dorsiflexion and inversion with toes extended and end in plantar flexion and eversion with toes flexed.
- D2 flexion: Start in plantar flexion and inversion with toes flexed and end in dorsiflexion and eversion with toes extended.
- D2 extension: Start in dorsiflexion and eversion with toes extended and end in plantar flexion and inversion with toes flexed.

patients with lateral ankle sprains, which will restrict dorsiflexion.[118] Performing an anterior to posterior talocrural glide joint mobilization technique can increase ankle dorsiflexion and reduce pain.[118]

Although joint mobilizations may be included in the physical therapist's POC, individual state practice acts indicate if an assistant is able to perform them. The physical therapist is responsible for delegating the task to the assistant when appropriate. To perform a posterior talocrural glide joint mobilization, the patient's leg should be supported on the table with the ankle off the edge. The clinician stands on the patient's affected side and positions the ankle in the resting position (about 10 degrees of plantar flexion) or the pain-free end range of available motion. The clinician palpates for the talus first (Figure 13-29A), then places the palmar part of their web space, using the hand closer to the patient's head, over the talus. The opposite forearm supports the patient's foot to maintain proper joint position, and the fingers firmly grasp the sides of the calcaneus (Figure 13-29B). The clinician then gently applies a caudal distraction of the calcaneus and passively dorsiflexes the ankle until slight resistance is felt (see Figure 13-29B). With the proximal hand, the clinician gently presses the talus posteriorly with gentle oscillations or a sustained hold. The number of oscillations and/or hold times should be determined by the physical therapist. The clinician should feel the talus "give" slightly, and the patient should not complain of pain during the treatment. Passive motion along with the posterior glide can be performed simultaneously. After the technique, the patient should perform active dorsiflexion to determine the effectiveness of the treatment.

Neuromuscular training should be initiated as early and safely as possible during this phase.[108,119] PNF ankle strengthening (Box 13-2) can be performed in pain-free ranges and progressed to full ROM with more resistance. To manually resist the flexion patterns, the clinician's palm should be placed on the dorsum of the foot with the fingers extended to resist toe extension. To manually resist extension patterns, wrap the hand around the metatarsal heads (ball of the foot) with the fingers extended across the plantar surface of the foot. Resistance bands can be added once the patient learns the patterns. The combined use of resistance bands and proprioceptive exercises reduces the risk of reinjury; these are effective tools to improve functional performance.[119]

During the final rehabilitation phase, small BOS balance activities (ie, tandem stance and Romberg tests) with eyes opened and closed on varied surfaces, single-leg balance training, and hopping stabilization activities can be introduced and progressed based on the patient's prior level of function. When working with athletes, hop stabilization can be used to improve stability and balance during dynamic activities.[119] During this test, the clinician must observe to ensure proper mechanics (vertical shin with no genu valgus) are used during hopping skills. The trunk should be positioned with the core engaged and a straight spine, with flexion occurring at the hips, not the lumbar spine. The foot should be positioned with the toes straight ahead and the heel down with the ankle dorsiflexed during

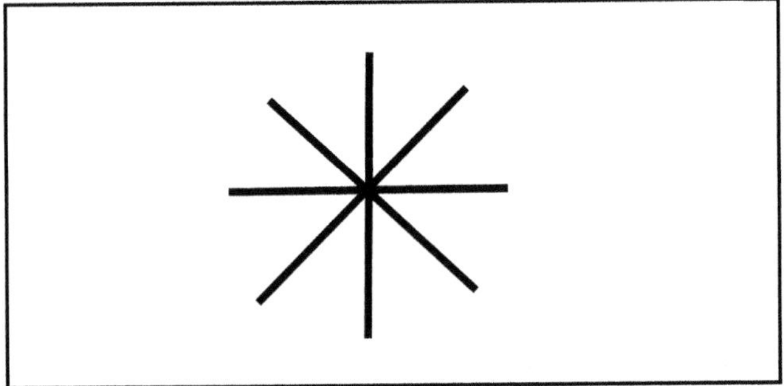

**Figure 13-30.** Tape pattern for the SEBT.

the initial takeoff and final landing. Correct positioning is critical for joint proprioception and functional performance as one accelerates and decelerates during hopping activities. A progression sequence for this activity includes the following: (1) take a small hop forward, control, and hold the landing; (2) take a small hop forward (control and hold the landing), then add another small hop forward, and then add a small hop backward and hold; (3) progress to sequential hops forward and back; and (4) then progress to sequential hops of 5 on one leg and then on the other while taking off and landing on a line painted on the floor. This progression improves strength, muscle endurance, balance, proprioception, and performance. As the individual improves, larger jumps and varied directions (lateral or diagonal) can be added.

Strength, performance, and balance tests should be performed before an athlete returns to sports. The side hop test and the Star Excursion Balance Test (SEBT) are tools to assess the patient's balance and functional performance. The patient's ability to perform well on these tests indicates regained functional ability and a reduced risk for reinjury. The skills performed in these tests can be used as part of the rehabilitation program during the return-to-function phase.[119]

When performing a side hop test, the patient hops laterally on the involved limb for 10 repetitions as fast as possible and then repeats the test on the uninvolved leg. Each hop must be greater than 11.8 in (30 cm) for 10 repetitions and performed as fast as possible. Each trial is timed with a stopwatch and then compared to determine if there is a difference in time between legs.[119]

When performing the SEBT, the patient stands barefoot in the middle where lines on the floor intersect (Figure 13-30). While standing on the involved lower extremity, the patient reaches out as far as possible with the opposite leg in each direction (along the line) and lightly touches down with the toes. Record the distance achieved in each direction. The patient returns to the starting position and assumes bilateral standing in the center following a reach in each direction. The test is then performed on the uninvolved side. Difficulty maintaining balance or achieving an appropriate distance (equal to that of the uninvolved leg) in any direction can be used to identify individuals/athletes who are at greater risk of ankle instability and/or lower extremity injuries (eg, ACL injury).[119] Test results indicate deficits that the therapy team can address with exercise, balance retraining, and graded functional task progressions. Other screenings and tests for athletes are discussed in Chapter 23.

## Conservative and Postoperative Rehabilitation Management for Ankle Fractures

Treatment and prognosis for ankle fractures are primarily dependent on whether the fracture is stable (ie, nondisplaced lateral malleolus or base of the fifth metacarpal avulsion) or unstable (ie, bimalleolar or trimalleolar fractures). Assuming medical clearance, patients with stable fractures can gradually increase weight-bearing status at 4 to 6 weeks and may progressively wean off the brace once FWB is achieved. Unstable fractures require surgical interventions to stabilize the fracture site, and surgeons typically perform ORIF with plates and/or screws. In the case of unstable fractures, FWB may be delayed up to 10 to 14 weeks, especially with grade III ligament tears and repair. Weight-bearing status and time frames vary significantly between surgeons; the assistant should follow the physician's protocol and POC. Most patients are placed in a boot, splinted, braced, or casted after an ankle fracture.[111,112]

Older patients or those with comorbidities tend to have a poorer prognosis after an ankle fracture. There is a 1-year mortality rate of 12% postoperatively for those who are 65 years and older, with an increase up to 50% for those who are older than 95 years old. Full recovery for postoperative fractures may take up to 1 to 2 years.[111]

Dorsiflexion and plantar flexion may be encouraged initially, but inversion and eversion are usually contraindicated early in the rehabilitation process because these motions are consistent with the common MOI causing the fractures. The patient should be instructed on normal gait mechanics, with an emphasis on maintaining prescribed weight-bearing precautions. The exercise progressions described for persons with ankle sprains are consistent with those applied after ankle fractures; however, the phase timelines are significantly longer after fractures. The assistant must consider the patient's prior level of function when progressing mobility and exercise interventions.

**Considerations for the Physical Therapist Assistant**

The assistant should be aware of possible hardware loosening or signs of infection after ORIF. The signs and symptoms of hardware loosening include increased pain and/or swelling, crepitus, and/or abnormal motion, especially with ankle strengthening. The signs and symptoms of infection include redness along the incision or around the joint, pain, swelling, and warmth to the touch. If either of these are suspected, the assistant should stop treatment immediately and notify the therapist because these may require immediate physician attention.

## *Conservative and Postoperative Rehabilitation Management for Achilles Tendon Injuries*

Achilles tendon ruptures can be surgically repaired or conservatively immobilized, and there is no clear consensus as to which treatment protocol has the best outcome. Nonsurgical patients are immobilized in a walking boot with a 1.5-cm (or approximately 0.5-in) wedge that keeps the patient in slight plantar flexion for 6 weeks with unrestricted weight bearing.[115] Both interventions have advantages and disadvantages.

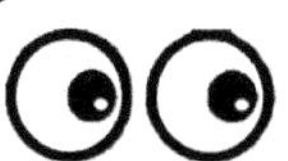

**Eye on the Research: Achilles Tendon Rehabilitation Management**

A 2019 review reported that the rerupture rate after surgical Achilles tendon repair (5%) was less than the nonsurgical rate (7%), but there was only a small difference of about 1.6% between the 2 interventions. The postoperative risk of complications (ie, DVT, infection, or nerve injury) varied from 16% to 21%. Researchers reported a decline in surgical repair interventions over the past decade due to comparable outcomes between the 2 options.[117]

Two other studies found no difference in the rerupture rate between postoperative or conservative interventions with early or late weight bearing; however, early weight bearing was associated with earlier return to work and ADLs.[115,117] One study reported that early FWB and ROM postoperatively were safe and effective.[115] There was no significant difference in the rerupture rate when early ROM and accelerated functional rehabilitation programs were implemented, and these accelerated programs resulted in increased strength and improved function.[115,117]

Most physicians have their own protocols regarding weight-bearing status, the angle of plantar flexion set in a controlled ankle motion walker or boot, and the amount of ROM that is permitted. These protocols should be strictly followed to protect the Achilles tendon. The physical therapist assistant should refer to the healing times and principles of tendon tissue healing for conservative or operative Achilles ruptures. Pain and swelling should be controlled using modalities as needed during the initial phase of rehabilitation. Table 13-26 provides suggested rehabilitation guidelines for these patients.

Prescribed weight-bearing status is very variable. Nonoperative patients may be NWB for the first 2 weeks, whereas some postoperative patients may be permitted WBAT. Weight bearing is advanced based on the physician's protocol, and the angle of plantar flexion in the brace is gradually decreased to neutral usually by week 6 to 8. Patients are progressed to FWB and weaned from use of the boot between 6 and 8 weeks after surgery. Nonoperative patients may take more than 8 weeks to achieve FWB and a normalized gait pattern. All patients should be reminded to avoid making sudden, ballistic movements on the involved lower extremity and to avoid aggressive stretching into dorsiflexion and full active plantar flexion contractions at least through week 8.[115,117]

Patients can usually perform active plantar flexion and dorsiflexion (with the boot off), but the range is often limited to no more than neutral for the first 2 to 4 weeks. Pain-free inversion and eversion can be performed with the foot in slight plantar flexion. Submaximal pain-free isometrics can be initiated in a protected range during phase 1.[117]

**Considerations for the Physical Therapist Assistant**

The criteria to progress the patient from one phase to another is dependent on the rate of tissue healing, pain level, amount of swelling, and the patient's response to exercise. Careful monitoring of the patient's exercise performance is very important during weeks 6 through 14 to reduce the risk of rerupture. It may take anywhere from 6 to 8 months for nonoperative patients to return to sports, whereas patients with operative repairs may return sooner.[115,117]

The highest risk of rerupture is between 8 and 14 weeks, so only low-velocity and controlled activities should be performed during this period. During phases 2 and 3, patients should be progressed gradually because of tissue healing constraints. It may take up to 6 to 8 months for nonoperative athletes to return to sports after Achilles tendon ruptures.[115,117]

## Table 13-26

### Suggested Rehabilitation Guidelines After Achilles Tendon Ruptures

| Acute Stage/Phase 1<br>Maximum Protection (Day 1 to 6 Weeks) | Subacute Stage/Phase 2<br>Moderate Protection (6 to 12 Weeks) | Return to Function/Phase 3<br>Minimal Protection (12 to 16+ Weeks) |
|---|---|---|
| Goals<br>• Tendon protection, control pain and swelling, and PRICE; abide by weight-bearing restrictions<br>• Maintain core, hip strength for both lower extremities, and knee strength for uninvolved side; knee ROM and strengthening in CAM for the involved side<br>• Initiate pain-free ROM to neutral with ankle dorsiflexion and submaximal isometrics as per physician's protocol<br>Exercises<br>• OKC: Pain-free AROM all directions out of CAM; after about week 2, toe curl towel crunches or marble pick-ups, pain-free submaximal ankle inversion/eversion isometrics<br>• CKC: Single-leg heel raises, partial squats on uninvolved leg but hold on for balance and safety; pool exercises as per weight-bearing restrictions and dorsiflexion not past neutral<br>• Stretching: Hips; *avoid* gastrocnemius/soleus stretches in CKC<br>• Additional exercises: Core strengthening, OKC hip strength for both lower extremities; knee strengthening uninvolved side; knee ROM and strengthening in CAM for involved side<br>Aerobics: UBE, stationary bike in CAM no resistance, deep water running with aqua vest (after wound heals) | Goals<br>• Progress ROM to 15 degrees dorsiflexion to 50 degrees plantar flexion by week 10 to 12 to progress to phase 3<br>• FWB and walking progressed to no use of CAM and normalized gait<br>• Uncompensated squats to 30 degrees of knee flexion and controlled SLS for > 10 seconds<br>Note: Patient at higher risk of rerupture during this phase. *Avoid* ballistic movements; controlled motion/exercise only.<br>Exercises<br>• OKC: Active ankle ROM, pain-free ankle strengthening with resistance bands all directions, manual resistance D1/D2 flexion/extension; knee strengthening on the involved side<br>• CKC: Pain-free seated heel raises, BAPS, partial ROM for squats, lunges, side stepping; initiate 2-in step-ups/downs at week 12 to 14 and pain free<br>• Stretches: Seated gentle gastrocnemius/soleus stretching progress to standing<br>• Additional exercises: Progress core and bilateral hip strengthening in OKC and CKC within parameters<br>Balance: Static balance exercises bilateral standing, then progress to Romberg, then on foam/rocker board, and then SLS on firm surface first and progress; perform eyes opened and closed<br>Aerobics: Progress to elliptical and walking progression on treadmill, no elevation | Goals: Get physician clearance to progress and return to sport/work<br>• Uncompensated squatting to 70 degrees at about week 16 or 18 (nonoperative).<br>• Criteria to return to sport/work: Pain-free full ROM, minimal joint swelling, 5/5 MMT, jump/hop tests at 90% compared with uninvolved and pain-free, sport-related skills.<br>Note: Progressing to more dynamic/plyometric activities may vary due to operative (12 to 14 weeks) or nonoperative interventions (16 to 20 weeks).<br>Exercises<br>• OKC: Continue with increasing resistance bands difficulty for all directions; work muscle strength and endurance<br>• CKC: SLS heel raises are progressed from 2 legs concentric involved leg eccentric to SLS concentric/eccentric heel raises; easy, small jumps, progress to alternating feet before hopping on involved leg; start with low-velocity, single-plane activities and progress to higher velocity and then to multiplane activities with good control<br>Balance: Progress from phase 2 and challenge patients with caution<br>Aerobics: Easy jogging on treadmill progress to straight-line running on ground as symptoms dictate |

CAM = controlled ankle movement.

## *Mechanisms of Injury and Signs and Symptoms for Foot Pathologies*

Plantar fasciitis is the most common source of foot pain, and it occurs in more than 1 million people in the United States each year.[21,120-122] It affects individuals of all ages and is found in both athletic and nonathletic populations. Plantar fasciitis was considered a chronic inflammatory condition, but current research indicates that it is more likely a degenerative process.[122,123] There is an increased risk of plantar fasciitis because the amount of ankle dorsiflexion decreases in nonathletic individuals. (Achilles tendon tightness is present in 80% of the cases.[120,122]) Seventy percent of people who are nonathletic and have plantar fasciitis are overweight.[122] Approximately 10% of runners report experiencing plantar fasciitis; it is the third most common musculoskeletal injury in runners.[21,121] Wearing improper footwear, overtraining (or overuse), and poor running mechanics are contributing factors for developing this condition.[21,123] Excessive pronation is a risk factor for plantar fasciitis.[121,122] Excessive pronation is caused by talar flexion and adduction, which create an increase in calcaneal eversion and flattening of the medial arch in standing, thus increasing tension of the plantar fascia.[121] Patients complaining of plantar fasciitis appear to have excessive pronation statically (81% to 86%), but there is conflicting evidence if there is any association between static pronation and what occurs during dynamic foot motion.[122]

Individuals commonly report a sharp pain located at the proximal attachment on the plantar surface of the calcaneus. Pain occurs with the first few steps after getting out of bed in the morning or after a long period of rest (eg, a long car ride). The pain usually subsides after a few minutes of walking but can get worse with prolonged standing or weight bearing later in the day.[21,120-123]

The plantar fascia prevents the separation of the calcaneus and the metatarsals as it maintains the medial longitudinal arch. When the MTP joints extend during the propulsive or preswing (heel off) phase of the gait cycle, the plantar fascia acts like a tight cable and shortens the distance between the calcaneus and metatarsals as it elevates the medial longitudinal arch; this is referred to as the **windlass mechanism** (Figure 13-31).[21] The windlass test assesses for plantar fasciitis. To perform the test in a NWB position, the ankle is placed in a neutral position; the clinician then passively extends the great toe at the MTP joint. The clinician palpates the plantar fascia where it attaches to the calcaneus. The test is considered positive if heel pain is reproduced. To perform the test in weight bearing, the patient stands on a stool with weight evenly distributed on both feet and the metatarsal heads just off the edge of the stool. The clinician will passively extend the great toe; if this elicits pain, the test is positive.[120] These tests have a specificity rate of 100% (the ability of a test to correctly identify plantar fasciitis) but a low sensitivity rate of 32% (limited ability to effectively rule out plantar fasciitis as the only cause of symptoms).[120]

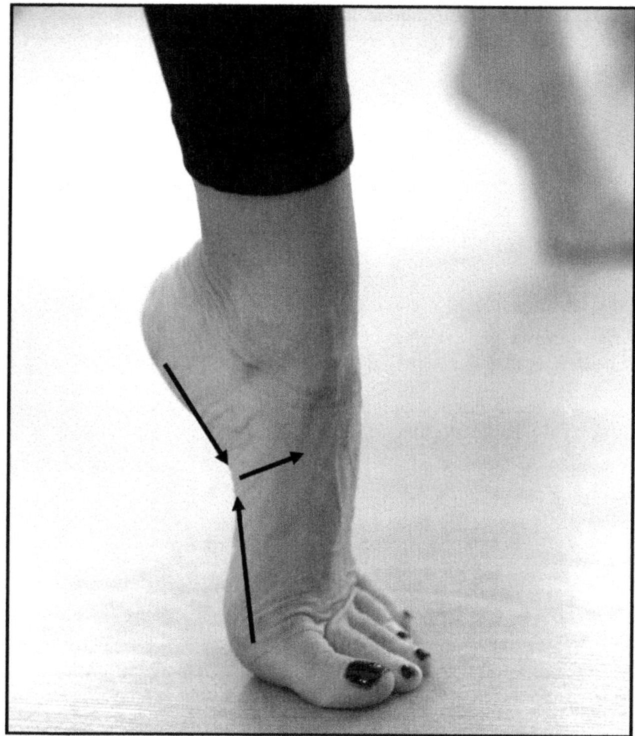

**Figure 13-31.** Windlass mechanism: The arch is lifted as the plantar fascia shortens (Angela Bragato/Shutterstock.com).

Foot fractures can occur due to a traumatic event or overuse. Calcaneal and talar fractures usually occur due to falling or jumping from a height (eg, off a roof). Stress fractures are microscopic cracks in bone (common in the feet) that occur when the bone is unable to handle the loads or stresses placed on it. Stress fractures are commonly seen in athletic and military populations due to repetitive overuse activities such as running and marching. These fractures are usually seen in the second or third metatarsals (17% to 35% occurrence), the calcaneus (21% to 28% occurrence) and navicular bones, and/or the sesamoid bones of the great toe.[124]

Patients report pain with palpation over the site of the fracture and a dull achy pain (occasionally sharp in some patients) that is worse in weight bearing and diminished in NWB. The presence and amount of swelling is dependent on the location of the fracture. With metatarsal fractures, swelling is located on the dorsum of the foot over the metatarsals.[124]

## *Conservative Management for Plantar Fasciitis*

The APTA clinical practice guidelines–recommended treatments include plantar fascia stretching, gastrocnemius/soleus stretching, manual therapy, night splints, and the use of a heel lift and/or taping to support the medial arch (especially during the first week to 10 days).[120-122] Low-dye taping using athletic tape is illustrated in Figure 13-32. Kinesiotaping techniques have also been used to reduce plantar fasciitis pain. Soft tissue mobilization to the

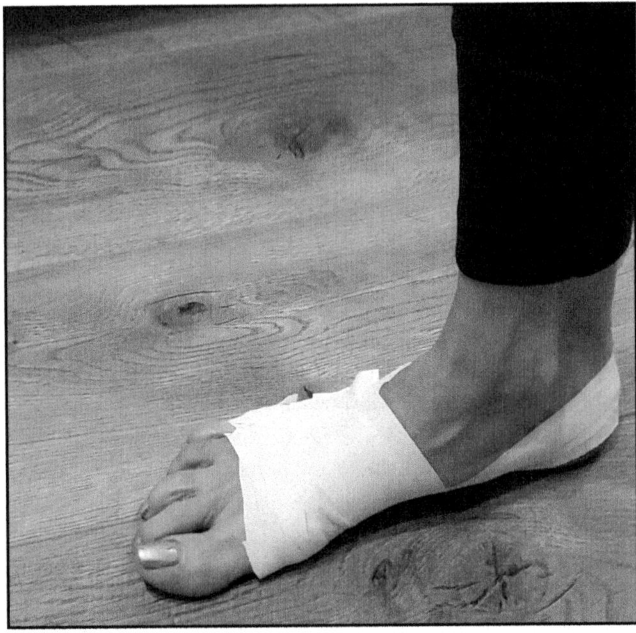

**Figure 13-32.** Low-dye taping for plantar fasciitis. Taping unloads the tension of the plantar fascia by stabilizing the calcaneus and supporting the arch.

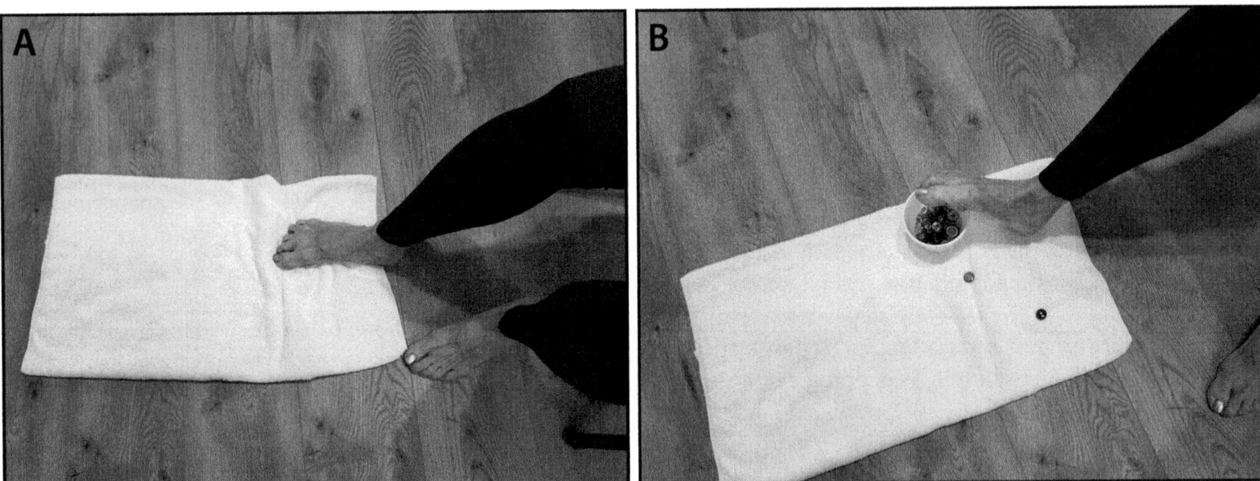

**Figure 13-33.** Exercises for plantar fasciitis. (A) Towel crunches. Strengthens the intrinsic muscles of the foot. (B) Marble pickups.

gastrocnemius/soleus complex to improve calf flexibility is recommended. Strengthening the intrinsic muscles of the foot may help support the arch. Picking up marbles with the toes or toe crunches with a towel (Figure 13-33) target those muscles. Ankle strengthening and balance exercises addressing specific muscle weaknesses should be implemented. A low-level laser can reduce patients' pain.[120] The guidelines report that ultrasound was not effective in reducing plantar fascia pain.[120]

Patients who stand for prolonged periods of time should be instructed to rotate their shoes often during the week. Rocker bottom–type shoes with an orthotic insert are helpful in controlling foot pain.[120] Patients who are obese should be encouraged to lose weight through exercise and diet; this education must be provided in a respectful manner.[120,122]

If patients do not get relief from physical therapy, a physician may decide to inject corticosteroids at the point of pain. Several studies have reported that extracorporeal shock wave therapy has also shown good results in reducing patients' pain and improving function over time.[123,125] Extracorporeal shock wave therapy is a noninvasive treatment that is Food and Drug Administration approved for use on chronic plantar fasciitis, Achilles tendonitis, tennis elbow, and other tendon conditions. This treatment creates new tissue cells in the damaged area, essentially "jump-starting" healing that gradually continues over days and weeks.[123,125]

## Conservative Management for Stress Fractures

During the acute phase, clinicians should follow the PRICE principle. Stress fractures take 6 to 12 weeks to heal depending on the severity and location of the fracture and the age of the patient. The physician may suggest modifying the weight-bearing status (ie, crutches, walker, and protected weight bearing) or prescribe a controlled ankle motion walker/boot to promote proper bone healing. OKC ROM, stretching, and strengthening for the entire lower quarter are recommended during phase 1 (day 1 through week 3 to 6). Patients should be progressed to WBAT per the POC and the physician's guidelines.

Modifying activities (ie, discontinue high- to moderate-impact activities) and transitioning to limited or NWB exercises (upper bike ergometer, stationary bike, swimming, or deep water running) are indicated to minimize symptoms while maintaining cardiovascular endurance. There should be a gradual return to the patient's prior level of function based on swelling and pain response to exercise.

During the second phase (week 3 to 6 to week 8 to 10), the patient can continue to progress to pain-free FWB once cleared by the physician. CKC exercises can be introduced, and the patient should be monitored for pain and swelling as these activities are increased. The criteria to progress to phase 3 should include the ability to complete single-leg hopping, 5/5 gastrocnemius strength, and the ability to walk or light jog with minimal to no pain or gait deviations.

Plyometrics and running can be introduced during phase 3 (week 6 to 12) as long as there is minimal to no pain or swelling during or after activities. The goal of this phase is to return the patient to their prior level of function, work, or sports participation.

## Pediatric Lower Quarter Orthopedic Conditions

A physical therapist assistant may see a variety of diagnoses when treating pediatric patients. Young patients can experience similar musculoskeletal injuries (ie, sprains, strains, and fractures) as adults, but they may need to be treated differently depending on their age and maturation. The treatment of pediatric patients is often provided by clinicians who specialize in pediatric physical therapy. However, it is important that all clinicians are aware of common diagnoses specific to the pediatric population. The ability of assistants to recognize and report signs and/or symptoms is vital to ensure safe and effective treatment.

### *Fractures in Children*

Epiphyseal fractures are commonly seen in young patients because of the mechanical properties of an immature skeleton. Open growth plates and immature bones are unable to handle higher loads or stress compared with adults, sometimes resulting in fractures rather than soft tissue injuries. Growth plate fractures account for 6% to 30% of all fractures in children.[126]

Fractures typically present with pain, weakness, and loss of ROM and decreased use of the affected limb. Pediatric fractures are stabilized the same way as adult fractures (ie, splinting, casting, or surgical fixators); however, the healing time tends to be shorter. Recovery and return to function also typically occur sooner. Most children regain full function and use of the affected extremity without the need for physical therapy.[127,128] Most epiphyseal fractures usually heal without complications, but deformities do occur due to severe injury to the epiphyseal plate (causing disruption of bone growth) in about 15% of the cases.[126]

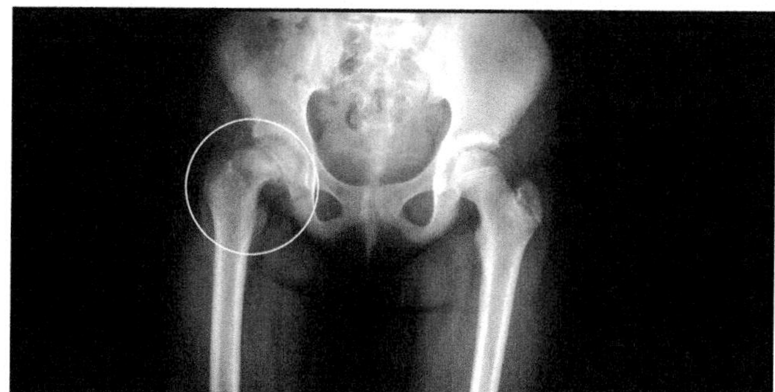

**Figure 13-34.** SCFE on the right femoral head (Yok_onepiece/Shutterstock.com).

### *Slipped Capital Femoral Epiphysis*

Slipped capital femoral epiphysis (SCFE) usually occurs in children 8 to 15 years old. It is the most common pediatric hip disorder with an occurrence of 10.8 in 100,000 adolescents; it is more common in boys than girls.[129] SCFE is a slipping of the proximal femoral epiphysis on the femoral neck at the site of the growth plate, but the femoral head remains in the acetabulum (Figure 13-34). This slippage can be stable or unstable. It is diagnosed by a physical examination and radiographs. A stable SCFE is more common and is present bilaterally in 18% to 50% of patients.[127,129]

Patients commonly report vague groin, hip, thigh, or knee pain. Patients present with an antalgic gait pattern with the involved hip externally rotated. Patients with a stable SCFE cannot usually attribute the pain to a specific acute event. However, patients with unstable SCFE may report experiencing a traumatic event (ie, falling) that resulted in the sudden inability to fully weight bear on the involved lower extremity due to pain. A key sign of SCFE is limited hip internal rotation. When the involved hip is passively flexed to 90 degrees, it will externally rotate. Both of these are positive tests for SCFE.[126,127,129]

**Considerations for the Physical Therapist Assistant**

If a pediatric patient is being seen for an orthopedic condition and they complain of unrelated groin pain, the assistant should notify the physical therapist immediately because SCFE can sometimes mimic hip adductor muscle pain, and adolescents rarely experience groin strains.[126,129]

The typical treatment for stable SCFE includes a surgical fixation with one screw through the growth plate to stabilize the femoral head. Stabilizing an unstable SCFE is a more complicated procedure and may increase future risk for developing osteonecrosis. Up to 50% of patients with unstable SCFE develop avascular necrosis of the femoral head, which increases future risk for degenerative hip OA.[127,129]

After surgery, patients have restricted weight-bearing status (NWB or TTWB) using crutches for about 6 to 8 weeks. It may take up to 3 to 4 months for the growth plate to fuse and full resumption of FWB. Physical therapy treatment typically includes ROM (focusing on internal rotation, flexion, and abduction), gradual strengthening (as per protocol/POC), and gait training with crutches (maintaining weight-bearing precautions). An upper bike ergometer or a stationary bike with no resistance can be implemented for aerobic conditioning. Once the patient is able to fully weight bear on the extremity, CKC strengthening and balance exercises should be initiated. Patients can return to play once cleared by the surgeon, but contact sports may not be an option.[126-129]

## Legg-Calve-Perthes Disease

Legg-Calve-Perthes (LCP) disease is idiopathic osteonecrosis of the femoral head and is a self-limiting disease. Femoral head deformation (flattening) is the primary complication with LCP disease. It takes several months for the blood supply to return to the femoral head. The blood supply allows reabsorption of necrotic bone and the development of new bone cells. This process can take 2 to 4 years for complete regeneration. Although LCP disease is rare, it most commonly occurs in children 3 to 12 years old and occurs more often in boys.[127,128,130]

The child typically presents with complaints of vague dull groin, hip, or persistent thigh and knee pain (obturator nerve pain pattern) and decreased hip abduction and internal rotation. The child may ambulate with an intermittent Trendelenburg gait pattern and the involved leg externally rotated. Other symptoms include hip stiffness, pain with activity but relieved with rest, and thigh muscle atrophy.[126-128,130]

Medical treatment interventions vary, but the primary focus is to achieve/maintain a spherical femoral head using splints/braces. There is discussion as to whether treatment is indicated because of the eventual resolution of symptoms. In some cases, a femoral or pelvic osteotomy is performed to facilitate appropriate alignment/shaping of the femoral head. LCP disease can result in an increased risk of OA later in life, especially if the femoral head does not reshape spherically.[127,128,130]

Nonsurgical interventions are most common, and physical therapy is usually initiated for children with mild/moderate symptoms. The goals of therapy are to restore hip ROM, reduce pain and inflammation, and protect the healing joint. Improving hip ROM reduces joint stiffness, mobilizes synovial fluid, and encourages a spherical shape of the femoral head that will fit appropriately in the acetabulum. Daily ROM exercises (specifically internal rotation and abduction) are recommended during the healing process.[127,130]

## Developmental Dysplasia of the Hip

Developmental dysplasia of the hip (DDH) is a relatively common hip disorder affecting infants and children. It occurs more commonly in girls (about 85%) than boys. Approximately 10% of infants in the United States are born with congenital hip dislocations.[127,131] There are 3 types/degrees of DDH. In unstable hip dysplasia, the hip is positioned normally but can be dislocated due to a shallow socket. Hip subluxation occurs when the head of the femur is in contact with the acetabulum but is partially displaced. In cases with a complete dislocation, the femoral head is positioned outside of the acetabulum.[127,131]

Signs of DDH in infants include asymmetries in hip ROM, extra thigh skinfolds, leg length discrepancy or asymmetry in the gluteal fold (higher on affected side), and a positive Barlow or Ortolani test.[131] Signs/symptoms in an ambulatory child include a Trendelenburg gait pattern, decreased hip extension on the affected side, and increased lumbar lordosis.

Splinting/bracing with a hip Pavlik harness for 3 to 9 months is a common treatment for infants. A closed reduction and adductor release procedure followed by the application of a spica cast is a common treatment for ambulatory children. Splinting/bracing occurs with the hips positioned in flexion, external rotation, and abduction to promote appropriate realignment of the femoral head within the acetabulum. Care must be taken to ensure that the appropriate joint angles are maintained with splinting or in the harness. Positioning that creates hip flexion greater than 120 degrees or abduction greater than 70 degrees can increase the risk of avascular necrosis.[131] The physical therapy team educates the patient's parents regarding proper mobility and harness use. The therapy team provides therapeutic interventions that promote motor milestone acquisition.[131]

## *Juvenile Osteochondritis Dissecans*

Juvenile osteochondritis dissecans (JOCD) can be a cause of knee pain. JOCD is more common in boys.[132,133] The incidence of JOCD of the knee is more prevalent in those 12 to 19 years old (21.8/100,000) compared with children 6 to 12 years old (8.7/100,000). A potential cause of knee osteochondritis dissecans is repeated microtrauma paired with vascular impairment on the lateral aspect of the medial femoral condyle. This area of the condyle repeatedly comes in contact with the tibial spine, causing this condition.[132] A decrease in the vascular supply to the bone results in cracking of subchondral bone and articular cartilage, causing bone surface fragmentation. Fragments may become unstable and break away or stay attached to the condyle (a stable lesion), which may heal on its own.[132,133]

Patients initially report varying amounts of vague pain and swelling. If the lesion goes undiagnosed and progresses, patients complain of the knee joint giving way, locking, or catching in the joint as the result of bone fragment movement within the joint space.[132]

Medical treatment options include conservative methods (nonsurgical) or a variety of surgical arthroscopic interventions (ie, subchondral drilling, fragment debridement, or stabilization). Children with open growth plates tend to have a good prognosis for healing using conservative (nonsurgical) methods.[132,133]

The physical therapy team is often involved in conservative management and postoperative management. Treatment includes gait training with instruction regarding protected weight-bearing status, progressive ROM, and strengthening exercises based on the healing status of the lesion. Patients may be immobilized in a long leg cast or hinged brace and/or will need to use crutches. If the patient is PWB, they can maintain aerobic conditioning using a stationary bike, deep water running, or swimming (but no breaststroke).

There are not widely accepted rehabilitation protocols or clinical guidelines for treating patients with JOCD.[133] During the initial phase, it is important to control swelling and pain and work toward normal ROM to promote healing. PROM, AAROM, and stretching are encouraged during this phase, and AROM can be initiated once full passive range is achieved. OKC strengthening can begin in the second phase and when cleared by the physician, the patient can be progressed to FWB, bilateral CKC, and balance activities. Running and gradual progression in higher-impact and sport-specific activities are considered after normal quadriceps control and strength are evident and the physician provides clearance.[133]

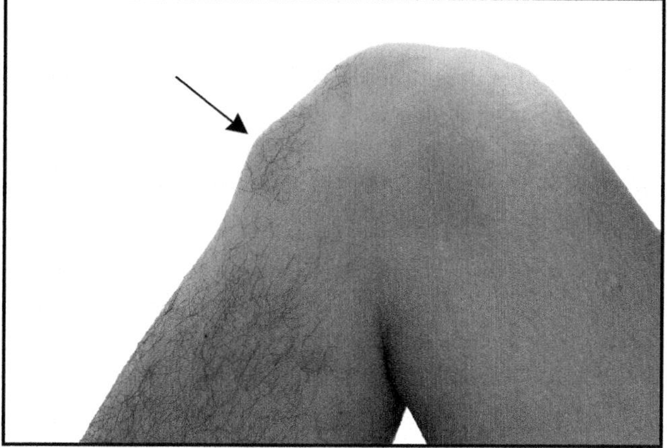

**Figure 13-35.** Bony formation of the tibial tuberosity of a male patient who had Osgood-Schlatter disease when younger (sutisakphoto14/Shutterstock.com).

## *Osgood-Schlatter Disease*

Osgood-Schlatter disease is a self-limiting traction apophysitis affecting the tibial tuberosity. It is a common cause of anterior knee pain in adolescent boys (ages 10 to 15 years) and girls (ages 8 to 13 years). It affects boys more than girls (3:1), and its onset often coincides with growth spurts.[131] It is seen in young athletes who commonly participate in basketball, volleyball, gymnastics, and running and is considered an overuse injury.[134]

Repetitive forceful contractions of the quadriceps muscle (ie, jumping and sprinting) stress the apophysis of the tibial tubercle (via the patellar tendon), resulting in small avulsion fractures. A compensatory response increases bone formation in the area, resulting in a visible bump at the site of the tibial tubercle (Figure 13-35). Fusion of the apophysis and proximal tibial epiphysis to the shaft of the proximal tibia occurs at 18 years or older.[134]

Patients typically complain of a dull ache at the tibial tubercle that increases with activity and subsides with rest (and icing). Pain is reproduced with resisted or active knee extension. The episodic pain can last for a few weeks to a few months, so aggravating sports and activities should be significantly restricted. Activities should be self-limited by pain until healing at the apophysis occurs (which may take 6 to 12+ months). Poor hamstring and quadriceps flexibility or extensor mechanism issues are also predisposing factors for Osgood-Schlatter disease and can be addressed in physical therapy.[134]

## Lower Extremity Exercises

This section presents various ROM, stretching, strengthening, and neuromuscular control exercises that can be used to treat various lower extremity diagnoses. Tables 13-13 through 13-26 list various exercises and general exercise progression for each diagnosis.

### *Hip Exercises*

Hip ROM and stretching exercises are illustrated in Figures 13-36 through 13-43, and hip strengthening exercises are shown in Figures 13-44 through 13-48.

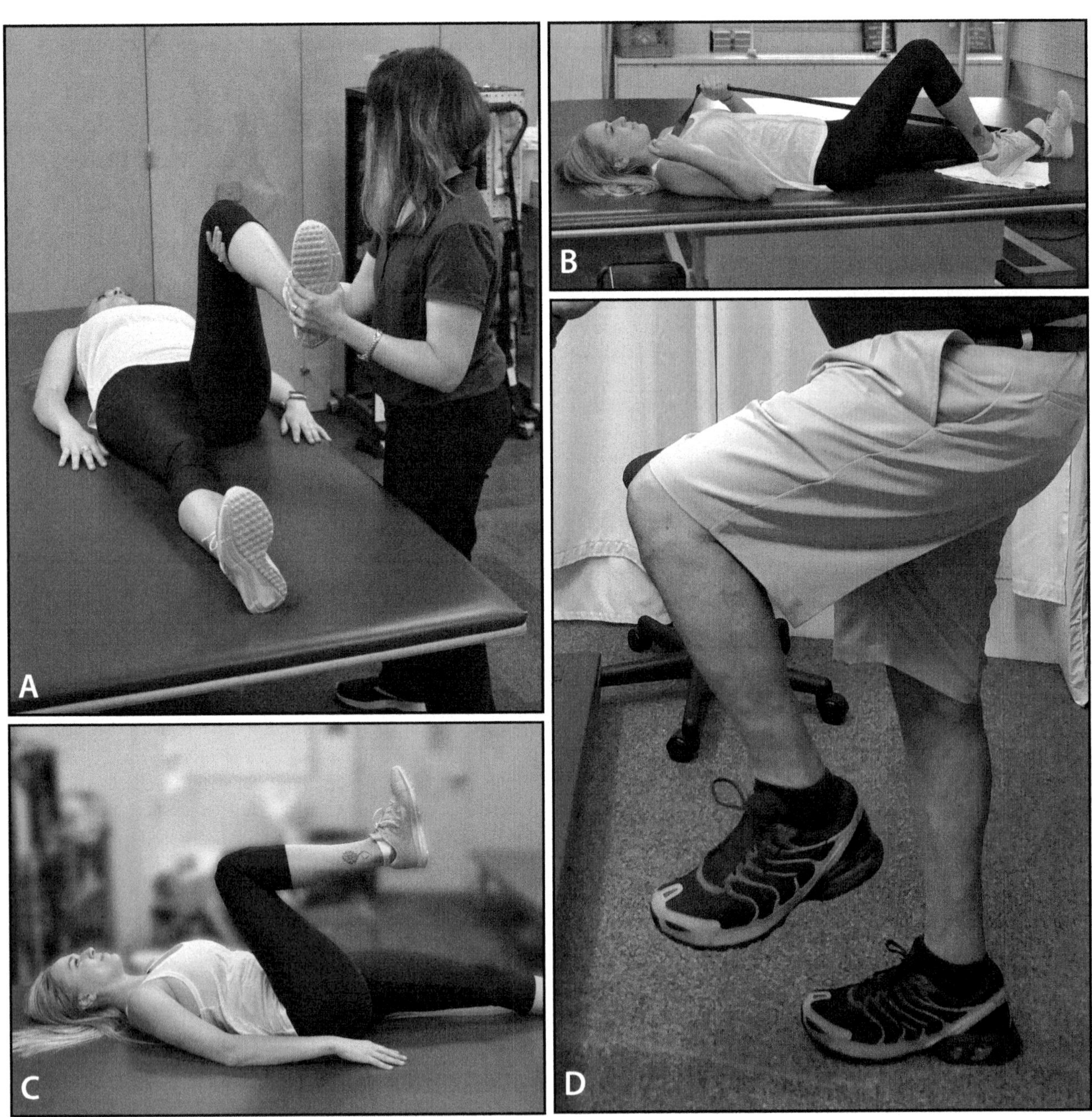


**Figure 13-36.** Hip flexion ROM exercises. (A) Hip flexion passive or AAROM by clinician. (B) Supine hip and knee flexion AAROM. Using a strap assists with improving both hip and knee motion. (C) Supine active hip flexion. The patient should be progressed to standing and then sitting. (D) Standing hip flexion on the left leg (against gravity). Have the patient hold on for support.

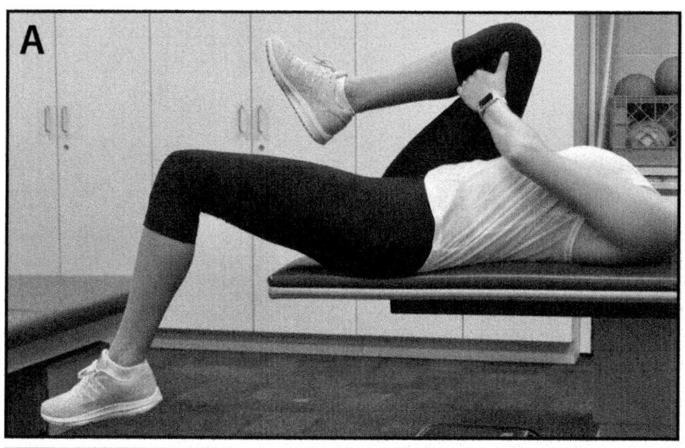


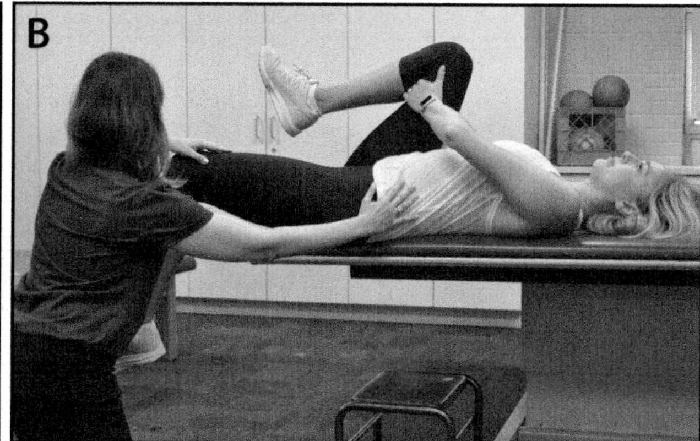


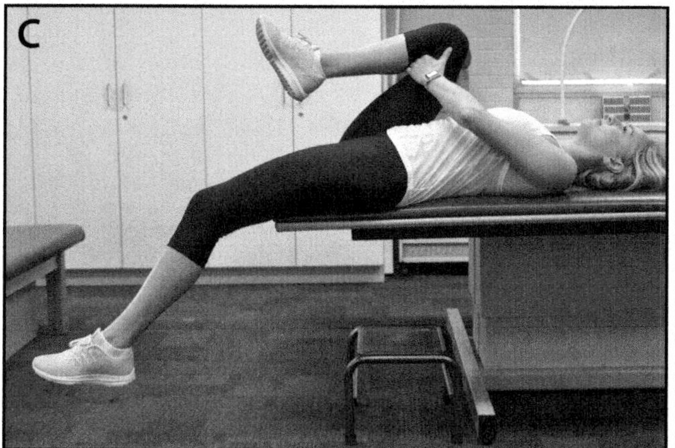


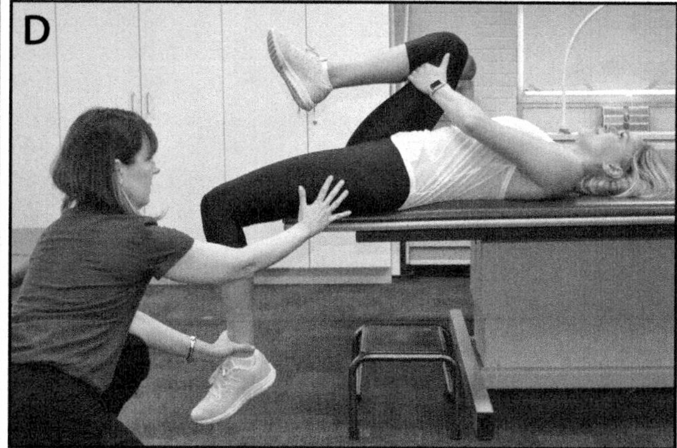


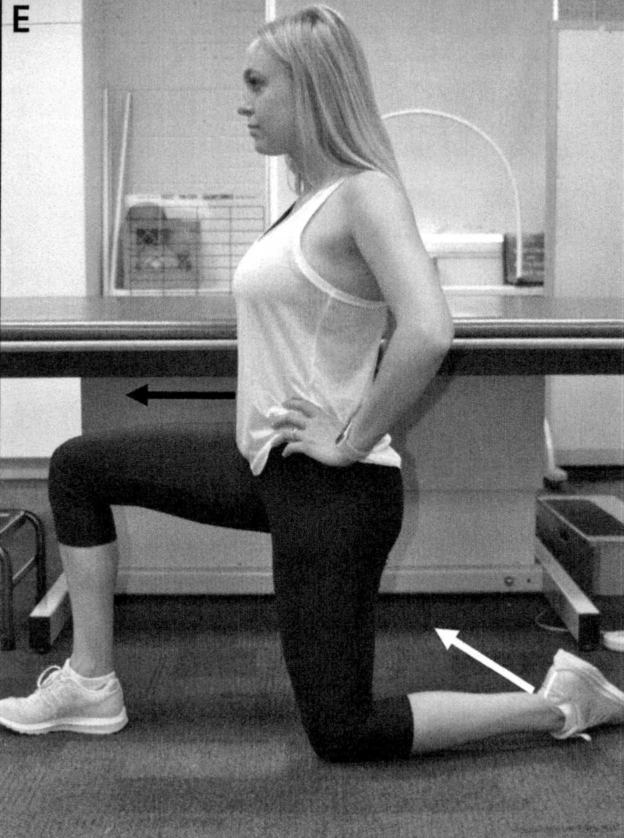


**Figure 13-37.** Hip flexor muscle stretches. (A) A hip flexor stretch (Thomas test position). The patient has tight hip flexors. (B) The clinician assists the patient to stretch the tight hip flexor muscles by gently pushing the thigh downward. (C) The Thomas test position. The knee is not able to flex to 90 degrees because of rectus femoris tightness. (D) The clinician assists the patient to stretch the rectus femoris by flexing the knee gently. (E) An active hip flexor stretch. To stretch the left hip flexors, the patient will keep the trunk upright and shift forward over the right leg (black arrow). To stretch the rectus femoris, the patient can reach back with the left hand grasping the ankle and flexing the knee (white arrow). A strap can be used around the foot if the patient is unable to reach. Make sure the patient is holding on with the right hand for balance and support.

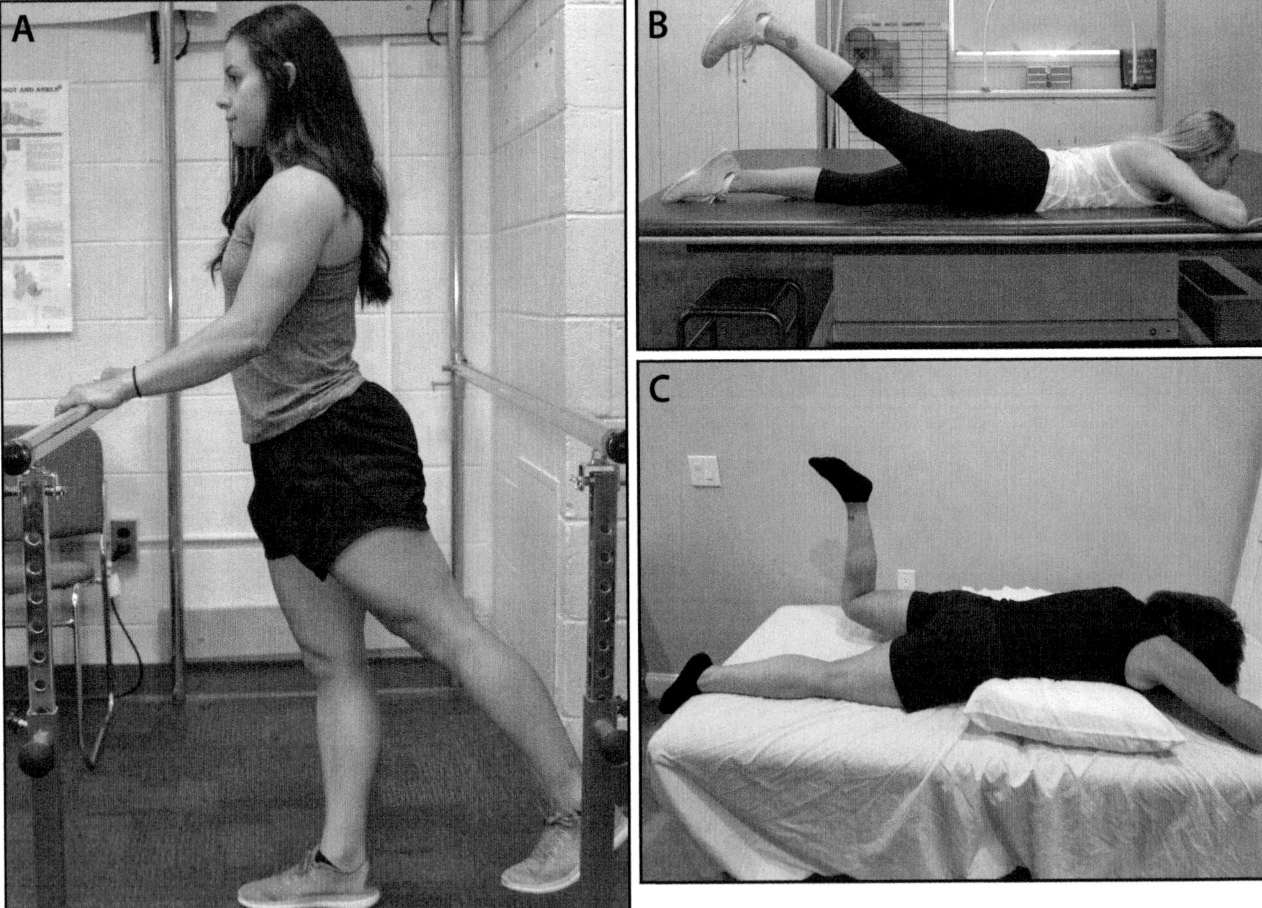


**Figure 13-38.** Hip extension ROM. (A) Standing hip extension AROM gravity minimized. Avoid lumbar extension. (B) Prone hip extension. The patient has good motion; check for excessive lumbar extension or pelvic rolling. (C) Prone hip extension with the knee flexed. The range is less due to rectus femoris passive insufficiency.

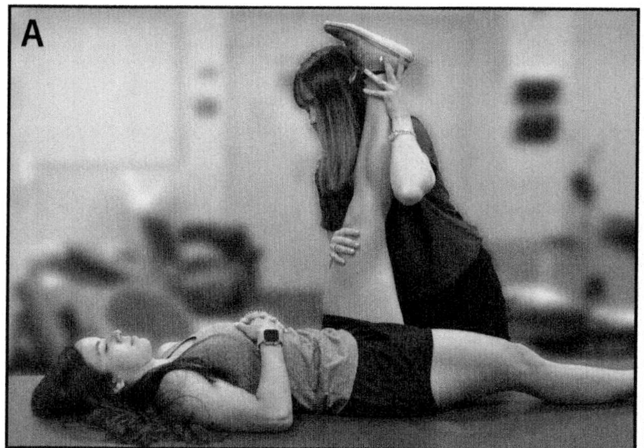


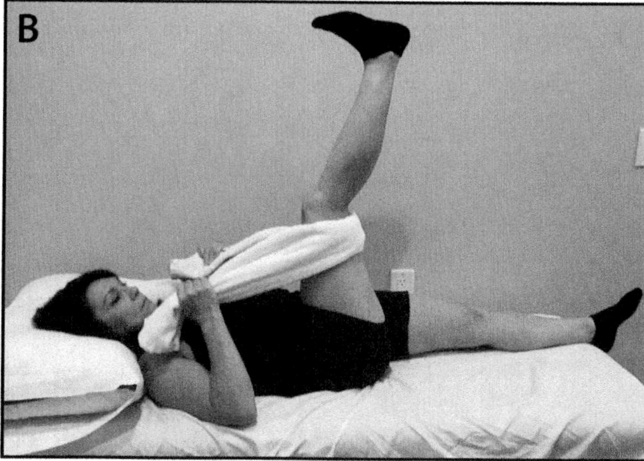


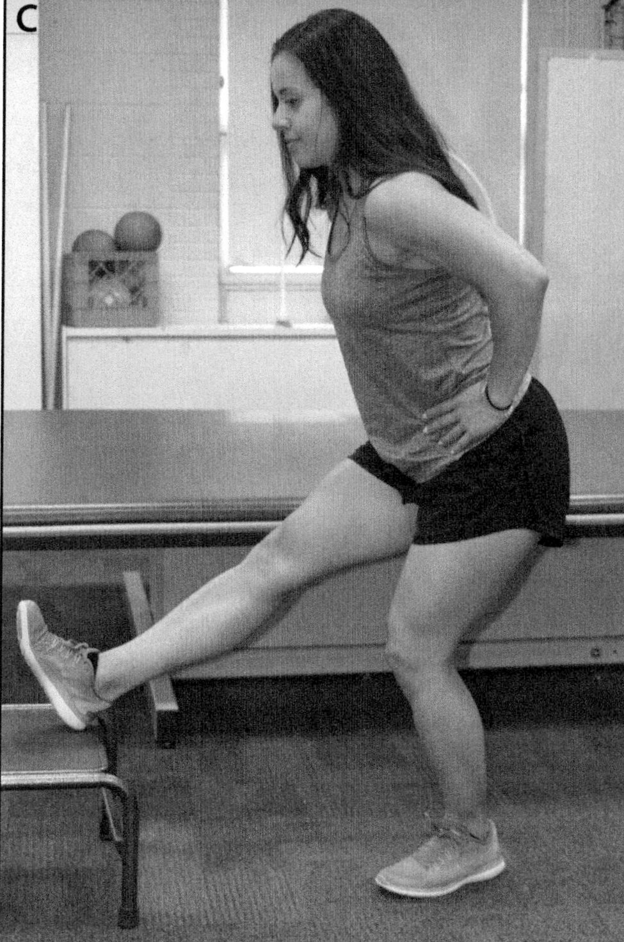


**Figure 13-39.** Hip extensor muscle stretches. (A) A supine hamstring stretch passively performed by the clinician. Notice the support of the lower leg. (B) A supine hamstring stretch. Instruct the patient to place the towel around thigh when positioned at 90 degrees and slowly extend the lower leg until stretch is felt. (C) A standing hamstring stretch. The patient keeps the spine straight and flexes at the hip. *(continued)*

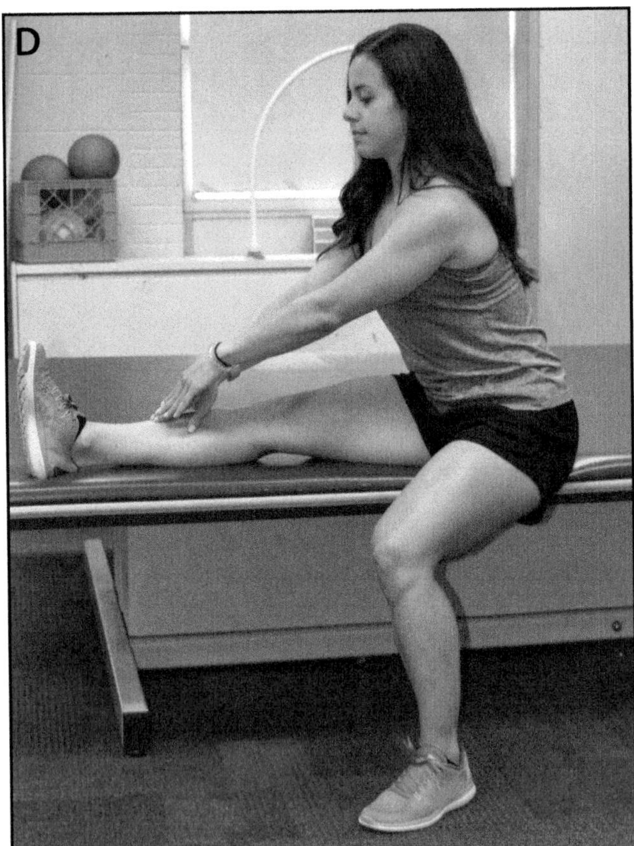


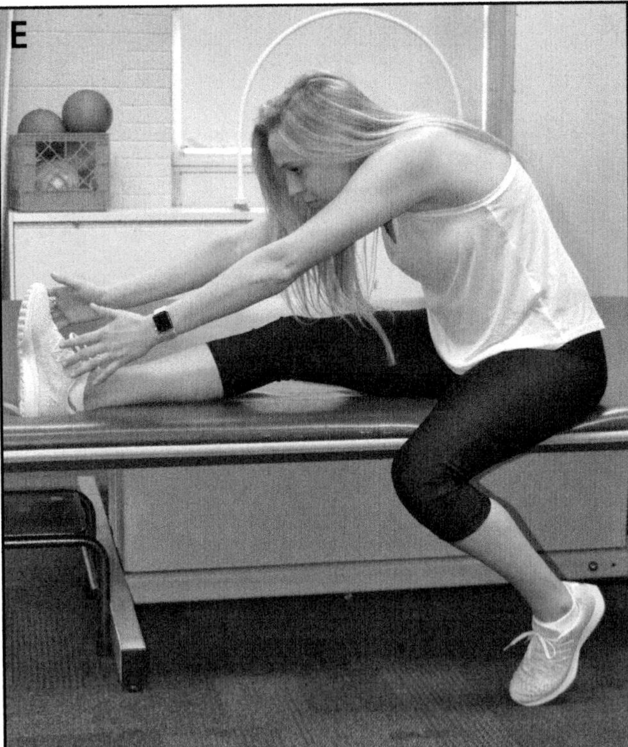


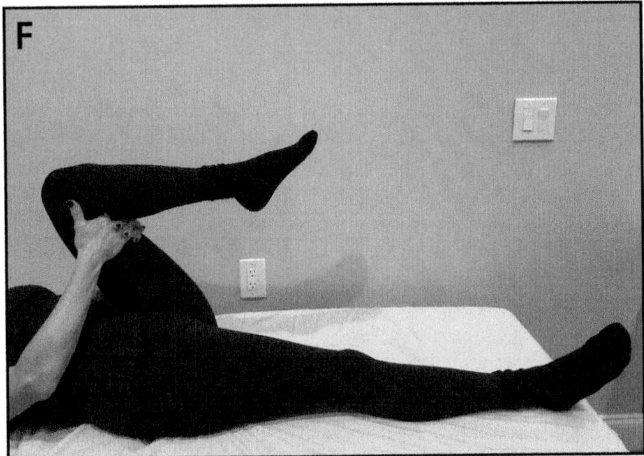


**Figure 13-39 (continued).** (D) A hamstring stretch with the leg supported. Notice the back is straight and the patient flexes at the hip. (E) A hamstring stretch using improper form with the back rounded, the knee flexed, and the left foot not flat on the floor. (F) Bringing the knee toward the chest in supine on the left leg targets the gluteal muscles. This is called the *single knee to chest exercise.*

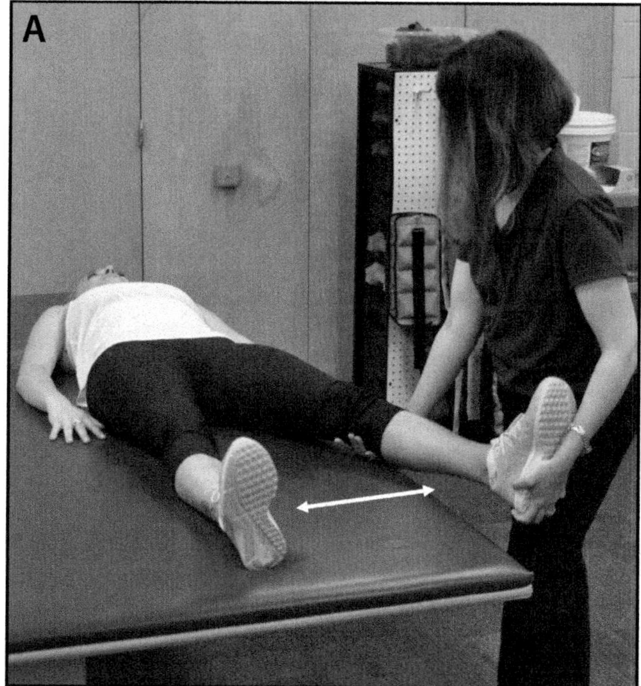

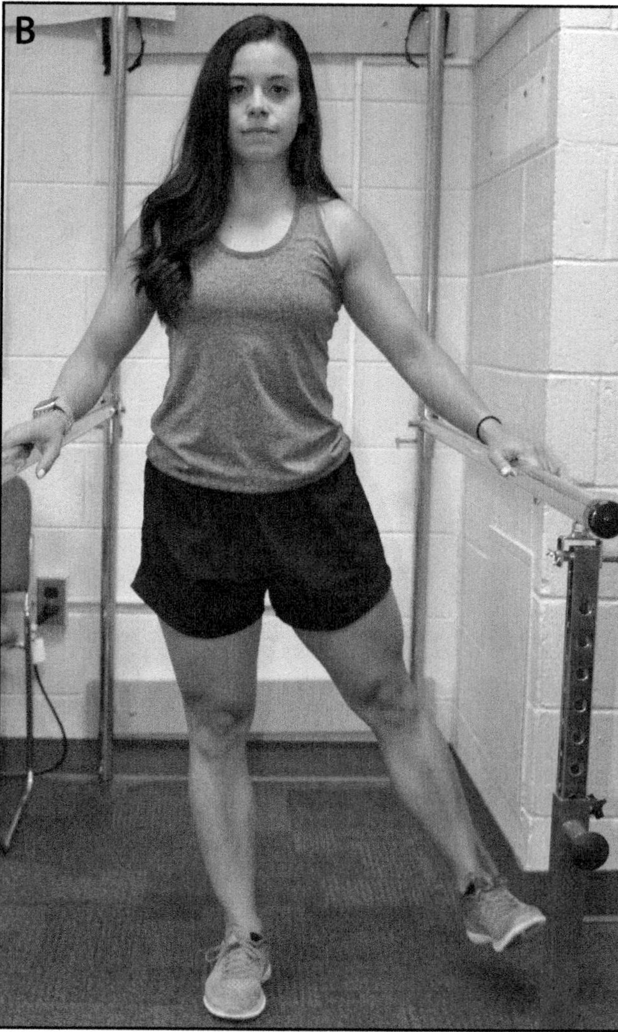

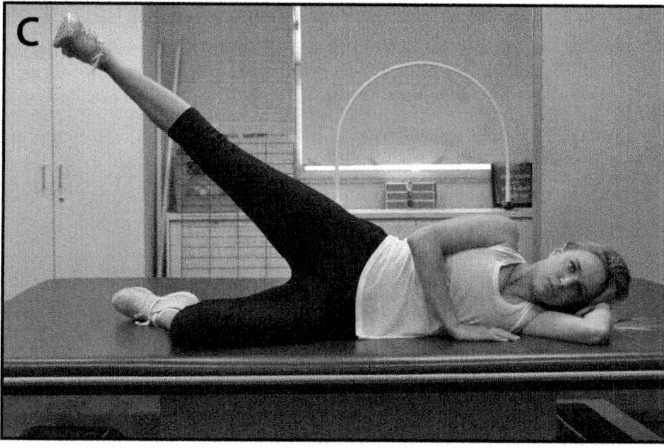

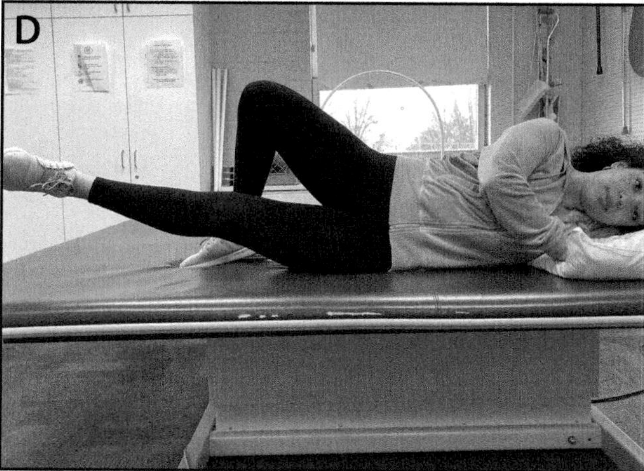

**Figure 13-40.** Hip abduction and adduction ROM. (A) Clinician-assisted hip abduction and adduction AAROM. The patient can also perform the exercise by placing a small towel under the left heel and sliding the leg on the table. The primary goal is for the patient to perform the exercise actively and then progress to a standing position and, finally, a side-lying position. (B) Hip abduction and adduction AROM standing. Progress to side lying. (C) Hip abduction AROM side lying. This position can be used when strengthening by adding ankle weights. (D) Hip adduction AROM side lying. The bottom leg is lifted (adducted) toward the top leg against gravity. The flexed knee provides stability and prevents the patient from rolling during the exercise.

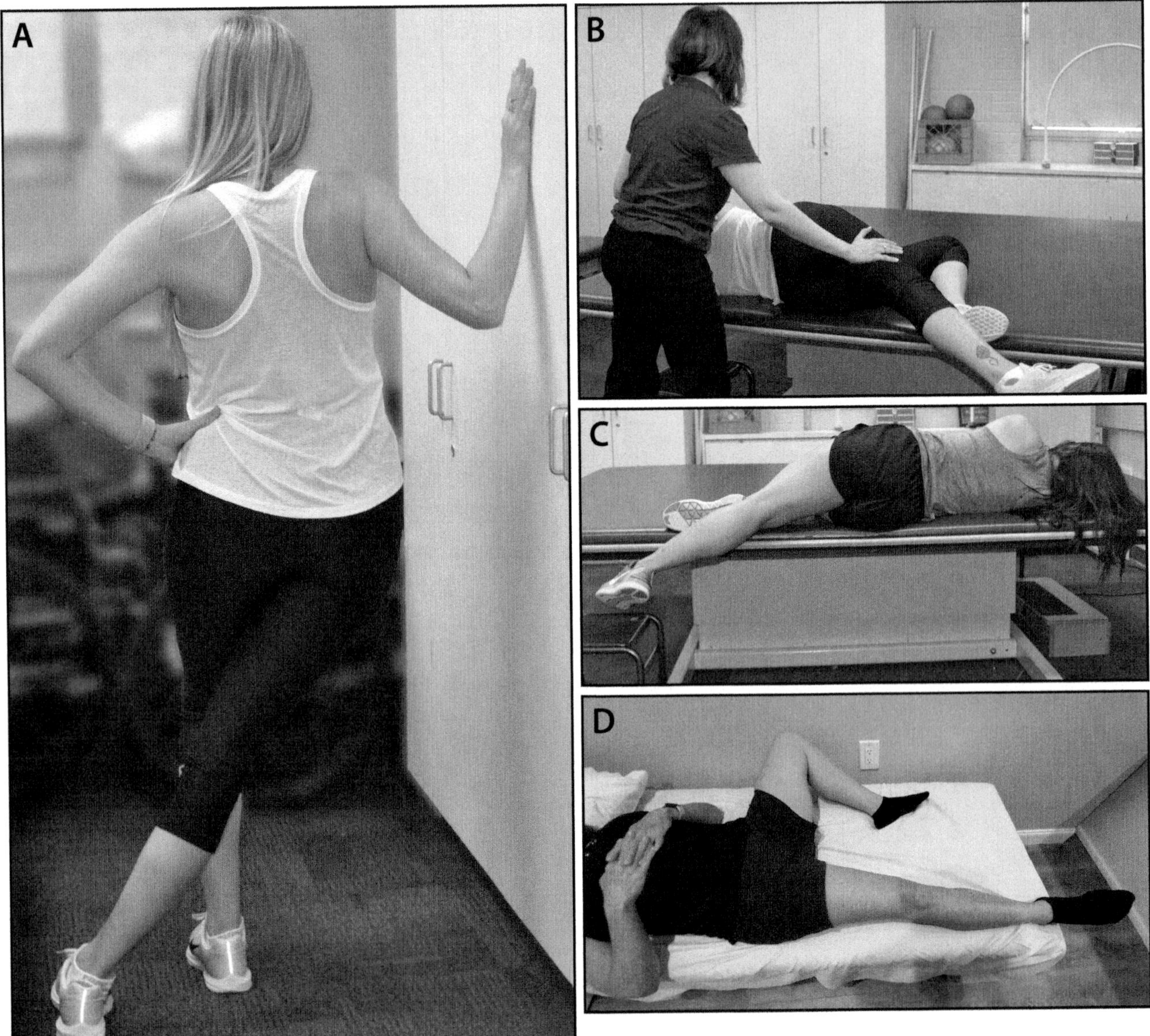


**Figure 13-41.** Hip abductor and adductor stretches. (A) The hip abductor muscle and ITB stretch for the right leg in standing. The pelvis is kept level as it is shifted toward the wall using the left hand. (B) The hip abductor stretch side lying with the clinician assisting in the Ober test position. (C) Independent hip abductor and ITB stretch side lying in the Ober test position. (D) The hip adductor stretch with active hip external rotation. The foot is first placed in an abducted position, and then the knee is rolled out to the side. *(continued)*

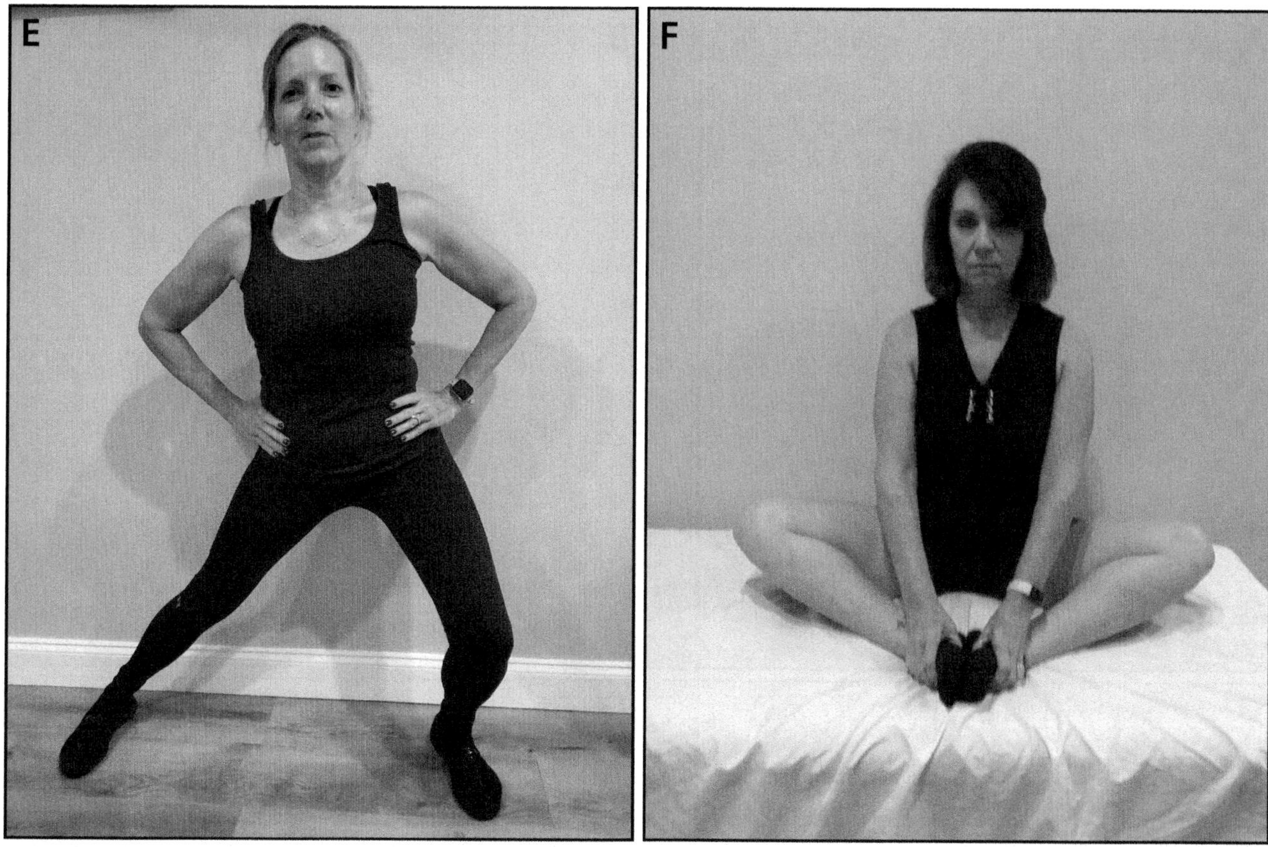


**Figure 13-41 (continued).** (E) The hip adductor stretch for the right hip in standing. (F) The hip adductor stretch bilaterally. This is also called the *butterfly stretch*.

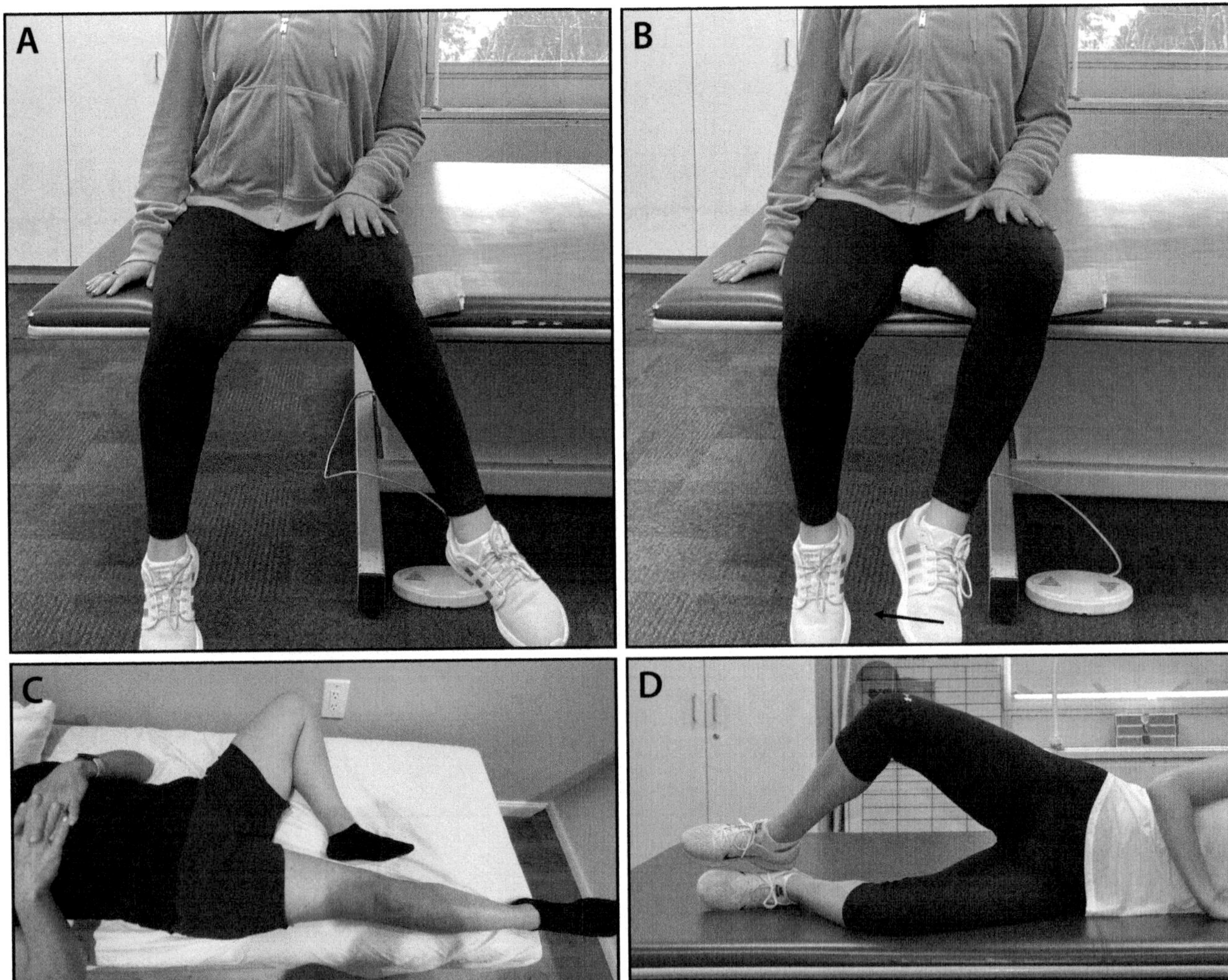

**Figure 13-42.** Hip internal and external ROM. (A) Seated hip internal rotation AROM. A resistance band can be used for strengthening. (B) Seated hip external rotation AROM. (C) Supine independent hip internal/external rotation. Start with the foot flat and knee flexed; roll the knee out to the side and back to the starting position. (D) Side-lying active hip external rotation (clamshells) against gravity. Start with the knees together and rotate the top leg upward as shown.

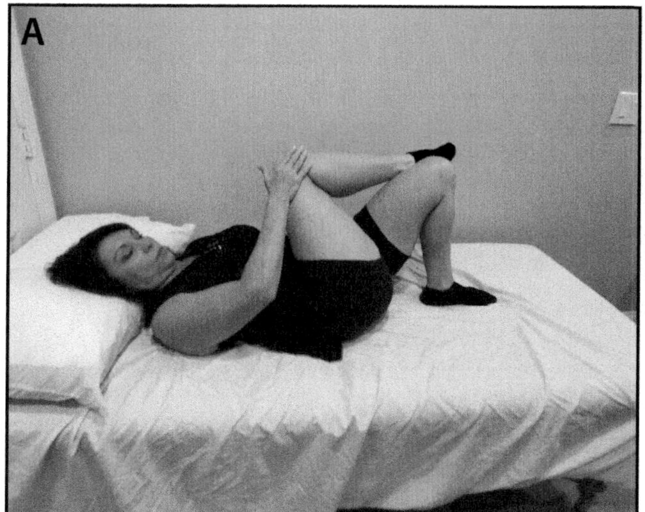


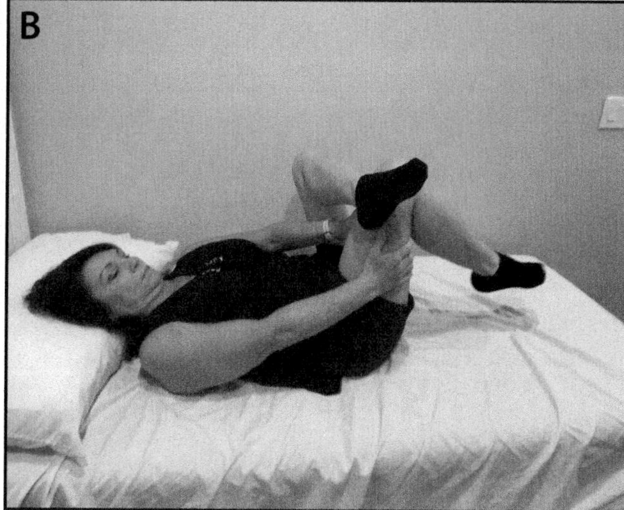


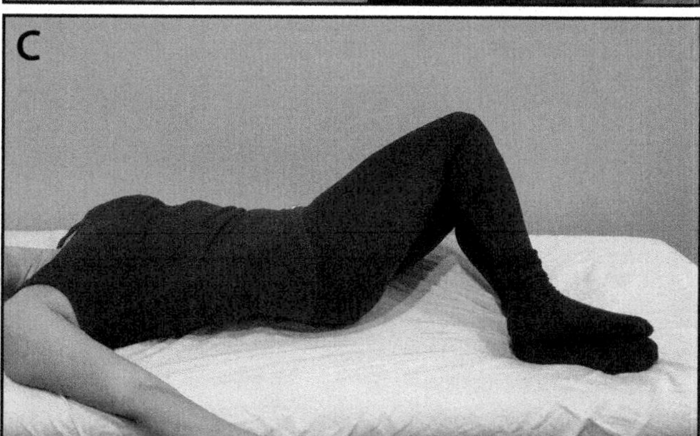


**Figure 13-43.** Hip external rotator muscle stretches including the piriformis muscle. (A) Bring the right knee to the opposite shoulder. The stretch is felt deep in the right buttocks area. (B) Hip external rotation figure-4 stretch for the left hip. Grasp and pull the right thigh toward the chest; the stretch is felt in the left buttocks area. (C) Bilateral hip rotation to the left stretches the right hip external rotators. Repeat to the right side to stretch the left hip external rotators. This also stretches the lumbar spine.

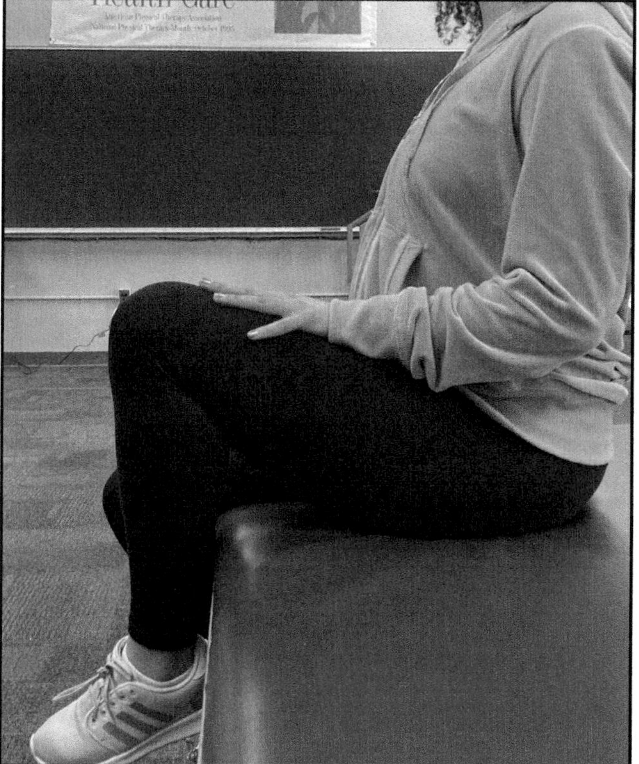

**Figure 13-44.** Hip flexion isometric strengthening seated. This can be performed with the patient supine and the hip and knee at 90 degrees and then progress to sitting. The patient can be progressed using ankle weights or a resistance band in standing or seated.

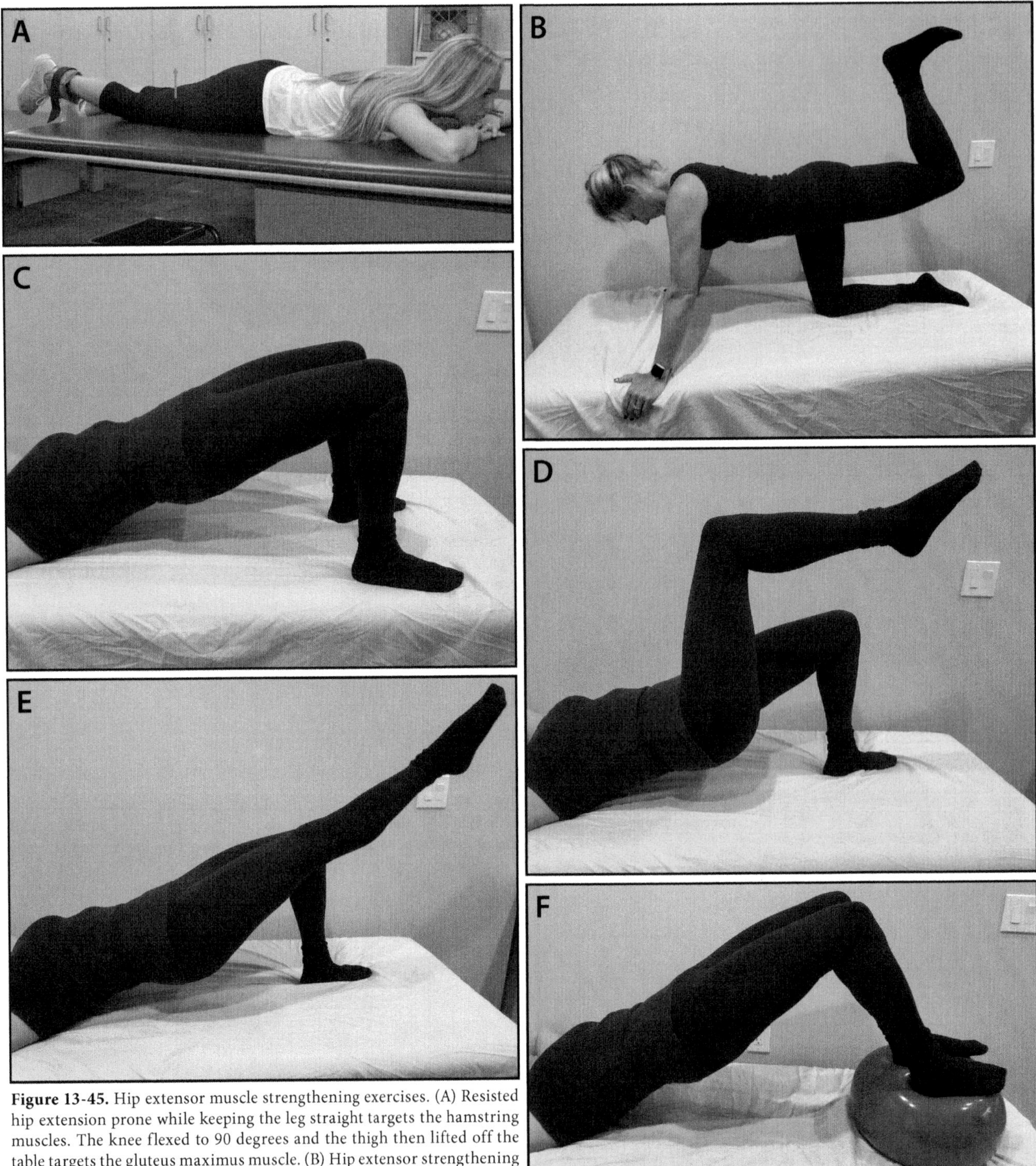


**Figure 13-45.** Hip extensor muscle strengthening exercises. (A) Resisted hip extension prone while keeping the leg straight targets the hamstring muscles. The knee flexed to 90 degrees and the thigh then lifted off the table targets the gluteus maximus muscle. (B) Hip extensor strengthening in quadruped. Start on all fours, and extend the hip with the knee flexed. (C) Bridges for hip extensor strengthening is a CKC exercise that can be used as an initial exercise. (D) Bridging progression 2—Single-leg bridge hip and knee flexed. Pelvis should be level. (E) Bridging progression 3—Single-leg bridge knee straight. Pelvis should be level. (F) Bridges on compliant surface (ball). This can be progressed to single-leg bridging as an advanced exercise.

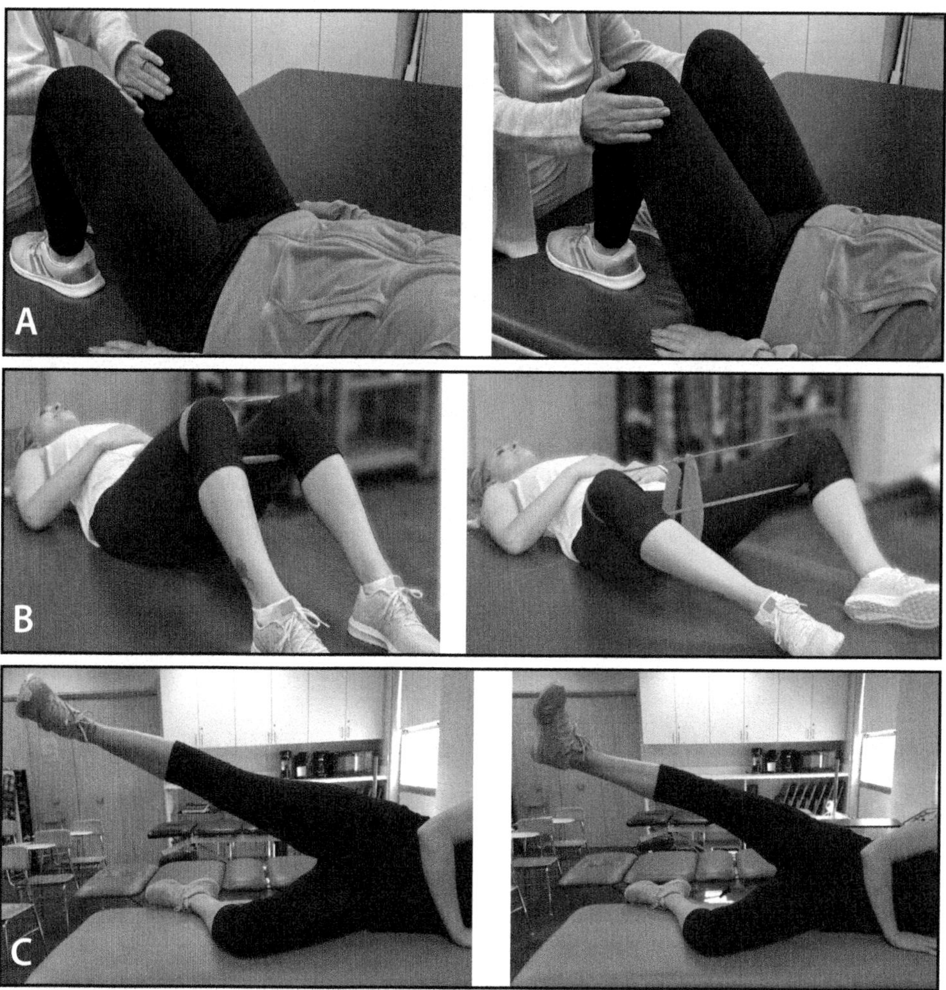

**Figure 13-46.** Hip abduction and adduction strengthening exercises. (A) Manual resistance isometric hip adduction (on left) and abduction (on right). These exercises can also be performed in sitting. (B) Supine resistance band hip abduction. Place the band just above the knees and start with feet flat about 5 to 6 in apart. Slowly move the knees away from the midline, hold momentarily, and then slowly return to the starting position. (C) Side-lying hip abduction strengthening for the gluteus medius and tensor fasciae latae. The patient on the left has the toes pointed straight ahead. This exercise targets the gluteus medius muscle. When the hip is externally rotated (patient on the right), the tensor fasciae latae muscle is targeted. Ankle weights or a secured resistance band can increase strength for the specific muscle. *(continued)*

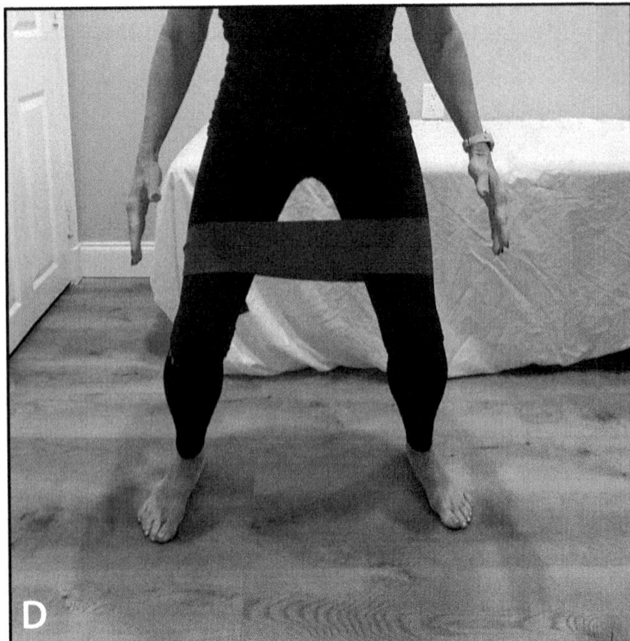

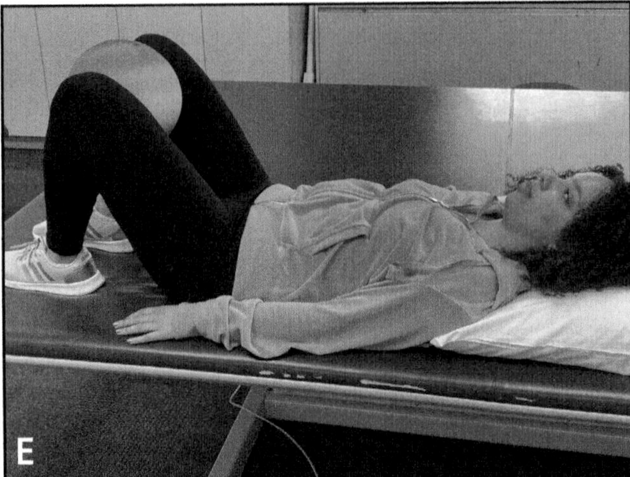

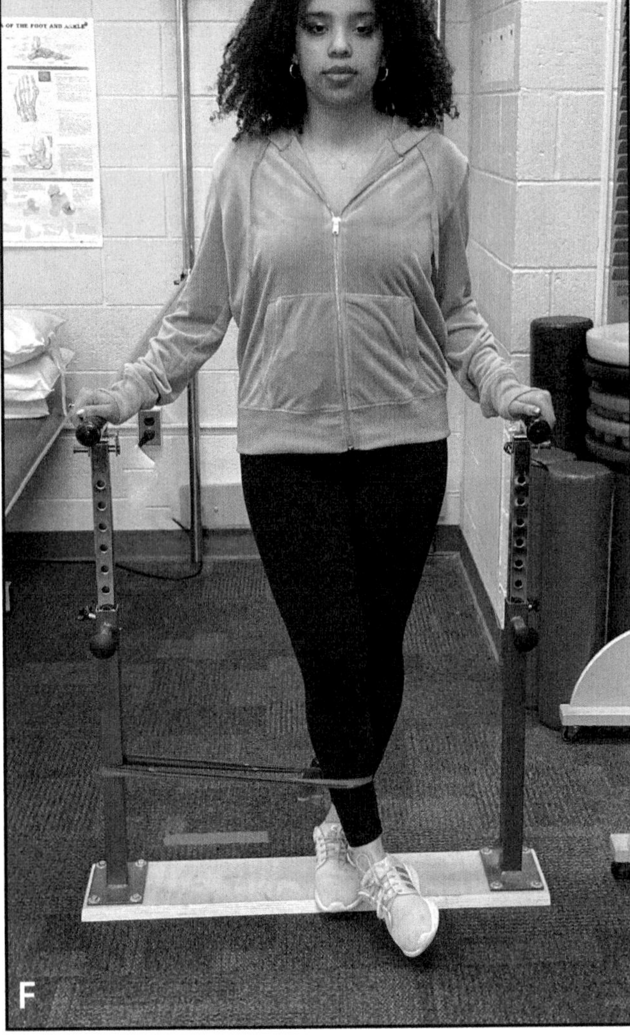

**Figure 13-46 (continued).** (D) Resistance band side stepping. (E) Ball isometric squeezes in the supine hook-lying position. This exercise can also be performed with both legs extended or seated for hip adductor strengthening. (F) Hip adduction standing with a resistance band.

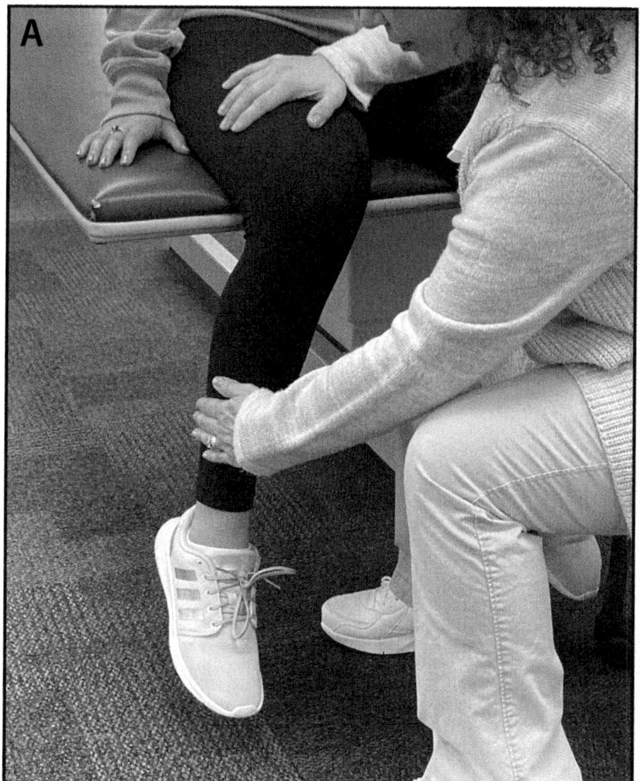


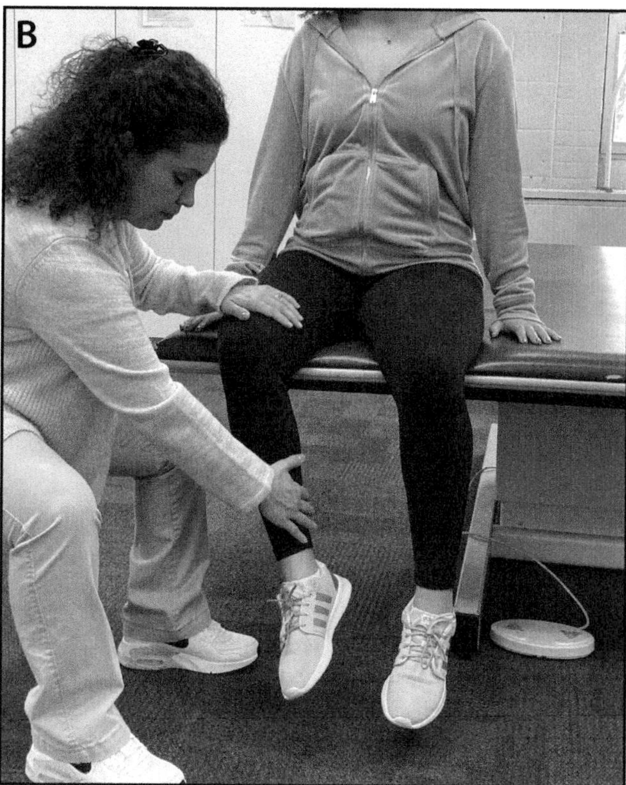


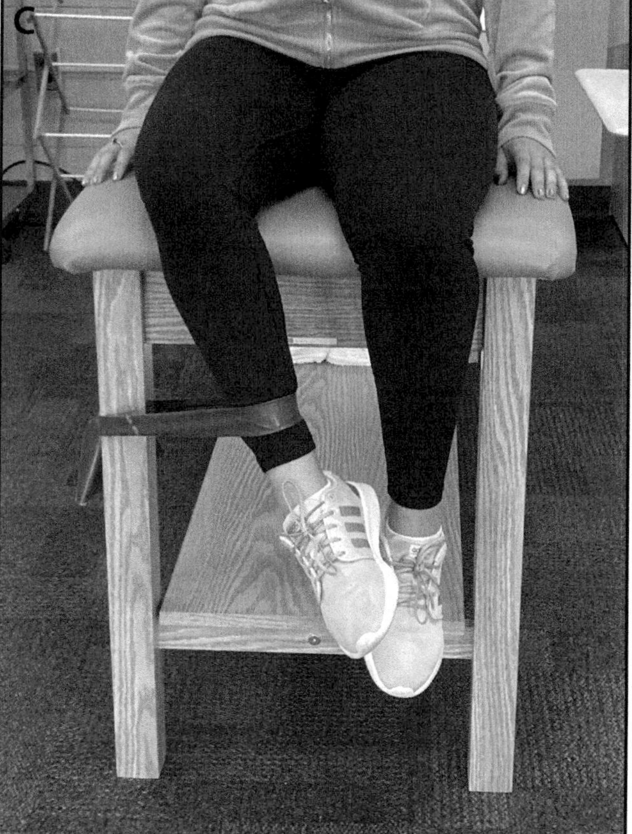


**Figure 13-47.** Hip internal and external rotation strengthening exercises. (A) A seated unilateral internal rotation manual resistance isometric contraction. Progress to active rotation using a resistance band. (B) A seated unilateral external rotation isometric contraction. (C) A seated unilateral hip external rotation using a resistance band. To progress the patient, place the band just above the knees when side lying as an alternative position for strengthening.

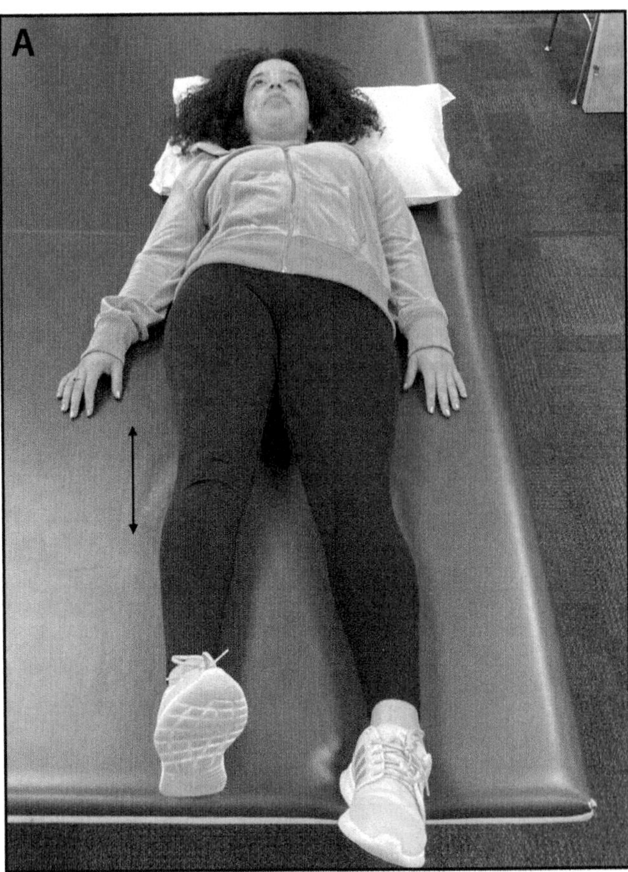


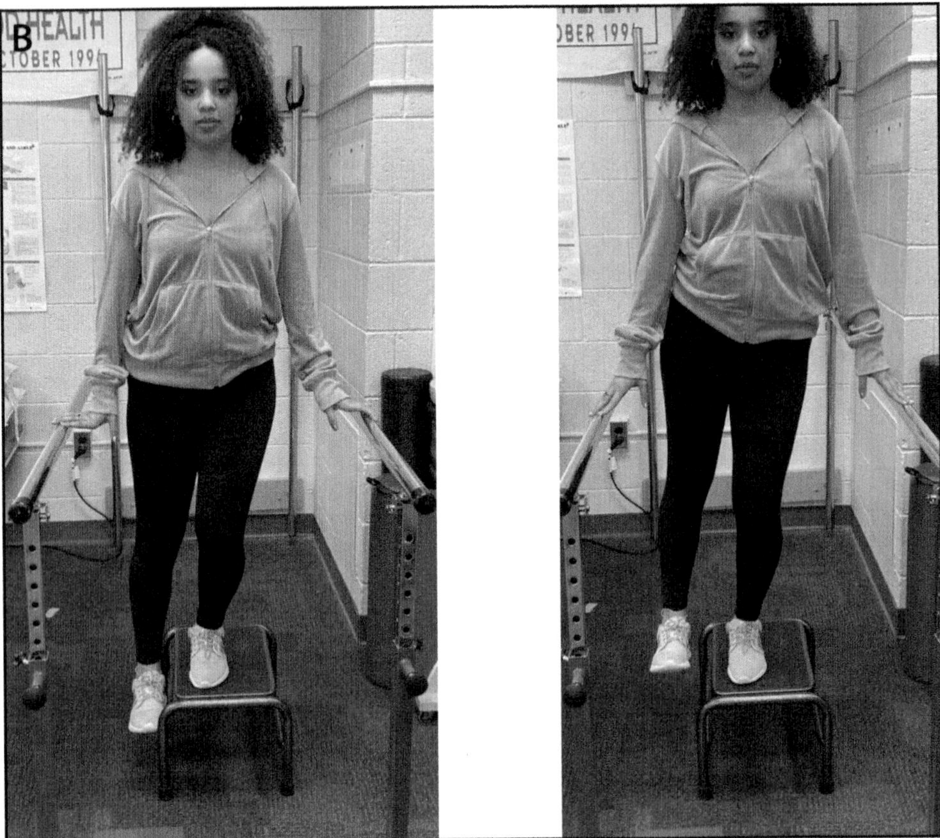


**Figure 13-48.** Hip hike and pelvic drop. (A) Supine hip hike and pelvic drop on the right lower extremity. This exercise targets the left gluteus medius to isometrically stabilize the left pelvis as quadratus lumborum contracts lifting the right pelvis. (B) Performing a right hip hike while standing on a stool with the left leg strengthens the left gluteus medius during this CKC exercise. This is a more advanced exercise.

## Knee Exercises

Knee ROM and stretching exercises are shown in Figures 13-49A through 13-49E. Knee strengthening exercises are illustrated in Figures 13-50 and 13-51.

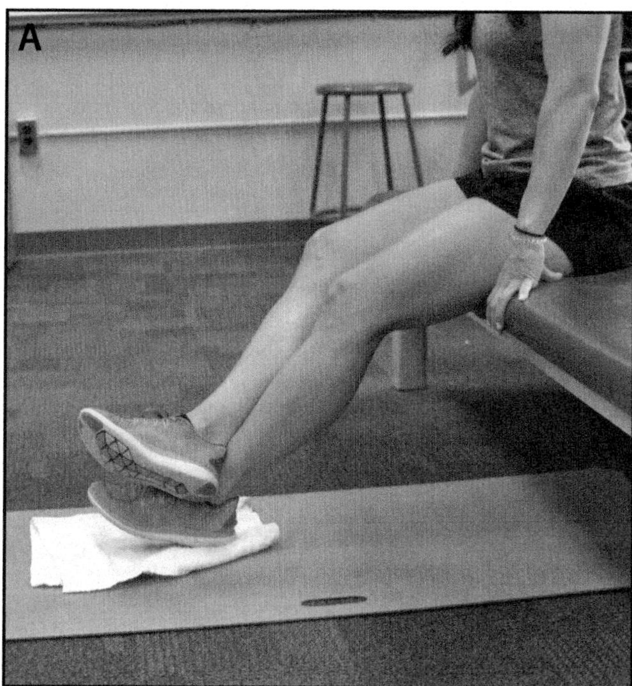


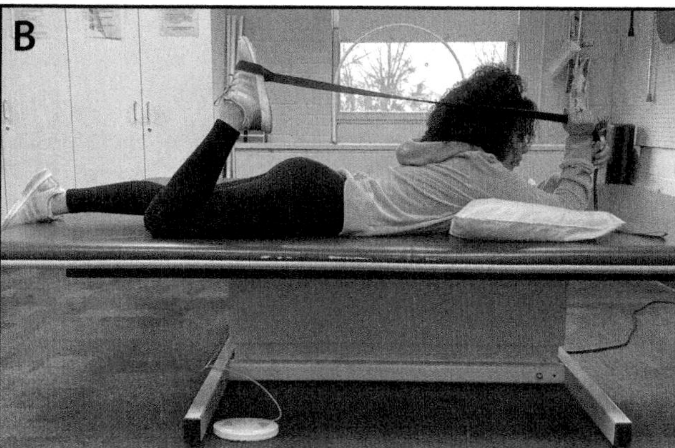


**Figure 13-49.** Knee ROM and stretching exercises. (A) Knee flexion AAROM seated. The patient uses the right foot to assist with increasing left knee flexion ROM. This can also be performed with the patient supine using a strap. (B) Prone AAROM knee flexion. Place a strap around the foot, and gently pull the lower leg to increase knee flexion. Make sure the patient keeps the pelvis flat on the table. This can also be used to stretch the quadricep muscles. (C) Standing active knee flexion. The hamstrings are working against gravity. *(continued)*

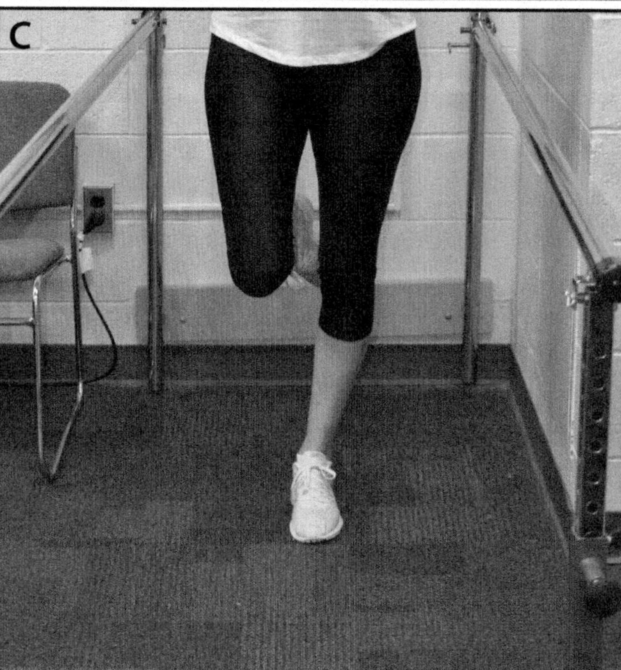

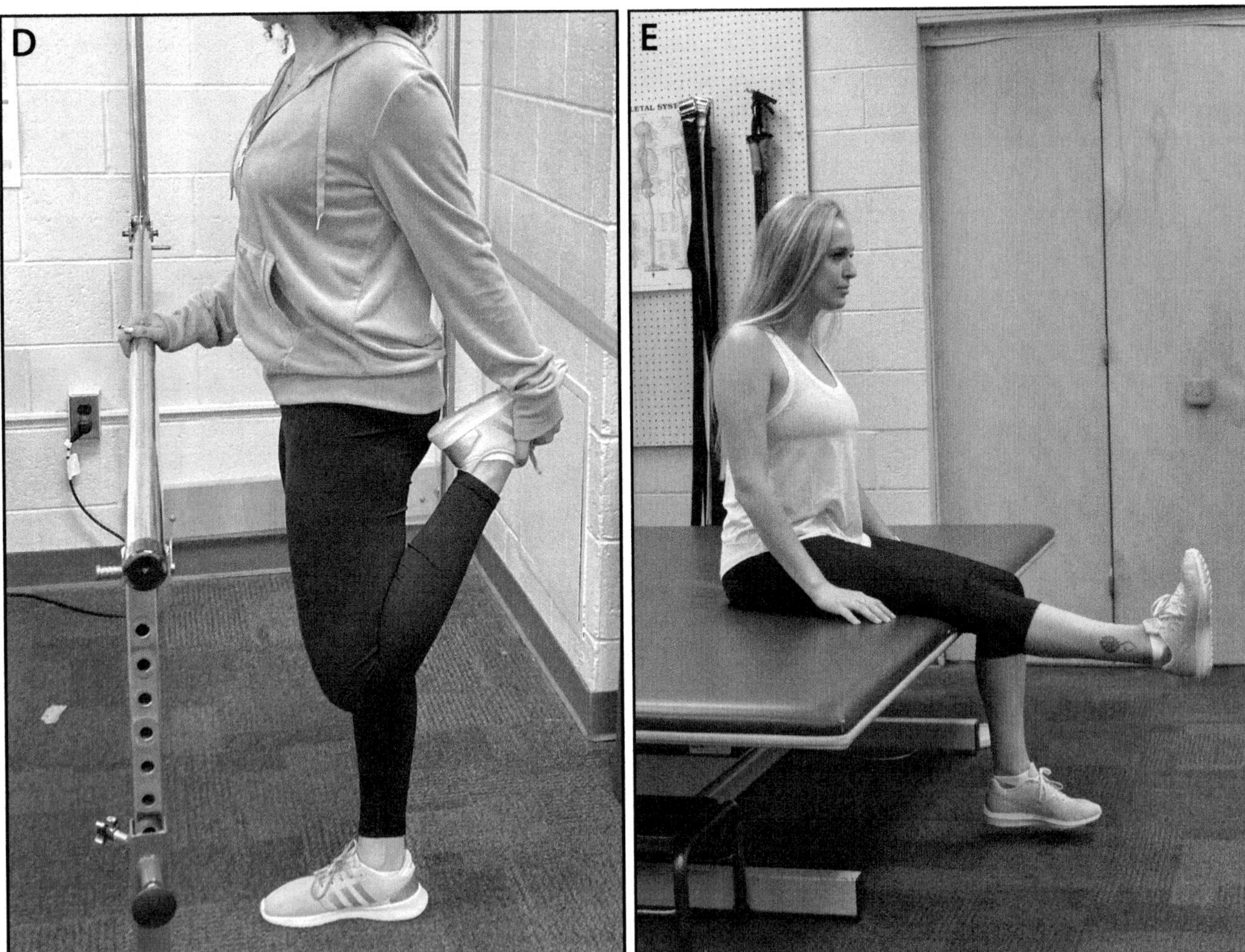


**Figure 13-49 (continued).** (D) Standing quadriceps muscle stretch. If the patient is unable to reach their ankle, a towel can be used around the ankle to pull the lower leg so the patient's heel moves closer to the buttocks. Have the patient hold on with the opposite hand for balance and safety. (E) Active knee extension seated. This can also stretch the hamstring muscles on the right leg. These stretches will help to increase knee extension. Adding ankle weights makes this a quadriceps muscle strengthening exercise.

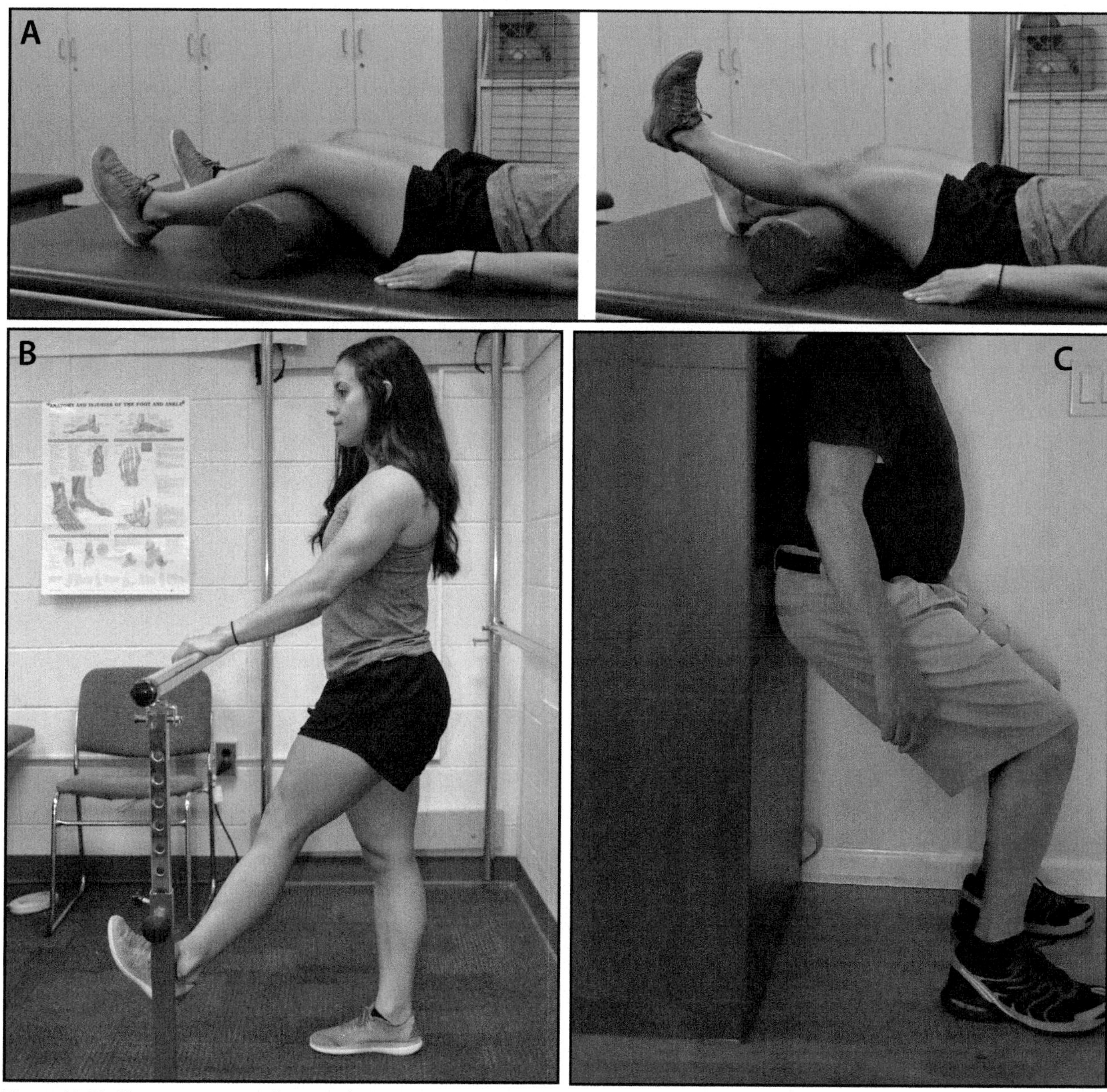


**Figure 13-50.** Knee extensor muscle strengthening exercises. (A) TKE promotes active knee extension and quadriceps muscle strength when adding ankle weights. Before performing this exercise, the patient should be able to perform a quadriceps set effectively. This exercise can also be performed in the CKC either in prone or standing. (B) Standing SLRs gravity minimized. This position should be used first when the patient is unable to perform an SLR correctly when supine (see Figure 13-39). (C) Partial squat wall slides for quadriceps muscle strengthening. The patient slides down the wall and holds that position for 10 to 30 seconds and then slides back to a standing position. A ball can also be placed between the knees when completing this exercise. The goal is for the patient to be able to slide down to 90 degrees of knee flexion maintaining a vertical shin and hold the position. *(continued)*

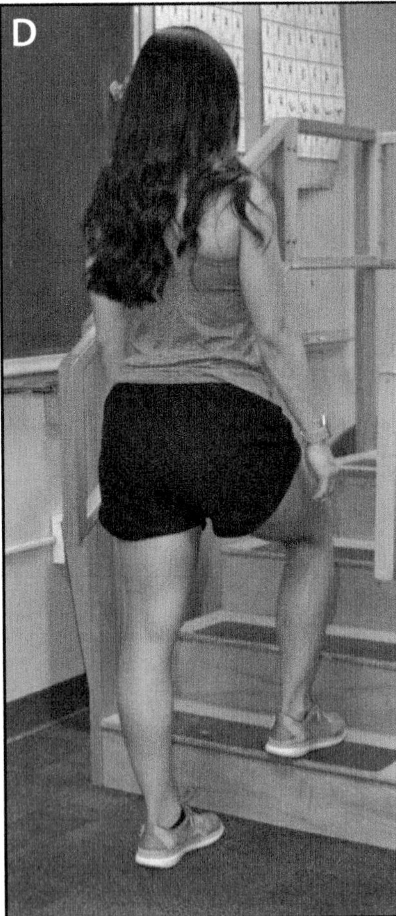


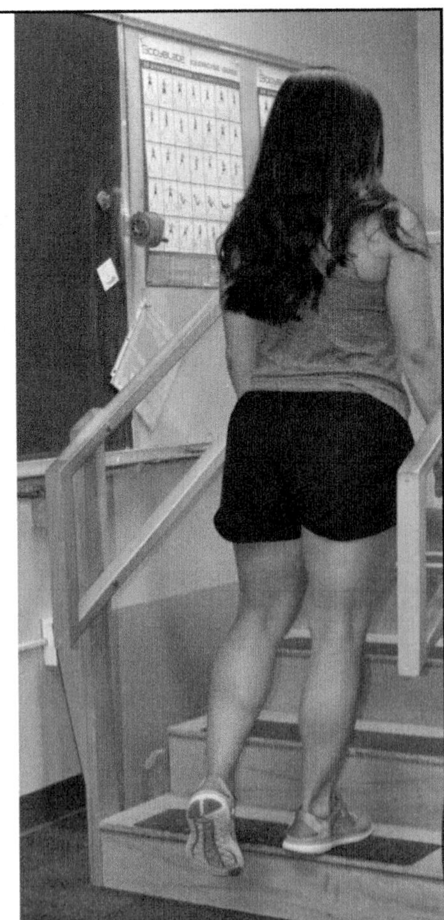

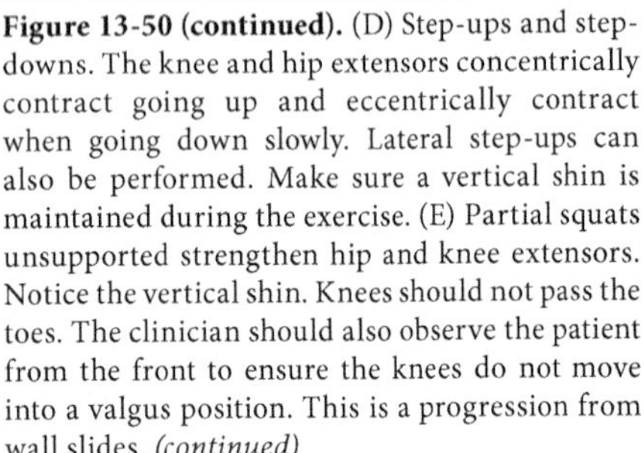

**Figure 13-50 (continued).** (D) Step-ups and step-downs. The knee and hip extensors concentrically contract going up and eccentrically contract when going down slowly. Lateral step-ups can also be performed. Make sure a vertical shin is maintained during the exercise. (E) Partial squats unsupported strengthen hip and knee extensors. Notice the vertical shin. Knees should not pass the toes. The clinician should also observe the patient from the front to ensure the knees do not move into a valgus position. This is a progression from wall slides. *(continued)*

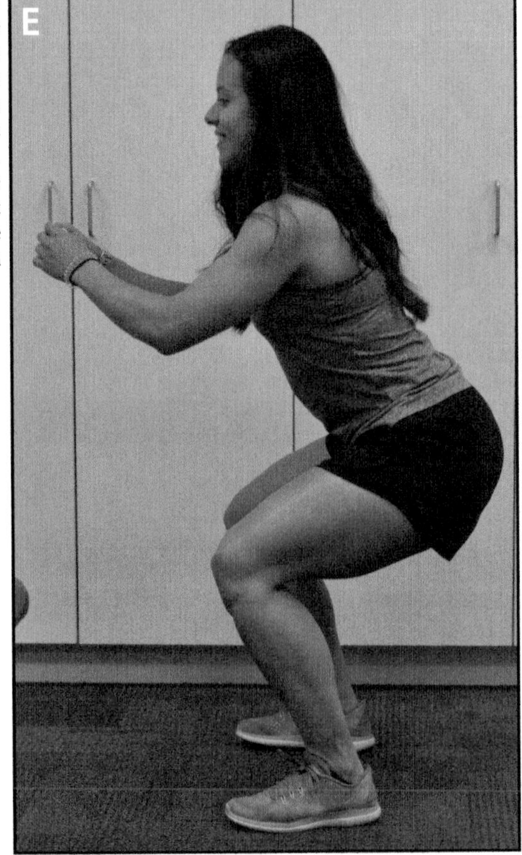

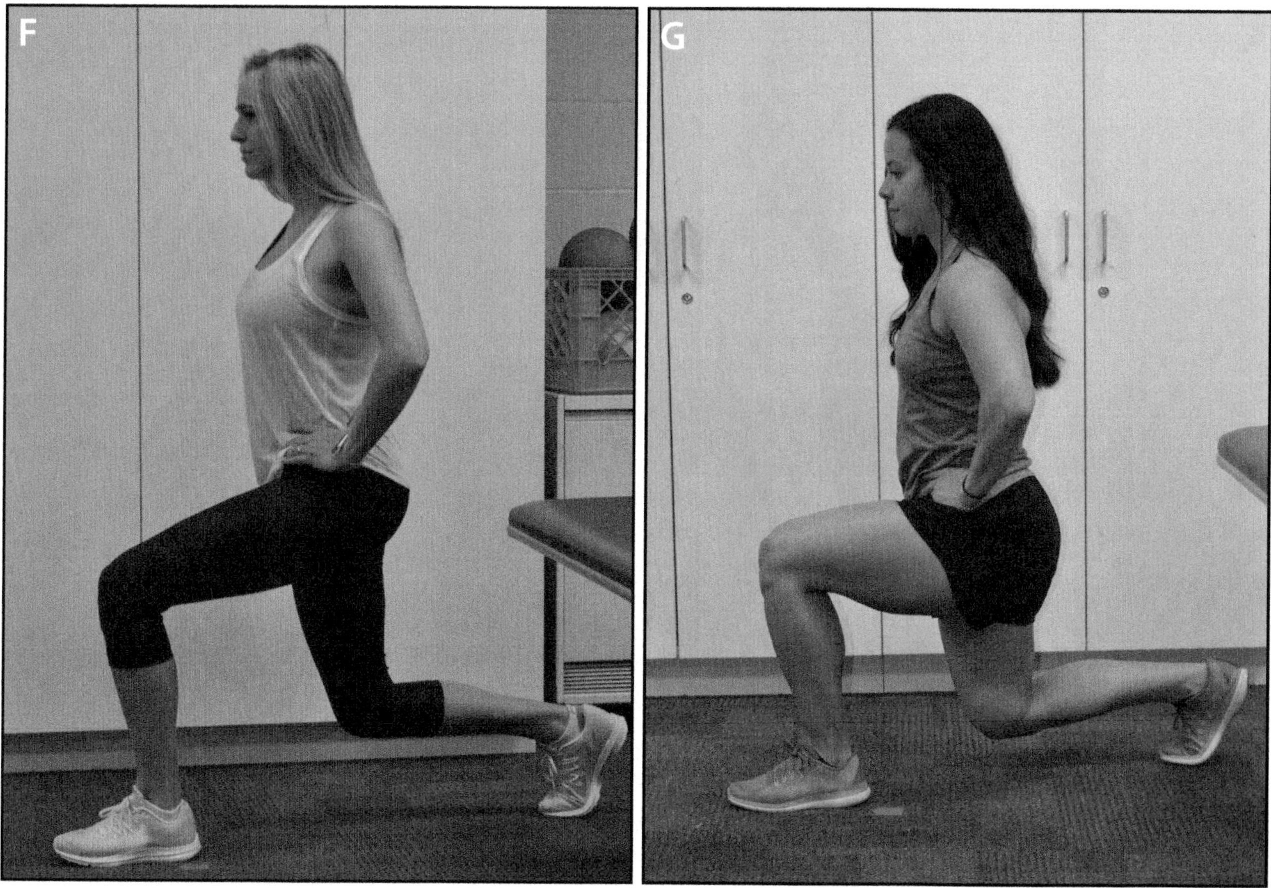


**Figure 13-50 (continued).** (F) Half forward lunges performed in a series along the floor strengthen hip and knee extensors and increase muscle endurance and balance. If performed in place, they can be performed forward or backward. (G) A full forward lunge exercise is a progression from half forward lunges.

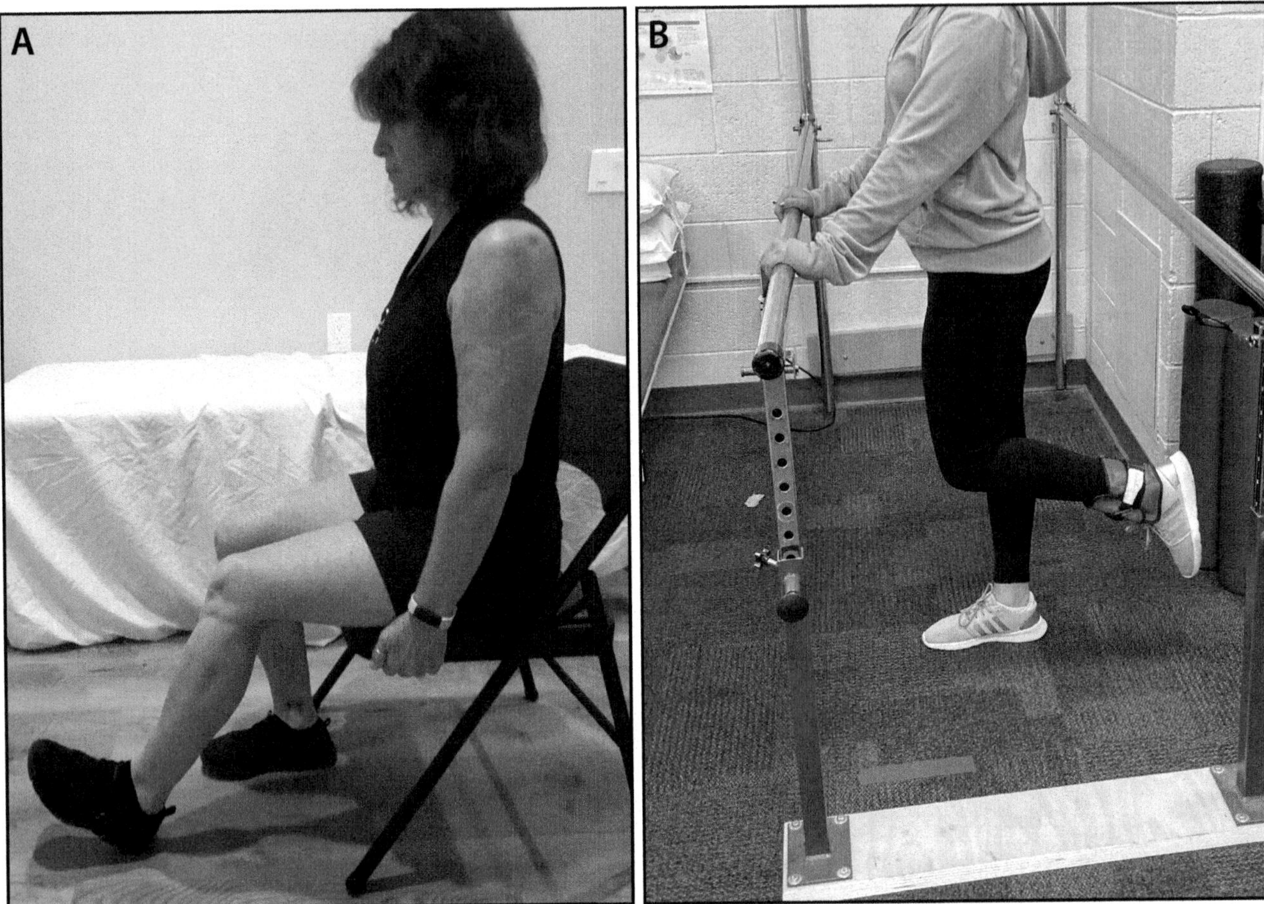


**Figure 13-51.** Knee flexor muscle strengthening exercises. (A) Heel digs. Isometric contractions can be performed at several points within the range (multiangle) progressing toward 90 degrees of knee flexion. A 6- to 10-second isometric hold facilitates hamstring strengthening at different angles throughout the patient's available range. Heel digs and quadriceps muscle sets with the knee flexed can also be used for cocontraction isometrics simultaneously. (B) Standing knee flexion with ankle weights to target the hamstring muscles. Have the patient hold on for safety.

## *Ankle and Foot Exercises*

Ankle ROM and stretching exercises are shown in Figures 13-52A through 13-52G and ankle strengthening exercises in Figures 13-53A through 13-53E. Advanced lower extremity strengthening, balance, and plyometric exercises are illustrated in Figures 13-54 and 13-55.

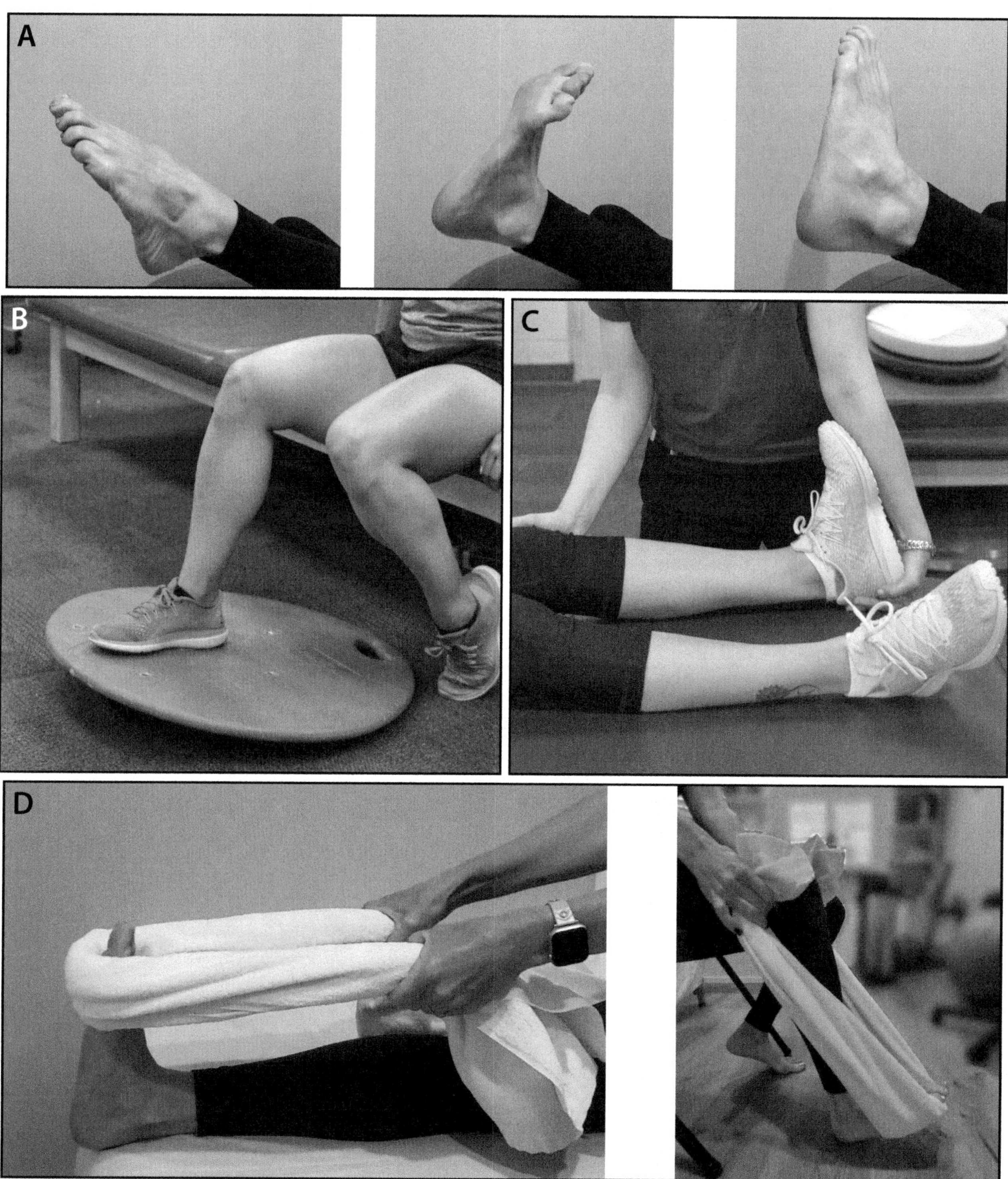

**Figure 13-52.** (A) AROM exercises. The patient can perform all single-plane motions that are pain free and then progress with writing the alphabet in capital and lowercase letters to achieve repetitive active ankle motions. This can be performed with the foot elevated to help reduce swelling. The patient can also perform arch and toe exercises. (B) Ankle AROM CKC using the BAPS board. All edges of the board should touch the floor as the ankle is moved through ROM. The larger the ball attachment on the bottom of the board, the greater the ROM. Start with the smaller ball and progress to a larger one. This can also be performed in standing as a progressive exercise. (C) Passive gastrocnemius stretches performed by the clinician. (D) The towel stretch for the gastrocnemius and soleus muscles. The knee should be kept straight during the gastrocnemius stretch (shown on the left). This stretch can also aid to facilitate knee extension because this muscle crosses 2 joints. To stretch the soleus muscle, the patient can sit in a chair with the knee flexed and use the towel to pull the ankle into dorsiflexion (right). Each stretch should be held for 20 to 30 seconds and repeated 2 to 3 times. *(continued)*

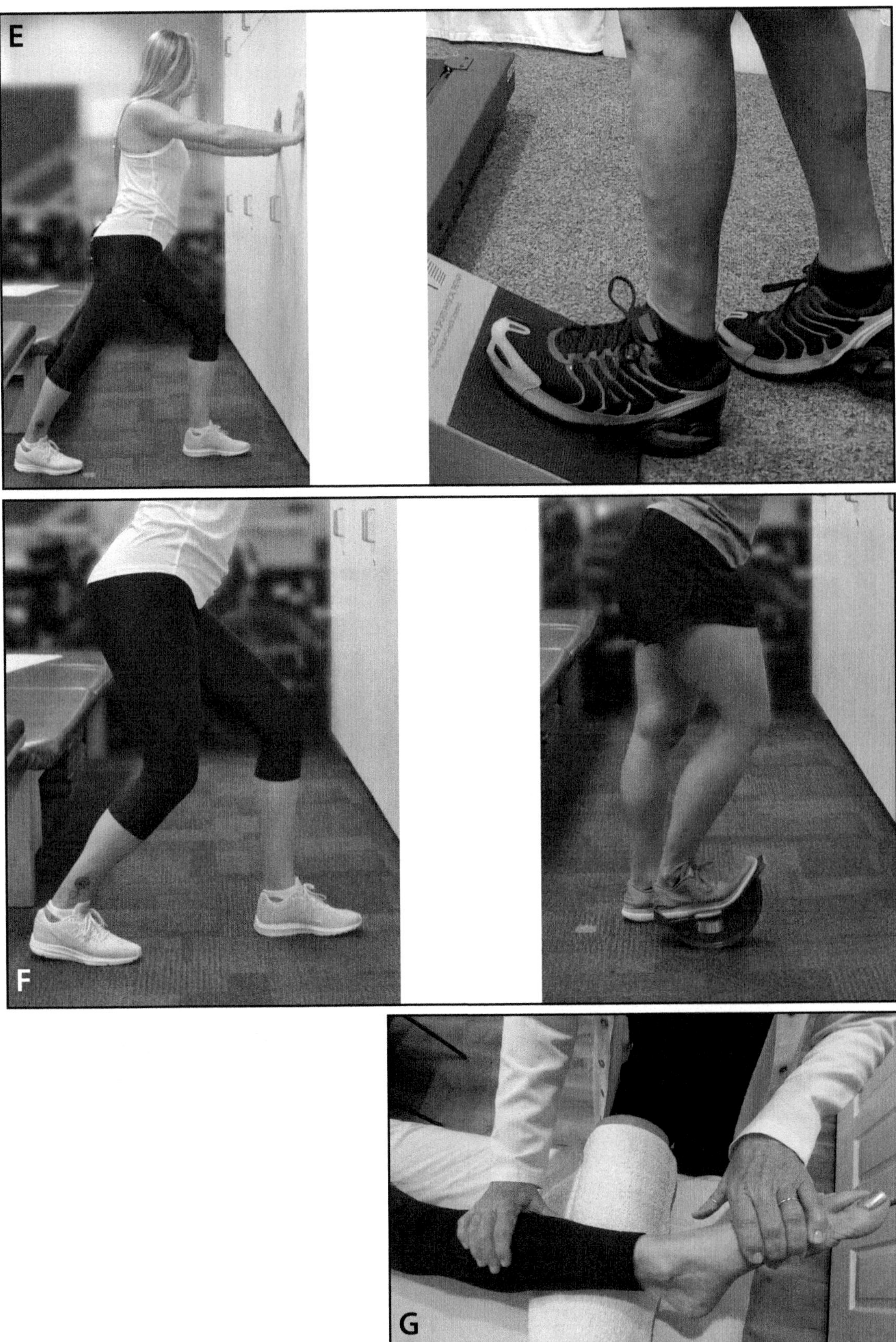


**Figure 13-52 (continued).** (E) The standing gastrocnemius stretch. The photograph on the left is usually given as a home exercise because most patients do not have a slant board (shown on the right). The important thing is to ensure that the patient keeps the knee straight during the stretch. Each stretch should be held for 20 to 30 seconds and repeated 2 to 3 times. (F) The standing soleus muscle stretch. To stretch the soleus, the knee is bent with the heel on the floor (left). Whether using an ankle rocker device (shown on right) or slant board, the knee still must be bent to target this muscle because it is a one-joint muscle. (G) To stretch the tibialis anterior, the clinician plantar flexes and everts the foot, which is the position opposite to that of the muscle's actual function. The patient can be taught to perform the stretch when seated.

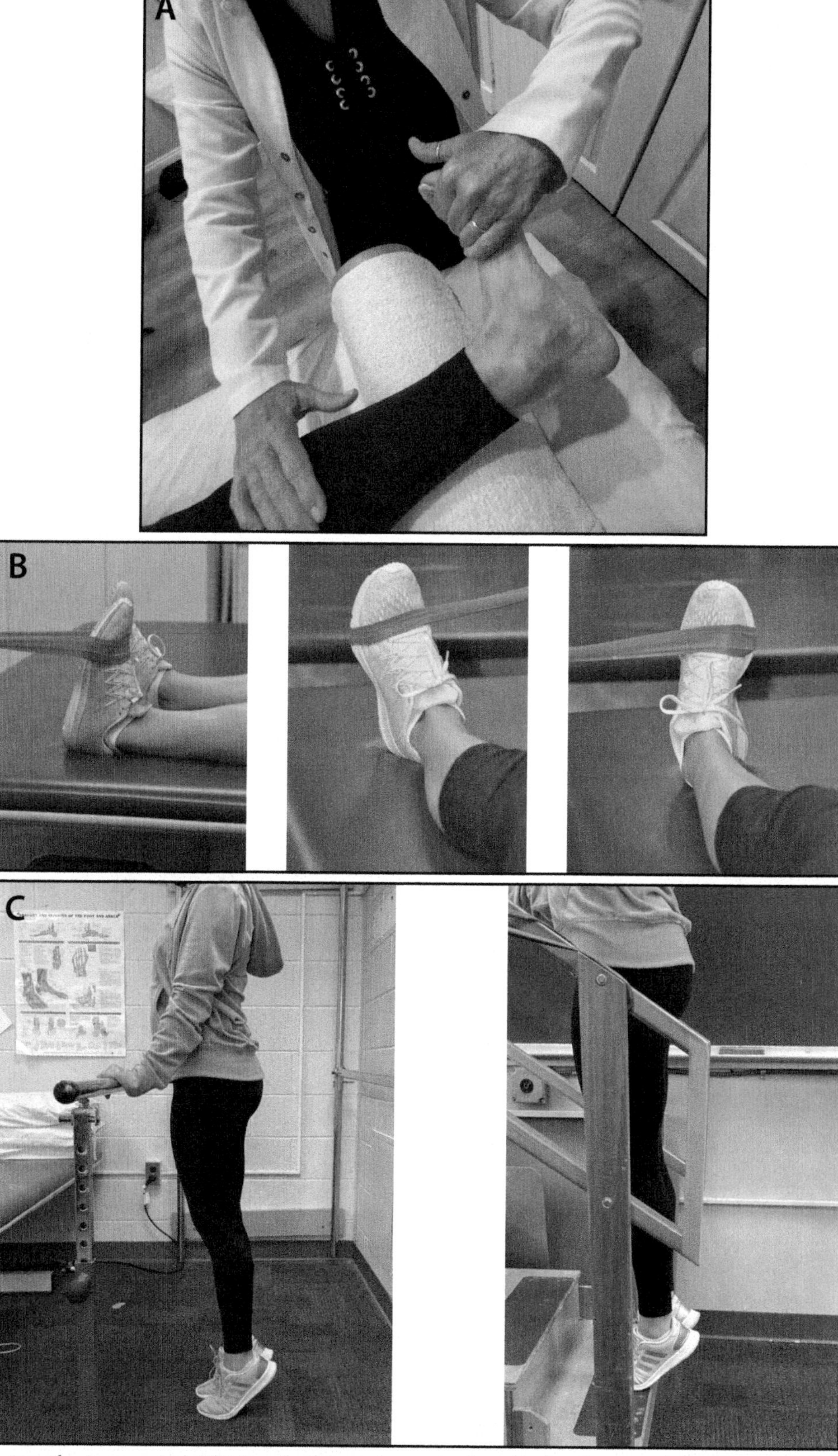

**Figure 13-53.** Ankle strengthening exercises. (A) Manual resistance isometrics for ankle dorsiflexion with the foot in a neutral position. This is an initial pain-free strengthening exercise that should be performed. The clinician applies the appropriate amount of manual resistance so that the patient does not experience pain. The manual resistance can be applied in all directions (ie, eversion, inversion, and plantar flexion). (B) Resistance band strengthening for dorsiflexion (left), eversion (center), and inversion (right). The patient should move through the pain-free ROM. Start with a lighter resistance band and progress to a heavier resistance band. This exercise is a progression from the isometric contraction exercises. (C) Bilateral heel raises. Performing heel raises with the knees straight targets the gastrocnemius muscle. Start by standing with both feet on the floor and go up on the toes, lifting the heels as high as possible. If the patient has difficulty performing the exercise with the weight evenly distributed on both legs, then have the patient first shift more of the weight on to the uninvolved side and then go up on the toes. Then, shift some of the weight back on to the involved leg and lower slowly. Progress exercise by performing on a step and then on one leg. *(continued)*

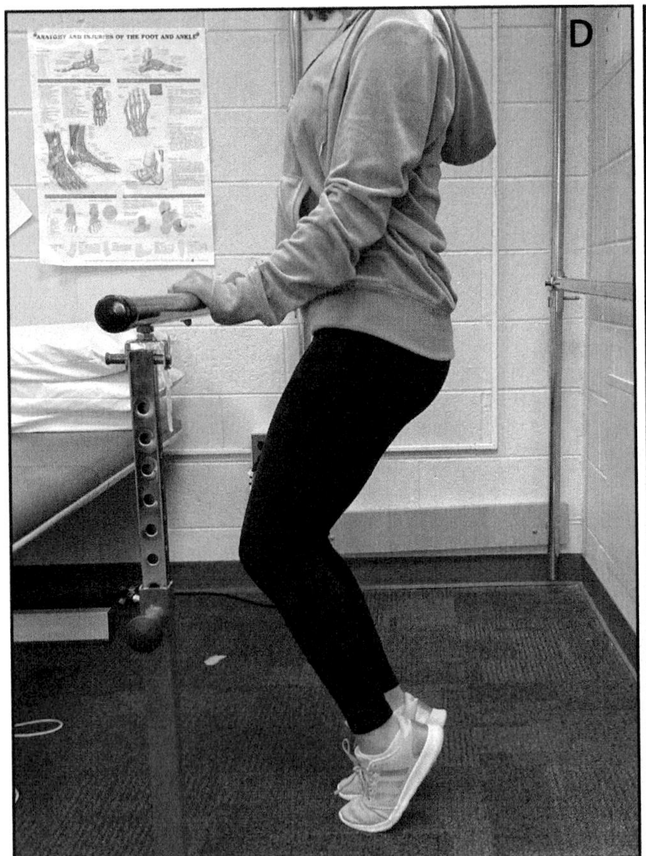


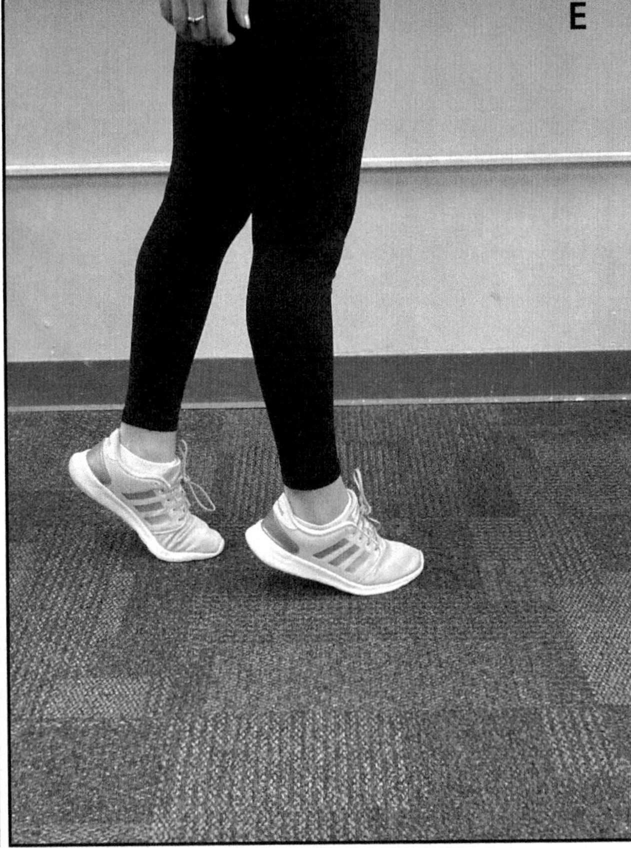


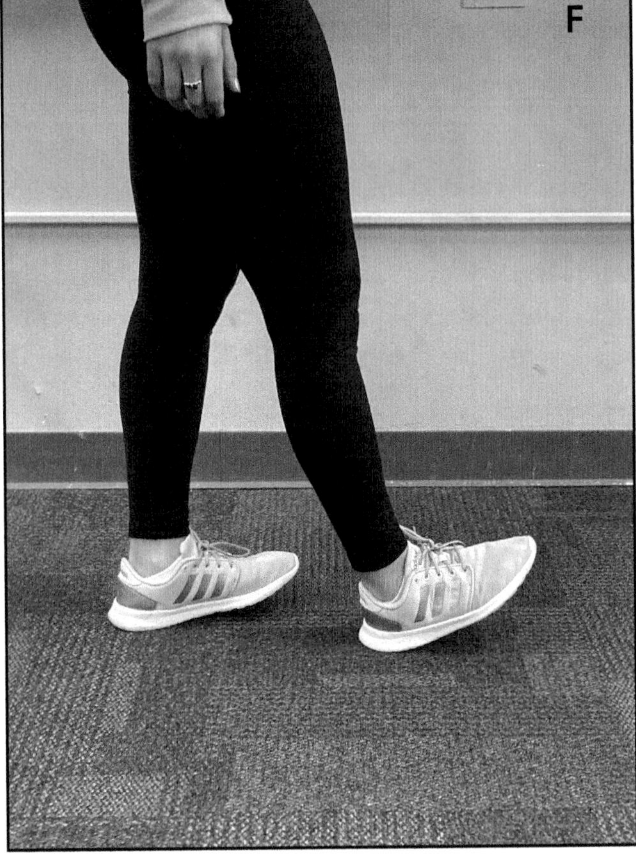


**Figure 13-53 (continued).** (D) Soleus muscle strengthening with the knees flexed. (E) Toe walking. (F) Heel walking.

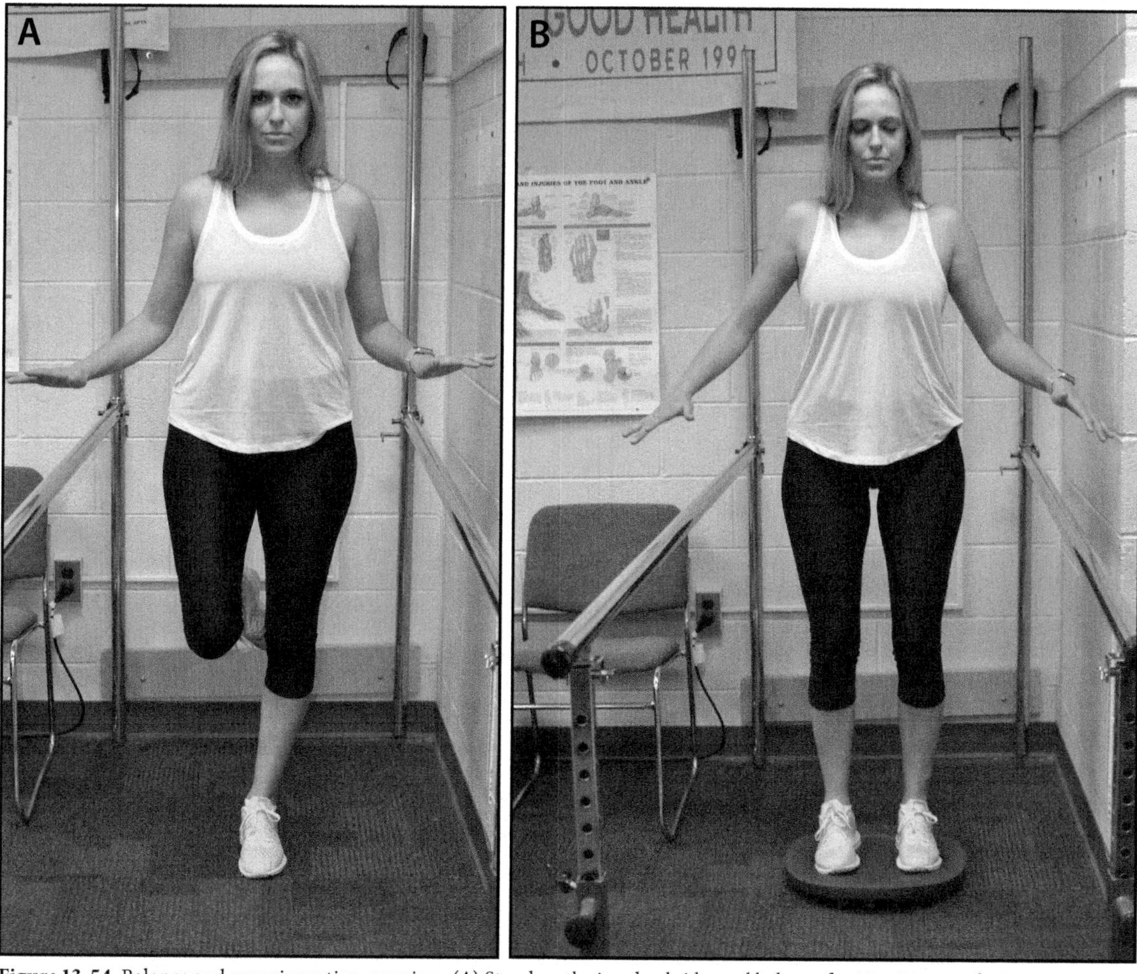


**Figure 13-54.** Balance and proprioception exercises. (A) Stand on the involved side, and balance for 10 to 30 seconds. Progress to eyes closed. (B) Balance on a compliant surface (foam) with eyes opened and closed for proprioception. Progress by moving feet together, and then progress to tandem standing and finally to standing on one foot.

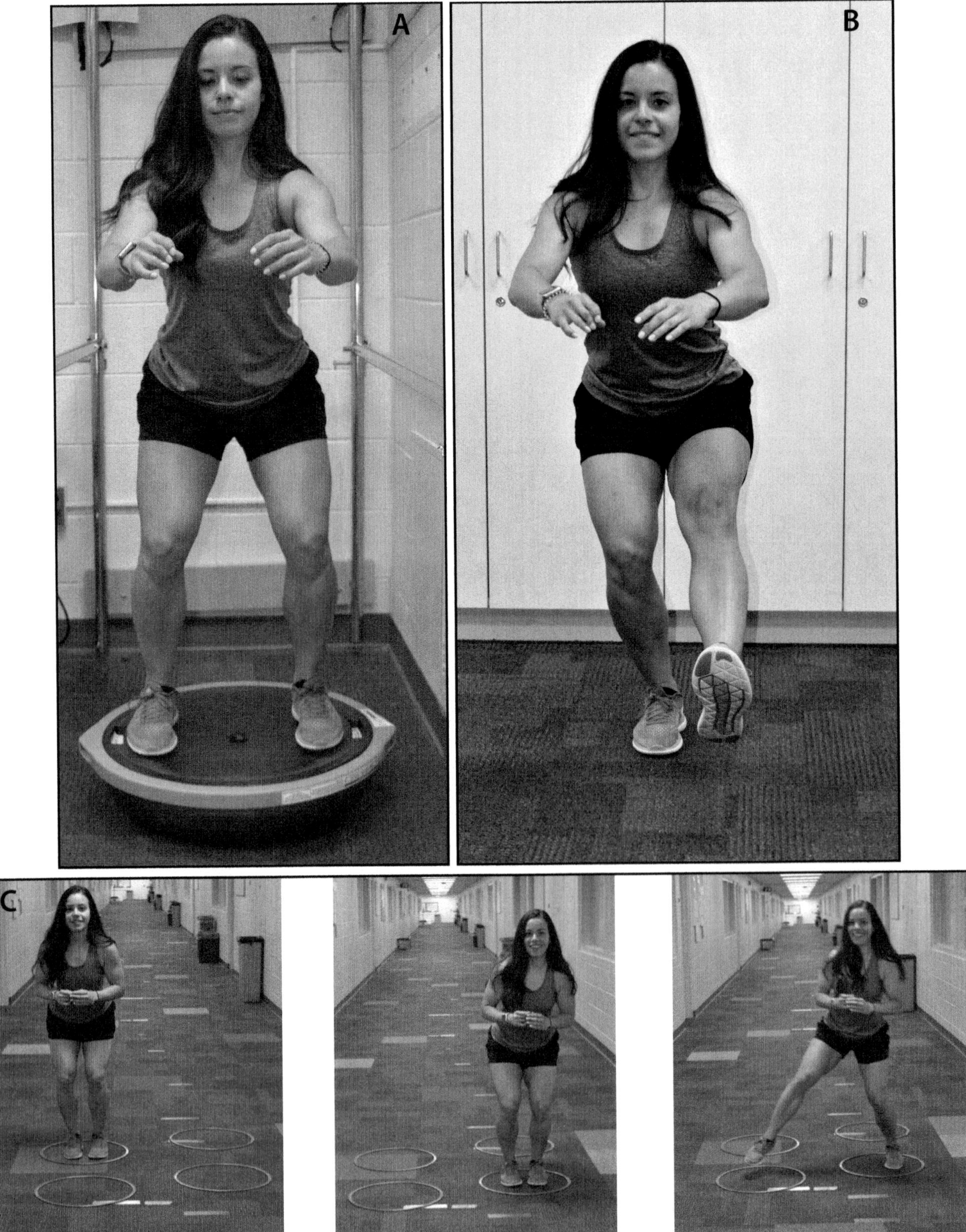


**Figure 13-55.** Advanced and plyometric lower extremity exercises. (A) Partial squats on BOSU Balance Trainer for strength and balance. Perform with feet apart and then with a narrow BOS and progress to single-leg standing. (B) Single-leg partial squats. Make sure the patient's shin is vertical and their knees do not pass the toes. Progress to single-leg deep squats for increasing strength and balance. (C) Plyometric jumping and hopping activities. Can be performed forward, backward, and on diagonals.

## Conclusion

Physical therapist assistants treat many patients with lower extremity diagnoses. The clinician should be able to understand the physical therapy examination and evaluation results and identify the primary source of a patient's symptoms or complaints. An assistant needs a comprehensive understanding of joint biomechanics, normal/abnormal movement patterns, and typical tissue healing times for conservative and postoperative diagnoses. This knowledge guides the assistant in the implementation of effective interventions that can facilitate optimal patient outcomes. This knowledge promotes accurate clinical decision making. Screening and ongoing monitoring will ensure that the clinician provides safe evidence-based treatments and intervention progressions.

## Review Questions

1. List 3 general treatment interventions that are most important to implement for a patient during the acute stage of healing. What activity is contraindicated during this phase?
2. List at least 2 exercises that are appropriate to include in the return-to-function phase of healing for a patient with a meniscal repair.
3. What characteristics are associated with hip labral tear?
4. Which special tests are most likely to be positive in a person with an ACL tear?
5. Describe an appropriate treatment progression (acute through return to function) for a person with a hip adductor strain.
6. What are the precautions for a patient after an Achilles tendon repair?
7. A patient presents with a weak hip abductor. Which muscles may need to be stretched? Which muscles should be strengthened? What substitution patterns would the assistant expect to see when observing the patient walk?
8. A patient presents with tight hip flexors. Which muscles need to be stretched? Which muscles should be strengthened? What special monitoring for form/substitutions will the assistant likely need to complete?
9. Describe an appropriate treatment progression for a patient with TKA. Is gait training indicated? Is an assistive device indicated? Consider the progression from postoperative day 1 through the return-to-function phase.
10. A patient presents with a diagnosis of hip OA. What information in the initial evaluation should the assistant review to determine the most appropriate treatment plan for the patient?

## Case Study 1

### *Part 1*

A 22-year-old basketball player had a grade II ankle sprain after rolling the left ankle when landing from a rebound 5 days ago. The physician ruled out a fracture and referred the patient to physical therapy. Currently, the patient is on crutches WBAT and wearing a brace. The patient reports 6 to 7/10 pain with movement.

The physical therapy initial evaluation includes the following:

- AROM: Dorsiflexion 5 degrees, plantar flexion 30 degrees, and inversion and eversion 5 degrees
- MMT: Dorsiflexion 3/5 available ROM, plantar flexion 3/5, and inversion and eversion 2/5

The patient is being treated in an outpatient clinic, and this is the first treatment session after the evaluation.

1. List 2 of each of the following: ROM, strengthening, and stretching exercises that are most appropriate for the patient addressing the injury during this visit after the evaluation.
2. Provide patient education as to what the patient should do at home (indications/contraindications).
3. What exercises (excluding ankle exercises) can the patient perform that will help the patient eventually return to play? List 4 exercises.

## Part 2

You have been seeing the patient 2 to 3 times per week for the last 4 weeks. The patient's gait is normal and pain free, and the patient is walking without crutches.

The physical therapy re-evaluation after 4 weeks of treatment is as follows:

- Left ankle AROM: Dorsiflexion 20 degrees, plantar flexion 50 degrees, inversion 10 degrees slight pain at end range, and eversion 35 degrees
- MMT: Dorsiflexion 4/5, plantar flexion 5/5, and inversion and eversion 4/5

1. Progress the patient and list 2 of each: ROM, stretching, and strengthening/dynamic stabilization exercises in order to progress the patient toward a long-term goal of return to play.

## Part 3

The patient is now starting week 7 of physical therapy and should be progressed to meet the following goals. List 6 exercises or activities that are appropriate for the athlete to perform without using the brace.

The physical therapy re-evaluation goals to be met by week 8 are as follows: (1) balance training and dynamic ankle stabilization and proprioception without brace; (2) increase functional ankle strength 5/5, power, and endurance so patient can return to sport beginning week 9; and (3) begin plyometrics if straight-line slow jog is pain free.

# Case Study 2

A 38-year-old female patient presents with right anterior knee pain superior and medial to the patella. There are no other complaints of pain. The patient is 6-week postoperative arthroscopy with no repair reported. The patient had physical therapy before surgery and completed 3 weeks of physical therapy after surgery. The original onset of pain was approximately 1 year ago. The patient states that she had just completed a 5-hour plane flight yesterday. The patient rates her pain as follows: 0/10 at rest, 3/10 currently, and 6/10 with stretching (which is worse than prior symptoms). She also states that she works from home, and the residence has 2 stories with stairs.

The physical therapy initial evaluation includes an unremarkable past medical history. Medications include birth control and Advil (ibuprofen) as needed. The patient's vitals are within normal limits.

Tests and measurements: The knee, lower leg, and foot appear slightly swollen. There is no report of calf tenderness. Circumference measurements on the right leg calf are 2 cm larger than prior measurements of the right lower extremity (measured 10 cm distal to the tibial tuberosity) without pitting edema and foot/ankle 3 cm larger (than prior measurements of right lower extremity).

Right AROM: Flexion 110 degrees with anterior knee pain, PROM 112 degrees with anterior knee pain and soft capsular end feel, and extension within normal limits with no significant hyperextension. Decreased weight-bearing and stance time are noted on right lower extremity during gait.

1. List and justify the possible causes of the patient's symptoms. What do you think is the least likely cause and why?
2. Which activity do you think would be the *most* difficult for the patient to perform?
3. List 2 stretching and 3 strengthening exercises in addition to one activity to improve the patient's gait pattern that would be *most* beneficial for this patient based on the information provided.

# Case Study 3

## Part 1

A 68-year-old had a left THA 3 weeks ago. The patient is going to outpatient therapy to work on increasing strength, balance, and mobility. The patient is anxious to return to playing tennis with her partner. The patient is WBAT and is cleared for FWB and walks with a forward flexed posture with a slight antalgic but normal pace using a rolling walker. The patient reports 5/10 pain during ambulation.

The physical therapy initial evaluation includes the following:

- ROM:
  - Right hip 0 to 120 degrees, knee 0 to 130 degrees, and ankle dorsiflexion 0 to 20 degrees
  - Left hip: 0 to 90 degrees, knee 10 to 90 degrees, and ankle dorsiflexion 0 to 5 degrees
- MMT: Right 4+/5 for hip knee and ankle motions and left hip flexion 3–/5 due to less than 90 degrees, extension 3+/5, hip abduction 3/5 knee flexion and extension 3+/5, and ankle dorsiflexion

You are seeing the patient for the first time after the initial evaluation. Based on the information provided, answer the following items.

1. List 2 of each of the following: ROM, strengthening, and stretching exercises that are most appropriate for the patient during this visit after the evaluation.
2. Provide patient education information regarding safety and fall prevention strategies.
3. What other exercises (other than hip exercises) can the patient perform that will help the patient eventually return to playing tennis? List 4 exercises.

## *Part 2*

You have seen the patient 2 times per week for the last 4 weeks. The patient now uses a cane only for community distances and has no pain and walks with a more erect posture.

The re-evaluation after 4 weeks of treatment includes the following:

- Right hip ROM: Within normal limits; left hip ROM: 0 to 90 degrees, knee 0 to 110 degrees, and ankle dorsiflexion 0 to 15 degrees
- MMT: Right 4+/5 for hip knee and ankle motions, left hip flex 4/5 in available range limit, extension 4/5, hip abduction 4/5 knee flexion and extension 4/5, and ankle dorsiflexion 3/5

1. Progress the patient and list 3 activities that are appropriate for each of the following: ROM, stretching, strengthening, balance exercises, and functional activities in order to meet the physical therapy re-evaluation goals.

The physical therapy re-evaluation goals to be met by week 12 (patient now 7 weeks status post THA) are as follows: (1) increase AROM to within functional limits so the patient can walk independently without an assistive device safely for community distances; (2) increase functional knee and ankle strength (5/5) to perform ADLs and gait activities without an assistive device safely by week 8; (3) begin balance and proprioception activities to reduce fall risk and improve mobility; (4) a negative Trendelenburg to improve patient's mobility and function week 7; and (5) by week 12, begin work on exercises/activities so the patient can return to tennis once cleared by the physician by week 16.

# Suggested Resource

Many of the outcomes assessment tools can be accessed from this link: https://www.sralab.org/rehabilitation-measures

# References


1. Brown MD, Gomez-Marin O, Brookfield KFW, Stokes Li P. Differential diagnosis of hip disease versus spine disease. *Clin Orthop Relat Res.* 2004;419:280-284.
2. Dibra FF, Prieto HA, Gray CF, Parvataneni HK. Don't forget the hip! Hip arthritis masquerading as knee pain. *Arthroplast Today.* 2017;4(1):118-124. doi:10.1016/j.artd.2017.06.008
3. Lesher J, Dreyfuss P, Hager N, Kaplan M, Furman M. Hip joint pain referral patterns: a descriptive study. *Pain Med.* 2008;9(1):22-25. doi:10.1111/j.1526-4637.2006.00153.x
4. Geersing GJ, Zuithoff NP, Kearon C, et al. Exclusion of deep vein thrombosis using the Wells rule in clinically important subgroups: individual patient data meta-analysis. *BMJ.* 2014;348:g1340. doi:10.1136/bmj.g1340
5. Modi S, Deisler R, Gozel K, et al. Wells criteria for DVT is a reliable clinical tool to assess the risk of deep venous thrombosis in trauma patients. *World J Emerg Surg.* 2016;11:24. doi:10.1186/s13017-016-0078-1
6. McLaughlin N, Heard H, Kelham S. Acute and chronic compartment syndromes: know when to act fast. *JAAPA.* 2014;27(6):23-26. doi:10.1097/01.JAA.0000446999.10176.13
7. Raff AB, Kroshinsky D. Cellulitis: a review. *JAMA.* 2016;316(3):325-337. doi:10.1001/jama.2016.8825
8. Barelds I, Krijnen WP, van de Leur JP, van der Schans CP, Goddard RJ. Diagnostic accuracy of clinical decision rules to exclude fractures in acute ankle injuries: systematic review and meta-analysis. *J Emerg Med.* 2017;53(3):353-368. doi:10.1016/j.jemermed.2017.04.035
9. LeBlanc KE, Muncie HL Jr, LeBlanc LL. Hip fracture: diagnosis, treatment, and secondary prevention. *Am Fam Physician.* 2014;89(12):945-951.
10. Hassan AS, Rao A, Manadan AM, Block JA. Peripheral bacterial septic arthritis: review of diagnosis and management. *J Clin Rheumatol.* 2017;23(8):435-442. doi:10.1097/RHU.0000000000000588
11. Neumann DA. Hip. In: Standring S, ed. *Gray's Anatomy: The Anatomical Basis of Clinical Practice.* 41st ed. Elsevier; 2016.
12. Muscolino J. *Kinesiology: The Skeletal System and Muscle Function.* Mosby Elsevier; 2006.
13. Norkin C, White D. *Measurement of Joint Motion.* 4th ed. FA Davis; 2009.
14. Samuels V. *Foundations in Kinesiology and Biomechanics.* FA Davis; 2018:266-267.
15. Loudon JK. Biomechanics and pathomechanics of the patellofemoral joint. *Int J Sports Phys Ther.* 2016;11(6):820-830.
16. Kisner C, Colby L, Borstad J. The knee. In: Kisner C, Colby L, Borstad J, eds. *Therapeutic Exercise Foundations and Techniques.* 7th ed. FA Davis; 2018:770-775.
17. Abulhasan JF, Grey MJ. Review anatomy and physiology of knee stability. *J Funct Morphol Kinesiol.* 2017;2(4):34. doi:10.3390/jfmk2040034
18. Kisner C, Colby L, Rose J, Borstad J. The ankle and foot. In: Kisner C, Colby L, Borstad J, eds. *Therapeutic Exercise Foundations and Techniques.* 7th ed. FA Davis; 2018:849-854.
19. Chan CS, Rudins A. Foot biomechanics during walking and running. *Mayo Clin Proc.* 1994;69:448-461.
20. Ranchos Los Amigos Medical Center. *Observational Gait Analysis.* Rancho Los Amigos Medical Center; 2001.
21. Bolgla LA, Malone TR. Plantar fasciitis and the windlass mechanism: a biomechanical link to clinical practice. *J Athl Train.* 2004;39(1):77-82.
22. Cibulka MT, White DM, Woehrle J, et al. Hip pain and mobility deficits--hip osteoarthritis: clinical practice guidelines linked to the international classification of functioning, disability, and health from the orthopaedic section of the American Physical Therapy Association. *J Orthop Sports Phys Ther.* 2009;39(4):A1-A25. doi:10.2519/jospt.2009.0301
23. Roos EM, Lohmander LS. The Knee injury and Osteoarthritis Outcome Score (KOOS): from joint injury to osteoarthritis. *Health Qual Life Outcomes.* 2003;1:64. doi:10.1186/1477-7525-1-64
24. Beutel BG, Trehan SK, Shalvoy RM, Mello MJ. The Ottawa knee rule: examining use in an academic emergency department. *West J Emerg Med.* 2012;13(4):366-372. doi:10.5811/westjem.2012.2.6892

25. Gould SJ, Cardone DA, Munyak J, Underwood PJ, Gould SA. Sideline coverage: when to get radiographs? A review of clinical decision tools. *Sports Health*. 2014;6(3):274-278. doi:10.1177/1941738114529701
26. Foye PM, Stitik TP. Hip osteoarthritis. In: Frontera WR, Silver JK, Rizzo TD Jr, eds. *Essentials of Physical Medicine and Rehabilitation Musculoskeletal Disorders, Pain and Rehabilitation*. 3rd ed. Elsevier/Saunders; 2015:285-290.
27. Wilson JJ, Furukawa M. Evaluation of the patient with hip pain. *Am Fam Physician*. 2014;89(1):27-34.
28. Sutlive TG, Lopez H, Scknitker D, et al. Development of a clinical prediction rule for diagnosing hip OA in individuals with unilateral hip pain. *Phys Ther*. 2008;38(9):542-550.
29. Chruściak T. Subjective evaluation of the effectiveness of whole-body cryotherapy in patients with osteoarthritis. *Reumatologia*. 2016;54(6):291-295. doi:10.5114/reum.2016.64904
30. Kisner C, Colby L, Rose J, Borstad J. The hip. In: Kisner C, Colby L, Borstad J, eds. *Therapeutic Exercise Foundations and Techniques*. 7th ed. FA Davis; 2018:714-751.
31. Wahoff M, Dischiavi S, Hodge J, Pharez JD. Rehabilitation after labral repair and femoroacetabular decompression: criteria-based progression through the return to sport phase. *Int J Sports Phys Ther*. 2014;9(6):813-826.
32. Garrison JC, Osler MT, Singleton SB. Rehabilitation after arthroscopy of an acetabular labral tear. *N Am J Sports Phys Ther*. 2007;2(4):241-250.
33. Groh MM, Herrera J. A comprehensive review of hip labral tears. *Curr Rev Musculoskelet Med*. 2009;2(2):105-117. doi:10.1007/s12178-009-9052-9
34. Domb BG, Sgroi TA, VanDevender JC. Physical therapy protocol after hip arthroscopy: clinical guidelines supported by 2-year outcomes. *Sports Health*. 2016;8(4):347-354. doi:10.1177/1941738116647920
35. Pivec R, Johnson J, Mears SC, Mont MA. Hip arthroplasty. *Lancet*. 2012;380(9855):1768-1777. doi:10.1016/S0140-6736(12)60607-2
36. Knight SR, Aujla R, Biswas SP. Total hip arthroplasty - over 100 years of operative history. *Orthop Rev (Pavia)*. 2011;3(2):e16. doi:10.4081/or.2011.e16
37. Dreinhöfer KE, Dieppe P, Stürmer T, et al. Indications for total hip replacement: comparison of assessments of orthopaedic surgeons and referring physicians. *Ann Rheum Dis*. 2006;65(10):1346-1350. doi:10.1136/ard.2005.047811
38. Bottner F, Pellicci PM. Review: posterior soft tissue repair in primary total hip arthroplasty. *HSS J*. 2006;2(1):7-11. doi:10.1007/s11420-005-0134-y
39. Berstock JR, Blom AW, Beswick AD. A systematic review and meta-analysis of complications following the posterior and lateral surgical approaches to total hip arthroplasty. *Ann R Coll Surg Engl*. 2015;97:11-16. doi10.1308/003588414X139461849040
40. Hwang SK. Experience of complications of hip arthroplasty. *Hip Pelvis*. 2014;26(4):207-213. doi:10.5371/hp.2014.26.4.207
41. Bitar AA, Kaplan RJ, Stitik TP, Shih VC, Vo AN, Kamen LB. Rehabilitation of orthopedic and rheumatologic disorders.3. total hip arthroplasty rehabilitation. *Arch Phys Med Rehabil*. 2005;86(suppl 1):S56-S59.
42. Melloh M, Eggli S, Busato A, Roder C. Predictors of early stem loosening after total hip arthroplasty: a case-control study. *J Orthop Surg (Hong Kong)*. 2011;19(3):269-273.
43. Klestil T, Röder C, Stotter C, et al. Impact of timing of surgery in elderly hip fracture patients: a systematic review and meta-analysis. *Sci Rep*. 2018;8(1):13933. doi:10.1038/s41598-018-32098-7
44. Guzon-Illescas O, Perez Fernandez E, Crespí Villarias N, et al. Mortality after osteoporotic hip fracture: incidence, trends, and associated factors. *J Orthop Surg Res*. 2019;14:203. doi:10.1186/s13018-019-1226-6
45. Pouresmaeili F, Kamalidehghan B, Kamarehei M, Goh YM. A comprehensive overview on osteoporosis and its risk factors. *Ther Clin Risk Manag*. 2018;14:2029-2049. doi:10.2147/TCRM.S138000
46. Giordano V, Giordano M, Aquino R, Grossi JO, Senna H, Koch HA. How do orthopedic surgeons manage displaced femoral neck fracture in the middle-aged patient? Brazilian survey of 78 orthopaedic surgeons. *Rev Bras Ortop (Sao Paulo)*. 2019;54(3):288-294.
47. Choi JY, Sung YB, Kim JH. Comparative study of bipolar hemiarthroplasty for femur neck fractures treated with cemented versus cementless stem. *Hip Pelvis*. 2016;28(4):208-216. doi:10.5371/hp.2016.28.4.208
48. Martin R, Martin HD, Kivlan BR. Nerve entrapment in the hip region: current concepts review. *Int J Sports Phys Ther*. 2017;12(7):1163-1173.
49. Martin HD, Khoury A, Schröder R, Palmer IJ. Ischiofemoral impingement and hamstring syndrome as causes of posterior hip pain: where do we go next? *Clin Sports Med*. 2016;35(3):469-486. doi:10.1016/j.csm.2016.02.010
50. Zhang Y, Jordan JM. Epidemiology of osteoarthritis. *Clin Geriatr Med*. 2013;26(3):355-369. doi:10.1016/j.cger.2010.03.001
51. Hsu H, Siwiec RM. *Knee Osteoarthritis*. StatPearls Publishing; 2020. https://www.ncbi.nlm.nih.gov/books/NBK507884/
52. Heidari B. Knee osteoarthritis prevalence, risk factors, pathogenesis and features: part I. *Caspian J Intern Med*. 2011;2(2):205-212.
53. Matzkin EG, Curry EJ, Kong Q, Rogers MJ, Henry M, Smith EL. Efficacy and treatment response of intra-articular corticosteroid injections in patients with symptomatic knee osteoarthritis. *J Am Acad Orthop Surg*. 2017;25(10):703-714. doi:10.5435/JAAOS-D-16-00541
54. Lee DC, Byun SJ. High tibial osteotomy. *Knee Surg Relat Res*. 2012;24(2):61-69. doi:10.5792/ksrr.2012.24.2.61
55. Kisner C, Colby L, Borstad J. The knee. In: Kisner C, Colby L, Borstad J, eds. *Therapeutic Exercise Foundations and Techniques*. 7th ed. FA Davis; 2018:775-840.
56. Jain RK, Neville LT, Ezzet KA, Sterling RS, Horwood RL, Colwell CW Jr. Two year follow-up of the preservation unicompartmental knee implant. *HSS J*. 2011;7(2):125-129. doi:10.1007/s11420-011-9205-4
57. Li X, Wang C, Guo Y, Chen W. An approach to developing customized total knee replacement implants. *J Healthc Eng*. 2017;2017:9298061. doi:10.1155/2017/9298061
58. Gandhi R, Tsvetkov D, Davey JR, Mahomed NN. Survival and clinical function of cemented and uncemented prostheses in total knee replacement: a meta-analysis. 2009. In: *Database of Abstracts of Reviews of Effects (DARE): Quality-assessed Reviews*. Centre for Reviews and Dissemination; 1995. https://www.ncbi.nlm.nih.gov/books/NBK77833/
59. Aalderink KJ, Shaffer M, Amendola A. Rehabilitation following high tibial osteotomy. *Clin Sports Med*. 2010;29(2):291-301, ix. doi:10.1016/j.csm.2009.12.005

60. Rossi R, Bonasia D, Amendola A. The role of high tibial osteotomy in the varus knee. *J Am Acad Orthop Surg.* 2011;19:590-599.
61. Amendola A, Bonasia DE. Results of high tibial osteotomy: review of the literature. *Int Orthop.* 2010;34(2):155-160. doi:10.1007/s00264-009-0889-8
62. Witjes S, Gouttebarge V, Kuijer PPFM, van Geenen RCI, Poolman RW, Kerkhoffs GMMJ. Return to sports and physical activity after total and unicondylar knee arthroplasty: a systematic review and meta-analysis. *Sports Med.* 2016;46(2):269-292. doi:10.1007/s40279-015-0421-9
63. Dagneaux L, Bourlez J, Degeorge B, Canovas F. Return to sport after total or unicompartmental knee arthroplasty: an informative guide for residents to patients. *EFORT Open Rev.* 2017;2(12):496-501. doi:10.1302/2058-5241.2.170037
64. Dávila Castrodad IM, Recai TM, Abraham MM, et al. Rehabilitation protocols following total knee arthroplasty: a review of study designs and outcome measures. *Ann Transl Med.* 2019;7(suppl 7):S255. doi:10.21037/atm.2019.08.15
65. Santoso MB, Wu L. Unicompartmental knee arthroplasty, is it superior to high tibial osteotomy in treating unicompartmental osteoarthritis? A meta-analysis and systemic review. *J Orthop Surg Res.* 2017;12:50. doi:10.1186/s13018-017-0552-9
66. Logerstedt DS, Scalzitti DA, Bennell KL, et al. Knee pain and mobility impairments: meniscal and articular lesions revision 2018. *J Orthop Sports Phys Ther.* 2018;48(2):A1-A50. doi:10.2519/jospt.2018.0301
67. Fox AJ, Wanivenhaus F, Burge AJ, Warren RF, Rodeo SA. The human meniscus: a review of anatomy, function, injury, and advances in treatment. *Clin Anat.* 2015;28(2):269-287.
68. Lento P, Akuthota V. Meniscal injuries. In: Frontera WR, Silver JK, Rizzo TD Jr, eds. *Essentials of Physical Medicine and Rehabilitation Musculoskeletal Disorders, Pain and Rehabilitation.* 3rd ed. Elsevier/Saunders; 2015:373-379.
69. Doral MN, Bilge O, Huri G, Turhan E, Verdonk R. Modern treatment of meniscal tears. *EFORT Open Rev.* 2018;3(5):260-268. doi:10.1302/2058-5241.3.170067
70. VanderHave KL, Perkins C, Le M. Weightbearing versus nonweightbearing after meniscus repair. *Sports Health.* 2015;7(5):399-402. doi:10.1177/1941738115576898
71. Lind M, Nielsen T, Faunø P, Lund B, Christiansen SE. Free rehabilitation is safe after isolated meniscus repair: a prospective randomized trial comparing free with restricted rehabilitation regimens. *Am J Sports Med.* 2013;41(12):2753-2758. doi:10.1177/0363546513505079
72. Lee YS, Lee OS, Lee SH. Return to sports after athletes undergo meniscal surgery: a systematic review. *Clin J Sport Med.* 2019;29(1):29-36. doi:10.1097/JSM.0000000000000500
73. Boden BP, Sheehan FT, Torg JS, Hewett TE. Noncontact anterior cruciate ligament injuries: mechanisms and risk factors. *J Am Acad Orthop Surg.* 2010;18(9):520-527. doi:10.5435/00124635-201009000-00003
74. Micheo W, Amy E, Sepúlveda. Anterior cruciate ligament tear. In: Frontera WR, Silver JK, Rizzo TD Jr, eds. *Essentials of Physical Medicine and Rehabilitation Musculoskeletal Disorders, Pain and Rehabilitation.* 3rd ed. Elsevier/Saunders; 2015:324-330.
75. Raj MA, Varacallo M. *Posterior cruciate ligament (PCL) knee injuries.* StatPearls Publishing; 2020. https://www.ncbi.nlm.nih.gov/books/NBK430726/
76. McCabe M, Khadavi M. Posterior cruciate injuries. Sports-Health. September 4, 2019. Accessed February 2, 2023. https://www.sports-health.com/sports-injuries/knee-injuries/symptoms-posterior-cruciate-ligament-pcl-tears
77. Andrews K, Lu A, Mckean L, Ebraheim N. Review: medial collateral ligament injuries. *J Orthop.* 2017;14(4):550-554. doi:10.1016/j.jor.2017.07.017
78. Bassett A, McCulloch PC. MCL knee injuries. *Ortho Bullets.* April 29, 2021. Accessed February 2, 2023. https://www.orthobullets.com/knee-and-sports/3010/mcl-knee-injuries
79. Macaulay AA, Perfetti DC, Levine WN. Anterior cruciate ligament graft choices. *Sports Health.* 2012;4(1):63-68. doi:10.1177/1941738111409890
80. Padua DA, Boling MC, Prentice WE. Rehabilitation of knee injuries. In: Prentice WE, ed. *Rehabilitation Techniques for Sports Medicine and Athletic Training.* 6th ed. SLACK Incorporated; 2015:639-709.
81. Marcacci M, Zaffagnini S, Iacono F, et al. Intra- and extra-articular anterior cruciate ligament reconstruction utilizing autogeneous semitendinosus and gracilis tendons: 5-year clinical results. *Knee Surg Sports Traumatol Arthrosc.* 2003;11:2-8. doi:10.1007/s00167-002-0323-x
82. Ferretti A. Extra-articular reconstruction in the anterior cruciate ligament deficient knee: a commentary. *Joints.* 2014;2(1):41-47.
83. Cavanaugh JT, Powers M. ACL rehabilitation progression: where are we now? *Curr Rev Musculoskelet Med.* 2017;10(3):289-296. doi:10.1007/s12178-017-9426-3
84. Van Grinsven S, Van Cingel REH, Holla CJ, Van Loo CJM. Evidence-based rehabilitation following anterior cruciate ligament reconstruction. *Knee Surg Sports Traumatol Arthrosc.* 2010;18:1128-1144. doi:10.1007/s00167-009-1027-2
85. Indorato D. A review of rehabilitation protocols following ACL reconstruction. *Inquiries J.* 2016;8:10. http://www.inquiriesjournal.com/a?id=1465
86. Gulick DT, Yoder HN. Anterior cruciate ligament reconstruction: clinical outcomes of patella tendon and hamstring tendon grafts. *J Sports Sci Med.* 2002;1(3):63-71.
87. Buckthorpe M, La Rosa G, Villa FD. Restoring knee extensor strength after anterior cruciate ligament reconstruction: a clinical commentary. *Int J Sports Phys Ther.* 2019;14(1):159-172.
88. Kruse LM, Gray B, Wright RW. Rehabilitation after anterior cruciate ligament reconstruction: a systematic review. *J Bone Joint Surg Am.* 2012;94(19):1737-1748. doi:10.2106/JBJS.K.01246
89. Logerstedt DS, Scalzitti D, Risberg MA, et al. Knee stability and movement coordination impairments: knee ligament sprain revision 2017. *J Orthop Sports Phys Ther.* 2017;47(11):A1-A47. doi:10.2519/jospt.2017.0303
90. Wang D, Graziano J, Williams RJ III, Jones KJ. Nonoperative treatment of PCL injuries: goals of rehabilitation and the natural history of conservative care. *Curr Rev Musculoskelet Med.* 2018;11(2):290-297. doi:10.1007/s12178-018-9487-y
91. Pierce CM, O'Brien L, Wohlt Griffin L, LaPrade RF. Posterior cruciate ligament tears: functional and postoperative rehabilitation. *Knee Surg Sports Traumatol Arthrosc.* 2013;21:1071-1084. doi:10.1007/s00167-012-1970-1
92. Senese M, Greenberg E, Todd Lawrence J, Ganley T. Rehabilitation following isolated posterior cruciate ligament reconstruction: a literature review of published protocols. *Int J Sports Phys Ther.* 2018;13(4):737-751.

93. DeGrace DM, Gill TJ IV, Gill TJ III. Analysis of medical collateral ligament injuries of the knee. *Harv Orthop J.* 2013;15:13-24.
94. Wijdicks CA, Griffith CJ, Johansen S, Engebretsen L, LaPrade RF. Injuries to the medical collateral ligament and associated medial structures of the knee. *J Bone Joint Surg Am.* 2010;92:1266-1280. doi:10.2106/JBJS.I.01229
95. Willy RW, Hoglund LT, Barton CJ, et al. Patellofemoral pain: clinical practice guidelines linked to the International Classification of Functioning, Disability and Health from the Academy of Orthopaedic Physical Therapy of the American Physical Therapy Association. *J Orthop Sports Phys Ther.* 2019;49(9):CPG1-CPG95. doi:10.2519/jospt.2019.0302
96. Malliaras P, Cook J, Purdam C, Rio E. Patellar tendinopathy: clinical diagnosis, load management, and advice for challenging case presentations. *J Orthop Sports Phys Ther.* 2015;45(11):887-898. doi:10.2519/jospt.2015.5987
97. Jibri Z, Jamieson P, Rakhra KS, Sampaio ML, Dervin G. Patellar maltracking: an update on the diagnosis and treatment strategies. *Insights Imaging.* 2019;10(1):65. doi:10.1186/s13244-019-0755-1
98. Tsai CH, Hsu CJ, Hung CH, Hsu HC. Primary traumatic patellar dislocation. *J Orthop Surg Res.* 2012;7:21. doi:10.1186/1749-799X-7-21
99. Alba-Martín P, Gallego-Izquierdo T, Plaza-Manzano G, Romero-Franco N, Núñez-Nagy S, Pecos-Martín D. Effectiveness of therapeutic physical exercise in the treatment of patellofemoral pain syndrome: a systematic review. *J Phys Ther Sci.* 2015;27(7):2387-2390. doi:10.1589/jpts.27.2387
100. Chen S, Chang WD, Wu JY, Fong YC. Electromyographic analysis of hip and knee muscles during specific exercise movements in females with patellofemoral pain syndrome: an observational study. *Medicine (Baltimore).* 2018;97(28):e11424. doi:10.1097/MD.0000000000011424
101. Chang WD, Huang WS, Lai PT. Muscle activation of vastus medialis oblique and vastus lateralis in sling-based exercises in patients with patellofemoral pain syndrome: a cross-over study. *Evid Based Complement Alternat Med.* 2015;2015:740315. doi:10.1155/2015/740315
102. Respizzi S, Cavallin R. First patellar dislocation: from conservative treatment to return to sport. *Joints.* 2014;2(3):141-145. doi:10.11138/jts/2014.2.3.141
103. Ekstrom RA, Donatelli RA, Carp KC. Electromyographic analysis of core trunk, hip, and thigh muscles during 9 rehabilitation exercises. *J Orthop Sports Phys Ther.* 2007;37(12):754-762. doi:10.2519/jospt.2007.2471
104. Herzog MM, Kerr ZK, Marshall SW, Wikstrom EA. Epidemiology of ankle sprains and chronic ankle instability. *J Athl Train.* 2019;54(6):603-610. doi:10.4085/1062-6050-447-17
105. Doherty C, Delahunt E, Caulfield B, Hertel J, Ryan J, Bleakley C. The incidence and prevalence of ankle sprain injury: a systematic review and meta-analysis of prospective epidemiological studies. *Sports Med.* 2014;44(1):123-140. doi:10.1007/s40279-013-0102-5
106. Mauntel TC, Wikstrom EA, Roos KG, Djoko A, Dompier TP, Kerr ZY. The epidemiology of high ankle sprains in national collegiate athletic association sports. *Am J Sports Med.* 2017;45(9):2156-2163. doi:10.1177/0363546517701428
107. Lynch SA. Assessment of the injured ankle in the athlete. *J Athl Train.* 2002;37(4):406-412.
108. Polzer H, Kanz KG, Prall WC, et al. Diagnosis and treatment of acute ankle injuries: development of an evidence-based algorithm. *Orthop Rev (Pavia).* 2012;4(1):e5. doi:10.4081/or.2012.e5
109. Norkus SA, Floyd RT. The anatomy and mechanisms of syndesmotic ankle sprains. *J Athl Train.* 2001;36(1):68-73.
110. Lötscher P, Lang TH, Zwicky L, Hintermann B, Knupp M. Osteoligamentous injuries of the medial ankle joint. *Eur J Trauma Emerg Surg.* 2015;41(6):615-621. doi:10.1007/s00068-015-0548-2
111. Wire J, Slane VH. *Ankle Fractures.* StatPearls Publishing; 2020. Accessed April 16, 2020. https://www.ncbi.nlm.nih.gov/books/NBK542324/
112. McAlister FJ, So E. Keys to deltoid ligament repair after ankle fracture. *Podiatry Today.* 2018;31(10):44-52. Accessed February 2, 2023. https://www.podiatrytoday.com/keys-deltoid-ligament-repair-after-ankle-fracture
113. Elsoe R, Ostgaard SE, Larsen P. Population-based epidemiology of 9767 ankle fractures. *Foot Ankle Surg.* 2018;24(1):34-39. doi:10.1016/j.fas.2016.11.002
114. Lemme NJ, Li NY, DeFroda SF, Kleiner J, Owens BD. Epidemiology of Achilles tendon ruptures in the United States: athletic and nonathletic injuries from 2012 to 2016. *Orthop J Sports Med.* 2018;6(11):2325967118808238. doi:10.1177/2325967118808238
115. Pedowitz D, Kirwan G. Achilles tendon ruptures. *Curr Rev Musculoskelet Med.* 2013;6(4):285-293. doi:10.1007/s12178-013-9185-8
116. Lewis T, Cook J. Fluoroquinolones and tendinopathy: a guide for athletes and sports clinicians and a systematic review of the literature. *J Athl Train.* 2014;49(3):422-427. doi:10.4085/1062-6050-49.2.09
117. Ochen Y, Beks RB, van Heijl M, et al. Operative treatment versus nonoperative treatment of Achilles tendon ruptures: systematic review and meta-analysis. *BMJ.* 2019;364:k5120. doi:10.1136/bmj.k5120
118. Landrum EL, Kelln CB, Parente WR, Ingersoll CD, Hertel J. Immediate effects of anterior-to-posterior talocrural joint mobilization after prolonged ankle immobilization: a preliminary study. *J Man Manip Ther.* 2008;16(2):100-105. doi:10.1179/106698108790818413
119. Hall EA, Chomistek AK, Kingma JJ, Docherty CL. Balance- and strength-training protocols to improve chronic ankle instability deficits, part i: assessing clinical outcome measures. *J Athl Train.* 2018;53(6):568-577. doi:10.4085/1062-6050-385-16
120. Martin RL, Davenport TE, Reischl SF. Heel pain—plantar fasciitis-revision 2014: clinical practice guidelines linked to the International Classification of Functioning, Disability, and Health from the orthopaedic section of the American Physical Therapy Association. *J Orthop Sports Phys Ther.* 2014;44(11):A1-A23. doi:10.2519/jospt.2014.0303
121. Hyland MR, Webber-Gaffney A, Cohen L, Lichtman SW. Randomized controlled trial of calcaneal taping, sham taping, and plantar fascia stretching for the short-term management of plantar heel pain. *J Orthop Sports Phys Ther.* 2006;36(6):364-371. doi:10.2519/jospt.2006.2078
122. Tahririan MA, Motififard M, Tahmasebi MN, Siavashi B. Plantar fasciitis. *J Res Med Sci.* 2012;17(8):799-804.

123. Petraglia F, Ramazzina I, Costantino C. Plantar fasciitis in athletes: diagnostic and treatment strategies. A systematic review. *Muscles Ligaments Tendons J.* 2017;7(1):107-118. doi:10.11138/mltj/2017.7.1.107
124. Pitrin Z. All about foot stress fractures. September 19, 2019. Accessed February 2, 2023. https://www.sports-health.com/sports-injuries/ankle-and-foot-injuries/all-about-foot-stress-fractures
125. Sun J, Gao F, Wang Y, Sun W, Jiang B, Li Z. Extracorporeal shock wave therapy is effective in treating chronic plantar fasciitis: a meta-analysis of RCTs. *Medicine (Baltimore).* 2017;96(15):e6621. doi:10.1097/MD.0000000000006621
126. Merkel DL, Molony JT Jr. Recognition and management of traumatic sports injuries in the skeletally immature athlete. *Int J Sports Phys Ther.* 2012;7(6):691-704.
127. Dutton M. Special populations. In: Dutton M, ed. *Dutton's Orthopaedics Examination, Evaluation and Intervention.* 3rd ed. McGraw-Hill Companies; 2012:1401-1419.
128. Helgeson K. Soft tissue, joint and bone disorders. In: Goodman CC, Fuller KS, eds. *Pathology: Implications for the Physical Therapist.* 4th ed. Elsevier; 2015:1285-1370.
129. Peck DM, Voss LM, Voss TT. Slipped capital femoral epiphysis: diagnosis and management. *Am Fam Physician.* 2017;95(12):779-784.
130. Joseph B. Management of Perthes' disease. *Indian J Orthop.* 2015;49(1):10-16. doi:10.4103/0019-5413.143906
131. Helgeson K. Genetic and developmental disorders. In: Goodman CC, Fuller KS, eds. *Pathology: Implications for the Physical Therapist.* 4th ed. Elsevier; 2015:1153-1210.
132. Zanon G, Di Vico G, Marullo M. Osteochondritis dissecans of the knee. *Joints.* 2014;2(1):29-36.
133. Eismann EA, Pettit RJ, Wall EJ, Myer GD. Management strategies for osteochondritis dissecans of the knee in the skeletally immature athlete. *J Orthop Sports Phys Ther.* 2014;44(9):665-679. doi:10.2519/jospt.2014.5140
134. Smith JM, Varacallo M. *Osgood Schlatter's Disease (Tibial Tubercle Apophysitis).* StatPearls Publishing; 2020. Accessed February 2, 2023. https://www.ncbi.nlm.nih.gov/books/NBK441995/

Chapter 14

# Management of Cervical and Thoracic Spine Orthopedic Conditions

*Patricia A. Crane, PT, DPT, MBA, OCS, Cert MDT*

**KEY TERMS** Joint position sense | Protrusion | Radiculopathy | Referred pain | Retrusion | Rocabado 6 × 6 | Spinal stenosis | Thoracic outlet syndrome

## Chapter Objectives

1. Recall the basic anatomical structures of the cervical spine, thoracic spine, and temporomandibular joint (TMJ).
2. Identify the common red flags warranting referral for further medical management of the cervical spine, thoracic spine, and TMJ.
3. Identify and describe common injuries to the cervical spine, thoracic spine, and TMJ.
4. Describe the use of the *International Classification of Functioning, Disability and Health (ICF)* classification system to guide physical therapy management of orthopedic cervical spine conditions.
5. Identify the commonly used special tests a physical therapist assistant will see in a physical therapist's evaluation of the cervical spine, thoracic spine, and TMJ.
6. Discuss the concept of regional interdependence as it applies to treatment of the cervical and thoracic spine.
7. Discuss the common treatment interventions used to address TMJ and cervical and thoracic spinal diagnoses/clinical presentations.
8. Given a physical therapy diagnosis and plan of care (POC), design and progress a basic exercise and intervention program to rehabilitate common cervical, thoracic, and TMJ injuries.

Patients with neck and upper back pain have varying presentations, and the treatment approaches used must match those presentations. Physical therapy management of the spine differs from management of the extremities because it focuses on treatment-based classification systems rather than a pathoanatomical approach. As described in Chapter 11, the aim of a treatment-based classification system is to apply treatment strategies based on the patient's clinical presentation to achieve optimal outcomes. Conversely, the pathoanatomical model uses an approach that identifies a specific anatomical tissue as the likely cause of the patient's pain and dysfunction (ie, signs/symptoms consistent with cervical stenosis). Regional interdependence (described in Chapter 11) should be considered when treating persons with cervical pain.[1,2] Neck pain accounts for up to 25% of all patients seen in outpatient physical therapy settings[3-5] and is the fourth leading cause of disability and work loss



Kopack JK, Cascardi KA.
*Principles of Therapeutic Exercise for the Physical Therapist Assistant* (pp 463-509).

in the United States.[6] The average reported incidence of neck pain is 37.5%,[7] with a higher prevalence in women compared with men.[3,4,8] Some studies have reported the prevalence of neck pain (at some point in life) to be as high as affecting 75% of the population[9] and peaking in the fifth decade of life.[7,10]

There are a number of comorbidities associated with neck pain, including but not limited to headache, shoulder pain, whiplash-associated disorders (WADs), back pain, and depression.[10-12] The majority of patients who experience neck pain usually recover quickly, but a reported 2.4% to 37.5% of these patients develop chronic symptoms.[10,13] The financial burden of medical expenses and the time lost at work due to neck pain are second only to the costs to treat low back pain in the United States.[5] Costs to treat spinal pain in the United States in 2005 were estimated at $85.9 billion.[14] Physical therapy can play an important role in containing these costs and improving function for patients with cervical pain. According to Horn et al,[15] patients treated following the clinical practice guidelines (CPGs) showed comparable improvement in disability outcomes compared with those whose care did not follow the guidelines. Patients receiving care that followed CPGs achieved comparable improvements in 3.6 fewer physical therapy visits and accrued fewer costs/charges. Additionally, there were fewer visits to other health care providers, a decreased use of prescription drugs, and 43% fewer diagnostic imaging tests compared with those who received care not following CPGs.[15]

Patients with neck pain are not a homogenous group, and there is often a lack of correlation between imaging findings and symptom presentation in patients with neck pain, resulting in debate about the reliance on a pathoanatomical approach to physical therapy management of spinal pain.[6] In recent years, there has been a transition from the pathoanatomical model to a treatment-based classification model that includes consideration of the impact of regional interdependence. Current CPGs advocate for the use of treatment-based classification systems or the *ICF* model to effectively and efficiently manage patients with neck pain.[16,17]

As evidence-based research continues to evolve, studies reveal that pathoanatomical diagnoses often present with variable symptoms and impairments in unrelated areas of the body; this supports the concept of *regional interdependence*, a term coined by Robert Wainner (refer to Chapter 11). Interventions that target one area of the body can often affect other areas unrelated to the source of the patient's symptoms.[2] For example, the thoracic spine is not typically a primary source of pain in patients receiving physical therapy. However, the thoracic spine has been linked to pain and dysfunction in relation to adjacent regions/joints, such as the neck and shoulder. Physical therapy treatment that includes thoracic mobilization has been linked to favorable outcomes in the management of neck pain[5,18] and improved shoulder range of motion (ROM) in patients with shoulder impingement syndrome.[19] Effective treatment of the cervical spine occurs when clinicians thoroughly screen for the involvement of other structures in the surrounding regions, including the thoracic spine, shoulders, and TMJ.

According to the American Physical Therapy Association, head, maxillofacial, craniomandibular, and temporomandibular dysfunction (TMD) account for 3% of all patient referrals to outpatient physical therapy.[20] TMD can occur as a result of trauma (eg, whiplash) or from microtrauma due to overuse such as clenching the teeth or bruxism (grinding the teeth) or osteoarthritis. Common complaints include pain, reduced ROM (ie, the inability to close or laterally deviate the jaw), clicking, and/or difficulty chewing. When examining a patient with TMD, the physical therapist will screen the cervical spine because the jaw is a common site of referred pain for cervical conditions. Similarly, screening of the TMJ should be performed when treating patients with upper cervical symptoms. However, the TMJ may not be thoroughly assessed if the patient's symptoms or medical diagnosis do not indicate a TMJ-related dysfunction. The physical therapist assistant should recognize the common symptoms present with TMD so the physical therapist can be notified for further assessment when indicated.

## Cervical, Thoracic Spine, Rib Cage, and Temporomandibular Joint Anatomy and Function

Cervical spine pain is a common reason for people to seek out physical therapy. Therefore, physical therapist assistants should understand the anatomy; joint mechanics; and the inter-relationship between the cervical spine, thoracic spine, and TMJ. The assistant will review the initial evaluation for any postural deviations and referred pain patterns documented by the therapist before treatment.

There are 7 cervical vertebrae (C1-C7). The cervical spine articulates with the skull superiorly and the thoracic spine inferiorly. The thoracic spine, made up of 12 vertebrae, is the only spinal region that attaches to the ribs. The thoracic spine is relatively strong and stable with less available ROM compared with the cervical and lumbar spines. This region is prone to compression fractures, especially in patients with osteoporosis.

The TMJ is the articulation between the mandible and maxilla, connecting the jawbone to the skull. According to current research, TMD is commonly associated with cervical spine disorders and headaches.[21]

### *Upper and Lower Cervical Spine Anatomy and Function*

The cervical spine is often subdivided into the upper cervical spine (articulations between the occiput, C1, C2, and C3) and the lower cervical spine (articulations between C3 through C7).[22] This distinction is made because of changes in bony morphology, movement patterns, and the function of each region. Cervical spinal movement is highly variable, and the true coupling of movements is not fully understood. Comprehending how general movement patterns occur in the upper and lower cervical spine helps create a basic understanding of this variability.

C1 (atlas) and C2 (axis) are atypical vertebrae, and they lack an intervertebral disk. The atlas lacks a vertebral body and spinous process, and the axis has a long superior projection called the *dens*. These structural differences allow for a great deal of movement in the upper cervical spine. Approximately 50% of cervical flexion and extension occur at the occiput and C1 (the atlanto-occipital [AO] joint), whereas rotation occurs at C1-C2 (the atlantoaxial [AA] joint).[22] This increased mobility leads to the potential for decreased stability.

Because of the potential for instability and the proximity of the upper cervical spine to vital vascular structures, it is important for the physical therapist to perform a thorough screening of these structures, particularly after a report of cervical trauma. The cervical spine creates a pathway for the vertebral artery, which arises from the subclavian artery, enters the cervical spine below the vertebral body of C6 through the intervertebral foramen, and travels superiorly through each of the cervical vertebrae via the transverse foramen into the foramen magnum of the skull where it becomes the basilar artery. These arteries supply blood to the spinal cord, brain stem, cerebellum, and the posterior portion of the brain. Vascular ischemia (or cervical arterial dysfunction) affecting these vessels can be severe or fatal. Because of the proximity of the vertebral artery to the vertebral bodies and facet joints, clinicians must be cautious when performing manual therapy and exercising this region.[23] The physical therapist should perform a vascular screen of the upper cervical spine consisting of blood pressure monitoring, upper cervical ligamentous screening (the alar ligament test, transverse ligament test, and Sharp-Purser), upper motor neuron testing (Hoffmann, Babinski, and Clonus tests and deep tendon reflexes), palpation of the carotid artery for symmetry, and a cranial nerve examination.[23] Positive findings on any of these tests warrant further evaluation by the therapist and possible referral for further medical management. The physical therapist assistant should be familiar with vascular screening tests and should monitor vital signs when treating patients with cervical spine pain. The physical therapist assistant monitors patients during treatment, looking for signs or symptoms that are red flags (Table 14-1). If red flags are present, the assistant must notify the physical therapist immediately to assess and possibly refer the patient out for further testing and/or medical management.

The vertebrae of the lower cervical spine (C3-C7) are traditional vertebrae with a vertebral body, spinous process, transverse processes, and an intervertebral disk. The facet joint is located between the lamina and pedicle, and the superior facet of the vertebra below articulates with the inferior facet on the vertebra above; this configuration allows for movement between the facets, but it also prevents excessive motion and provides stability. The facet joints are a common area for the degenerative changes that are associated with cervical spondylosis.[21]

## Muscles and Nerves of the Cervical Spine

The muscles of the cervical spine are listed in Table 14-2. There are 4 deep anterior cervical spine muscles (often called the *prevertebral muscles*[24]): the rectus capitis anterior and lateralis, the longus capitis, and the longus colli. These 4 muscles form the deep neck flexors (DNFs; also called the *deep cervical flexors*). Recent literature has focused on rehabilitation for impaired strength, endurance, and motor control of the DNFs as it relates to neck pain and disability.[12,25-27] Testing and retraining of the DNFs are described later in this chapter.

The superficial anterior muscles of the cervical spine include the sternocleidomastoid (SCM) and the anterior, middle, and posterior scalene muscles. In addition to the primary actions related to neck motion described in Table 14-2, the SCM assists the scalene muscles during forced inspiration.[24] The scalene muscles lie deep to the SCM. When the neck is stationary (fixed), the anterior and middle scalene muscles elevate the first rib (in a reversal of muscle action), and the posterior scalene muscle elevates the second rib.[22,24]

The deep posterior muscles of the cervical spine include the splenius capitis, the splenius cervicis, the suboccipital muscles, and the transversospinalis muscles (ie, the semispinalis capitis, semispinalis cervicis, multifidus, and rotatores). Generally, these muscles extend the head and neck when they contract bilaterally. The semispinalis capitis is the largest and most superior part of the semispinalis muscle. The semispinalis cervicis makes up the middle portion of the muscle, and the semispinalis thoracis makes up the lowest portion. This group lies deep to the splenius muscles and medial to the longissimus muscles. The upper trapezius, levator scapulae, and rhomboid minor lie superficial to these deep muscles, and all have some attachment to the posterior cervical spine and/or occipital bone (refer to Chapter 12).

The suboccipital muscles are a group of 4 small muscles situated inferior to the occipital bone; they include the rectus capitis posterior major, rectus capitis posterior minor, obliquus capitis inferior, and obliquus capitis superior. These muscles only cross 1 or 2 vertebrae and lie deep to the semispinalis and splenius muscles. Collectively, the suboccipital muscles extend the head in a rocking, nodding, or tilting motion at the AO joint. The rectus capitis posterior and obliquus capitis inferior major have a secondary role; they perform ipsilateral rotation of the atlas (C1) around the odontoid process of C2.[22,24]

### Clinical Tip

The suboccipital muscles act as stabilizers when the head moves. The rectus capitis posterior major, rectus capitis posterior minor, and obliquus capitis superior stabilize the occiput on the atlas (AO joint), and the obliquus capitis inferior stabilizes the atlas on the axis (AA joint).[24]

**Table 14-1**

**Red Flags for Physical Therapy Management of the Cervical Spine**

| Red Flag | Rationale |
|---|---|
| Trauma that fails the Canadian C-spine rule[32] | Possible fracture or upper cervical ligamentous instability |
| Age >50 years, prior history of cancer, unexplained weight loss, failure of conservative therapy | Possible cancer |
| Positive alar ligament test, positive transverse ligament test, positive Sharp-Purser | Possible cervical instability |
| Age >45 years, gait dysfunction, positive inverted supinator sign, positive Hoffmann sign, positive Babinski sign | Possible cervical myelopathy |
| Fever, chills, night sweats | Possible infection |
| History of smoking, left shoulder pain with compression, miosis, ptosis, anhidrosis | Possible Pancoast tumor |
| Pain in the C3 distribution of the upper extremity | Possible heart disease |
| Dizziness, diplopia, drop attack, dysarthria, dysphagia, nystagmus, numbness, nausea | Possible cervical arterial dysfunction or neurologic involvement |
| Multilevel nerve root involvement | Possible cancer, infection, or neurologic involvement |
| Cranial nerve alterations | Possible central nervous system involvement |
| Recent onset of severe headache | Possible subarachnoid hemorrhage or carotid/vertebral artery dissection (Refer to Neck Pain With Headaches section for headache red flags) |

The cervical plexus innervates the cervical muscles and is formed by the communication of the anterior divisions (anterior rami) of C1-C4 nerves. This plexus lies under the SCM, opposite the C1-C4 vertebrae, resting on the levator scapula and middle scalene muscles. The phrenic nerve (branches of C3, C4, and C5) is part of the cervical plexus and innervates the diaphragm. The 5 spinal nerves from C5 through T1 form the brachial plexus, which was discussed in more detail in Chapter 12.[22,24] Nerve root compression involving either plexus can be associated with cervical radiculopathy, which causes pain, numbness, tingling, or weakness along the sensory or motor distribution of the nerve.

**Clinical Tip**

An easy way to remember the nerve innervation for the diaphragm is C3, C4, C5 keep the diaphragm alive!

## *Thoracic Spine and Thorax: Anatomy and Function*

The thoracic cage is composed of the 12 thoracic vertebrae (T1-T12), ribs, costal cartilage, and the sternum. There is an intervertebral disk between each level, and the vertebral body shapes and spinous process lengths vary throughout the thoracic spine, but the spinous processes are oriented downward. The inferior articular process (facet) of each superior thoracic vertebra articulates with the superior articular process of the thoracic vertebra of the thoracic vertebrae below. The 10 superior thoracic vertebrae articulate with the ribs at the transverse costal facets (forming the costotransverse joint), and the costal facets (or demi facets) form the costovertebral joint. The last 2 thoracic vertebral bodies (T11 and T12) begin to resemble that of a lumbar vertebra; they do not have transverse costal facets, and their spinous processes are slightly more horizontal compared with the thoracic vertebrae above these levels.[28,29]

**Table 14-2**

Cervical Spine, Thoracic Spine, and Trunk Muscles[24,29]

| Muscle | Primary Action | Origin | Insertion | Innervation |
|---|---|---|---|---|
| ***Anterior Cervical Muscles*** | | | | |
| Rectus capitis anterior (prevertebral muscles) | Unilaterally: Assists with ipsilateral side bending<br>Bilaterally: Cervical flexion at AO joints | C1 (atlas) | Occipital bone | Anterior rami C1, C2 |
| Rectus capitis lateralis (prevertebral muscles) | Unilaterally: Ipsilateral side bending<br>Bilaterally: Stabilizes AO joints | Transverse process C1 | Occipital bone | Anterior rami C1, C2 |
| Longus capitis (prevertebral muscles) | Cervical flexion | Transverse processes C3-C6 | Occipital bone | Anterior rami C1-C3 |
| Longus colli (prevertebral muscles) | All parts flex cervical spine | Upper: Transverse processes C3-C5<br>Middle: Vertebral bodies C5-T3<br>Lower: Vertebral bodies T1-T3 | Upper: Anterior tubercle C1<br>Middle: Vertebral bodies C2-C6<br>Lower: Transverse processes C5-C6 | Anterior rami C2-C6 |
| SCM | Unilaterally: Ipsilateral side bending and contralateral rotation<br>Bilaterally: Cervical flexion | Manubrium of sternum and medial portion of clavicle | Mastoid process | Accessory nerve (cranial nerve XI) |
| Scalene muscles | Anterior and middle<br>Unilaterally: Ipsilateral side bending<br>Bilaterally: Flexion of cervical spine; elevates first rib<br>Posterior<br>Unilaterally: Ipsilateral side bending<br>Bilaterally: Flexion of cervical spine; elevates second rib | Anterior: Transverse processes C3-C6<br>Middle: Transverse processes C2-C7<br>Posterior: Posterior transverse processes C5-C7 | Anterior: Inner border of first rib<br>Middle: Inner border of first rib<br>Posterior: Inner border of second rib | Anterior rami C5-C6<br>Anterior rami C3-C8<br>Anterior rami of C6-C8 |

(continued)

**Table 14-2 (continued)**

Cervical Spine, Thoracic Spine, and Trunk Muscles[24,29]

| Muscle | Primary Action | Origin | Insertion | Innervation |
|---|---|---|---|---|
| ***Posterior Cervical Muscles*** | | | | |
| Splenius capitis | Unilaterally: Ipsilateral side bending and rotation to same side<br>Bilaterally: Extends neck and head | Lower half of ligamentum nuchae C4-C6 and spinous process C7-T3 | Lateral aspect of occipital bone and mastoid process | Dorsal rami C3-C6 |
| Splenius cervicis | Unilaterally: Rotates head to same side<br>Bilaterally: Extends cervical spine | Spinous processes T3-T6 | Posterior tubercle of transverse processes C1-C3 | Dorsal rami C5-C8 |
| Rectus capitis posterior major (suboccipital group) | Rocks/tilts head at AO joint into extension<br>Rotates head to same side | Spinous process C2 (axis) | Inferior nuchal line of the occiput | Suboccipital nerve |
| Rectus capitis posterior minor (suboccipital group) | Rocks/tilts head at AO joint into extension | Tubercle of posterior arch C1 (atlas) | Inferior nuchal line of the occiput | Suboccipital nerve |
| Oblique capitis superior (suboccipital group) | Rocks/tilts head at AO joint into extension<br>Lateral flexion of the head to the same side | Transverse process C1 (atlas) | Between the nuchal lines of the occiput | Suboccipital nerve |
| Oblique capitis inferior (suboccipital group) | Rocks/tilts head at AO joint into extension<br>Rotates head to same side | Spinous process C2 (axis) | Transverse process C1 (atlas) | Suboccipital nerve |

*(continued)*

**Table 14-2 (continued)**

Cervical Spine, Thoracic Spine, and Trunk Muscles[24,29]

| Muscle | Primary Action | Origin | Insertion | Innervation |
|---|---|---|---|---|
| ***Erector Spinae Group, Transversospinalis Group, and Other Trunk and Abdominal Muscles*** | | | | |
| Spinalis (erector spinae group) | Unilaterally: Lateral flexion of the vertebral column to the same side<br>Bilaterally: Extends vertebral column | Cervicis: Ligamentum nuchae, spinous process of C7<br>Thoracis: Spinous processes of upper lumbar and lower thoracic vertebrae | Cervicis: Spinous processes of cervical vertebrae, except C1<br>Thoracis: Spinous processes of upper thoracic | Spinal nerve |
| Longissimus (erector spinae group) | Unilaterally: Lateral flexion vertebral column to the same side<br>Bilaterally: Extends the vertebral column<br>Capitis only<br>Unilaterally: Head/neck lateral flexion and rotation to same side<br>Bilaterally: Extension of the head and neck | Capitis: Transverse processes C4-T5<br>Cervicis: Transverse processes T1-T5<br>Thoracis: Spinous and transverse processes L1-L5, posterior sacrum, posterior iliac crest, lumbar aponeurosis | Capitis: Mastoid process<br>Cervicis: Transverse processes C2-C6<br>Thoracis: Transverse processes T1-T12, angles of ribs 7 through 12 | Spinal nerve |
| Iliocostalis (erector spinae group) | Unilaterally: Lateral flexion vertebral column to the same side<br>Bilaterally: Extends the vertebral column | Cervicis: Angle of ribs 3 through 6<br>Thoracis: Angle of ribs 7 through 12<br>Lumborum: Lateral crest of sacrum, medial iliac crest, thoracolumbar fascia | Cervicis: Transverse processes C4-C6<br>Thoracis: Posterior surface of ribs 1 through 6<br>Lumborum: Transverse processes L1-L4, posterior surface angle of ribs 6 through 12, thoracolumbar fascia | Spinal nerve |
| Semispinalis capitis (transversospinalis group) | Extends the neck and head | Transverse processes C4-T5 | Between superior and inferior nuchal lines of the occiput | Dorsal rami C2-C3 |
| Semispinalis cervicis (transversospinalis group) | Unilaterally: Ipsilateral side bending and rotation to opposite side<br>Bilaterally: Extends the neck/head | Transverse processes T1-T6 | Spinous processes C2-C5 | Dorsal rami |

(continued)

**Table 14-2 (continued)**

Cervical Spine, Thoracic Spine, and Trunk Muscles[24,29]

| Muscle | Primary Action | Origin | Insertion | Innervation |
|---|---|---|---|---|
| Multifidi and rotatores (transversospinalis group) | Unilaterally: Trunk rotation to opposite side in small segments<br>Bilaterally: Extends vertebral column<br>Unilaterally: Trunk rotation to opposite side in small segments<br>Bilaterally: Extends vertebral column | Multifidi: Sacrum and transverse processes of lumbar through cervical vertebrae<br>Rotatores: Transverse process of lumbar through cervical vertebrae | Spinous processes of lumbar vertebrae through the second cervical vertebra<br>(Multifidi span 2 to 4 vertebrae)<br>(Rotatores span 1 to 2 vertebrae) | Spinal nerve |
| Diaphragm | Draws down the central tendon of the diaphragm; increases the volume of the thoracic cavity during inhalation | Costal attachment: Inner surface of the lower 6 ribs<br>Lumbar attachment: Upper 2 or 3 lumbar vertebrae<br>Sternal attachment: Inner part of xiphoid process | Central tendon of the diaphragm | Phrenic C3-C5 |
| Internal and external intercostals | External intercostals: Drawing ribs superiorly (increases space of thoracic cavity); assists with inhalation<br>Internal intercostals: Drawing ribs inferiorly (decreases space of thoracic cavity); assists with exhalation | Inferior border of the rib above | Superior border of the rib below | Thoracic nerve |
| Serratus posterior superior | Elevates ribs during inhalation | Spinous processes of C7-T3 | Posterior surface of ribs 2 through 5 | T1-T4 |
| Serratus posterior inferior | Depresses ribs during exhalation | Spinous processes of T12-L3 | Posterior surface of ribs 9 through 12 | T9-T11 (T12) |
| Intertransversarii | Unilaterally: Lateral flexion of vertebral column to the same side.<br>Bilaterally: Extends vertebral column | Cervical: Spans transverse processes of C2-C7<br>Lumbar: Spans transverse processes of L1-L5 | Cervical: Spans transverse processes of C2-C7<br>Lumbar: Spans transverse processes of L1- L5 | Spinal nerve |
| Interspinales | Extend the neck and trunk | Cervical: Spans spinous processes of C2-T3<br>Lumbar: Spans spinous processes of T12-L5 | Cervical: Spans transverse processes of C2-C7<br>Lumbar: Spans transverse processes of L1-L5 | Spinal nerve |

*(continued)*

**Table 14-2 (continued)**

Cervical Spine, Thoracic Spine, and Trunk Muscles[24,29]

| Muscle | Primary Action | Origin | Insertion | Innervation |
|---|---|---|---|---|
| *Abdominal Muscles* | | | | |
| Rectus abdominis[a] | Flexes vertebral column<br>Tilts pelvis posteriorly | Pubic crest, pubic symphysis | Cartilage of ribs 5 to 7 and xiphoid process | T5, T6, T7-T11, T12 intercostal nerves |
| External oblique[a] | Unilaterally: Lateral flexion vertebral column to same side; rotates vertebral column to opposite side<br>Bilaterally: Flexion of vertebral column; compresses abdominal contents | External surfaces of ribs 5 to 12 | Anterior part of iliac crest, abdominal aponeurosis to linea alba | (T5, T6), T7-T11, T12; iliohypogastric and ilioinguinal |
| Internal oblique[a] | Unilaterally: Lateral flexion vertebral column to the same side; rotation to the same side<br>Bilaterally: Flexes vertebral column; compresses abdominal contents | Lateral inguinal ligament, iliac crest, and thoracolumbar fascia | Internal surface of the lower 3 ribs, abdominal aponeurosis to linea alba | T7, T8, T9-T12, L1, iliohypogastric and ilioinguinal, ventral rami |
| Transverse abdominis[a] | Compress abdominal contents | Lateral inguinal ligament, iliac crest, thoracolumbar fascia, and internal surface of the lower 6 ribs | Abdominal aponeurosis to linea alba; pubic crest | T7-T12, L1, iliohypogastric and ilioinguinal, ventral rami |
| Pyramidalis | Tenses the linea alba | Pubic symphysis | Linea alba | 12th thoracic nerve |

[a]These muscles are discussed in more detail in Chapter 15.

Physical therapist assistants should be able to locate and identify each vertebra in the spine by palpating bony landmarks, but this is more challenging when palpating bony landmarks in the thoracic spine. Palpation is performed to determine symmetry, pain provocation, and segmental mobility. Clinicians commonly use the "rule of threes" for locating the level of the transverse processes relative to their corresponding spinous processes. According to the rule, the thoracic spine is divided into 4 sections of 3 vertebrae. The first 3 spinous processes of T1 through T3 are located at the same level as their respective transverse processes. The spinous processes of T4 through T6 are located one-half of a vertebral level below their respective transverse processes, and the spinous processes of T7 through T9 are a full level below the transverse processes. The spinous processes of T10 through T12 are located at the same vertebral level as their transverse processes.[30,31] Although the rule of threes is the most common method for palpating the thoracic spine, Geelhoed's rule has been shown to be more accurate in locating a specific vertebral level.

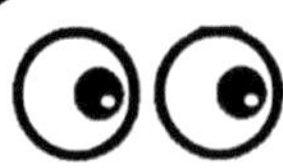

### Eye on the Research: The Rule of Threes Versus Geelhoed's Rule

The rule of threes has not been anatomically validated in the research. Geelhoed et al[30] proposed a potentially more accurate relationship between the thoracic spine transverse processes and spinous processes. They determined that the transverse processes of each thoracic vertebra were located at approximately the same level as the spinous process of the superior vertebra. The investigators noted that it was more difficult to predict the location of the transverse processes of T11 and T12 because of the variability of their position.

Oakley et al[31] examined 44 cadavers and compared the 2 rules to determine which one was more anatomically accurate and concluded that Geelhoed's rule was more accurate. Both studies concluded that the thoracic transverse processes can be found laterally to the most prominent point of the spinous process of the vertebra just above.[30,31]

### Clinical Application

To accurately palpate a specific thoracic vertebra, first locate the most prominent point of the spinous process of the vertebra above the level you want to palpate. Then, move the fingers laterally; they should now be on the transverse processes of the desired thoracic vertebra.

The ribs protect the organs of the thorax and have a role in breathing, allowing for chest expansion during inhalation. There are 12 pairs of ribs that articulate with the 12 thoracic vertebrae posteriorly. The first 7 ribs are called *true ribs* because they attach directly to the sternum. Ribs 8 through 10 are called *false ribs* because of their attachment to the sternum via the seventh rib's costal cartilage. Finally, ribs 11 and 12 are referred to as *floating ribs* because they do not attach to the sternum at all. Ribs are described as typical or atypical. Ribs 3 through 9 are typical ribs because they consist of a head, neck, and body. Ribs 1, 2, 10, 11, and 12 are considered atypical ribs. Atypical ribs have at least one feature that varies from a typical rib.[28,29] The articular surface of the tubercle on a rib articulates on each side of a thoracic vertebra. Anteriorly, the articulation between a rib and the costal cartilage is called the *costochondral joint*, and the ribs are joined to the sternum via the costal cartilage at the sternocostal joint. The articulation between the thoracic spine and the rib cage allows for significant stability but still allows for varying amounts of movement to increase lung volume during inspiration.

## Muscles and Nerves of the Thoracic Spine and Thorax

There are several muscles that attach to the thoracic spine and the ribs (see Table 14-2). Posteriorly, the erector spinae muscle group is located bilaterally, adjacent to the entire spinal column, crossing several spinal levels. The erector spinae muscles assist with maintaining erect posture, extending and rotating the spine. Other muscles that attach to the cervical and thoracic vertebra (including the upper and middle trapezius and the rhomboid muscles) are discussed in Chapter 12.

The diaphragm separates the abdominal cavity from the thoracic cavity. It attaches to the xiphoid process, the lower 6 ribs, and the upper lumbar vertebrae, creating a thin circular muscle shape. When the diaphragm contracts during inspiration, it pulls downward, increasing the size of the thoracic cavity. During expiration, the diaphragm relaxes, decreasing the size of the thoracic cavity. Anteriorly, the 11 internal and external intercostal muscles lie between the ribs on oblique angles within the intercostal space; the external intercostals are superficial to the internal intercostal muscles. The internal intercostal muscles depress the ribs during expiration, and the external intercostal muscles elevate the ribs during inspiration.[28,29] The pectoralis major and minor and the serratus anterior have their attachments on the ribs; their functions are discussed in Chapter 12.

The 12 thoracic spinal nerves are divided into the anterior (ventral) rami (also referred to as the *intercostal nerves*) and the posterior (dorsal) rami. Both the anterior and posterior rami have a cutaneous and a muscular branch. The superior portion of the intercostal nerve of T1 forms part of the brachial plexus. The central spinal canal between T4 and T9 is narrow compared with the rest of the thoracic spine; this area is referred to as the *critical zone*. This region of the spinal canal is vulnerable to central cord compression.

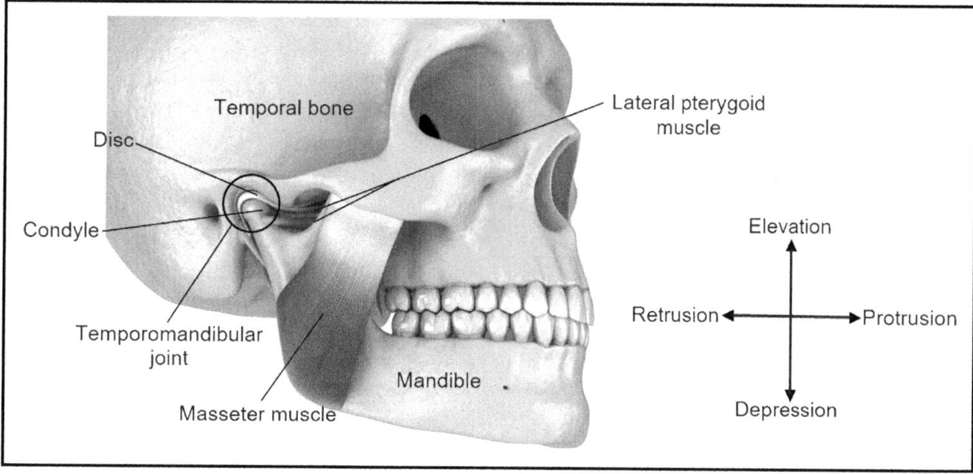


**Figure 14-1.** The TMJ (Alex Mit/Shutterstock.com).

## *Temporomandibular Joint Anatomy and Function*

The TMJ is a diarthrodial synovial joint formed by the articulation between the temporal bone and the mandibular bone (Figure 14-1). The joint is positioned anterior to the external auditory meatus and contains a fibrocartilaginous disk, ligaments, and a joint capsule. The temporal bone forms the superior portion of the TMJ, and the mandible is the distal, mobile bone of the joint. The disk divides the joint into 2 cavities, and these superior and inferior articular cavities are lined with separate synovial membranes.

When the jaw opens, the mandible moves down, the condyle rotates forward, and the disk moves forward and downward. The temporomandibular ligament, collateral ligaments, and accessory ligaments are structures that support and limit the motion of the TMJ.

### Temporomandibular Joint Muscles and Nerves

The muscles that perform chewing actions include the masseter, temporalis, medial pterygoid, suprahyoid, and lateral pterygoid. The masseter, temporalis, medial pterygoid, and superior fibers of the lateral pterygoid elevate the mandible to close the mouth. The inferior fibers of the lateral pterygoids and the suprahyoid depress the mandible to open the mouth. **Protrusion** (moving the mandible forward) occurs through the action of the medial pterygoid, the lateral pterygoid, and the superficial fibers of the masseter. The temporalis, suprahyoid, and deep fibers of the masseter are responsible for **retrusion** of the mandible (moving the mandible posterior). The contralateral medial and lateral pterygoid and the ipsilateral temporalis and masseter perform lateral deviation of the mandible.

The TMJ is innervated primarily by the trigeminal nerve (cranial nerve III). The deep temporal nerve and the masseteric nerve innervate the anterior and medial TMJ, whereas the auriculotemporal nerve innervates the posterior and lateral joint. For more in-depth information regarding TMJ anatomy and function, refer to kinesiology textbooks.

# Cervical Spine Diagnoses and Critical Assessment Tools

The physical therapist will take a detailed patient history to screen for the appropriateness of physical therapy and to guide the initial examination and selection of treatment interventions. This section discusses the assessment tools used by physical therapists that are of critical importance in determining if treatment is warranted or if patients should be referred back to the physician for alternative care. Physical therapist assistants need to be familiar with these tools in case any findings arise during treatment that may lead an assistant to believe that continued treatment would be detrimental to the patient's health.

Some diagnoses and clinical presentations warrant a referral for further diagnostic testing or additional medical management due to nonmusculoskeletal origins or because of a potential risk for harm if not managed medically. Some of these diagnoses include a cervical fracture, cervical myelopathy, cancer, upper cervical instability, cervical arterial dysfunction, or inflammatory disease processes. It is vital for the physical therapist assistant to recognize the potential red flags listed in Table 14-1; these red flags can be indicative of nonmusculoskeletal causes of the patient's neck pain. If the presence or new onset of a red flag sign or symptom is found or reported, the assistant should immediately consult with the therapist. Open lines of communication between physical therapy team members are essential, especially when any unexpected changes in patient presentation occurs during treatment or if the patient is not progressing as expected.

Cervical arterial dysfunction and upper cervical instability can mimic musculoskeletal conditions, but they are potentially harmful or even fatal in some incidents. For this reason, the physical therapist's examination should minimally include the following: vital signs, ligamentous stability special tests including the Sharp-Purser Test (for AA joint instability), transverse and alar ligament tests, cranial nerve examination, and upper motor neuron testing (ie, the Babinski sign, Clonus test, and Hoffmann sign).[23]

Ligament and instability testing should only be performed by the physical therapist. However, the therapist and assistant should monitor these patients for dizziness, dysphagia, dysarthria, diplopia, drop attacks, ataxia, anxiety, nausea, nystagmus, and numbness. These signs and symptoms are commonly referred to as the *5Ds And 3Ns*. New signs or symptoms consistent with this list can be indicative of a neurovascular problem and warrant immediate consultation with the supervising physical therapist.

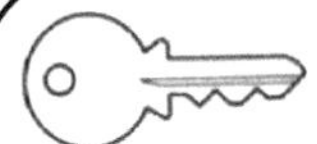

**Key Safety Considerations: Contact the Physical Therapist if the Patient Reports or You Observe Any of the 5Ds And 3Ns**

**5Ds**

- Dizziness
- Drop attacks
- Diplopia (double vision)
- Dysarthria (difficulty forming words, slurred speech)
- Dysphagia (difficulty swallowing)

**And**

- Ataxia
- Anxiety

**3Ns**

- Nausea
- Numbness
- Nystagmus

In the presence of a blunt traumatic injury involving the cervical spine, the physical therapist should screen the patient using the Canadian C-Spine Rule to determine if the patient should be referred out for further imaging to rule out a cervical fracture.[32] This tool is used with patients who are alert and medically stable and have experienced blunt trauma affecting the cervical spine. There are 3 parts of the Canadian C-Spine Rule: the high-risk factor questions (ie, 65+ years, dangerous mechanism of injury [MOI], or paresthesia in the extremities), the low-risk factor questions, and the patient's ability to perform active cervical rotation. A dangerous MOI includes a fall from 3 feet or higher (ie, from a ladder or 5 or more stairs), a high-speed or rollover motor vehicle accident (MVA), being ejected from a vehicle, axial loading to the head (ie, a diving accident), or a bicycle/recreational vehicle collision.[32] A yes response to any of the high-risk factor questions indicates the need for a radiograph before continuing with the examination. If the patient does not present with high-risk factors, the therapist will then assess for lower-risk factors, such as experiencing a less serious MVA (ie, a slow-speed rear-ended accident), the ability to perform prolonged sitting, the ability to ambulate at any time, delayed onset of neck pain, or the absence of midline cervical spine tenderness. If the patient answers no to any of these questions, a radiograph should be performed before proceeding. If the patient answers yes to all lower-risk factor questions, then the patient is asked to actively rotate their head to the right and left. If they are unable to perform the active range of motion (AROM) past 45 degrees, then they should be referred for a radiograph.[32] It is important that physical therapist assistants continue to question patients and be alert to any changes or new events that may increase suspicion of a possible fracture; all findings should be reported to the therapist.

Compression fractures are caused by axial compression or flexion forces but are more commonly seen in the thoracic and lumbar spine; they respond well to a multimodal physical therapy treatment approach.[33] As stated earlier, these fractures are more prevalent in patients with osteoporosis or osteopenia and rarely show neurologic deficits.

Cervical myelopathy is a gradual degenerative process of the spinal canal that may be associated with spinal trauma, spinal stenosis, spinal infection, or disk herniation resulting in spinal cord compression. A diagnosis of cervical myelopathy may warrant further diagnostic testing or medical management. A clinical prediction rule for ruling in cervical myelopathy was developed by Cook et al[34] in 2010. The study determined that 5 specific clinical signs/tests (ie, gait deviation, Babinski sign, Hoffmann sign, inverted supinator sign, and age 45 years or older) completed together best determine the presence or absence of cervical myelopathy. A positive Babinski sign is characterized by great toe extension and fanning of toes 2 through 5 while stroking the plantar surface of the foot with a blunt object. A positive Hoffman sign is described by adduction of the thumb and/or finger flexion with flicking of the third digit nail bed, and a positive inverted supinator sign results with finger flexion during brachioradialis deep tendon reflex tapping. A positive result for any 3 of the 5 tests/signs yielded a 94% probability, and 4 of 5 yielded a 99% probability to rule in cervical myelopathy.[34]

Predictors of cancer include a previous history of cancer, unexplained weight loss, pain at rest or at night, age older than 50 years or younger than 17 years, and failure to improve over the predicted time interval after treatment. Screening for inflammatory processes or systemic conditions include monitoring vital signs and the presence of a fever.[35]

## *Forward Head Posture and Cervical Impairments*

Posture plays a key role in physical therapy management of the cervical spine; therefore, an initial postural assessment is usually performed by the physical therapist. As discussed in Chapter 7, the physical therapist assistant should be able to reassess, treat, and document changes or improvements for postural deviations noted in an initial evaluation. Forward head posture is the most common postural impairment. It results from the combination of prolonged upper cervical spine extension and lower cervical flexion. In this position, the DNFs are not at their optimal muscle length to efficiently contract so they become weak and lengthened, whereas the upper cervical posterior musculature becomes shortened and inefficient. Chapter 7 (see Table 7-4) provides additional information on various postural deviations and their associated compensations and muscle adaptations. Several common impairments related to forward head posture include the following:

- DNF weakness, altered motor control, and/or decreased muscle endurance lead to poor posture, cervical pain, headaches, and reduced activity tolerance (eg, driving, computer use, reading).
- Altered cervical joint mobility limits ROM and function (ie, the inability to rotate the head when driving).
- Radicular symptoms into the upper extremity lead to decreased positional tolerance throughout the day and during sleep.
- Shortened anterior chest wall musculature (ie, the pectoralis major and minor muscles) leads to rounded shoulders and an increased use of accessory muscles when breathing negatively impacts the cardiovascular system by limiting tidal volume.
- Lengthened and weak lower trapezius and rhomboid muscles contribute to scapular protraction and an increased potential for shoulder pain/impingement.
- Shortened posterior upper cervical musculature and the SCM contribute to an increased risk of headaches.
- Altered resting position of the TMJ contributes to deviations during mouth opening and pain with chewing and speaking.

## Common Cervical Spine Diagnoses and *International Classification of Functioning, Disability and Health* Classification System Categories

Neck pain that interferes with daily activities affects 20% to 70% of all adults at some time during their life,[36] and about 54% have experienced neck pain within the last 6 months.[37] There are several risk factors associated with developing chronic neck pain such as being older than 40 years; "coexistence of low back pain, a long history of neck pain, cycling as a regular activity"[36]; loss of hand strength; a "worrisome attitude"[36]; poor quality of life; and decreased vitality.[36,37] A prior history of neck pain and being female are the strongest risk factors for a new onset of neck pain in the general population and in office workers.[36]

The medical diagnoses associated with cervical pain that commonly result in referral to physical therapy include degenerative disk disease, disk herniation, cervical stenosis, postural dysfunction, cervical radiculopathy, cervical fracture, WAD, sprain/strain, spondylolisthesis, spondylosis, myelopathy, scoliosis, cervicalgia, rheumatoid arthritis, facet syndrome, mechanical neck pain, contusion, cervicogenic headache (CGH), and cervicogenic dizziness. Although the cause of neck pain may be consistent with the findings on diagnostic imaging, the actual tissue causing the pain is often unknown. For this reason, the physical therapist will assess the function of all structures (ie, the muscles, connective tissue, and nerves) most likely associated with the injured tissues.[37]

The medical diagnoses on the referring physician prescriptions may be classified into an *ICF* category based on the physical therapy examination findings.[36,37] A POC is then created based on the initial findings. During the evaluation, the physical therapist assesses the patient for cervical and thoracic ROM limitations, the presence or absence of CGHs, a history of trauma, and the presence of upper extremity radiating pain. The therapist then classifies the patient based on the patient's presentation and examination findings while considering the medical diagnosis. The physical therapist assistant will then treat the patient based on the evaluation findings, the patient's goals, and the treatment plan outlined in the initial evaluation.

**Considerations for the Physical Therapist Assistant**

Regardless of the patient's diagnosis or *ICF* category, the assistant should continually monitor patients for the 5Ds and 3Ns and red flag signs during treatment.

The *ICF* guidelines are the recommended classification system for categorizing patients with neck pain. The primary goal for using this classification system is to determine the most appropriate treatment approach to ensure the best outcome for each patient. The *ICF* classification system has identified 4 categories of neck pain with functional impairments[36,37]:

1. Neck pain with mobility deficits
2. Neck pain with headaches
3. Neck pain with movement coordination impairments
4. Neck pain with radiating pain

Each category has testing techniques and interventions that are specific to their classification (Table 14-3). The impairments identified during the evaluation are the key areas that the physical therapist assistant should address during treatment interventions. For example, if a patient has limited ROM due to decreased flexibility or weakness, then specific stretching or strengthening techniques/exercises should be incorporated to target those muscles. Postural deficits should be addressed by stretching shortened tissues, strengthening lengthened tissues, improving motor control, and increasing muscular endurance in an optimal postural position.

**Table 14-3**

*International Classification of Functioning, Disability and Health* Categories, Associated Symptoms, Testing, and General Treatment Guidelines

| Neck Pain With Mobility Deficits (Cervicalgia) | Neck Pain With Headaches (Cervicogenic) | Neck Pain With Movement Coordination Impairments (Sprain/Strains, Whiplash-Associated Disorder) | Neck Pain With Radiating Pain (Spondylosis and Diskogenic With Radicular Symptoms) |
|---|---|---|---|
| Common symptoms[36]<br>• Limited cervical movement that consistently reproduces neck pain<br>• Neck pain located on one side and/or located in the center<br>• Referred pain possibly into the shoulder girdle or upper extremity | Common symptoms[36,37]<br>• Noncontinuous unilateral neck pain that is associated with a headache<br>• Headache caused or aggravated by cervical motions, sustained positions, or postures; can be associated with bilateral/unilateral neck pain causing bilateral/unilateral headaches<br>• CGHs are usually unilateral starting with neck or suboccipital area pain that moves up to the front of the head[37] | Common symptoms[36]<br>• Reported MOI linked to whiplash or trauma<br>• Neck pain with/without upper extremity pain symptoms<br>• Headaches, fatigue, dizziness, vertigo, irritation to light/noise, cognitive functional changes, radicular pain, poor concentration | Common symptoms[36]<br>• Neck pain with radicular pain in the upper extremity<br>• Upper extremity myotomal muscle weakness and/or dermatomal paresthesia or numbness |
| Specific tests[36]<br>• Cervical AROM limited<br>• + Cervical flexion-rotation test (CFRT; for AA joint mobility)<br>• + Cervical and thoracic segmental mobility tests | Specific tests[36,50,51]<br>• Cervical AROM limited<br>• + CFRT (for AA joint mobility)<br>• + Upper cervical segmental mobility: Headaches reproduced with provocation of involved upper cervical segments<br>• Note: Cervical flexion test was suggested in the 2008 CPGs[16] | Specific tests[36,58]<br>• Cervical AROM limited: Pain in midrange that becomes worse at end ROM<br>• + DNF endurance test<br>• + Cranial cervical flexion test<br>• Altered cervical joint position sense (+ joint position error test)<br>• Sensorimotor impairments may include altered muscle activation patterns, proprioceptive deficit, impaired postural control or balance | Specific tests[36,64]<br>• Cervical rotation AROM to involved side < 60 degrees<br>• + Upper limb tension test (ULTT) 1/A[64]<br>• + Spurling test<br>• + Cervical distraction test<br>• Possible reflex, sensory, or strength deficits in involved upper extremity |

*(continued)*

**Table 14-3 (continued)**

*International Classification of Functioning, Disability and Health* Categories, Associated Symptoms, Testing, and General Treatment Guidelines

| Neck Pain With Mobility Deficits (Cervicalgia) | Neck Pain With Headaches (Cervicogenic) | Neck Pain With Movement Coordination Impairments (Sprain/Strains, Whiplash-Associated Disorder) | Neck Pain With Radiating Pain (Spondylosis and Diskogenic With Radicular Symptoms) |
|---|---|---|---|
| Treatment guidelines<br>Initial: Gentle cervical ROM exercises, gentle stretching of shortened muscles, and strengthening of scapulothoracic muscles; postural education; begin DNF muscle strengthening<br>Progression: Improve cervical/scapulothoracic endurance, neuromuscular coordination, proprioception, postural retraining stretching, strengthening exercises, aerobic conditioning | Treatment guidelines<br>Soft tissue mobilization of upper cervical and suboccipital muscles, gentle manual traction, increase cervical rotation, and stretches for suboccipital muscles and other muscles indicated as shortened in initial evaluation<br>Progression: DNF strengthening, upper quarter, scapulothoracic strengthening; patient education for proper cervical positioning with activities (eg, reading, computer work, sleeping) | Treatment guidelines<br>Stretching of suboccipital muscles, scalene muscles, upper trapezius, levator scapulae, and pectoralis major and minor; strengthening DNF muscles, middle trapezius, lower trapezius, and serratus anterior; and joint positioning sense retraining. Address dizziness if indicated (refer to Chapter 8).<br>Progression: Improve cervical/scapulothoracic and DNF muscle strengthening and endurance, neuromuscular, coordination, proprioception, postural retraining exercises, improve balance | Treatment guidelines<br>Goal: Centralize the pain; chin tucks (cervical retraction), postural and occupational/activity patient education; intermittent cervical traction, manual therapy, nerve glides, and/or joint mobilization for cervical and thoracic region<br>Progression: Strengthening and endurance training of DNF, cervical extensors, and upper quarter muscles (ie, scapular retraction) and aerobic training; stretching of lower cervical and upper thoracic muscles (upper trapezius, levator scapulae, and pectoralis major)[37] |

There is often an overlap among categories, so patients may be placed in more than one category; these classifications are intended to guide treatments. Not all diagnoses fit clearly into a specific category, so a patient may transition from one category to another throughout the course of their care. As patient presentations change, the physical therapist assistant should discuss them with the supervising physical therapist because this may warrant a re-evaluation or a change in the POC.

All patients should complete a self-report questionnaire because it can provide valuable information about a patient's status during the initial evaluation and the patient's progress during the course of therapy. The Neck Disability Index (NDI) is commonly used in outpatient clinics; it can provide information about pain level and disability in patients who fall into any of the 4 cervical pain categories. The NDI is a validated 10-item questionnaire that includes questions about pain intensity and disability during self-care, lifting, reading, headaches, concentration levels, work, driving, sleeping, and recreational activities. NDI scores of 10% to 28% indicate mild disability, 30% to 48% indicate moderate disability, 50% to 68% indicate severe disability, and 72% or higher complete disability.[36,38]

Physical therapist assistants may see POCs reflective of the evaluating physical therapist's training/experience, regional practice patterns, and/or treatment philosophy (ie, diagnosis and stage of healing, the treatment classification system, a mechanical diagnosis, or a movement system impairment). The treatment-based classification system provides a beneficial guide to clinical decision making because interventions are based on the patient's current signs and symptoms.[37] This promotes a focus on improving joint mechanics, mobility, strength, and muscle endurance by targeting the underlying joint, soft tissue, and/or neural mobility that produces the patient's neck pain. Joint compression or traction (manual or mechanical) may help reduce and centralize radicular symptoms. Research regarding cervical pain treatments continues to evolve, so it is important to stay current on evidence-based practice interventions that improve patient outcomes.

## *Neck Pain With Mobility Deficits*

Patients with acute or chronic neck pain whose primary limitation is decreased ROM are classified in the neck pain with mobility deficits category. The most common characteristics of this subgroup include individuals younger than 50 years old, acute neck pain for less than 12 weeks, symptoms isolated to the neck, and restricted cervical ROM.[16,17] Many diagnoses can fall into this category. These patients usually do not have imaging issues or present with any red flag signs or symptoms.[36] When performing AROM, these patients tend to report pain that is usually localized to the neck and do not report radicular symptoms.[37]

### Assessing Neck Pain With Mobility Deficits

First, an initial screening examination to rule out serious complications (ie, cervical fracture, myelopathy, instability, cancer, and arterial dysfunction) should be completed by the physical therapist. Once deemed safe, AROM is assessed. Normal ROM for the cervical spine includes 80 degrees of flexion, 70 degrees of extension, 20 to 45 degrees of lateral flexion, and a maximum of 90 degrees of rotation.[39] Thoracic spine flexion and extension are between 20 and 45 degrees in each direction and between 20 and 40 degrees of lateral flexion (when measured using a goniometer).[30]

Before taking measurements, ensure the patient is sitting in a good postural position. Both cervical and thoracic spine AROM should be assessed in all directions for motion restrictions and/or movement compensation or substitutions. AROM assessment provides valuable information about available motion and left-to-right symmetry as well as the patient's symptom irritability level, willingness to move, and the quality of movement. Note the patient's pain with movement as well as the points in the range where the pain occurs. According to the 2017 CPGs, a goniometer and inclinometer are the most commonly used tools for measuring cervical ROM; however, a tape measure is also a reliable and valid tool.[36] Physical therapist assistants should be able to replicate the measurement techniques used in the initial evaluation to track the patient's progress. Cervical spine AROM can also be included as part of an exercise program (Figure 14-2).

**Quick Class Activity**

Sit in a slumped position, and then flex, extend, side bend, and rotate your head to both sides. Take note of the available ROM. Next, sit up straight, and repeat the motions. What is the difference in the available cervical ROM in each of these postures?

Having the patient sit in an erect position when measuring AROM helps to standardize the technique and increases the reliability of the measurements. In addition to ROM measurements, the therapist typically completes quadrant testing during an initial examination. Quadrant testing is a combination of active cervical extension with ipsilateral side bending and rotation to determine if a facet issue and/or nerve root impingement is present. If AROM is pain free, the physical therapist provides slight overpressure in each plane in an attempt to reproduce symptoms and determine the source of pain. The absence of pain with overpressure helps the therapist to rule out each of the tissues being stressed as the source of a patient's pain. The therapist considers the end feel when performing overpressure at the end of the patient's available range. The normal end feel for the cervical spine is firm.

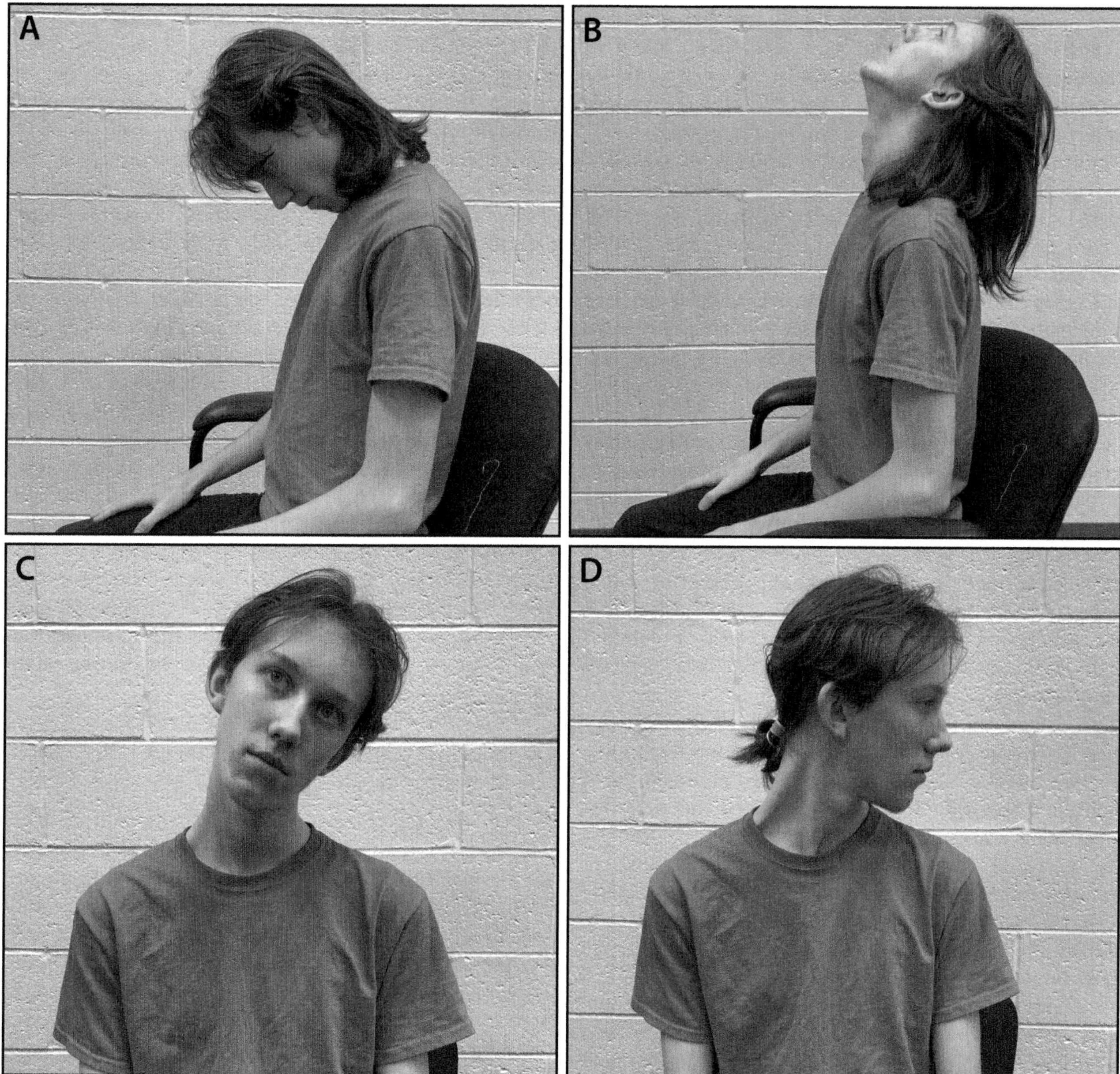


**Figure 14-2.** (A) Cervical AROM flexion. (B) Cervical AROM extension. (C) Cervical AROM lateral flexion. (D) Cervical AROM rotation.

The physical therapist performs manual muscle testing to assess muscle strength, and the assistant uses this information to determine which muscles should be stretched and which should be strengthened. The assistant can passively stretch shortened muscles and instruct patients on proper stretching exercises targeting those muscles so stretching can be performed at home. Strengthening is initiated for those muscles that were identified as being weak. Specific exercises are found at the end of this chapter, and the associated upper quarter muscle stretching and strengthening exercises are described in Chapter 12.

Physical therapists perform special tests during the initial evaluation. The 2017 CPGs suggest the CFRT (to assess AA joint mobility) and cervical and thoracic segmental mobility tests are best to use in order to determine the presence or absence of neck pain with mobility deficits.[36] To perform the CFRT, the patient is positioned supine, and the clinician passively flexes the cervical spine as far as possible and then passively rotates the head to the left and right. The amount of ROM is recorded when the patient initially reports the onset of pain or when the clinician feels a firm resistance. The clinician can visually estimate the patient's available range to each side, and a 10-degree reduction is considered a positive test result. During cervical and thoracic segmental mobility testing, the therapist assesses each vertebral segment in the cervical and thoracic spine to determine pain intensity and individual vertebral mobility (graded as normal mobility, hypermobile, or hypomobile).[16]

## Interventions for Neck Pain With Mobility Deficits

Generally, acute, subacute, and chronic staging for patients with neck pain tends to be time based and dependent on the irritability of the patient's condition (ie, SINSS [Severity, Irritability, Nature, Stage, Stability]). In the acute stage, the patient's condition is highly irritable, and pain is experienced at rest and/or pain occurs with initial to midrange movement of the cervical spine when no tissue resistance is felt. During the subacute phase, the patient usually has no pain at rest but exhibits moderate irritability and pain during midrange that worsens at end-range movement and into tissue resistance. A condition is considered chronic if it is present for more than 3 months or if pain increases with sustained end-range movements/positions and with overpressure into the tissue resistance. This is very important for the physical therapist assistant to remember because the patient's level of irritability must be considered in order to implement the most appropriate interventions because this determines the tissue's ability to accept the stress placed on it.[36]

Interventions for patients with neck pain with mobility deficits include joint mobilizations and therapeutic exercise for pain control and to improve cervical mobility. These interventions are initiated early and within the patient's pain tolerance. When treating patients with neck pain, the physical therapist assistant should review the initial evaluation for shoulder region or thoracic spine issues and address any of those findings (ie, decreased mobility/strength) because they may be contributing to the patient's symptoms (regional interdependence).[1]

Clinicians can apply a test-retest method during treatment to determine which interventions are most appropriate. This method incorporates identifying an impairment, choosing a specific intervention to address the identified impairment, and retesting the impairment to see if changes have occurred after implementing the intervention. For example, a patient who has limited right cervical lateral flexion is instructed to stretch the left upper trapezius to address the limitation. After the stretch, the clinician remeasures right-side bending. If improvement is noted, the intervention chosen is deemed effective and should become part of the patient's home exercise program if it can be performed independently and correctly. If no change is observed, other interventions should be explored.

**Considerations for the Physical Therapist Assistant**

The test-retest method helps the assistant facilitate effective and efficient clinical decision making to improve patient outcomes.

## Joint Mobilization Techniques for the Cervical Spine

Performing joint mobilization techniques to the cervical spine and/or thoracic spine is done to reduce pain and muscle guarding (grades I and II) or to increase mobility of the specific spinal segment being mobilized (grades III or IV). Spinal joint mobilizations are not considered entry-level practice for the physical therapist assistant, but the physical therapist will incorporate these when appropriate to maximize patient outcomes. Joint mobilization of the cervical spine can be applied from a posterior to anterior fashion both centrally and unilaterally with varying levels of force and speed.[40] The therapist considers regional interdependence when selecting joint mobilizations for those with neck pain.[41] There is evidence to support that patients with neck pain treated with a combination of cervical and thoracic mobilization and exercise (or a multimodal treatment approach) had superior outcomes compared with those treated with only cervical mobilization and exercise.[42] A Cochrane review of mobilization of the cervical spine found that thrust and nonthrust mobilizations alone were not as beneficial as thrust and nonthrust techniques performed with exercise in reducing pain and improving patient satisfaction.[43] Joint mobilization of this region is not well studied, and there are rare incidents of adverse events occurring in patients who received thrust mobilizations to the cervical spine.[36,44] The assistant will complete exercise interventions after the therapist performs mobilizations, and the assistant should observe and report changes in a patient's status.

## Therapeutic Exercises for Neck Pain With Mobility Deficits

The goal for patients with neck pain and mobility deficits is to restore cervical spine movement, allowing for normal function and maintaining properly aligned postures. ROM deficits can be addressed using a multimodal approach including ROM exercises, AROM with overpressure, stretching, and strengthening (see Table 14-3). Gentle contract-relax stretching techniques can be used to specifically increase ROM for lateral flexion and rotation. This technique should only be performed if pain-free submaximal isometric contractions can be achieved. Postural re-education should be incorporated into the muscle strengthening, muscle endurance, motor control, and proprioception portions of the rehabilitation program. Exercises can be performed in various positions (supine, seated, or standing), but proper erect posture should be achieved before performing any cervical or thoracic motion exercises.

One systematic review found that there were minimal differences in short-and long-term benefits for patients with acute and chronic neck pain who performed exercises vs those who received cervical joint mobilizations, but the results were limited because there was variability in the treatment interventions and outcome assessment tools.[45] Several studies have reported that the inclusion of scapulothoracic and upper extremity endurance exercises was beneficial during the acute and chronic phases.[36]

### *Deep Neck Flexor Muscle and Strengthening Progression*

The DNF muscles are intrinsic muscles, and strengthening them is necessary to normalize cervical flexion mechanics; therefore, the use of a low level of resistance is suggested. In normal cervical flexion joint mechanics, the head and upper cervical spine (craniocervical spine) should flex before the lower cervical spine. The DNF muscles are responsible for initiating upper cervical spine flexion and should be active through the full ROM.[25,46] Patients who complain of neck pain and present with forward head posture tend to have limited active cervical flexion. This limitation is usually due to tight upper cervical extensors and weak DNF muscles; these muscles are weak because they are not in an optimal position to contract effectively.[25,46]

The best way to tell if the DNFs are firing appropriately is to have the patient positioned supine and perform active cervical flexion. If the chin does not tuck first and move down toward the sternum as the head leaves the surface and the neck flexes, then those muscles are not engaged and/or are weak. The clinician may see the SCM and anterior scalene muscles (which are superficial) contracting on both sides, indicating they are initiating the motion and not the DNFs. The clinician should observe the patient's ability to complete the ROM and monitor proper mechanics and motor control. The inability to perform proper cervical flexion mechanics through the normal range is due to DNF muscle weakness or poor motor control.

If a patient is unable to effectively fire the DNF muscles, the clinician will educate the patient regarding how to complete a chin tuck, which will help cue a contraction of the appropriate muscles. The clinician instructs the patient to sit erect with the cervical spine relaxed in a neutral position (Figure 14-3A). The patient should gently bring the chin in a slight downward motion toward the sternum (eg, performing a slight nod "yes" in a short range). The patient can assist the motion by gently using 2 fingers to apply slight overpressure (Figure 14-3B). During this motion, the upper cervical spine lengthens, and the lordosis flattens. Once the patient can actively perform this exercise correctly without assistance, the patient can perform the exercise isometrically. To perform a DNF isometric exercise, the patient should be positioned supine with the neck relaxed (Figure 14-3C), and then the clinician can instruct the patient to slowly and gently press the back of the head straight into the surface by gently tucking the chin and retracting the cervical spine (Figure 14-3D). If the physical therapist assistant sees the SCM muscles contracting during the exercise, it is being performed incorrectly.[46] The firing of the SCM muscles is usually due to an exaggerated chin tuck, and the patient must learn to generate the amount of force necessary to contract the DNFs and not facilitate the SCM muscles. To determine SCM activation, the patient can palpate the muscle (on the anterolateral side of the neck) during the exercise. The assistant should continually monitor and provide feedback (extrinsic and then intrinsic) so that the patient learns to limit SCM muscle activation during the exercise because the key to this isometric exercise is to control the movement (motor control). DNF muscle contractions should be modulated and gradually increased but only if SCM activation is kept at a minimum. A sphygmometer (ie, Chattanooga Stabilizer Pressure Biofeedback [DJO, LLC] shown in Figure 15-9 in Chapter 15) can be placed behind the head just below the occiput and inflated to 20 mm Hg while the patient relaxes. The device provides feedback regarding the amount of pressure the patient can generate and maintain for 10 seconds during the chin tuck exercise. The patient should progress the exercise by gradually increasing the force on the device by 2 mm Hg. At each stage, the patient should maintain an isometric hold for 10 seconds followed by a 10-second rest. The goal is for the patient to be able to increase strength and generate 30 mm Hg pressure while sustaining the isometric contraction for 10 seconds with minimal activation of the SCM. This exercise is often performed during the initial evaluation as a special test, which is called the *craniocervical flexion test*. The test is positive if the patient is unable to generate an increase pressure of at least 6 mm Hg during the activity, is unable to sustain the position for 10 seconds, substitutes using superficial cervical musculature to obtain the position, or substitutes using cervical extension to the increase pressure.[16,25,46]

Once the patient can correctly perform the chin tuck exercise, the patient should be progressed to a controlled AROM into cervical flexion exercise to improve motor control throughout the range. The purpose of this exercise is to improve the coordination of the muscle firing sequencing between the DNFs and the superficial muscles (ie, the SCM and anterior scalene muscles). The DNF muscles should initially contract with craniocervical spine flexion followed by superficial muscle firing with lower cervical spine flexion. This exercise should first be performed in sitting or standing (gravity-minimized positions) with the initial goal of completing proper sequencing during full AROM cervical flexion and with a minimal SCM contraction (Figure 14-4). The patient can palpate the SCM during the exercise to feel for muscle activation. Once the patient can successfully perform the exercise in a gravity-minimized position, the patient can be placed in a semireclined position to increase the resistance of gravity and perform the slight "yes" nodding (or chin tuck) with a head lift exercise first targeting the upper cervical spine and then incorporating the lower cervical spine muscles. The patient can then be progressed to a supine position and instructed to repeat the chin tuck–head lift exercise, again with limited SCM activation (Figure 14-5A). The exercise can be held for 10 seconds and repeated 10 times. Progression is determined by the patient's ability to maintain the retracted cervical spine position during the sustained head lift. If the patient's chin protracts during the exercise, either the muscles are fatigued or the position is too difficult for the patient to perform the exercise correctly. If this occurs, the

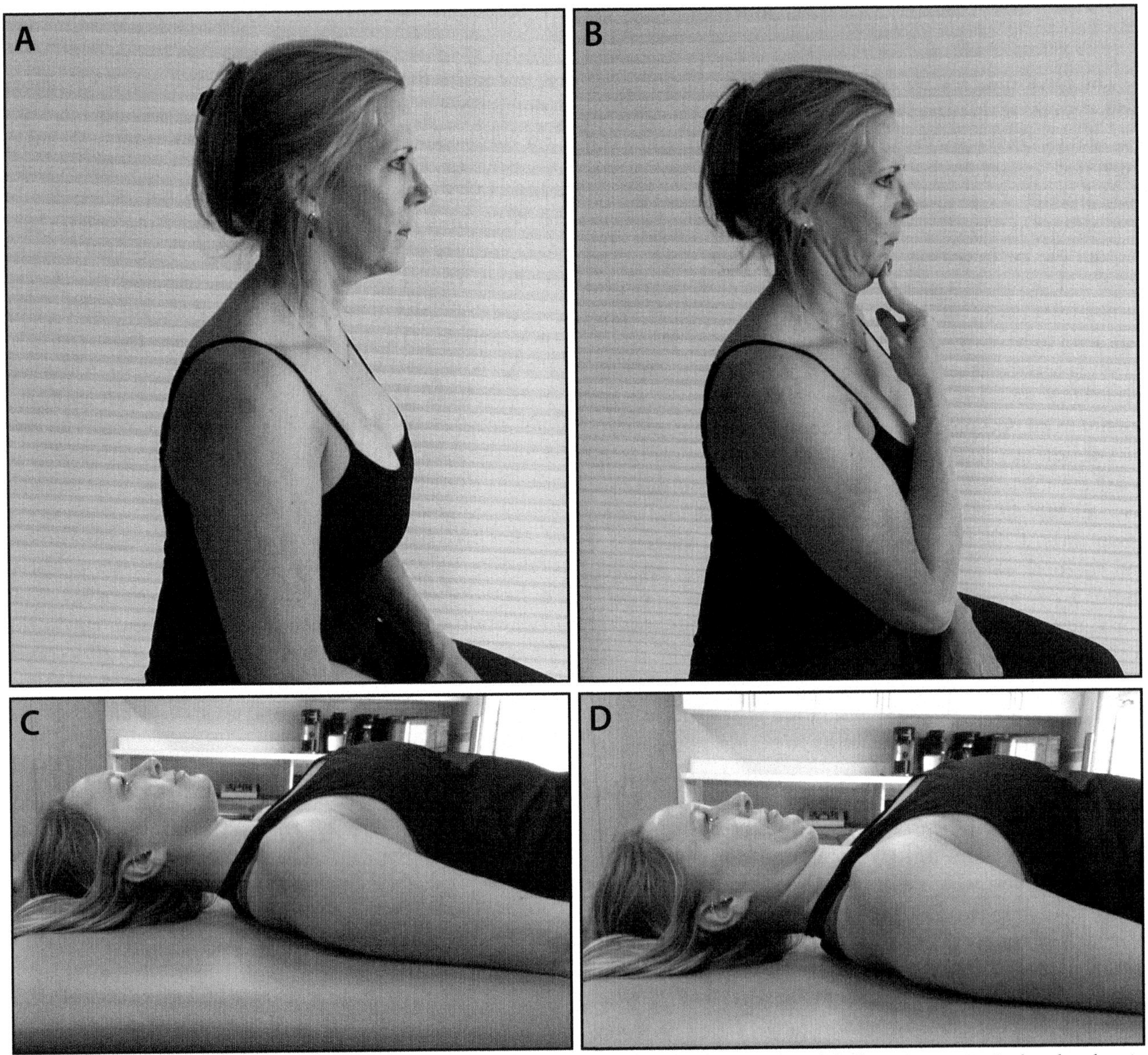

**Figure 14-3.** (A) The patient is relaxed in the neutral position. (B) A chin tuck with assisted overpressure. (C) The patient supine in the relaxed position. (D) The chin tuck exercise: Supine isometric contraction to initiate DNF muscles.

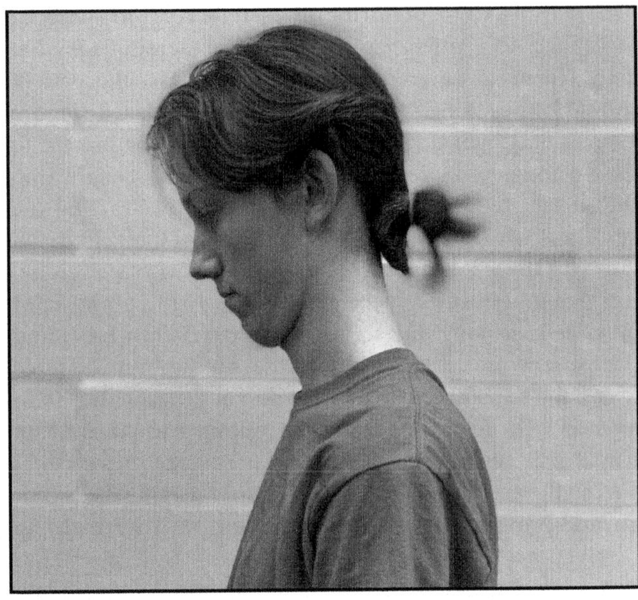

**Figure 14-4.** Notice that the SCM muscles are not contracting. The patient can palpate the muscle for feedback.

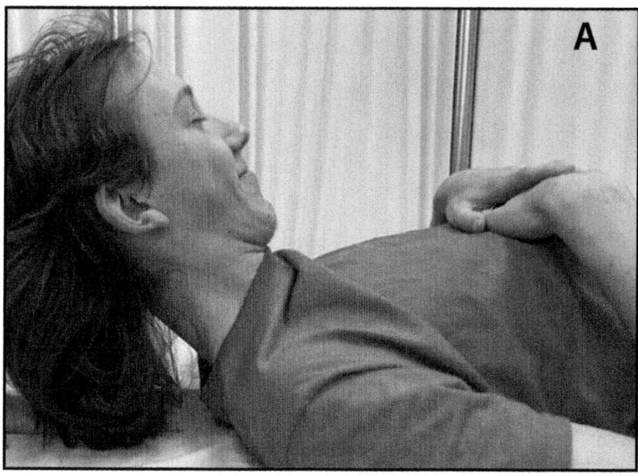


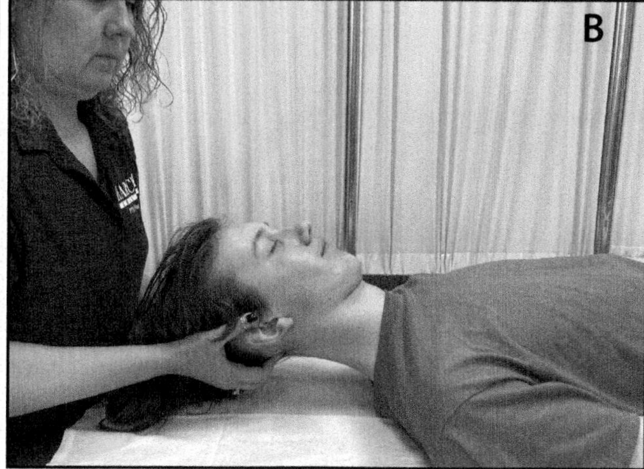


**Figure 14-5.** (A) The patient is able to maintain the chin tuck during the head lift exercises. If the chin protracts during the exercise, the muscles are fatigued. (B) The clinician can assist the patient during the head lift exercise if the exercise is too difficult.

patient can be moved into a position where gravity is less resistant or be assisted by the clinician (Figure 14-5B), or the patient can use one hand behind the head to actively self-assist with the head lift.

Once the patient can correctly perform these exercises in a supine position, the patient can attempt cervical extension in the quadruped or prone position (Figure 14-6). The correct sequencing of the exercise is to perform a chin tuck first to maintain good craniocervical spine position followed by lower cervical extension. There should be no movement of the craniocervical spine during neck extension of the lower cervical spine. This exercise reinforces neuromuscular control of the DNFs while targeting the neck extensors.

Isometric cervical strengthening for flexion, extension, lateral flexion, and rotation can be added if indicated by the POC; these exercises are demonstrated in Figure 14-7. The physical therapist assistant should have the patient perform these exercises in front of a mirror first to ensure that the patient's head is straight and in proper alignment (avoiding forward head posture). The head position should be maintained during a 10-second isometric contraction. The patient should be instructed to gradually increase the force (during the first 2 seconds) to a maximal pain-free contraction and then hold the maximal contraction for the next 6 seconds followed by a slow muscle force release over the last 2 seconds. The patient should rest for 5 to 10 seconds, repeat the exercise, and progress up to 2 sets of 8 to 10 repetitions.

Endurance training and/or strengthening can be addressed by applying low loads of resistance using lightweight resistance bands or a ball (Figures 14-8 and 14-9). If the patient cannot accurately perform the exercise or uses muscle substitution (ie, cervical protraction), this indicates that the muscles are fatigued; the exercise should be terminated to allow the muscles to rest. Training these muscles should reduce neck pain and improve neuromuscular coordination.[25,46]

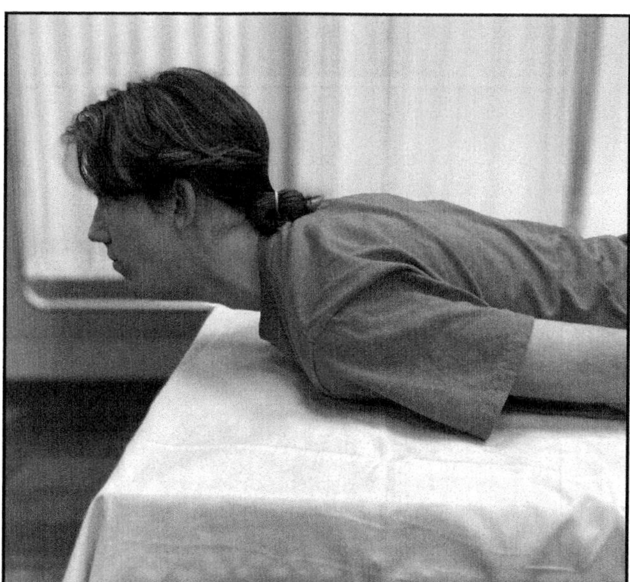

**Figure 14-6.** Prone cervical extension. The patient performs cervical retraction followed by extension.

### Clinical Tip

DNF muscle strengthening and endurance training are beneficial in reducing pain and improving neuromuscular coordination in patients with any cervical dysfunction diagnosis or *ICF* category.

## *Neck Pain With Headaches*

The International Headache Society has classified 14 different types of headaches that are categorized as being of primary (ie, a vascular migraine or muscular tension type) or secondary (resulting from head/neck injury or inflammation) origin.[47] CGHs are considered a type of secondary headache.[48] A CGH is defined as a classification of headache in which pain is referred from the

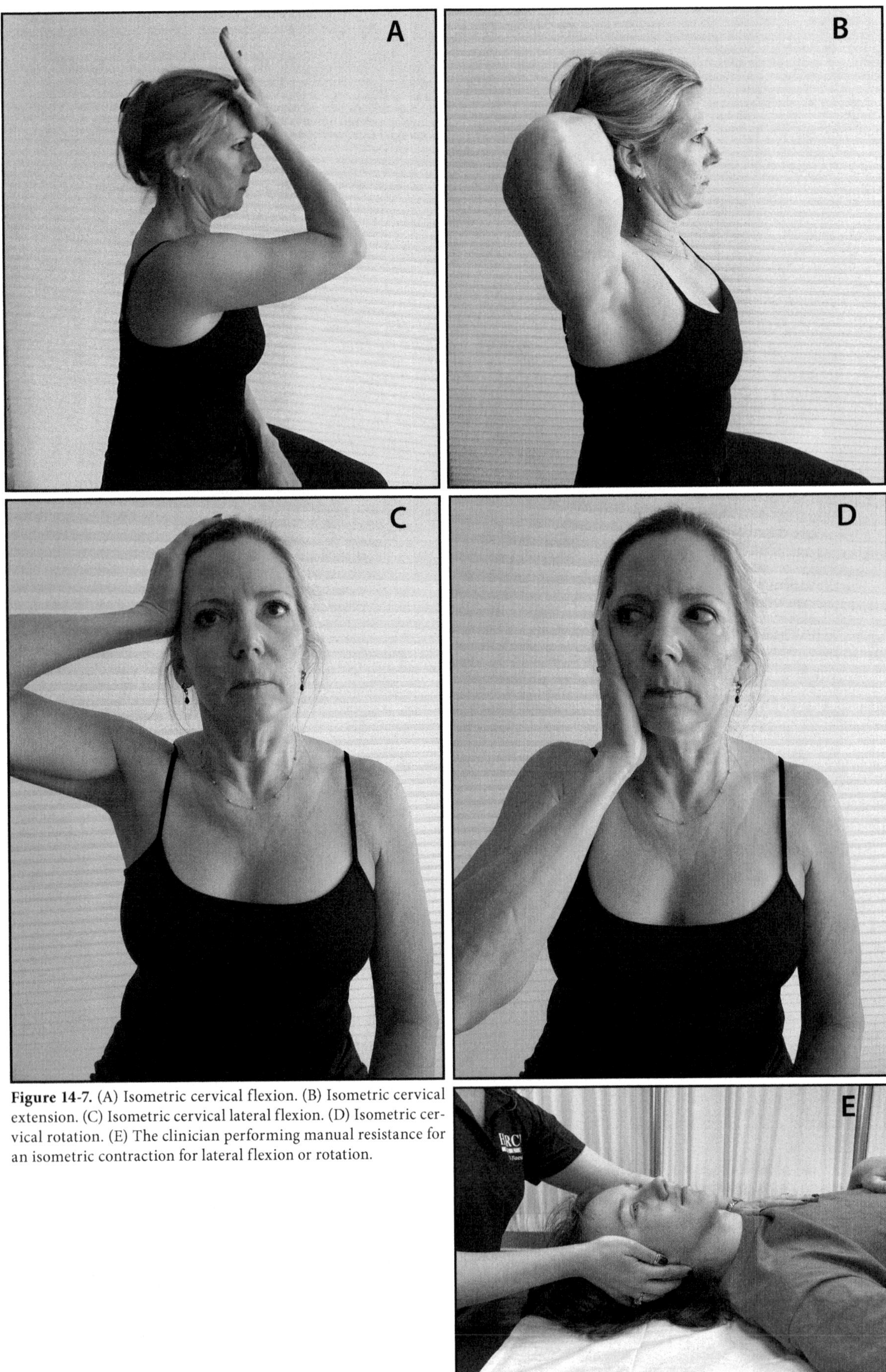


**Figure 14-7.** (A) Isometric cervical flexion. (B) Isometric cervical extension. (C) Isometric cervical lateral flexion. (D) Isometric cervical rotation. (E) The clinician performing manual resistance for an isometric contraction for lateral flexion or rotation.

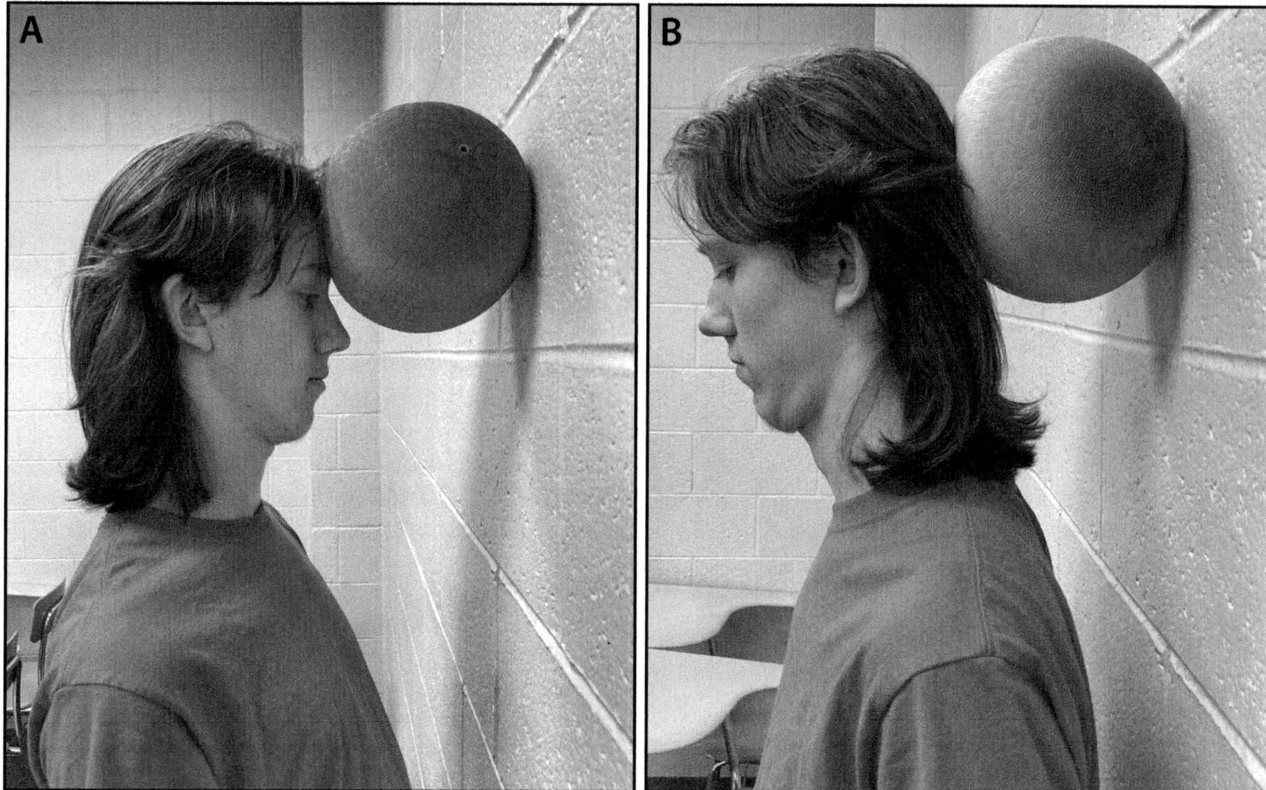


**Figure 14-8.** (A) Cervical isometric strengthening and muscle endurance for neck flexion using a ball. (B) Cervical retraction and extension isometrics for increasing muscle strength and endurance.

cervical spine. There is a great deal of overlap among the categories of headache. The physical therapist will determine the appropriateness of physical therapy for the management of a patient's headaches. Careful evaluation and accurate differential diagnosis are important when making this determination. If headache symptoms do not appear to be cervicogenic in nature, the therapist will refer the patient for further medical follow-up.

CGH symptoms change with cervical spine motions. Specific muscle imbalances are common in patients with CGHs. The most common muscle imbalance is called the *upper crossed syndrome*, which includes muscle tightness of the suboccipital muscle group, the levator scapulae, and the upper trapezius muscles paired with weakness of the DNFs. These patients may also present with tightness in the scalene muscles, SCM, and pectoralis major and minor muscles.[38] Clinical findings commonly associated with CGHs include unilateral headaches precipitated by neck movement; maintaining prolonged positions or postures; external pressure over the upper cervical or occipital region; restricted neck ROM; ipsilateral neck, shoulder, or arm pain; and a lack of response to migraine medications. Common impairments associated with CGHs include cervical ROM restrictions, palpable restrictions and pain in the craniocervical spine, and a positive CFRT. When all 3 impairments are present during testing, there is 100% specificity of ruling in CGHs.[36,49,50]

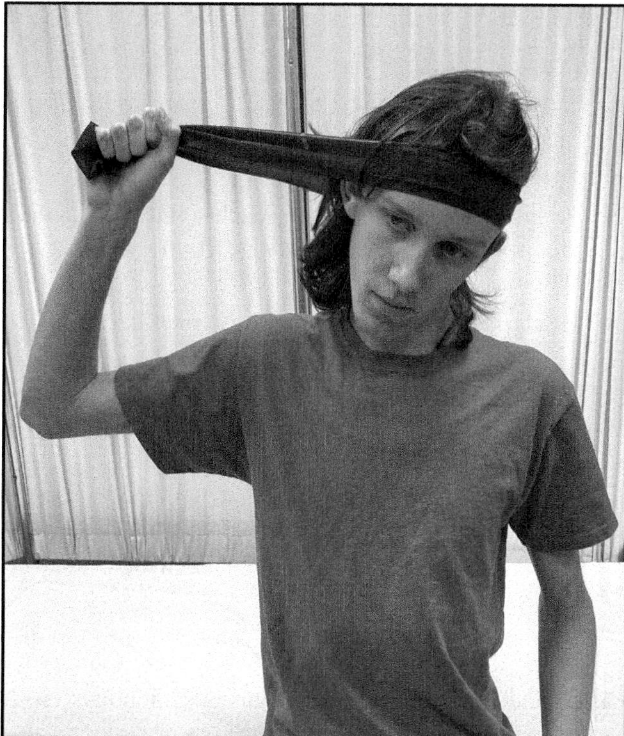

**Figure 14-9.** Lateral flexion strengthening using a resistance band. This exercise can be used in any direction.

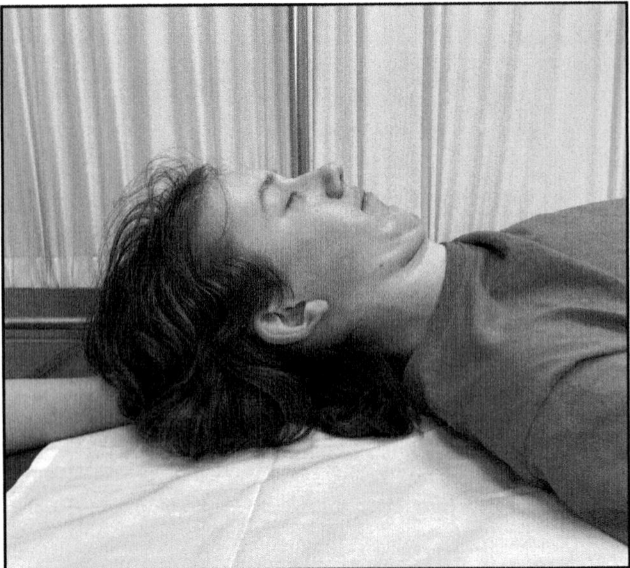

**Figure 14-10.** The DNF endurance test. The patient lifts their head 1 in off the surface. The clinician's hand is placed on the table to cue the patient if the head touches the clinician's hand.

## Assessing Neck Pain With Headaches

There are many nonmusculoskeletal conditions with headaches as a symptom, so the physical therapist will complete a thorough and careful examination (including all indicated screenings) of patients who present with this symptom. Physical therapist assistants should also be aware of the following red flags associated with headaches when treating these patients:

- Severe headache with sudden onset (can indicate subarachnoid hemorrhage or carotid/vertebral artery dissection)
- Progressively worsening headache without obvious predisposing factors (can indicate a tumor or giant cell arteritis)
- Headache with fever, neck stiffness, or skin rash
- History of cancer or human immunodeficiency virus
- Any systemic illness
- Headache associated with focal neurologic symptoms
- Moderate to severe headache triggered by cough, exertion, or bearing down (can indicate an aneurysm)
- New onset of headache during pregnancy (may be associated with preeclampsia)[51]

There are a cluster of tests that can assist with the differential diagnosis of CGHs including cervical AROM, the CFRT, and the upper cervical segmental mobility test.[36] Patients with CGHs typically have decreased cervical rotation during the CFRT compared with those with migraine headaches.[52,53] The CFRT was found to correctly differentiate between those with CGHs vs other types of headaches 85% of the time.[53] The purpose of the CFRT is to assess the amount of available rotation at C1 and C2 either by using a goniometer or visual estimation. To perform the test, the patient is positioned in supine in a hook-lying position, and the clinician passively flexes the patient's head maximally to end range. While maintaining this position, the clinician then passively rotates the patient's head to the right and then the left. According to the research, the average rotation ROM was 39 to 45 degrees in healthy adults and 20 to 28 degrees in patients with CGHs. A ROM finding of less than 32 degrees or a difference between the 2 sides of 10 degrees is considered a positive test. This test has excellent test-retest and inter-rater reliability (92%), a sensitivity of 90% to 95%, and a specificity of 90% to 97%.[36] Patients who suffer from headaches with C1-C2 dysfunction average 17 degrees less rotation than normal subjects.[53]

Other recommended special tests include the craniocervical flexion test[16] and the DNF endurance test. The DNF endurance test provides a timed baseline score for DNF muscle endurance so progress can be tracked. The test is completed with the patient positioned in supine in a hook-lying position. The patient performs a chin tuck and then lifts the head 1 inch (in) off the surface and holds the position (Figure 14-10). The clinician slides one hand under the patient's head while observing for anterior neck skinfold changes, substitution by the anterior cervical musculature, and contact from the patient's head with the clinician's hand. The clinician can provide one verbal corrective cue. The test is terminated, and the time recorded once the patient uses muscle substitution for a second time or the patient's head touches the therapist's hand for more than 1 second.[54,55] Normative data indicate that hold times are 38.95 seconds for those without neck pain and 24.1 seconds for those with neck pain.[16,54,55]

## Interventions for Neck Pain With Headaches

Patients with CGHs commonly have limited upper cervical mobility, so implementing exercises is important to restoring motion. These patients experience headaches because of prolonged misaligned postures due to weak DNFs and tight upper cervical spine muscles. Patient education for proper positioning (eg, sitting and sleeping), correcting faulty posture, and restoring normal ROM are the primary goals during the initial phase of treatment to reduce CGHs. Scapulothoracic strengthening and anterior shoulder muscle stretching should be targeted to improve muscle endurance and neuromuscular conditioning for the upper quarter and cervicothoracic spine.[36]

Stretching the suboccipital muscles is beneficial for patients with headaches because these stretches target the limited upper cervical motion. To stretch these muscles, the patient passively performs and maintains a chin tuck with one hand and places the other hand so the pads of the fingers are on the occiput (Figure 14-11). Gently flex the head on the neck until a stretch is felt in the upper cervical area. Hold the stretch for 20 to 30 seconds, and then relax and repeat 3 to 4 times. After the stretching exercise, the patient should perform a chin tuck and active cervical retraction (with or without overpressure) and then rotate the head

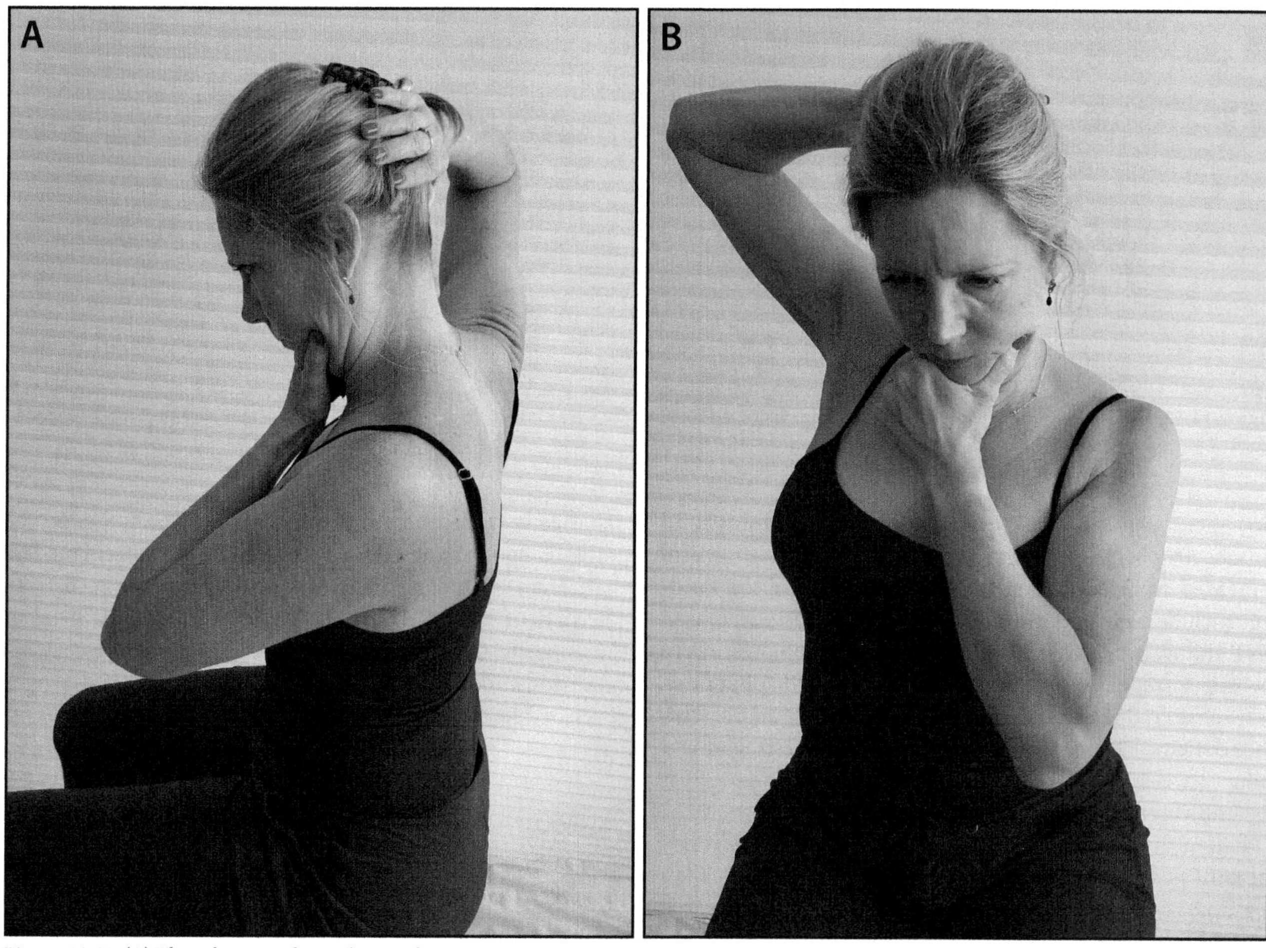


**Figure 14-11.** (A) The suboccipital muscle stretching starting position. (B) Suboccipital muscle stretching; the patient pulls downward with the hand on the occiput to stretch these muscles.

slowly to each side. The patient should use a mirror as feedback to ensure proper cervical alignment is maintained (ie, the chin tuck) before performing the rotation exercise.

DNF strengthening should be initiated early in the rehabilitation process. Performing DNF strengthening after suboccipital stretching and cervical AROM exercises allows these intrinsic muscles to be better positioned to effectively contract, thus reducing the chances of activating the superficial anterior muscles (the SCM).

Generally, all tight/shortened muscles affecting proper postural alignment or mobility in the upper quarter that attach to the skull (ie, the upper trapezius), cervical spine (ie, the levator scapula), ribs (ie, the pectoralis major), and/or scapula should be stretched. All weak (or antagonist) muscles should be strengthened.

## *Neck Pain With Movement Coordination Impairments*

Neck pain with movement coordination impairments is a large classification of patients and the most common category. It includes those with WAD. Between 42% and 50% of these patients will experience long-term or chronic symptoms.[56,57] Annual costs in the United States associated with WAD exceed $29 billion.[57]

Whiplash occurs because of sudden hyperflexion, hyperextension, or lateral flexion motions, which apply excessive shear and tensile forces on the cervical spine. This energy transfer is due to a quick acceleration-deceleration mechanism, such as one commonly associated with nonfatal car accidents. Because the incident happens so quickly, individuals are not able to react by voluntarily contracting their muscles.[57] Commonly reported signs and symptoms in patients with WAD include high-intensity neck pain (6/10 or greater), headache (commonly suboccipital), a high NDI score (15/50 or higher), and low back pain (at any level of intensity). When these findings are present at the onset, there is an increased risk of persistent pain and disability.[56,57] Other symptoms associated with WAD are listed in Table 14-3.[36]

### Assessing Neck Pain With Movement Coordination Impairments

There is a great deal of overlap in the physical therapy examination for those with neck pain with movement coordination impairments and those in other neck pain categories. Clinical presentations for patients in this category include decreased cervical ROM with reports of increased pain at end ranges, altered cervical and upper quarter

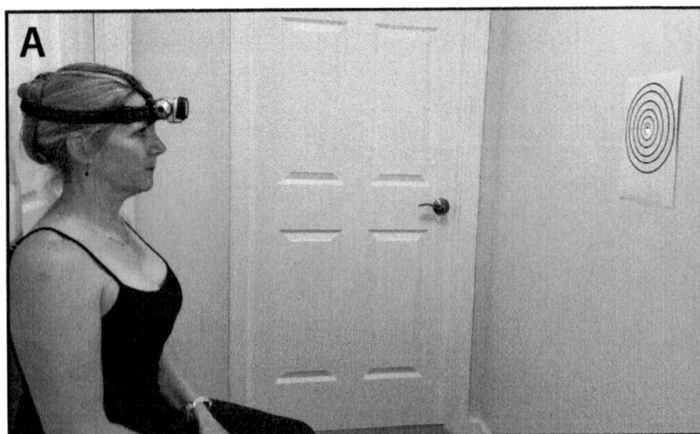


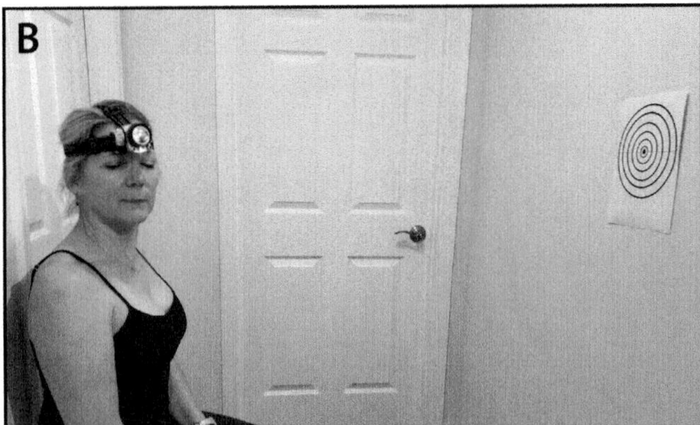


**Figure 14-12.** (A) The joint position error test starting position. (B) With the eyes closed, the head is rotated to one side and then back to center where a mark is placed on the target.

movement patterns due to limitations in flexibility and muscle atrophy/weakness, reduced DNF motor control, and decreased muscle endurance. Common positive test findings include a positive craniocervical flexion test, decreased DNF endurance, and localized pain with applied pressure to the upper trapezius muscles, abnormal cervical spine position sense, reduced postural or motor control, and/or balance deficits. These patients often report pain lasting longer than 12 weeks.[16,36,56,57] Balance testing (see Chapter 8) is also indicated for patients in this classification.

Patients in this category often present with altered cervical **joint position sense** (proprioception deficits), which is a key finding in patients with WAD. Research indicates that patients with WAD who also report dizziness have greater joint position errors than those who report no dizziness.[58] There is preliminary acceptance that cervical spine impairments are associated with the cause of dizziness in these patients.[59] Joint position sense is defined as the ability of an individual to accurately return the head to a neutral posture after active flexion/extension and/or rotation of the cervical spine. Testing for joint position error is important because this is a common finding unique to this category of neck pain.[60] Altered joint position sense is measured using a joint position error test, and this can also be used as an intervention to retrain the patient.[58,59] To perform this test, the patient is seated in a chair with back support with a laser pointer secured to the top of the patient's head. A target (40 cm in diameter with 1-cm concentric circle intervals) is placed 90 cm (or about 35 in) away from the patient. While the patient is in their resting head position with the eyes opened, the laser should be aligned with the center of the target (Figure 14-12A). The patient is asked to close their eyes (or a blindfold can be used) to block their vision. The patient is then instructed to rotate the head one time to either side (the right or left) as far as possible in a slow and steady motion and then return the head back to the center start position (Figure 14-12B). A mark is placed on the target at the patient's final position. The patient is then instructed to open their eyes, recenter the laser on the center target again, and repeat the task. Another mark is placed on the patient's end position. This is repeated 3 times. The distance is measured from the center of the target to the patient's end position for each trial. A measurement less than 7 cm is an acceptable margin of error for each trial. The patient should repeat the test by rotating the head to the opposite side. The test can include performing cervical extension and flexion.[59,60] Joint position sense retraining is described in the following section.

## Interventions for Neck Pain With Movement Coordination Impairments

It is best to use a multimodal treatment approach that includes strengthening exercises, endurance exercises, and manual therapy for patients with WAD.[36,61] This approach yielded superior outcomes with regard to pain reduction and patient satisfaction compared with those treated with manual therapy alone.[36,61] General treatment guidelines are listed in Table 14-3, but the physical therapist assistant should always refer to the POC for specific guidance. The assistant may include many of the stretching and strengthening interventions that have been discussed in this chapter as well as those included in Chapter 12 for the scapulothoracic region and the upper quarter.

Joint position errors (proprioception deficits) can be addressed through joint position sense retraining activities. To perform this intervention, the patient is seated with the same setup described previously in the joint position error testing procedure (see Figure 14-12A). The intervention can simulate the actual test but should be performed first with the patient's eyes open and progressed to eyes closed. Once the task is mastered in sitting, joint position sense retraining can be progressed while standing on a firm surface, standing on foam, and then with the single-leg stance. Head movements must remain slow and steady to facilitate joint proprioception; if the head moves too quickly, the vestibular system (specifically the vestibulo-ocular reflex) will be stimulated instead. To improve kinesthetic responses, the patient can use the laser (with their eyes open) to trace various intricate patterns or shapes on a wall.[61,62]

If the patient has segmental mobility limitations, the physical therapist will likely perform joint mobilization techniques to the hypomobile and painful cervicothoracic segments before the physical therapist assistant initiates any other treatment interventions.

## *Neck Pain With Radiating Pain*

Cervical radiculopathy is a referring diagnosis that accounts for a large portion of the neck pain population managed with physical therapy[63] and is included in the classification group of neck pain with radiating pain. This pain is often associated with diskogenic herniation or protrusion, degenerative disk disease, or spinal stenosis. **Radiculopathy** can be due to compression, traction, or inflammation of a spinal nerve, resulting in symptoms along the distribution of a specific nerve. The physical therapist will evaluate the integrity of myotomes and dermatomes during the initial examination. A pattern of sensory innervation of a single spinal nerve is called a *dermatome*, and a *myotome* is a group of muscles innervated by a single spinal nerve. Radicular symptoms follow a dermatomal and/or myotomal pattern and may result in lower motor neuron signs, including weakness in a myotomal pattern, hypotonia, fasciculations, atrophy, and hyporeflexia (see Appendix F for dermatome patterns).

**Spinal stenosis** is a degenerative narrowing of the spinal canal, and the incidence increases with increased age. The condition may result in spinal cord compression and/or myelopathy. Cervical stenosis is usually confirmed by radiography because some people with this diagnosis do not experience symptoms. It is important to remember to treat patients based on individual examination findings. In addition to the symptoms associated with cervical radiculopathy, cervical stenosis may also present with lower extremity weakness, gait deviations, balance deficits, and/or falls. As the stenosis progresses, the patient may present with upper motor neuron signs, including spasticity, a positive Babinski test, clonus, an increased deep tendon reflex response, and a positive Hoffmann sign.[64]

Radicular or radiating pain differs from referred pain. **Referred pain** is a more generalized pain pattern where pain is generated from one anatomical source and is felt in a distal location (or structure); it does not follow a dermatomal and/or myotomal pattern. Referred pain originating from the cervical spine is also included under the *ICF* classification of neck pain with radiating pain. Symptoms in the upper extremity, scapula region, and/or upper trapezius region can be caused by compression, traction, or inflammation of a cervical nerve. These symptoms originating from the cervical spine are considered referred pain because this pain pattern does not follow a specific nerve distribution.[65] Treatments must address the cervical spine to successfully manage neck pain symptoms and the referred upper extremity pain. Referred pain symptoms are variable and include pain, numbness, tingling (paresthesia), burning, feeling of warmth, shooting, sharp, or stabbing pain. The presence of distal symptoms can occur as a result of a central lesion or injury. The physical therapist must determine the correct differential diagnosis because referred pain and radiculopathy can be mistaken for pain seen with isolated shoulder, elbow, wrist, or hand pathology.

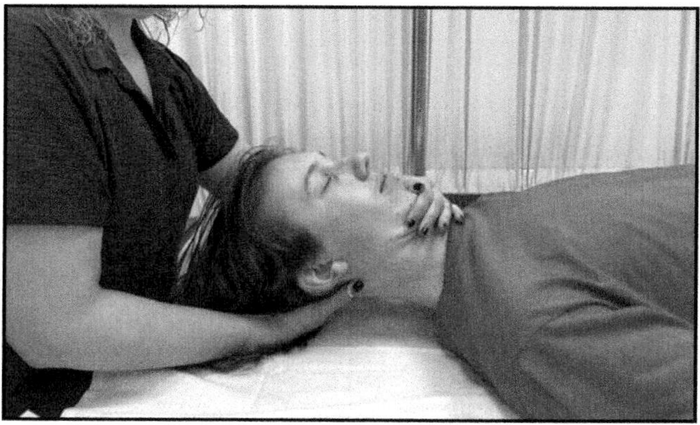

**Figure 14-13.** The distraction test can also be used as a treatment if it reduces symptoms.

### Assessing Neck Pain With Radiating Pain

Patients with positive clinical findings for the cervical spine rotation AROM test, ULTT, distraction test, and Spurling test are considered to have a cervical radiculopathy diagnosis.[16,36,63] A cervical spine rotation AROM test is positive if a patient has less than 60 degrees of active cervical rotation to the involved side. An ULTT (see Chapter 11) for the median nerve (ULTT 1 or A) is considered positive when symptoms are reproduced, if the difference in elbow extension (in a bilateral comparison) is greater than 10 degrees, or when ipsilateral cervical lateral flexion decreases symptoms and/or contralateral cervical lateral flexion increases symptoms.[63] The distraction test (Figure 14-13) is completed with the patient in supine; the clinician grasps the chin and occiput and then applies a distraction force equivalent to approximately 14 pounds. If the patient's symptoms are reduced, the test is considered to be positive. This test can also be used as a treatment intervention. During the Spurling test, the patient is seated, and the clinician passively laterally flexes the head approximately 20 degrees to the involved side and then applies a 15-pound (7-kg) compressive force through the patient's head. The reproduction of symptoms indicates a positive test.[63] If 3 of 4 of these tests are positive, the specificity is 94%, and if 4 of 4 tests are positive, the specificity rate is 100% accurate for ruling in a diagnosis of cervical radiculopathy.[63]

Deep tendon reflex, dermatome, and myotome tests are also performed during the initial evaluation. These tests assess reflex response (normal, hyporeflexia, or hyperreflexia) and sensory loss and/or weakness associated with a specific spinal level (Table 14-4).

After assessing AROM, the physical therapist will have the patient perform repeated motions in neck flexion, neck extension, and right and left side bending. The therapist is monitoring symptom presentation/changes (which motions centralized symptoms to the neck or peripheralized symptoms distally) with these repeated motions to guide the selection of treatment interventions. Not all patients with radiating symptoms will report centralization or a directional preference, but those who do report centralization of

**Table 14-4**

**Deep Tendon Reflex, Dermatome, and Myotome Testing and Associated Cervical Spine Levels**

| Deep Tendon Reflex Testing | Dermatome Testing | Myotome Testing[68] |
|---|---|---|
| • Biceps brachii: C5, C6<br>• Brachioradialis: C5, C6<br>• Triceps: C7 | • C5: Mid-deltoid<br>• C6: Radial aspect of the second metacarpal<br>• C7: Dorsal aspect of the middle finger<br>• C8: Ulnar aspect of the fifth metacarpal<br>• T1: Medial forearm | • C3 neck lateral flexion: Longus capitis, longus cervicis, and trapezius, middle scalene<br>• C4 shoulder elevation: Trapezius, levator scapulae, and scalene muscles (anterior and middle)<br>• C5 shoulder abduction: Deltoid, rhomboid major and minor, supraspinatus, infraspinatus, teres minor, and biceps<br>• C6 elbow flexion and wrist extension: All 3 scalene muscles, serratus anterior, latissimus dorsi, pectoralis major clavicular head, subscapularis, teres major, coracobrachialis, biceps, brachialis, brachioradialis, supinator, and extensor carpi radialis longus<br>• C7 elbow extension and wrist flexion: Latissimus dorsi, pectoralis major sternal head, pectoralis minor, triceps, pronator teres, flexor carpi radialis, extensor carpi radialis longus and brevis, flexor digitorum superficialis, and extensor digitorum<br>• C8: Thumb abduction and ulnar deviation; triceps, flexor carpi ulnaris, pronator quadratus, flexor, extensor and abductor pollicis longus, and extensor and abductor pollicis brevis<br>• T1: Finger intrinsic and second and third finger adduction; intrinsic hand muscles, except for pollicis muscles |

symptoms with exercises in one direction will benefit from including and progressing exercises in the directional preference.[66,67] Patient presentation with a diskogenic pathology often includes centralization of symptoms with cervical retraction and/or neck extension movements. Patients with spinal stenosis may have symptom reduction with neck flexion. However, this is not always true, so physical therapist assistants should have the patient perform those exercises or activities in the specific directional preference that reduces peripheral symptoms and centralizes their pain.

**Considerations for the Physical Therapist Assistant**

Some patients with cervical myelopathy who are not surgical candidates are treated with physical therapy. Assistants should monitor for the presence of weakness in multiple muscles within a myotome and the progression of weakness; this warrants follow-up with the physical therapist for further examination.

## Interventions for Neck Pain With Radiating Pain

Interventions for patients with neck pain with radiating symptoms are based on an impairment-based approach with the goal of centralizing and then reducing/eliminating symptoms and restoring normal mobility and function. Exercises should address the key impairments identified in the physical therapy evaluation. The 2008 CPGs reported that nerve glides, intermittent traction, and exercise combined with manual therapy and strengthening exercises are successful in reducing peripheral and cervical pain and improving function in patients with radicular symptoms. The 2017 guidelines added recommendations to include patient education to maximize efficiency for work and exercise activities.[16,36] The goal is to eliminate the radicular symptoms, then reduce the neck pain intensity, and then restore normal mobility and function. Specific interventions include directional preference exercises, joint mobilization, DNF and scapulothoracic strengthening and endurance exercises, and stretching exercises of the upper cervical and thoracic areas.

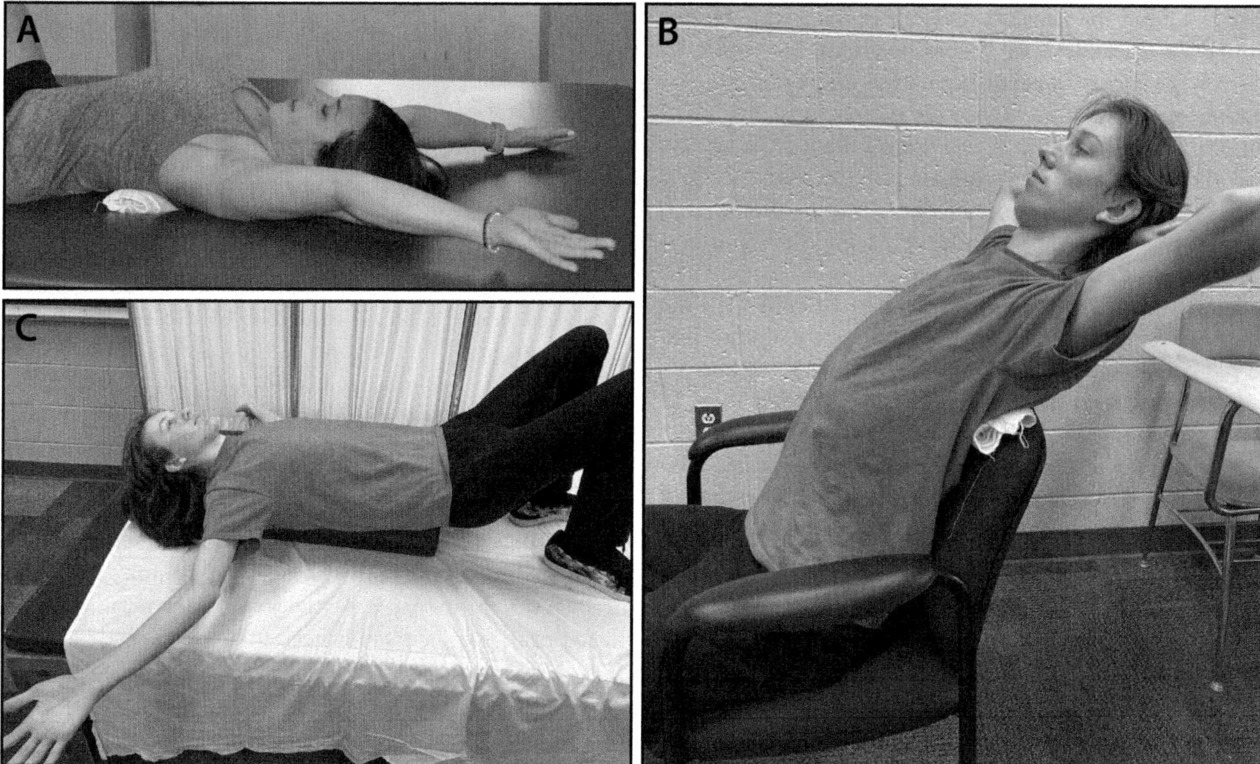

**Figure 14-14.** (A) The end position. Lift both arms up over the head during an exhalation. Once overhead, inhale and bring the arms back down to the side. (B) Seated thoracic extension for self-mobilization of the thoracic spine. (C) A patient using a foam roll to improve thoracic spine alignment and mobility.

As stated earlier, the physical therapist may perform joint mobilizations to hypomobile and/or painful joint segments of the cervical and thoracic spine. Patients can be instructed on self-mobilization for the thoracic spine to increase mobility as part of a home program. A tightly rolled towel is placed horizontally at a level of hypomobility along the thoracic spine with the patient supine and in a hook-lying position. The patient takes a deep breath at the starting position with the arms at the sides of the trunk. As the patient slowly exhales, they actively lift the arms overhead into a "V" (Figure 14-14A). This exercise should be performed for 5 to 10 repetitions several times a day to improve and maintain thoracic mobility. The towel roll can be relocated at various points along the thoracic spine and the exercise repeated. A similar self-mobilization exercise can be performed while sitting in a chair (Figure 14-14B). A foam roll can be used to improve mobility and alignment (Figure 14-14C). These stretching exercises can improve thoracic spine and rib cage mobility.

Patients who report that cervical retraction or extension reduces radicular pain and centralizes their symptoms will benefit from the early inclusion of a chin tuck progression program followed by global extension exercises.[66,67] Once symptoms are centralized, additional strengthening and muscle endurance exercises can be introduced in all directions. Combined treatment interventions should be attempted if they centralize and reduce the patient's pain and improve function. Physical therapist assistants should implement no more than 1 or 2 interventions/exercises at a time so the effectiveness of each intervention/exercise can be determined.

A common impairment for patients with neck pain with radiating symptoms is altered neurodynamics. As a nerve becomes less mobile, compression, traction, or irritability of the nerve can occur, resulting in pain and radiating symptoms. A nerve glide (nerve flossing) is an intervention that can improve and restore neurodynamics of the specific nerve by restoring its ability to glide/slide through the sheath (refer to Chapter 11). Patients can be instructed in self-management techniques to reinforce the manual nerve glide. There is the potential to further irritate the nerve if the technique is performed too aggressively or progressed too quickly. The clinician must be mindful of the patient's response and any changes in symptoms. When performing a nerve glide, the clinician should move the patient slowly and rhythmically, gently moving one segment in and out of a position just to the point where tissue resistance is met or when the patient reports symptoms. The clinician will gradually add components to the movement pattern and should stop movement progression when symptoms are reported by the patient. For example, when a clinician performs a median nerve glide (ULTT 1 or A), the patient's shoulder is first depressed and abducted to 110 degrees while keeping the elbow bent at 90 degrees. The patient's wrist and all of the fingers are then extended while maintaining the shoulder and elbow position. The clinician passively performs forearm supination and then external rotation of the shoulder. Once the patient is in this position, the clinician should slowly extend the patient's elbow until the patient reports symptoms or the clinician feels tissue resistance. At that point, the clinician should stop extending the elbow and should adjust the elbow position into a couple degrees less of elbow extension. Finally, the clinician should instruct the patient to laterally flex the neck to the contralateral side. If symptoms are reproduced, the patient should then laterally flex the neck toward the ipsilateral side, and the assistant should ask the patient to report any changes in the symptoms. Laterally flexing the neck toward the test (or ipsilateral) side places the nerve on slack, and the symptoms should be reduced. The patient does not need to move through the full movement excursion at each joint during neurodynamic testing/treatment. Movement progression is stopped at the point where the patient reports symptoms. The goal of this technique is to progressively advance the positioning until the patient can maintain shoulder, wrist, and finger positioning with full elbow extension without radicular symptoms.

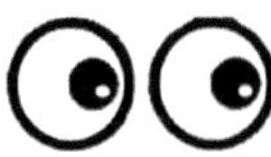

### Eye on the Research: Cervical Traction

Cervical traction is an effective intervention for some patients with neck pain, in addition to exercise.[69] Cervical traction can be applied either manually or mechanically. Raney et al[69] developed a clinical prediction rule that identified subgroups of patients with neck pain who are most likely to benefit from cervical traction and exercise. Five variables were identified:

1. Age 55 years or older
2. Patient-reported peripheralization of symptoms with lower cervical spine mobility testing
3. Shoulder abduction test produces reduced symptoms (while seated, the patient is instructed to place the hand of the affected extremity on the head in order to support the extremity while in the scapular plane)
4. Positive ULTT 1 or A
5. Positive distraction test

Exercises included cervical and scapula retraction and DNF strengthening. The researchers concluded that treatment success was correlated to the number of patient presentation variables. Patients presenting with 3 of the 5 variables had a 79.2% likelihood of successful outcomes when treatment included traction and exercise, and there was a 94.8% likelihood of successful outcomes if patients presented with 4 or more variables.[69] Although these study outcomes have the potential to help clinicians make better clinical decisions for patients with cervical pain and radicular symptoms, further research is needed to validate these results.[69] A 2014 randomized controlled trial found lower long-term disability and pain after including mechanical traction and exercise for patients with cervical radiculopathy.[70]

## Cervical Spine Surgical Procedures and Physical Therapy Management of the Postoperative Patient

Indications for an immediate surgical intervention include acute injury/trauma that results in instability or spinal cord compromise, nontraumatic injuries such as a tumor or infection causing neurologic compression, or degenerative conditions that lead to progressive spinal cord compression and reduced function.[71] Patients may choose elective surgical intervention of the cervical spine due to failed conservative management of symptoms. Reasons for surgical intervention include reducing neck and radicular pain, improving cervical spine stability and alignment, and preserving as much ROM as possible. Surgery may include removing osteophytes (bone spurs) and/or disk material, which reduces pressure on the nerve roots and creates more space for nerves to pass through the spinal canal and/or intervertebral spaces. If the joints become unstable, a fusion of the segments may need to be performed.

### Common Types of Cervical Spine Procedures to Address Cervical Radiculopathy

There are 3 surgical procedures commonly performed to treat cervical radiculopathy: anterior cervical discectomy and fusion (ACDF), posterior cervical foraminotomy (PCF), and/or cervical disk arthroplasty (CDA) or replacement.[72,73] Advantages and disadvantages for an anterior or posterior surgical approach are found in Table 14-5.

ACDF is a common procedure that involves removing the problematic disk or bone spurs and then stabilizing the segment using a cage. The cage has a hollow center filled with bone-promoting material or a bone graft (often harvested from the patient's hip), and it acts as a space holder between the segments. This allows bone to grow through the cage and fuse the vertebrae together to heal as a single unit (Figure 14-15). The fusion eliminates motion between the fused segments. Patients often experience pain from the autograft harvest site (ie, the hip), so physical therapist assistants should consider this during the rehabilitation process.

PCF is performed using a posterior approach, and a burring tool is used first to thin the lamina and create a larger space to access the involved nerve. Tissues (ie, bone spurs and disk material) that compress the nerve root are removed. This procedure can be performed as an open or minimally invasive procedure.

CDA includes an anterior approach to remove the degenerated disk followed by the placement of an artificial disk between the 2 vertebral segments (Figure 14-16). This procedure allows the patient to maintain normal cervical spine motion.

**Table 14-5**

**Anterior and Posterior Cervical Surgical Approaches: Advantages and Disadvantages[72]**

| Approach | Advantages | Disadvantages |
|---|---|---|
| Anterior | • Easier exposure of intervertebral space<br>• Less patient discomfort | • Symptomatic adjacent disk disease<br>• Instrumentation failure<br>• Possible complications: Dysphagia, hematoma, and recurrent laryngeal palsy |
| Posterior | • Potential avoidance for anterior approach complications<br>• Potential for nerve decompression without fusion | • Higher rates of postoperative neck pain<br>• Increased blood loss<br>• Damage to the dorsal cervical musculature |

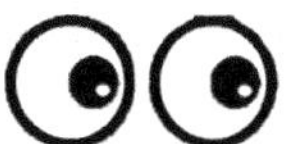

### Eye on the Research: Comparing Surgical Interventions for Cervical Radiculopathy

A review compared the outcomes of ACDF with PCF and concluded that both procedures were safe and effective. A primary difference was the cost of the procedures; the PCF procedure was the more cost-effective option for treating patients with cervical radiculopathy.[72]

A meta-analysis determined that CDA was superior to ACDF for treating symptomatic cervical disk disease in terms of overall success and postoperative NDI scores. There were lower rates of surgery- or implant-related serious adverse events and a statistically significant difference in long-term functional outcomes in favor of the patients with CDA.[73]

A recent meta-analysis examined clinical outcomes and complications for PCF procedures compared with ACDF in patients with cervical radiculopathy without myelopathy and concluded that minimally invasive PCF is a safe, effective alternative to ACDF for this group of patients.[74]

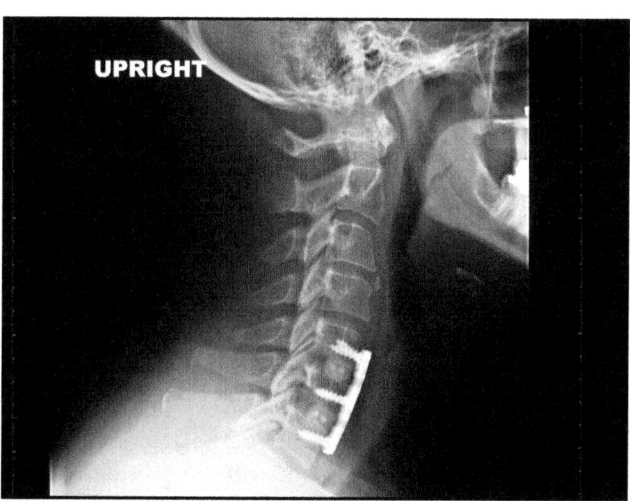


**Figure 14-15.** ACDF using a cage (Anthony Ricci/Shutterstock.com).

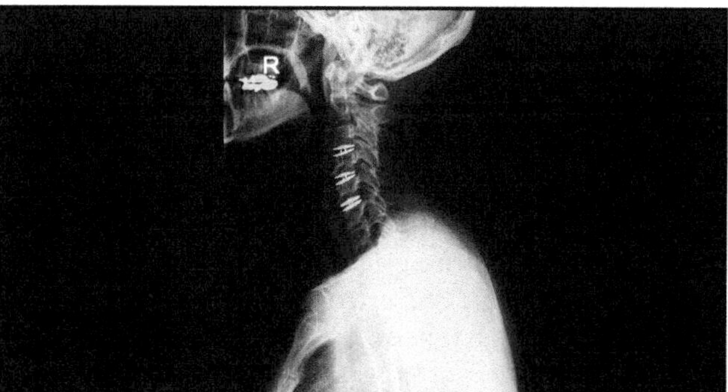

**Figure 14-16.** The lateral view showing multilevel artificial cervical disk replacement (Yok_onepiece/Shutterstock.com).

## Postoperative Considerations

Although postoperative rehabilitation protocols are surgeon specific (which creates some variability), many postoperative protocols include the use of cervical bracing and activity limitations during the initial postoperative phase of rehabilitation. The initial postoperative period is focused on protection and healing. Table 14-6 lists the signs and symptoms that require immediate medical follow-up for postoperative cervical spine patients. During the second stage of rehabilitation, patients can be weaned from cervical collar use and can usually begin AROM, postural re-education, and gentle stretching. Cervical and scapulothoracic strengthening begins during the third rehabilitation phase, and returning to functional activities is the goal of the final phase. Treatment guidelines established in postoperative protocols use time frames based on physiological healing. Patient progression is modified based on individual patient's presentation and the physician's protocol. Changes in symptoms warrant a follow-up with the physical therapist or surgeon depending on the nature of those changes.

**Table 14-6**

Red Flags After Cervical Spine Surgery

- Persistent fever > 101 °F
- Persistent headache worse when sitting and better when lying down
- Bleeding or increasing drainage from the incision (ie, yellow or green or with a foul odor)
- Increased swelling, redness, or tenderness around the incision
- Separation of incision edges
- New onset of bowel and/or bladder issues
- Problems swallowing or breathing
- New onset of numbness or tingling in hands or fingers
- New onset of weakness in upper or lower extremities
- Gait instability or ataxia

## *Thoracic Outlet Syndrome: Classifications and Assessments*

The thoracic outlet is the area between the cervical spine and the upper chest region that contains the pathway of the brachial plexus. The thoracic outlet spans from the interscalene triangle to the lateral border of the pectoralis minor muscle (Figure 14-17). The anterior and middle scalene muscles and the first rib form the interscalene triangle; this is where the brachial plexus enters the thoracic outlet. The subclavian artery passes posteriorly to the anterior scalene, and the subclavian vein passes anteriorly to the anterior scalene. These vessels and the brachial plexus travel together, passing posteriorly and inferiorly to the clavicle and superiorly to the first rib (the costoclavicular space); they continue to pass below the coracoid process and posteriorly to the pectoralis minor muscle (the subcoracoid or subpectoral space).[75-77] Irritation or compression to the brachial plexus and/or vascular structures (the neurovascular bundle) is called **thoracic outlet syndrome (TOS).** This irritation or compression commonly occurs in the interscalene triangle, but it can also occur at the costoclavicular or subcoracoid spaces.[75-77] TOS is a complex condition. There are different types of TOS, but the 3 most common types are neurogenic or true neurogenic thoracic outlet syndrome (NTOS), arterial, and venous.[75,77] NTOS is the most common type and accounts for more than 90% of the cases, whereas arterial TOS is rare but can result in significant morbidity. TOS is 3 to 4 times more common in women and is most common in individuals between 20 and 50 years of age.[75-77] Although TOS commonly has a radiating pain presentation similar to cervical radiculopathy, there are some differences in the distribution of the pain pattern depending on where the compression or irritation occurs and the type of TOS. A physician may order various imaging studies to rule in or out a TOS diagnosis including radiographs, magnetic resonance imaging, electromyography, and/or arteriography/venography to determine the presence of a congenital anomaly, cervical rib, vascular compression location, and/or brachial plexus nerve compression.

Trauma (due to high-velocity impact), repetitive or overuse injury, and anatomic or congenital variations (the presence of a cervical rib) can cause TOS. The signs and symptoms of TOS are listed in Table 14-7. NTOS commonly occurs from neck trauma (eg, whiplash injury), repetitive overuse injury, and postural deficits. Patients commonly report neck, trapezius, and shoulder discomfort and experience paresthesia at night when the arm is positioned in an elevated or overhead position.[7] Venous TOS can occur from an MVA or work-/sport-related overuse activities resulting in subclavian vein compression in the costoclavicular space. It is most common in younger physically active individuals who perform repetitive overhead activities or heavy lifting. Pulmonary embolism is a complication that can occur in 10% to 20% of these patients.[77] Arterial TOS occurs when a cervical rib compresses the subclavian artery, which can result in complications of an arterial embolus or thrombus with arterial damage. The patient may experience claudication due to arterial obstruction and may report pain in the upper extremity at rest that worsens when the arm is elevated overhead. The pain tends to be localized in the upper extremity, not in the cervical region.[75,77]

An accurate physical therapy diagnosis is important. Patient symptoms and clinical findings will guide the physical therapy treatment plan. A number of special tests have been historically used to assess for TOS, but some of these tools may not reliably corroborate the diagnosis. The research is still conflicted as to which tests are most accurate. When used alone, the Adson test and the elevated arm stress test have a specificity of 76% and 30%, respectively, but when the tests are used as a cluster test, the specificity increases to 82%.[75,78] Another study indicated that the Exaggerated Military Brace Test (the Halstead maneuver),

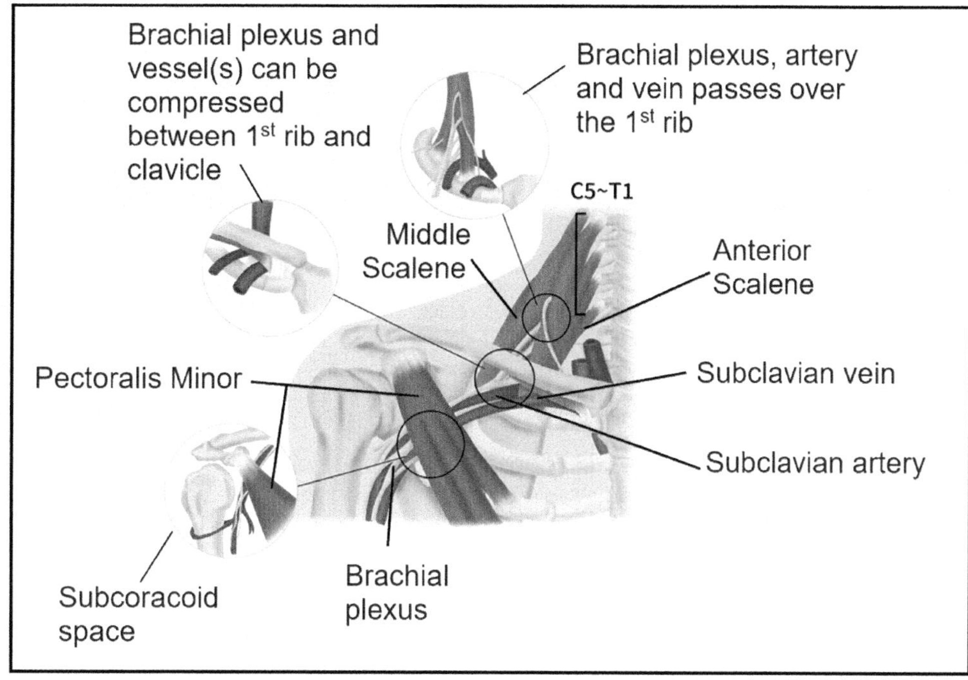


**Figure 14-17.** TOS (Chu KyungMin/Shutterstock.com).

**Table 14-7**

**Thoracic Outlet Syndrome Signs and Symptoms[75-77]**

| Characteristic | Arterial | Venous | Neurogenic |
|---|---|---|---|
| Digital ischemia/ulceration | X | | |
| Claudication | X | | |
| Pallor | X | | |
| Coldness | X | | |
| Pain in the hand | X | | |
| Paresthesia | X | X | X |
| Swelling of the arm | | X | |
| Cyanosis | | X | |
| Distended superficial veins over the chest wall and shoulder | | X | |
| Upper extremity weakness | | | X |
| Neck pain/occipital headaches | | | X |
| Raynaud disease | X | | X |

Wright Test (or hyperabduction test), Cyriax Release Test, and supraclavicular pressure test have good diagnostic accuracy, with these researchers suggesting that the Adson and Roos tests should not be used for the differential diagnosis of TOS.[79] Some therapists use ULTT (for the median nerve) testing to determine if a stretch applied to the brachial plexus will reproduce the patient's symptoms. A physical therapist assistant should monitor the patient for changes associated with each type of TOS (Table 14-8).[75-77]

## Physical Therapy Management for Thoracic Outlet Syndrome

Medical management is indicated for venous and arterial TOS. Physical therapy management for NTOS includes an impairment-based approach. As with cervical radiculopathy and stenosis, physical therapy management of TOS and referred pain originating from TOS compression addresses symptom reduction first and then functional improvement.

**Table 14-8**

Thoracic Outlet Syndrome Additional Findings[75]

| Type | Additional Findings |
|---|---|
| Arterial TOS | • Blood pressure difference between arms > 20 mm Hg |
| Venous TOS | • Upper limb swelling<br>• Cyanosis<br>• Deep pain in the upper limb, chest, and shoulder at rest or with movement |
| Neurogenic TOS | • Interscalene and/or subcoracoid tenderness with palpation<br>• Upper plexus (C5-C7): Sensory disturbance of arm; weakness/atrophy of deltoid, biceps, and brachialis<br>• Lower plexus (C8-T1): Sensory disturbance of the ulnar aspect of the forearm and hand; weakness/atrophy of intrinsic hand muscles, weak wrist and finger flexors, abductor pollicis brevis, hypothenar, and interossei muscles |

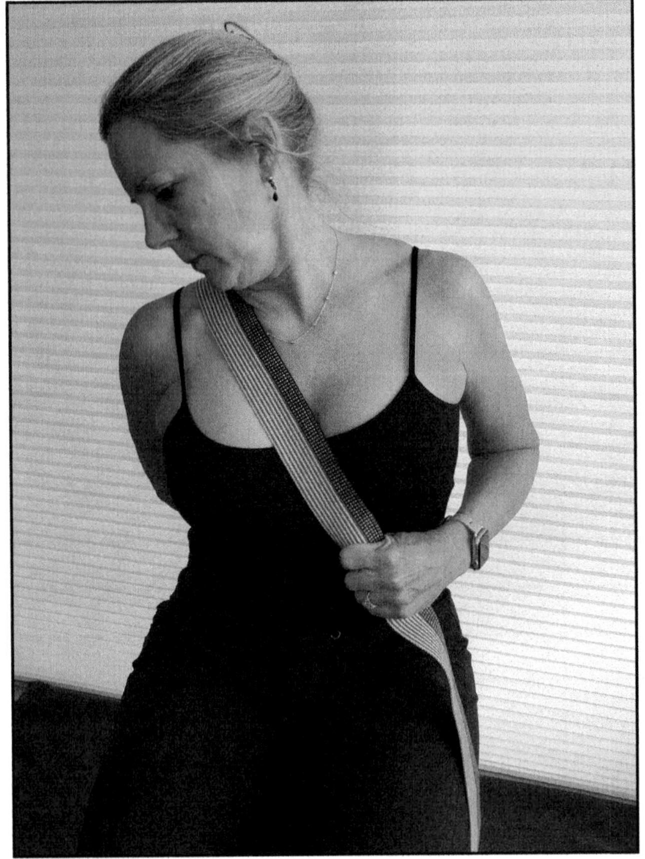

**Figure 14-18.** First rib mobilization. The patient should pull down toward the left thigh and then side bend the head to the right or involved side.

Conservative physical therapy treatment for NTOS has been shown to be effective, and it may include soft tissue and joint mobilization, cervical traction, postural retraining, stretching, strengthening, and patient education for ergonomic/behavioral modifications.[80] There is no consensus on a specific protocol, but a multimodal rehabilitation approach is suggested in the research.[77,80] The physician may also suggest nonsteroidal anti-inflammatory medications.

After controlling the patient's symptoms, the primary treatment goals include restoring normal joint arthrokinematics and nerve mobility (by decreasing nerve compression) and correcting muscle imbalances (stretching/strengthening). The combination of soft tissue mobilization to tight muscles (ie, scalene, upper trapezius, and pectoralis minor muscles), ULTT intervention, and first rib mobilization have been effective in addressing these goals.[77,80]

Mobilizing the first rib will restore mobility and increase the costoclavicular space, which reduces the compressive load on the neurovascular structures. Patients can be instructed to perform this technique. With the patient seated, place a tightly rolled long towel (eg, beach towel, gait belt) over the involved shoulder, close to the base of the neck. The towel/belt should be positioned across the front of the body (similar to the way a seat belt is worn) and secured with the opposite hand (Figure 14-18). The other end of the belt/towel should hang down behind the patient (close to the seat of the chair), and the patient will grasp it with the involved hand (behind the back) to secure it. Alternately, the patient can lean back against the back of the chair to secure that end of the belt/towel using pressure from the torso. Once the patient is correctly positioned, the clinician should provide the following instructions and monitor the patient's response to the exercise:

- Maintain a firm grasp with the hand in the back (to stabilize the towel/belt).
- Pull down and on an angle laterally with the hand in the front of the body until pressure is felt under the belt.
- Laterally side bend the neck toward the involved side (to relax the scalene muscles on that side).

- Instruct the patient to inhale fairly deeply and hold momentarily (about 2 seconds).
- As the patient exhales, instruct them to maintain the tension with the hand in the back and to pull down harder with the hand in the front of the body to create more pressure at the base of the neck. Hold for 20 to 30 seconds.

The exercise should be repeated 3 to 5 times and can be performed throughout the day. This exercise should reduce the patient's symptoms, but the physical therapist assistant should monitor the patient for adverse reactions and ensure the exercise is being performed correctly before allowing the patient to perform it independently at home. The patient should be instructed to discontinue the exercise immediately if the exercise reproduces or worsens their symptoms or creates a headache. Adverse reactions should be reported to the physical therapist.

Stretching the upper trapezius, scalene, and pectoralis minor muscles can help reduce symptoms, increase muscle extensibility, and increase the space where the neurovascular bundle passes through. To stretch the middle scalene muscle, perform the exercise shown in Figure 14-19. To target the anterior scalene muscle, maintain the cervical side-bending stretch but rotate the head up toward the ceiling, and to stretch the posterior scalene rotate the head downward toward the armpit. Upper trapezius and pectoralis muscle stretches are described in Chapter 12. Thoracic spine mobility and postural alignment exercises are also indicated.

## Other Considerations and Interventions for the Thoracic Spine and Rib Cage

Because the thoracic spine and viscera have shared nerve innervations, the pain a patient may experience in the thoracic area may be referred from a regional organ vs a musculoskeletal structure (see Appendix G). The physical therapist screens for nonmusculoskeletal causes of thoracic pain during the evaluation, and the physical therapist assistant continues to monitor symptoms and patient presentations during treatment (Table 14-9). Generally, pain of a visceral origin does not change when testing ROM or strength and does not mirror typical musculoskeletal pain patterns. If the patient's symptoms cannot be reproduced with musculoskeletal testing, the assistant should follow up with the therapist; a medical referral may be indicated.

### Considerations for the Physical Therapist Assistant

If symptoms cannot be reproduced during ROM or strength testing, report findings to the physical therapist before continuing with treatment.

Although the incidence of primary thoracic spine pathology is low, addressing the thoracic spine when treating the shoulder and cervical spine should be considered. The concept of regional interdependence has been studied for interventions (particularly manual therapy) that target the thoracic spine.[41,81] Thoracic mobilization and exercise have been found to be an effective management strategy for those with shoulder pain including diagnoses such as shoulder pain, impingement syndrome, and rotator cuff tendinopathy.[81] Hypomobility of the cervical and thoracic spine may be a primary impairment that contributes to shoulder pain.

Thoracic AROM exercises such as seated thoracic self-extension mobilization (see Figure 14-14), thoracic rotation stretch and self-mobilization (Figure 14-20), and the side-lying thoracic arm sweep (Figure 14-21) are excellent exercises to improve thoracic and rib cage mobility. To effectively perform the thoracic arm sweep, the patient is instructed to make an entire circle with the top arm while attempting to maintain hand contact with the mat surface/floor during the exercise. This exercise is also good for improving or maintaining scapulothoracic and glenohumeral shoulder ROM. If the patient cannot perform the thoracic arm sweep, then side-lying horizontal abduction with trunk rotation exercise (Figure 14-22) or quadruped active thoracic rotation (Figures 14-23 and 14-24) can be used initially until mobility increases. Performing trunk lateral side bending in standing with hands overhead stretches the latissimus dorsi muscle and increases lateral thoracic joint mobility (Figure 14-25).

Exercises that target the thoracic spine will also affect the rib cage because of the anatomical relationship and articulations between the 2 areas. Incorporating breathing techniques such as diaphragmatic breathing exercises (refer to Chapter 18) will affect the pulmonary system as well as improve mobility of the thoracic spine and rib cage. Breathing techniques can also be incorporated during postural exercises to reinforce upright posture and relax the accessory muscles.

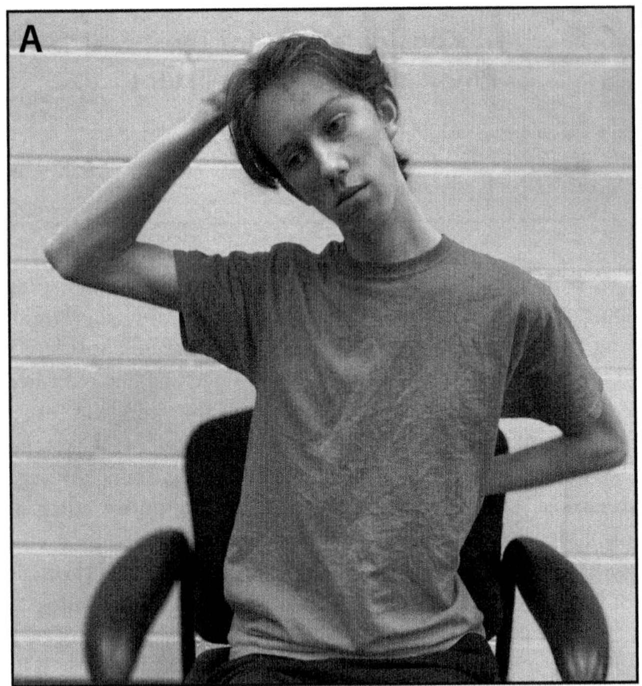

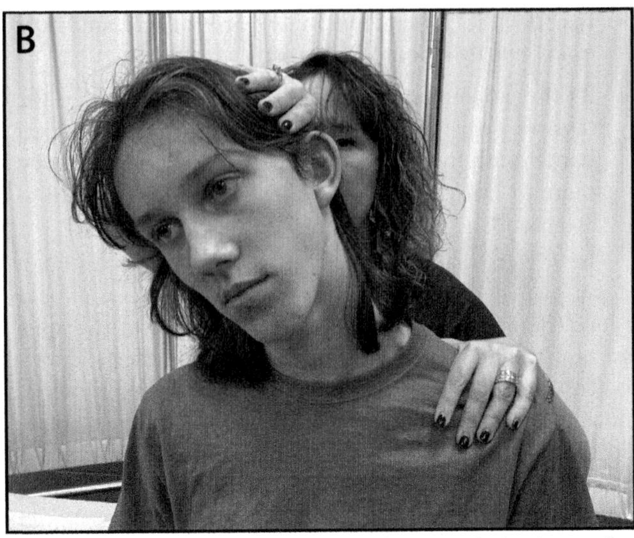

**Figure 14-19.** (A) The middle scalene stretch. Rotate the head upward to stretch the anterior scalene, and rotate the head down toward the armpit to stretch the posterior scalene muscle. (B) Clinician-assisted lateral flexion stretching with overpressure for the middle scalene muscle.

**Table 14-9**

**Referred Pain Patterns or Characteristics and Originating Pain Source**

| Pain Source | Pain Referral Pattern or Characteristics |
|---|---|
| Myocardial infarction | Pain in the anterior chest and upper back and heaviness with or without nausea; cardiac signs/symptoms not relieved with nitroglycerin |
| Peptic ulcer | Pain in the midthoracic spine and increases with food intake |
| Dissecting thoracic aortic aneurysm | Unrelenting chest pain that radiates to the back and has a sudden onset |
| Lung cancer metastasis | Pain to the first rib |
| Compression fracture, risk increases with history of osteoporosis | New/increased thoracic kyphosis with bruising or pain |
| Renal colic | Flank pain with lower abdominal pain that spreads to the labia or testicles |
| Pericarditis | Sharp or stabbing pain that changes with respiration; pain increases with left side lying and decreases with trunk flexion |
| Pneumothorax | Recent trauma with new onset of chest pain associated with respiration |
| Pneumonia | Pleuritic pain, shoulder pain, fever, and productive cough |
| Pulmonary embolus | Dyspnea, tachycardia, and tachypnea in patients with risk factors for deep vein thrombosis |
| Gallbladder | Pain in the right upper quadrant and inferior scapula region |
| Ankylosing spondylitis | Morning stiffness > 30 minutes; decreased pain with exercise but not rest; awakening due to back pain during the second half of the night only, alternating buttock pain, and the presence of HLA-B27 in blood |

HLA-B27 = human leukocyte antigen B27.

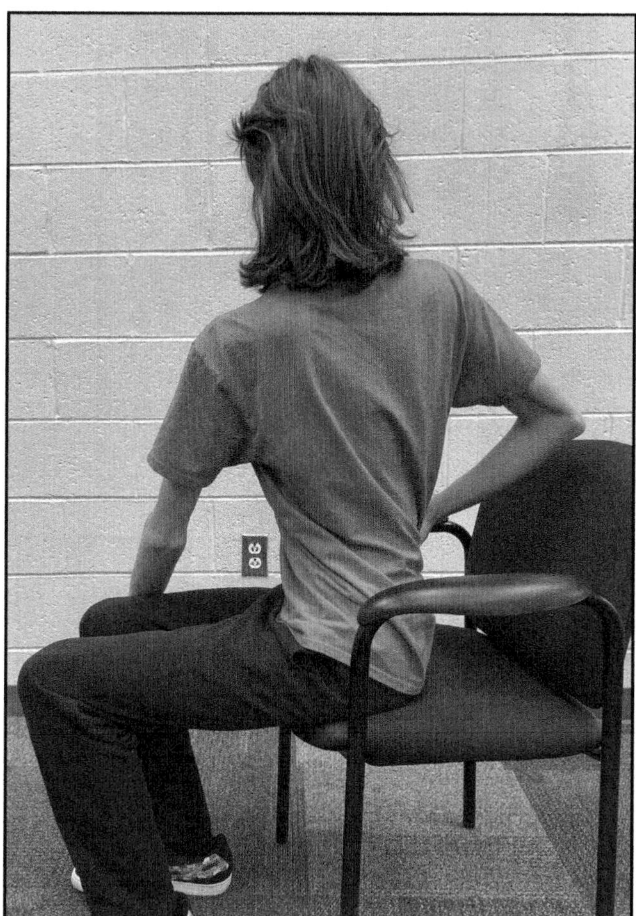

**Figure 14-20.** The thoracic rotation self-stretch and mobilization.

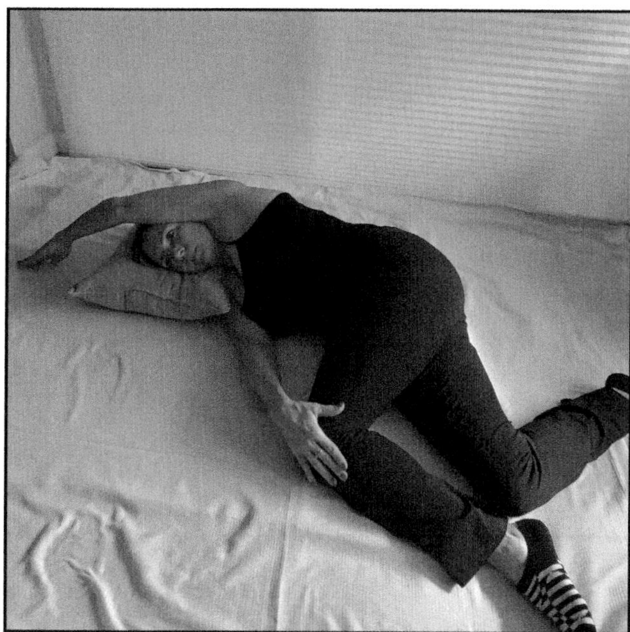

**Figure 14-21.** The thoracic arm sweep for thoracic and rib cage mobility.

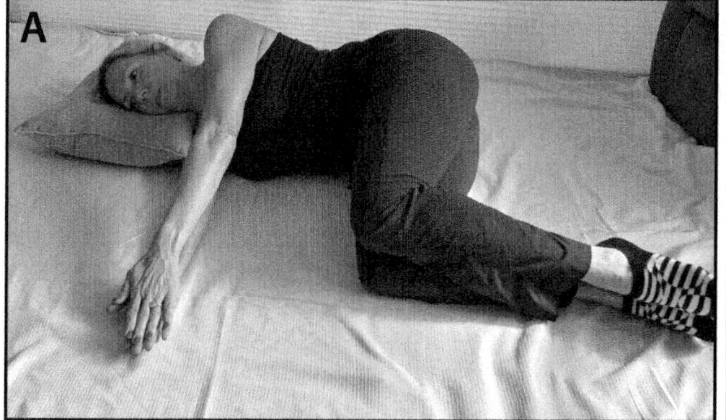


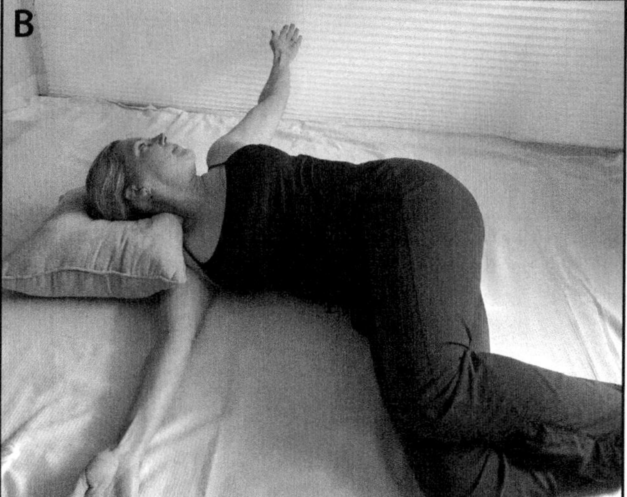


**Figure 14-22.** (A) The starting position for shoulder horizontal abduction with thoracic spine rotation. (B) The end position. Notice the head and trunk rotation.

**Figure 14-23.** The quadruped thoracic rotation stretch.

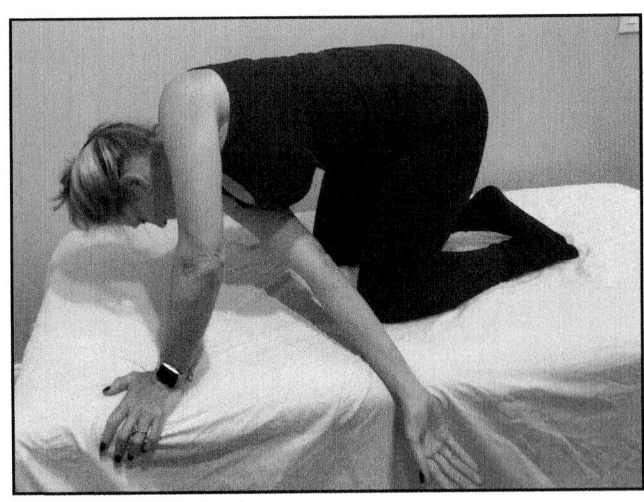

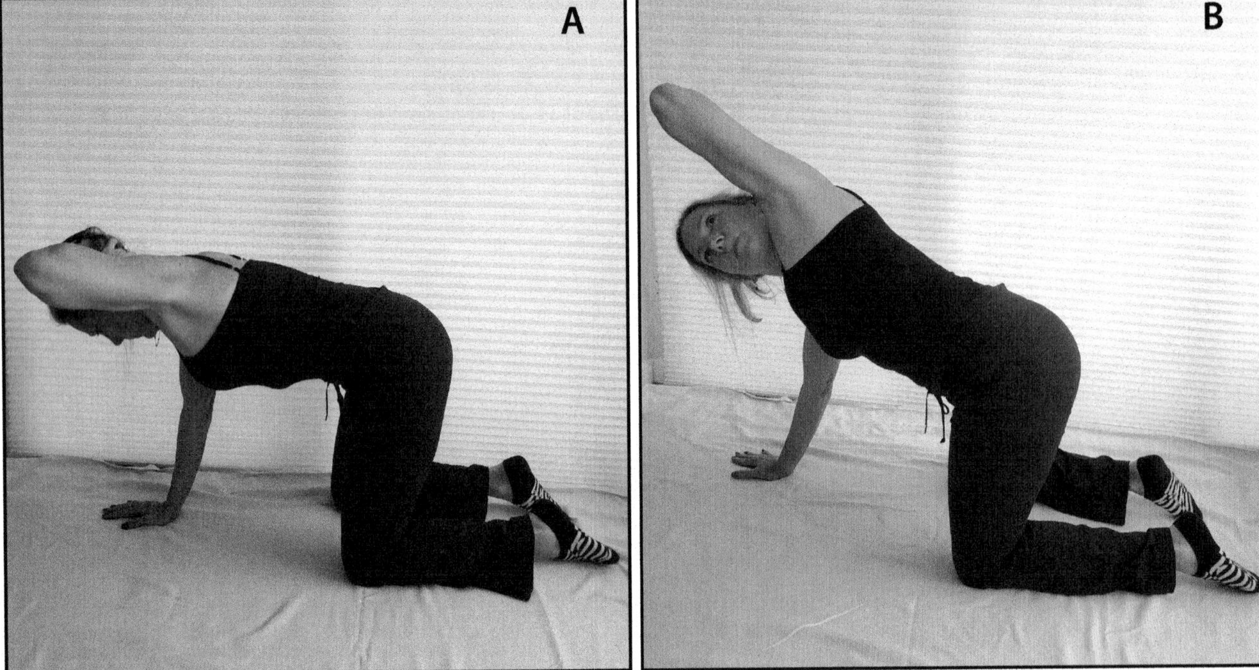

**Figure 14-24.** (A) The quadruped active thoracic spine rotation starting position to increase mobility. (B) The active thoracic spine rotation end position.

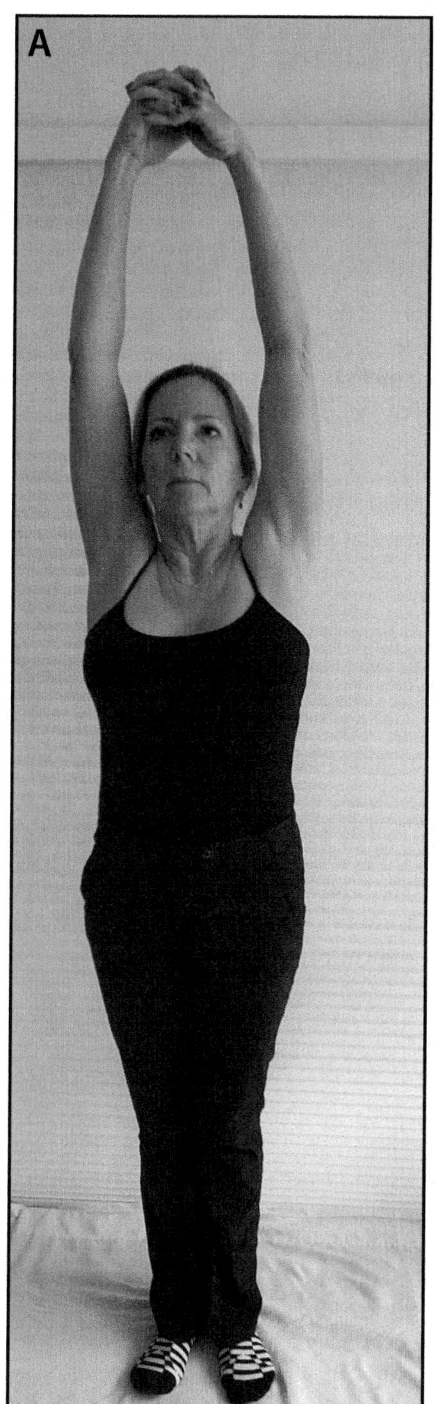


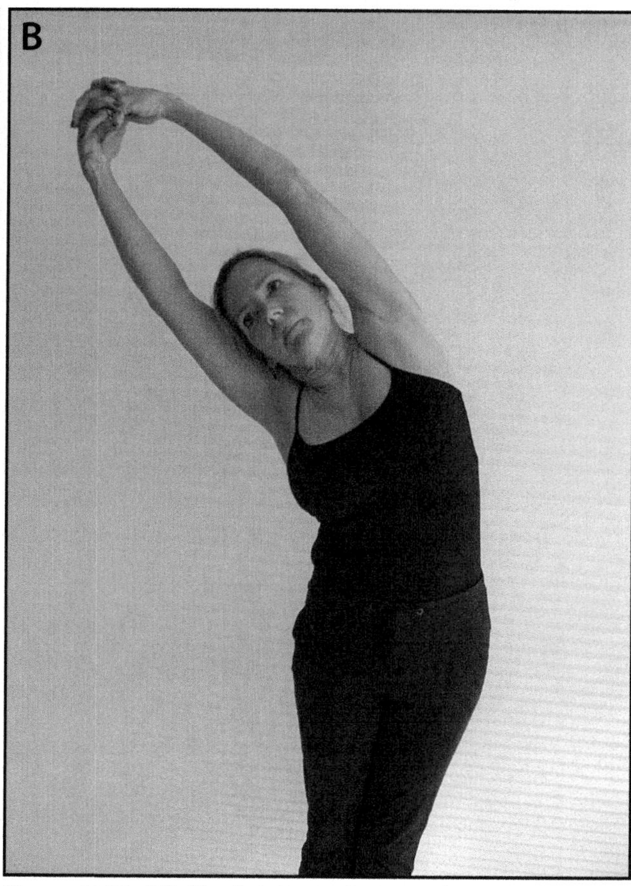


**Figure 14-25.** (A) The latissimus dorsi stretch starting position. (B) Stretching the latissimus dorsi muscle also improves lateral thoracic mobility.

## Temporomandibular Joint Disorders

Temporomandibular pain is more prevalent in women, is commonly seen in young and middle-aged adults, and occurs in 10% to 25% of the US population.[82,83] Temporomandibular joint disorders (TMJD or TMD) involve the TMJ and masticatory (chewing) muscles. TMD is considered a chronic repetitive motion condition that causes pain that is usually increased with chewing and/or speaking; it is also associated with a history of chronic stress or trauma. TMJ pain, clicking noises, and/or locking can result in a patient self-limiting their mouth opening motion due to apprehension and the occurrence of these symptoms. An abnormal hypertrophy of masticatory muscles can occur resulting in poor jaw motion mechanics.[82-84] Research indicates that there is an association between TMJ and cervical spine disability with changes in DNF strength and bite position in patients with TMD.[82]

The following are ways to prevent and reduce TMD[84]:

- Avoid biting into and chewing hard or chewy items, such as apples, gummies, taffy, and chewing gum.
- Eat soft foods.
- Avoid clenching or grinding (bruxing) the teeth.

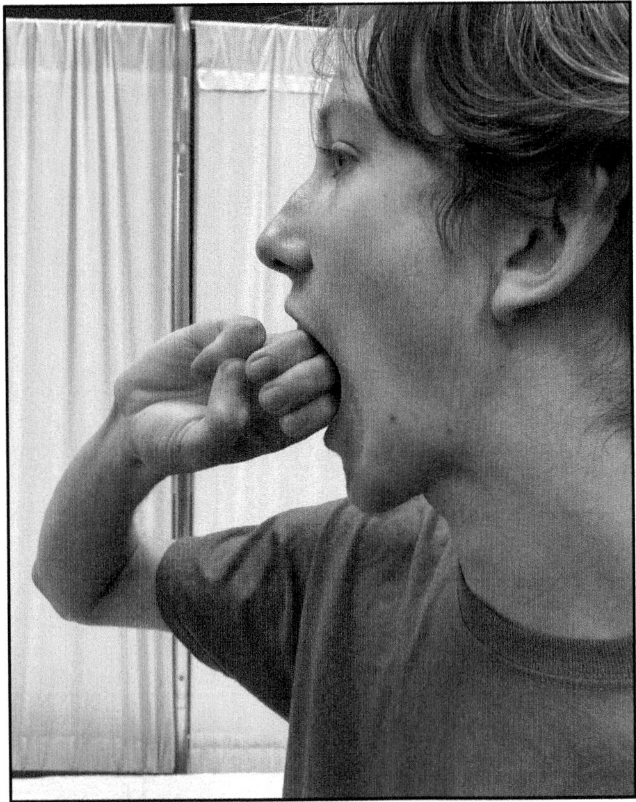

**Figure 14-26.** The knuckle test to determine if the patient can functionally open the mouth.

- Do not chew the tongue or on the cheek inside of the mouth.
- Chew on both sides of the mouth.
- Avoid yawning with a wide-opened mouth.

## *Assessing the Temporomandibular Joint Disorders*

The initial evaluation of TMJD begins with observation of the patient's posture, breathing pattern, and speech. Forward head posture causes a posterior rotation of the cranium on the cervical spine and alters the resting position of the TMJ. The therapist needs to inquire about the patient's oral parafunctional habits such as nail biting, cheek/tongue biting, thumb sucking, and/or teeth grinding or clenching. The presence of these habits cues the therapist to the potential of overuse microtrauma of the TMJ as a potential source of pain and dysfunction.[84]

Motion of the TMJ (mandible depression and lateral excursion) can be measured using a ruler or disposable paper measuring tool. Reduced ROM can indicate muscular tightness, joint hypomobility, capsular tightness, or self-limited movement due to pain or anticipation of pain. To determine a patient's ability to functionally open the mouth, the knuckle test (using 2 or 3 fingers) can be performed (Figure 14-26). TheraBite (Atos Medical) ROM tools can be used to obtain objective, repeatable measurements. If the patient cannot perform this test, the TMJ is hypomobile.[85]

Normally, the jaw moves in a straight line during opening and closing, so the therapist should observe the movement pattern of a patient's mandible for deviations such as a "C" curve or an "S" curve. A C curve is an abnormal movement pattern that occurs during mandibular depression (opening the mouth) in which the mandible deviates to one side during midopening and returns to the center at the end of the movement. This pattern is a common indicator of a capsular restriction. An S curve occurs when the mandible deviates in the shape of an S during mouth opening. In the absence of pain during movement, this typically is indicative of a muscular imbalance or coordination deficit. If pain is present, this deviation may indicate disk or joint capsule involvement. Patients with ipsilateral disk involvement may exhibit mandibular deflection, which occurs when the mandible deviates to one side during opening and does not return to the center when fully open.[85]

Palpation of the joint with the fingers placed in the external auditory meatus allows the clinician to feel for joint crepitus and deviation. Palpation of the muscles of mastication is performed both intra- and extraorally. Intraoral palpation is required for the medial and lateral pterygoid. Extraoral palpation of the masseter, temporalis, and suprahyoid can be performed to assess for the presence of pain or tightness.

## *Conservative Management of Temporomandibular Joint Disorders*

Treatment principles for other joints can be applied when treating TMJDs. Physical therapy goals usually include decreasing pain, increasing muscle relaxation by reducing muscle hyperactivity, and restoring normal joint mobility and function.[86] Joint mobilization techniques are only performed by experienced TMJ physical therapists. Soft tissue mobilization for painful or tight masticatory and cervical musculature is indicated for patients experiencing pain and muscular impairments. Exercise, joint conservation, and resting the muscles are interventions used to treat a painful TMJD (Figures 14-27 through 14-29). Joint conservation is achieved through diet modification (ie, soft diet) and education to avoid parafunctional habits. Patients should be instructed on maintaining the proper TMJ resting positioning. This is achieved by keeping the tip of the tongue on the palate with the teeth slightly apart and the lips together. Some patients may benefit from using a mouth guard/appliance, which is typically provided by a dentist.

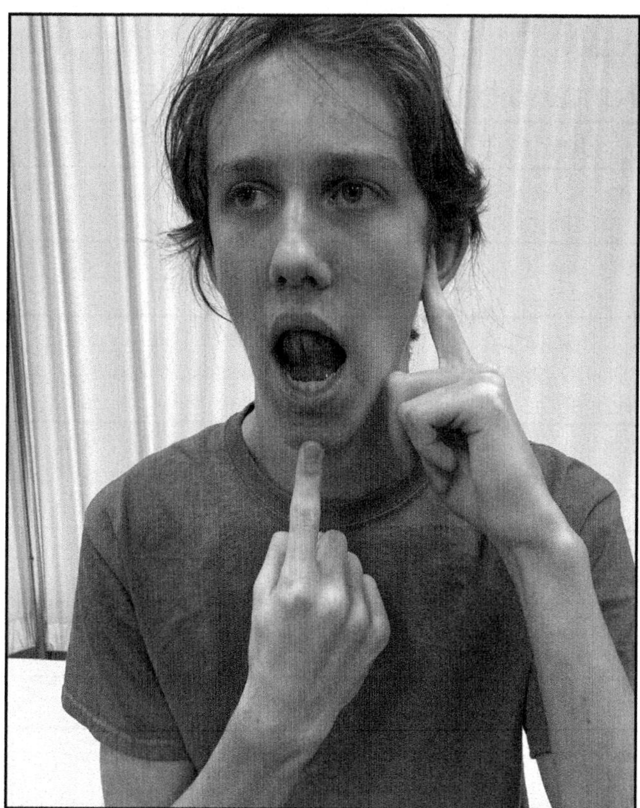

**Figure 14-27.** Controlled opening. Place one finger on the TMJ joint and the other on the chin to maintain a straight opening and closing.

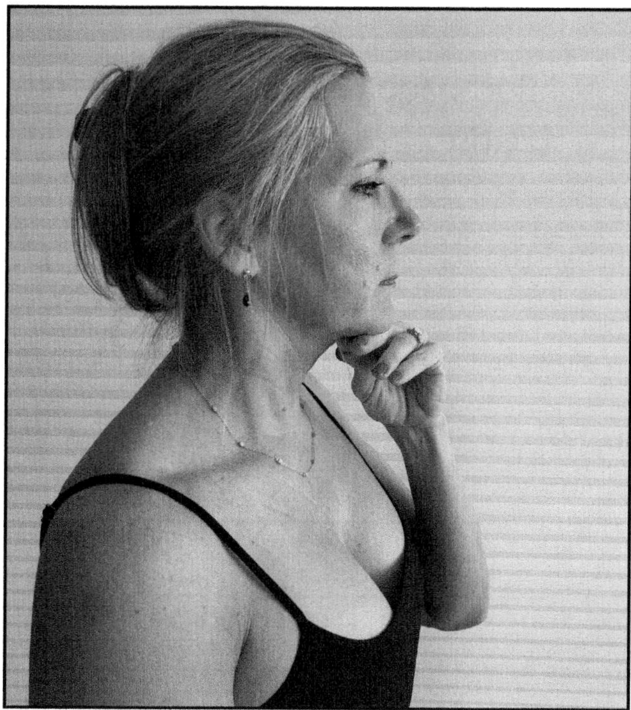

**Figure 14-28.** An isometric mandibular depression exercise while maintaining a normal resting jaw position.

Mariano Rocabado, PT, DPT, contributed to TMJD evaluation and treatment through the development of an exercise program called the **Rocabado 6×6** (Table 14-10). The Rocabado 6×6 includes 6 exercises performed for 6 repetitions 6 times per day.[87,88] To increase AROM and neuromuscular control, some physical therapists use a stack of several tongue depressors (bound together with rubber bands) and place them in the patient's mouth between the teeth to gradually increase pain-free motion during opening. This technique can also be used to improve lateral excursion. TMJ exercise progression is described in Table 14-11.

Research indicates that manual therapy in conjunction with exercise has the best results in reducing pain and improving TMJ motion. Patients with TMD may present with limited cervical ROM and strength deficits, and exercises that address cervical spine postural deviations (ie, forward head) and TMD should be included in the patient's rehabilitation program.[82,83,86,89] Patient education should include techniques to promote muscle relaxation of tight over-recruited masticatory muscles, tips to reduce TMJ stress, and the importance of mouth guard/appliance compliance if prescribed.[84,89]

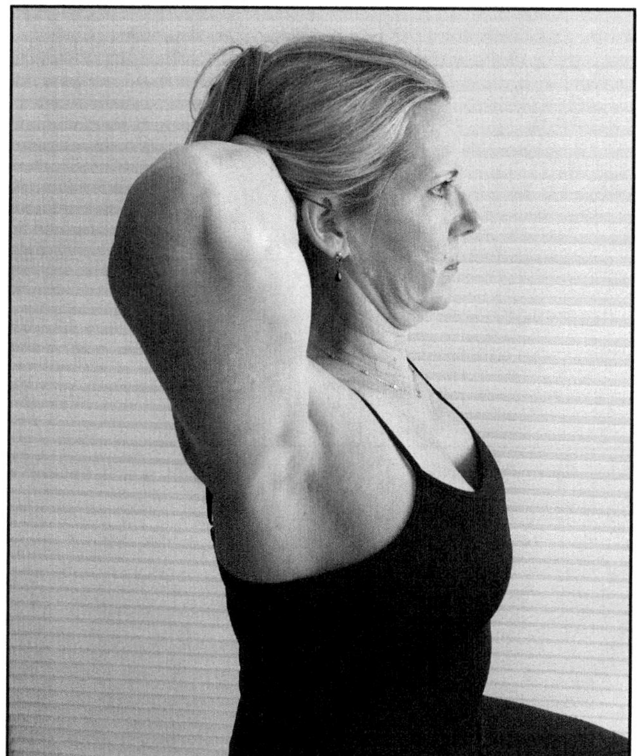

**Figure 14-29.** Upper cervical distraction.

**Table 14-10**

**Rocabado 6x6 Exercises for Temporomandibular Joint Disorders[87-89]**

| Exercise | Description |
|---|---|
| Tongue clucking | Position the tongue against the hard palate with the mouth in the proper resting position for the TMJ. Then, make a clucking sound with the tongue. |
| Controlled TMJ opening | Position the tip of the tongue on the palate while opening and closing the jaw (see Figure 14-27), maintaining a straight path. |
| Mandibular rhythmic stabilization | The patient applies gentle isometric resistance to the mandible while in the normal TMJ resting position and while opening (see Figure 14-28). This exercise can be repeated with closing and lateral deviation. |
| Upper cervical distraction | The patient performs upper cervical flexion and stabilizes the lower spine with their hands clasped behind the neck. The cervical flexion distracts the occiput from the atlas (see Figure 14-29). |
| Axial extension of the cervical spine | Cervical retraction is performed by flexing the upper cervical spine and extending the lower cervical spine as shown in Figure 14-6. |
| Scapula retraction | Retracting and depressing the scapulae (back and down) while maintaining good head position improves posture. |

**Table 14-11**

**Temporomandibular Joint Range of Motion and Neuromuscular Re-Education Exercise Progression**

| | |
|---|---|
| Tongue depressor opening | • Patient performs maximal pain-free mouth opening.<br>• A stack of tongue depressors bound together with rubber bands is placed between the maxillary and mandibular teeth.<br>• Maintain this position for 30 seconds.<br>• Add tongue depressors as AROM improves. |
| Tongue depressor lateral excursion | • A stack of tongue depressors is placed between the maxillary and mandibular teeth.<br>• Patient translates the stack side to side.<br>• The number of tongue depressors varies based on the amount of available opening. |
| Condylar remodeling | • Place a piece of surgical tubing between the maxillary and mandibular center incisors.<br>• Perform lateral deviation while maintaining the surgical tubing between the teeth.<br>• If movement is pain free, bite down on the tubing in the deviated position and release the contraction before returning to neutral.<br>• Progression: Maintain biting contraction when deviated and return back to neutral. |

## Conclusion

There is a close relationship between the TMJ and the cervical and thoracic spines, so when patients present with pain or dysfunction in any of these regions, interventions should target all areas identified in physical therapist evaluation. Vascular and neurologic structures in these regions may be compromised, and physical therapist assistants should monitor for a change in symptoms and red flag items throughout treatment. Patients reporting neck pain, TMD, and/or thoracic pain can benefit from physical therapy treatments that are applied within a treatment-based classification system. A review of the initial evaluation and continual assessment of patient presentation will guide the assistant's selection of the most appropriate exercises for the patient in real time. Patient education for proper posture and positioning with static and dynamic activities will also improve patient outcomes.

## Review Questions

1. Describe the typical presentation of a person in a neck pain with mobility deficits category. What are the common clinical findings? List the appropriate treatment interventions for a patient with this treatment classification.
2. Which special tests are likely positive for a patient who has neck pain with radiating symptoms? What medical/pathoanatomical diagnoses often present with radiating symptoms? List the appropriate treatment interventions that may be included for a patient with this treatment classification.
3. Describe the clinical significance of the following special tests: the alar ligament test, Sharp-Purser test, transverse ligament test, Babinski sign, and Hoffmann sign.
4. List at least 5 potential red flags that the assistant should be aware of when treating a patient with neck pain.
5. What are the 5Ds and 3Ns? What is the clinical significance of these signs/symptoms?
6. Compare and contrast the role of the superficial and DNF muscles. What exercises increase strength and muscle endurance for these muscles?
7. Describe the potential impact forward head posture has on the TMJ and the cervical and thoracic structures.
8. List 3 exercises that can address thoracic spine hypomobility.
9. Compare and contrast the 3 types of TOS. List 3 interventions used to treat NTOS.
10. Describe 3 interventions that can be included for a patient who presents with TMJ pain due to muscle tightness.

## Case Study 1

Maria is a 45-year-old woman who was involved in an MVA 1 week ago. Maria (the driver) reported being stopped at a red light when her car was rear-ended at a slow speed. She was wearing a seat belt at the time of the accident and denies loss of consciousness but reported minor stiffness that was alleviated with over-the-counter nonsteroidal anti-inflammatory drugs. The next morning she reported posterior neck pain, stiffness, and ROM limitations. She denies numbness, tingling, or upper extremity symptoms but reports increased pain with sitting, driving, and texting. Pain is alleviated with lying down. After seeing her primary care physician, Maria was referred to physical therapy with a diagnosis of "neck pain." No diagnostic testing was performed, and she works full time as a high school teacher.

1. List any red flags that are in the history or patient presentation or state if none are present.

The following objective measures were found on evaluation:

- Vital signs: Stable
- Pain: 6/10
- NDI: 60%
- Posture: Forward head and rounded shoulders
- Negative Sharp-Purser, alar ligament test, transverse ligament test, and Hoffman Sign
- Active ROM: Cervical flexion and extension 35 degrees and painful to central cervical spine
- Cervical rotation: 60 degrees right and 80 degrees left
- Cervical side bend: 25 degrees right and 45 degrees left
- Flexibility testing: Reduced pectoralis major and minor, right SCM
- Bilateral upper extremity strength testing 5/5 throughout the shoulder, elbow, wrist, and hand

2. Based on the findings and patient presentation, which *ICF* classification is most representative of this patient?
3. Outline a treatment intervention for this patient.

Three weeks later, Maria reports a new onset of right-sided headaches with prolonged computer use. Her clinical examination findings pretreatment include the following:

- Vital signs: Stable
- Pain: 4/10
- NDI: 28%
- Active cervical rotation: 60 degrees right and 80 degrees left
- Negative cranial nerve assessment and cervical instability test
- Positive craniocervical flexion test

- DNF endurance testing: 14 seconds
- Positive craniocervical rotation test: Right 28 degrees and left 44 degrees

4. What should the assistant do next? Why?
5. Which *ICF* classification now appears to best coincide with the patient's presentation?
6. Outline a treatment plan based on the current findings.

## Case Study 2

Michael is a 50-year-old man with a 4-month history of central neck pain and left scapula and upper arm pain that began during accounting season. Michael is an accountant and reports that during that time he worked 16-hour days 6 days a week on the computer. Pain is relieved temporarily with moving his neck or sitting upright. He denies any type of trauma or a prior history of neck pain. Pain has gradually worsened over time and limits his ability to sleep or use the computer for longer than 1 hour. Michael saw an orthopedist who ordered magnetic resonance imaging, which revealed degenerative disk disease and a small disk herniation at C6-7. The patient was referred to physical therapy with a diagnosis of "chronic neck pain." Michael is an avid cyclist and is unable to cycle currently because of neck pain. He continues working full time as an accountant but is considering obtaining a standing desk due to pain with prolonged computer use. The physical therapy examination indicated the following:

- Vital signs: Stable
- Pain: 5/10
- NDI: 46%
- Posture: Forward head, rounded shoulder, and increased thoracic spine kyphosis
- Upper cervical instability screening tests: Negative
- AROM cervical spine: Within functional limits, except for cervical extension, which is 35 degrees and painful
- AROM thoracic spine: Thoracic extension limited to 25%
- Thoracic flexion and rotation within functional limits
- Negative cervical radiculopathy cluster
- Positive craniocervical flexion test
- DNF endurance: 8 seconds
- Positive joint position error testing: A 25-cm margin of error
- Manual muscle testing
    - Shoulder flexion, extension, and internal rotation: 5/5 bilateral
    - Shoulder external rotation: 4/5 right 3+/5 left
    - Middle and lower trapezius: 3/5 bilateral
- Flexibility testing: Reduced flexibility of the pectoralis major and minor and suboccipital muscles
- Joint mobility: Hypomobile upper and midthoracic spine with posterior to anterior forces

1. Based on these findings and the patient presentation, what *ICF* classification is most consistent with the patient presentation?
2. Create a treatment intervention for this patient

## References


1. Wainner RS, Whitman JM, Cleland JA, Flynn TW. Regional interdependence: a musculoskeletal examination model whose time has come. *J Orthop Sports Phys Ther.* 2007;37(11):658-660. doi:10.2519/jospt.2007.0110
2. Sueki DG, Cleland JA, Wainner RS. A regional interdependence model of musculoskeletal dysfunction: research, mechanisms, and clinical implications. *J Man Manip Ther.* 2013;21(2):90-102. doi:10.1179/2042618612Y.0000000027
3. Miller MB. The cervical spine: physical therapy patient management utilizing current evidence. In: Wilmarth MA, ed. *ISC 21.2.6, Current Concepts of Orthopaedic Physical Therapy.* 3rd ed. Orthopaedic Section, APTA; 2011.
4. Miller MB. The cervical spine: the physical therapy patient management utilizing current evidence. In: Hughs C, ed. *ISC 21.2.6, Current Concepts of Orthopaedic Physical Therapy.* 4th ed. Orthopaedic Section, APTA; 2016.
5. Cleland JA, Childs JD, McRae M, Palmer JA, Stowell T. Immediate effects of thoracic manipulation in patients with neck pain: a randomized clinical trial. *Man Ther.* 2005;10(2):127-135.
6. Côté P, van der Velde G, Cassidy JD, et al. The burden and determinants of neck pain in workers: results of the bone and joint decade 2000–2010 task force on neck pain and its associated disorders. *Spine.* 2008;33(suppl):S60-S74. doi:10.1097/BRS.0b013e3181643ee4
7. Fejer R, Kyvik KO, Hartvigsen J. The prevalence of neck pain in the world population: a systematic critical review of the literature. *Eur Spine J.* 2006;15(6):834-848. doi:10.1007/s00586-004-0864-4
8. Croft PR, Lewis M, Papageorgiou AC, et al. Risk factors for neck pain: a longitudinal study in the general population. *Pain.* 2001;93(3):317-325. doi:10.1016/s0304-3959(01)00334-7
9. Rajala U, Keinänen-Kiukaanniemi S, Uusimäki A, Kivelä SL. Musculoskeletal pains and depression in a middle-aged Finnish population. *Pain.* 1995;61(3):451-457. doi:10.1016/0304-3959(94)00206-t
10. Hogg-Johnson S, van der Velde G, Carroll LJ, et al. The burden and determinants of neck pain in the general population: results of the Bone and Joint Decade 2000–2010 Task Force on Neck Pain and Its Associated Disorders. *Eur Spine J.* 2008;17(suppl 1):39-51. doi:10.1007/s00586-008-0624-y
11. Fernández-de-las-Peñas C, Hernández-Barrera V, Alonso-Blanco C, et al. Prevalence of neck and low back pain in community-dwelling adults in Spain: a population-based national study. *Spine.* 2011;36(3):E213-E219. doi:10.1097/BRS.0b013e3181d952c2
12. Jull G, Sterling M, Falla D, Treleaven J, O'Leary S. Whiplash-associated disorders. In: Jull G, Sterling M, Falla D, Treleaven J, O'Leary S, eds. *Whiplash, Headache, and Neck Pain: Research-Based Directions for Physical Therapies.* Churchill Livingston Elsevier Health Sciences; 2008:101-115.

13. Côté P, Cassidy JD, Carroll L, Kristman V. The annual incidence and course of neck pain in the general population: a population-based cohort study. *Pain.* 2004;112(3):267-273.
14. Martin BI, Deyo RA, Mirza SK, et al. Expenditures and health status among adults with back and neck problems. *JAMA.* 2008;299(6):656-664. doi:10.1001/jama.299.6.656
15. Horn ME, Brennan GP, George SZ, Harman JS, Bishop MD. Clinical outcomes, utilization, and charges in persons with neck pain receiving guideline adherent physical therapy. *Eval Health Prof.* 2016;39(4):421-434. doi:10.1177/0163278715583510
16. Childs JD, Cleland JA, Elliott JM, et al. Neck pain: Clinical practice guidelines linked to the International Classification of Functioning, Disability, and Health from the Orthopedic Section of the American Physical Therapy Association [published correction appears in J Orthop Sports Phys Ther. 2009;39(4):297]. *J Orthop Sports Phys Ther.* 2008;38(9):A1-A34. doi:10.2519/jospt.2008.0303
17. Fritz JM, Brennan JP. Preliminary examination of a proposed treatment-based classification system for patients receiving physical therapy interventions for neck pain. *Phys Ther.* 2007;87(5):513-524. doi:10.2522/ptj.20060192
18. Bergman GJ, Winters JC, Groenier KH, et al. Manipulative therapy in addition to usual medical care for patients with shoulder dysfunction and pain: a randomized, controlled trial. *Ann Intern Med.* 2004;141(6):432-439. doi:10.7326/0003-4819-141-6-200409210-00008
19. Boyles RE, Ritland BM, Miracle BM, et al. The short-term effects of thoracic spine thrust manipulation on patients with shoulder impingement syndrome. *Man Ther.* 2009;14:375-380. doi:10.1016/j.math.2008.05.005
20. APTA Specialty Council on Orthopedic Physical Therapy. *Orthopaedic Physical Therapy Description of Specialty Practice.* 2014:17. Accessed February 3, 2023. http://aptaapps.apta.org/SpecialistCertification/Files/KIT-ORTHO.pdf
21. Silveira A, Gadotti IC, Armijo-Olivo S, Biasotto-Gonzalez DA, Magee D. Jaw dysfunction is associated with neck disability and muscle tenderness in subjects with and without chronic temporomandibular disorders. *Biomed Res Int.* 2015;2015:512792. doi:10.1155/2015/512792.
22. Drake RL, Vogl AW, Mitchell AWM. *Gray's Anatomy for Students.* 2nd ed. Churchill Livingston/Elsevier Health Sciences; 2009.
23. Rushton A, Rivett D, Carlesso L, Flynn T, Hing W, Kerry R. International framework for examination of the cervical region for potential of cervical arterial dysfunction prior to orthopaedic manual therapy intervention. *Man Ther.* 2014;19(3):222-228. doi:10.1016/j.math.2013.11.005
24. Lippert L. Neck and trunk. In: Lippert L, ed. *Clinical Kinesiology and Anatomy.* 6th ed. FA Davis Company; 2017:239-262.
25. Blomgren J, Strandell E, Jull G, Vikman I, Röijezon U. Effects of deep cervical flexor training on impaired physiological functions associated with chronic neck pain: a systematic review. *BMC Musculoskelet Disord.* 2018;19(1):415. doi:10.1186/s12891-018-2324-z
26. Suvarnnato T, Puntumetakul R, Uthaikhup S, Boucaut R. Effect of specific deep cervical muscle exercises on functional disability, pain intensity, craniovertebral angle, and neck-muscle strength in chronic mechanical neck pain: a randomized controlled trial. *J Pain Res.* 2019;12:915-925. doi:10.2147/JPR.S190125
27. Kim JY, Kwag KI. Clinical effects of deep cervical flexor muscle activation in patients with chronic neck pain. *J Phys Ther Sci.* 2016;28(1):269-273. doi:10.1589/jpts.28.269
28. Lippert L. *Clinical Kinesiology and Anatomy.* 6th ed. FA Davis Company; 2017:267-269.
29. Dutton M. The thoracic spine. In: Dutton M, ed. *Dutton's Orthopaedic Examination, Evaluation and Intervention.* 3rd ed. McGraw-Hill Companies; 2012:1229-1243.
30. Geelhoed MA, McGaugh J, Brewer PA, Murphy D. A new model to facilitate palpation of the level of the transverse processes of the thoracic spine. *J Orthop Sports Phys Ther.* 2006;36(11):876-881. doi:10.2519/jospt.2006.2243
31. Oakley CK, Janssen SAK, Pankratz JP, McCumber TL, Treffer KD, Olinger AB. Validity of the rule of threes and anatomical relationships in the thoracic spine. *J Am Osteopath Assoc.* 2018;118(10):645-653. doi:10.7556/jaoa.2018.143
32. Stiell IG, Clement CM, McKnight RD, et al. The Canadian C-spine rule versus the NEXUS low-risk criteria in patients with trauma. *N Engl J Med.* 2003;349(26):2510-2518.
33. Bennell KL, Matthews B, Greig A, et al. Effects of an exercise and manual therapy program on physical impairments, function and quality-of-life in people with osteoporotic vertebral fracture: a randomised, single-blind controlled pilot trial. *BMC Musculoskelet Disord.* 2010;11:36. doi:10.1186/1471-2474-11-36
34. Cook C, Brown C, Isaacs R, Roman M, Davis S, Richardson W. Clustered clinical findings for diagnosis of cervical spine myelopathy. *J Man Manip Ther.* 2010;18(4):175-180. doi:10.1179/106698110X12804993427045
35. Henschke N, Maher CG, Refshauge KM. Screening for malignancy in low back pain patients: a systematic review. *Eur Spine J.* 2007;16(10):1673-1679.
36. Blanfied PR, Gross AR, Elliott JM, et al. Neck pain revision 2017: clinical practice guidelines linked to the International Classification of Functioning, Disability, and Health from the Orthopedic Section of the American Physical Therapy Association. *J Orthop Sports Phys Ther.* 2017;47(7):A1-A83. doi:10.2519/jospt.2017.0302
37. Childs JD, Fritz JM, Piva SR, Whitman JM. Proposal of a classification system for patients with neck pain. *J Orthop Sports Phys Ther.* 2004;34(11):686-700. doi:10.2519/jospt.2004.34.11.686
38. Macdermid JC, Walton DM, Avery S, et al. Measurement properties of the neck disability index a systematic review. *J Orthop Sports Phys Ther.* 2009;39(5):400-417.
39. Swartz EE, Floyd RT, Cendoma M. Cervical spine functional anatomy and the biomechanics of injury due to compressive loading. *J Athl Train.* 2005;40(3):155-161.
40. Maitland FW. *The Constitutional History of England: A Course of Lectures Delivered.* The Lawbook Exchange, Ltd; 2001.
41. McDevitt A, Young J, Mintken P, Cleland J. Regional interdependence and manual therapy directed at the thoracic spine. *J Man Manip Ther.* 2015;23(3):139-146. doi:10.1179/2042618615Y.0000000005
42. Masaracchio M, Cleland JA, Hellman M, Hagins M. Short-term combined effects of thoracic spine thrust manipulation and cervical spine nonthrust manipulation in individuals with mechanical neck pain: a randomized clinical trial. *J Orthop Sports Phys Ther.* 2013;43(3):118-127.

43. Gross AR, Hoving JL, Haines TA, et al. A Cochrane review of manipulation and mobilization for mechanical neck disorders. *Spine (Phila Pa 1976).* 2004;29(14):1541-1548. doi:10.1097/01.brs.0000131218.35875.ed
44. Carlesso LC, Miller J, D'Sylva J, et al. Adverse events associated with the use of cervical manipulation and mobilization for the treatment of neck pain in adults: a systematic review. *Man Ther.* 2010;15(5):434-444.
45. Schroeder J, Kaplan L, Fischer DJ, Skelly AC. The outcomes of manipulation or mobilization therapy compared with physical therapy or exercise for neck pain: a systematic review. *Evid Based Spine Care J.* 2013;4(1):30-41. doi:10.1055/s-0033-1341605
46. Durall CJ. Therapeutic exercise for athletes with nonspecific neck pain: a current concepts review. *Sports Health.* 2012;4(4):293-301. doi:10.1177/1941738112446138
47. Page P. Cervicogenic headaches: an evidence-led approach to clinical management. *Int J Sports Phys Ther.* 2011;6(3):254-266.
48. Sjaastad O, Fredriksen TA, Pfaffenrath V. Cervicogenic headache: diagnostic criteria. The Cervicogenic Headache International Study Group. *Headache.* 1998;38(6):442-445.
49. Jull G, Amiri M, Bullock-Saxton J, Darnell R, Lander C. Cervical musculoskeletal impairment in frequent intermittent headache. Part 1: subjects with single headaches. *Cephalalgia.* 2007;27(7):793-802.
50. Amiri M, Jull G, Bullock-Saxton J, Darnell R, Lander C. Cervical musculoskeletal impairment in frequent intermittent headache. Part 2: subjects with concurrent headache types. *Cephalalgia.* 2007;27(8):891-898.
51. Hall T, Briffa K, Hopper D. Clinical evaluation of cervicogenic headache: a clinical perspective. *J Man Manip Ther.* 2008;16(2):73-80.
52. Ogince M, Hall T, Robinson K, Blackmore AM. The diagnostic validity of the cervical flexion–rotation test in C1/2-related cervicogenic headache. *Man Ther.* 2007;12(3):256-262.
53. Hall TM, Robinson KW, Fujinawa O, Akasaka K, Pyne EA. Intertester reliability and diagnostic validity of the cervical flexion-rotation test. *J Manipulative Physiol Ther.* 2008;31(4):293-300. doi:10.1016/j.jmpt.2008.03.012
54. Harris KD, Heer DM, Roy TC, et al. Reliability of a measurement of neck flexor muscle endurance. *Phys Ther.* 2005;85(12):1349-1355.
55. Domenech MA, Sizer PS, Dedrick GS, McGalliard MK, Brismee JM. The deep neck flexor endurance test: normative data scores in healthy adults. *PM R.* 2011;3(2):105-110.
56. Walton DM, Macdermid JC, Giorgianni AA, Mascarenhas JC, West SC, Zammit CA. Risk factors for persistent problems following acute whiplash injury: update of a systematic review and meta-analysis. *J Orthop Sports Phys Ther.* 2013;43(2):31-43. doi:10.2519/jospt.2013.4507
57. Elliott JM, Noteboom JT, Flynn TW, Sterling M. Characterization of acute and chronic whiplash-associated disorders. *J Orthop Sports Phys Ther.* 2009;39(5):312-323.
58. Treleaven J, Jull G, Sterling M. Dizziness and unsteadiness following whiplash injury: characteristic features and relationship with cervical joint position error. *J Rehabil Med.* 2003;35(1):36-43.
59. Jull G, Falla D, Treleaven J, Hodges P, Vicenzino B. Retraining cervical joint position sense: the effect of two exercise regimes. *J Orthop Res.* 2007;25(3):404-412. doi:10.1002/jor.20220
60. Treleaven J, Jull G, LowChoy N. The relationship of cervical joint position error to balance and eye movement disturbances in persistent whiplash. *Man Ther.* 2006;11(2):99-106.
61. Sutton DA, Côté P, Wong JJ, et al. Is multimodal care effective for the management of patients with whiplash-associated disorders or neck pain and associated disorders? A systematic review by the Ontario Protocol for Traffic Injury Management (OPTIMa) Collaboration. *Spine J.* 2016;16(12):1541-1565. doi:10.1016/j.spinee.2014.06.019
62. Clark NC, Röijezon U, Treleaven J. Proprioception in musculoskeletal rehabilitation. Part 2: Clinical assessment and intervention. *Man Ther.* 2015;20(3):378-387. doi:10.1016/j.math.2015.01.009
63. Wainner RS, Irrgang JJ, Boninger ML, Delitto A, Allison S. Reliability and diagnostic accuracy of the clinical examination and patient self-report measures for cervical radiculopathy. *Spine.* 2003;28(1):52-62.
64. Raja A, Hanna A, Hoang S, Mesfin FB. Spinal stenosis. Accessed February 3, 2023. https://www.ncbi.nlm.nih.gov/books/NBK441989/
65. Arendt-Nielsen L, Svensson P. Referred muscle pain: basic and clinical findings. *Clin J Pain.* 2001;17(1):11-19. doi:10.1097/00002508-200103000-00003
66. Yarznbowicz R, Wlodarski M, Dolutan J. Classification by pain pattern for patients with cervical spine radiculopathy. *J Man Manip Ther.* 2020;28(3):160-169. doi:10.1080/10669817.2019.1587135
67. Edmond SL, Cutrone G, Werneke M, et al. Association between centralization and directional preference and functional and pain outcomes in patients with neck pain. *J Orthop Sports Phys Ther.* 2014;44(2):68-75. doi:10.2519/jospt.2014.4632
68. Magee DJ. *Orthopedic Physical Assessment.* 6th ed. Elsevier; 2014:177.
69. Raney NH, Petersen EJ, Smith TA, et al. Development of a clinical prediction rule to identify patients with neck pain likely to benefit from cervical traction and exercise. *Eur Spine J.* 2009;18(3):382-391. doi:10.1007/s00586-008-0859-7
70. Fritz JM, Thackeray A, Brennan GP, Childs JD. Exercise only, exercise with mechanical traction, or exercise with over-door traction for patients with cervical radiculopathy, with or without consideration of status on a previously described subgrouping rule: a randomized clinical trial. *J Orthop Sports Phys Ther.* 2014;44(2):45-57. doi:10.2519/jospt.2014.5065
71. Carragee EJ, Hurwitz EL, Cheng I, et al. Treatment of neck pain: injections and surgical interventions: results of the Bone and Joint Decade 2000–2010 Task Force on Neck Pain and Its Associated Disorders. *Eur Spine J.* 2008;17(suppl 1):153-169. doi:10.1007/s00586-008-0632-y
72. Liu WJ, Hu L, Chou PH, Wang JW, Kan WS. Comparison of anterior cervical discectomy and fusion versus posterior cervical foraminotomy in the treatment of cervical radiculopathy: a systematic review. *Orthop Surg.* 2016;8(4):425-431. doi:10.1111/os.12285
73. Hu Y, Lv G, Ren S, Johansen D. Mid- to long-term outcomes of cervical disc arthroplasty versus anterior cervical discectomy and fusion for treatment of symptomatic cervical disc disease: a systematic review and meta-analysis of eight prospective randomized controlled trials. *PLoS One.* 2016;11(2):e0149312. doi:10.1371/journal.pone.0149312

74. Sahai N, Changoor S, Dunn CJ, et al. Minimally invasive posterior cervical foraminotomy as an alternative to anterior cervical discectomy and fusion for unilateral cervical radiculopathy: a systematic review and meta-analysis. *Spine (Phila Pa 1976).* 2019;44(24):1731-1739. doi:10.1097/BRS.0000000000003156
75. Povlsen S, Povlsen B. Diagnosing thoracic outlet syndrome: current approaches and future directions. *Diagnostics (Basel).* 2018;8(1):21. doi:10.3390/diagnostics8010021
76. Hooper TL, Denton J, McGalliard MK, Brismée JM, Sizer PS Jr. Thoracic outlet syndrome: a controversial clinical condition. Part 1: anatomy, and clinical examination/diagnosis. *J Man Manip Ther.* 2010;18(2):74-83. doi:10.1179/106698110X12640740712734
77. Jones MR, Prabhakar A, Viswanath O, et al. Thoracic outlet syndrome: a comprehensive review of pathophysiology, diagnosis, and treatment. *Pain Ther.* 2019;8(1):5-18. doi:10.1007/s40122-019-0124-2
78. Gillard J, Pérez-Cousin M, Hachulla E, et al. Diagnosing thoracic outlet syndrome: contribution of provocative tests, ultrasonography, electrophysiology, and helical computed tomography in 48 patients. *Joint Bone Spine.* 2001;68(5):416-424. doi:10.1016/s1297-319x(01)00298-6
79. Hixson KM, Horris HB, Valovich McLeod TC, Welch Bacon CE. The diagnostic accuracy of clinical diagnostic tests for thoracic outlet syndrome. *J Sport Rehabil.* 2016;26(5):459-465. doi.org/10.1123/jrs.2016-0051
80. Hooper TL, Denton J, McGalliard MK, Brismée JM, Sizer PS Jr. Thoracic outlet syndrome: a controversial clinical condition. Part 2: non-surgical and surgical management. *J Man Manip Ther.* 2010;18(3):132-138. doi:10.1179/106698110X12640740712338
81. Haik MN, Alburquerque-Sendín F, Silva CZ, Siqueira-Junior AL, Ribeiro IL, Camargo PR. Scapular kinematics pre- and post-thoracic thrust manipulation in individuals with and without shoulder impingement symptoms: a randomized controlled study. *J Orthop Sports Phys Ther.* 2014;44(7):475-487. doi:10.2519/jospt.2014.4760
82. Cuenca-Martínez F, Herranz-Gómez A, Madroñero-Miguel B, et al. Craniocervical and cervical spine features of patients with temporomandibular disorders: a systematic review and meta-analysis of observational studies. *J Clin Med.* 2020;9(9):2806. doi:10.3390/jcm9092806
83. Murphy MK, MacBarb RF, Wong ME, Athanasiou KA. Temporomandibular disorders: a review of etiology, clinical management, and tissue engineering strategies. *Int J Oral Maxillofac Implants.* 2013;28(6):e393-e414. doi:10.11607/jomi.te20
84. Wright EF, North SL. Management and treatment of temporomandibular disorders: a clinical perspective. *J Man Manip Ther.* 2009;17(4):247-254. doi:10.1179/106698109791352184
85. Magee DJ. Temporomandibular joint. In: Magee DJ, ed. *Orthopedic Physical Assessment.* 6th ed. Elsevier; 2014:234-239.
86. Armijo-Olivo S, Pitance L, Singh V, Neto F, Thie N, Michelotti A. Effectiveness of manual therapy and therapeutic exercise for temporomandibular disorders: systematic review and meta-analysis. *Phys Ther.* 2016;96(1):9-25. doi:10.2522/ptj.2014054
87. Rocabado M, Johnston BE Jr, Blakney MG. Physical therapy and dentistry: an overview. *J Craniomandibular Pract.* 1982;1(1):46-49. doi:10.1080/07345410.1982.11677818
88. Mulet M, Decker KL, Look JO, Lenton PA, Schiffman EL. A randomized clinical trial assessing the efficacy of adding 6 x 6 exercises to self-care for the treatment of masticatory myofascial pain. *J Orofac Pain.* 2007;21(4):318-328.
89. Shaffer SM, Brismée JM, Sizer PS, Courtney CA. Temporomandibular disorders. Part 2: conservative management. *J Man Manip Ther.* 2014;22(1):13-23. doi:10.1179/2042618613Y.0000000061

Chapter 15

# Lumbar Spine and Sacroiliac Joint

## Common Diagnoses and Orthopedic Management

*Jacki Klaczak Kopack, PT, DPT and Karen A. Cascardi, PhD, MS, ATC, PTA*

**KEY TERMS** Counternutation | Directional preference | Global muscles | Herniated disk (protrusion) | Local muscles | Lumbar neutral spine position | Nutation | Spondylolisthesis | Spondylolysis | Spondylosis

## Chapter Objectives

1. Recall the basic anatomical structures of the lumbar spine and the sacroiliac (SI) joint.
2. Identify and describe common sprains, strains, and injuries to the lumbar spine/SI joint.
3. Describe the impact of structural or muscle weakness/tightness on posture, pain, and function.
4. Identify the common special tests used in a physical therapy evaluation for the low back/pelvic region.
5. Discuss the common treatment interventions used to address spinal diagnoses.
6. Given a patient diagnosis and plan of care (POC), design and progress a basic exercise/intervention program to rehabilitate common low back/pelvic diagnoses.

Low back pain (LBP) causes higher rates of global disability than any other condition.[1] The highest incidence of LBP occurs in individuals in their 30s and continues to be prevalent until the sixth decade of life when incidence begins to decrease. Many individuals who have activity-limiting LBP experience recurrent episodes of pain. The estimated recurrence rate in the first year after the initial onset of pain is 24% to 80%.[1]

Back pain is characterized as either specific or nonspecific, with nonspecific back pain comprising the majority of the cases. Specific LBP is caused by a specific/known pathology or mechanism of injury (eg, ankylosing spondylitis, osteoporosis, disk herniation, infection, arthritis). Nonspecific LBP is the diagnosis issued when specific pathologies are ruled out, and there is no clear cause of symptoms or history of injury.[2]

Treatment approaches should not only address patient presentations and complaints of pain but also biomedical and psychosocial factors.[3-5] Treating LBP often focuses on reducing pain and the resultant decreases in motion and strength. Trunk and core strengthening exercises, aerobic conditioning, flexibility exercises, and postural education have been found to be effective at preventing low back injury and/or injury reoccurrence.[3,5]

Patient education is a vital part of the rehabilitation process when treating patients with LBP. Clinicians need to identify any negative feelings/thoughts that a patient with LBP is experiencing and then work to guide and redirect the patient to thoughts that are more positive. Education also



Kopack JK, Cascardi KA.
*Principles of Therapeutic Exercise for the Physical Therapist Assistant* (pp 511-559).

**Table 15-1**

Referred Pain Patterns in the Lumbopelvic Region

| Source of Pain | Possible Referred Pain Pattern |
|---|---|
| Hip joint | Groin |
| SI joint | Posterior superior iliac spine (PSIS), iliac fossa, low back, superior lateral and posterior hip or thigh, posterior gluteal region, or groin |
| Trigger points | Rectus abdominis to posterior pelvis; quadratus lumborum to lateral ilium, greater trochanter, or groin |
| L4-L5 facet joints, ipsilateral interspinous ligaments L3-S2 | Sacrum |

focuses on ways to improve the patient's ability to cope with stress, pain, and daily problems that occur because of their pain. Patients who understand pain physiology tend to have better outcomes. It is important for patients to understand that inactivity has a negative effect on pain (making it worse) and that exercise will reduce their pain, allowing them to return to their prior level of function sooner.[4,5]

A physical therapist evaluates patients to determine the most accurate diagnosis, which is critical for developing an effective treatment POC and achieving optimal outcomes. There is an intimate relationship between the lumbar spine and pelvis, so all surrounding regions should also be examined. The therapist will assess the patient's postural alignment; spinal range of motion (ROM) and strength; and lower extremity (hip and knee, ankle/foot) alignment, flexibility, and strength to determine the true cause of their symptoms. Muscle imbalances (weakness/tightness) in any of these areas can affect spinal alignment and mobility, which can contribute to LBP or pelvic/SI symptoms and dysfunction. Faulty posture affects alignment up and down the kinetic chain, which increases stress on static structures, decreases muscle efficiency during motion, and increases the risk of overuse syndromes and pain (refer to Chapter 7).

Identifying the source of symptoms is a priority for the physical therapist during the evaluation. Pain can be referred to the back from other organs or regions (Table 15-1).[6-8] Physical therapist assistants must be aware of these pain patterns during treatment so that any changes in a patient's pain patterns (or pain intensity) can be documented in the medical record and reported to the therapist.

The stresses and forces exerted on the lumbar spine, pelvis, and hips vary with motion and task performance (ie, exercise, activities of daily living [ADLs], lifting, sitting, and standing). It is probable that a patient's symptoms will evolve and/or change throughout the day. The physical therapist assistant should monitor the patient's response to a variety of activities (eg, sitting, standing, walking) and look for patterns that increase or decrease pain in response to specific exercises and motions during treatment. The assistant is responsible for gathering data, screening for and identifying red flags regarding nonspecific LBP (Table 15-2),[9] and tracking patient presentation and progress. As discussed in Chapter 11, the assistant should modify treatment as appropriate based on the stage of healing and monitor patient responses and presentations (SINSS [Severity, Irritability, Nature of complaint, Stage, Stability]; refer to Table 11-1) during every session. Any adverse changes in patient presentation or lack of progress should be brought to the physical therapist's attention for reassessment.

### Considerations for the Physical Therapist Assistant: Treating Patients With Low Back Pain

The assistant needs to recognize and acknowledge the patient's negative psychosocial responses regarding their pain and guide the patient by turning those thoughts into positive ones with honest, easy-to-understand education on pain physiology and explain how exercises will help reduce their symptoms.

The use of the treatment-based classification system for managing patients with LBP has been common practice for several years and is useful when making evidence-based treatment decisions. Three general treatment approaches (ie, symptom modulation, movement control, and functional optimization) are used when treating patients with LBP. This approach aligns with the American Physical Therapy Association's vision.[3,5] Determining the appropriate treatment approach depends on the patient's disability (high, medium, or low), symptom status (volatile, controlled, or stable), and pain level (high, moderate, or low to none).[3]

In conjunction with the treatment-based classification systems, pathoanatomical factors (a specific anatomic tissue/pathology causing a patient's pain and dysfunction) and movement patterns have to be considered when treating

**Table 15-2**

**Low Back Pain Red Flags**

- Bowel dysfunction: May be due to spinal cord injury or blocked colon
- Bladder dysfunction: Incontinence, change in frequency, retention, or hematuria may be due to infection (kidney or urinary tract) or cauda equina syndrome
- History of cancer: LBP may be due to increased risk of cancer-related causes
- Resting night pain not related to movement or repositioning: Increased risk of cancer, infection, or an abdominal aortic aneurysm
- History of trauma, motor vehicle accident (MVA), fall, or heavy lifting: May denote fracture, especially in older patients or patients with osteoporosis
- Saddle anesthesia: Absence of sensation or tingling along the inner thighs and groin and/or perianal or genital areas (second to fifth sacral nerve roots), cauda equina syndrome
- Severe or progressive lower extremity neurologic deficit: May indicate cauda equina syndrome
- Recent infection: Recent urinary tract infection may cause LBP
- Night sweats, fever, or chills: May denote infection or increased risk of cancer
- Age 50 years or older: LBP may be due to an infection, fracture, abdominal aortic aneurysm, or cancer
- Unexplained weight loss > 10 pounds in 3 months: Increased risk of cancer

patients with LBP.[4] The inclusion of nonpharmaceutical and noninvasive treatments (eg, physical therapy interventions) to address LBP is strongly supported in the research. One randomized controlled trial concluded that "In chronic [LBP], the physical therapy exercise approach remains a first line treatment, and should routinely be used."[10] Another randomized controlled trial found that if patients with acute LBP began physical therapy early, there was a reduced risk of developing chronic low back symptoms.[5]

Physical therapist assistants may see treatment plans generated based on different treatment philosophies, such as those based on a pathoanatomical diagnosis and stages of healing, a mechanical diagnosis (ie, the McKenzie Method of Mechanical Diagnosis and Treatment [MDT]), a treatment classification,[5] or movement system impairment. The treatment-based classification system allows the integration of key aspects of these philosophies into the treatment plan. Treatment plans should address pathoanatomical issues and stage of healing; mechanical or movement impairments (ie, McKenzie); joint, soft tissue, or neural hyper- or hypomobility (ie, Travell et al[7]); and/or joint compression or radicular symptoms (ie, mechanical/manual traction). Although there are times when treatments may be selected based on the physical therapist's training and regional practice patterns, the application of current evidence-based practice treatment options can maximize patient outcomes.[3-5,7,10] Research continues to emerge, and dedication to lifelong learning will promote continued exploration and evolution of research findings. It is a clinician's responsibility to attend evidence-based continuing education courses and apply new knowledge.

## Lumbar Spine, Pelvis, and Sacroiliac Joint: Anatomy and Biomechanics

Because LBP is prevalent, it is important to have a solid understanding of anatomy; joint mechanics; and the interrelationship of the lumbar spine, pelvis, and SI joint. The biomechanical relationship between the pelvis and the hip was discussed in detail in Chapter 13. Various lumbar spinal deviations, compensatory motions, and muscle adaptations were discussed in Chapter 7.

### *The Lumbar Spine Anatomy and Biomechanics*

The lumbar spine consists of 5 lumbar vertebrae, and their bodies are thicker and wider than the cervical or thoracic vertebrae, allowing them to sustain and transmit higher loads. The segment between L5-S1 is the spinal level that bears the most load, and it is the most common site of injury.[11]

An intervertebral disk separates each lumbar vertebra, and the disk assists with shock absorption. The disk absorbs much of the compressive force and allows for movement between the bony segments. When an individual flexes forward, the intervertebral disks migrate posteriorly, and the disks migrate anteriorly with extension. The intervertebral disk is made up of the annulus fibrosus (a tough, outer fibrocartilaginous ring) and a central portion called the *nucleus pulposus*, which is composed of 85% to 90% of water. The fluid content decreases approximately 65% with age. This loss results in disk height loss, changes in facet joint load bearing, and decreases in the ability of the annulus fibers to withstand compressive forces. The facet joints (also called the *zygapophyseal joints*) are supported by ligaments that assist with managing compressive joint loads during prolonged weight bearing, with midrange spinal extension, and when extension and rotation occur together.[11,12] The inferior facet of the vertebra above articulates with the superior facet of the vertebra below to create the facet joint. When a normal disk is intact, facet joints bear about 25% of the axial load, but this load increases to 70% with a degenerated disk.[11] The least amount of intervertebral disk pressure occurs when a patient is positioned supine, prone, or side lying; however, there is some conflicting research regarding which posture creates the greatest intervertebral disk pressure (sitting vs standing).[11,13,14]

## Clinical Note: Does Spinal Position Affect Forces on the Intervertebral Disks?

Researchers agree that pressures increase significantly on the disks in both sitting and standing. There is a significant increase in disk pressure during sitting and standing with forward flexion, and these forces are increased even more when flexion and rotation are combined in these positions.[13,14] The physical therapy team prioritizes educating patients regarding proper body mechanics and lifting, including instruction to avoid combined motions of trunk flexion with rotation (or bending, lifting, and twisting). Chapter 22 provides an overview of proper body mechanics and lifting recommendations.

Three spinal ligaments provide trunk stability and control mobility by limiting specific motions: the anterior longitudinal ligament (ALL), the posterior longitudinal ligament (PLL), and the ligamentum flavum. The ALL is a broad flat ligament that spans the anterior aspect of the vertebral bodies. It limits excessive extension in the lumbar spine and prevents the disk from migrating too far forward during extension. The PLL spans the posterior aspect of the vertebral bodies, just anteriorly to the spinal cord. It limits lumbar flexion and is important in preventing disk migration posteriorly when bending forward. The ligamentum flavum is a broad, elastic structure that attaches to the laminae and lies posterior to the PLL. It protects the posterior aspect of the spinal cord, resists excessive lumbar flexion, and prevents the lamina from separating during flexion. Each of these structures span the entire length of the vertebral column.[15]

Understanding the location, function, and nerve innervations of the muscles that support and move the spine is important (Table 15-3).[15] There are functional differences between global and local muscles in the lumbar spine. **Local muscles** are small deep/intrinsic muscles that attach directly or via a fascia attachment to the lumbar vertebrae; they provide intervertebral segmental stability. The transverse abdominis (TrA), internal obliques, multifidi, and rotatores are considered local stabilizers. **Global muscles** are larger, superficial muscles that cross many vertebral segments and generate movement. These muscles include the rectus abdominis, external obliques, quadratus lumborum, and the erector spinae group.[16] Appropriate muscle activation and coordination combined with adequate strength of the lumbar (local) stabilizers are key to reducing LBP and improving function. Oftentimes, when a patient presents with lumbar or SI dysfunction, the local (deep) muscle stabilizers are not functioning correctly. If they are weak, their ability to activate quickly during coordinated gross spine or extremity movement is diminished. This inability to adequately control motion is a contributing factor to increased pain. Spinal stabilization exercises produce better patient outcomes compared with general exercises alone. These deep local muscles need to stabilize each segment of the spine while maintaining proper spinal alignment, which allows the superficial global muscles to work efficiently in providing overall trunk stability and mobility. TrA and multifidi are the primary spinal stabilizers, and strengthening these muscles early in the rehabilitation process should be initiated for those patients with LBP and SI pain to reduce their pain and improve function.[16-19] Specific spinal stabilization exercises, which are discussed later in this chapter, should be initiated very early during the rehabilitation process to facilitate appropriate muscle activity.

The primary motions available at the lumbar spine are flexion and extension (lower lumbar segments), small amounts of side bending (midlumbar segments), and minimal amounts of rotation. The availability of motion in each direction is a result of the orientation of the lumbar facet joints.[12] Lumbar spine active range of motion (AROM) averages include flexion of 40 to 60 degrees (5 to 7 inches [in] using the modified Schober test), extension of 20 to 35 degrees (1 to 3 in using the modified Schober test), lateral flexion of 15 to 25 degrees, and rotation of 3 to 18 degrees (but isolated ROM is difficult to assess). Having patients perform combined active motions will help clinicians assess which of these combined movements increase the signs/symptoms compared with straight plane motions. For example, pain (eg, hip and buttocks or pain above the knee) that occurs with lumbar extension and rotation is commonly associated with facet problems.[11]

The dorsal spinal roots carry afferent sensory fibers to the spinal cord, and the ventral spinal roots carry efferent motor fibers away from the spinal cord to the motor end plates on the muscles. There are 5 pairs of lumbar spinal nerves that innervate the lower extremities. Spinal nerves are located at each vertebral level, and the dorsal (sensory) and ventral (motor) nerves converge (synapse) within the intervertebral foramen. One pair of nerves exit the intervertebral foramina from each side of the vertebra, below the vertebral segment. These nerves travel down and merge to form the lumbar and lumbosacral plexuses. When a nerve root is compressed, entrapped, injured, or irritated (ie, disk involvement or muscle spasms), sensory and/or motor deficits can occur.[11] Dermatome and myotome innervations are listed in Table 15-4. If the patient reports pain or numbness along a nerve's sensory distribution, the clinician should also test the muscles that are innervated by these levels.

**Table 15-3**

Muscles of the Lumbar Spine

| Muscle | Action | Origin | Insertion | Innervation |
|---|---|---|---|---|
| Rectus abdominis (G) | Flexes the vertebral column<br>Tilts pelvis posteriorly | Pubic crest, pubic symphysis | Cartilage of fifth, sixth, and seventh ribs and xiphoid process | T6-T12 |
| External oblique (G) | Unilaterally: Laterally flexes vertebral column to the same side, rotates vertebral column to the opposite side<br>Bilaterally: Flexes vertebral column, compresses abdominal contents | External surfaces 5th to 12th ribs | Anterior part of iliac crest, abdominal aponeurosis to linea alba | T7-T12 |
| Internal oblique (L) | Unilaterally: Laterally flexes and rotates vertebral column to the same side<br>Bilaterally: Flexes vertebral column, compresses abdominal contents | Lateral inguinal ligament, iliac crest, and thoracolumbar fascia | Internal surface of lower 3 ribs, abdominal aponeurosis to linea alba | Ventral rami<br>T7-T12, L1 |
| TrA (L) | Compresses abdomen (runs transversely around the trunk and draws abdomen toward the spine) | Lateral inguinal ligament, iliac crest, thoracolumbar fascia, and internal surface of lower 6 ribs | Abdominal aponeurosis to linea alba | Ventral rami<br>T7-T12, L1 |
| ***Erector Spinae Group*** | | | | |
| Spinalis thoracis (G) | Unilaterally: Laterally flexes vertebral column to the same side<br>Bilaterally: Extends vertebral column | Spinous processes upper lumbar and lower thoracic vertebrae | Spinous processes of upper thoracic | Spinal<br>L1-L3 |
| Longissimus (G) | Unilaterally: Laterally flexes vertebral column to the same side<br>Bilaterally: Extends the vertebral column | Common tendon | Lower 9 ribs, transverse processes thoracic vertebrae | Spinal<br>L1-L5 |
| Iliocostalis lumborum (G) | Unilaterally: Laterally flexes vertebral column to the same side<br>Bilaterally: Extends vertebral column | Common tendon | Transverse processes of lumbar vertebrae 1 to 3 and posterior surface of ribs 6 to 12 | Spinal<br>L1-L3 |

*(continued)*

**Table 15-3 (continued)**

Muscles of the Lumbar Spine

| Muscle | Action | Origin | Insertion | Innervation |
|---|---|---|---|---|
| ***Transversospinalis Group*** | | | | |
| Multifidi (L) | Unilaterally: Rotates vertebral column to the opposite side<br>Bilaterally: Extends vertebral column (segmentally stabilizes the spine with the rotator) | Sacrum and transverse processes of lumbar through cervical vertebrae | Spinous processes of lumbar vertebrae through second cervical vertebra: Span 2 to 4 vertebrae | Spinal<br>L1-L5 |
| Rotatores (L) | Unilaterally: Rotates vertebral column to the opposite side<br>Bilaterally: Extends vertebral column | Transverse process of lumbar through cervical vertebrae | Spinous processes of lumbar vertebrae through second cervical vertebra: Span 1 to 2 vertebrae | Spinal<br>L1-L5 |
| Semispinalis (G) | Unilaterally: Rotates vertebral column to the opposite side<br>Bilaterally: Extends vertebral column and head | Transverse process of lower thoracic through cervical vertebrae | Spinous processes of lumbar vertebrae through second cervical vertebra: Spans 5 or more vertebrae | Spinal nerves |
| ***Other*** | | | | |
| Interspinales (L) | Trunk and head extension | Spinous process below | Spinous process above | Spinal nerves |
| Intertransversarii (L) | Trunk and head lateral bending to the same side | Transverse process below | Transverse process above | Spinal nerves |
| Quadratus lumborum (G) | Unilaterally: Lateral lumbar flexion or hip hike (pelvic elevation)<br>Bilaterally: Lumbar extension | Superiorly to the 12th rib and transverse processes of L1-L4 | Inferiorly to iliolumbar ligament and iliac crest | T12, L1-L4 |

G=global (superficial) muscles; L=local (deep) muscles.

**Table 15-4**

Dermatome and Myotome Testing

| Nerve Root | Dermatome Testing (Sensory) | Muscle Actions | Patient Position and Myotome Isometric Testing (Motor) |
|---|---|---|---|
| L1-L2 | L1: Inguinal crease<br>L2: Around greater trochanter | Hip flexion and hip adduction | Supine: Position knee at 90 degrees and hip at about 40 degrees with heel off the table; resist hip flexion |
| L3 | Medial knee | Knee extension | Supine: Position knee at 25 to 30 degrees of knee flexion; resist knee extension<br>Test patellar reflex |
| L4 | Medial ankle | Ankle dorsiflexion and inversion | Attempt heel walking. If unable to perform position supine, place ankles in neutral; resist dorsiflexion |
| S1 | Lateral foot | Ankle plantar flexion, eversion, and hip extension | Attempt toe walking or standing plantar flexion; if unable to perform position prone, resist plantar flexion<br>Test Achilles tendon reflex |
| S2 | Posterior medial knee | Hip extension and knee flexion | Prone: Flex knee to 90 degrees; resist knee flexion |

Note: Any new onset of weakness, decreased sensation, decreased reflexes, any change in bowel or bladder function (or new incontinence issues), and/or saddle paresthesia should be immediately reported to the physical therapist/physician. See Table 15-2 for red flags.

### Considerations for the Physical Therapist Assistant: Radicular Pain Versus Referred Pain in Patients With Low Back Pain

Radicular and referred pain patterns were defined and described in Chapter 14. Each organ in the body has a specific region where pain may refer to if a pathologic problem exists in the organ. For example, a patient with a kidney problem can have referred pain to the flank area, resulting in LBP. A kidney stone can present with acute, sharp LBP, and a thorough examination by the physical therapist should distinguish pain whose source is not musculoskeletal in origin. These patients would be referred back to the physician for further medical workup. Remember, if we cannot reproduce the pain, we should not be treating it. See Appendix F for dermatome patterns and Appendix G and Table 15-1 for referred pain patterns.

Radicular pain along the sciatic nerve causing pain down the posterior/lateral aspect of the leg into the foot can occur with an L4-L5 disk herniation with compression of the nerve root. Muscles innervated by this nerve root can be affected; ankle dorsiflexion and great toe extension may be weak with L4-L5 diskogenic problems. The ability to differentiate between radicular and referred pain allows the assistant to recognize possible red flags and modify treatment appropriately. The assistant should contact the supervising therapist with significant changes in the patient's pain pattern.

The normal resting position of the lumbar spine while standing should be in slight lumbar lordosis. This is the midway position between extreme lordosis and a flat back posture and is referred to as the **lumbar neutral spine position** (also referred to as neutral spine). The pelvis is in a neutral position when the anterior superior iliac spine (ASIS) and pubic symphysis are oriented in the same vertical line. The ASIS is about 2 fingers lower than the PSIS when the pelvis is in neutral.[11,12] Pelvic positioning has a direct effect on the position of the spinal column (and vice versa), and improper positioning of either structure will contribute to postural deviations (refer to Chapter 7). A patient who presents with an increased anterior pelvic tilt in standing has an increased shift of the ASIS anteriorly and inferiorly (as the pelvis rotates anteriorly around a fixed hip joint), and this position results in an increase in lumbar extension. Individuals who have an anterior pelvic tilt tend to present with adaptively shortened hip flexors and lumbar erector spinae and weak abdominals. A patient who presents with a posterior pelvic tilt (PPT) in standing has the ASIS shifted superiorly and posteriorly (as the pelvis rotates posteriorly around a fixed hip joint), with a resultant increase in lumbar flexion. A PPT posture often results in adaptively shortened hip extensors (hamstrings/gluteal muscles) and lengthened hip flexors/lumbar extensors (refer to Chapter 13). Pelvic tilt exercises are often prescribed to retrain the postural muscles to improve posture. The performance of appropriate pelvic tilt exercises can reduce symptoms in patients with LBP. For example, anterior pelvic tilts may alleviate symptoms due to disk herniation, and PPTs may be recommended for patients diagnosed with spinal stenosis.

**Table 15-5**

Ligaments of the Sacroiliac Joint

| Ligaments | Attachments | Function |
|---|---|---|
| Sacrospinous | Sacrum to ischial spine | Lowers ischium in relation to sacrum |
| Sacrotuberous | Sacrum to ischial tuberosities | Restricts nutation |
| Anterior/posterior SI (interosseous) | Sacrum to ilium; anterior ligament is not well defined and is thinnest of SI ligaments; prone to injury and pain | Stabilizes SI joint |
| Long dorsal SI | PSIS to third and fourth sacral segments; strongest SI ligament | Resists counternutation |
| Iliolumbar | Iliac crest to transverse process of fifth lumbar vertebra | Restricts nutation and side bending |
| Supraspinous | Spinous process to spinous process of each vertebra | Helps prevent flexion and rotation of the ilium |

**Clinical Note and Questions for Thought**

What are the postural implications of sitting too much? Which stretches are most appropriate for the person to perform to correct pelvic positioning? Prolonged sitting can result in hip flexor muscle shortening and contributes to increased anterior pelvic tilting. Hip flexor and lumbar paraspinal stretching should be initiated to address this tightness.

## *The Sacroiliac Joint Anatomy and Function*

The pelvis consists of the ilium, ischium, pubis (which are fused), and the sacrum. The 2 SI joints join the pelvis posteriorly, and the pubic symphysis connects both sides of the pelvis anteriorly. The SI joints are stabilized by ligaments (Table 15-5) and muscles that cross the joint (refer to Chapter 21).

The SI joint is a stable diarthrodial joint; yet, it accommodates motion as it transmits weight from the head, arms, and trunk through the pelvis to the lower extremities. During walking, the SI joints assist with shock absorption for the spine, and forces are transmitted up the kinetic chain from the lower extremities. There is a small amount of accessory motion occurring at the SI joints during lower extremity movement, spinal motion, and stabilization activities. Excessive motion or instability at an SI joint can lead to dysfunction and pain. Sacral movement occurs between the SI joints and the base of the sacrum and L5; this affects the movement between the disks and vertebrae of the lumbar spine. Technically, the sacrum can flex/extend, rotate, and side bend. It is beyond the scope of this text to discuss these movements in detail (refer to kinesiology textbooks for additional details); a basic summary is provided here.

The 2 primary motions of the sacrum are **nutation** and **counternutation** (Figure 15-1). The strong ligamentous support at the SI joints promotes stability and limits the available motion, so these motions are subtle. During nutation, the base of the sacrum moves/tilts in an anterior and inferior direction, and the coccyx moves posteriorly as the ilium rotates posteriorly. During counternutation, the base of the sacrum tilts in a posterior and superior direction, and the coccyx moves anteriorly as the ilium rotates anteriorly.[20] Nutation and counternutation can occur bilaterally, but these motions occur unilaterally during reciprocal tasks (eg, walking). During bilateral motion (eg, lifting), both SI joints move in the same direction, and L5 will move in the opposite direction to that of the sacrum. Lumbar extension is accompanied by nutation, and lumbar flexion is accompanied by counternutation. Proximally, cervical and lumbar curves increase, and the thoracic curve decreases.[21] However, during unilateral reciprocal motion, one SI joint is in nutation, whereas the opposite SI joint is in counternutation. For example, during gait, as the left limb prepares for the loading response, the sacrum tilts into nutation as the left ilium rotates posteriorly. Simultaneously, the right hip is in extension, and the sacrum tilts into counternutation on the right as the right ilium rotates anteriorly.[21] Nutation and counternutation occur during open chain hip motions as well as closed chain pelvic tilting and trunk motions.

In addition to sacral motion, sacral positioning contributes to the stability of the pelvis and SI joints. Static pelvic stability is called *form closure* and is achieved when the iliac surfaces interlock with the articular surfaces of the sacrum during nutation.[15,20] Nutation is the closed-pack position for the SI joint; this position creates SI ligamentous

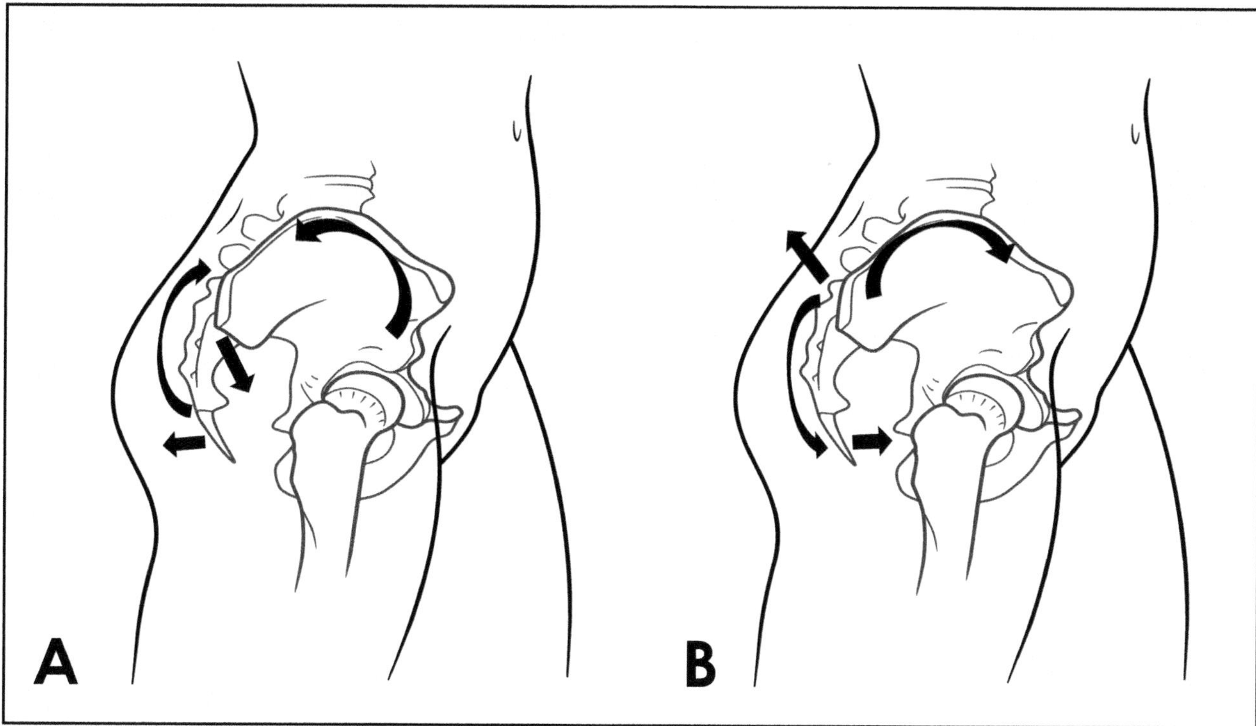


**Figure 15-1.** Nutation and counternutation. (A) Nutation: The base of the sacrum (which articulates with L5) tilts anteriorly and inferiorly as the coccyx moves posteriorly, creating a posterior rotation of the ilium. (B) Counternutation: The base of the sacrum tilts posterior and superiorly as the coccyx moves anteriorly, creating an anterior rotation of the ilium (juliawhite/Shutterstock.com).

tension and increases joint stability. Force closure occurs as other forces (ligaments, muscles, and thoracolumbar fascia) create tension at the SI joint, increasing joint compression and stability during movement.[15,20] Force closure creates dynamic stability, and it is dependent on the ability of the sacrum to nutate, especially during unilateral loading with walking. Appropriate sacral positioning and adequate force closure minimize the shearing forces between the iliac bones and sacrum, which allows an effective transfer of load/forces between the trunk, pelvis, and lower extremities.[20] The ligaments that contribute to force closure are described in Table 15-5.[20,22] The muscles that contract to increase SI stability include the pelvic floor muscles, TrA, multifidi, gluteal muscles, erector spinae, latissimus dorsi, internal/external obliques, piriformis, obturator externus, and hip adductors. Functional movements such as trunk flexion greater than 60 degrees, hip hyperextension, and long sitting (especially in patients with tight hamstrings) create counternutation.[21,23] Counternutation decreases the dynamic stability as the sacrum becomes "unlocked" (SI joint open-packed position).[21,23] Nutation initially occurs with trunk flexion, but then the sacrum counternutates at about 60 degrees when the deep posterior muscles and thoracolumbar fascia become tight. Inaccurate movement patterns, poor body mechanics, and/or muscle weakness can reduce the efficiency of the force closure mechanism, resulting in decreased dynamic SI joint stability and increased risk for potential injury.

## Objective Measurements for the Lumbar and Sacroiliac Joints

During normal functional activities and gait, the pelvis, low back, and SI joints work together to allow controlled, coordinated motion and appropriate transmission of weight-bearing forces. Any areas of imbalance can alter the biomechanics in these joints and can lead to improper muscle activation, increased joint stresses, pain, and excess instability.

A comprehensive physical therapy examination and evaluation provide the physical therapist assistant with information needed to create effective treatment interventions for patients with back pain. The physical therapist will examine the patient's pelvis, SI, and low back (locally and regionally) during the initial evaluation. During treatments, the assistant should continue collecting data to determine if selected interventions are effective in reducing pain, improving core stabilization, and rebalancing muscle strength/endurance and flexibility in all targeted areas. Patient education for LBP diagnoses include symptom reduction techniques, proper positioning (ie, sleeping, sitting, and standing), modality use, normalizing movement patterns, and using proper body mechanics during ADLs to reduce the chance of reinjury.

During the initial evaluation, the physical therapist will obtain information about the patient's pain, pain pattern, and those activities that make their pain better or worse. Sensory testing (dermatome) and muscle strength (myotome) testing are used to assess for patterns indicating a neurologic source of the patient's symptoms. In addition to

**Table 15-6**

Special Tests for Lumbar Spine and Sacroiliac Joint Diagnoses

| Diagnosis | Special Tests |
|---|---|
| Disk with/without nerve root involvement | • SLR or crossed SLR (specificity 89%)[11,24]<br>• Slump test (sensitivity 84%)[11,24]<br>• Centralization of symptoms is positive for disk pathology<br>• 3 of 4 positive tests: Dermatome pain associated with a specific nerve root, sensory deficits, abnormal reflexes (patella/Achilles), and motor weakness associated with specific nerve root[24] |
| Spinal stenosis | • History: 3 of 5 positive indicators: ≥48 years, bilateral symptoms, more leg than LBP, increased pain with standing/walking, and seated pain relief[24]<br>• Pain relief with forward flexion or "shopping cart sign" |
| Facet (zygapophyseal) joint involvement | • 3 of 5 positive indicators/tests: ≥50 years, symptoms least with walking, symptoms least with sitting, paraspinal pain, quadrant test (lumbar extension and rotation; 85% sensitivity and 91% specificity)[28] |
| Ankylosis spondylitis | • Positive Schober test (This test can also be positive with other LBP diagnoses.)<br>• More common in men<br>• Decreased chest expansion, decreased lumbar lordosis, SI joint point tender, modified Stoke Ankylosing Spondylitis Spine Score<br>• History: 4 of 5 positive indicators/tests: <30 years, morning stiffness, less discomfort with exercise, gradual onset, and pain for at least 3 months[15] |
| Spondylolisthesis | • Functional flexion/extension radiography is the gold standard[24]<br>• Low midline sill sign at L4-L5[24] (sensitivity 81.3% and specificity 89.1%)[29]<br>• Passive lumbar extension test for degenerative spondylolisthesis in older patients[24] |
| Lumbar instability[a] | • Passive lumbar extension test (sensitivity 84% and specificity 90%)[29]<br>• Interspinous gap change during lumbar flexion-extension motion[25] (sensitivity 82.2% and specificity 60.7%)[29]<br>• Special test/diagnostic cluster: positive prone instability test and posterior shear test |
| SI joint | • No centralization of symptoms<br>• Pain with palpation to sacral sulcus (medial to PSIS)<br>• 3 of 5 positive indicators/tests: SI compression, SI distraction, Gaenslen's, sacral spring, and thigh thrust tests[24] |

[a]Note: Interspinous gap change used for lumbar instability can also be used for spondylolisthesis.
Crossed SLR test is performed on the unaffected/uninvolved leg.
SLR = straight leg raise.

dermatome and myotome testing, there are several special tests the therapist can perform to determine the patient's source of LBP. The physical therapist assistant should also be familiar with the tests performed during the initial evaluation because they may be repeated during treatment sessions to determine patient progress. Table 15-6 provides the commonly used special tests for various low back and SI diagnoses.

The physical therapist will first assess the patient's available ROM in all directions. Then, the patient will be asked to perform several repetitions of lumbar flexion, extension, and left/right lateral flexion while standing. During these repeated motions, the therapist is monitoring for reports of centralization of pain (lumbar spine) or increased radicular symptoms (ie, numbness, tingling, or pain) that peripheralize pain distally. Based on the patient's reports of what positions make their pain better or worse, the therapist may have the patient lie prone propped up on their forearms into lumbar extension or lie supine and bring the knees to the chest to create trunk flexion. Sustaining those respective positions for a period of time helps determine which position best centralizes symptoms.

Patients with diskogenic pathology often present with symptoms that centralize with trunk extension, resulting in a decrease in radicular symptoms (decreased peripheralization); this is referred to as *extension bias*. Patients with spinal stenosis tend to have symptom reduction when performing trunk flexion and are referred to as having *flexion bias*. The direction of motion that centralizes the patient's symptoms is called **directional preference**. This is further discussed in the Treatment-Based Classification System: Rehabilitation Approaches and Treatments for Low Back Pain section of this chapter.

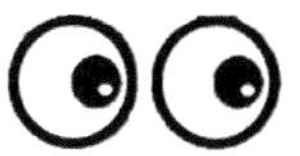

### Eye on the Research: Cluster Testing to Better Identify the Source of Low Back Pain and Sacroiliac Pain

Research indicates that a physical examination that includes the use of a validated cluster of tests is more reliable to predict both the spinal diagnosis and effective interventions than the use of a single test alone. For example, a positive straight leg raise or crossed straight leg raise test together with dermatome testing, reflex testing, and manual muscle testing better determines disk herniation and nerve root involvement compared with using a single assessment.[24] Additional studies assessed the effectiveness of the individual tests commonly used to diagnosis SI dysfunction and determined that many of the commonly used tests had low sensitivity and specificity when used alone.[25] The distraction test, compression test, thigh thrust/posterior shear, sacral thrust, and resisted hip abduction were the only tests to have a specificity and sensitivity greater than 60%.[25] Researchers determined that cluster testing generates more reliable results; if at least 3 of 5 of the following provocation tests (SI compression, SI distraction, Gaenslen's, sacral spring, or thigh thrust) were positive, then the SI joint is the probable source of the pain.[24,26]

It is useful to have patients complete a functional assessment scale to determine their perception of their abilities/limitations. Some commonly used tests include the Oswestry Disability Index, the Quebec Back Pain Disability Scale, and the Roland-Morris Questionnaire. The Oswestry is commonly used to assess a patient's perspective on their ability to perform ADLs. The Roland-Morris Questionnaire is a short (yes or no and checkoff answers) form that can be used to determine how patients are progressing with their pain and function.[11] These 2 tools are validated and are recommended to determine both a baseline and changes in status according to current clinical practice guidelines.[5] Other tools that may be used include the Fear Avoidance Back Questionnaire Physical Activity, Waddell Disability Index, and the STarT Back Screening Tool (refer to the Suggested Resources at the end of the chapter).

## *Yellow Flags: Pain and Fear Avoidance Behaviors*

It is important to carefully review a patient's initial evaluation to understand their presentation. If a patient's pain has been present for an extended period of time, it may affect their psychosocial behaviors, their ability to cope, and their ability to progress in therapy. Back pain often creates fear and apprehension in patients. Patients presenting with high fear avoidance behaviors have an increased risk of catastrophizing and tend to have poor outcomes. Understanding a patient's perception is important because it influences how to best educate patients.

The physical therapy team can assist patients by providing education that encourages and assists with putting pain into perspective.[11] Appropriate education can improve the effectiveness of treatment and patient outcomes. Refer to Chapter 11 for specific information related to the neuroscience of pain.

### Clinical Tips: Communicating With Patients and Fear Avoidance Behaviors

- If the patient states, "I'm not going to be able to ..." (eg, take care of my children, do my job, earn a paycheck, enjoy my retirement), the assistant's response should be as follows: "The exercises and information I give you will help reduce your pain so you can back to your normal activities. You need to tell me which positions or activities make you better or worse, so together we can work on controlling your pain and addressing your concerns."
- If the patient states, "My x-ray or MRI (magnetic resonance imaging) was abnormal," "I have a herniated/bulging disk," or "The doctor said I have major arthritis ... bone on bone," the assistant's response should be the following: "Many people have the same condition as you and don't know it and don't have symptoms. As we get older, some of these changes can occur, but they can also affect younger people. The exercises I give you will help reduce your pain and the things I teach you will help you to work smarter."
- If the patient states, "I'm afraid the exercises will make me worse," the assistant's response should be as follows: "Your back may be more sensitive at first, but the more you move, the better you'll feel. The more you focus on or worry about your pain, the worse it seems. The exercises I give you will help you move easier without pain and get you stronger. That is why I always ask you how you feel when you are doing the exercises and I make sure you are doing them correctly."

# Introduction to Rehabilitation Management for Lumbar Spine and Sacroiliac Joint

There are 3 phases/stages of healing, and the associated time frames are based on the original onset of LBP. The acute phase is considered to be less than 1 month from onset/injury (0 to 4 weeks), the subacute phase can span from week 4 to week 12, and the chronic or return-to-function phase can last from 3 months or longer.[5] In addition to the patient's current phase of healing, the therapy team needs to consider the patient's pain, level of disability, diagnosis, and any other medical factors when treating patients with lumbar or SI dysfunction. In order to provide a high level of evidence-based treatments, physical therapist assistants should understand which interventions are appropriate based on the patient's diagnosis and pain location or distribution pattern. When designing an effective treatment program for a patient with LBP or SI dysfunction, the assistant needs to consider the following: the severity and irritability of the signs/symptoms and the directional preference that reduces symptoms (positional or movement), pain-free spinal AROM, trunk/core muscle strength/stability (targeting local and then global muscle endurance), spinal and lower extremity flexibility, and prior level of cardiovascular fitness.

The lumbar spine, SI joints, and pelvis are often observed and treated simultaneously. Monitoring SINSS throughout each treatment session is imperative and allows the assistant to immediately modify patient positioning and/or exercises based on the patient's symptom tolerance and pain presentation. When treating patients with LBP, there is no "one-size-fits-all" or evidence of "one best treatment regimen"; there are only guidelines.[5] The core muscles impact respiration, maintain postural alignment, and stabilize the lumbar spine and SI joints during walking, lifting, and other everyday activities. The demands placed on these muscles need to be considered in patients presenting with LBP. Physical therapist assistants will treat a significant number of patients with diagnoses of specific LBP (eg, disk herniation or spondylolisthesis) as well as those with nonspecific LBP. Clinicians benefit from ongoing continuing education and active mentoring by experienced physical therapy team members to help develop strong treatment skills and sound clinical decisions when treating these patients.

Patient education is an integral part of treating patients with a lumbar or SI diagnosis. Reducing pain is a top priority, especially with sleeping and getting in/out of bed. Sleeping positions to reduce stress on the lumbar spine should be addressed very early in the rehabilitation process. The patient should sleep on a firm mattress to provide adequate support. Depending on the patient's preferred sleeping position (side lying or supine), the clinician should ensure that the cervical and lumbar spines are properly aligned by using pillows for support to maintain a neutral position (Figure 15-2A). Patients should be instructed on the proper way to get into and out of bed to reduce low back stress/LBP (Figure 15-2B). Patients should demonstrate these positions and movements during the treatment session to determine if the symptoms are reduced/controlled and to ensure they are using correct movement patterns. Physical therapist assistants can provide alternative recommendations for positioning/movements that are individualized and that minimize stress on the lumbar spine. Education and training on proper body mechanics for lifting and workstation and ergonomic modification are indicated after the symptoms are better controlled (refer to Chapter 22).

The acuity of the patient's presentation is the first factor physical therapist assistants must consider when initiating treatment. The type of injury and degree of inflammation/irritation will guide treatment decisions. Encouraging compliance with therapy interventions is important, but helping patients cope with their pain and coaching them to consistently perform exercises can be challenging for clinicians. Current research indicates that patients with acute LBP may experience more pain relief and demonstrate functional improvement by staying active vs resting in bed.[27]

### Clinical Tips: Coping Strategies for Patients With Low Back Pain[28]

- Provide positive coping skill strategies (eg, meditation or relaxation techniques, do things to distract from pain, pray, walk, perform gentle exercises).
- Provide education about back pain and guide the patient to accept their current level of pain and that it can be managed.
- Encourage the patient to be hopeful, think positively, and self-reflect to better manage their pain.
- Encourage patients to take an active role in the rehabilitation process and to be open to different treatment approaches. "We will find a treatment that works best for you. Initially your back may feel sensitive (stiff, sore), but the more you move, the better you will feel."

When progressing a patient's treatment program, a goal is to minimize the risk of symptom exacerbation. The physical therapist assistant should ensure that (1) only 1 or 2 exercises are given to the patient at a time, (2) exercises are not added until the patient is able to stabilize the spine/core efficiently with lower-level exercises, and (3) exercises/activities are not performed too aggressively. Patients who are feeling better and progressing well may experience an exacerbation as they attempt new activities or overdo those activities that they previously performed (eg, gardening, house cleaning) if the activities are currently beyond their physiological capabilities. Exacerbations are most commonly due to poor core muscle endurance and the inability to control and stabilize the spine/trunk during those activities. If this occurs, the clinician should readjust treatment interventions accordingly to reflect the change in patient acuity/irritability. Patients must be reminded of their

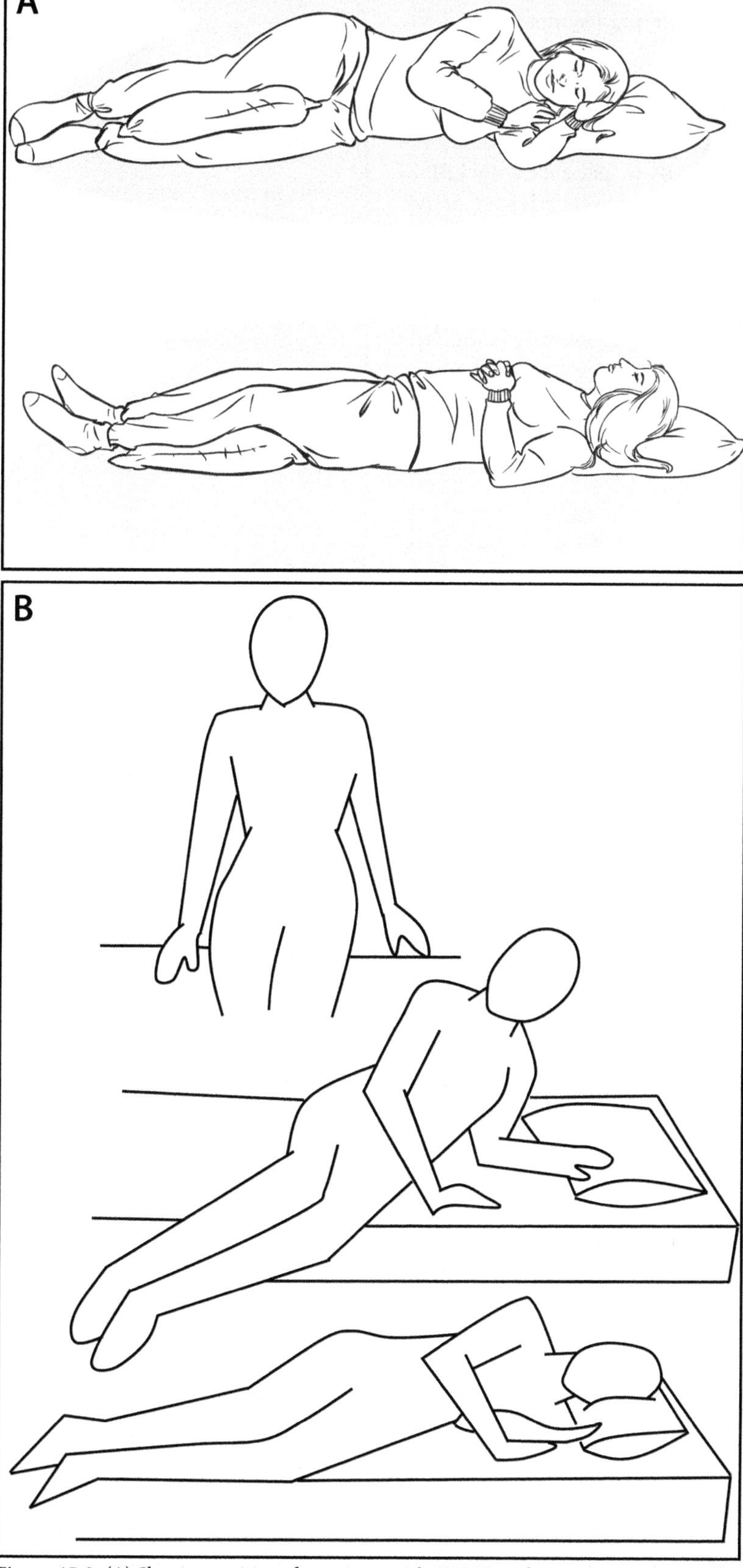


**Figure 15-2.** (A) Sleeping positions for patients with LBP. Note that patients with a smaller waist and wider hips may benefit from placing a small pillow or towel at the waist level to keep the spine straight when lying on their side (Drp8/Shutterstock.com). (B) The proper way to get out of bed. The patient first rolls to a side-lying position. The patient will move the legs off the bed and push up into a sitting position, maintaining a straight spine to protect the low back. (Graphic created by John Kopack.)

current/temporary limitations and re-educated on how to control, reduce, or reverse their pain/symptoms quickly and effectively.

Long-term goals typically focus on increasing ROM and muscle strength/endurance, normalizing motion, and promoting independent and full return to prior functional activities. To achieve these goals in patients with LBP/SI diagnoses, assistants should progressively advance activities that focus on improving the following:

- Independent and coordinated joint mobility/flexibility (of the spine, pelvis, and upper and lower extremities)
- Muscle endurance and strength (address local and then global core muscles and hip musculature)
- Kinesthetic awareness to improve the patient's ability to demonstrate appropriate postural alignment and muscle recruitment during various activities
- Cardiopulmonary performance (address respiration patterns that may be impacted with spinal pain/diagnoses if indicated)
- Functional task performance without pain and reduced stress on the lumbar spine (eg, proper body mechanics, ergonomic training, and adaptations)

General suggestions for treatment interventions that reflect the progressions of acuity/healing are included in Table 15-7. Note the parallels between interventions based on the stages of healing and the treatment-based classifications (Table 15-8). Treatment interventions are selected based on the treatment-based classification, diagnosis, and individual patient presentation. Treatment modifications are based on diagnosis-specific precautions, stage of healing, and the patient's presentation during each session (ie, SINSS). The templates found in Appendices A and B can help guide new clinicians in developing a treatment plan.

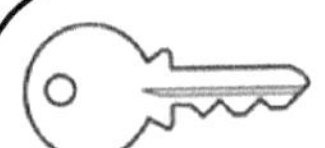

**Key Safety Considerations**

- Monitor vital signs for appropriate response to activity.
- Monitor general signs/symptoms that indicate the need to terminate exercise.
- If symptoms cannot be reproduced, treatment should not be initiated. If medical red flags are present, refer out!
- If patients present with traits consistent with more than one treatment-based classification, the physical therapist will prioritize presentation and select the most appropriate classification for the initial treatments.
- Patients can have changes in presentation as treatments progress; this will warrant a review and potential change to the treatment classification/intervention plan. The goal is to centralize and then reduce symptoms.
- Monitor for appropriate positions at rest and proper form/mechanics with exercise and activities.
- Adjust interventions based on the stage of healing and the irritability of the symptoms.
- Education is important! Incorporate education regarding pain neuroscience; a neutral spine; and the use of drawing-in/abdominal bracing maneuvers, body mechanics, and positional changes/bias positions/exercises.

## Low Back Pain and Sacroiliac Joint Diagnoses, Causes, Signs, and Symptoms

It is important to understand the causes and signs/symptoms of various LBP and SI diagnoses. Initially, the physical therapist will assess for underlying causes of a patient's symptoms and perform various tests (motor function, neurologic, and special tests) to ensure that the treatment plan targets all of the involved structures. Each diagnosis has a typical pattern/presentation, so the therapist will carefully assess the patient to appropriately rule in or out varied diagnoses.

**Table 15-7**

**Intervention Suggestions for Patients With Low Back Pain Based on Acuity/Stages of Healing**

| Acute Phase |
|---|
| Patient typically presents with acute pain, guarded posture, limited ROM, difficulty completing ADLs/IADLs, difficulty finding a comfortable position, and possible radiculopathy. |
| Treatment goals: Decrease acute symptoms and promote healing (pain/inflammation/muscle spasms), demonstrate safe postures/positions/mobility patterns/ADLs/movement transitions, increase pain-free ROM, and initiate neuromuscular control exercises (stabilization). |
| Instruct patients to use passive positioning to decrease symptoms. Positions will be dependent on the patient's diagnosis and symptoms. |
| Possible treatment interventions: Modalities; passive positioning (position of comfort or functional position depending on the pathologic condition (flexion bias, extension bias, or a non–weight-bearing/traction bias positions/exercises); patient education for postural education/training, body mechanics, and stabilization exercises; passive or active stretching to tight lower extremity muscles that contribute to poor posture or increased symptoms (modify or hold exercises if symptoms increase). |
| Key exercises: Pelvis neutral position, drawing-in (hollowing) and/or abdominal bracing maneuvers, PPT, multifidi contraction, hip and lower extremity stretching as tolerated. Instruct proper breathing techniques. Emphasize the importance of correct form/quality of motion. |
| **Subacute Phase** |
| Patient typically presents with pain at end of available ROM (where injured tissue/structure is stressed), deconditioned, decreased muscle strength/endurance, difficulty completing some IADLs (especially for a prolonged period of time), decreased postural awareness, and poor body mechanics. Patients may express apprehension with increasing mobility due to fear of pain or reinjury. |
| Treatment goals: Promote independence in self-management of pain and appropriate postural control at rest and with activity. Increase AROM, muscle strength, muscle endurance, and aerobic conditioning. Promote relaxation/stress reduction, and promote proper body mechanics independently. |
| Treatment interventions can include patient education, practice proper postures/body mechanics, and postural correction/bias exercises reducing symptoms with increasing activity levels. Lumbar/thoracic joint mobilizations, spinal endurance exercises, spinal ROM exercises, low-/moderate-intensity aerobic conditioning, neuromuscular re-education (with appropriate core contractions with activity), segmental trunk movements in opposite direction of preference bias,[a] increasing stabilization exercises to improve muscle endurance), and extremity strengthening with stable spine. |
| Key exercises: Core stability progression, extremity stretching/strengthening, maintaining good posture, aerobic conditioning, and spinal ROM (intersperse bias exercise to minimize symptoms). |
| *(continued)* |

| Table 15-7 (continued) Intervention Suggestions for Patients With Low Back Pain Based on Acuity/Stages of Healing |
|---|
| Chronic Phase |
| The patient typically reports pain with repetitive motions or long duration positioning in vulnerable postures, continued deconditioning (especially during high-intensity activities), muscle strength imbalances, difficulty completing high-intensity activities for long periods, and decreased postural control during high-intensity activities (plyometrics, sports, and drills). |
| Treatment goals: Complete resolution of pain (or minimal amount if resolution is not possible), full pain-free spinal ROM, ability to maintain core stability with all upper and lower extremity motions, functional tasks, and recreational/sports activities. Improve muscle performance, coordination, and endurance. Maximize aerobic conditioning. Independent with stress reduction techniques and postural correction at rest and during activity. Safely return to high-level activity/sports/all IADLs. |
| Treatment interventions can include stretching, progressive trunk/extremity resistance exercises in various postures on stable and compliant surfaces, aerobic exercises (increase intensity), ergonomic recommendations, activity/sport-specific training/drills/plyometrics, and patient education. |
| Key exercises: Core stability progressions in challenging positions on stable and compliant surfaces (ie, a physioball and planks) with upper and/or lower extremity movements, extremity strengthening and plyometrics, aerobic conditioning, trunk lower extremity strengthening, activity/sport-specific training, spinal/trunk control, endurance, and coordination progressions. |
| [a]If a patient continues to display an extension or flexion bias, continue to focus exercises in that direction but gradually attempt to move in the opposite direction without increasing symptoms.<br>IADLs = instrumental activities of daily living. |

Lumbar disk herniations commonly occur because of stresses on the disk (trauma) or due to degenerative changes as the water content of the disk decreases. Disk herniation is more common in people under the age of 50 years. There are 4 types of disk herniation. A **herniated disk (protrusion)** occurs when the nucleus pulposus pushes outward but does not completely rupture the annulus; herniation most commonly occurs posteriorly or posterolateral. The layperson's term for this condition is a *bulging disk*. A prolapsed disk occurs when the nucleus pulposus bulges into the annulus and the outermost fibers prevent the nucleus material from moving into the epidural space. A disk extrusion is more severe; the nucleus pulposus breaches the annulus fibrosis and moves into the epidural space. Any of these conditions can put pressure on a nerve root. If the disk herniation increases pressure on a spinal nerve root level, the patient may present with pain, paresthesia, decreased reflexes, and weakness in the affected dermatome/myotome. Pain can be located in the low back and can radiate down into the lower extremity if a nerve root is impinged/compressed. Anterior protrusions may present with pain but no neurologic symptoms. Posterior and posterolateral disk injuries usually respond better to extension exercises because this motion tends to centralize the disk material back toward the center of the disk. A sequestrated disk occurs when fragments of the nucleus pulposus of a herniated disk material break off and migrate into the spinal canal. This can lead to pressure on the spinal cord, causing myelopathy or creating pressure on the cauda equina (called *cauda equina syndrome*), which may cause saddle anesthesia (S3, S4, or S5 nerves) or bowel/bladder problems. A sequestrated disk can also create compression on nerve roots.[11,15]

During the initial evaluation, the physical therapist will assess for the underlying cause of the radicular symptoms to ensure that treatments target the appropriate structures; this is important when a patient presents with sciatica (ie, pain along the sciatic nerve distribution). Sciatica can be caused by a disk herniation, but an alternate source of the pain can be more distal nerve compression in which the nerve passes through a tight piriformis muscle.

**Table 15-8**

Treatment-Based Classification System: Approaches for Low Back Pain[3,31]

| | Symptom Modulation | Movement Control | Functional Optimization |
|---|---|---|---|
| Patient presentations or reports: Clinical findings | Pain: High/moderate<br>Symptom status: Volatile (easily irritated/aggravated by minor movements)<br>Disability: High | Pain: Moderate/low<br>Symptom status: Stable<br>Disability: Moderate | Pain: Low/none<br>Symptom status: Controlled<br>Disability: Low |
| Goals | Reduce/control pain. Centralize symptoms. Determine directional preference. | Improve motor control.<br>Deep muscle–independent activation and isolation; disassociated coordinated motion of thoracic/lumbar spine, lumbopelvic, and pelvis/hip motions with various activities.<br>Effective transition/assimilation of learned skills with functional activities. | Increase muscle strength, power and endurance.<br>Return to sport or work activities without fear/anxiety. |
| Treatment interventions | Active rest: Perform activities pain free; do not increase symptoms<br>Traction: Mechanical/manual, positional traction, or nonweighted positions<br>Joint mobilization performed by physical therapist<br>Direction preference exercises and positioning<br>Flexion, extension, neutral spine<br>Modalities<br>Patient education | Muscle activation<br>Activate/isolate: Drawing-in maneuver, abdominal bracing, multifidi contractions in neutral spine position<br>Skill acquisition: Initiate cocontractions and alternating trunk perturbations to increase core stability.<br>Perform neutral spine unilateral exercises and single-plane exercises with upper or lower extremity motions progress by changing positions using 2 extremities simultaneously.<br>Improve balance and motor control.<br>Initiate transitional stabilization controlled movement from one position to another<br>Assimilation: Perform exercises simulating functional activities (eg, squats for lifting and resisted trunk rotation for mopping) | Introduce high-level challenging exercises to increase strength, endurance, and power (eg, quadruped or planks on foam rolls, side planks with upper extremity/lower extremity movements, prone/supine activities on therapy balls, twisting exercises on various surfaces with weighted ball, squats/lifting activities).<br>Address any observable impairments in the movement system that occur with activity progression. |

Spinal stenosis is a narrowing of a canal (spinal or intervertebral foramina) that can result in nerve root or spinal cord compression. It is often a result of osteoarthritis affecting the vertebral body and/or facet joints (Figure 15-3A). Patients usually experience LBP (with/without radicular symptoms) with lumbar extension, standing, and/or walking. Symptoms often improve with sitting, lying down, or forward bending.

**Spondylosis**, degenerative joint disease, and osteoarthritis are more common in adults older than 45 years of age; these terms are used interchangeably. Both the intervertebral disks and facet joints are subject to wear and tear over time, and bone spurs (osteophytes) can also form on the vertebral body and/or facets (Figure 15-3B). Faulty posture, prolonged immobilization, and severe or repetitive trauma can cause irritation to these structures. Spinal stenosis, degenerative joint disease, and facet irritation usually respond better with exercises that are flexion bias, but clinicians need to determine which directional preference relieves pain or centralizes the symptoms best.[11,15]

Ankylosing spondylitis is an inflammatory disease that can affect thoracic, lumbar spines, and SI joints (and, in some cases, proximal extremity joints). In the progressive later stages, it results in the fusing of the vertebrae, which is referred to as a *bamboo spine* (Figure 15-4). This condition affects men more often than women and appears in adolescents and young adults. Patients usually walk with a stooped posture, and extension exercises should be encouraged to maintain spinal mobility.[15]

**Spondylolysis** is a stress fracture of the pars interarticularis (Figure 15-5). **Spondylolisthesis** occurs when the fractured pars interarticularis separates and the fractured vertebra shifts forward on the vertebra directly below it; this most commonly occurs at L5-S1 (but can also occur at L4-L5). Spondylolisthesis is typically caused by spondylolysis. Both conditions are most commonly observed in adolescents who participate in sports in which repetitive lumbar extension forces are greatest. Degenerative spondylolisthesis is less common and occurs in older adults (more than 40 years); it presents with LBP that increases with activity, muscle spasms, and tenderness with palpation and may present with skin creases posteriorly or on the abdomen. Spondylolisthesis can progress to lumbar instability. Patients with lumbar instability often report "clicking/clunking," "locking," or "catching" and pain with transitional activities or sustained postures.[15] Patients may report a frequent need to self-manipulate their spine. Lumbar instability, spondylolysis, and spondylolisthesis are best addressed in a neutral spine position with strengthening of the local deep muscles.[15,29]

Lumbar facet joint syndrome/zygapophyseal joint dysfunction presents with LBP and muscle guarding in all motions, exacerbated especially with lumbar hyperextension or lateral bending. The patient presents with decreased mobility. Treatment includes a mobilization-based focus, which often includes joint manipulations, flexibility exercises, and correction of movement impairments.

Lumbar compression fractures are often associated with osteoporosis and occur more commonly in older women (more than 70 years). Some causes include falls, a direct blow to the spine, or a MVA. Prolonged use of corticosteroids is also a risk factor for sustaining compression fractures without a traumatic event. These fractures are common in the thoracic spine and are associated with kyphosis. Common symptoms include increased pain with weight bearing and point tenderness over the fracture site.[5,24] Physical therapist assistants should immediately report any of the symptoms stated previously because they are considered a red flag.[24] Burst fractures are the most dangerous type of compression fracture because bone fragments can scatter and migrate toward the spinal cord causing severe injury. Because the vertebral body is the structure most commonly fractured, forward flexion or combined flexion and rotation exercises should be avoided for these patients.

Lumbar strain or sprain usually occurs as a result of acute injury/trauma or repetitive stresses. During the acute phase, patients typically report limited ROM and localized pain that increases with activity or sleeping. Treatment typically focuses on pain control (education, positioning, and modalities as indicated), with an early emphasis on the importance of movement vs full rest. AROM, resistance exercises, stretching, patient education, and body mechanics training are all typically included during the treatment progressions.

Patients referred for physical therapy immediately after spinal surgery require additional consideration. Physical therapist assistants need to carefully review the physical therapy evaluation, medical diagnosis, orthopedic stabilization procedure, and the surgeon's postoperative protocol and restrictions before treatment. Treatments typically include pain control, back protection, and/or proper donning/doffing of a brace; positioning; bed mobility and transfer training; and functional mobility retraining (with assistive devices as indicated). Progressions are based on physician orders/protocols for ROM, resistance exercise, and stretching. Clinicians should include interventions (if medically appropriate) to decrease the risk of postoperative complications, such as early movement (vs bed rest), breathing exercises/incentive spirometer, ankle pumps, and deep vein thrombosis prevention.

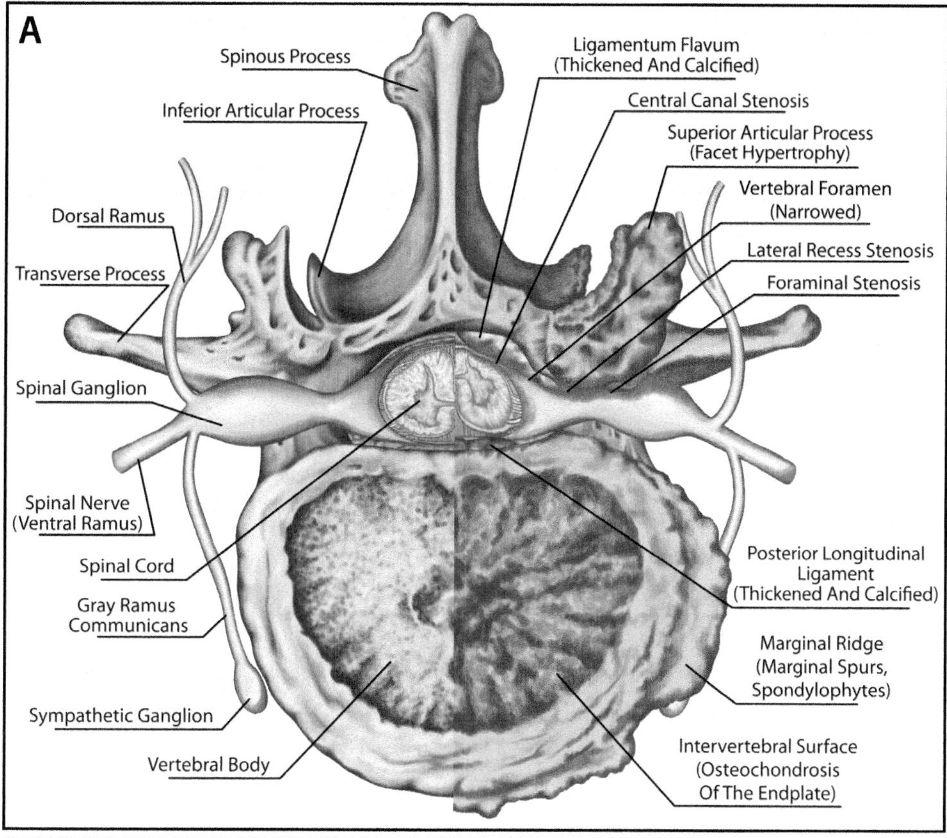


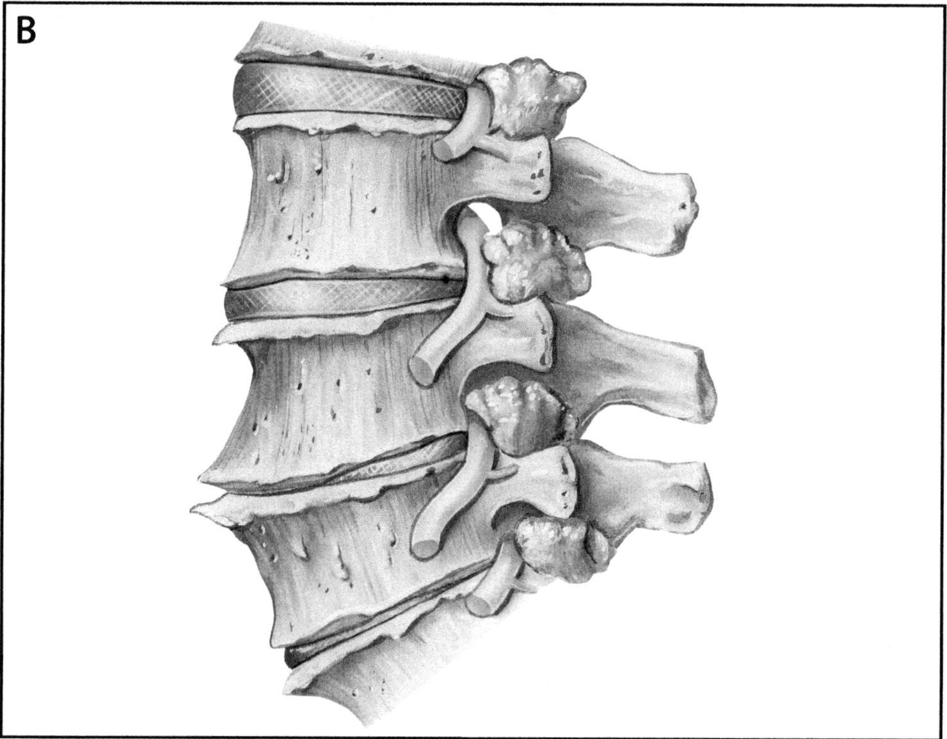


**Figure 15-3.** (A) The overhead view. The left side is normal, and the right side illustrates spinal stenosis with canal narrowing and degenerative changes (stihii/Shutterstock.com). (B) The lateral view. Spondylosis and facet joint osteoarthritis (osteophytes), intervertebral foramina narrowing with nerve compression, decreased disk height, and bony outgrowth of vertebral bodies (Medical Art Inc/Shutterstock.com).

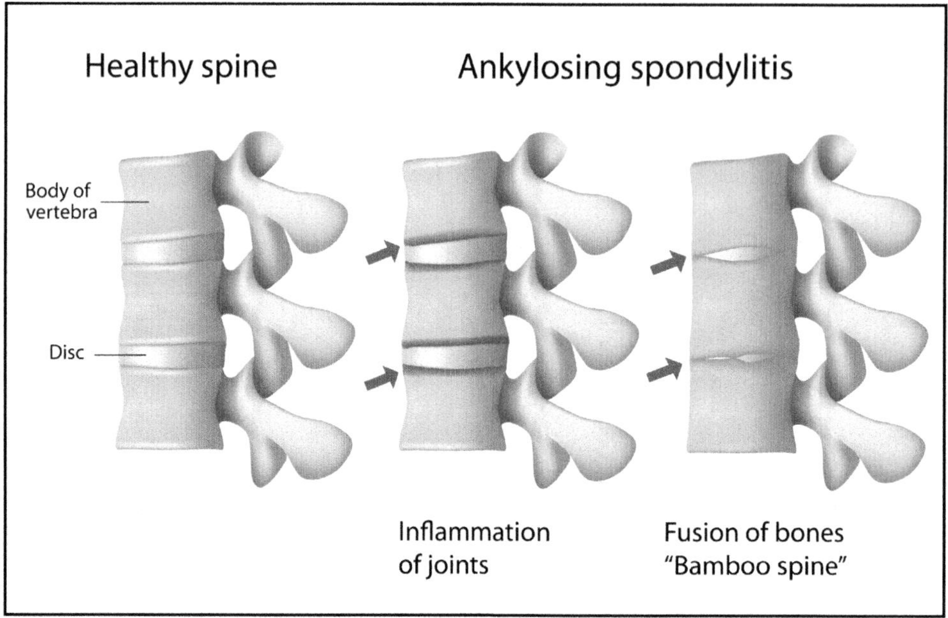


**Figure 15-4.** Ankylosing spondylitis disease progression (Alila Medical Media/Shutterstock.com).

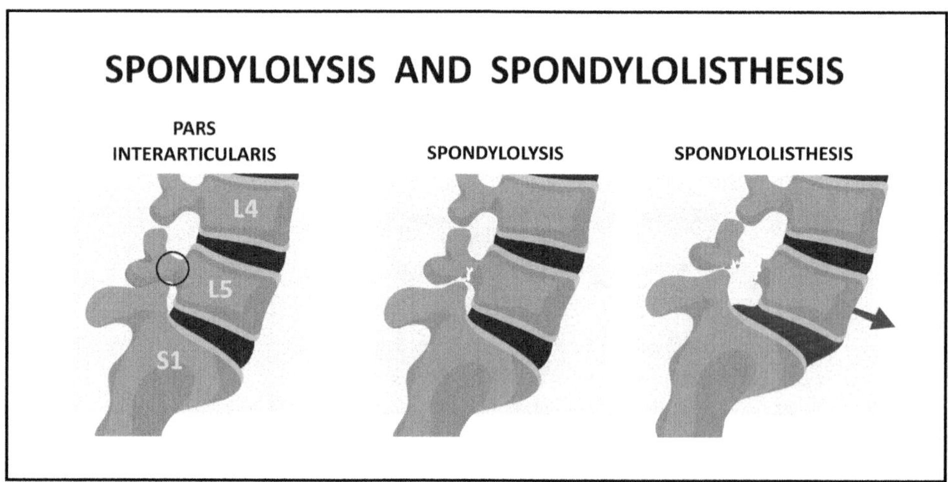


**Figure 15-5.** Spondylolysis and spondylolisthesis. Note that the pars interarticularis is a portion of the lamina between the superior and inferior facets (logika600/Shutterstock.com).

The mechanism of injury for SI pain/dysfunction may be due to a sudden event such as a fall (on the buttocks), an MVA, or landing hard on one or both feet, but this is not always true. Repetitive rotation with or without axial loading such as bending, twisting, lifting, or participating in sports (eg, golf, baseball, soccer) can also create SI pain. As many as 27% of all cases of LBP may originate from the SI joint.[22] Patients with LBP originating from the SI joint often present with symptoms that are worse when moving from sitting to standing, sitting or standing for prolonged periods, and/or stair climbing. Other symptoms may include unilateral sacral area pain (lateral and inferior to the PSIS) or LBP (but no radicular pain distal to the knee), referred pain into the buttocks that may include sharp pain that wakes a person after rolling in bed, pain with the single-limb stance on the involved side, or pain/limited motion with trunk extension/ipsilateral lateral bending. Pregnancy or having a leg length discrepancy are additional risk factors.[22,30] Some patients report pain relief when in non–weight-bearing positions. Hip stretches and pelvic floor and core muscle strengthening paired with patient education for pain reduction and increasing stability can improve symptoms.

## Treatment-Based Classification System: Rehabilitation Approaches and Treatments for Low Back Pain

The treatment-based classification system approach is useful to guide selection of the most appropriate treatment interventions (see Table 15-8). The clinician should provide education that is focused on maximizing outcomes, including encouraging early mobility, addressing fear avoidance or pain apprehension behaviors, and providing advice to stay active. The physical therapist generates a POC and establishes the best treatment approach based on the patient's examination/evaluation results and the level of disability (high, medium, or low), symptom status (volatile, controlled, or stable), and pain level (high, moderate, or low to none).[3,27,31] The 3 approaches include symptom modulation, movement control, and functional optimization. The goal is to progress the patient to functional optimization/return-to-function phase. Although patients may move between approaches/phases, the clinician should implement treatment interventions to minimize the likelihood of patients reverting to a lower level of function.

The physical therapist assistant must understand that there are many philosophies of treatment and interventions that can be used when treating patients with LBP diagnoses. These treatment-based classification system approaches can be looked at in parallel terms with the phases of healing (acute, subacute, and return to function); each approach addresses the level of pain and disability as the patient progresses along the continuum and return to function.

## *Symptom Modulation Approach*

Each approach within the treatment-based classification system includes interventions focused on achieving appropriate goals based on the patient's presentation. Understanding the goals for each approach helps to guide clinical decision making. The goal during the symptom modulation phase (early after onset) is controlling severe pain and symptoms (which may be volatile). These patients often present with increased pain during minimal lumbar spine motions in small ranges and usually report that the pain severely limits their activities and ability to move. Treatment interventions usually include active rest, traction, joint mobilizations, and directional preference exercises.[3,31] Modalities and various manual techniques are often used to reduce pain and muscle guarding and to increase tissue mobility.

Active rest activities can include light exercises, walking on land or in a pool, and modifying ADLs. Activities should not increase pain or symptoms. Staying active promotes healing and decreases the intensity of symptoms compared with bed rest.[27] For patients with acute LBP, there is often one position of motion (flexion or extension) that is most comfortable and that minimizes pain and reduces stress/pressure on the inflamed tissues. This directional preference is used to determine appropriate management strategies during treatment. Directional preference and the patient's response should be continually monitored during each treatment session. The centralization of pain (toward the center of the spine) and a reduction/decrease in radicular symptoms (less pain, tingling, or numbness in the leg/foot) is a primary treatment goal in this phase.

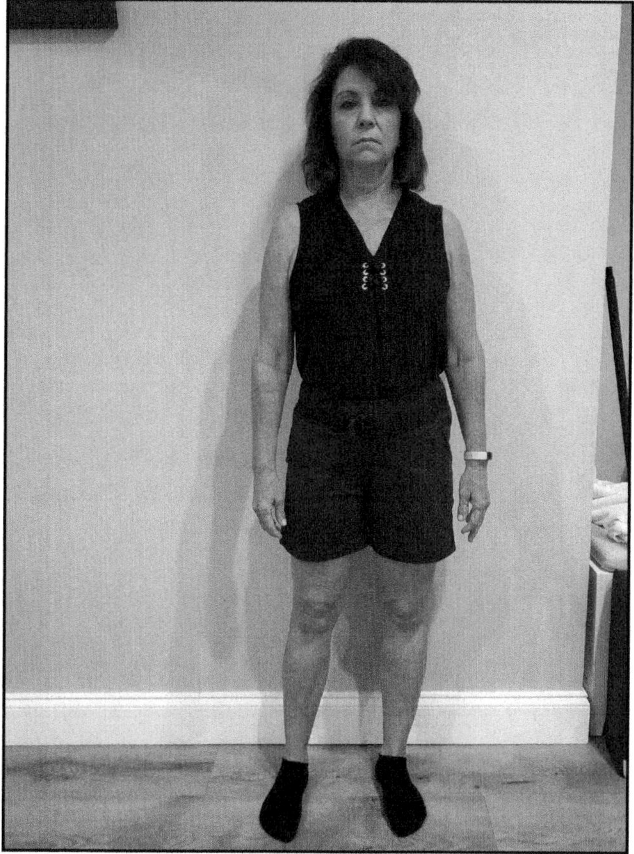

**Figure 15-6.** The patient demonstrates a left lateral shift of the pelvis due to laterally flexed lumbar vertebrae to the right.

Any motion that increases radicular symptoms (peripheralization of symptoms) should be avoided.[18,32]

The key to determining a patient's directional preference is to consider the diagnosis found in the initial evaluation and to listen to the patient's responses as to what movements or positions centralize their pain and reduce the radicular symptoms. The goal is to centralize the pain and then eventually eliminate the patient's symptoms. If the patient's symptoms increase or peripheralize, the assistant should consult the physical therapist before starting/resuming treatment.

Patients with a diagnosis of intervertebral diskogenic involvement (a posterior or posterolateral herniated disk) or forward flexed posture without a lateral shift often benefit from an extension bias approach. Lumbar extension positions or extension exercises reduce the radicular symptoms and centralize the pain into the low back (this is the desired response) for these patients. However, if the patient presents with a lateral shift (Figure 15-6), this *must* be corrected before performing lumbar extension positioning or exercises. The clinician can correct the lateral shift (Figure 15-7A), but patients should also learn to self-correct the shift (Figure 15-7B).

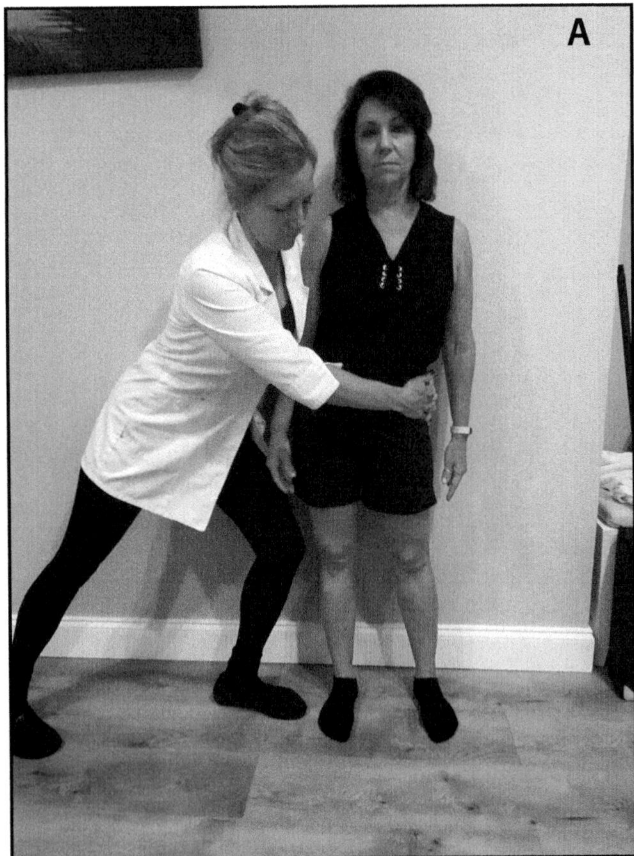


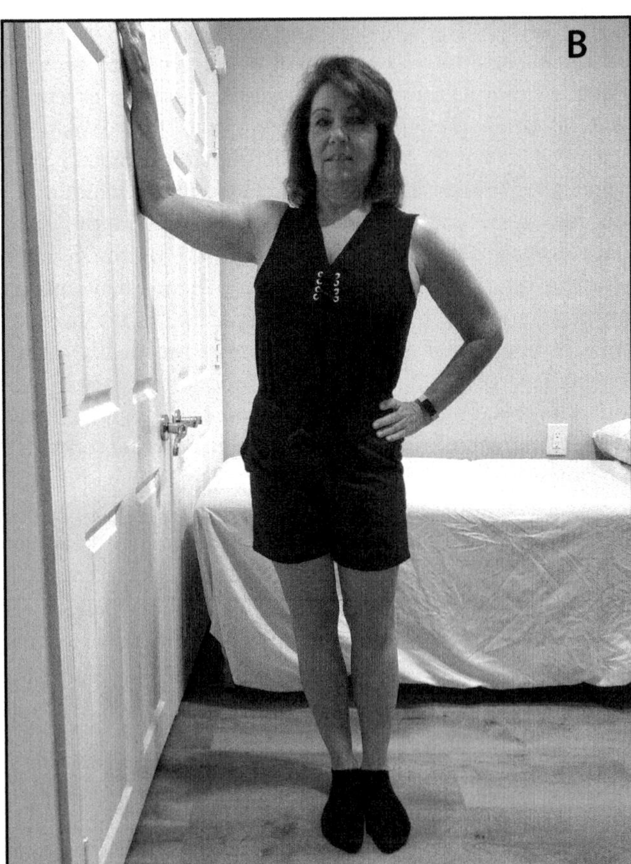


**Figure 15-7.** (A) The therapist applies over-presure to the left pelvis while stabilizing the right shoulder to correct for the lateral shift shown in Figure 15-6. (B) The patient demonstrates lateral shift self-correction. Note the right upper extremity is fixed as over-pressure is applied to the shifted pelvis.

### Considerations for the Physical Therapist Assistant: Identifying a Lateral Shift

A lateral shift is named based on the direction of translation of the shoulders. The pelvis is positioned opposite to the named shift. The lateral shift should be corrected first, and then extension exercises can be implemented. Always monitor the patient's pain level and peripheralization of symptoms throughout the treatment.

It is imperative that patients understand that they should experience an increase in LBP initially as the symptoms centralize and the radicular symptoms dissipate. Inform the patient that the LBP will decrease as well, but it is important that it stays centralized in the low back region and does not radiate.

MDT is a method of assessment and treatment in which a patient is asked to perform different movements repetitively and to assume certain positions for a period of time to determine the directional preference that centralizes and/or reduces symptoms (discussed in Chapter 11). The goal of MDT interventions is to progressively abolish lower extremity symptoms in a distal to central direction; many patients experience centralization with extension bias exercises, especially during the initial phase of rehabilitation.[18,32] Examples of these exercises/positions include lying prone, prone on elbows (supported on forearms), prone press-ups, and standing lumbar extension. Illustrations of these exercises are provided later in this chapter.

Patients with spinal stenosis, spondylosis, facet irritation, or excessive lumbar lordosis tend to have symptom reduction when performing trunk flexion or hip flexion exercises and are considered to have a flexion bias. These exercises are sometimes referred to as *Williams flexion exercises*; illustrations of these exercises are provided later in this chapter. Some of these exercises include PPT, single and double knee to chest, partial sit-up, and hamstring stretches. Hip flexor stretches and squats address flexibility and strength deficits often seen in patients with these diagnoses.

Some patients may report an increase in symptoms during weight bearing (standing or walking) or with movements in any direction but a reduction in symptoms when the spine is unweighted or in non–weight-bearing positions (lying down), especially during the acute phase. This is referred to as non–weight-bearing (or traction) bias. Treatment options that may relieve pain in these patients include spinal traction (mechanical or manual) or unweighting positions, such as vertical suspension in a pool by holding on to the sides or supported by a noodle or aqua vest.

Regardless of the diagnosis or directional preference, the eventual goal is to restore symptom-free full spinal motion. Muscle activation of the deep/local muscles can be initiated during the acute stage if contractions are performed in a position of preference/comfort or neutral spine and if the contraction reduces symptoms (or keeps pain centralized). These muscles assist in stabilizing the spine during transitional movements (eg, rolling in bed, sitting to standing). Table 15-9 lists diagnoses and general treatment intervention suggestions, and Table 15-10 presents a list of exercises/progressions differentiated by directional preference, neutral spine stabilization, or transitional exercises. Neutral spine and directional preference exercise progressions are illustrated in Figures 15-14 through 15-23. As the patient progresses through later phases, additional spinal motions will gradually be added, and the assistant should continue to monitor that the centralization of symptoms is maintained.

## *Movement Control Approach*

Goals for movement control include normalizing joint and soft tissue mobility and neuromuscular control to improve lumbar movement quality. This is achieved through implementing core stabilization and stretching exercises and restoring normal postural and motor movement patterns.[3] Progressing from directional bias exercises to core stabilization occurs after a patient's pain is reduced and the patient demonstrates the ability to centralize symptoms. Once the symptoms are controlled, the patient can begin to resume activities that do not increase pain or the radicular symptoms. However, if symptoms do increase, then directional bias exercises/positions should be initiated immediately to centralize and reduce symptoms.

The mobility of adjacent soft tissue/joint and nerve tissues of the lumbar spine is referred to as *local mobility*.[3,31] Nerve mobility can be assessed using a slump or straight leg raise test, and limitations can be treated using nerve glides/flossing. If joint mobility is hyper- or hypomobile or soft tissue extensibility is limited, normal posture or associated movements cannot be achieved. Various manual therapy techniques can be used to help improve/restore joint or soft tissue mobility, increase ROM, and normalize movement.[3,31] Manual therapy interventions are usually performed by physical therapists and selected based on the patient's diagnosis and clinical presentation.

The local spinal stabilizers are deep muscles that contract to stabilize the lumbar spine and trunk. The global spinal stabilizers activate to perform coordinated movements of the spine, which is necessary to perform trunk motions/activities without compensation or substitution. Exercises should focus on improving motor control through muscle activation of the stabilizers first followed by improving skill acquisition while increasing movement assimilation (in this order).[3] Lumbar spine and trunk muscles need to actively contract to provide stability (local spinal stabilizers) and mobility (global spinal stabilizers) in the trunk region, whereas other regional muscles attaching to the hip/pelvis contract to allow for coordinated actions between the spine and those joints.

> **Clinical Tips**
>
> Local mobility and global stability interventions can be implemented concurrently. The deep local stabilizers (ie, TrA, pelvic floor, and multifidus) need to be activated as early as possible in a spinal position that keeps pain/symptoms centralized and at a moderate to low level. Remember, the goal is to first acquire proximal stability, which is necessary to allow for pain-free distal mobility while maintaining a neutral spine.

Patient education is critical to prevent symptom recurrences. Initial education focuses on ensuring that patients have a good understanding of those spinal positions that reduce radicular symptoms and on how to activate the TrA muscle to stabilize the spine. Education should also focus on instructing the patient to immediately use the appropriate directional preference exercise/position any time symptoms occur. Physical therapist assistants should inform patients to limit prolonged static positions to no more than 30 minutes (ie, standing or sitting) and interrupt those positions often (ie, initially every 10 minutes or at the onset of symptoms) with directional bias exercises. In addition, any exercises performed in the opposite direction of their directional preference should be introduced as early as possible during the rehabilitation process but should always be followed by directional preference exercises/positioning. For example, if a patient with a disk herniation is able to keep symptoms centralized with extension bias exercises, they should be instructed to interrupt (prolonged) sitting with standing lumbar extension and repeat lumbar extension after performing trunk flexion exercises (ie, partial sit-ups).

### Muscle Activation

Muscle activation of local spinal stabilizers is essential for controlling pain and providing segmental and core stability.[3,16,17,19,24,29,31-33] Core muscle training for stability mirrors the principles of motor control by progressing through the stages of stability, mobility, controlled mobility, and skill. The ability to isolate and activate TrA and multifidi muscles is imperative, but it can be challenging for patients initially. These muscles are often weak and/or inhibited in this population, and patients usually require tactile and verbal cuing during exercises initially. TrA weakness and poor timing of its activation are associated with an increase of injury recurrence because it affects spinal stabilization.[16,33-35] TrA muscle activation can be initiated during the acute stage (or symptom modulation approach) only if the exercises centralize and/or decrease the patient's symptoms.

**Table 15-9**

General Intervention Suggestions for Various Diagnoses

| Diagnosis | General Treatment Suggestions for Intervention |
|---|---|
| Ankylosing spondylitis | Exercises: Increase spinal extension, pain control, correct movement impairments, postural education, and diaphragmatic breathing exercises/respiratory muscle strengthening<br>Stretch: Hip flexors and pectoralis major; promote thoracic extension/rotation<br>Strengthen: Trunk/core stabilization, latissimus dorsi, scapula muscles, hip muscles, and body mechanics training<br>Encourage positioning/stretching into extension |
| Compression fracture | Core and scapular stabilization exercises, correct movement impairments, postural education/body mechanics/ergonomic training, and encourage weight-bearing exercises as tolerated<br>Stretch antagonist muscles (ie, hip flexors and hip internal rotators)<br>Avoid trunk flexion exercises (ie, sit-ups) or activities that combine trunk flexion and rotation |
| Diskogenic conditions | Extension bias (based on presentation), address lateral shift first if indicated; nerve glides/flossing (if appropriate), manual or mechanical traction (if symptoms are centralized), stabilization exercises, correct movement impairments, postural education, and body mechanics/ergonomic training |
| Lumbar instability | Core stabilization, correct movement impairments; target hip flexibility and strengthening |
| Lumbar facet joint syndrome/ zygapophyseal joint dysfunction | Flexion bias exercises (based on presentation), joint mobilizations (performed by therapist), correct movement impairments, core stabilization in neutral spine or PPT, stretch lumbar extensors |
| Spinal stenosis | Flexion bias exercises, stabilization exercises, aerobic exercise/graded ambulation program, correct movement impairments, postural education, balance exercises; stretch hip flexors and lumbar paraspinals |
| Spondylolysis, spondylolisthesis | Pain control, stabilization exercises in neutral spine, resistance exercises, planks, correct movement impairments, add trunk rotation exercises, postural education, and aerobic exercises; stretch hamstring, hip flexors rotators, and gluteal muscles<br>Avoid lumbar hyperextension exercises/activities |
| Spondylosis (degenerative disk disease, degenerative joint disease, arthritis) | Pain control; bias based on presentation; stabilization exercises, resistance trunk exercises, correction of movement impairments, and postural education<br>Stretch hamstrings and hip flexors<br>Avoid high-impact activities and excessive lumbar hyperextension |
| SI dysfunction | General treatment: Core, lumbar, and pelvic floor stabilization exercises in neutral spine; stretch hip flexors, hip strengthening (ie, adduction, extension, and external rotation)<br>SI hypermobility: Consider a pelvic/SI brace, core stabilization exercises, and strengthen weak core muscle to create balance between opposing muscle groups<br>SI ligament/joint strain: Directional preference positioning; core stabilization exercises followed by hip/trunk strengthening<br>SI rotation/torsion: MET to correct innominate rotation; follow with stretching and/or strengthening based on individual presentation |

Note: Refer to Table 15-2 for red flags and Table 15-10 for exercises and progression.
MET = muscle energy technique.

**Table 15-10**

Directional Preference, Neutral Spine, and Transitional Exercises and Progressions

| Extension Bias Exercises | Flexion Bias Exercises | Neutral Spine Stabilization and Plank Exercises | Transitional Exercises (Moving From Flexion to Extension) |
|---|---|---|---|
| Patient positioning:<br>• Supine with a towel/lumbar roll in low back<br>• Prone with pillow under the chest<br>Exercises:<br>• Lateral shift correction (perform before extension)<br>• Prone on elbows/forearms<br>• Prone press-up<br>• Standing back extension<br>• Prone hip extension<br>• Prone opposite arm and leg lifts<br>• Prone active lumbar extension on physioball (add arm positions: At side, overhead)<br>• Prone extension on floor<br>• Prone Superman<br>• Quadruped with an anterior pelvic tilt<br>• Progress to quadruped posterior to anterior tilting (cat/camel)<br>• Quadruped lateral trunk/pelvic flexion (dog wagging its tail)<br>• Quadruped trunk rotation (upper extremity reaches to opposite lower extremity side) | Patient positioning:<br>• Supine with pillow under thighs/knees; hips and knees at 90/90 degrees; hook lying<br>• Prone with pillow under the stomach<br>Exercises:<br>• PPT<br>• Single knee to chest<br>• Double knee to chest<br>• Hamstring stretches<br>• Hip flexor stretches<br>• Prayer stretches<br>• Lower trunk rotation supine<br>• Seated trunk flexion<br>• Partial curl ups (crunches)<br>• Partial/deep squats<br>• Quadruped cat<br>• Progress to cat and camel<br>• Quadruped lateral trunk/pelvic flexion<br>• Quadruped trunk rotation | Deep muscle activation:<br>• Drawing-in maneuver<br>• Abdominal bracing<br>• Multifidus facilitation<br>• Kegel's pelvic floor<br>*Once patients can successfully perform drawing-in (hollowing) maneuver, multifidi contraction, and abdominal bracing, progressions can be initiated (based on patient presentation/SINSS).* | • Prayer stretch to press-up<br>• Kneeling trunk chops<br>• Bridging progression<br>• Pain-free bridging available ROM with feet flat<br>• Full bridging feet flat<br>• Bridge with ankles dorsiflexed<br>• Bridging with alternating knee lifts (marching); alternating knee flexion/extension<br>• Single-leg bridging one knee flexed<br>• Single-leg bridging straight leg raise<br>• Bridges on physioball: First calves and then ankles; progress to moving ball in and out, and then attempt moving legs laterally with legs straight |

*(continued)*

**Table 15-10 (continued)**

Directional Preference, Neutral Spine, and Transitional Exercises and Progressions

| Extension Bias Exercises | Flexion Bias Exercises | Neutral Spine Stabilization and Plank Exercises | Transitional Exercises (Moving From Flexion to Extension) |
|---|---|---|---|
| | | Stabilization exercise progression[a]:<br>• Supine<br>• Single-arm flexion<br>• Bilateral arm flexion<br>• Unilateral heel slides<br>• Independent hip rotation (3 positions)<br>• Alternating straight leg raise<br>• Dead bugs: Reciprocal arm and leg lifts (start in heel slide position/lower extremity supported and then progress to leg lift/lower extremity unsupported)<br>• Quadruped<br>• Single-arm flexion<br>• Single-leg extension (start sliding leg into hip extension; progress to hip extension lift)<br>• Opposite arm/leg lifts (bird dog)<br>• Opposite arm/leg moves with weights<br>• Single-hip abduction knee flexed<br>• Single-hip abduction with knee flexion and extension<br>Note: to increase difficulty have patient perform on balance discs, foam rolls, or 65-cm/85-cm physioball. | |

*(continued)*

**Table 15-10 (continued)**

Directional Preference, Neutral Spine, and Transitional Exercises and Progressions

| Extension Bias Exercises | Flexion Bias Exercises | Neutral Spine Stabilization and Plank Exercises | Transitional Exercises (Moving From Flexion to Extension) |
|---|---|---|---|
| | | Plank exercise progression[a]<br>Prone:<br>• On forearms and knees<br>• On forearms and toes<br>• Plank with arms and legs extended<br>• Plank with added hip extension<br>• Plank hip/knee flexion/extension<br>• Plank on physioball<br>• Plank with arm walk outs with legs on a physioball<br>• Plank on physioball/balance discs add opposite arm/leg lifts and/or trunk rotation<br>Side:<br>• On knees and forearm<br>• Legs straight on forearm<br>• Legs straight with a straight arm<br>• Then with shoulder abduction, progress to shoulder horizontal abduction/trunk rotation and then with hip and shoulder abduction then flexion/extension | |

*(continued)*

**Table 15-10 (continued)**

Directional Preference, Neutral Spine, and Transitional Exercises and Progressions

| Extension Bias Exercises | Flexion Bias Exercises | Neutral Spine Stabilization and Plank Exercises | Transitional Exercises (Moving From Flexion to Extension) |
|---|---|---|---|
| | | Standing:<br>• Partial squats (hitching at hips)<br>• Squats double leg to lunges to single-leg squats<br>• Squats with handheld weights | |
| *Contact the physical therapist emergently for reassessment when pain does not change with a change in position or reports of saddle paresthesia or bowel/bladder changes. Avoid motions, activities, exercises, or interventions that create/increase peripheralization of symptoms.* | | | |

[a]Neutral spine position with deep/local muscles engaged. Clinician to initially use verbal and tactile cuing when performing any new exercise to reinforce muscle engagement. Patients needs to develop kinesthetic awareness of the neutral spine position.

There are 2 ways to contract core stabilizers (specifically, the TrA): one method is the drawing-in (abdominal hollowing) maneuver, and the other is abdominal bracing. The drawing-in maneuver involves contraction of the TrA, and during abdominal bracing, the TrA and the oblique muscles perform a cocontraction.

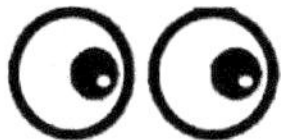

## Eye on the Research: Comparing Drawing-In Versus Abdominal Bracing Maneuvers

Research indicates that core stability exercises are more effective than general exercises in decreasing pain and increasing functional status in persons with back pain.[34,35] There are several studies examining the role of the TrA and the methods used to activate and create tension in this muscle. The TrA is a deep muscle of the anterior abdominal wall; it plays a significant role in spine stabilization. There has been discussion of whether the drawing-in/hollowing maneuver or abdominal bracing maneuver is better to create tension and provide core stability.

Several studies reported that the inward movement of the lower abdominal wall in supine (drawing-in or hollowing maneuver) produced greater activity of the TrA (vs the internal or external obliques or rectus abdominis).[19,32,33] One study reported that the abdominal drawing-in maneuver facilitates the deep muscles and more effectively stabilizes the trunk compared with other lumbar stabilization exercises.[36] Other research indicated that abdominal bracing exercises can result in greater TrA activation and spine stabilization compared with hollowing.[33,34] Park and Yu[33] noted a statistically significant relationship between pain reduction (based on the Oswestry Disability Index) and increased TrA muscle thickness using a drawing-in maneuver. They also reported increased thickness of the internal obliques using core stabilizing exercises. However, investigators noted that abdominal bracing creates better spinal stability against sudden trunk perturbations.[33] Another study revealed the cross-sectional area of the TrA was greater in the drawing-in group but that the bracing group showed a statistically significant increase in the cross-sectional area in the bilateral internal and external oblique muscles in middle-aged healthy women, thereby also increasing core stability.[37] Moghadam et al[34] compared both techniques in supine, hook lying, bridging, and quadruped opposite arm/leg exercises and found the highest activation of the TrA occurred during bridging using abdominal bracing. These researchers concluded that abdominal bracing could be beneficial in increasing core stability in healthy subjects, and they suggested that the drawing-in maneuver may be more useful in patients with spinal instability or altered muscle

Patients often struggle to understand how to complete core stability exercises; careful instruction and verbal and tactile cues can guide the patient to perform these exercises correctly. The clinician and patient (together) can use tactile cues to help the patient activate the TrA using a drawing-in (abdominal hollowing) maneuver (Figure 15-8). The patient is first positioned supine in hook lying and instructed to move the low back into a position of comfort or into a neutral spine position. To find the position of comfort or neutral spine, the patient should perform an anterior pelvic tilt and then move slowly into a PPT position and then again move the pelvis anteriorly slowly until they achieve a pain-free or neutral spine position. The pelvis should not be held in a full PPT because a PPT activates the rectus abdominis, not the TrA. Once the pelvis is positioned, the clinician should have the patient place their hands just medially to the ASIS with the fingers flat and pointing toward the midline and the thumbs circling the waist with one hand on each side for feedback. The assistant can place one hand behind the lumbar spine and the other over one of the patient's hands as an additional cue. The patient is then instructed to "draw your belly toward your spine" or "suck in your stomach"[39] and hold for 10 seconds. The patient should also be instructed to count to 10 aloud to avoid the Valsalva maneuver. Alternately, they can exhale during the drawing in. The spine and pelvis should remain stationary, but the muscle contraction should be palpable. If available, the assistant can use the Stabilizer Pressure Biofeedback Unit (DJO, LLC; Figure 15-9) and place it under the lumbar spine. The device is pumped up to about 40 mm Hg, and the patient is instructed to increase the pressure to 42 to 44 mm Hg during the maneuver. Again, the patient is instructed to hold the isometric contraction for 10 seconds and to count aloud to facilitate breathing. A goal of several sets (5 to 7) and repetitions (10) with a 5-second rest between repetitions should be performed, but the sets should be gradually increased to improve stability and muscle endurance.[36] Eventually, patients should maintain the hollowing maneuver while performing all other exercises as the patient progresses.

Abdominal bracing activates a cocontraction of the TrA and internal/external oblique muscles.[36] The patient should not draw in or extend the abdomen by pushing out. Patient positioning and hand positioning are the same as described previously for the drawing-in maneuver. When performing abdominal bracing, the patient is instructed to "take a deep breath, then slowly blow out as if you are blowing up a balloon" (Figure 15-10). The patient should feel the muscles press outward toward the fingers that are positioned just medially to the ASIS. The balloon blowing maneuver eliminates the risk of the Valsalva maneuver. The patient should eventually be able to perform abdominal bracing without

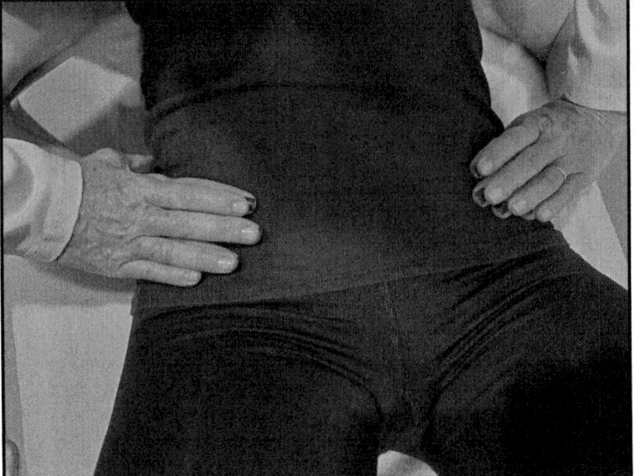

**Figure 15-8.** The drawing-in or hollowing maneuver with palpation.

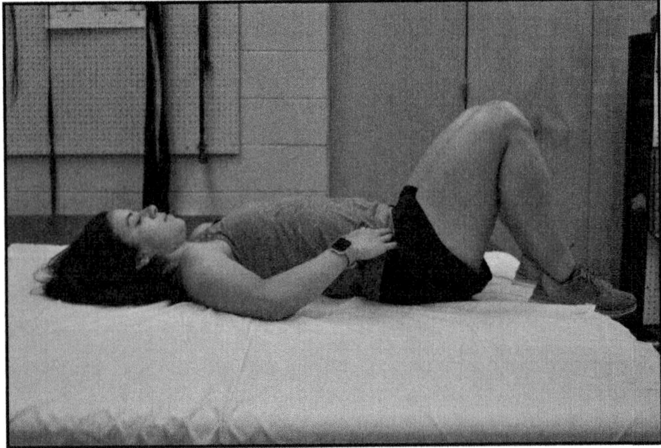

**Figure 15-10.** An abdominal bracing exercise with palpation.

these instructions. The act of coughing or laughing also engages these muscles and can be used as another method of cuing for abdominal bracing.

## Clinical Tips

To help the patient understand how to maintain a neutral spine position, the physical therapist assistant can say, "Pretend I put a grape under your low back. When you draw in or perform abdominal bracing, don't squish the grape."

The multifidi muscles provide spinal segmental stability; yet, these muscles are usually inhibited in patients with LBP. Patients need to understand how these muscles work so they can learn to voluntarily contract them. These muscles are very small and lie deep to the paraspinals, but they can be palpated when contracted. To palpate these muscles, the patient should be positioned prone and with a neutral spine. Placing a pillow under the patient's stomach may help the muscles relax and make it easier to palpate them when contracted. Multifidi are more developed in the

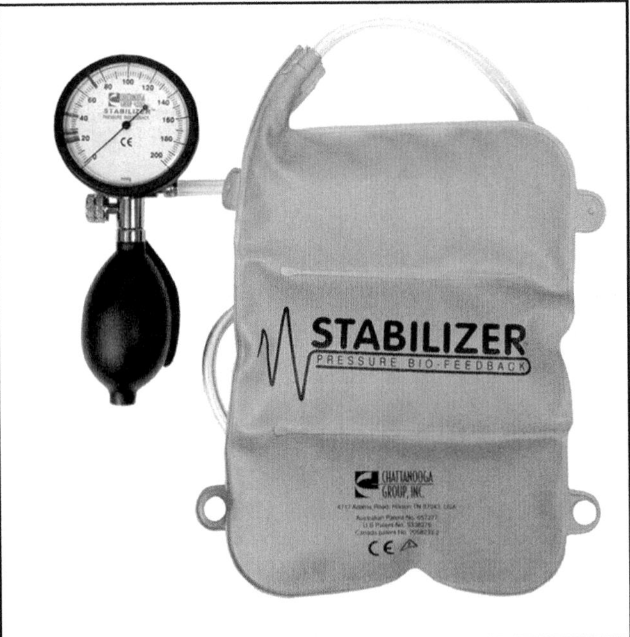


**Figure 15-9.** The Chattanooga Stabilizer Pressure Biofeedback. (DJO and Chattanooga are registered trademarks of DJO, LLC in the U.S. and/or other countries. ©2020 DJO, LLC. Used with permission from DJO, LLC. All rights reserved.)

lumbar spine, progressively increasing in size from L1 to L5. It is helpful to palpate each level to determine muscle activation at each level, in addition to each side (left or right).[40] To palpate the muscles, the clinician should place 2 fingers (or thumbs) just lateral to the spinous processes on either side of the lumbar spine and let them sink down into the muscles (Figure 15-11A). Place a small, rolled towel under the left ASIS and then instruct the patient to "push down into the towel with 20% effort." Because these muscles also rotate, the clinician should feel the multifidus on the right contract (Figure 15-11B). Then, repeat on the other side. Patients should be able to activate and isolate these stabilizing muscles in a neutral spine position while using normal breathing patterns before progressing to the next level (skill acquisition).

## Considerations for the Physical Therapist Assistant: When Is It Best to Initiate Muscle Activation

The drawing-in maneuver, abdominal bracing, multifidi muscle contraction, and/or pelvic floor activation should be initiated as soon as possible as long as the symptoms are not increased. Training to complete these exercises is initiated in the acute phase of the rehabilitation process within the first or second week if possible. The clinician should determine which of these activation techniques is best suited for the patient. Muscle activation is initially performed in the patient's position of comfort or directional preference, but the goal is to perform contractions in a neutral spine position (without any increase in symptoms).

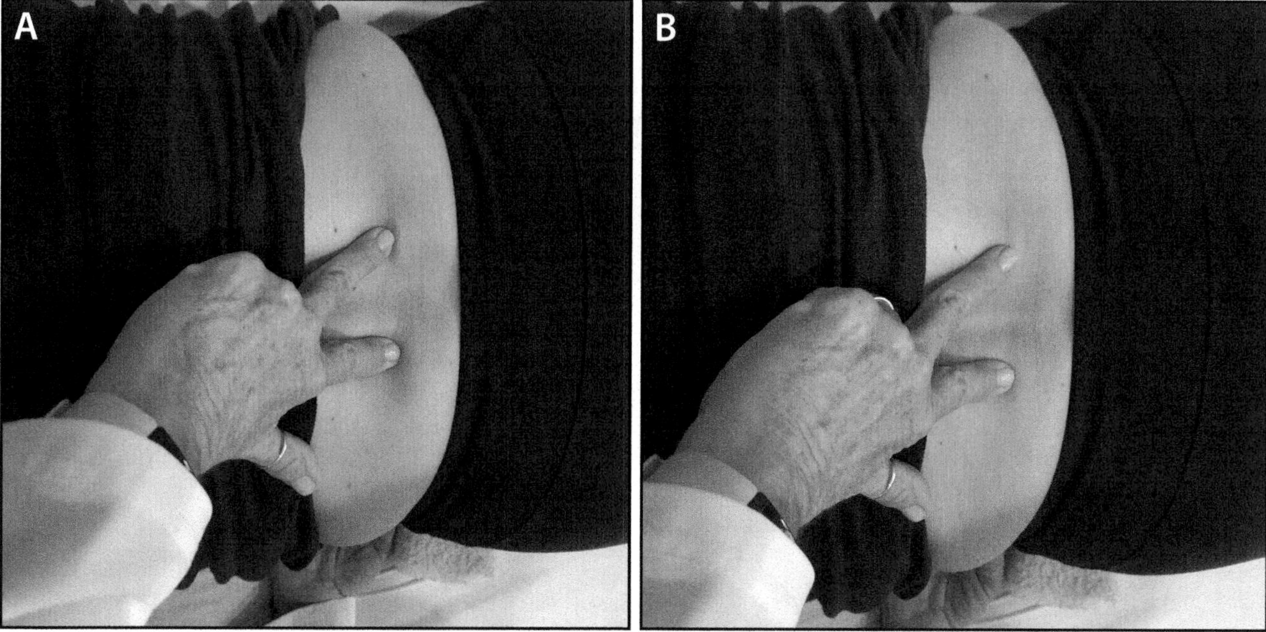


**Figure 15-11.** (A) The multifidi muscles are relaxed. Observe the clinician's finger location and how they are sunken into the tissue. (B) Right multifidi muscles are contracting. Observe the clinician's right hand under the left ASIS cuing the patient to push down into it.

## Skill Acquisition Approach

The goal of skill acquisition is for patients to disassociate and coordinate thoracic/lumbar spine, pelvis, and hip motions while performing single-plane cocontraction exercises. Prone active hip extension or a supine straight leg raise can be used to test the patient's ability to perform these exercises correctly with the core engaged. A patient should be able to maintain a supine neutral spine position while lifting both arms overhead or performing a straight leg raise without increasing/decreasing lordosis, rocking the pelvis, or using compensatory rotary movements. If the patient is unable to perform these exercises correctly, then the clinician needs to provide cuing and guidance until the skill (or exercise) is acquired. Those exercises should not become part of their home exercise program until they learn how to perform them correctly while maintaining good spinal position.[3] Exercises should be progressed to include active spinal movements in all directions regardless of their initial directional preference. After a patient is able to isolate and maintain the local deep stabilizing muscles in a posture with activity, exercise difficulty can be progressed. A general progression for stabilization exercises includes moving one and then both upper extremities, moving one and then both lower extremities, and then combining opposite arm and leg exercises. These exercises can be performed first in supine (sometimes called the *dead bug exercise*), then progressed to quadruped on a firm surface, and then progressed to completing the exercises on an unstable surface (ie, a therapy ball, half or full foam rolls, or balance discs); progressions are dependent on the patient's goals. Alternating isometric contractions and rhythmic stabilization (manual perturbation in sitting and then standing) should be initiated and progressed. Once muscle strength and endurance are established, patients can be progressed to more challenging transitional tasks/exercises (ie, moving from one position to another) and balance and coordination exercises on a stable surface and then progressed to unstable surfaces.

MET is a manual therapy technique that uses a patient-controlled submaximal isometric muscle contraction to normalize joint motion and reduce lumbopelvic or SI pain. The technique has been shown to be effective in correcting asymmetrical pelvic alignment (or rotation) and muscle imbalances in the lumbopelvic region and in reducing patient-reported LBP.[41] Table 15-11 explains the appropriate technique to test and realign the pelvis/SI joints for an anterior innominate rotation using MET,[23,41] and Figure 15-12 illustrates the technique. There are other variations of this technique that can be used.

Motor control interventions improve optimal muscle recruitment strategies of the TrA, pelvic floor, and multifidi muscles during static and dynamic activities because larger (global) muscles produce smooth and coordinated motions. Motor control exercises should target and correct movement impairments that limit the patient's motion or ability to complete tasks and ADLs. The ability to complete these exercises successfully and to progress through an exercise sequence will allow the patient to resume ADLs with little to no pain.[3,42]

A patient's ability to maintain a neutral spine position during mobility and fitness exercises results in reduced symptoms.[42] The movement system impairment approach uses motor skill training to correct movement and alignment impairments. Research shows that this approach results in less symptoms than the isolated use of strengthening and flexibility exercises in patients with chronic LBP.[42]

## Table 15-11

## Muscle Energy Technique: Testing and Intervention to Reduce Pelvic and Sacroiliac Asymmetries Due to Innominate Rotation

Testing for anterior/posterior innominate rotation

- Patient lies supine and performs a bridge first to make sure the trunk and pelvis are straight/level.
- Have the patient straighten both legs, and the clinician checks bilateral ASISs to determine if they are even. If the left ASIS is more prominent, then there may be an anterior rotation on that side or a posterior rotation on the right (see Figure 15-12A).
- After checking ASIS levels, check medial malleoli levels while still supine. With an anterior rotation, the left leg will appear longer, or they may appear equal when supine, but with long sitting this may change (see Figure 15-12B).
- Once the patient long sits, see how the malleoli have changed (see Figure 15-12C). If the left side appears to have shortened, then that confirms that the left side is rotated anteriorly (see Figure 15-12D). If the longer side stays long or appears to get longer, then it would be a posterior innominate on that side.

To correct for an anterior innominate

- Have the patient lie supine with their buttocks partially off the treatment table, and place the left leg (the anterior rotated side) over or on the clinician's right shoulder and the right leg in a Thomas test position (see Figure 15-12E).
- Instruct the patient to "gently push (the flexed leg) down into my shoulder" and "push (the extended leg) up into my hand with the opposite leg simultaneously without pain." Resist the submaximal isometric contractions for 5 to 6 seconds (see Figure 15-12F).
- The patient should relax, and the clinician can then push the flexed leg into more flexion and the extended leg into more extension.
- Recheck the level of the malleoli to see if they are equal (see Figure 15-12G).
- If not level, have the patient relax for 5 seconds and repeat the technique 2 to 3 more times. Recheck to determine treatment effectiveness after each technique.

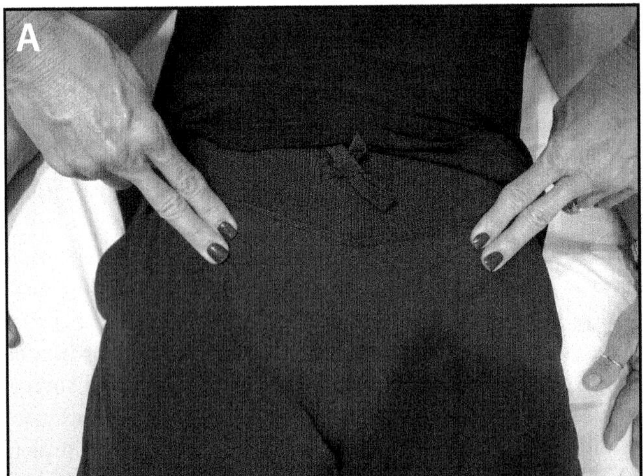


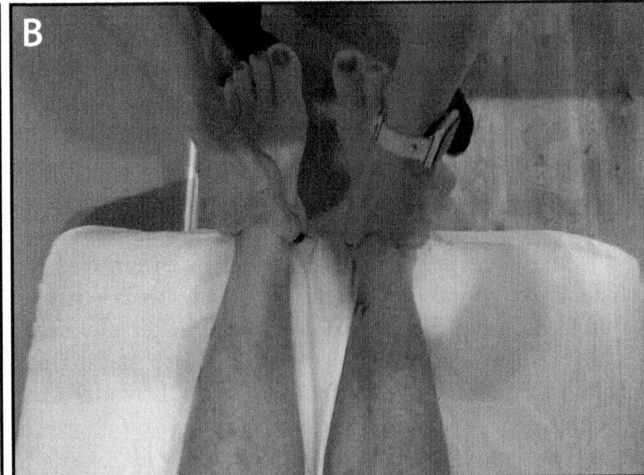


**Figure 15-12.** SI MET to correct for a left anterior rotation. (A) MET technique. First have the patient perform a bridge to level the pelvis. Then extend the legs and check both ASIS to see if they are level. Here the left ASIS is more prominent due to an anterior rotation on that side. (B) Note the left leg (malleolus) looks longer (more distal) than the right. *(continued)*

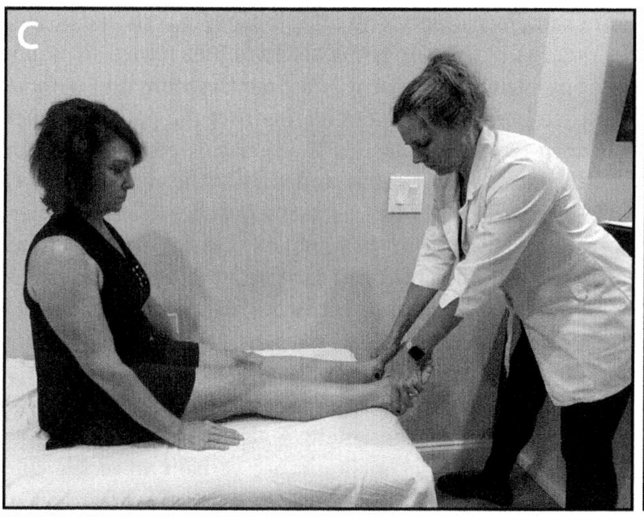


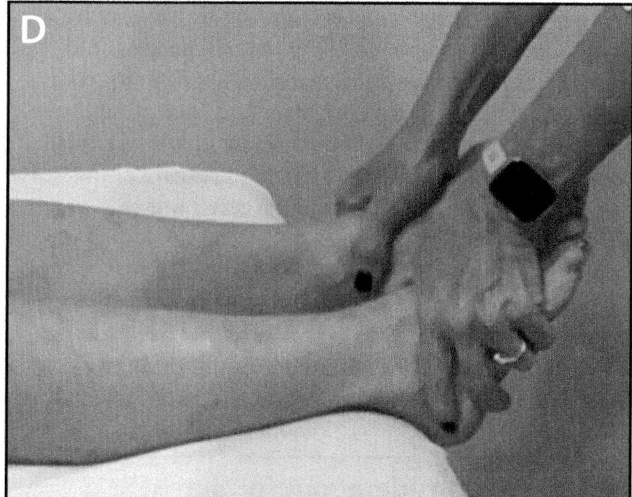


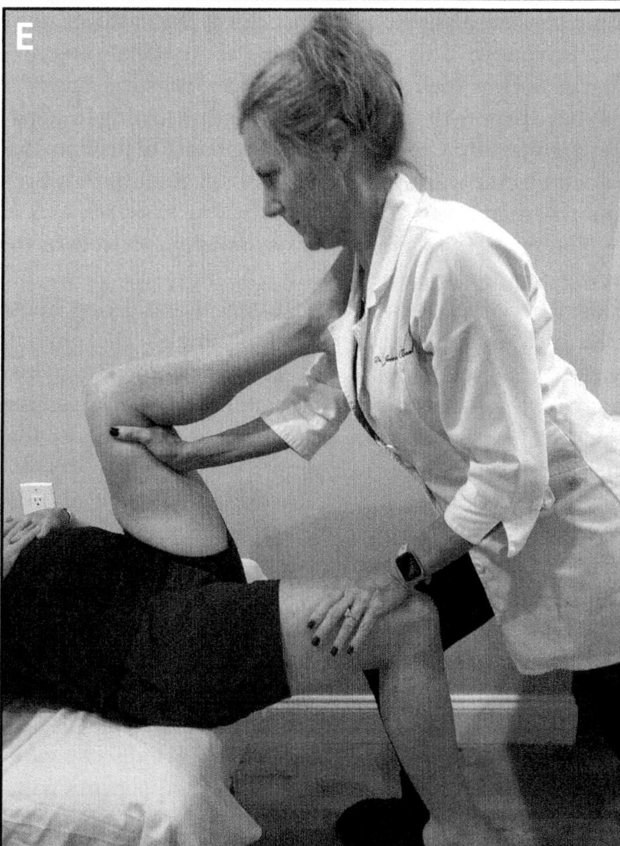


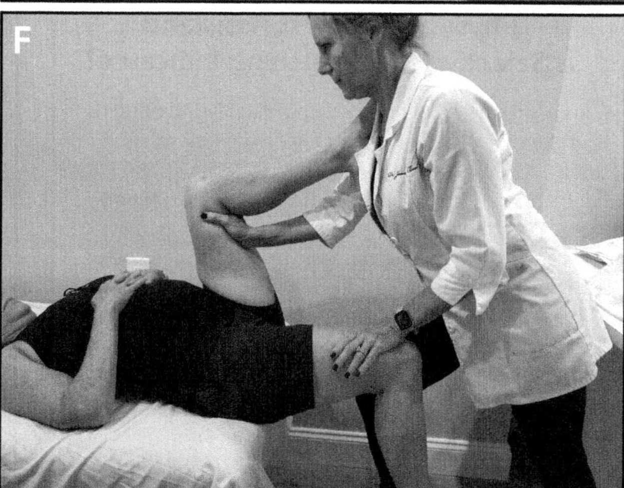


**Figure 15-12 (continued).** (C) Have the patient sit up and check the level of the malleoli. (D) The left malleolus appears to be slightly shorter than the left after sitting. (E) Position the patient to correct the left (anterior rotation) side. The clinician will resist as the patient completes a submaximal isometric contraction of the hip extensors on the left and hip flexors on the right. The gluteal muscles will help rotate the left side by pulling it posteriorly to correct for the anterior rotation. (F) After the isometric contraction, stabilize the left leg posteriorly, and stretch the right hip into extension. After the technique, have the patient perform a bridge, and recheck the malleoli levels to ensure they are even. (G) The malleoli are even after the technique.

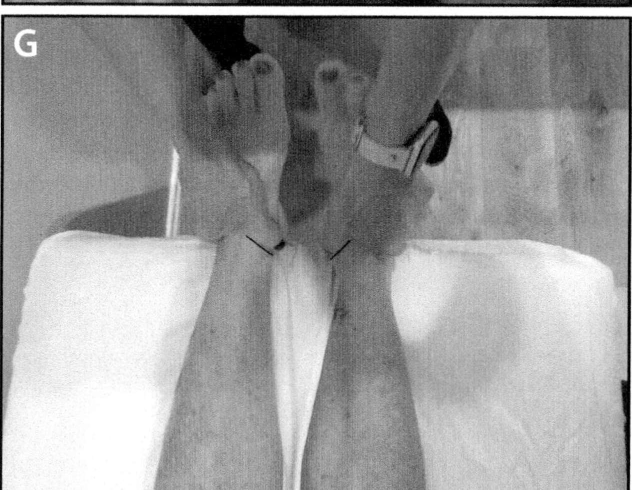

A patient's available ROM, the ability to accurately move/sequence movements of the joints/segments, and the ability to activate muscle firing with appropriate timing and force is critical to reducing pain and correcting abnormal movement patterns. The clinician should verify that thoracic spine, lumbar spine, hip joint mobility, and soft tissue extensibility are all within normal limits to perform all exercises (refer to Chapter 13). Patients with lumbar instability may have limited hip mobility. One study found that patients with chronic LBP and lumbar instability who performed hip exercises in addition to low back exercises had better outcomes and reduced levels of disability compared with those who just performed low back exercises.[43]

### Considerations for the Physical Therapist Assistant: Is Selective Hip Stretching Indicated?

Common patterns of tightness that can lead to ongoing back pain symptoms include tight hip flexors or hamstrings. Assessment to determine if hip flexor or hamstring tightness is present is an important part of the physical therapy examination. If a patient presents with spinal stenosis and hip flexor tightness and symptoms centralize with flexion bias exercises, the physical therapist assistant will need to use selective stretching for the hip flexors. The assistant will use care to maintain a neutral spine/limit excessive lumbar extension when stretching the hip flexors. Similarly, patients with diskogenic conditions who respond well to extension bias exercises, but who also have tight hamstrings will need selective stretching of the hamstrings. Selective stretching of the hamstrings is performed while maintaining a neutral spine or lumbar lordosis during stretches.

## Movement Assimilation

Early in the subacute phase (around week 5 or 6) as a patient's ROM increases, the patient may complain of pain at the end of the available range when the injured tissue/structure is stressed. Patients are usually deconditioned and often present with decreased muscle strength and endurance, difficulty completing some IADLs (especially for prolonged periods of time), decreased postural awareness, and poor body mechanics. The patient may also express apprehension regarding increasing mobility due to fear of increasing pain or causing reinjury. It is the clinician's responsibility to explain that by correcting movement impairments the risk of reinjury can be significantly reduced.

The treatment goal is for patients to be able to move in the opposite direction of their directional preference bias. For example, patients with an extension bias should be able to eventually flex the trunk forward and return to standing one vertebral segment at a time (segmentally) without pain. To perform this activity, instruct the patient to tuck the chin first and then flex the cervical spine followed by the thoracic spine flexion and finally the upper to lower lumbar segments. The reverse sequence should be performed (starting from the lumbar spine up) to return to an upright position. Clinicians can use a motorized treatment table to help the patient perform this activity. Start with the table up as high as possible when the person is standing erect with the hands on the tabletop. Slowly lower the table and guide the patient so they understand how to move into trunk flexion segmentally. Raise the table to return to standing. The clinician should use verbal and tactile cues to ensure the activity is performed correctly. After fear or apprehension dissipates, patients can perform this activity independently. This activity helps the patient recognize that as long as their core stabilizers are engaged, they will not have pain with flexing forward and returning to standing segmentally. Clinicians should reiterate to patients that bending at the waist puts significant stress on the low back and will increase pain.

The purpose of movement assimilation is to take the newly acquired (learned) skills and integrate them into more dynamic activities and ADLs/IADLs (ie, lifting, house cleaning, reaching, and pushing/pulling).[3] The physical therapist assistant should first determine which activities increase the patient's symptoms and then select exercises that break down and simulate the functional activity that aggravates symptoms. For example, if a patient reports having increased symptoms while washing the floor on their hands and knees but states symptoms disappear when the activity is stopped, the clinician should first check to see if the patient can maintain core stabilization in quadruped. The clinician should then add subtask training while in quadruped; have the patient initiate lateral pelvic motions while maintaining core stabilization or attempt to slide one arm forward and back (or side to side) with a stable core. An exercise to target trunk rotation might include having the patient first start in a standing position and perform trunk rotation with the arm out straight and then add a resistance band to make the exercise more difficult. As a progression, have the patient perform the exercise with the trunk flexed while supported on one arm and moving the other arm horizontally with slight resistance. Clinicians often need to be creative to break down and simulate activities a patient needs to perform. The key to success is continuous reinforcement to activate and maintain core stability while gradually increasing repetitions/time, thereby increasing muscle endurance for a new task.

### Considerations for the Physical Therapist Assistant: Monitor Trunk and Pelvis Position

Movement or a dip/drop of the pelvis on one side during an exercise/activity indicates the patient's inability to maintain trunk control. Using the Stabilizer for biofeedback can provide input regarding core stability and muscle endurance while the patient is learning basic or new spinal stabilization exercises. During quadruped or squatting exercises, using a dowel placed along the spine can provide tactile and visual feedback to ensure a neutral spine position is maintained during exercise (Figure 15-13). If a patient is in a good postural alignment, they should be able to squat down by flexing at the hips, and the core muscles should automatically contract. If the patient is unable to maintain core stability with a challenging exercise, modify the progression by altering the position or revert to a less challenging exercise but make it slightly more difficult by adding weights or changing body positions.

## *Functional Optimization Approach*

The functional optimization approach focuses on increasing muscle strength, power, and endurance in order to meet the higher demands of functional performance necessary for patients to return to prior levels of function for work/sport. Patients entering this phase are usually asymptomatic when performing ADLs. Patients are usually discharged from physical therapy at this point, but those who have not reached their prior level of function or are returning to high physically demanding activities can benefit from the expertise of the physical therapy team in this phase of recovery. Advanced strength/conditioning and aerobic exercises are implemented during this phase. Clinicians should be aware of and address the psychological factors (ie, fear and/or anxiety of injury recurrence) that may present themselves during this phase while preparing to return to sport or work.[3,31]

### Clinical Tips

As patients progress (increasing muscle strength, endurance, and control), physical therapist assistants must consider their current functional abilities and long-term goals. To promote a full return to the highest level of function, exercises should be progressed from single-plane stability exercises to multiplanar dynamic exercises. Exercise training on various surfaces that require core and postural stability during extremity loading and/or plyometrics should be incorporated (based on the POC/patient's goals). As patients progress, ongoing education to emphasize core stability while maintaining a neutral spine position is critical. Patients must be kinesthetically aware of spinal position changes during all activities and make the automatic adjustments to correct deviations.

## Patient Education to Control Symptoms During Activities

Patient education begins during the initial evaluation and is continually reinforced in each treatment session. To minimize symptoms during the acute phase, education and training should focus on protecting the low back during normal activities or on modifying those activities. Key educational components include proper positioning (ie, sleeping and standing) and instruction on bed mobility and transfers while maintaining a neutral spine and engaging core musculature to reduce symptoms. The use of directional preference positions and exercises should encourage the patient to continue these postures/exercises between sessions to reduce symptoms. They should also be instructed to change positions frequently to avoid an increase in symptoms. Maintaining a neutral spine by practicing the drawing-in maneuver during walking and checking spine position during gait should be encouraged.

Sitting or driving long distances (greater than 30 minutes) should be interrupted by standing because this tends to significantly reduce stress on the spine and decrease patient symptoms. Teaching patients to properly get into and out of a vehicle, the use of a lumbar roll for proper positioning (if indicated), frequent stops to interrupt sitting by walking around, and performing directional preference exercises are very important. To get in/out of the vehicle, the patient should move the body as one unit to avoid twisting motions. To enter the car, have the patient move the seat as far back as possible while contracting the TrA and flexing at the hips to lower the buttocks down into the seat and then in one motion turn the spine and lower extremities into the seat facing forward. Reverse the process to get out of the car.

As symptoms decrease, the patient should be able to maintain a neutral spine position at rest, with general mobility, and while completing ROM and strengthening exercises because these activities will eventually promote return to full function. Ongoing patient education regarding muscle endurance with core stabilization in a neutral spine position is important as the patient's activity level increases. The patient's work space should be modified to ensure that they are able to work in an environment that is safe and efficient (refer to Chapter 22). Workplace modifications based on an individual's diagnosis/presentation and job requirements may be indicated, including a limitation in or elimination of repetitive activities such as lifting, pulling, bending, and reaching. Work simulation and practice of higher-level work-related tasks can be initiated once the patient is asymptomatic. Progressions are described in Chapter 22.

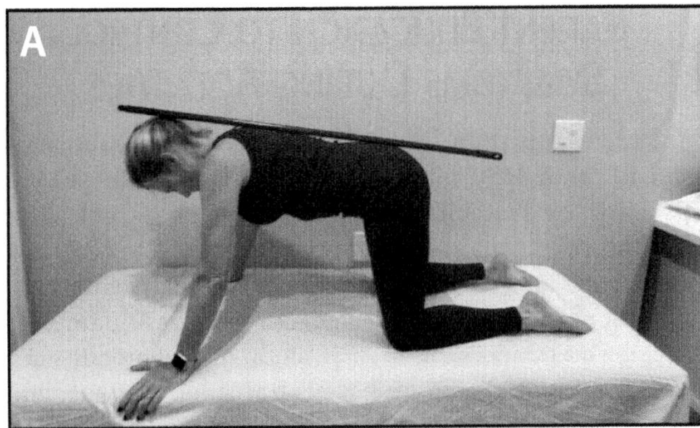


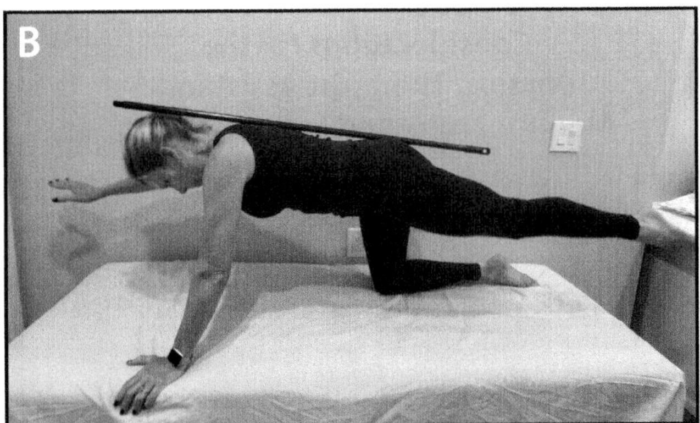


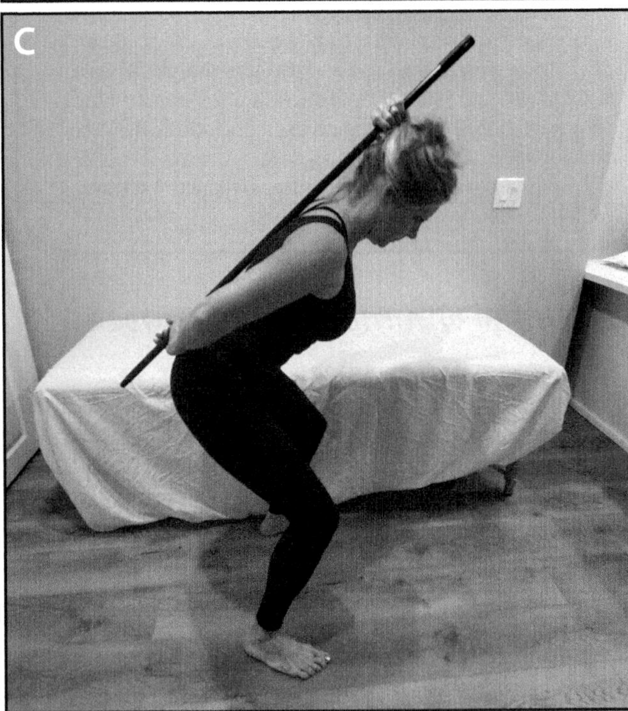


**Figure 15-13.** The use of a dowel for tactile feedback. (A) The use of a dowel to provide feedback with a neutral spine in quadruped. (B) The use of a dowel to provide feedback with a neutral spine in quadruped with reciprocal extremity motion. (C) The use of a dowel to provide feedback with a neutral spine during a squat.

## Clinical Tips

Focusing on patient education is key! The patient must become independent in self-monitoring for maintenance of a neutral spine position and engaging/maintaining core/spine stabilizers for the duration of an exercise or activity while using good movement sequencing. Patients must also learn to terminate an activity when there is a loss of postural control, muscle fatigue, or deviation from the neutral spine position.

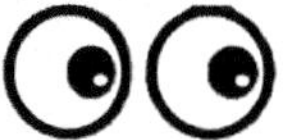

### Eye on the Research: Other Treatment Options and Considerations

The American College of Physicians' clinical recommendations for noninvasive treatment of LBP noted that patients with acute or subacute LBP have been shown to improve over time regardless of treatment and that initial interventions should include nonpharmacologic treatment. Treatments could include superficial heat, massage, acupuncture, or spinal manipulation (there was a lower quality of evidence for this intervention). If pharmacologic treatment was selected, nonsteroidal anti-inflammatory drugs or skeletal muscle relaxants are preferred vs narcotics/opioids. The initial treatment should include exercise, multidisciplinary rehabilitation, acupuncture, mindfulness-based stress reduction, tai chi, yoga, motor control exercise, progressive relaxation, electromyography biofeedback, low-level laser therapy, operant therapy, cognitive behavioral therapy, or spinal manipulation (lower-quality evidence). If medications must be considered, the use of nonsteroidal anti-inflammatory drugs should be a first-line therapy, and tramadol or duloxetine should be the second-line therapy. Opioids should only be considered for patients who have failed the first 2 recommendations and only if the potential benefits outweigh the risks for the individual patient (after a discussion of the known risks and realistic benefits).[44]

The use of a nonpharmacologic exercise-first treatment is also supported by a 2018 study by Alhakami et al[18] that also concluded that exercise interventions provide better outcomes for chronic LBP than passive methods such as rest and medication. A 2018 study by Frogner et al[45] followed patients for 1 year after a new diagnosis of LBP and concluded that when patients went to physical therapy first, there was a lower use of opioid medications and that physical therapy was a more cost-effective method of treatment that reflected a "lower utilization of high-cost medical services." Some patients in drug rehabilitation centers for detoxification often need physical therapy treatments to decrease their pain and improve function. Physical therapy can reduce pain, decreasing the risk of an opioid medication relapse. There are new opportunities for physical therapists and physical therapist assistants to play a supportive role in patient recovery.

## Pediatric Considerations

Adolescent idiopathic scoliosis is the most common type of scoliosis, affecting 2% to 4% of the adolescent population between 10 and 18 years of age. A Cobb angle of 10 degrees or more is indicative of adolescent idiopathic scoliosis. Scoliosis is characterized by a lateral curvature of the spine, often with associated vertebral rotation.[46] The curve usually develops during rapid growth periods, and physical therapy can be prescribed as an intervention for persons with smaller curves. There is no definitive evidence that physical therapy can help correct the curves associated with scoliosis; however, it can be used to strengthen the weak muscles on the convex side of the curve and stretch tight muscles on the concave side. Exercises may improve spinal alignment and breathing. Physicians determine if bracing is indicated for patients with curves greater than 20 degrees; therapy may also be prescribed to support a bracing intervention.

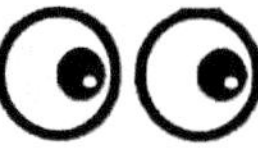

### Eye on the Research: Idiopathic Scoliosis

A small pilot study with 15 participants reported that patients with idiopathic scoliosis presented with postural instability due to paraspinal muscle weakness on the concave side of the curve. Patients with a right "C" thoracic scoliotic curve were found to have left paraspinal muscle weakness (which was weak and shortened). The exercise technique used in the study is called *asymmetric spinal stabilization exercises (ASSEs)*.[46] ASSEs were performed in prone, quadruped, and side lying in order to reduce the angle of the curve by strengthening the weak muscles on the concave side. The researchers noted that muscle function not only creates motion but also may shape and maintain spinal alignment. Scoliosis develops in a standing resting position. Investigators suggest that the weakened paraspinal muscles may not support the spine in a straight line due to a decrease in the number of slow-twitch muscle fibers. The investigators surmised that due to muscle weakness (and fewer fibers) on the concave side, the spine was migrating laterally toward the convex side. These investigators found that based on surface electromyographic and radiographic findings, a personalized paraspinal muscle strengthening program for the muscles on the concave side using ASSEs was shown to reduce the severity of the curve. They noted that this is a preliminary study, and larger randomized controlled trials are needed to support these claims.[46] This study may provide early evidence that an individualized and targeted exercise program may provide positive outcomes for persons with mild scoliosis.[46]

## Spinal and Core Stabilization Exercise Progression

Extension bias exercise progression is shown in Figure 15-14, flexion bias exercise progression is shown in Figure 15-15, and core stabilization progressions are depicted in Figures 15-16 and 15-17. Bridging exercise progression is illustrated in Figures 15-18 and 15-19. Plank progression is demonstrated in Figure 15-20 and side plank progression in Figure 15-21. Figure 15-22 illustrated quadruped progressions, and more advanced trunk extensor strengthening exercises are portrayed in Figure 15-23.

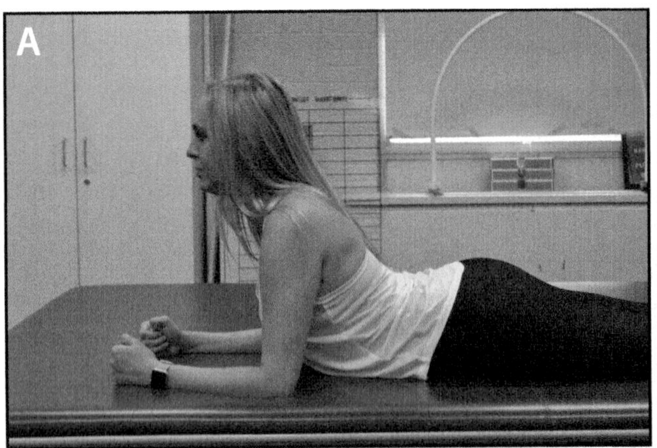


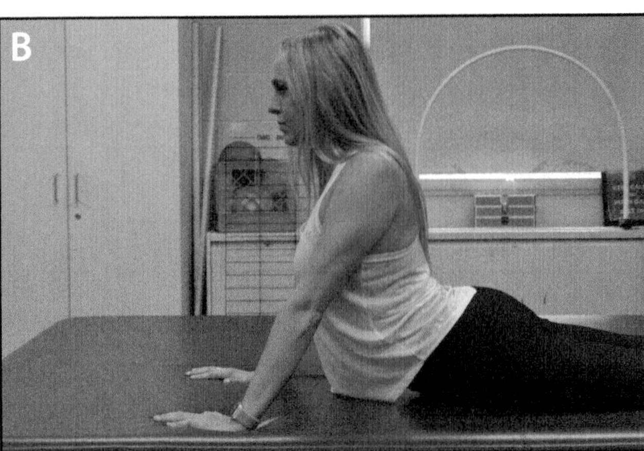


**Figure 15-14.** Extension bias exercise sequence. (A) Prone on the elbows (forearms). (B) A prone press-up. (C) Standing lumbar extension.

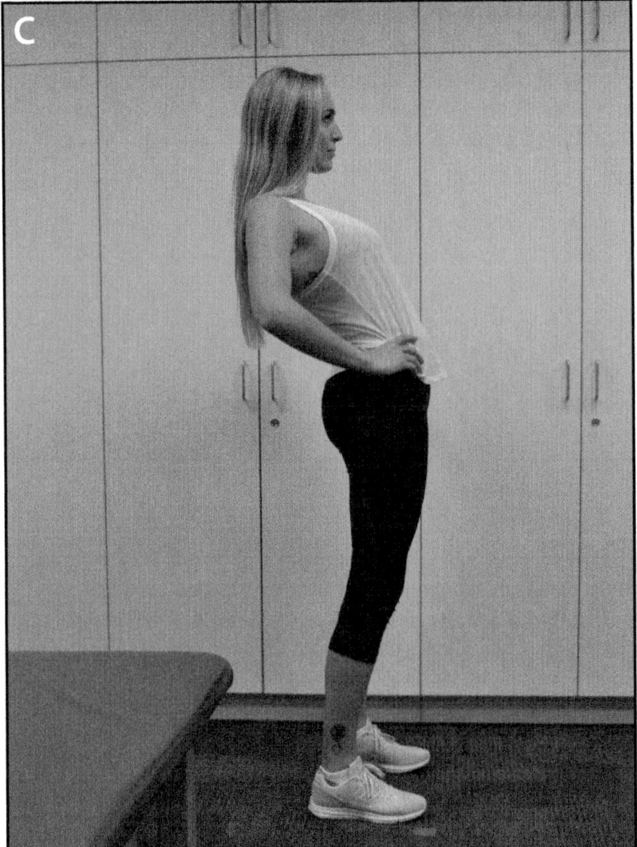

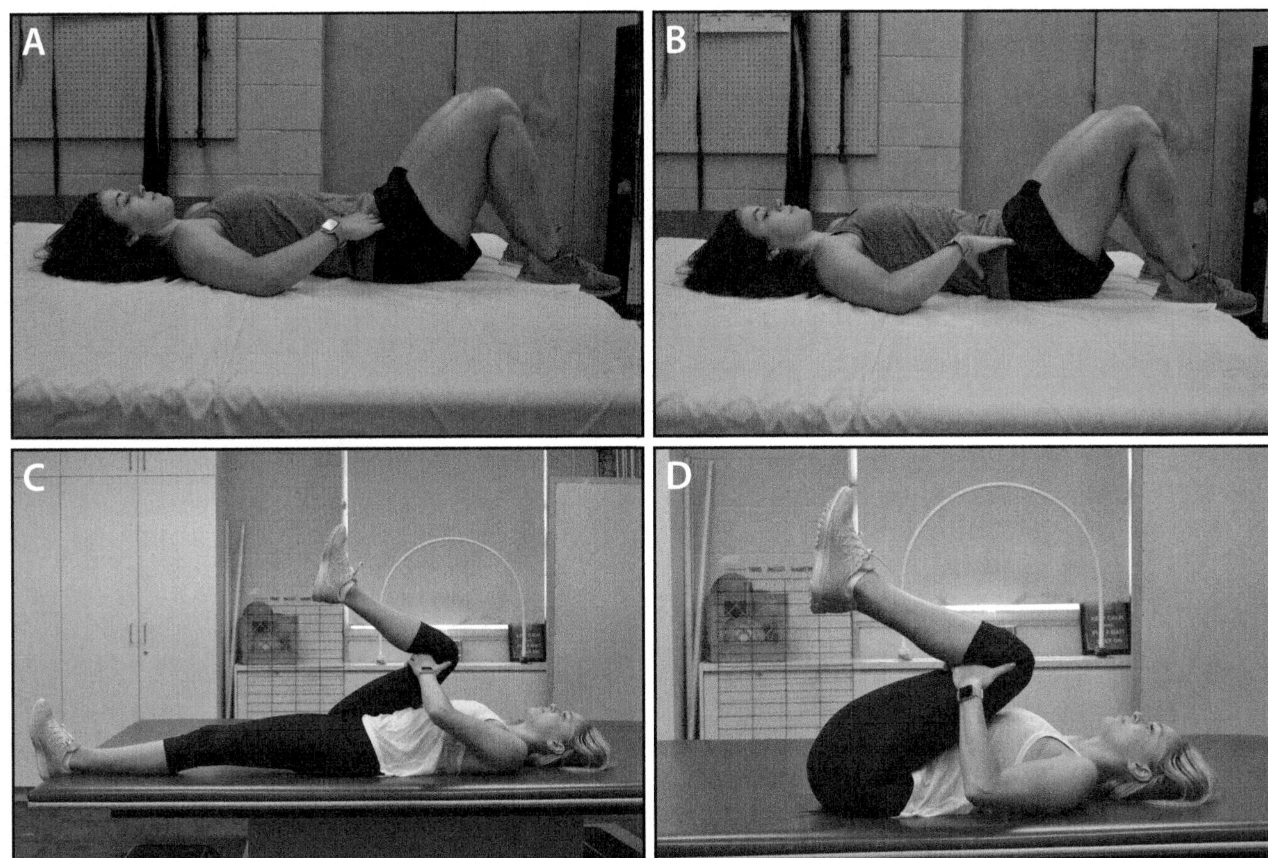


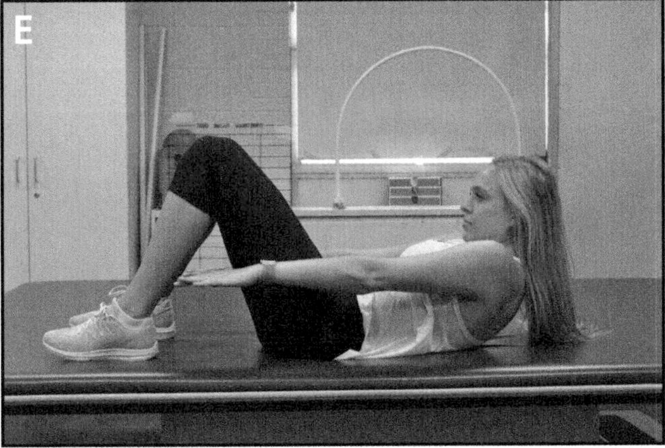


**Figure 15-15.** Flexion bias exercise sequence. (A) The PPT starting position. (B) The PPT end position. (C) Single knee to chest. (D) Double knee to chest. (E) Crunch/partial sit-up. Note just the head and shoulders are lifted off the table. Crossing the arms on the chest or placing hands behind the head will make this exercise more difficult.

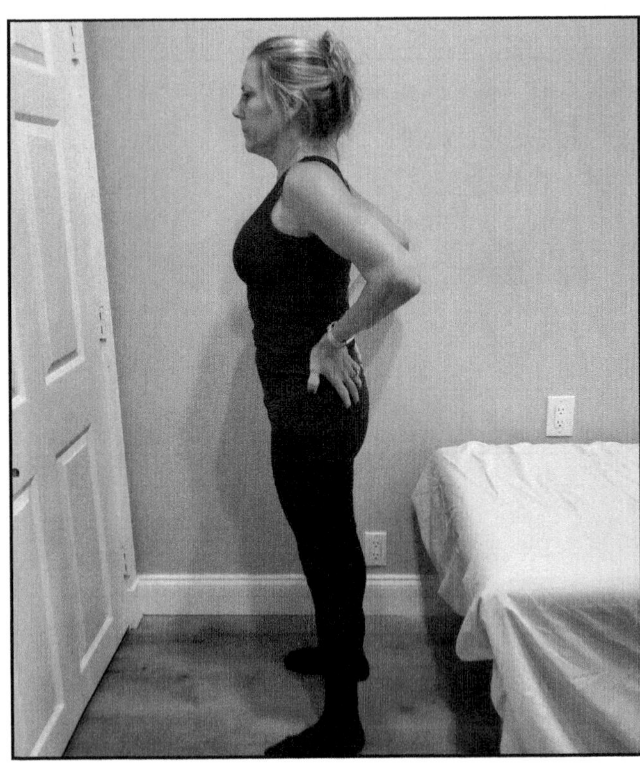

**Figure 15-16.** Core stabilization in standing in neutral spine with abdominal bracing or the drawing-in maneuver.

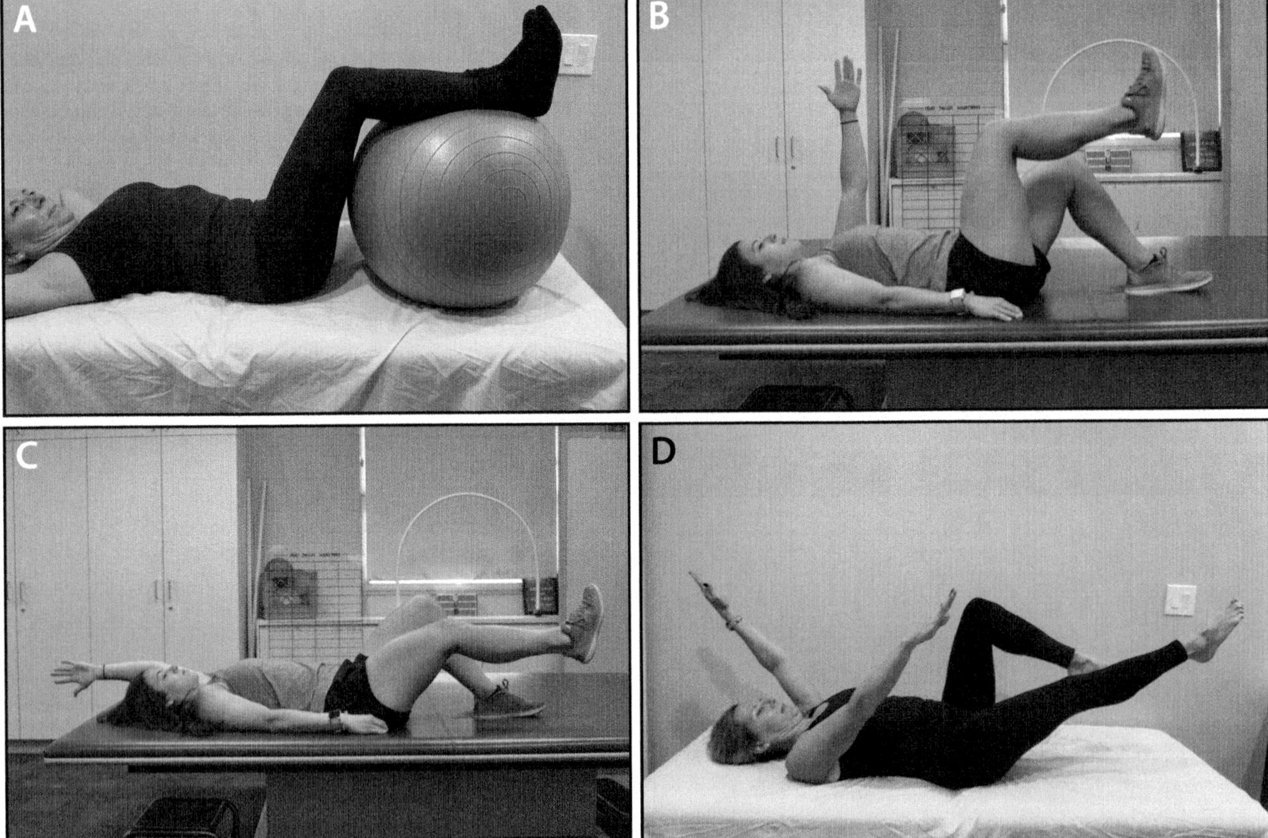


**Figure 15-17.** (A) Core stabilization using abdominal bracing and drawing-in maneuver in neutral spine or a PPT on a ball. (B) Core stabilization supine with small reciprocal upper extremity and lower extremity motions. First start moving one extremity at a time while keeping the core engaged and then add both extremities. (C) Core stabilization in supine with large reciprocal upper extremity and lower extremity motions. (D) Progress to supine reciprocal upper extremity and lower extremity motion unsupported.

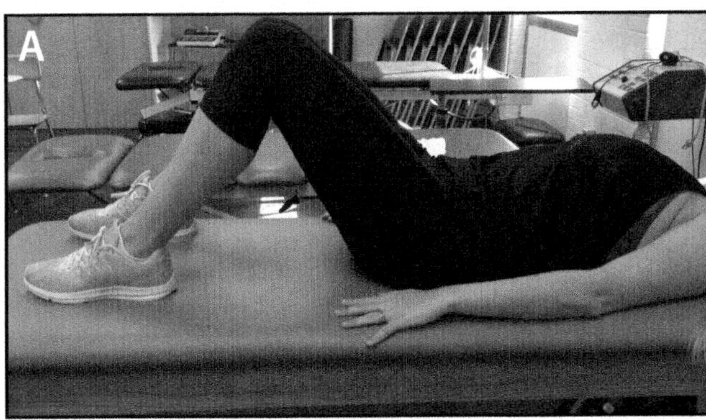


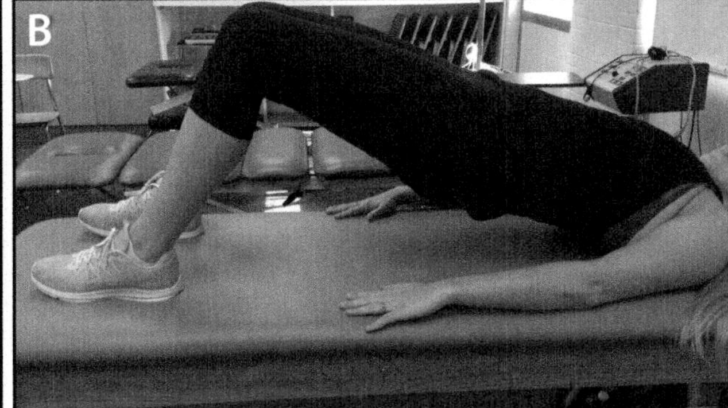


**Figure 15-18.** Bridging. (A) The hook-lying starting position to (B) bridging with the core muscles engaged.

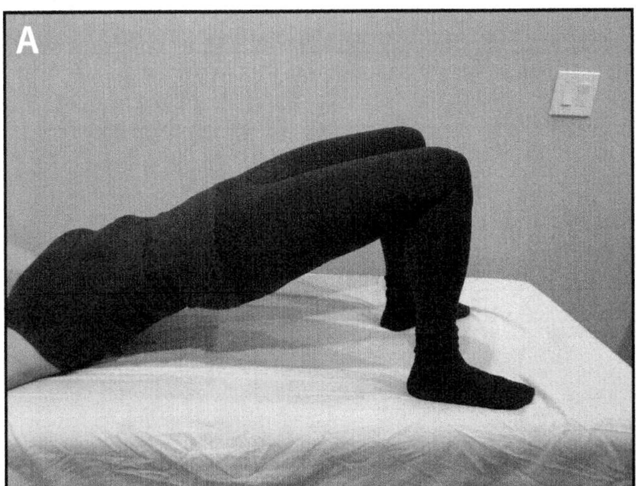


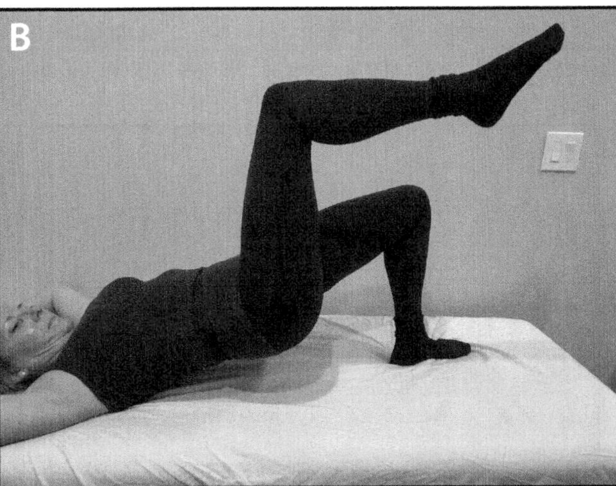


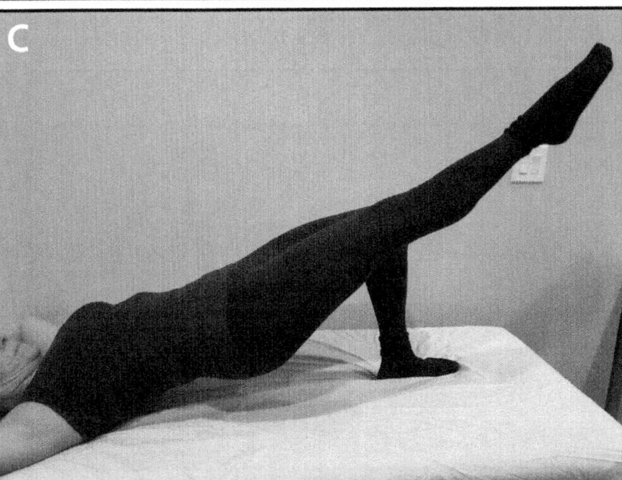


**Figure 15-19.** Bridging progressions. (A) The patient can perform hip abduction and adduction while maintaining the bridge as a progression. (B) Bridging with one lower extremity flexed. The patient can perform marching while maintaining a bridge as a progression. The clinician must ensure the pelvis stays up and level during these exercises. (C) Bridging with one lower extremity extended. *(continued)*

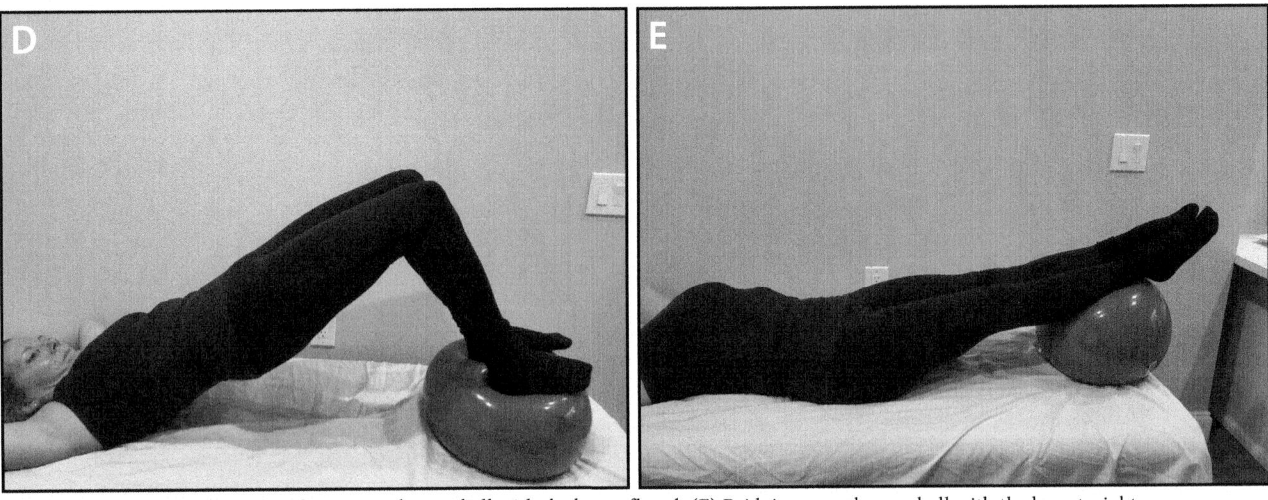

**Figure 15-19 (continued).** (D) Bridging on a therapy ball with the knees flexed. (E) Bridging on a therapy ball with the legs straight.

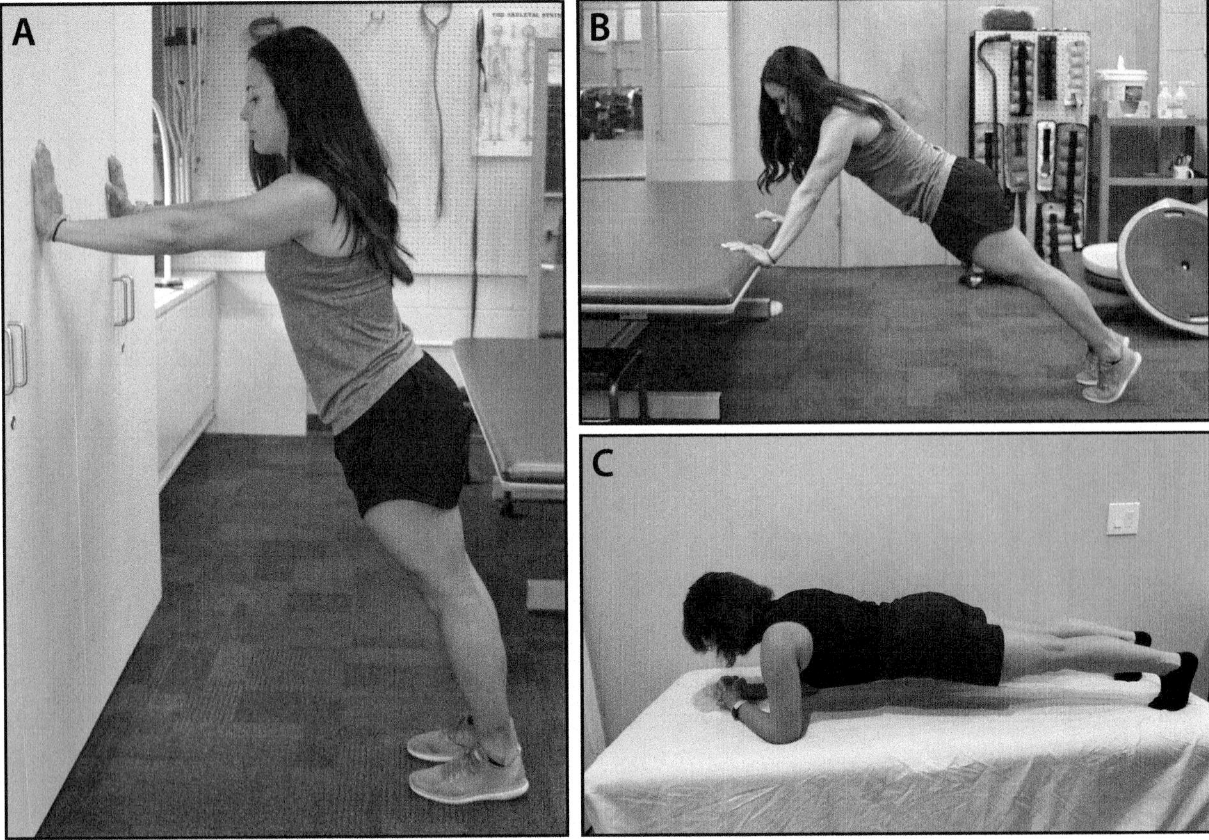

**Figure 15-20.** Plank progressions. (A) A plank modified at the wall. Can be progressed to a wall push-up. (B) A plank modified on plinth. Can be progressed to a push-up. (C) A plank on forearms. *(continued)*

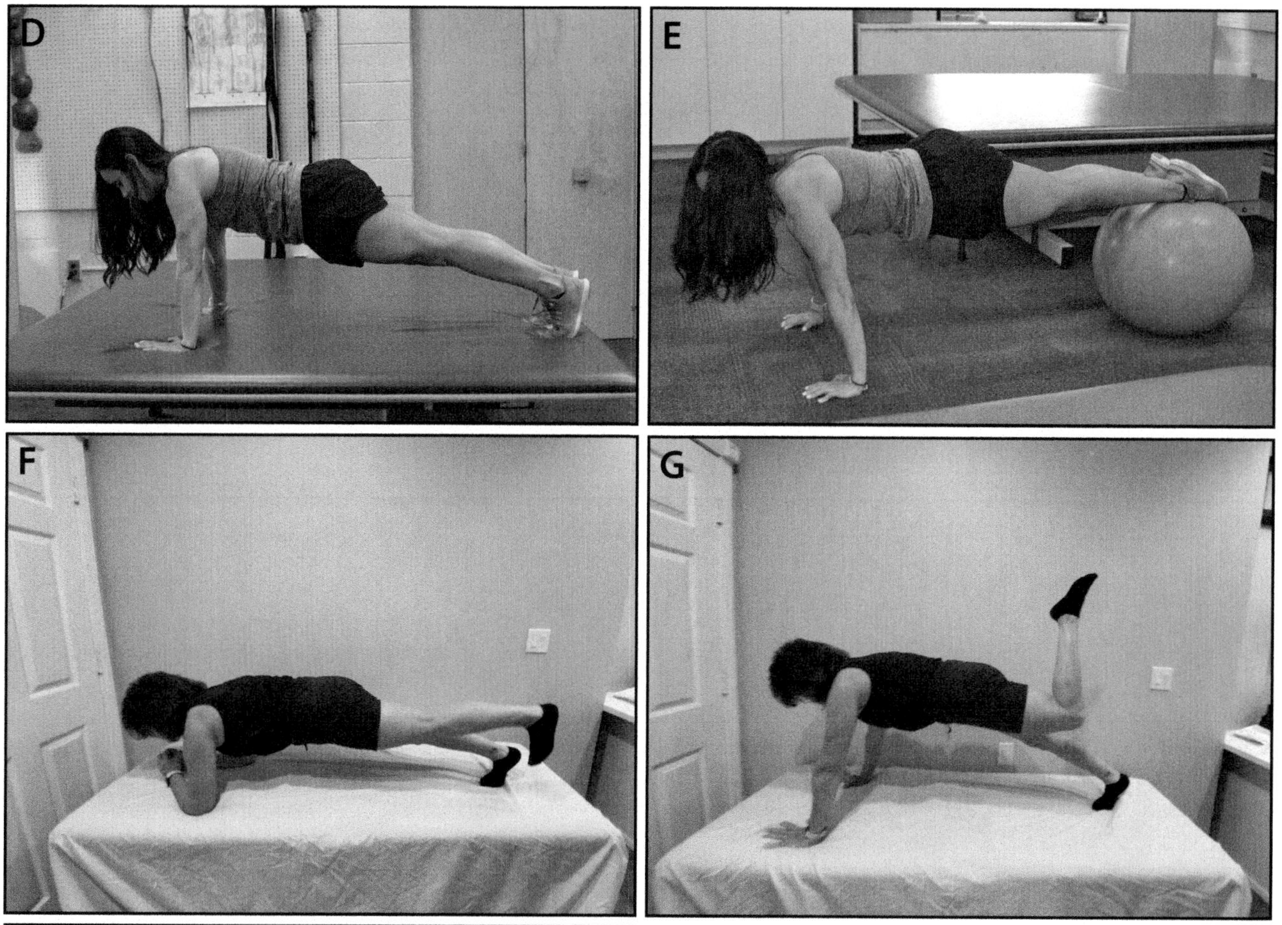

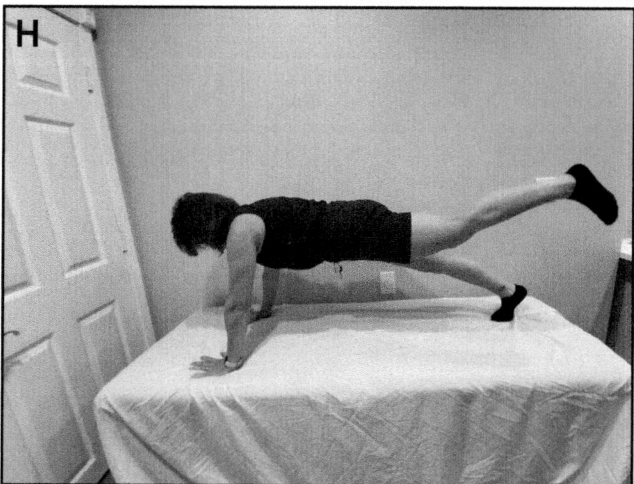

**Figure 15-20 (continued).** (D) A plank with arms straight. (E) A plank with the lower extremities on a physioball. (F) A plank on forearms with one lower extremity minimally extended. (G) A plank with hip extension and knee flexion. Can also be performed on a therapy ball. (H) A plank with the lower extremity extended. Can also be performed on a therapy ball.

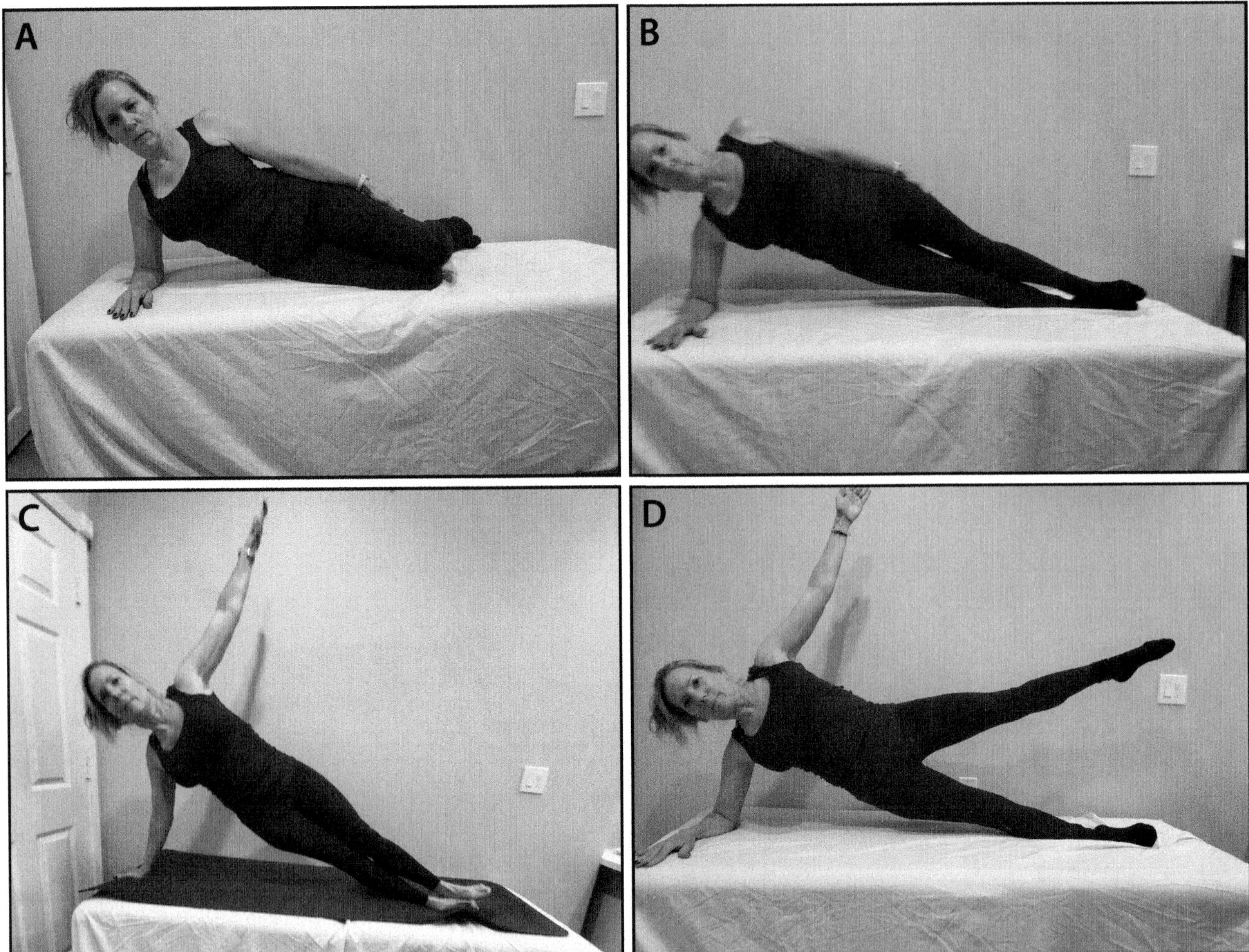


**Figure 15-21.** (A) A side plank on the knees. (B) A side plank on the forearm with the legs straight. (C) A side plank full. (D) A side plank with upper and lower extremity abduction.

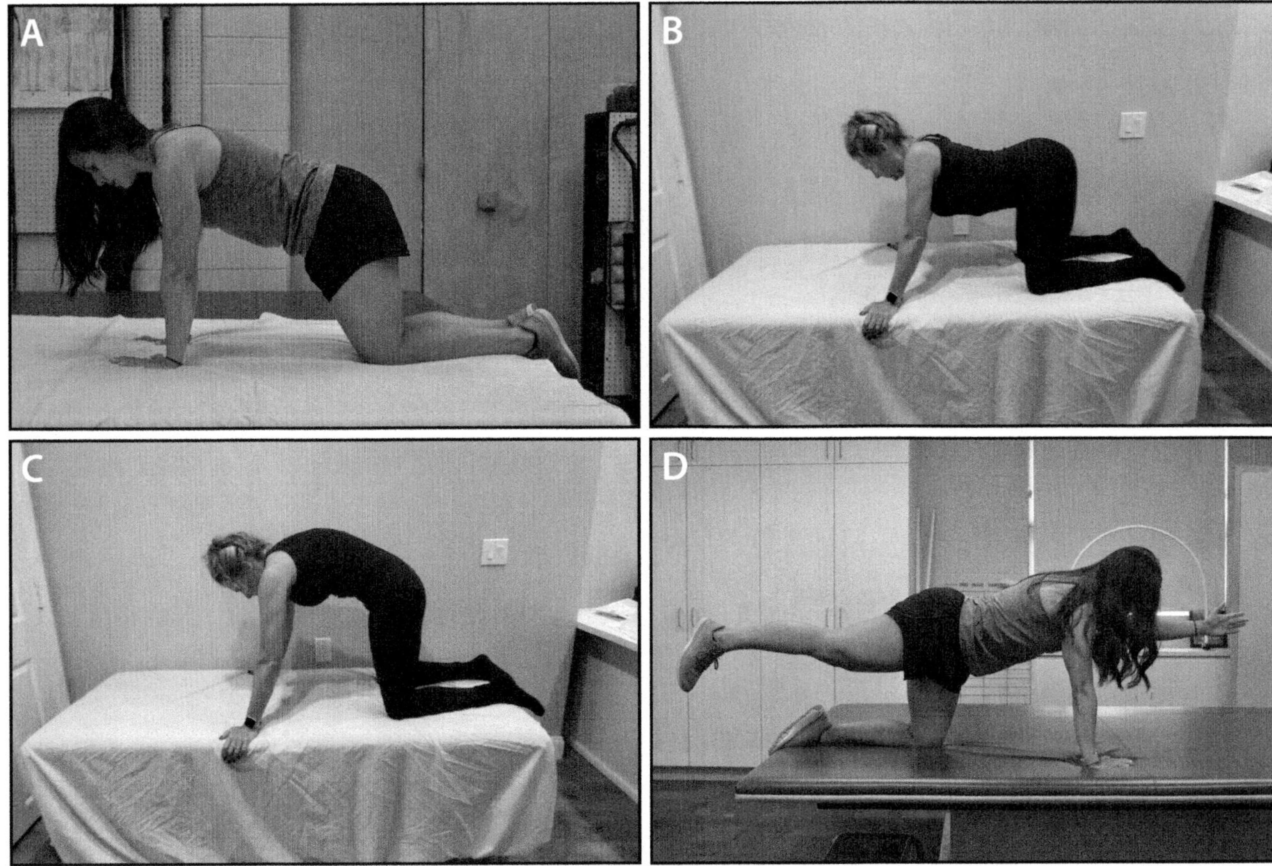


**Figure 15-22.** (A) Quadruped. (B) Quadruped anterior pelvic tilt: Camel position. (C) Quadruped cat position: Trunk flexion. (D) In quadruped, first start with lifting of one upper extremity; progress to lifting one lower extremity at a time and then reciprocal arm and leg motions as shown.

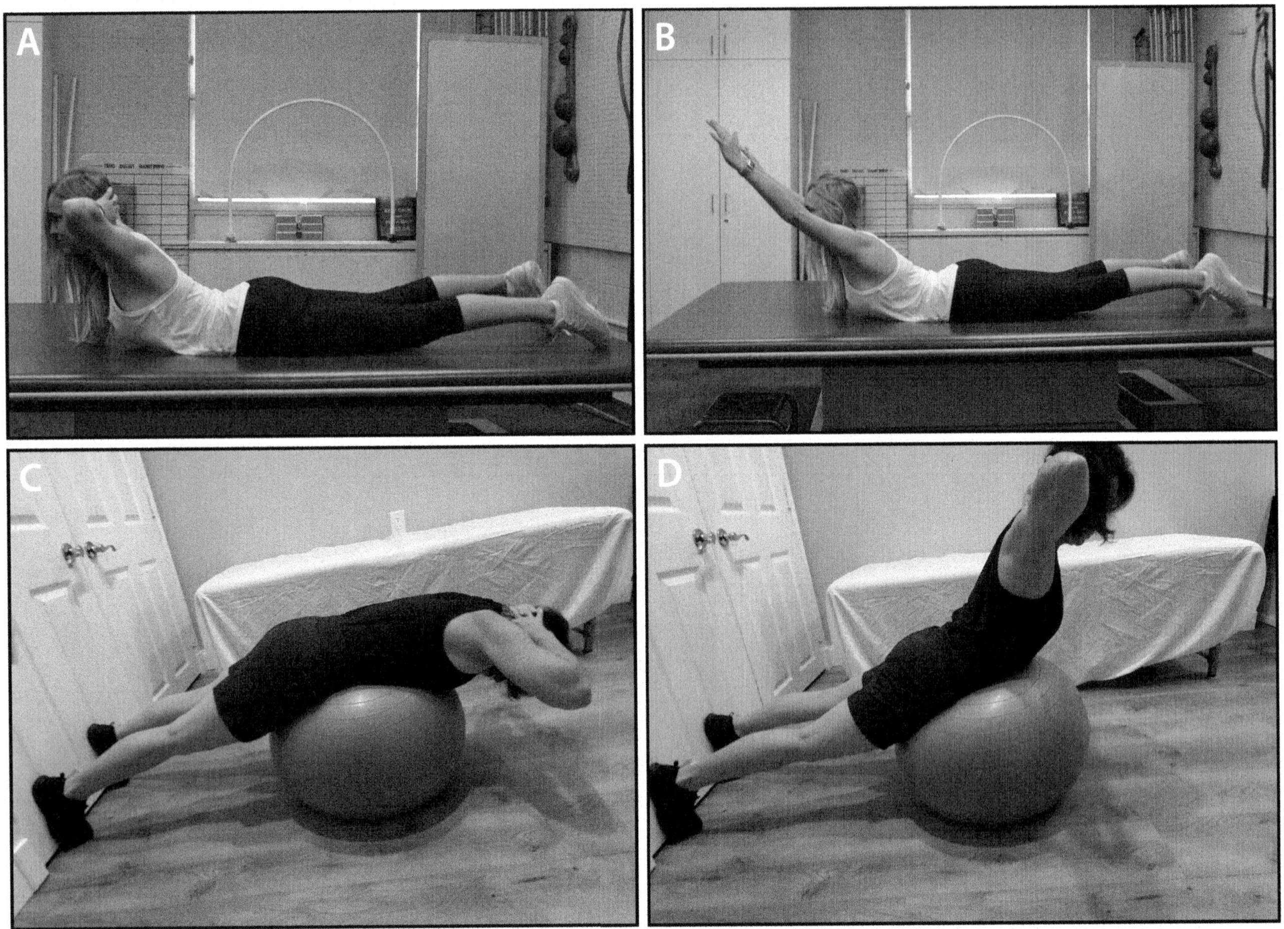

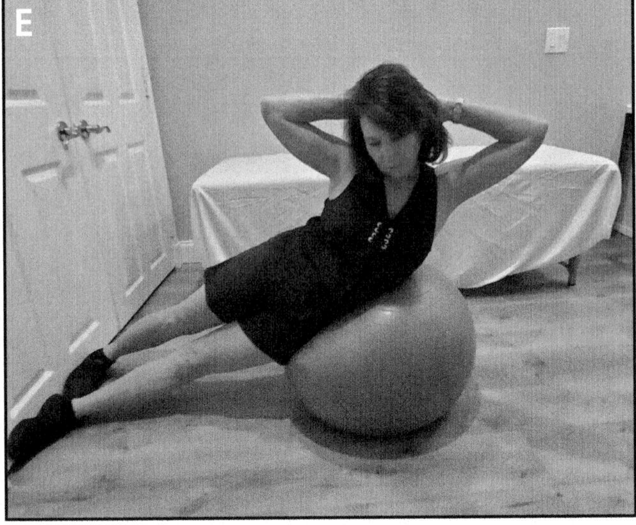

**Figure 15-23.** (A) Strengthening trunk extension prone. (B) Strengthening trunk extension prone with the upper extremity extended. (C) Strengthening trunk extensors on a physioball: Starting position. (D) Strengthening trunk extension on a physioball: End position. (E) Lateral flexion side lying on a physioball for strengthening.

## Conclusion

Physical therapy is an effective way to treat patients who experience LBP, and the treatment-based classification system is useful when generating an effective treatment plan for these patients. The information from the physical therapy evaluation and the patient's presentation should guide the selection of the most appropriate exercises. Therapeutic exercises are important interventions that are used to reduce patient symptoms, improve trunk stability and mobility, and promote the return to the prior level of function for all patients with low back and SI diagnoses. Physical therapist assistants must be alert to any changes in patient symptoms that may be red flags and report them to the physical therapist immediately. Physical therapist assistants should provide reassurance to patients to address their concerns about their LBP. Assistants must be confident that patients are kinesthetically aware of all positions or movements that affect their LBP. One goal for patients is to feel confident in performing all spinal movements without symptoms. However, if symptoms do occur, patients should be able to reverse the symptoms immediately using directional preference interventions independently. Patients should also be able to independently demonstrate proper bed mobility, transfers, and body mechanic techniques and recognize ergonomic conditions that may be present at work.

## Review Questions

1. Compare and contrast patient presentation for a herniated disk (posterior lateral) and spinal stenosis. Which special tests would most likely be positive with each diagnosis?
2. Describe the typical presentation for a lumbar strain.
3. Define directional preference exercise, and list the 2 categories. Which diagnoses are typically treated using directional preference exercises?
4. List 3 exercises that are appropriate for a patient with a posterior lateral disk herniation to perform to reduce radicular symptoms.
5. List the local/deep muscles that stabilize the trunk and low back.
6. List 3 exercises that are contraindicated for a patient after vertebral compression fracture.
7. Describe the components of the motor control approach based on the treatment-based classification system.
8. List 4 exercises that would be most appropriate for a patient who is in the final phase of rehabilitation and planning to return to baseball after spondylolisthesis.
9. List 4 red flag items that should alert a physical therapist assistant to contact the physical therapist immediately when treating a patient with LBP.
10. Describe the treatment technique that is effective for treating an SI innominate where the patient appears to have a longer leg when supine and a shorter leg with long sitting.

## Case Study 1

A 76-year-old patient presents with a diagnosis of spinal stenosis. The patient describes pain that increases with walking greater than 150 feet and requires standing rest, such as leaning on a grocery cart to decrease the pain. The patient's goal is to be able to return to walking 1 mile without pain and return to gardening.

1. Is this presentation consistent with the typical presentation of spinal stenosis?
2. Based on the treatment-based classification system, which rehabilitation approach should be initiated for this patient? List 5 exercises that are most appropriate to initiate when treating this patient.
3. List 3 activities the patient should avoid at this time.
4. Develop an appropriate exercise progression to promote achievement of the goals.

## Case Study 2

A 28-year-old patient presents with a report of acute LBP after helping a friend move to a new apartment last weekend. The patient states that the pain is 7/10 and that it originates in the right lumbar area and radiates posteriorly down the right leg to the midcalf. The patient's pain increases with forward bending to tie shoes, and the leg pain decreases in standing. The physical therapy evaluation notes that the lower extremity pain increases with lumbar flexion and prolonged sitting and that the pain centralizes with trunk extension AROM. The patient's goal is to return to work as a computer programmer and to play softball again with the company team.

1. Which diagnosis is most consistent with this presentation?
2. Which is the most appropriate treatment-based classification system approach initially for this patient? What is the patient's directional preference? List 4 exercises that are most appropriate to initiate when treating this patient on the first visit.
3. List 4 patient education items that are most appropriate for this patient at this time.
4. Problem solve and develop an appropriate exercise progression so it is possible for the patient to achieve the goals in the scenario.

## Suggested Resources

American Academy of Orthopaedic Surgeons. Owesetry Low Back Disability Questionnaire. Accessed April 19, 2023. https://aaos.org/globalassets/quality-and-practice-resources/patient-reported-outcome-measures/spine/oswestry-2.pdf

Chaitow L. *Muscle Energy Techniques.* 3rd ed. Churchill-Livingstone; 2006.

McKenzie R, May S. *The Lumbar Spine: Mechanical Diagnosis and Therapy.* 2nd ed. Spinal Publications New Zealand Ltd; 2003.

Orthotoolkit. Oswestry Disability Index--OrthoToolKit. 2023. Accessed April 19, 2023. https://www.orthotoolkit.com/oswestry/

Rehabilitative Care Alliance. The Roland-Morris Low Back Pain and Disability Questionnaire. Accessed April 19, 2023. https://mississaugahalton.rehabcareontario.ca/Uploads/ContentDocuments/Roland-Morris-Questionaire.pdf

Shirley Ryan AbilityLab. Fear-Avoidance Beliefs Questionnaire. Updated June 26, 2014. Accessed April 19, 2023. https://www.sralab.org/rehabilitation-measures/fear-avoidance-beliefs-questionnaire

Shirley Ryan AbilityLab. STarT Back Screening Tool. Updated April 12, 2016. Accessed April 19, 2023. https://www.sralab.org/rehabilitation-measures/start-back-screening-tool

Transport Accident Commission. The Quebec Back Pan Disability Scale. Accessed April 19, 2023. https://www.tac.vic.gov.au/files-to-move/media/upload/quebec_scale.pdf

## References


1. Hoy D, March L, Brooks P, et al. The global burden of low back pain: estimates from the Global Burden of Disease 2010 Study. *Ann Rheum Dis.* 2014;73:968-974.
2. Maher C, Underwood M, Buchbinder R. Non-specific low back pain. *Lancet.* 2017;389(10070):736-747. doi:10.1016/S0140-6736(16)30970-9
3. Alrwaily M, Timko M, Schneider M, et al. Treatment-based classification system for patients with low back pain: the movement control approach. *Phys Ther.* 2017;97(12):1147-1157. doi:10.1093/ptj/pzx087
4. Ford JJ, Hahne AJ. Pathoanatomy and classification of low back disorders. *Man Ther.* 2013;18(2):165-168. doi:10.1016/j.math.2012.05.007
5. Delitto A, George SZ, VanDillen L, et al. Low back pain: clinical practice guidelines linked to the International Classification of Functioning, Disability and Health from the Academy of Orthopaedic Physical Therapy of the American Physical Therapy Association. *J Orthop Sports Phys Ther.* 2012;42(4):A1-A57. doi:10.2519/jospt.2012.42.4.A1
6. Jung JH, Kim HI, Shin DA, et al. Usefulness of pain distribution pattern assessment in decision-making for the patients with lumbar zygapophyseal and sacroiliac joint arthropathy. *J Korean Med Sci.* 2007;22(6):1048-1054.
7. Travell J, Simons D, Simons L. *Myofascial Pain and Dysfunction: The Trigger Point Manual.* 2nd ed. Lippincott, Williams & Wilkins; 1999.
8. Bogduk N. On the definitions and physiology of back pain, referred pain, and radicular pain. *Pain.* 2009;147(1-3):17-19. doi:10.1016/j.pain.2009.08.020
9. Leerar PJ, Boissonnault W, Domholdt E, Roddey T. Documentation of red flags by physical therapists for patients with low back pain. *J Man Manip Ther.* 2007;15(1):42-49. doi:10.1179/106698107779109010
10. Shipton EA. Physical therapy approaches in the treatment of low back pain. *Pain Ther.* 2018;7(2):127-137. doi:10.1007/s40122-018-0105-x
11. Magee DJ. Lumbar spine. In: Magee DJ, ed. *Orthopedic Physical Assessment.* 6th ed. Elsevier; 2014:551-641.
12. Nordin M, Weiner SS. Biomechanics of the lumbar spine. In: Nordin M, Frankel VH, eds. *Basic Biomechanics of the Musculoskeletal System.* Lippincott, Williams and Wilkins; 2012.
13. Nachemson AL. Disc pressure measurements. *Spine (Phila Pa 1976).* 1981;6(1):93-97.
14. Sato K, Kikuchi S, Yonezawa T. In vivo intradiscal pressure measurement in healthy individuals and in patients with ongoing back problems. *Spine.* 1999;24(23):2468-2474.
15. Dutton M. Lumbar spine. In: Dutton M, ed. *Dutton's Orthopaedic Examination, Evaluation and Intervention.* 3rd ed. The McGraw-Hill Companies, Inc; 2012:1273-1355.
16. Kolber MJ, Beekhuizen K. Lumbar stabilization: an evidence-based approach for the athlete with low back pain. *Strength Cond J.* 2007;29(2):26-37.
17. Akhtar MW, Karimi H, Gilani SA. Effectiveness of core stabilization exercises and routine exercise therapy in management of pain in chronic non-specific low back pain: a randomized controlled clinical trial. *Pak J Med Sci.* 2017;33(4):1002-1006. doi:10.12669/pjms.334.12664
18. Alhakami AM, Davis S, Qasheesh M, Shaphe A, Chahal A. Effects of McKenzie and stabilization exercises in reducing pain intensity and functional disability in individuals with nonspecific chronic low back pain: a systematic review. *J Phys Ther Sci.* 2019;31(7):590-597. doi:10.1589/jpts.31.590
19. Richardson CA, Snijders CJ, Hides JA, Damen L, Pas MS, Storm J. The relation between the transversus abdominis muscles, sacroiliac joint mechanics, and low back pain. *Spine.* 2002;27(4):399-405. doi:10.1097/00007632-200202150-00015
20. Vleeming A, Schuenke MD, Masi AT, Carreiro JE, Danneels L, Willard FH. The sacroiliac joint: an overview of its anatomy, function and potential clinical implications. *J Anat.* 2012;221(6):537-567.
21. Serola R. Unilateral and bilateral nutation and counternutation. *Serola Biomechanics.* January 20, 2020. Accessed February 3, 2023. https://www.serola.net/research-entry/reciprocating-unilateral-motion/
22. Wong M, Sinkler M, Kiel J. *Anatomy, Abdomen and Pelvis, Sacroiliac Joint.* StatPearls; 2020. https://www.ncbi.nlm.nih.gov/books/NBK507801/
23. Magee DJ. Pelvis. In: Magee DJ, ed. *Orthopedic Physical Assessment.* 6th ed. Elsevier; 2014:649-681.
24. Petersen T, Laslett M, Juhl C. Clinical classification in low back pain: best-evidence diagnostic rules based on systematic reviews. *BMC Musculoskelet Disord.* 2017;18(1):188. doi:10.1186/s12891-017-1549-6
25. Stuber KJ. Specificity, sensitivity, and predictive values of clinical tests of the sacroiliac joint: a systematic review of the literature. *J Can Chiropr Assoc.* 2007;51(1):30-41. PMC1924656.
26. Laslett M, Young SB, Aprill CN, McDonald B. Diagnosing painful sacroiliac joints: a validity study of a McKenzie evaluation and sacroiliac provocation tests. *Aust J Physiother.* 2003;49(2):89-97.
27. Dahm KT, Brurberg KG, Jamtvedt G, Hagen KB. Advice to rest in bed versus advice to stay active for acute low-back pain and sciatica. *Cochrane Database Syst Rev.* 2010;6:CD007612. doi:10.1002/14651858.CD007612.pub2
28. Cabak A, Dąbrowska-Zimakowska A, Truszczyńska A, Rogala P, Laprus K, Tomaszewski W. Strategies for coping with chronic lower back pain in patients with long physiotherapy wait time. *Med Sci Monit.* 2015;21:3913-3920. doi:10.12659/msm.894743

29. Ahn K, Jhun HJ. New physical examination tests for lumbar spondylolisthesis and instability: low midline sill sign and interspinous gap change during lumbar flexion-extension motion. *BMC Musculoskelet Disord.* 2015;16:97. doi:10.1186/s12891-015-0551-0
30. Carlson SW, Magee S, Carlson WO. An algorithm for the evaluation and treatment of sacroiliac joint dysfunction. *S D Med.* 2014;67(11):445-449, 451.
31. Alrwaily M, Timko M, Schneider M, et al. Treatment-based classification system for low back pain: revision and update. *Phys Ther.* 2016;96(7):1057-1066.
32. May S, Aina A. Centralization and directional preference: a systematic review. *Man Ther.* 2012;17(6):497-506. doi:10.1016/j.math.2012.05.003
33. Park SD, Yu SH. The effects of abdominal draw-in maneuver and core exercise on abdominal muscle thickness and Oswestry disability index in subjects with chronic low back pain. *J Exerc Rehabil.* 2013;9(2):286-291. doi:10.12965/jer.130012
34. Moghadam N, Ghaffari MS, Noormohammadpour P, et al. Comparison of the recruitment of transverse abdominis through drawing-in and bracing in different core stability training positions. *J Exerc Rehabil.* 2019;15(6):819-825. doi:10.12965/jer.1939064.352
35. Coulombe BJ, Games KE, Neil ER, Eberman LE. core stability exercise versus general exercise for chronic low back pain. *J Athl Train.* 2017;52(1):71-72. doi:10.4085/1062-6050-51.11.16
36. Lee JS, Kim DY, Kim TH. The comparison of abdominal muscle activation on unstable surface according to the different trunk stability exercises. *J Phys Ther Sci.* 2016;28(3):1003-1006. doi:10.1589/jpts.28.1003
37. Koh HW, Cho SH, Kim CY. Comparison of the effects of hollowing and bracing exercises on cross-sectional areas of abdominal muscles in middle-aged women. *J Phys Ther Sci.* 2014;26(2):295-299. doi:10.1589/jpts.26.295
38. Vera-Garcia FJ, Elvira JL, Brown SH, McGill SM. Effects of abdominal stabilization maneuvers on the control of spine motion and stability against sudden trunk perturbations. *J Electromyogr Kinesiol.* 2007;17(5):556-567. doi:10.1016/j.jelekin.2006.07.004
39. Lynders C. The critical role of development of the transversus abdominis in the prevention and treatment of low back pain. *HSS J.* 2019;15:214-220. doi:10.1007/s11420-019-09717-8
40. Hodges PW, Jull GA. Spinal segmental stabilization training. In: Liebenson C, ed. *Rehabilitation of the Spine: A Practitioner's Manual.* 2nd ed. Lippincott Williams & Wilkins; 2007:585-611.
41. Selkow NM, Grindstaff TL, Cross KM, Pugh K, Hertel J, Saliba S. Short-term effect of muscle energy technique on pain in individuals with non-specific lumbopelvic pain: a pilot study. *J Man Manip Ther.* 2009;17(1):E14-E18.
42. Hides JA, Donelson R, Lee D, Prather H, Sahrmann SA, Hodges PW. Convergence and divergence of exercise-based approaches that incorporate motor control for the management of low back pain. *J Orthop Sports Phys Ther.* 2019;49(6):437-452. doi:10.2519/jospt.2019.8451
43. Lee SW, Kim SY. Effects of hip exercises for chronic low-back pain patients with lumbar instability. *J Phys Ther Sci.* 2015;27(2):345-348. doi:10.1589/jpts.27.345
44. Qaseem A, Wilt TJ, McLean RM, Forciea MA; Clinical Guidelines Committee of the American College of Physicians. Noninvasive treatments for acute, subacute, and chronic low back pain: a clinical practice guideline from the American College of Physicians. *Ann Intern Med.* 2017;166(7):514-530. doi:10.7326/M16-2367
45. Frogner BK, Harwood K, Andrilla CH, Schwartz M, Pines JM. Physical therapy as the first point of care to treat low back pain: an instrumental variables approach to estimate impact on opioid prescription, health care utilization, and costs. *Health Serv Res.* 2018;53(6):4629-4646. doi:10.1111/1475-6773.12984
46. Addai D, Zarkos J, Bowey AJ. Current concepts in the diagnosis and management of adolescent idiopathic scoliosis. *Childs Nerv Syst.* 2020;36(6):1111-1119. doi:10.1007/s00381-020-04608-4
47. Ko JY, Suh JH, Kim H, Ryu JS. Proposal of a new exercise protocol for idiopathic scoliosis: a preliminary study. *Medicine (Baltimore).* 2018;97(49):e13336. doi:10.1097/MD.0000000000013336

# Section III

# Specific Applications of Therapeutic Exercise

Chapter 16

# Exercise Considerations for Persons With Neurologic Diagnoses

*Jacki Klaczak Kopack, PT, DPT*

**KEY TERMS** Compensatory training | Function-induced recovery | Neuroplasticity | Reference of correctness | Spasticity | Synergy pattern

## Chapter Objectives

1. Explain the potential impact of the common impairments associated with the following neurologic pathologies on mobility and the ability to exercise: cerebrovascular accident (CVA), traumatic brain injury (TBI), spinal cord injury (SCI), Parkinson disease (PD), amyotrophic lateral sclerosis (ALS), multiple sclerosis (MS), and epilepsy.
2. Describe the common pediatric neurologic conditions and their impact on mobility and the ability to exercise.
3. Differentiate between function-induced recovery and compensatory training.
4. Identify the common tests and measures for patients with common neurologic disorders.
5. Distinguish between the treatment interventions to increase and decrease muscle tone.
6. Explain the impact tonal changes and fatigue can have on physical therapy interventions.
7. Recommend the appropriate modifications a physical therapist assistant can make to maximize patient performance and outcomes in persons with neurologic diagnoses.
8. Summarize the appropriate monitoring needed to maximize safety when increasing activity levels/exercise with patients with various neurologic diagnoses.
9. Discuss the indications, precautions, and contraindications to exercise interventions for patients with various neurologic pathologies.
10. Given a patient scenario and plan of care (POC), develop an appropriate treatment intervention plan for a patient with a selected neurologic diagnosis.

## Introduction to Neurologic Disorders

Neurologic disorders are diseases that affect the central nervous system (CNS) and/or peripheral nervous system (PNS), including diseases that affect the brain, spinal cord, nerves, or the neuromuscular junction. Some of the more common neurologic diseases include epilepsy, cerebrovascular disease (stroke), MS, PD, and brain injury. Hundreds of millions of people worldwide are affected by neurologic disorders.[1] The impairments associated with each disease have a predictable presentation based on the



Kopack JK, Cascardi KA. *Principles of Therapeutic Exercise for the Physical Therapist Assistant* (pp 563-594).

pathophysiology of the disease and the affected nervous system structures; however, each patient with a given disorder will likely present somewhat differently. The physical therapist assistant will use knowledge of the disease presentation to develop an appropriate exercise program. The exercise program/parameters should be modified based on each patient's presentation to allow the patient to get the optimal benefit from each exercise. Exercise is traditionally viewed in the context of healthy people, but physical activity and exercise can provide the same benefits for patients with neurologic disease. The physical therapy team is uniquely qualified to assist these patients in all aspects of rehabilitation, including exercise interventions.

Understanding the anatomy and the normal function of the neurologic system allows the clinician to predict a patient's presentation, including likely impairments based on the location of neurologic damage or injury. Table 16-1 provides an overview of the nervous system anatomy and function. The CNS includes the brain and spinal cord. The brain is divided into 4 lobes: the frontal, parietal, temporal, and occipital lobe. The PNS includes the nerves and ganglia outside of the CNS.

The nervous system includes pathways for communication between the CNS and PNS that are critical for normal muscle movement and resting muscle tone. Upper motor neurons direct the lower motor neurons to produce muscle movements. Lower motor neurons send messages to individual muscles in the body. Upper motor neurons relay information within the brain and spinal cord. Motor information is relayed from the brain (upper motor neurons) to the anterior (ventral) horn of the spinal cord (where lower motor neurons originate). The motor nerve cells that exit the spinal cord (lower motor neurons) synapse with the peripheral nerves and end at the muscle, releasing neurotransmitters and creating a voluntary muscle contraction. There is an alternate communication pathway to the lower motor neuron that allows the body to respond to painful or dangerous stimuli rapidly. This pathway is called a *reflex arc*, and it allows a local response to a sensory stimulus (eg, pain). In the presence of a noxious stimulus (eg, a person touches a hot stove), sensory information is perceived by sensory receptors in the skin. This information is transmitted via afferent neurons and travels to the posterior (dorsal) horn of the spinal cord where it synapses with a motor nerve or interneuron. The interneuron synapses with a lower motor neuron in the anterior (ventral) horn of the spinal cord; this lower motor neuron relays information via a peripheral motor nerve (efferent nerves) to the muscles so they quickly contract to move the limb away. Neurologic disorders can disrupt these pathways, resulting in movement and/or muscle tone abnormalities.

## Common Presentations in Patients With a Neurologic Diagnosis

Therapeutic exercise programs typically target strength deficits, cardiorespiratory impairments, balance deficits, and/or postural deviations/malalignment. In patients with neurologic deficits or diseases, some or all of these impairments may be present. Impaired voluntary motion and decreased coordination are common. Patients may present with paralysis (complete loss of muscle strength and function) or paresis (partial loss of muscle strength or weakness). Weakness or paralysis may prevent the ability to ambulate, or this impairment may increase energy demands during walking, decreasing the quality and functional effectiveness of gait. Damage to the CNS can result in changes in muscle tone, which can affect functional abilities and the ability to participate in an exercise or training program. Upper motor neuron damage/lesions can result in spasticity, hyperactive reflexes, and paralysis or paresis. If an upper motor neuron is injured, inhibitory messages from the motor cortex that travel via the upper motor neurons to the lower motor neurons are not sent. When lower motor neurons are not receiving inhibitory signals, it results in muscle stiffness (spasticity) and overactive reflexes. **Spasticity** is a condition characterized by muscle tightness due to increased involuntary muscle tone paired with a velocity-dependent resistance to range of motion (ROM). Spasticity increases with higher-velocity motions, and, when persistent, it results in the development of contractures. The presence of spasticity can make voluntary movements slow and difficult, resulting in difficulty with ambulation and self-care activities.

A patient with a lower motor neuron lesion presents with flaccid paralysis or paresis due to a loss of muscle tone (hypotonia). Reflexes will be decreased or absent. When the muscles do not receive signals from the lower motor neurons, they begin to weaken and shrink in size (muscle atrophy). The muscles may also start to spontaneously twitch (fasciculations) below the surface of the skin.

Examples of upper and lower motor lesion diagnoses are listed in Table 16-2. Some neurologic conditions can affect both upper and lower motor neurons (eg, ALS). Early symptoms of ALS (also called *Lou Gehrig disease*) may include weakness, stiff or tight muscles, and fasciculations resulting from damage to both the upper and lower motor neurons.

**Table 16-1**

## Anatomy/Physiology and Function of the Nervous System

| The CNS includes the brain and spinal cord; nerves in these areas are considered to be upper motor neurons. | |
|---|---|
| Brain | The cerebral cortex is composed of a right and left hemisphere, each divided into 4 lobes. Each side of the body is controlled by the opposite hemisphere of the brain. |
| Frontal lobe | The primary motor cortex is responsible for controlling motor function and expressive language. Broca's area is linked to the ability to speak. A deficit in language production is referred to as *Broca's* or *expressive aphasia*. The prefrontal area is located in the most anterior portion of the frontal lobe; this area is responsible for control of the executive functions (behavior, judgment, abstract thinking, goal planning, and higher-level thought processes). |
| Temporal lobe | The primary auditory cortex is responsible for receptive language. Wernicke's area allows for interpretation and speech comprehension. A deficit in this area is referred to as *Wernicke's* or *receptive aphasia*. This lobe contributes to visual perception and music discrimination. The hippocampus is located here; it plays an important role in the formation of memories. |
| Parietal lobe | The primary sensory cortex is responsible for processing sensory information (eg, light touch, pressure, pain). |
| Occipital lobe | The primary visual cortex; responsible for interpreting visual information. |
| Thalamus | Acts as a relay station, accepting, processing, and transmitting sensory information and motor information (from the cerebellum and the basal ganglia) to the cerebral cortex. |
| Basal ganglia | Regulates posture and muscle tone and controls/coordinates body motions. The basal ganglia and substantia nigra contain dopamine-producing neurons. |
| Hypothalamus | Plays a role in the control of hunger, thirst, emotion, and body temperature. The hypothalamus plays a regulatory role over the pituitary gland (thereby playing a role in many body functions). |
| Cerebellum | Plays a role in the control of posture, balance, and the coordination of voluntary movements. |
| Brainstem | Includes the midbrain, pons, and medulla oblongata. Midbrain: Relay between spinal cord and cerebrum. Houses reflex centers that respond to visual, auditory, and tactile stimuli. Pons: Stimulates breathing and controls sleep cycles. Medulla oblongata: Controls heart rate, breathing, and blood pressure (autonomic functions) and coordinates involuntary reflexes (cough, sneeze, vomit). |
| Spinal cord | Transmits motor nerve impulses from the cerebral cortex and sensory information from the periphery to the parietal lobe. Coordinates reflexes and contains reflex arcs. Information travels in tracts (white matter/myelinated neurons) and synapses in the gray matter, centrally in the cord, at each level. |
| The PNS: These nerves are considered to be lower motor neurons. | |
| PNS | All peripheral nerves lie outside the spinal cord and travel via the ventral root from the anterior horn of the spinal cord to the muscles. These include cranial nerves, spinal nerves, nerve roots and branches, peripheral nerves, and neuromuscular junctions. Ventral (motor) and dorsal (sensory) roots are located at each spinal cord level and combine to form the spinal nerves. |

**Table 16-2**

Upper and Lower Motor Neuron Lesion Diagnoses

| Upper Motor Neuron Lesion Diagnoses | Lower Motor Neuron Lesion Diagnoses | Diagnoses With Both Upper and Lower Motor Neuron Involvement |
|---|---|---|
| • CVA<br>• Huntington disease<br>• MS<br>• PD<br>• SCI<br>• TBI | • Guillain-Barré<br>• Postpolio syndrome<br>• Myasthenia gravis<br>• Spinal muscular atrophy | • ALS |

Certain neurologic diseases can cause tremors. Tremors are defined as involuntary muscle contractions that are rhythmic in nature and result in the shaking of a body segment. They are often observed in the hands but can also occur in the upper or lower extremities, head, or trunk and may even be evident in a patient's voice (due to vocal cord tremors). The most common types are resting and intention tremors. Resting tremors can be observed in patients when the extremity is supported with muscles at rest. This type of tremor is often noted in patients with PD when their hands and fingers can be observed moving rhythmically (referred to as a *pill-rolling tremor*). Intention tremors are observed when a patient reaches for an object or target (eg, when reaching for a glass of water, the closer to the glass, the worse the shaking [tremors] will appear). These tremors are common in patients diagnosed with cerebellar conditions or MS. Rigidity may be present in patients with a neurologic condition; it is commonly associated with PD. Cogwheel rigidity is a jerky or ratchetlike movement when a patient's extremity is passively moved. Lead-pipe rigidity is a continuous resistance to passive motion throughout the ROM.

## Quick Review: Motor Learning, Feedback, Practice, and Treatment Suggestions

Cognitive changes or neurologic damage can affect a person's ability to participate in therapy, learn, and/or relearn purposeful movements. Knowledge and the application of techniques that support learning allow the clinician to effectively guide patients in a program designed to meet the patients' goals.

Motor control is the ability of the CNS to produce and modulate coordinated, purposeful motion.[2] Motor control describes the process the brain uses to preplan, initiate, and modify muscle movement (providing stability or mobility) during various activities in different environments. Motor control theories continue to evolve. As defined in Chapter 2, motor learning is the process of skill acquisition and retention through repetitive practice. Treatment suggestions to enhance learning are summarized in Table 16-3. The therapy team works with patients to promote motor learning, guide recovery, and improve functional abilities to maximize the patient's ability to complete the desired tasks. Optimal selection of practice schedules and the type of feedback can enhance and optimize patient outcomes and can assist a patient with transitioning through the stages of motor learning for task and skill acquisition.[3]

A common goal is to promote the patient's ability to develop strategies to complete a task efficiently and effectively. Early in the rehabilitation process, this often requires the clinician to demonstrate the task/activity correctly. This demonstration establishes a **reference of correctness** (ie, an internal cognitive map/plan for how the task should look) for the patient. The clinician may need to manually guide the patient through the task or motions initially to assist the patient with establishing this reference of correctness. Verbal and tactile cues can be provided but should be reduced as early as possible to prevent the patient from being dependent on them.[3] It is often said that "practice makes perfect," but only *perfect* practice makes perfect. Practicing a task incorrectly interferes with learning. This is why establishing a reference of correctness and monitoring performance during learning are important.

The practice schedule can be manipulated to promote early learning and then to enhance skill retention/acquisition later in the training program. The physical therapist assistant should modify practice schedules based on the stage of motor learning, the patient's presentation, and skill performance. Blocked part practice may be used initially (during the cognitive stage), but blocked order whole practice of the skill should be encouraged as quickly as possible to enhance early acquisition. As the patient fine-tunes task performance (during the autonomous stage), practice should become more randomized with added distractions.

Initial feedback, which is provided in the cognitive stages of learning, should be precise yet brief, targeting the critical components of the task. Attempting to provide feedback for all components of the task will overwhelm the patient.

**Table 16-3**

**Treatment Suggestions to Enhance Learning in Each Stage of Learning**

| Cognitive → | Associative → | Autonomous |
|---|---|---|
| • Demonstrate task so patient has a reference for correct performance.<br>• Review critical components of task.<br>• Have patient verbalize steps.<br>• Let patient visually watch motions. Provide concurrent or immediate terminal augmented feedback about performance when errors are consistent.<br>• Use manual guidance early on if needed; remove as soon as appropriate.<br>• Limit distractions (work in a closed environment).<br>• Use blocked and part practice as needed. Progress to whole practice. | • Emphasize attention to how the task "feels."<br>• Encourage learner to self-assess performance.<br>• Minimize manual guidance and augmented feedback. Transition to delayed and summary feedback.<br>• Transition from blocked practice to a serial and random order practice.<br>• Begin working in an open environment. Increase task complexity.<br>• Focus on good outcomes/results of task performance. | • Instruct patient to self-monitor performance; encourage self-assessment.<br>• Provide minimal delayed feedback only when errors are evident and not identified by patient's self-assessment.<br>• Increase practice in various environments and with increased complexity and distractions.<br>• Integrate tasks into activities of daily living (ADLs) and instrumental ADLs. |

As the patient becomes more proficient at performing a task, the clinician can redirect the patient's focus to intrinsic kinesthetic feedback so the patient can self-correct and refine skill performance. The clinician should initially provide extrinsic (augmented) feedback to assist the patient with learning and then refining task performance, with a goal of transitioning the patient to intrinsic (internal) feedback as early as possible during skill acquisition. Allowing a brief delay before providing feedback after task completion allows the patient the opportunity to self-correct errors first.

**Clinical Tip**

Provide feedback and assistance as much as necessary but as little as possible.

## Interventions for the Neurologic Patient: Restoration of Function or Compensation?

The nervous system is responsible for the initiation of muscle contraction, movement, and coordination. Neurologic damage can impact motion and function. The primary goals of therapy are to restore function and to maximize independence using interventions such as strength training, coordination retraining, sensory stimulation, tone management techniques, positioning, cognitive training activities, aerobic exercise/endurance training, balance training, and patient/caregiver education. The desired outcomes of treatment often include increased strength, endurance, and functional independence; decreased care needs; decreased risk of secondary impairments; increased levels of alertness and attention; improved coordination, balance, posture, and gait; increased motor learning capabilities; increased health or well-being and fitness; and better quality of life (QOL) and personal satisfaction.

If there is an injury to the CNS, the damaged nerve cells do not regenerate (conversely, peripheral nerve cells do have the ability to regenerate). Recovery after brain injury (eg, ischemic stroke) can occur as a result of spontaneous recovery, function-induced recovery, and/or compensation. Some recovery is facilitated by early medical care. For example, with an ischemic stroke, if a patient is given a thrombolytic medication (eg, a tissue plasminogen activator) within 3 hours of the onset of stroke symptoms, the amount of brain damage can be limited. This treatment works by restoring blood flow (and oxygen supply) to the affected area of the brain.

Spontaneous recovery refers to the neuronal changes that result from the repair processes occurring in the cells immediately surrounding the injured area. This restores some neural function that may have appeared lost immediately postinjury. Spontaneous recovery rates for neurologic function vary for each individual. Recovery rates also vary based on the affected region of the brain and the activity/task. For example, most motor function improvements usually occur within the first 3 months, whereas visuospatial, memory, and/or language improvements may continue over several months to years poststroke.[4]

**Function-induced recovery** (use-dependent cortical reorganization) results when a patient performs a motion or task postinjury similarly to how task completion occurred preinjury; it relies on adaptation within the CNS. **Neuroplasticity** is the brain's ability to form and reorganize neuronal (nerve cell) connections in the remaining/undamaged areas of the brain. It allows the neurons to compensate and adapt to CNS injury or disease by adjusting their function to allow completion of the needed skills. Neuroplasticity is an important factor in maximizing recovery, and it is dependent on having an appropriate learning environment.[3,5,6]

Compensation is the use of a new or different movement pattern (compared with that used preinjury) or the use of a substitution motor pattern to perform a skill or task that the patient was initially unable to complete after the CNS injury. **Compensatory training** includes task training that uses substitution (ie, training a patient to complete tasks in a new way). Compensatory training is appropriate to implement early in the rehabilitation process when there is no reasonable expectation of recovery of the affected skill. An example of clinically appropriate compensatory training is teaching a patient with a complete (American Spinal Injury Association Classification [ASIA] A) thoracic SCI to complete transfers using the head-hips relationship. According to the classification definition, this patient has no motor or sensory function below the level of the injury.[3,5] Compensatory training is sometimes initiated postinjury as an attempt to increase early function and independence, but this may be detrimental to maximal recovery.[6] Early use of compensatory strategies (eg, increased use of the unaffected arm after a stroke to complete feeding and ADLs) can result in less use of the affected limb, fewer opportunities to develop new motor pathways in the brain, and a phenomenon called *learned nonuse*. Learned nonuse occurs when the brain progressively decreases the use of the affected limb.[7] Facilitating task-specific training and focused use of the impaired limbs may encourage function-induced recovery. Delaying the start of compensatory training and delaying the use of assistive devices may also encourage function-induced recovery.

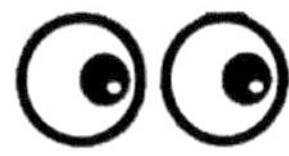

### Eye on the Research: Reducing Learned Nonuse

Constraint-induced movement therapy (CIMT) is effective in treating learned nonuse and promoting increased use of the affected limbs, but the high intensity of typical CIMT protocols makes compliance and adherence difficult.[8] Newer research indicates that the improvement in limb motion achieved with CIMT is not always associated with decreased disability in these patients.[9]

Reinforcement-induced movement therapy (RIMT) incorporates practicing amplified goal-oriented movements in a virtual reality setting. Preliminary research indicates that RIMT has the ability to restore motor function by maximizing limb use.[10] Motions are selected to replicate the desired movements/patterns that the patient wants to improve. Although the control group and the RIMT group both demonstrated improved upper extremity function, only the RIMT group exhibited a significant increase in arm use and continued gains in later follow-up.[10]

When working with patients with neurologic diagnoses, the physical therapist assistant should implement interventions that encourage function-induced recovery (Table 16-4).[11] To do this effectively, the physical therapist assistant must merge their knowledge of exercise application with the specific treatment principles that promote function-induced recovery. With neurologic recovery, overstimulation, lack of appropriate rest, and excessive practice can be detrimental to healing but so can a lack of exercise or an environment that is poor in stimulation and opportunities for social interaction. Neuroplasticity and adaptability are more prevalent/likely in the young. The clinician may see less plasticity (and less improvement) in older patients, but plasticity may also depend on a patient's cognitive reserve (ie, the mind's resistance to damage of the brain or the ability of the brain to be resilient after injury/damage to the brain). Higher cognitive reserve is associated with greater neuroplasticity. Increased cognitive reserve is associated with participation in a diverse number of lifestyle activities, healthy diet, higher intelligence quotient, and increased levels of occupational complexity.[6]

**Table 16-4**

**Factors That Promote Function-Induced Recovery**

- **Use it or lose it.** Incorporate practice of key motor skills/tasks (to discourage learned nonuse).
- **Practice.** Use repetition wisely (build repetition of task training into therapy session, caregiver interactions, and home exercise program; practice enhances performance).
- **Intensity matters.** Sufficient intensity induces improvement. Practice at an appropriate intensity. Monitor the patient carefully for signs of fatigue/overwork, but ensure that the environment provides adequate stimulation/opportunities for social interaction and build in appropriate rest periods.
- **Timing matters.** Initiate activities at an appropriate time during the patient's recovery (aggressive therapy implemented too early can inhibit recovery, but delaying implementation of therapy can result in learned nonuse).
- **Relevance matters.** Select appropriate stimuli to generate the desired response.
- **Specificity is important.** Practice skills and functional tasks that are relevant to the patient; include task training that specifically and clearly relates to the patient's personal goals.
- **Improve it.** Modify and advance skill training as the patient improves (continually address areas where the patient is improving by increasing the intensity or parameters of the task).
- **Engage the patient.** Promote attention to the task and confirm that the patient will "give their all!" Tie the task to rewards that are important to the patient and elicit patient feedback after task completion to promote transition to autonomous performance).
- **Provide appropriate feedback.** Use an appropriate fading schedule and use knowledge of performance and knowledge of feedback only as needed to improve task performance (limit manual guidance).

## *Addressing Muscle Tone*

Patients with neurologic involvement often present with changes in muscle tone. The goal of treatment interventions is to normalize tone, maintain ROM, and promote the ability to complete functional tasks with the affected limb. Flaccidity (hypotonicity) is often present early after a CVA, TBI, SCI, and other neurologic injuries. Those who present with flaccidity do not have the ability to actively move the affected limbs. The physical therapist assistant needs to address positioning of the affected limb to protect the limb and to maintain tissue length (Figure 16-1). Three key things to remember when positioning patients with hemiplegia are as follows:

1. Avoid prolonged shoulder adduction, internal rotation, elbow flexion, and finger and wrist flexion.
2. Avoid prolonged hip external rotation, hip/knee flexion, and ankle inversion and plantar flexion.
3. Maintain the patient's head and trunk in normal alignment.

Patients with a flaccid upper extremity are at risk of shoulder subluxation, so care must be taken to reduce the risk of injury. In the supine position, the affected arm should be supported by a pillow with the shoulder positioned in slight abduction and external rotation, the elbow extended, the forearm and wrist in neutral, and the fingers in extension. Before performing upper extremity passive range of motion (PROM), the clinician should assess the scapulothoracic joint to ensure adequate scapular mobility, and then the glenohumeral joint should be externally rotated during shoulder flexion and abduction PROM to prevent impingement. The patient should not complete self–active assisted ROM or use pulleys if the upper extremity is flaccid. The flaccid upper extremity may be placed in a sling during functional mobility and gait training to prevent a sulcus sign (ie, dropping of the humeral head in the glenoid fossa) or subluxation.

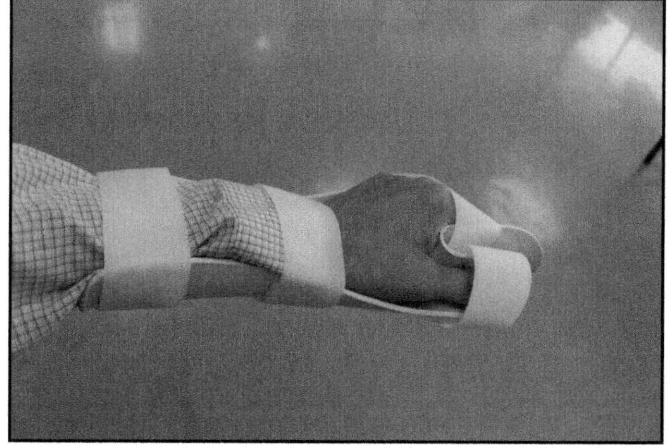

**Figure 16-1.** A resting hand splint (CactusG/Shutterstock.com).

Most patients (except those with tetraplegia or paraplegia) regain some use of the lower extremity early in the recovery process. The assistant should consider the strength deficits; the patient may need bracing during functional mobility and gait training. An appropriately selected ankle-foot orthosis can accommodate for the inability to actively dorsiflex and can also be used to limit knee hyperextension in stance (Figure 16-2). The physical

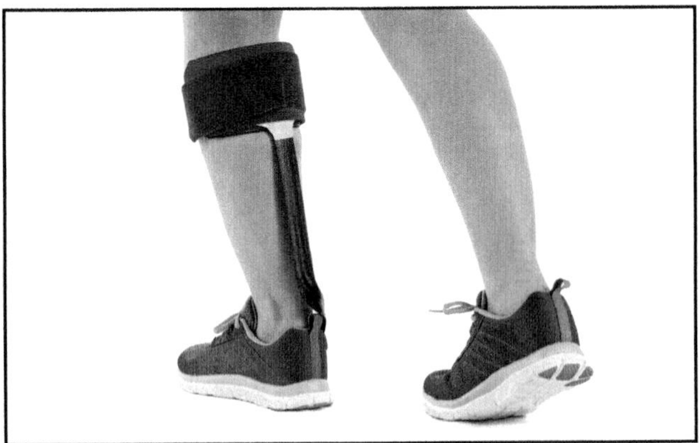

**Figure 16-2.** A type of ankle-foot orthosis to prevent knee hyperextension and to maintain ankle dorsiflexion in patients with hemiparesis (belushi/Shutterstock.com).

## Study Tip

Students often struggle when trying to learn the motions that occur in each of the spasticity and synergy patterns. Put motor learning to work for you; as you study the list of terms, place your limb in the full spasticity or synergy pattern that you are studying. Each time you study the terms for a pattern, place your limb in the joint positions included in that pattern. Use blocked practice first; state "upper extremity flexor spasticity pattern," and then move all of your upper extremity joints into their respective positions. Relax and do it again and again until the pattern seems familiar. Then, complete the same steps with the next pattern. Once you can complete each pattern easily in blocked practice, progress to random practice, alternating which pattern you will practice.

therapist assistant may need to implement techniques to facilitate muscle tone in patients who present with hypotonia or flaccid limbs (Table 16-5).[12]

Spasticity is associated with upper motor neuron disorders. Spasticity is a velocity-dependent increase in muscle tone that presents with abnormal muscle tightness due to prolonged muscle contraction. Persons with spasticity commonly exhibit poor voluntary control of the spastic limb. Significant spasticity increases the likelihood of contracture development in the affected limb. The characteristic spasticity pattern for the upper extremity is a flexion (flexor) spasticity pattern, and the lower extremity pattern is an extension (extensor) spasticity pattern. Table 16-6 provides a description of the joint positions associated with each spasticity pattern.

Some patients exhibit synergy patterns after neurologic injury. A **synergy pattern** is a primitive pattern of movement that interferes with normal coordinated motion (Table 16-7).[13] It often occurs when the patient is attempting volitional motion, but it can also occur reflexively (eg, when a patient coughs or sneezes). After a stroke, the most common pattern is a flexion synergy pattern in the affected upper extremity and an extension synergy pattern in the lower extremity (Figure 16-3). Synergy patterns can interfere with the completion of functional mobility and ADLs (eg, eating, dressing, walking). Positioning, weight bearing, the use of reflex inhibiting postures, and tone reduction techniques are used when treating patients with spasticity and synergy patterns.

Although it is important for the patient to use the affected limb, excessive effort may result in an increase in tone. Exercise modification and specific tone management techniques are indicated if the patient exhibits an increase in tone during the intervention.[12] Activity modifications to reduce increased tone include decreasing the intensity of the task, decreasing the speed of the motion the patient is performing, or adding a weight-bearing component to the task. These patients may also be taking medication to help control the spasticity.

Therapy interventions are applied to normalize movement patterns and facilitate postural alignment during tasks. Muscle strength/functional return after a CVA typically occurs from proximal to distal. Strengthening exercises and task-specific functional training are important and should address the patient's impairments. For example, if a patient exhibits a flexor synergy pattern and strength less than 3/5, appropriate interventions can include gravity-minimized or active assisted ROM exercises, the use of reflex inhibiting postures (to lengthen shortened muscles), weight bearing through the limb (with the elbow/wrist extended), and facilitation techniques to the weak muscles (stabilizers and extensors). Gentle joint traction may also reduce spasticity and improve joint movement.[13]

**Table 16-5**

Treatment Techniques to Address Altered Muscle Tone (Hypotonia and Hypertonia)

| | |
|---|---|
| Techniques That Facilitate an Increase in Tone for Persons With Hypotonia or Flaccidity | • Weight bearing and joint approximation to facilitate joint awareness and contraction in the stabilizing muscles<br>• Active assisted ROM or exercises in gravity minimized<br>  ○ Use caution to ensure appropriate biomechanics at each joint<br>  ○ Avoid overstretching joints<br>• Quick stretch<br>• Quick tapping over muscle belly or tendon<br>• Brisk or quick icing strokes<br>• Light resistance to promote additional motor unit firing<br>• Use of rapid, staccato commands<br>• Use of air splints to provide sensory input and stabilization of joints |
| Techniques That Facilitate a Decrease in Tone for Persons With Hypertonia or Spasticity | • Weight bearing and joint approximation, especially in a reflex inhibiting posture<br>• Patient should be positioned out of spasticity patterns<br>  ○ Position upper extremity in scapular protraction, slight shoulder flexion, elbow/wrist/finger extension, and thumb abduction<br>  ○ Position lower extremity in pelvic protraction, slight knee flexion, and ankle neutral<br>• Use of neutral warmth (air splints)<br>• Trunk or limb rhythmic rotation or rocking<br>• Slow sustained manual joint compression or traction<br>• Serial casting or adjustable or dynamic (splinting) orthoses<br>• Prolonged/sustained stretches<br>• Use of deep pressure over the spastic muscle tendon<br>• Cold pack applied over the spastic muscle<br>• Neuromuscular electric stimulation to the antagonist muscles<br>• Exercises to focus on weak antagonists (eg, triceps, hamstrings)<br>• Use of soothing, slow verbal commands |

**Table 16-6**

Spasticity Patterns

| Upper Extremity | Lower Extremity |
|---|---|
| • Scapular retraction<br>• Shoulder adduction and internal rotation<br>• Elbow flexion<br>• Wrist flexion and radial deviation<br>• Finger flexion<br>• Thumb adduction/flexion | • Pelvic retraction (hip hiking)<br>• Hip internal rotation, adduction, and extension<br>• Knee extension<br>• Ankle plantar flexion and inversion<br>• Clawed toes (MCP ext, PIP flex, DIP ext) |

DIP ext = distal interphalangeal extension; MCP ext = metacarpophalangeal extension; PIP flex = proximal interphalangeal flexion.

**Table 16-7**

**Synergy Patterns for Upper and Lower Extremities**

| Upper Extremity | Lower Extremity |
|---|---|
| Flexion: Scapular retraction, shoulder abduction and external rotation, elbow flexion, forearm supination, and wrist and finger flexion | Flexion: Hip flexion, abduction and external rotation, knee flexion, and ankle dorsiflexion |
| Extension: Scapular protraction, shoulder adduction and internal rotation, elbow extension, forearm pronation, and wrist and finger flexion | Extension: Hip extension, adduction and internal rotation, knee extension, ankle plantar flexion and inversion, and toe flexion |

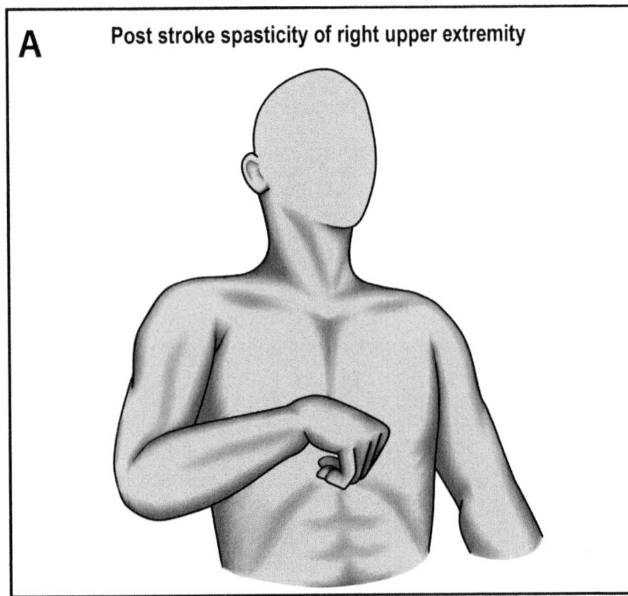


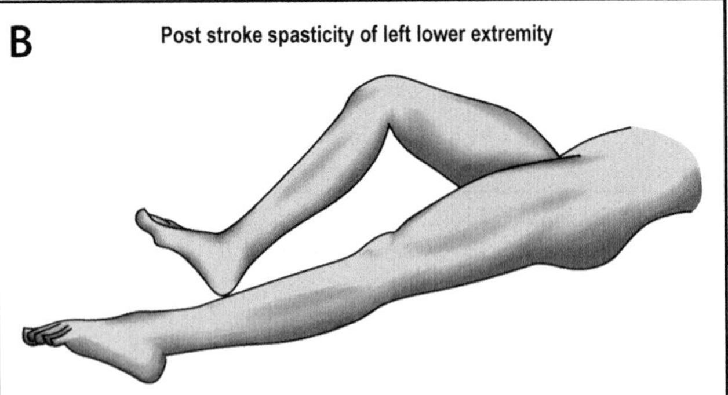


**Figure 16-3.** (A) Right upper extremity flexion spasticity pattern (Songkram Chotik-anuchit/Shutterstock.com). (B) Left lower extremity extension spasticity pattern (Songkram Chotik-anuchit/Shutterstock.com).

> **Clinical Tip**
>
> Inhibit abnormal tone and encourage repetition of normal responses once they are elicited.

## *Developmental Postures*

Patients who have deficits in strength, motor control, and balance may benefit from interventions addressing these deficits in postures that initially have a large base of support (BOS) and a low center of mass (COM). The assistant should select functional postures based on the patient's presentation and goals. For example, if a patient's hip extensors are weak, gluteal and hip extension strengthening is initiated in a position that is safe but challenging to those muscles (ie, bridging in the hook-lying position). As the patient shows improvement in symmetrical weight bearing, strength, motor control, and balance, the assistant will select postures that are more challenging (decreasing the BOS and raising the height of the COM; Table 16-8). Developmental postures include prone on elbows, quadruped, hook lying (with bridging), sitting, half kneeling, kneeling, modified plantigrade, and standing (Figure 16-4).[12] The assistant should select exercises to improve stability within each posture by strengthening those muscles that provide stability in that posture. Interventions that target stability can include static holding, alternating isometrics, and rhythmic stabilization. To address balance, dynamic strength, and stability, the assistant can include weight shifting, functional reaching, strengthening exercises, and practice moving into and out of the posture. In sitting, kneeling, and standing, the patient can practice active range of motion (AROM) and strengthening for the limbs as well as bilateral extremity movement patterns, such as proprioceptive neuromuscular facilitation (PNF) patterns (Figure 16-5). PNF exercises include rotational components, promote limb motions that cross the midline, and challenge postural and balance responses.

The physical therapist assistant should initially provide as much assistance and cuing as needed so the patient correctly performs the activity/exercise while guarding the patient appropriately. Manual guidance is used to facilitate desired movements, provide trunk or limb stabilization, and/or prevent undesired movement patterns. The assistant should reduce the assistance as soon as it is safe to do so. This diminishes the patient's dependence on the clinician's feedback and encourages active control of the movements, kinesthetic awareness, and intrinsic feedback.[12] The goal is

**Table 16-8**

Developmental Postural Positions:
Progressively Decreasing Base of Support and Higher Center of Mass

| | Postural Position | Indications for Use |
|---|---|---|
| Large BOS<br>Low COM | Prone on Elbows | Promotes head, neck, upper trunk, and upper extremity control; stretches hip flexors; and improves stability and strength in shoulder and scapular muscles. Can be progressed to arms extended for weight bearing into upper extremities. |
| Moderate BOS and COM height | Quadruped | Promotes head, neck, trunk, and lower extremity and upper extremity control. Inhibits tone in quadriceps and finger/wrist flexors via prolonged weight bearing and during weight shifting through all extremities. Promotes improved stability and strength in trunk, hip, shoulder muscles, and elbow extensors. |
| Moderate BOS and low COG height | Hook lying (bridging exercises) | Promotes lower trunk/pelvis and lower extremity control. Inhibits tone in the quadriceps and plantar flexors due to positioning out of the spasticity pattern and weight bearing through lower extremities. Promotes improved strength in the hip extensors and abductors and ankle stabilizer muscles. |
| | Sitting | Promotes head, neck, and trunk control. Important for upright balance and precursor to standing balance tasks. Allows symmetrical weight bearing through trunk and lower extremities, and upper extremity weight bearing can be included for tone modification. Can be progressed with weight shifting/reaching activities. |
| | Half kneeling (large BOS)<br>Kneeling (small BOS) | Promotes head, neck, trunk, and pelvic/lower extremity control. Inhibits tone in quads via prolonged weight bearing and promotes improved stability and strength in trunk and hip muscles. Progression from half kneeling to (tall) kneeling increases the challenge to a person's balance. |
| Large BOS<br>High COM | Modified plantigrade | Promotes head, neck, trunk, lower extremity, and upper extremity control. Inhibits tone in finger/wrist flexors via prolonged weight bearing and encourages improved stability and strength in elbow extensors. Knee extension is facilitated due to the extensor moment at knee. Allows supported practice/transition to standing. |
| High BOS<br>Small COM | Standing | Promotes head, neck, trunk, and lower extremity control in a full upright posture. Allows for symmetrical weight bearing and weight shifting in all directions. |

task completion with little to no errors and limited external/augmented feedback.

## *Other Treatment Interventions for the Neurologically Involved Patient*

The experienced clinician will often use specialized treatment interventions such as PNF (refer to Chapter 6), neurodevelopmental treatment (or the Bobath approach), or the Rood approach when treating the neurologic population. This section provides brief descriptions of various techniques that have been shown to be effective for patients with neurologic conditions. Some of these interventions are used early in the rehabilitation process to either facilitate or inhibit muscle tone and are less appropriate to use once the patient is demonstrating active motion and control of the affected extremities. A common theme with neurologic treatment approaches is the relationship between sensory input and motor function output. Karel Bobath (physician) and Bertha Bobath (physical therapist) developed an approach to treat children with cerebral palsy (CP) and adults who sustained a stroke. They believed that function could improve by changing (or modifying) abnormal

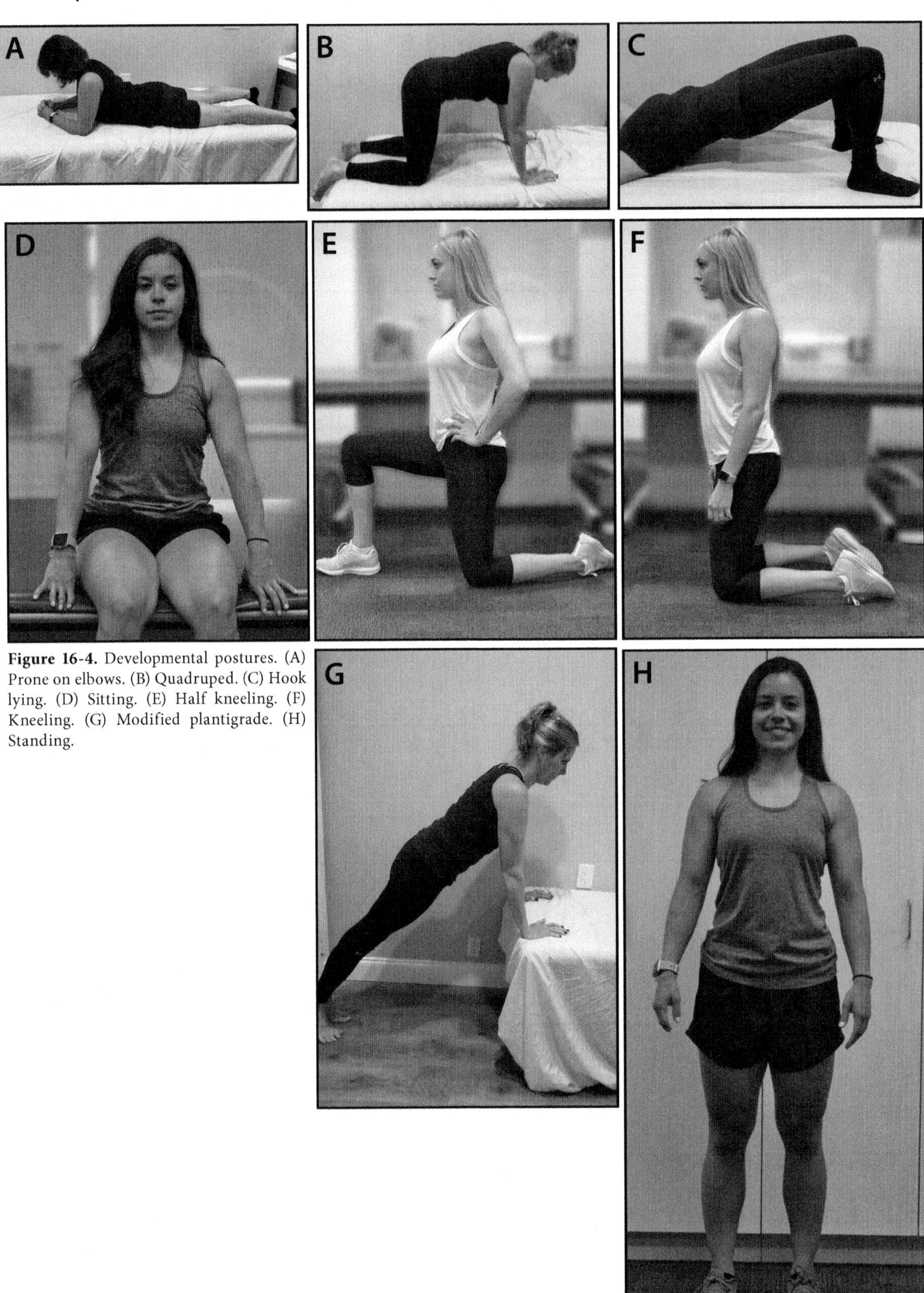


**Figure 16-4.** Developmental postures. (A) Prone on elbows. (B) Quadruped. (C) Hook lying. (D) Sitting. (E) Half kneeling. (F) Kneeling. (G) Modified plantigrade. (H) Standing.

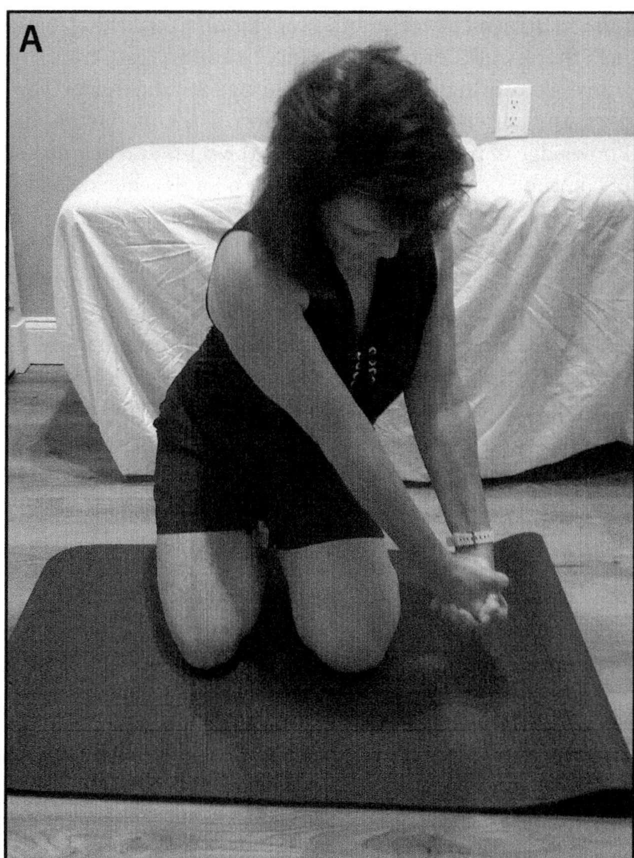


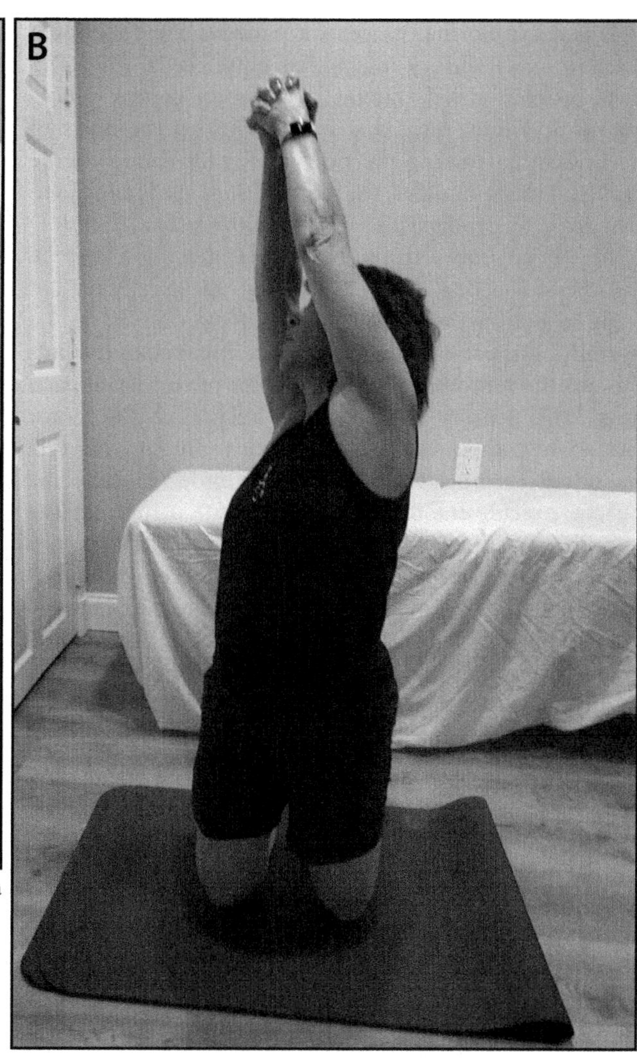


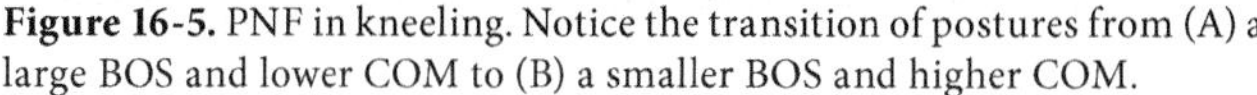
**Figure 16-5.** PNF in kneeling. Notice the transition of postures from (A) a large BOS and lower COM to (B) a smaller BOS and higher COM.

movement patterns. This approach is referred to as *neurodevelopmental treatment techniques.* Neurodevelopmental treatment primarily focuses on using sensorimotor function (sensory input/motor output) to promote CNS neuroplasticity and adaptation, and it includes neuromuscular and functional re-education and practice.[12] It is guided by motor learning principles. The goal of neurodevelopmental treatment is to facilitate and maintain proper postural alignment and then progress to sequential movement patterns that target the affected side using progressive developmental positioning and functional activities/exercises. Treatment is functional and task specific based on the goals outlined in the POC. The ability to differentiate between normal/abnormal postures and the desired/unwanted movement patterns allows the assistant to guide the patient toward appropriate movement patterns using tactile or verbal cues and feedback.

The Rood approach was developed by Margaret Rood (a physical therapist) in the 1940s; the goal was to normalize muscle tone and improve function by using purposeful repetitive movements. Rood believed that sensory mechanisms were inter-related with motor function and that stimulating the sensory receptors of the primitive reflexes resulted in specific motor patterns.[14] Some patients may need sensory stimulation (ie, semicomatose patients or patients with flaccidity), whereas others may require sensory inhibiting techniques (ie, patients with TBI who are agitated or highly aroused and those with hypersensitivity or spasticity). Sensory stimulation can facilitate a patient response in several ways, including the use of quick/loud verbal cues, quick brushing, and noxious smells. Interventions that reduce sensory stimulation include pleasant smells, rocking, constant pressure, and swaddling (see Table 16-5).

When peripheral nerves regenerate, patients may report a tingling feeling and hypersensitivity in the area where numbness was originally experienced. To accommodate for these sensations, the clinician can rub various textured materials (eg, cotton swab, washcloth, sandpaper) for a few minutes over the area to desensitize it and reduce the uncomfortable sensations. Sensory retraining is another technique that can help the brain recognize or discriminate between various sizes, shapes, weights, and textures of objects held in the patient's involved hand (without visual cues) that were recognizable before the injury (eg, a stroke). Sensory retraining for the lower extremity (and feet) can include walking on various surfaces or inclines to regain more kinesthetic awareness.[12,15]

To achieve normal movement patterns and functional mobility, multisensory integration must occur. The CNS must process visual, tactile, and proprioceptive information and then relay that information to the areas of the brain that initiate the output of information (nerve impulses) to the muscles; the muscles then need to respond accurately to produce the desired movements or task.[15] If there is an injury to the brain, task execution may be unsuccessful. Consider the following example: A patient needs to button their pants when getting dressed in the morning. The patient first needs to see and feel for the button and the buttonhole (determine the proximity to each other); this sensory information is relayed to the motor cortex where the message is then sent to the muscles (via the spinal cord/peripheral nerves) in order to have the muscles execute the task (ie, put the button through the buttonhole). If the patient is unable to process the sensory information, perform all of the steps in order, or cannot manipulate the button and buttonhole at the correct angle due to poor muscle control (dexterity), the patient will not be able to button their pants. The motor cortex not only produces the command for movement, but after task practice, it also experiences plasticity, leading to a reduction in the number of errors and an improvement in motor skill accuracy. Performing motor learning skills, incorporating appropriate feedback, and good skill practice are important to regaining normal movement.

### *Addressing Fatigue*

It is important to create treatment plans that challenge the patient while preventing fatigue. Gradual increases in activity level, adequate warm-up and cooldown, appropriate rest periods, and close monitoring of the patient can all be beneficial in minimizing fatigue. Individuals with neurologic diagnoses may perform activities/exercises with an increased number of errors, and they may present with a decline in functional ability when fatigued. Fatigue can also increase aggressive behaviors as sometimes observed in patients with TBI. It is not uncommon to have a patient who does well in therapy one day and then the next day struggles to complete their program. Fatigue can reduce the patient's motivation level and can negatively affect progress.[12] Monitoring each patient's presentation and actively observing patient responses guide the clinician to appropriately modify each treatment session.

## Treatment Considerations for Various Neurologic Diagnoses

Physical therapy is indicated for patients with neurologic diagnoses throughout the continuum of care. Many neurologically involved patients will receive physical therapy in each treatment setting, including the intensive care unit (ICU), acute care, acute rehabilitation hospital, skilled nursing facility, home health, and the outpatient clinic. Rehabilitation interventions often include muscle tone management techniques, positioning, splinting/bracing, therapeutic exercise, balance training, gait training, transfer training, cognitive training, psychological support, and patient/caregiver education. The clinician applies knowledge of pathophysiology and the signs and symptoms of common neurologic conditions as a guide when developing treatment programs, individualizing the plan based on each patient's presentation.

The physical therapist's evaluation provides an overview of the patient's abilities and impairments. The assessment of ROM is important, especially if altered tone is present, indicating that a stretching program may be appropriate to prevent contractures and improve function. Tone reduction techniques (see Table 16-5) are useful before initiating exercises. For example, lower trunk rotation in hook lying or with legs over a ball can be useful to break up tone, as can rhythmic rotation of a limb before initiating ROM exercises. Physical therapy interventions often focus on balance, functional mobility, and movement transitions/transfers. The incorporation of developmental postures allows the patient to practice movement transitions with the benefit of addressing tone and weakness (ie, transitioning from supine hook lying to side lying or quadruped into side sitting). Appendix B provides a useful template to guide the assistant in developing an appropriate treatment plan.

**Documentation Tip**

For consistency of care, it is useful to document both the sequence and the purpose of all exercise interventions. For example, if the therapist is completing exercises for tone reduction before completing ROM exercise, delineate that in the treatment note. Documentation could state the following:

Patient presents in bed with R LE in full extensor spasticity position. Tone reduction: Supine, passive rhythmic rotation to R hip IR/ER × 10 reps followed by PROM for lower trunk rotation completed with LE supported on T-ball, with gentle approximation into B hips, 10 reps (mod A to assist patient into hip and knee flexion over a therapy ball in supine).

ROM: Patient assisted (min A) into side lying on L, and powder board placed under R LE. Patient completed 2 × 8 reps of R hip flexion AROM, reported fatigue, requiring a 3-minute rest between sets. Knee extension AROM 2 × 8 reps with tapping applied to quadriceps to facilitate full ROM.

### *Multiple Sclerosis*

MS is a chronic disease that causes demyelination of nerve cells in the CNS. MS is a chronic disease that is believed to impact 2.3 million people in the United States.[16] MS affects women more than men, and the typical onset is between 20 and 40 years of age. MS presentation can vary greatly from person to person as well as within an individual's disease progression over time. There are 3 different major MS disease courses: relapsing-remitting, primary progressive, and secondary progressive MS.[17] Relapsing-remitting MS is the most common type; it accounts for 85% of cases on initial diagnosis, and presentation is characterized by periods of exacerbations (or relapses) and remissions. During an exacerbation, there are new or increased neurologic symptoms. During remission (a period of partial or complete recovery), all symptoms may disappear, or some symptoms may remain, resulting in a decline in functional status. There does not appear to be a progression of the disease during periods of remission. Primary progressive MS accounts for approximately 15% of cases on initial diagnosis, and these patients present with a continuous worsening of neurologic function and increasing functional loss/disability. Secondary progressive MS is diagnosed after a person with an initial diagnosis of relapsing-remitting MS presents with a progressive worsening of neurologic function and a progressive decline in functional ability over time.[17]

Each person's disease progression is individualized. Oftentimes, the first presentation of MS is an episode of neurologic symptoms (lasting longer than 24 hours). This type of episode is called *clinically isolated syndrome*. It is not solely diagnostic of MS; however, when it is paired with evidence of lesions in the CNS, there may be an increased likelihood of a future episode and a future diagnosis of MS. A definitive diagnosis of MS is issued only with evidence of CNS lesions and symptom presentation that occurs at 2 separate points in time.[16]

**Considerations for the Physical Therapist Assistant**

Report any new or different neurologic signs or symptoms that the patient reports or that you observe to the physical therapist.

Common signs and symptoms of MS include visual disturbances, sensory changes, pain, short-term memory loss, weakness, spasticity, fatigue, balance impairments, impaired gait, bowel and bladder dysfunction, depression, cognitive changes, speech or swallowing deficits, and sexual dysfunction (Table 16-9). Overheating or excessive fatigue can result in a transient increase in symptoms (Uhthoff's phenomenon). Patient presentation is individualized; a patient may exhibit any of the signs/symptoms but is not likely to present with all of them.[16]

Specific assessment tools that are commonly used for persons with MS include the Kurtzke Expanded Disability Status Scale, the Minimum Record of Disability, the MS Functional Composite, the MS QOL-54, and the Multiple Sclerosis Impact Scale (29 items). These instruments have better responsiveness than tools used for the general population. Scoring on these tools can be useful to track changes over time, especially when monitoring for the effectiveness of therapy interventions. Other functional assessment tools can be useful within sessions to track specific functional parameters based on an individual patient's goals and the selected physical therapy interventions. The Timed 25-Foot Walk Test, Timed Up and Go Test, Four-Square Test, and Dynamic Gait Index have been shown to be valid when used with people with MS, and these tools can be useful to track progress as well as for predicting fall risk.[16,18-20]

The medical and pharmacologic management of MS can be complex and continues to change as medical advances are made. The management of MS typically includes a number of medications that are used to manage the disease (disease-modifying therapeutic agents), address acute exacerbations, and help manage the symptoms of MS. The clinician will need to become familiar with the medications a patient is taking and be alert to possible adverse reactions. Refer to the Suggested Resources section at the end of the chapter for a list of medical treatments used for patients with MS.

### Rehabilitation for Patients With Multiple Sclerosis

People with MS who are educated and self-aware about their condition tend to be invested and engaged with their treatment.[21] Physical therapy interventions focus on maximizing function and safety as well as preventing complications (deconditioning, pressure ulcers, weakness, and contractures secondary to spasticity). Regular exercise can help achieve these goals. Physical therapy interventions may emphasize gait training; stretching/strengthening exercises; postural exercises; balance training; pelvic floor exercises (if bladder issues are present); and interventions to normalize tone, address pain and fatigue, and provide patient/caregiver education. Many people with MS are heat sensitive; research indicates that heat and humidity tend to aggravate MS symptoms. Maintaining lower body temperature through the use of cooling vests has been shown to lessen the negative effects of heat in a person with MS.[16]

Recent research shows that people with MS prioritize maintaining wellness. Treatment focus is shifting to a holistic approach including diet, exercise, and emotional health as opposed to a pure pharmacologic approach.[21] During periods of remission, aerobic training, resistance exercise, and flexibility exercises can be resumed. Aerobic exercise at a rate of perceived exertion (RPE) at a level of 12 to 15 out of 20 for 2 to 5 days per week and resistance training twice a week at 60% to 80% of a one-repetition maximum (1RM) up to 2 sets of 10 to 15 repetitions are considered safe for the patient. A recumbent stepper or bike are options if balance is a concern. Aquatic exercise is another option as long as the pool temperature is appropriate.[22]

**Table 16-9**

**Common Signs and Symptoms of Multiple Sclerosis**

| | |
|---|---|
| Visual Disturbances | Diplopia (double vision), optic neuritis (severe eye pain, blurring/graying of vision), scotoma (dark spot in the central vision), nystagmus (involuntary eye movements) |
| Sensory Changes | Paresthesia, impaired sense of kinesthesia, impaired vibratory sense |
| Pain | Trigeminal neuralgia, headache, Lhermitte's sign (neck flexion causes electric shock–like sensations into lower extremity), hyperpathia (hypersensitivity to minor stimuli), neuropathic pain (often described as a burning-type pain) |
| Cognitive Changes | Short-term memory loss; decreased attention, concentration, and processing; decreased visuospatial functions |
| Motor Changes | Muscle weakness, decreased endurance, spasticity (may also see increased deep tendon reflexes and clonus), ataxia, tremor, balance and gait impairments |
| Bowel and Bladder Changes | Spastic, flaccid bladder or bladder dyssynergia (bladder contraction and sphincter relaxation are not coordinated); these can result in incontinence, constipation, diarrhea, and bowel incontinence (less typical) |
| Emotional Changes | Depression, pseudobulbar affect (involuntary emotional expressions) |
| Speech and Swallowing Disorders | Dysarthria (slurred or poorly articulated speech), diminished verbal fluency, dysphonia (changes in vocal quality: Harshness, breathiness), dysphagia (difficulty swallowing) |

Activities should be progressed gradually and should not cause overheating or excessive fatigue. Frequent rests should be encouraged. Consider the use of cooling vests during exercise or keep the environment cooler. During exacerbations (depending on the severity), exercise intensity should be decreased or halted, and the intervention focus should be shifted to functional mobility training with the goal of maintaining function. The clinician can use the Modified Fatigue Impact Scale to monitor fatigue.[23] The physical therapist assistant should be aware of a patient's cognitive or short-term memory deficits. The clinician may need to provide additional education to ensure that the patient and/or caregiver understands the exercises, and a written exercise program should always be provided.

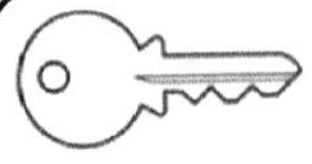

**Key Safety Considerations: Tips to Avoid Triggering Exacerbations for Patients With Multiple Sclerosis**

- Avoid overheating
- Avoid fatigue
- Focus on a gradual progression of exercise

## *Cerebrovascular Accident*

A CVA or stroke is the sudden onset of neurologic signs/symptoms that result from a disruption of blood supply to the brain. Strokes are the result of an occlusion in the brain (ischemic stroke) or a bleed in the vasculature of the brain (hemorrhagic stroke). Ischemic strokes are the most common type and account for approximately 87% of all stroke types. Stroke kills about 140,000 Americans each year and is a leading cause of long-term disability in the United States. Each year, about 800,000 Americans experience a stroke. The risk of stroke increases with age, but people of any age can experience a stroke.[24]

Patient presentation after a stroke is dependent on the location of the affected vessel, the extent of damage to the brain, and the potential for neuroplasticity. The patient presents with impairments on the side of the body opposite to the hemisphere in the brain where the stroke occurred. The middle cerebral artery (MCA) is the most common site for a blockage or occlusion to occur. Significant damage can occur due to the large area of the brain (including portions of the frontal, temporal, and parietal lobes, as well as portions of the caudate, internal capsule, and thalamus) the MCA supplies.[25] A patient with MCA stroke commonly presents with contralateral hemiparesis/hemiplegia of the face, upper extremity, and lower extremity, with the upper extremity typically more affected than the lower extremity. If the left or dominant hemisphere of the brain is injured, the patient may also experience a speech impairment, such as Broca's (expressive) aphasia, Wernicke's (receptive) aphasia, or global aphasia, that affects both the frontal and temporal lobes (see Table 16-1). Patients may also experience visual or perceptual disturbances on one side called *hemispatial* or *unilateral neglect*. If a patient had a CVA in the right (nondominant) hemisphere, they might experience left-side neglect, meaning that the patient ignores the left side because of visual or perceptual deficits.

A specific assessment tool that is commonly used for persons with stroke is the Fugl-Meyer Assessment of motor recovery after stroke. This 50-item tool measures balance, sensation, joint motion, and pain.[26-28] This instrument is time consuming to complete, but it has good validity and reliability. A shorter form with 12 items was developed and appears to be easier to complete in the clinic; this version demonstrates good reliability and validity.[27,28] A patient's scores on these tools can help track changes and progress over time. Other functional assessment tools can be useful within sessions to track specific functional parameters; the Berg Balance Scale, the 5-Step Test, and the Dynamic Gait Index have been shown to be valid when used with patients with stroke.[29,30]

The medical and pharmacologic management of stroke varies depending on the type of stroke and the patient's premorbid health status and disease history. It is relatively common to observe comorbidities in persons with stroke; these often include hypertension, diabetes mellitus, and atherosclerotic cardiovascular disease.[24] The clinician should become familiar with all medications a patient is taking and be alert to any possible adverse reactions (refer to Appendix E for an overview of the commonly seen medication classes). The assistant will monitor the patient (vital signs and RPE) during each treatment session; new signs or symptoms should be reported to the physical therapist.

## Rehabilitation for Patients After a Stroke

Decreased functional mobility, decreased endurance, and sedentary behaviors are more common after stroke. The American Heart Association recommends physical activity and exercise across all stages of recovery.[31] Most patients with a stroke will begin physical therapy in the acute care, acute rehabilitation hospital, or skilled nursing settings. Rehabilitation typically focuses on promoting return to the highest feasible level of function. Interventions are selected based on patient presentation and cognition and often include tone management, therapeutic exercise, balance training, gait training, bed mobility, transfer training, and patient education.

In the acute/early recovery phases, the physical therapist assistant must be alert to changes in all aspects of the patient's medical status, monitoring the level of alertness/consciousness, vital signs, oxygen saturation levels, pain level, and changes in skin color or temperature. The patient may have speech or processing deficits and may require increased time to respond. The assistant should speak in a slow normal tone using short direct phrases. The assistant should be patient when waiting for a response.

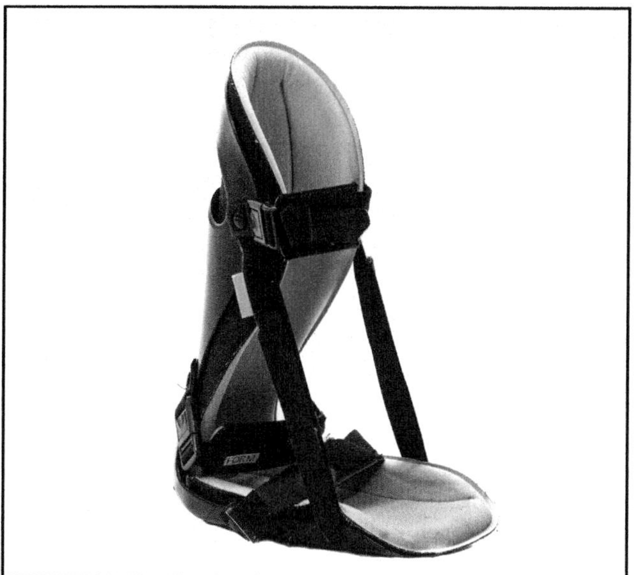

**Figure 16-6.** A multipodus boot (Blaj Gabriel/Shutterstock.com).

### Considerations for the Physical Therapist Assistant

Regardless of the treatment environment, the assistant always monitors patients for potential medical emergencies and complications such as cardiac events (eg, heart attack), deep venous thrombosis, fluctuating blood pressure readings, and subsequent stroke signs/symptoms. These all require immediate medical attention.

Many patients with a stroke exhibit poor or limited upper extremity control. Interventions that address tone and weight-bearing activities are important to improving function, but the physical therapist assistant must also protect the shoulder joint because it is prone to subluxation. Decreased grasp strength is common, so adaptations for upper extremity exercises are indicated (eg, wrist cuffs to add resistance vs hand weights). Careful attention to the biomechanics at each joint during activity execution is important. The clinician should ensure appropriate scapular mobility is available before performing shoulder ROM to prevent impingement.

It is important to use proper patient positioning to reduce the impact of synergies and spasticity. When in bed, the patient's head/neck should be in a neutral position, the scapula protracted, and the upper extremity in extension with slight abduction. For patients who exhibit lower extremity extension tone, the pelvis should be protracted with the lower extremity positioned with the hip in slight abduction and external rotation, the knee in slight flexion, and the ankle dorsiflexed to neutral. Early use of splinting may be beneficial (eg, a resting hand splint, multipodus boot; Figure 16-6) in assisting to reduce tone and prevent contractures.

Facilitation techniques and strengthening should target the antagonist muscles (the muscles opposite of those contracting in the synergistic pattern). The clinician should guard/stand on the affected side and encourage the patient to look to that side during tasks. Cuing the patient to pay attention to the affected side when they are performing exercises or activities and during completion of bilateral motions and motions that cross the midline is beneficial. These patients tend to weight shift to the unaffected side in sitting and standing, which can increase their risk for falling. Activities that promote normal upright posture, symmetrical weight bearing, use of bilateral limbs concurrently, and unilateral or bilateral exercises that cross the midline (ie, PNF patterns) should be encouraged. Strengthening exercises for the core and any weak muscles that are causing gait deviations should be included in the rehabilitation program.

As the patient transitions to the outpatient or home care setting, the clinician continues to progress the patient and focus interventions on more functional activities to increase independence. Exercise testing and prescription are tailored to the patient based on their physical abilities and impairments. Exercises should include aerobic conditioning at a low to moderate intensity and muscle strengthening/stretching. The American College of Sports Medicine (ACSM) recommends aerobic exercise 3 to 5 days per week at an RPE level of 11 to 14 out of 20.[22] Sessions can be broken down into 10-minute sessions to improve tolerance. A recumbent stepper or bike are good options if balance is a concern. Resistance training is recommended twice a week with 1 to 3 sets of 8 to 15 repetitions at 50% to 70% of 1RM.[22] Patients should also be encouraged to reduce their sedentary behavior and manage their risks for a subsequent stroke.[31]

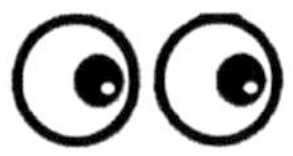

### Eye on the Research: Cerebrovascular Accident Rehabilitation

Poststroke rehabilitation often includes balance training. Sorinola et al[32] completed a meta-analysis that supported the addition of specific trunk exercises to conventional early stroke rehabilitation to significantly improve standing balance and mobility after stroke; the study offered (weak) support for the effect of additional trunk exercises on trunk performance and in functional independence. The addition of core stability exercises can significantly improve outcomes (trunk control, dynamic sitting balance, standing balance, gait, and ADLs) compared with conventional therapy alone.[33] Longer-term outcomes indicated continued improved performance in patients who completed core exercises in addition to conventional rehabilitation.[34] A recent pilot study (14 patients) demonstrated preliminary support for the addition of scapulohumeral rehabilitation exercises in addition to conventional arm rehabilitation, with results showing improved trunk control, especially during static and dynamic tasks.[35] A Cochrane review summarized that there was not one best rehabilitation approach, so physical therapy should include individualized treatments based on the patient's specific presentation.[36]

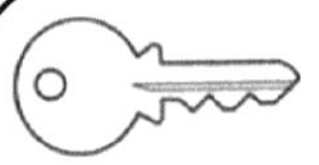

### Key Safety Considerations: Tips for Treating a Patient With a Stroke

- Monitor vital signs and RPE.
- Address tonal changes.
- Avoid traction forces and protect from a flaccid upper extremity.

## Parkinson Disease

PD is a chronic, progressive neurologic disease that currently affects more than 1 million Americans and 7 to 10 million people globally. The incidence for PD is about 20 in 100,000 people a year, and it is one of the most common degenerative neurologic diseases.[37] Although the disease is more prevalent in people over the age of 60 years, younger people can also be affected. The disease progresses at variable rates from person to person. PD is caused by damage to the dopamine pathways in the substantia nigra and the basal ganglia, resulting in reduced amounts of dopamine and subsequent movement disorders.[37,38]

The cardinal features of PD are bradykinesia, rigidity, tremors, and postural instability. Other clinical features of PD may include depression, dysphagia, micrographia (ie, progressively smaller handwriting), fatigue, gait abnormalities, bradyphrenia (ie, slow thinking/processing), sleep disorders, and dementia (Table 16-10).[37,39] As symptoms progress, patients have decreased arm swing and progressive difficulty with walking, transferring, and completing ADLs. Further disease progression tends to lead to retropulsion (ie, loss of balance backward) due to increasing postural instability. The patient begins to assume a forward-leaning posture during gait. The patient's COG moves anteriorly toward the toes beyond the BOS, and the patient demonstrates a festinating gait; these small, quick steps and inadequate balance responses increase fall risk.[39]

There is currently no cure for PD, and the primary treatment intervention is pharmaceutical. The most common medication used is Sinemet (carbidopa-levodopa)/Atamat (carbidopa-levodopa). Levodopa functions like dopamine in the brain, and carbidopa prevents the breakdown of levodopa so more levodopa can be used by the brain. Despite its significant benefit, medication effectiveness begins to diminish over time and is often associated with an "on-off" effect (meaning the medication does not work as well or as long) as the disease progresses. The long-term use of levodopa/carbidopa is also associated with the development of dyskinesia and dystonia. The patient may also be taking anticholinergics (to address tremor and rigidity), amantadine, dopamine receptor agonists, monoamine oxidase-B inhibitors, and catechol-O-methyltransferase inhibitors. The therapist should be familiar with the specific medications the patient is taking. Finding the best medication regimen is challenging for this patient population.[40]

**Table 16-10**

Signs and Symptoms of Parkinson Disease

| | |
|---|---|
| Bradykinesia | Cardinal feature of disease, slowness of movement |
| Tremor | Cardinal feature of disease, resting tremor (tremor is present at rest only) |
| Postural Instability | Cardinal feature of disease, exacerbated by the typical flexed posture associated with advancing disease: Trunk flexion, hip, and knee flexion. The posture shifts the COM anterior to the BOS. |
| Rigidity | Cardinal feature of disease, resistance to passive motion; can present as cogwheel or lead-pipe rigidity |
| Bradyphrenia | Slowness of thought, can contribute to bradykinesia |
| Akinesia | Lack of spontaneous movement |
| Hypomimia | Masked facial expression |
| Freezing | Sudden stops in movement, often seen during gait |
| Hypokinesia | Slowed/reduced movements |
| Gait Disturbances | Festinating gait pattern: Decreased step length and increased cadence; a shuffling-type gait; freezing episodes (inability to move) during gait, often seen when trying to turn/change direction |

Deep brain stimulation (DBS) is a surgical intervention used to disrupt or block abnormal brain activity that causes PD symptoms. Although most patients still need to take medication, DBS can reduce the dosage amount of levodopa and can decrease dyskinesia (a side effect of levodopa). DBS has also been shown to help alleviate fluctuations of symptoms and to reduce tremors, slowness of movements, and gait problems.[41]

### Rehabilitation Interventions for Patients With Parkinson Disease

Physical therapy treatment for patients with PD is based on disease progression and how the patient's symptoms present (ie, early/mild, moderate, or late/advanced). The modified Hoehn and Yahr Scale is used to describe the severity of the disease (Table 16-11). As the disease progresses, the focus shifts from maximizing ROM, strength, and function to maintaining these functions and then to compensatory strategies.

The specific assessment tool commonly used for persons with PD is the Unified Parkinson's Disease Rating Scale (UPDRS). Scoring on this tool is useful to track changes in patients with PD over time. Another functional assessment tool that can be useful within sessions to track specific functional parameters is the Mini-Balance Evaluation Systems Test. The Berg Balance Scale, Timed Up and Go Test, Falls Efficacy Scale International, and the Activities-Specific Balance Confidence Scale are reliable, valid tools to assess balance and fall risk for persons with PD.[43]

Therapy interventions early in the disease process should focus on maximizing flexibility, balance, and strength in the extensor musculature. Patients with PD typically have a number of impairments that should be addressed. The assistant should prioritize and combine treatment activities because the patient may not tolerate extensive treatment sessions. The patient will participate better during the medication "on" time, and therapy should be scheduled accordingly. Fall precautions and appropriate guarding are indicated during all interventions.

Persons with PD are prone to develop a forward flexed posture, so it is important to include interventions that maximize trunk extension, cervical extension, and hip and knee extension ROM and strength. The use of prone lying (if tolerated), upper extremity diagonal 2 flexion and lower extremity diagonal 1 extension PNF patterns, pectoralis corner stretches, bridging, and deep breathing exercises can be useful to reduce a flexed trunk.

Tone management techniques can be a useful pretreatment intervention to address rigidity, and specific exercises that can assist with reducing rigidity can include lower trunk rotation, segmental rolling, rhythmic rotation applied proximally on the limbs (eg, hips/pelvis and scapular/shoulder), and the incorporation of PNF diagonal patterns.

Balance training should be task specific and should mimic environmental demands. Static balance with postural cues in sitting and standing using a mirror to provide feedback is a good starting point. Cues should guide the patient to attend to where their COM is in relation to the BOS both statically and dynamically with weight shifting (throughout the limits of stability). The use of a computerized balance machine provides additional feedback that can improve the effectiveness of this training. (The Nintendo Wii Balance Board is a relatively low-cost option.) This can be progressed to weight shifts in all directions and on compliant surfaces to further challenge the limits of stability.

**Table 16-11**

Modified Hoehn and Yahr Scale[42]

| Stage | Description of Stage |
|---|---|
| 0 | No signs of disease |
| 1 | Unilateral involvement only |
| 1.5 | Unilateral and axial involvement |
| 2 | Bilateral involvement without impairment of balance |
| 2.5 | Mild bilateral disease; able to recover on pull test |
| 3 | Mild to moderate bilateral disease; some postural instability; physically independent |
| 4 | Severe disability; still able to walk or stand unassisted |
| 5 | Wheelchair bound or bedridden unless aided |

Typical balance training progressions can be used (refer to Chapter 8). Additional treatment modifications that can be helpful for this population include the use of developmental postures, the addition of rotation-type motions during reaching tasks, the use of PNF patterns to create dynamic challenges, and tasks that focus on achieving faster initiation of motions. External perturbation training may be counterproductive for this population because it can increase rigidity.

Other intervention considerations and techniques to maximize function that are specific to persons with PD include the following:

- The use of auditory cues to facilitate improved gait (music with a strong beat or a metronome). Have the patient count out a rhythmic beat to minimize freezing episodes.
- Ambulate using Nordic walking poles/sticks to increase/maintain an upright posture.
- Use verbal cues that target posture, step length, and arm swing. Cues that are brief (eg, "big steps," "stand tall," and "swing big" for arm swing) are more helpful than lengthy cues.
- Step length training using markers on the floor to increase step length.
- Step height training starting with lower-height steps and progressing to a higher height.
- High marching in place (also useful if patient has "freezing" episodes).
- Use visual markers on the floor (eg, red tape) for freezing episodes, or consider a Parkinson Walker with Laser (U-Step 2, In-Step Mobility Products) or the LaserCane (In-Step Mobility Products).

The ACSM exercise guidelines recognize that exercise parameters will be dependent on the stage/severity of disease. They propose general guidelines including (as tolerated/appropriate given the patient's presentation) aerobic exercise 3 days per week at a moderate intensity (12 to 13 RPE) for 30 minutes; resistance training 2 to 3 days per week at 40% to 50% of 1RM (beginners) to 60% to 70% of 1RM for 1 to 2 sets of 8 to 12 repetitions (or 10 to 15 repetitions for beginners); and slow, static stretches for all major muscle groups.[22] The focus for stretching for persons with PD is on stretching the flexors; strengthening focuses on strengthening the postural muscles and the extensor muscles.

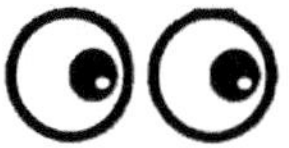

### Eye on the Research: Treatment Interventions for Parkinson Disease

LSVT (Lee Silverman Voice Treatment) LOUD (LVST Global) is a speech therapy treatment to improve the voice quality and volume in patients with PD. Using LSVT LOUD concepts, the LSVT BIG program (LSVT Global) was developed, and it integrates large-amplitude movement patterns into the exercise program. The BIG program has been shown to improve short-term motor function outcomes (UPDRS motor scores, Timed Up and Go Test, and 10-m walk scores) for persons with PD compared with traditional therapy interventions.[44] Physical therapist assistants can complete LSVT BIG training and certification through continuing education courses.

Whole-body vibration (WBV) is a treatment that might be useful for persons with PD due to its ability to elicit postural responses and to increase the effectiveness of muscle cocontraction. Researchers report significant variability (ie, the frequency of vibration, treatment time, rest periods, and number of sessions) in the manner in which WBV intervention was conducted across 6 randomized controlled trials. The majority of the studies appeared to show a favorable response after WBV for mobility and balance but not significantly better than other active interventions.[45] In a 2016 study by Kaut et al,[46] the researchers noted that there was improvement in postural stability, rigidity, bradykinesia, and the UPDRS III sum score in persons who participated in WBV; they concluded that there was a significant improvement in postural stability even in individuals with an increased risk of falling.

Schenkman et al[47] researched the feasibility and safety of high-intensity (80% to 85% maximum heart rate) treadmill exercise for patients diagnosed with PD (Hoehn and Yahr Scale 1 or 2) who were not taking medication and who were within 5 years of a diagnosis. The investigators determined that high-intensity treadmill exercise was safe for patients with PD, and they recommended an efficacy trial to determine whether high-intensity treadmill exercise could produce meaningful improvements in newly diagnosed PD. The use of high-intensity training is supported by a 2019 study in which the high-intensity interval training group showed statically significant improvements in immediate memory and attention. The researchers determined that high-intensity interval training appears to promote better cognitive function in people with PD compared with moderate-intensity continuous exercise. These findings are important because patients with PD often present with cognitive impairments that increase disability and negatively affect their QOL.[48]

## *Traumatic Brain Injury*

A blow to the head, skull penetration (eg, a bullet wound), or a violent shaking of the head can cause a TBI. Signs and symptoms of a TBI can vary and can affect a person's neurologic (sensory and motor autonomic systems) and cognitive function as well as create personality or behavioral changes. Approximately 2.8 million people annually require medical attention in the United States because of a TBI.[49] TBIs affect men (74%) about 3 times more than women (26%).[50] Vehicular accidents (50%) are the number one cause of TBIs, and falls (28%) are the second most common cause.[50,51] Deaths related to TBIs were highest in older adults (75 years or more).[50] Emergency room visits, hospitalizations, and deaths due to TBIs are increasing among older adults and are mostly attributed to falls. The most common cause of moderate or severe TBI in young adults is high-speed motor vehicle accidents; some injuries are the result of sport-related incidents.[49-51] TBIs can also affect deployed soldiers who may experience closed-head injuries as a result of the mechanical energy released during the blast waves of improvised explosive devices. This is a nonimpact type of TBI, but the neurologic effects are similar to impact-type injuries.[52]

A TBI is also referred to as an *acquired brain injury*. There are 3 degrees of TBIs (mild, moderate, and severe). A mild TBI is characterized by a brief loss of consciousness (less than 30 minutes) and normal brain images. A concussion is considered a mild TBI. A person with a moderate TBI has experienced loss of consciousness for 30 minutes to 24 hours and normal or abnormal brain imaging. Experiencing a loss of consciousness or being in a comatose state for longer than 24 hours with normal or abnormal imaging is considered a severe TBI. The Glasgow Coma Scale is commonly used (within the first 24 hours) to initially classify the degree of TBI severity. The Glasgow Coma Scale assesses the individual's best motor response, best verbal response, and eye-opening ability. The sum of the scores range from 3 to 15. A total score of less than 9 is indicative of a severe TBI, 9 to 12 is moderate, and 13 to 15 is associated with a mild TBI.[53] The Functional Independence Measure is also commonly used to determine the patient's level of independence in mobility, self-care, and cognition during rehabilitation. Any number of balance, vestibular, and gait tests can be used on patients who sustained a mild TBI. After being cleared by the physician, athletes should be reassessed before return to play using the Sport Concussion Assessment Tool 5.

### Rehabilitation Interventions for Patients After Traumatic Brain Injury

Physical therapists and assistants are members of a multidisciplinary team involved in rehabilitation after a TBI across the continuum of care. The main goal of rehabilitation is to maximize the patient's functional abilities, maximize QOL, and return to the community as independently as possible. Rehabilitation often begins in the ICU or acute care settings. Once the patient is medically stable, the goal for the unconscious patient with a TBI is to limit secondary complications (eg, deep vein thrombosis, pressure ulcers, contractures) due to the injury or early bed rest. The physical therapy team initiates early PROM and other interventions (positioning and splinting) to reduce the secondary effects. Initiating rehabilitation interventions early may improve patient recovery and possibly increase long-term survival.[54] Throughout the rehabilitation process, the physical therapist assistant may include tone management techniques, positioning, splinting/bracing, therapeutic exercise, balance training, gait training, transfer training, cognitive training, behavioral modification, and family/patient education. Patients may be transferred from the hospital to an acute rehabilitation hospital for more intensive physical therapy or to a skilled nursing facility; the goal is to achieve discharge back to home if feasible. Some patients will progress from an inpatient rehabilitation setting to a day program for community reintegration. Not all patients are able to return to community-level function (even with assistance/support); in these situations, the medical team guides the family in considering alternate discharge options (ie, a long-term care facility, group home, or home with 24-hour care).

There are additional factors to consider when treating patients with a TBI. The assistant must review the patient's comprehensive multidisciplinary care plan to ensure that selected interventions support the cognitive and behavioral plans for each patient. Careful monitoring of the patient's response to activity is of the utmost importance. Gradual, monitored activity progression is indicated. Exercise or activity that is too aggressive can result in cognitive decline, an altered mental status, or other red flag signs/symptoms. Integration of a symptom tracking log into the patient's daily journal can be an effective way to monitor for trends in performance related to activity level. Fatigue can increase patient frustration and increase aggressive behavior. Clinicians working with this patient population will pursue additional training in behavioral redirection and de-escalation techniques.

## *Spinal Cord Injury*

SCIs damage the spinal cord, and these injuries affect the nervous system and musculoskeletal and autonomic function; they can also affect the cardiopulmonary, gastrointestinal, genitourinary, and integumentary systems depending on the spinal level involved. As a result of traumatic injury, some patients transition from being fully independent to total paralysis in an instant. The psychological effects can be overwhelming because of the loss of function, increased dependence on others, and a change in self-image. According to the National Spinal Cord Injury Statistical Center, there are about 17,730 new SCI cases each year (about 54 out of each million Americans). Based on 2019 statistics, there are between 249,000 and 363,000 Americans living with SCIs. This number is significantly lower than the rate for TBIs, but the expense for treatment and continued support and care for each of these patients over their lifetime is between \$2.4 million for paraplegics and about \$5 million for quadriplegics. Although most cases involve men (78%) between the ages of 16 and 30 years (age 19 years has the highest frequency), the average is 43 years of age. Vehicular accidents (39.3%) and falls (31.8%) are the most common causes of injury. Other causes resulting in SCIs include violent incidents such as gunshot wounds (13.5%) and sport-related activities (8.0%).[55]

SCIs are described as either complete or incomplete lesions/injuries. A complete SCI is a total loss of motor and sensory function below the level of the lesion, and an incomplete SCI means that the person maintains some sensory and/or motor function below the level of the lesion. SCI is defined by the highest intact neurologic level. For example, a C7 complete SCI indicates that the patient has motor and sensory function intact from C1 to C7 but motor and sensory loss at C8 distally (caudally), including the loss of bowel and bladder function. A person with tetraplegia (or quadriplegia) has paralysis of all 4 extremities, the trunk/chest, and potentially the respiratory muscles (based on the level of injury) caused by injury to the cervical spine. Persons with paraplegia have paralysis of both lower extremities and part of the trunk caused by injury to the thoracic or lumbar spine. The percentage of individuals classified as paraplegic is 39.5%, and 59.9% are considered tetraplegic. An incomplete tetraplegic SCI occurs most frequently (47.6%) followed by complete paraplegic injury (19.9%) and then incomplete paraplegic injury (19.6%).[55]

According to the ASIA, there are classifications that provide an international standardization to classify SCIs. A complete spinal cord injury (ASIA A) results in the loss of motor, sensory, and autonomic nervous system functions below the level of the lesion. Patients with ASIA B SCI (sensory incomplete) have sensory function (but not motor function) below the level of the lesion. ASIA C (motor incomplete) indicates that motor function is maintained below the level of the lesion; less than half of the key muscles present with strength 3/5 or greater. ASIA D (motor incomplete) indicates that motor function is maintained below the level of the lesion, with one-half or more key muscles with strength $\geq 3/5$.[56]

### Rehabilitation Interventions for Patients After Spinal Cord Injury

Physical therapists and physical therapist assistants are involved in the extended rehabilitation process for persons with an SCI across the continuum of care. The goal is to maximize functional independence and to return to community-level function. Physical therapy is individualized based on the patient's presentation/level of injury and can include tone management techniques, positioning, splinting/bracing, therapeutic exercise, balance training, standing tolerance/supported weight bearing, transfer training, wheelchair training, gait training (with paraplegia patients), and patient/caregiver education. Physical therapy is initiated early while the patient is in the ICU or acute care setting. Care for patients with SCI requires an interdisciplinary approach, and the rehabilitation goals during this phase include maintaining or improving respiratory function, preventing joint contractures, reducing the risk of skin breakdown (pressure ulcers), and preventing other complications.[57] Physical therapist assistants should recognize the complications associated with SCIs. Some complications depend on the level of lesion—the higher the level of injury, the greater the chance of serious, life-threatening complications. Neurogenic shock (spinal shock) occurs in the acute period after injury. It is most common with severe trauma to the spinal cord above the level of T6 and presents with the absence of reflexes below the level of the lesion, bradycardia, and severe hypotension (systolic less than 90 mm Hg when supine). Patients with lesions above T6 may experience autonomic dysreflexia (AD) in the acute or chronic stage after injury. AD is a potentially life-threatening increase in blood pressure that occurs in response to a noxious stimulus.[58] Heterotopic ossification, defined as bone formation in the soft tissue around the joints, affects 10% to 53% of people with SCI; the hip joint is most commonly affected. The typical onset of heterotopic ossification is 2 to 3 weeks after the injury.[57,59] Bradycardia, hypotension, thermoregulation (hyper/hypothermia), deep vein thrombosis, respiratory complications, urinary tract infections, pressure ulcers, pain, and spasticity are other potential complications (especially in cervical or high thoracic SCI). Table 16-12 highlights key considerations when providing therapy for patients with SCI. The assistant should be able to identify and respond appropriately to new onset of symptoms in these patients.

### Considerations for the Physical Therapist Assistant

AD is a medical emergency, and the signs and symptoms include severe headache, blurred vision, profuse sweating, increased spasticity, skin flushing, and/or restlessness. An increase in the resting systolic blood pressure of 20 to 30 mm Hg is also indicative of AD.[58,59] Bladder distension is a common cause of AD.

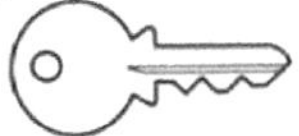

### Key Safety Considerations

If a physical therapist assistant suspects AD, the following course of actions should be taken immediately:

- Sit the patient up if supine.
- Check for bladder distension or other noxious stimuli; check the catheter and Foley bag; check for tight/constricting clothing.
- Immediately report any of these findings to nursing; nursing will assess for bladder distension or bowl impaction.

All patients with an SCI and caregivers should be educated in recognizing the signs and symptoms of AD and have a plan of action to handle this emergency.

During the acute phase of rehabilitation, proper positioning, splinting/bracing, and ROM exercises are important to protect the joints and maintain normal muscle length. PROM can be performed in the presence of either flaccidity or spasticity. However, there are situations when stretching must be avoided and PROM must be completed with careful modifications (see Table 16-12; refer to Chapter 5). The physical therapist assistant must take care when stretching patients with tetraplegia who do not have active wrist extension and finger flexion. These patients will rely on the resting tension in the long finger flexors to create a compensatory grasp called *tenodesis*. To maintain the potential for a tenodesis grasp, PROM to the finger extensors should be completed with the wrist in neutral, and wrist extension ROM should be completed with the fingers placed in flexion. Initiating strengthening of key muscles early will reduce the risk of muscle atrophy and osteopenia and will promote increased function. Breathing exercises are initiated during the acute phase to maintain or improve lung capacity (refer to Chapter 18).[57]

Once the patient is orthopedically and medically stable, the patient transfers to a rehabilitation hospital or specialized facility for intensive physical and occupational therapy. The use of developmental postures with patients with SCI is helpful as a progression to improve bed mobility, transfers, and walking (if this is a goal based on the patient's level of injury). Alternating isometrics and rhythmic stabilization can promote cocontraction around the joints, thus increasing stability. Weight bearing into both the upper extremity and lower extremity can reduce pain and spasticity in the respective joints. Patients should work on upper extremity strengthening and aerobic training as early as possible. The key muscles to target include (if available based on the level of lesion) the anterior deltoid, the serratus anterior, shoulder extensors, biceps and triceps, the latissimus dorsi, shoulder rotators, and scapula stabilizers. Strengthening of these muscles is necessary for transfers, wheelchair propulsion, and gait training. Aerobic training can include wheelchair propulsion and an upper body ergometer. The cardiac demand when using upper extremity muscles is higher than with lower extremity muscles, and upper extremity muscles will fatigue more quickly than lower extremity muscles.

Patients with T10 lesions or lower should be able to walk with appropriate braces and assistive devices.[57,60] Patients who are ASIA C have a better prognosis for ambulation.[60] Core exercises and pelvic stabilization exercises are indicated. Patients will begin with standing, weight shifting, and balance activities in parallel bars, wearing necessary back and leg braces. Functional neuromuscular stimulation can be used to activate muscles.[60] The use of robotic gait training devices (Figure 16-7) may reduce complications (eg, the perception of pain and spasticity) and can improve walking.[61] Standing and walking (when feasible based on the level of injury) can reduce the potential for complications and can improve psychological well-being.[60,61]

**Table 16-12**

Special Considerations for Patients With Spinal Cord Injuries[3]

| Concern | Description | Intervention |
|---|---|---|
| Orthopedic restrictions | Until physician provides clearance, during the poststabilization healing period, for patients with paraplegia, limit straight leg raise to 60 degrees and hip flexion to 90 degrees.<br>For patients with tetraplegia, avoid head/neck ROM and no shoulder flex/abduction > 90 degrees. | Maintain compliance with restrictions per physician orders. |
| Tenodesis grasp | Persons with tetraplegia with intact wrist extensors (but no active finger flexion) can use tenodesis (passive finger flexion occurs with active wrist extension) to create a functional grasp. | Use of an intrinsic plus splint. Maintain finger flexion during mobility tasks that include wrist extension.<br>Avoid stretching into the wrist and finger flexion simultaneously. |
| Hamstring length/low back (erector spinae) tightness | To maintain long sitting, the patient needs about 110 degrees of straight leg raise, but tightness in the lumbosacral erector spinae can help with sitting balance. | Focus on manual stretching of hamstrings and maintaining a neutral pelvis (controlled/selective stretch completed in supine). Avoid having patient "self-stretch" in long sit because this may increase the posterior pelvic tilt and overstretch the low back muscles. |
| AD | Highest risk are persons with lesions above T6. Symptoms: Rapid/sudden increase in blood pressure, severe headache, and flushed/sweating above level of lesion; often triggered by noxious stimuli (full bladder, bowel impaction, pressure ulcer, tight/constricting clothing, and irritation below the level of the lesion). | Treat as medical emergency; contact physician/nurse.<br>Loosen clothing, check catheter is not kinked, and look for other triggers. Move patient into sitting and monitor vital signs. |
| Orthostatic hypotension | Drop in blood pressure (with increase in heart rate) with positional changes to more upright posture. Symptoms: Blurred vision, light-headedness, fainting. | Gradual acclimatization to upright; use of compression stockings and abdominal binder. |
| Deconditioning | Reduced exercise tolerance, reduced cardiac output. | Aerobic/fitness exercise. |
| Impaired temperature control | Loss of autonomic control of sweating and shivering below the level of the lesion. | Monitor temperature, maintain hydration, and use sunscreen; if participating in competition/high-level physical activity, consider the use of cooling vests. |
| Pressure sores | Decubitus ulcer/ulceration of soft tissue caused by unrelieved pressure or shearing forces. | Appropriate pressure relief, repositioning, and use of pressure-reducing cushions; regularly monitor skin in higher pressure areas. |
| Osteopenia | Decreased bone mineral density and increased fracture risk below the level of the lesion. | Avoid excess pressure with stretching; avoid forced motions with transfers and ADLs. |

### Eye on the Research: Fitness Training Programs for Persons After Spinal Cord Injury

Exercise improves fitness and cardiovascular metabolic health of adults with chronic SCI.[62] The incorporation of aerobic and strengthening exercise can improve patient outcomes, including cardiorespiratory fitness, muscle strength, and body composition, and reduce cardiovascular risk.[62] Recent exercise guidelines for persons with SCI include at least 20 minutes of moderate- to vigorous-intensity aerobic exercise twice a week and 3 sets of strengthening exercises for each major functioning muscle group at a moderate to vigorous intensity twice a week for cardiorespiratory fitness and muscle strength benefits.[63] Australian guidelines include recommendations for 30 minutes or more of moderate aerobic exercise 5 days per week or more or 20 minutes or more of vigorous aerobic 3 days per week or more, strength training 2 days per week or more (targeting the scapula stabilizers and posterior shoulder girdle muscles), and a flexibility program 2 days per week or more targeting shoulder internal and external rotators. The researchers recommended stratifying patients into categories of beginners, intermediate, and advanced to assist with appropriate application of the recommendations in clinical practice. Researchers recommended pre-exercise initial screening for AD, orthostatic hypotension, exercise-induced hypotension, thermoregulatory dysfunction, pressure sores, spasticity, and pain.[64]

## Amyotrophic Lateral Sclerosis

ALS (also known as *Lou Gehrig disease*) is a chronic, progressive neurologic disease that is fatal; there is no cure. ALS is a disease that causes degeneration of the upper and lower motor neurons. Progressive muscle weakness without sensory loss is the hallmark sign of ALS. Cognitive loss, once thought to be atypical for persons with ALS, is now believed to be present in 50% of all patients with ALS.[65] The average time from diagnosis to death is 2 to 5 years. The estimated prevalence rate for 2013 was 5.0 per 100,000 people, and ALS is more common in White men greater than 60 years of age.[66]

Persons with ALS are staged as having early, middle, or late ALS. In the early stages, muscle stiffness, weakness, atrophy, and fasciculations are most often noted distally, and treatment focuses on promoting independence and maximizing function. During the middle stage, mobility and ADL abilities decline, and the patient needs assistance and transitions to motorized mobility. Patients experience difficulty chewing and swallowing, increasing the risk for choking. Late-stage ALS is characterized by dependence for ADLs and mobility, severe dysphagia, and dysarthria. These patients will require mechanical ventilation and placement of a feeding tube to survive and are typically restricted to bed or specialized motorized seating systems. As the patient moves through the stages of disease, the therapy focus shifts from restorative to compensatory to palliative care. Education and interventions are targeted to prevent or minimize complications.

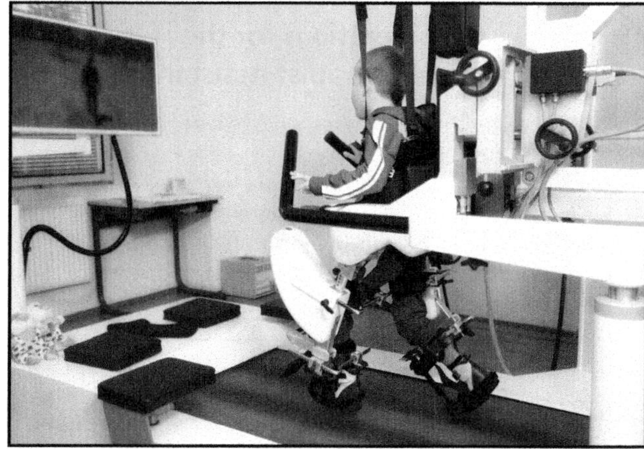

**Figure 16-7.** A robotic gait training machine (Olesia Bilkei/Shutterstock.com).

Despite the prevalence of muscle weakness in persons with ALS, there is the risk of disuse atrophy without regular exercise. Traditionally, physical therapy exercises were limited to functional mobility training, ROM, and stretching due to a belief that incorporating strengthening exercise would result in overuse weakness. However, one systematic review determined that there was a significant improvement in the Amyotrophic Lateral Sclerosis Functional Rating Scale measure of function in the patients who participated in exercise, but there were no statistically significant differences in QOL, fatigue, or muscle strength.[67] Although the researchers reported no adverse effects, such as increased muscle cramping, muscle soreness, or fatigue, they summarized that the studies were too small and that more research is needed.[67] In a larger randomized controlled trial by Lunetta et al,[68] researchers summarized that a strictly monitored exercise program might significantly reduce motor deterioration in patients with ALS.[68] Strengthening and endurance training programs are safe and do not worsen ALS outcomes, but inactivity leads to cardiovascular deconditioning and atrophy that exacerbates the weakness caused by ALS. A 2018 randomized controlled trial (N = 38) found that participation in an isometric strengthening and moderate-intensity aerobic exercise program was beneficial for patients with ALS, resulting in overall improvement of functional independence, reduced deconditioning, and a decrease in the muscle.[69]

There is evidence of positive patient outcomes with exercise and no reports of adverse effects. The physical therapist may determine (especially in the early stages of the disease) that general ROM and stretching could be combined with moderate levels of strengthening exercises and aerobic training. The therapy team will monitor the patient and adjust exercise intensity to prevent overuse or excessive fatigue. The signs and symptoms of overuse include excessive fatigue, pain, the inability to complete ADLs postexercise, increased muscle cramps, and increased muscle fasciculation. Any of these responses indicate the need to stop or modify the activity.

**Considerations for the Physical Therapist Assistant**

Always monitor the patient's response to exercises in order to avoid overuse and fatigue. Be alert to increased muscle cramping or fasciculation and dyspnea, which may occur due to exercise intolerance. Reduce intensity or terminate exercises and have the patient rest. Continue to monitor the patient, document the patient's responses, and notify the physical therapist.

## Seizures and Epilepsy

"A seizure is defined as a transient occurrence of signs and/or symptoms due to abnormal excessive or synchronous neuronal activity in the brain."[70] A seizure is considered as a single event, whereas epilepsy is a neurologic disorder in which 2 or more seizures occur that are unprovoked.[70] There are about 3.4 million people who have a diagnosis of epilepsy in the United States, including 3 million adults and 470,000 children.[71]

There are 2 broad categories of seizures: focal (partial) seizures and general seizures. Focal seizures start in one area of the brain, and generalized seizures affect a large area(s) of the brain.[70,71] Seizure symptoms can vary widely and depend on the type of seizure, but seizure episodes/types tend to be consistent for an individual with epilepsy. A person who has a simple focal seizure does not lose consciousness or memory but may report a strange change of smell and may experience muscle twitching or changes in sensation. A person who experiences a complex focal seizure may be confused or dazed and unable to respond to questions or commands. The patient may have an aura (or warning) that a seizure may be starting. Generalized types of seizures can be further classified as absence (formerly called *petit mal seizures*) or tonic-clonic seizures (grand mal seizures). An absence seizure occurs for just a few seconds where there is a short loss of consciousness and the person appears to be staring into space. During a tonic-clonic seizure, the person's muscles stiffen, causing the person to fall to the floor. They often bite their tongue or the side of their mouth. After the tonic phase, the clonic phase is evident by the jerky rhythmic shaking of the extremities. The patient will gradually stop shaking, and consciousness will slowly return.[72] Immediate initiation of the emergency medical system is indicated in the following situations: a seizure occurs that lasts longer than a patient's typical seizure or that lasts more than 5 minutes or the patient experiences 2 separate seizures that occur without the patient regaining consciousness between them.

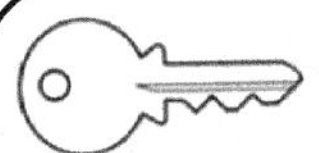

**Key Safety Considerations: Seizure Emergency First Aid Actions**

The physical therapist assistant should clear an area on the floor where the patient has collapsed. Observe the patient's condition and/or movements during the event, and time the length of the seizure. Whenever possible, roll the patient on their side and continue to monitor the patient. Always follow the facility protocols and report the incident to the physical therapist.

The clinician should always be aware of a patient's medical history; if the patient has a diagnosis of epilepsy, it is important to know if the seizures are controlled and the typical type and duration of the seizures that the patient experiences. Seizures often occur after activity, so the patient should be monitored both during and after activity. Persons with newly diagnosed epilepsy may have exercise restrictions until the doctor is confident that the seizures are medically managed. Patients with uncontrolled seizures should not participate in an aquatic exercise program.

## Conditions That Impact the Neuromuscular System in Children

### Cerebral Palsy

CP is a nonprogressive brain lesion (occurring before, during, or shortly after birth) that interferes with normal development and results in motor and coordination impairments as well as alterations in muscle tone and reflexes. Primitive reflexes (the asymmetrical tonic neck, symmetrical tonic neck, and tonic labyrinthine reflexes) tend to persist, creating additional barriers to normal movement patterns. The resultant impact on function is dependent on the location and size of the lesion, and presentation is extremely variable among patients. In addition to the motor deficits, cognitive impairments are also often present. Worldwide population studies have reported that the prevalence of CP is 1.5 to 4 per 1000.[73]

There are 4 general types of CP: spastic (about 80% of the cases), dyskinetic, ataxic, and mixed (a combination of spastic and dyskinetic). Spastic CP is characterized by increased tone, and the 2 most common types of spastic CP are spastic quadriplegic CP and spastic diplegic CP.[73] In people with diplegic CP, legs are more commonly affected compared with the upper extremities, which are either minimally or not affected. These patients usually have extremely tight hip muscles (especially adductors and flexors) and leg muscle tightness and stiffness, which causes them to walk with a scissoring gait pattern (Figure 16-8). Quadriplegic CP is the most severe spastic type because all extremities are affected, and most of these children have additional disabilities (ie, speech, vision, and seizures). Dyskinetic patients have involuntary, uncontrollable, and twisting (writhing) upper extremity and lower extremity movements, making it difficult to maintain sitting or standing postures. Examples of dyskinetic CP include athetoid, dystonic, and choreoathetoid.[73]

The severity of CP is typically graded using the Gross Motor Function Classification System–Expanded and Revised. This tool is a 5-level classification system that describes current gross motor function of children with CP based on self-initiated movements that include sitting, walking, and/or wheelchair mobility. This test can be administered by physical therapists or other health care providers, and it is also used to assess the child's need for additional or alternative assistive devices.[74]

Although CP is a nonprogressive condition, clinical presentations appear to worsen as the secondary impairments (ie, tone changes, coordination deficits, and weakness) impact developmental growth as the child ages. The impact of impairments is exacerbated by the increased environmental, functional, and/or social demands that occur during growth. Growth spurts can affect tone and muscle balance significantly, so treatments need to be modified and adjusted regularly. Changes in muscle tone and reflex activity decrease the efficiency of movement patterns and increase the energy demand for almost all activities the patient performs.

Physical therapy interventions typically focus on maximizing function and may include activities geared toward completion of developmental milestones, functional mobility training, tone management techniques, stretching/bracing/splinting, balance exercises, positioning to reduce the impact of tone, and therapeutic exercise. Tone management techniques are a key component of all therapy interventions for this patient population. Medical and pharmacologic interventions (ie, tendon lengthening procedures, implantation of a baclofen pump, and botulism injections) used to decrease tone or increase ROM may alter patient presentation and functional abilities. The physical therapist will re-evaluate these patients and revise the POC after these medical interventions before the assistant resumes treatment.

According to the ACSM guidelines, the FITT (frequency, intensity, time, type) principles may still apply to this patient population, but modification based on patient presentation is required. All exercise progressions should be gradual and monitored. The recommendation is to begin with frequent but short bouts of aerobic exercise at moderate intensity (RPE 12 to 13), with a goal of increasing (if appropriate) to 20 minutes. The mode of aerobic exercise should be determined based on the patient's motor ability, function, and balance (ie, the stationary bike, recumbent bike or step machine, upper extremity ergometer, and aquatic exercise).[22]

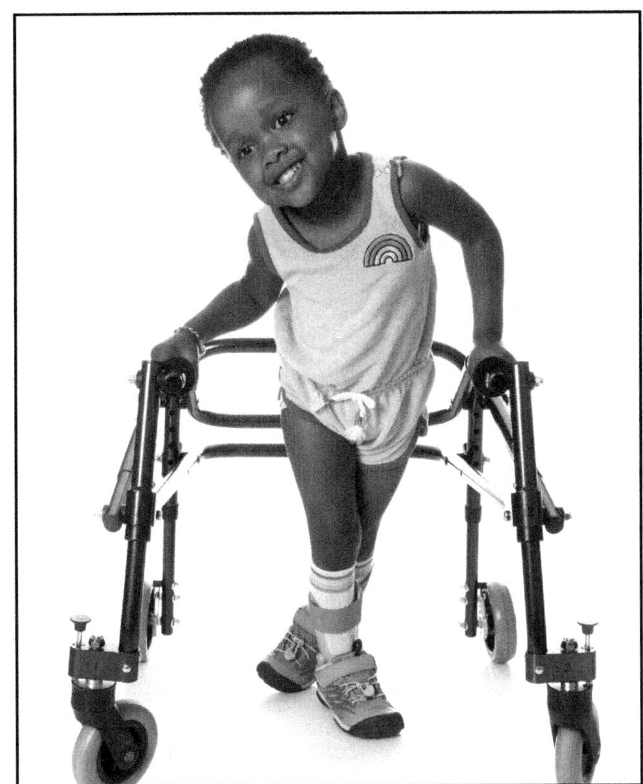

**Figure 16-8.** Diplegic CP scissoring gait pattern (Ahturner/Shutterstock.com).

Physical therapist assistants ensure that the patient's head, trunk, and joints (especially proximal ones) are positioned correctly before performing exercises. If the patient has difficulty holding dumbbell weights, Velcro gloves or straps can be used. Resistance exercise should target the weaker antagonist muscles in areas of increased tone. Slow-speed contractions are preferred over high speed to avoid eliciting increased tone due to stretch reflex activity. Closed kinetic chain exercises may allow better control and more normalized movement patterns. Eccentric training may be useful in decreasing cocontraction in hypertonic muscles. Slow sustained stretching for 30 seconds to the hypertonic muscles can improve antagonistic muscle contractions.[22] People with CP may fatigue easily due to the high energy expenditure required during movement production and exercise. Several short training sessions are recommended (compared with one longer one), especially for those with a high degree of muscle tone. It is helpful to use stretching and relaxation techniques throughout the session. When adding new exercises or activities, it is best to introduce them very early in the treatment session.[22]

## Muscular Dystrophy

Muscular dystrophies are the most common group of inherited (genetic) progressive neuromuscular diseases with an onset in childhood. They cause a progressive loss of muscle strength due to the wasting of muscles, and each type of muscular dystrophy affects different groupings of muscles. Duchenne muscular dystrophy (DMD) is the most common type, affecting men only. Onset is typically between 2 and 4 years of age, and a characteristic indicator is the presence of a positive Gowers sign (difficulty getting up off the floor) due to pelvic girdle and proximal lower extremity weakness.

Physical therapy focuses on maximizing function and facilitating compensatory techniques as well as recommending equipment and modifications to the home as the disease progresses. Eccentric and maximal exercise should be avoided because strenuous exercise may exacerbate the breakdown of muscle fibers. Because the respiratory muscles are also impacted, monitoring oxygen saturation levels with activity is recommended. Inspiratory muscle training may be beneficial in maintaining respiratory function and delaying intubation.

In recent years, several small studies demonstrated that low-intensity exercise is beneficial for some boys with DMD. Exercises should be monitored by physical therapy clinicians; patients should be educated that low-volume and low-intensity exercise should be self-limited based on symptoms.[75,76] One study found a statistically significant improvement in ambulation scores, proximal muscle strength, and arm function in a group who exercised using an arm ergometer compared with a control group who performed strengthening ROM exercises in patients with early-stage DMD.[77] These are small studies, and further research regarding the appropriate dosing of exercise is necessary because there are still many unknowns.

## Spina Bifida Occulta, Meningocele, and Myelomeningocele

Spina bifida occulta, meningocele, and myelomeningocele are categories of spina bifida. Spina bifida is a birth defect characterized by a neural tube defect in which the spine and spinal cord do not develop normally. Spina bifida occulta refers to a birth defect where the neural tube does not close completely; there is typically no visible evidence of the defect and no functional impairments. With a meningocele, the spinal cord meninges and cerebrospinal fluid protrude out through the defect in the vertebral column, but the spinal cord itself remains within the vertebral column. Although there is a saclike area present on the infant's back that must be surgically repaired, neurologic involvement is not common. With myelomeningocele, the spinal cord and meninges protrude through the defect in the vertebral column, and they develop outside the body. A surgical procedure to repair the defect is usually performed 1 to 2 days after birth. Myelomeningocele results in permanent neurologic deficits, and the severity of disability varies based on the spinal level of the defect.[78] The surgery to repair the defect does not restore neurologic function, and the patient typically has full motor and sensory loss below the level of the neural tube defect.

Persons with myelomeningocele are at an increased risk of developing hydrocephalus (increased fluid in the ventricles of the brain, resulting in compression of the brain tissue). Treatment of hydrocephalus is the surgical placement of a ventriculoperitoneal shunt that reduces the intracranial pressure. The worldwide incidence of the occurrence of a neural tube defect is about 1 for every 1000 pregnancies. Spina bifida can occur due to several genetic and environmental factors.[79] It affects 1500 to 2000 infants born in the United States each year.[80]

Physical therapy plays an important role in treating patients with spina bifida. The goal for young children is to maximize independence and mobility. As the child moves into adolescence, the goals shift to maintaining a healthy body weight and promoting independence and participation in physical activities.[80-82] Interventions vary based on the level of lesion but can include ROM, stretching (to prevent contractures), strengthening the innervated available muscles, age-appropriate developmental motor skills, balance training, assisted or independent gait training, and/or wheelchair mobility. Aquatics and hippotherapy may be good alternatives for these patients. Patients usually require ongoing orthotic/bracing and assistive device management as they age and grow.[80] Preteens and adolescents with spina bifida are at risk for obesity, diabetes, and heart disease because of inactivity. These patients should be encouraged to exercise and increase their cardiovascular fitness to reduce risk factors and maintain functional mobility.[81,82] The spina bifida physical activity guidelines found in the Suggested Resources section at the end of the chapter provide guidelines for all age groups.

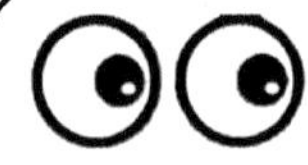

### Eye on the Research: Impact of Exercise on Other Neuromuscular Diseases

Research indicates that controlled, monitored exercise does not have harmful effects and may be beneficial in maintaining function for longer periods of time for persons with neuromuscular diseases. Appropriately prescribed exercise can improve muscle strength, ROM, cardiorespiratory fitness, efficiency of ambulation, and a patient's sense of well-being in persons with postpolio syndrome.[83]

Preliminary evidence (adult and animal models) indicates that progressive resistance training exercise programs are feasible, safe, and well tolerated in children with spinal muscular atrophy, although researchers acknowledge that further studies are warranted.[84]

Voet et al[85] summarized that there were no harmful effects with moderate-intensity strength training for persons with myotonic dystrophy and facioscapulohumeral muscular dystrophy or with aerobic exercise training for persons with dermatomyositis, polymyositis, and myotonic dystrophy type 1. Aerobic exercise combined with strength training for persons with mitochondrial myopathy appears to be safe and may be effective in increasing submaximal endurance capacity.

## Conclusion

Patients with neurologic diagnoses benefit from the inclusion of therapeutic exercise in their treatment programs to maximize function, mobility, and QOL. The physical therapy team will work with patients with neurologic diagnoses across the continuum of care; a skilled physical therapist assistant will use their knowledge of the varied diseases to develop appropriate exercise programs to maximize function and to appropriately monitor, adjust, and progress treatment plans. The physical therapy team works with medical professionals, the patient, and the patient's support system to promote the highest level of independence for patients with neurologic diagnoses.

## Review Questions

1. Explain the difference between function-induced recovery and compensatory training. Give one example of each. What role can therapeutic exercise play in each?
2. Compare and contrast the presentations of an upper motor neuron lesion and a lower motor neuron lesion. Describe how these different presentations affect the type of exercises the assistant would complete on the affected limb.
3. List 3 interventions to decrease muscle tone. List 3 interventions to increase muscle tone. Compare and contrast the types of exercise that would be appropriate to complete on a limb that is flaccid vs in a limb with increased tone.
4. Briefly describe the various treatment approaches that can be used when treating patients with neurologic conditions.
5. List 3 exercises that can be performed in quadruped, and state what the goal of each exercise is. List 3 exercises that can be performed in modified plantigrade, and state what the goal of each exercise is.
6. List 3 things that a physical therapist assistant should monitor or modify to prevent an exacerbation in patients with MS.
7. Which exercises are most appropriate to include when treating a patient with a diagnosis of PD? Provide a rationale for your selections.
8. Describe the general focus/goal for exercises for a patient with early stage ALS. List 5 appropriate exercises.
9. List 5 complications a physical therapist assistant needs to be aware of when treating a patient with SCI.
10. List 5 exercises that will be important when promoting function for a person with T10 paraplegia.

## Case Study

The patient is a 73-year-old who sustained a right CVA 2 weeks ago. She has moderate flexor synergy in her left upper extremity and some active return in her left lower extremity (hip flexion active ROM to 60 degrees, hip extension AROM to neutral, hip abduction AROM to 10 degrees, knee flexion to 70 degrees, and ankle dorsiflexion to 0 to 2 degrees). She has moderate proprioceptive loss in her left upper and lower extremity. She is performing transfers with moderate assist and has begun to ambulate with a left molded ankle-foot orthosis with a narrow base quad cane 100 feet with moderate assistance, requiring assistance for the swing phase of gait approximately 50% time. She completed stair training with the physical therapist on evaluation requiring moderate assistance (for advancement and placement of the left lower extremity). Static and dynamic sitting balance grades are good; static and dynamic standing balance is fair.

The physical therapy POC includes patient/caregiver education, therapy exercises, balance training, neurofacilitation interventions, bed mobility/transfer/gait training levels, and stairs; progress as appropriate.

Physical therapy short-term goal include the following: (1) increase left AROM hip flexion, abduction, and extension and knee flexion and extension by 10 degrees to promote improved gait quality; (2) improve left ankle AROM to 0 to 10 degrees to promote adequate foot clearance during gait; (3) improve sitting and standing balance by one grade to decrease the risk of falls; (4) improve all functional transfers to a minimal assistance level or better; (5) ambulate 200 ft with a single-point cane and left modified ankle-foot orthosis and minimal assistance/contact guard assistance, demonstrating consistent ability to perform the swing phase without assistance; and (6) ascend/descend 4 steps with minimal assistance.

1. Create a treatment plan that will address this patient's current status and goals.
2. Outline a list of therapeutic exercises that will promote increased AROM and strength.
3. List at least 3 interventions that can address the patient's tone.

## Suggested Resources

MS medications: https://www.nationalmssociety.org/Treating-MS/Medications

Spina bifida physical activity guidelines: https://www.spinabifidaassociation.org/resource/physical-activity/

# References


1. World Health Organization. Mental health: neurological disorders. May 2016. Accessed February 6, 2023. http://www.who.int/features/qa/55/en/
2. Latash ML, Levin MF, Scholz JP, Schöner G. Motor control theories and their applications. *Medicina (Kaunas).* 2010;46(6):382-392.
3. O'Sullivan SB, Schmitz TJ, Fulk GD. *Physical Rehabilitation.* 7th ed. FA Davis Company; 2019.
4. Cassidy JM, Cramer SC. Spontaneous and therapeutic-induced mechanisms of functional recovery after stroke. *Transl Stroke Res.* 2017;8(1):33-46. doi:10.1007/s12975-016-0467-5
5. Rugnetta M. Neuroplasticity. *Encyclopaedia Britannica.* Updated January 26, 2023. Accessed February 6, 2023. https://www.britannica.com/science/neuroplasticity
6. Hylin MJ, Kerr AL, Holden R. Understanding the mechanisms of recovery and/or compensation following injury. *Neural Plast.* 2017;2017:7125057. doi:10.1155/2017/7125057
7. Taub E, Uswatte G, Mark VW, Morris DM. The learned nonuse phenomenon: implications for rehabilitation. *Eura Medicophys.* 2006;42(3):241-256.
8. Sirtori V, Corbetta D, Moja L, Gatti R. Constraint-induced movement therapy for upper extremities in stroke patients. *Cochrane Database Syst Rev.* 2009;4:CD004433. doi:10.1002/14651858.CD004433.pub2
9. Corbetta D, Sirtori V, Castellini G, Moja L, Gatti R. Constraint-induced movement therapy for upper extremities in people with stroke. *Cochrane Database Syst Rev.* 2015;10:CD004433
10. Ballester BR, Maier M, San Segundo Mozo RM, Castañeda V, Duff A, Verschure PF. Counteracting learned non-use in chronic stroke patients with reinforcement-induced movement therapy. *J Neuroeng Rehabil.* 2016;13(1):74. doi:10.1186/s12984-016-0178-x
11. Kleim JA. Neural plasticity and neurorehabilitation: teaching the new brain old tricks. *J Commun Disord.* 2011;44(5):521-528. doi:10.1016/j.jcomdis.2011.04.006
12. O'Sullivan SB. Interventions to improve motor function. In: O'Sullivan SB, Schmitz T, eds. *Improving Functional Outcomes in Physical Rehabilitation.* 2nd ed. FA Davis; 2016:15-33.
13. The Free Dictionary. Synergy patterns. 2009. Accessed February 6, 2023. https://medical-dictionary.thefreedictionary.com/synergy+patterns
14. Bordoloil K, Deka RS. Scientific reconciliation of the concepts and principles of rood approach. *Int J Health Sci Res.* 2018;8(9):225-234.
15. Edwards LL, King EM, Buetefisch CM, Borich MR. Putting the "sensory" into sensorimotor control: the role of sensorimotor integration in goal-directed hand movements after stroke. *Front Integr Neurosci.* 2019;13:16. doi:10.3389/fnint.2019.00016
16. National Multiple Sclerosis Society. Accessed February 6, 2023. https://www.nationalmssociety.org/Symptoms-Diagnosis
17. Lublin FD, Reingold SC, Cohen JA, et al. Defining the clinical course of multiple sclerosis: the 2013 revisions. *Neurology.* 2014;83(3):278-286. doi:10.1212/WNL.0000000000000560
18. Kalron A, Givon U. Construct validity of the four square step test in multiple sclerosis. *Arch Phys Med Rehabil.* 2016;97(9):1496-1501. doi:10.1016/j.apmr.2016.04.012
19. Kalron A, Dolev M, Givon U. Further construct validity of the timed up and go test as a measure of ambulation in persons with multiple sclerosis. *Eur J Phys Rehabil Med.* 2017;53(6):841-847. doi:10.23736/S1973-9087.17.04599-3
20. Forsberg A, Andreasson M, Nilsagård YE. Validity of the dynamic gait index in people with multiple sclerosis. *Phys Ther.* 2013;93(10):1369-1376. doi:10.2522/ptj.20120284
21. Dunn M, Bhargava P, Kalb R. Your patients with multiple sclerosis have set wellness as a high priority-and the national multiple sclerosis society is responding. *US Neurol.* 2015;11(2):80-86. doi:10.17925/USN.2015.11.02.80
22. Protas EJ. Exercise testing and prescription for populations with other chronic diseases. In: Riebe D, Ehman JK, Liguori G, Magal M, eds. *ACSM's Guidelines for Exercise Testing and Prescription.* 10th ed. Wolters Kluwer; 2018.
23. Learmonth YC, Dlugonski D, Pilutti LA, Sandroff BM, Klaren R, Motl RW. Psychometric properties of the Fatigue Severity Scale and the Modified Fatigue Impact Scale. *J Neurol Sci.* 2013;331(1-2):102-107. doi:10.1016/j.jns.2013.05.023
24. Centers for Disease Control and Prevention. Stroke facts. September 6, 2017. Accessed February 6, 2023. https://www.cdc.gov/stroke/facts.htm
25. Nogles TE, Galuska MA. *Middle Cerebral Artery Stroke.* StatPearls Publishing; 2020.
26. Gladstone DJ, Danells CJ, Black SE. The Fugl-Meyer assessment of motor recovery after stroke: a critical review of its measurement properties. *Neurorehabil Neural Repair.* 2002;16(3):232-240.
27. Hsieh YW, Hsueh IP, Chou YT, Sheu CF, Hsieh CL, Kwakkel G. development and validation of a short form of the Fugl-Meyer motor scale in patients with stroke. *Stroke.* 2007;38(11):3052-3054. doi:10.1161/STROKEAHA.107.490730
28. Chen KL, Chen CT, Chou YT, Shih CL, Koh CL, Hsieh CL. Is the long form of the Fugl-Meyer motor scale more responsive than the short form in patients with stroke? *Arch Phys Med Rehabil.* 2014;95(5):941-949. doi:10.1016/j.apmr.2014.01.014
29. Blum L, Korner-Bitensky N. Usefulness of the Berg Balance Scale in stroke rehabilitation: a systematic review. *Phys Ther.* 2008;88(5):559-566. doi:10.2522/ptj.20070205
30. Ng SS, Tse MM, Tam EW, Lai CY. Reliability and convergent validity of the five-step test in people with chronic stroke. *J Rehabil Med.* 2018;50(1):16-21. doi:10.2340/16501977-2291
31. Billinger S, Arena R, Bernhardt J, et al. Physical activity and exercise recommendations for stroke survivors. *Stroke.* 2014;45:2532-2553. doi:10.1161/STR.0000000000000022
32. Sorinola IO, Powis I, White CM. Does additional exercise improve trunk function recovery in stroke patients? A meta-analysis. *NeuroRehabilitation.* 2014;35(2):205-213. doi:10.3233/NRE-141123
33. Cabanas-Valdés R, Bagur-Calafat C, Girabent-Farrés M, Caballero-Gómez FM, Hernández-Valiño M, Urrútia Cuchí G. The effect of additional core stability exercises on improving dynamic sitting balance and trunk control for subacute stroke patients: a randomized controlled trial. *Clin Rehabil.* 2016;30(10):1024-1033.
34. Cabanas-Valdés R, Bagur-Calafat C, Girabent-Farrés M, et al. Long-term follow-up of a randomized controlled trial on additional core stability exercises training for improving dynamic sitting balance and trunk control in stroke patients. *Clin Rehabil.* 2017;31(11):1492-1499. doi:10.1177/0269215517701804

35. Dell'Uomo D, Morone G, Centrella A, et al. Effects of scapulohumeral rehabilitation protocol on trunk control recovery in patients with subacute stroke: a pilot randomized controlled trial. *NeuroRehabilitation.* 2017;40(3):337-343. doi:10.3233/NRE-161421
36. Pollock A, Baer G, Campbell P, et al. Physical rehabilitation approaches for the recovery of function and mobility following stroke. *Cochrane Database Syst Rev.* 2014;4:CD001920. doi:10.1002/14651858.CD001920.pub3
37. National Institute of Neurological Disorders and Stroke. Parkinson's disease information page. Accessed February 6, 2023. https://www.ninds.nih.gov/health-information/disorders/parkinsons-disease
38. DeMaagd G, Philip A. Parkinson's disease and its management: part 1: disease entity, risk factors, pathophysiology, clinical presentation, and diagnosis. *P T.* 2015;40(8):504-532.
39. Nonnekes J, Giladi N, Guha A, Fietzek UM, Bloem BR, Růžička E. Gait festination in parkinsonism: introduction of two phenotypes. *J Neurol.* 2019;266(2):426-430. doi:10.1007/s00415-018-9146-7
40. Parkinson'sDisease.Net. Medications used to treat Parkinson's. Accessed February 6, 2023. https://parkinsonsdisease.net/medications/
41. National Institute of Neurological Disorders and Stroke. Deep brain stimulation for movement disorders. Accessed February 6, 2023. https://www.ninds.nih.gov/Disorders/Patient-Caregiver-Education/Fact-Sheets/Deep-Brain-Stimulation-Movement-Disorders-Fact
42. Goetz CG, Poewe W, Rascol O, et al. Movement disorder society task force report on the Hoehn and Yahr staging scale: status and recommendations. *Mov Disord.* 2004;19(9):1020-1028. doi:10.1002/mds.20213
43. Winser SJ, Kannan P, Bello UM, Whitney SL. Measures of balance and falls risk prediction in people with Parkinson's disease: a systematic review of psychometric properties. *Clin Rehabil.* 2019;33(12):1949-1962. doi:10.1177/0269215519877498
44. McDonnell MN, Rischbieth B, Schammer TT, Seaforth C, Shaw AJ, Phillips AC. Lee Silverman Voice Treatment (LSVT)-BIG to improve motor function in people with Parkinson's disease: a systematic review and meta-analysis. *Clin Rehabil.* 2018;32(5):607-618. doi:10.1177/0269215517734385
45. Sharififar S, Coronado RA, Romero S, Azari H, Thigpen M. The effects of whole body vibration on mobility and balance in Parkinson disease: a systematic review. *Iran J Med Sci.* 2014;39(4):318-326.
46. Kaut O, Brenig D, Marek M, Allert N, Wüllner U. Postural stability in Parkinson's disease patients is improved after stochastic resonance therapy. *Parkinsons Dis.* 2016;2016:7948721. doi:10.1155/2016/7948721
47. Schenkman M, Moore CG, Kohrt WM, et al. Effect of high-intensity treadmill exercise on motor symptoms in patients with de novo Parkinson disease: a phase 2 randomized clinical trial. *JAMA Neurol.* 2018;75(2):219-226. doi:10.1001/jamaneurol.2017.3517
48. Fiorelli CM, Ciolac EG, Simieli L, et al. Differential acute effect of high-intensity interval or continuous moderate exercise on cognition in individuals with Parkinson's disease. *J Phys Act Health.* 2019;16(2):157-164.
49. Garza N, Toussi A, Wilson M, Shahlaie K, Martin R. The increasing age of TBI patients at a single level 1 trauma center and the discordance between GCS and CT Rotterdam scores in the elderly. *Front Neurol.* 2020;11:112. doi:10.3389/fneur.2020.00112
50. Traumatic Brain Injury Model Systems National Data and Statistical Center. National Database: 2020 profile of people within the traumatic brain injury model systems. Accessed February 6, 2023. https://www.tbindsc.org/StaticFiles/Documents/2022%20TBIMS%20National%20Database%20Update.pdf
51. Peterson AB, Kegler SR. Deaths from fall-related traumatic brain injury — United States, 2008–2017. *MMWR Morb Mortal Wkly Rep.* 2020;69:225-230. doi:10.15585/mmwr.mm6909a2
52. Bryden DW, Tilghman JI, Hinds SR II. Blast-related traumatic brain injury: current concepts and research considerations. *J Exp Neurosci.* 2019;13:1179069519872213. doi:10.1177/1179069519872213
53. O'Neil ME, Carlson K, Storzbach D, et al. Complications of mild traumatic brain injury in veterans and military personnel: a systematic review. Department of Veterans Affairs; January 2013. Accessed February 6, 2023. https://www.ncbi.nlm.nih.gov/books/NBK189784/table/appc.t1/
54. Lendraitienė E, Petruševičienė D, Savickas R, Žemaitienė I, Mingaila S. The impact of physical therapy in patients with severe traumatic brain injury during acute and post-acute rehabilitation according to coma duration. *J Phys Ther Sci.* 2016;28(7):2048-2054. doi:10.1589/jpts.28.2048
55. Statistics for spinal cord injury based on NSCISC data 2019. Accessed June 11, 2020. https://www.sci-info-pages.com/spinal-cord-injury-facts-and-statistics/
56. American Spinal Cord Injury Association. International standards for Neurological Classification of Spinal Cord Injury (ISNCSCI). Accessed January 12, 2018. http://lms3.learnshare.com/Images/Brand/120/ASIA/International%20Standards%20Worksheet.pdf
57. Nas K, Yazmalar L, Şah V, Aydın A, Öneş K. Rehabilitation of spinal cord injuries. *World J Orthop.* 2015;6(1):8-16. doi:10.5312/wjo.v6.i1.8
58. Hou S, Rabchevsky AG. Autonomic consequences of spinal cord injury. *Compr Physiol.* 2014;4(4):1419-1453. doi:10.1002/cphy.c130045
59. Hagen EM. Acute complications of spinal cord injuries. *World J Orthop.* 2015;6(1):17-23. doi:10.5312/wjo.v6.i1.17
60. Scivoletto G, Tamburella F, Laurenza L, Torre M, Molinari M. Who is going to walk? A review of the factors influencing walking recovery after spinal cord injury. *Front Hum Neurosci.* 2014;8:141. doi:10.3389/fnhum.2014.00141
61. Holanda LJ, Silva PM, Amorim TC, Lacerda MO, Simão CR, Morya E. Robotic assisted gait as a tool for rehabilitation of individuals with spinal cord injury: a systematic review. *J Neuroeng Rehabil.* 2017;14(1):126. doi:10.1186/s12984-017-0338-7
62. van der Scheer JW, Martin Ginis KA, Ditor DS, et al. Effects of exercise on fitness and health of adults with spinal cord injury: a systematic review. *Neurology.* 2017;89(7):736-745. doi:10.1212/WNL.0000000000004224

63. Martin Ginis KA, van der Scheer JW, Latimer-Cheung AE, et al. Evidence-based scientific exercise guidelines for adults with spinal cord injury: an update and a new guideline. *Spinal Cord.* 2018;56(4):308-321. doi:10.1038/s41393-017-0017-3
64. Tweedy SM, Beckman EM, Geraghty TJ, et al. Exercise and Sports Science Australia (ESSA) position statement on exercise and spinal cord injury. *J Sci Med Sport.* 2017;20(2):108-115. doi:10.1016/j.jsams.2016.02.001
65. Ringholz GM, Appel SH, Bradshaw M, Cooke NA, Mosnik DM, Schulz PE. Prevalence and patterns of cognitive impairment in sporadic ALS. *Neurology.* 2005;65(4):586-590.
66. Mehta P, Kaye W, Bryan L, et al. Prevalence of amyotrophic lateral sclerosis — United States, 2012–2013. *MMWR Surveill Summ.* 2016;65(8):1-12. doi:10.15585/mmwr.ss6508a1
67. Dal Bello-Haas V, Florence JM. Therapeutic exercise for people with amyotrophic lateral sclerosis or motor neuron disease. *Cochrane Database Syst Rev.* 2013;5:CD005229. doi:10.1002/14651858.CD005229.pub3
68. Lunetta C, Lizio A, Sansone VA, et al. Strictly monitored exercise programs reduce motor deterioration in ALS: preliminary results of a randomized controlled trial. *J Neurol.* 2016;263(1):52-60.
69. Merico A, Cavinato M, Gregorio C, et al. Effects of combined endurance and resistance training in amyotrophic lateral sclerosis: a pilot, randomized, controlled study [published correction appears in Eur J Transl Myol. 2018;28(3):7842]. *Eur J Transl Myol.* 2018;28(1):7278. doi:10.4081/ejtm.2018.7278
70. Fisher RS, Cross JH, French JA, et al. Operational classification of seizure types by the International League Against Epilepsy: position paper of the ILAE Commission for Classification and Terminology. *Epilepsia.* 2017;58(4):522-530. doi:10.1111/epi.13670
71. Zack MM, Kobau R. National and state estimates of the numbers of adults and children with active epilepsy - United States. 2015. *MMWR Morb Mortal Wkly Rep.* 2017;66:821-825. doi:10.15585/mmwr.mm6631a1
72. Epilepsy Foundation. Types of seizures. Accessed February 6, 2023. https://www.epilepsy.com/learn/types-seizures
73. Centers for Disease Control and Prevention. What is cerebral palsy? Accessed February 6, 2023. https://www.cdc.gov/ncbddd/cp/facts.html
74. CanChild. Gross Motor Function Classification System, Expanded and Revised (GMFCS-E&R). Accessed February 6, 2023 https://canchild.ca/en/resources/42-gross-motor-function-classification-system-expanded-revised-gmfcs-e-r
75. Kostek MC, Gordon B. Exercise is an adjuvant to contemporary dystrophy treatments. *Exerc Sport Sci Rev.* 2018;46(1):34-41. doi:10.1249/JES.0000000000000131
76. Kostek M. Precision medicine and exercise therapy in Duchenne muscular dystrophy. *Sports (Basel).* 2019;7(3):64. doi:10.3390/sports7030064
77. Alemdaroğlu I, Karaduman A, Yilmaz ÖT, Topaloğlu H. Different types of upper extremity exercise training in Duchenne muscular dystrophy: effects on functional performance, strength, endurance, and ambulation. *Muscle Nerve.* 2015;51(5):697-705. doi:10.1002/mus.24451
78. Centers for Disease Control and Prevention. What is spina bifida? Accessed February 6, 2023. https://www.cdc.gov/ncbddd/spinabifida/facts.html
79. Apkon SD, Grady R, Hart S, et al. Advances in the care of children with spina bifida. *Adv Pediatr.* 2014;61(1):33-74. doi:10.1016/j.yapd.2014.03.007
80. Hart SM. Spina bifida: myelomeningocele. May 26, 2017. Accessed February 6, 2023. https://www.apta.org/patient-care/evidence-based-practice-resources/clinical-summaries/spina-bifida-myelomeningocele
81. Oliveira A, Jacome C, Marques A. Physical fitness and exercise training on individuals with spina bifida: a systematic review. *Res Dev Disabil.* 2014;35(5):1119-1136.
82. Crytzer TM, Dicianno BE, Kapoor R. Physical activity, exercise, and health-related measures of fitness in adults with spina bifida: a review of the literature. *P MR.* 2013;5(12):1051-1062.
83. Agre JC, Rodriquez AA. Muscular function in late polio and the role of exercise in post-polio patients. *NeuroRehabilitation.* 1997;8(2):107-118. doi:10.3233/NRE-1997-8205
84. Lewelt A, Krosschell KJ, Stoddard GJ, et al. Resistance strength training exercise in children with spinal muscular atrophy. *Muscle Nerve.* 2015;52(4):559-567. doi:10.1002/mus.24568
85. Voet NB, van der Kooi EL, Riphagen II, Lindeman E, van Engelen BG, Geurts AC. Strength training and aerobic exercise training for muscle disease. *Cochrane Database Syst Rev.* 2013;7:CD003907. doi:10.1002/14651858.CD003907

Chapter 17

# Therapeutic Exercise Considerations After Lower Extremity Amputation

*Jacki Klaczak Kopack, PT, DPT*

**KEY TERMS** Amputee mobility predictor | Phantom limb pain | Phantom limb sensation | Transfemoral amputation | Transtibial amputation

## Chapter Objectives

1. Explain the importance of regular exercise and activity after an amputation.
2. Discuss the indications, contraindications, and treatment focus for a patient who presents with a lower extremity amputation.
3. Describe the priority exercises for patients with a transtibial amputation (TTA) or transfemoral amputation (TFA).
4. Explain the treatment goals and primary treatment interventions for each stage of rehabilitation postamputation (postsurgical, preprosthetic, and prosthetic training phases).
5. Discuss additional monitoring that is indicated before, during, and after treatment for patients with acquired limb loss.
6. Given a patient scenario and plan of care, develop an appropriate treatment intervention plan for a patient with acquired limb loss.

Amputation or acquired limb loss (the loss of an upper or lower extremity) has the potential to result in disability for patients. There are a number of medical conditions (comorbidities) that increase the risk of limb loss.[1] Approximately 180,000 amputations occur in the United States annually, and the number of persons with limb loss is projected to reach 3.6 million by the year 2050. The most common causes of amputation in order of prevalence include dysvascular disease, trauma, and cancer.[2] Dysvascular causes of amputations include peripheral vascular disease and diabetes. Each year there are typically a larger number of lower extremity amputations due to diabetes and vascular disease than trauma; yet, the long-term survival rates for patients who are status post–trauma are higher. Young adults and adolescents tend to sustain amputations most commonly due to trauma, whereas vascular disease accounts for a larger percentage of amputations in older adults. The presence of diabetes or cardiovascular disease contributes to higher mortality rates and greater disability after amputation. Experts in the field describe a "50/50 rule" for persons with dysvascular causes for amputation—50% of persons with a dysvascular amputation die within 5 years, and 50% of survivors lose a portion of the opposite limb.[1,3]



Kopack JK, Cascardi KA.
*Principles of Therapeutic Exercise for the Physical Therapist Assistant* (pp 595-621).

**Table 17-1**

Descriptions of Various Levels of Amputation

| Level | Description |
|---|---|
| Partial toe | Excision of any part of one or more toes |
| Toe disarticulation | Disarticulation at the metatarsophalangeal joint |
| Partial foot/ray resection | Amputation of third, fourth, and fifth metatarsals and digits |
| Transmetatarsal | Amputation through the midsection of all metatarsals |
| Syme's | Ankle disarticulation with attachment of the heel pad to the distal end of the tibia; may include removal of malleoli and distal tibia/fibula |
| Long transtibial | More than 50% of tibial length remains |
| Transtibial | Between 20% and 50% of tibial length preserved |
| Short transtibial | < 20% of tibial length remains |
| Knee disarticulation | Amputation through knee joint; femur intact |
| Long transfemoral | More than 60% femoral length preserved |
| Transfemoral | 35% to 60% femoral length preserved |
| Short transfemoral | < 35% femoral length preserved |
| Hip disarticulation | Amputation through hip joint; pelvis intact |
| Hemipelvectomy | Resection through the lower half of the pelvis |
| Hemicorpectomy | Amputation of both lower limbs and pelvis below L4-L5 level |

Limb loss can result in a decline in functional mobility and ambulation. The strongest predictors of return to effective functional mobility and ambulation with a prosthesis include amputation level, age, physical fitness, and the presence of fewer comorbidities. These factors are considerations when determining the appropriate prosthetic device prescription and potential for functional performance (mobility).[4] Physical therapy interventions play a crucial role in maximizing functional outcomes for persons with acquired limb loss. Ambulation after an amputation requires a significant amount of effort and a significant increase in energy expenditure compared with a healthy person without an amputation. This increases the demand on the cardiovascular system with gait, and patients typically report higher rates of perceived exertion levels during mobility training.[5-7]

## Levels of Amputation

Amputations are defined by the anatomical location of the amputation and the length of the terminal bone in the residual limb (Table 17-1 and Figure 17-1). The most common lower extremity amputations are **TTAs** and **TFAs.** The surgeon considers the patient's overall medical status and typically amputates the limb at the lowest level possible to maximize future function. This determination is made with consideration of the vascular supply of the limb. More proximal amputation levels often have better potential for healing and fewer complications (related to vascular supply) but tend to result in lower levels of functional mobility.[4] The level of amputation affects prosthetic ambulation potential; patients with longer residual limbs and more intact joints in the affected limb are more likely to be functional prosthetic ambulators.[4]

## Phases of Rehabilitation After Limb Amputation

There are 3 phases of postamputation rehabilitation: the postsurgical phase, preprosthetic training, and the prosthetic training phase (each with different goals). The focus of the rehabilitation process is to maximize function and to promote the highest level of independent mobility possible. Early initiation of rehabilitation is pivotal to achieving the best outcomes. Delays in initiating rehabilitation increase the risk of contracture development, general debilitation, and depression. Throughout the rehabilitation process, the clinician will emphasize the importance of residual limb care, limb positioning, and monitoring. A well-healed, well-shaped residual limb with a nonadherent scar is easier to fit with a prosthesis. It is important to maintain normal knee and hip range of motion (ROM); full ROM will be critical for future lower extremity prosthesis use. The patient should perform therapeutic exercises and proper limb positioning to reduce the risk of contractures. The vascular status of the residual limb, the patient's physiological (not chronological) age, and the level of patient motivation all influence a patient's rehabilitation potential. Patient education that addresses the patient's individual presentation (medical and physiological), progression, goals, and rehabilitation potential is important to obtaining optimal outcomes.

The early phases of the rehabilitation program include pregait activities (ie, upper and lower extremity stretching/strengthening and balance training) and aerobic training to prepare the patient for the increased energy demands of ambulation. Later stages of the rehabilitation process focus on improving balance and gait and will include prosthesis fitting. Interventions to progress ambulation and functional use of the prosthesis are implemented to maximize patient safety with the prosthesis.

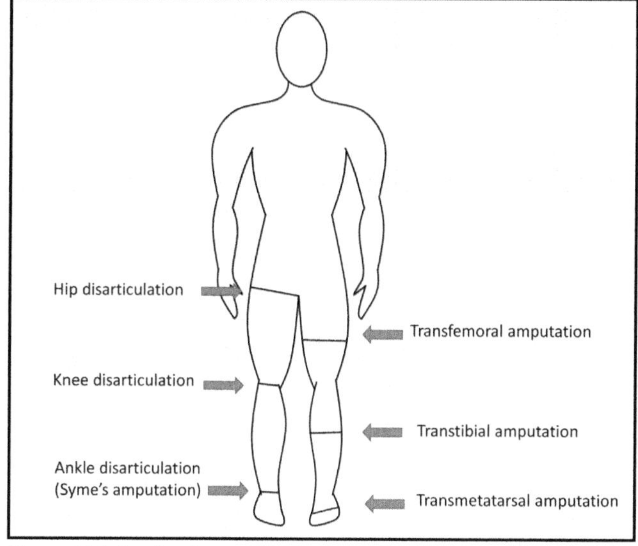


**Figure 17-1.** Levels of amputations.

## Postsurgical Phase: Interventions

The time between the surgery and discharge from the acute care hospital is the postsurgical phase of rehabilitation. Physical therapy is initiated day 1 postoperatively if the patient is medically stable and cleared for treatment. The physical therapist individualizes the patient's goals and plan of care based on clinical findings (ie, active range of motion [AROM], passive ROM, and manual muscle strength for all limbs including the residual limb), vascular status/health of the uninvolved limbs, current functional status (ie, activities of daily living [ADLs], transfers, bed mobility, sitting balance, standing balance, and gait), and prior level of function/activity. The physical therapist considers the patient's medical status (including all comorbidities, cognition, and cardiac status) because conditions such as diabetes, cardiovascular disease, renal disease, and impairments (ie, visual, ROM, and strength) can affect the patient's activity tolerance and rehabilitation potential. Some patients may need a cardiovascular stress test before initiating the inpatient rehabilitation process. The patient's emotional status and available social and psychological supports are assessed. The rehabilitation program addresses the physical skills (ie, strength, balance, and endurance) needed for eventual prosthetic rehabilitation while supporting emotional adjustment.

The patient is in the hospital for a short period, so the physical therapist assistant will provide patient education and interventions to prepare the patient for discharge. Interventions include patient education (ie, skin care, limb wrapping, and positioning), desensitization, therapeutic exercise, functional mobility retraining, and balance exercises. An early focus on limb positioning and the inclusion of specific exercises sets the stage for future prosthetic device training. Table 17-2 provides a list of goals and typical interventions for each rehabilitation phase.

## Patient Monitoring: Physiological and Psychological Status

The physical therapist assistant monitors the patient's response throughout the rehabilitation process, including the patient's coping skills. The loss of a limb is a significant event that can result in depression, anger, and grieving. The assistant should let the patient express their feelings while exhibiting compassion and empathy. Patient interaction with friends and family plays an important role in the healing process, and participation in support groups can be useful.

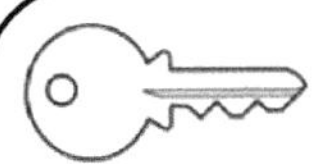

### Key Safety Considerations

Monitor:

- Vital signs
- The status of the residual limb and the uninvolved limb (skin color, temperature, pulses, and sensation)
- Medical comorbidities (pay special attention to monitoring the vascular status of both limbs if it was a dysvascular amputation, and pay attention to indications of blood sugar changes if the amputation was a complication of a diabetes)
- Healing (observe for early signs/symptoms of infection or delayed healing)
- Limb positioning (promote the prevention of contractures)

**Table 17-2**

## Postoperative Amputation Rehabilitation Phases

| Phase | Patient Goals | Therapy Interventions |
|---|---|---|
| Postsurgical (time between surgery and discharge from the hospital) | • Assist with residual limb care (wrapping, skin care, and positioning)<br>• Advance mobility/functional abilities; promote independence with toilet transfers as soon as possible<br>• Independent HEP: Residual limb, intact lower limb, and upper extremities<br>• Independent with care of residual limb<br>• Positioning: Maintain full ROM at key joints; contracture prevention<br>• Pain management<br>• Management of comorbidities/risk factors | • Patient education: Participation in limb wrapping/care, and positioning. Focus on shaping, edema control, skin inspection, and proper positioning to prevent contractures; initiate desensitization activities.<br>• Functional mobility training: Bed mobility and transfers. Stand pivot, transfer board, or lateral transfer (squat pivot) based on patient presentation.<br>• Gait training: Crutches are more functional than a walker if feasible given patient presentation.<br>• Therapeutic exercise: Supine, seated. Include ROM, isometrics, wheelchair push-ups, and modified bridging. Give patient HEP. Avoid tension/pulling on incision.<br>• Aerobic exercise: Wheelchair mobility, and upper bike ergometer<br>• Pain control: Mental practice, imagery, and desensitization techniques for the residual limb<br>• General postoperative prevention for deep vein thrombosis and pneumonia: Compression pumps and ankle pump exercise for nonaffected lower extremity, incentive spirometer, and mobilization out of bed |
| Preprosthetic training (time between hospital discharge to prosthetic fitting or the decision that the patient is not a prosthetic candidate) | • Independent with residual limb care (wrapping, skin care, and positioning)<br>• Independent mobility with assistive device<br>• Independent HEP<br>• Independent with care of unaffected lower extremity.<br>• Full ROM in lower extremity joints<br>• Increase strength in upper extremity and lower extremity<br>• Improve aerobic capacity | • Patient education: Participation in limb wrapping/care as needed. Continue and progress activities that were initiated in the postoperative period.<br>• Therapeutic exercise: Supine, seated, prone, standing; increase resistance (as tolerated)<br>• Balance: Weight shifting on to residual limb, standing on intact limb, challenge balance, and vary surfaces<br>• Progressive functional mobility training without prosthesis<br>• Aerobic exercise: Upper bike ergometer, swimming (if incision is healed), and wheelchair mobility for endurance<br><br>*(continued)* |

**Table 17-2 (continued)**

Postoperative Amputation Rehabilitation Phases

| Phase | Patient Goals | Therapy Interventions |
|---|---|---|
| Prosthetic training (time between delivery of prosthesis to maximal function with prosthesis) | • Independent with residual limb care (wrapping, skin care, and positioning)<br>• Independent mobility with assistive device<br>• Independent HEP<br>• Independent with care of remaining lower extremity | • Patient education: Skin integrity, sock management, and prosthesis education (parts and care)<br>• Progressive functional mobility training and balance activities with prosthesis<br>• Advanced therapeutic exercise: Progress to prosthetic training progressions as indicated.<br>• Aerobic exercise: Upper bike ergometer, walking with prosthetic, and swimming |

HEP = home exercise program.

Monitoring the intact limb is important, especially for persons with dysvascular amputations and diabetes; ensure that the patient is wearing a properly supportive and well-fitting shoe on that limb and monitor skin integrity (color, temperature, hair/nail growth, texture, and wounds/scars) and for the presence of any callus or fissures (pay attention to pressure-bearing areas). Monitor the lower extremity for any signs consistent with vascular issues (ie, hemosiderin staining or trophic changes in the lower extremity).

### Considerations for the Physical Therapist Assistant

Clinicians review the Ankle-Brachial Index (ABI), hemoglobin A1C, and albumin levels for persons with acquired limb loss. ABI values less than 1 indicate peripheral arterial disease, which may affect the potential for healing. Hemoglobin A1C levels greater than 8 indicate poor blood glucose control, which may also impact the potential for healing.[8] Serum albumin levels provide insight into nutritional status, which impacts healing. Comprehensive management may include consultation with the wound care team.

Addressing the intricacies of wound management is outside the scope of this text. Concerns regarding the incision, lower extremity skin integrity, or the healing process should be brought immediately to the physical therapist/medical team's attention.

## Types of Postsurgical Dressings and Wrapping the Residual Limb

Healing and positioning of the residual limb are priorities throughout the rehabilitation process. Edema reduction promotes healing and shaping of the residual limb and is achieved through the use of postsurgical dressings such as rigid or semirigid dressings or soft dressings. Soft dressings include elastic wraps or limb shrinker socks (compression socks, "shrinkers," or retention socks). Rigid dressings are made of plaster or fiberglass casting materials and are very effective for controlling edema. These are applied immediately after surgery or during the postsurgical phase, and they can be removed for wound inspection. Semirigid dressings are not commonly used (they tend to loosen and are not as effective as rigid dressings). Shrinkers are sock-like garments with rubber-reinforced cotton. Elastic wraps are commonly used for edema control after lower extremity amputations.

### Clinical Tip

Shrinkers are not recommended when sutures are intact, but some surgeons may consider early application of shrinkers if compliance with limb wrapping is a concern. In these cases, a nylon wrap is placed over the incision dressing, and shrinker donning is closely supervised.

For patients using elastic wraps for residual limb wrapping, the clinician should complete skin checks and rewrapping during each session. The goal for limb wrapping is to promote a cylindrical limb shape, which allows for a proper weight-bearing surface area and a better prosthesis fit. Table 17-3 provides tips for residual limb wrapping, and Figures 17-2 and 17-3 illustrate step-by-step wrapping techniques for persons with a TTA and TFA, respectively. Inappropriate application can result in damage to the residual limb. Learning to correctly apply residual limb wrapping using elastic bandages is a skill that takes considerable practice; proper application is critical to both patient (limb) safety and to maintaining optimal potential for prosthesis use.

## Table 17-3

### Tips for Wrapping the Residual Limb

- Complete a skin inspection pre- and postwrapping.
- Use slightly more pressure distally, decreasing the pressure as the wrap is applied proximally. Too much pressure can result in skin breakdown or a tourniquet effect.
- The wrap should be applied with diagonal wraps, no circumferential wrapping! Avoid wrinkles when applying the bandages. Overlap the layers of the bandages, and *do not* leave any open spaces around the residual limb. Make sure there are at least 2 layers of the bandage covering the residual limb. Avoid excess pressure over the tibial crest. Transfemoral wrapping: The wrap should extend high up into the groin area (to avoid risk of creation of an adductor roll because this will make prosthetic fitting and ambulation more difficult).
- Most limbs require 2 to 3 elastic bandages (4 and/or 6 inches wide) to complete the wrapping.
- The wrap should be removed and reapplied every 2 to 4 hours.
- Once the staples/sutures are removed and the incision is healed, the physician may prescribe a shrinker.

**Safety tip:** The elastic wrap or shrinker should *not* cause pain; if it does, it is likely too tight.

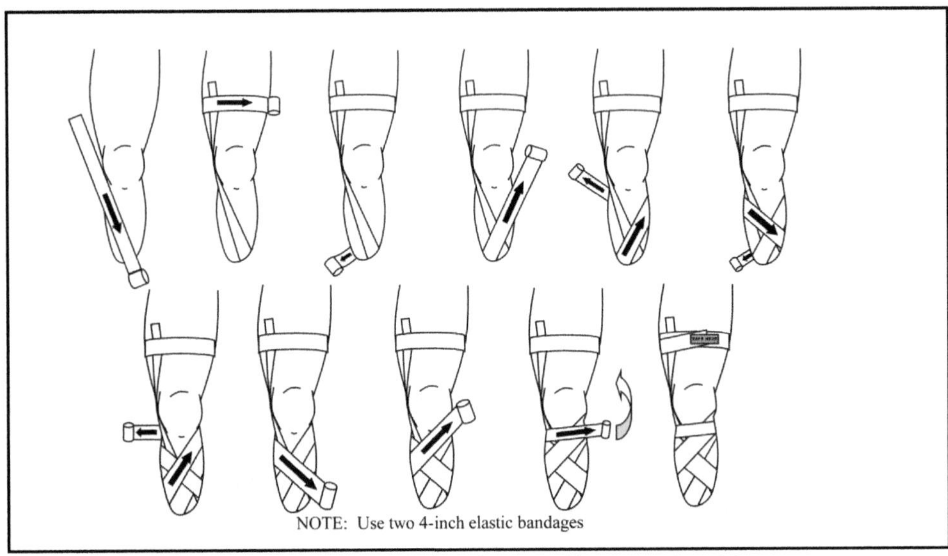


**Figure 17-2.** Transtibial residual limb wrapping. (Graphic created by Jimmy Kopack.)

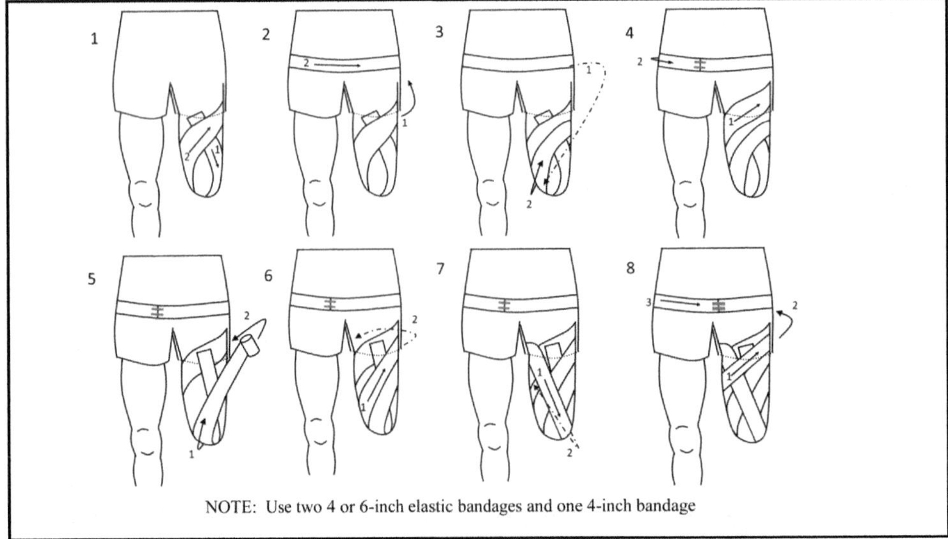


**Figure 17-3.** Transfemoral residual limb wrapping. (Graphic created by Jimmy Kopack.)

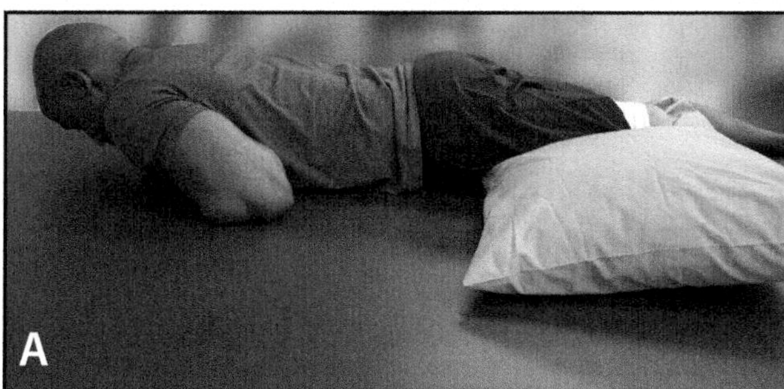


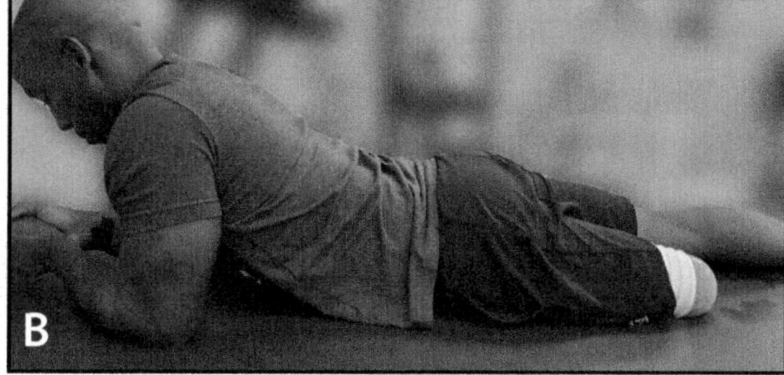


**Figure 17-4.** (A) Prone positioning prevents hip flexor contractures in people with TFAs. (B) Progress patient to prone on elbows.

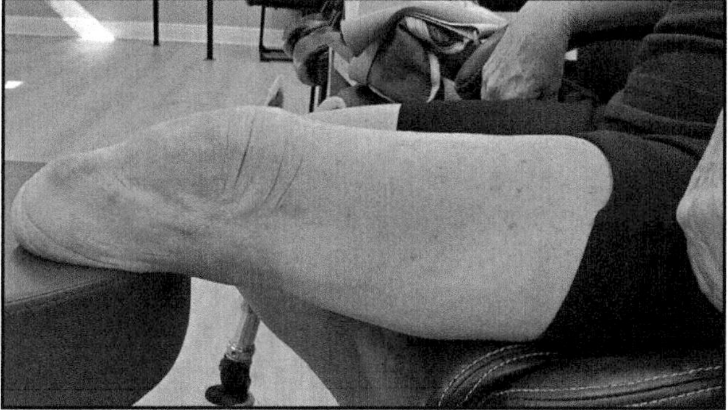

**Figure 17-5.** A patient with a TTA is positioned with the knee extended to prevent a knee flexor contracture in a seated position.

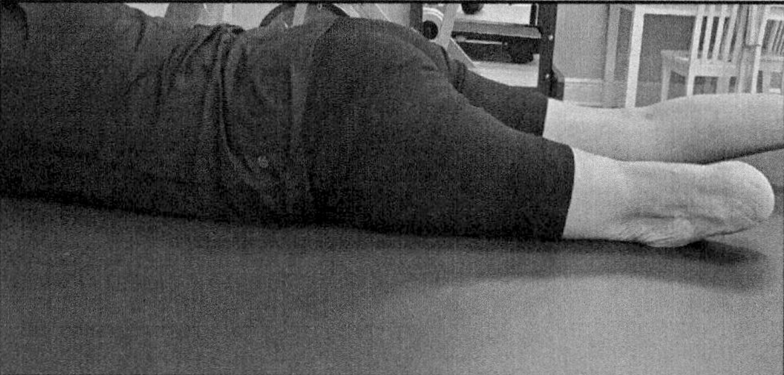

**Figure 17-6.** A patient with a TTA positioned prone to reduce hip and knee flexor contractures.

## Positioning and Skin Care

One of the greatest risks to effective prosthesis usage is the development of contractures at the hip or knee. Contractures are a result of muscle tightness, muscle imbalance, fascial tightness, or prolonged positioning of a joint in a "comfort position" (ie, hip flexion, hip abduction, or knee flexion). Patients tend to position their involved lower extremity with the hip flexed, abducted, and externally rotated. Knee flexion contractures are commonly observed in persons with TTAs, and hip flexion and abduction contractures are commonly noted in persons with TFAs. Normal hip extension ROM is necessary for an efficient gait pattern with any (lower extremity) prosthesis, and an efficient gait pattern results in less energy expenditure during ambulation. Patients with a TFA also need to maintain full hip adduction in the residual limb, and persons with a TTA also need full knee extension.

> **Considerations for the Physical Therapist Assistant**
>
> The minimal AROMs to facilitate full function include 20 degrees of hip extension, 0 degrees of knee extension, 100 degrees of knee flexion, and 10 degrees of ankle dorsiflexion. Higher-level instrumental ADLs require normal AROM in the intact joints.

The clinician will educate the patient on proper positioning and its relevance to the future ambulation ability. Persons with a TTA or TFA are instructed to lay prone as long and as often as possible and to avoid comfort positions (hip flexion, hip abduction, and knee flexion). Prone on elbows positioning is a useful position (to promote hip extension ROM; Figures 17-4A and 17-4B). The patient should avoid elevating the limb on pillows in bed (avoid flexion), and patients with a TFA should try to limit time spent sitting. Patients with a TTA should maintain knee extension when seated (this is especially important in the early days postamputation when the patient may be using a wheelchair for mobility). A posterior splint or an extension board adaptation for the wheelchair is applied to maintain knee extension ROM. The patient is instructed how to maintain knee extension while seated (Figure 17-5). Prone positioning is important for patients with a TTA (Figure 17-6), and the clinician should monitor for increased pressure on the patella; a small pad can be placed under the distal thigh if needed to reduce pressure on the patella. Additional positioning recommendations to reduce the risk of contractures in lower extremity amputees are illustrated in Figure 17-7. Although some prostheses can accommodate small knee contractures, they cannot easily accommodate for hip flexion contractures. The presence of any contracture alters the biomechanics of gait, decreasing efficiency and lowering the likelihood of the patient becoming a functional ambulator.

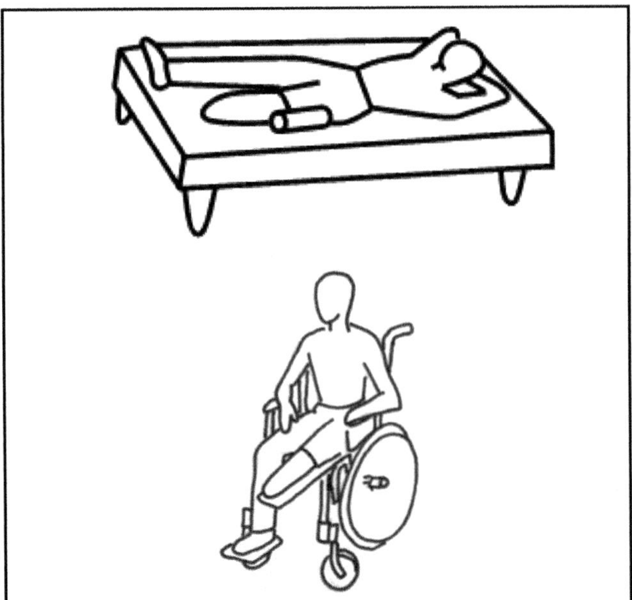

**Figure 17-7.** Additional proper positioning for patients with lower extremity amputations to prevent contractures: Supine with hip and knee extended and hip in adduction. Seated in a wheelchair with a knee extension board (used for people with TTAs). (Graphic created by Jimmy Kopack.)

### Clinical Tip

Consider measuring hip extension in a modified Thomas test position vs prone; document the patient's measurement position.

Patient education includes education about skin care and scar management. Table 17-4 provides a list of guidelines for residual limb skin care for patients. Residual limb desensitization should begin in the early postoperative phase. Desensitization includes gentle massage of the skin on the residual limb (Figure 17-8) followed by a sequence of massaging the limb with cloths/substances of increasing texture (ie, cotton ball, soft cotton cloth, corduroy, and then terry cloth). Gentle mobilization of the tissues surrounding the scar can begin day 1 postoperatively as long as the clinician approximates the incision surfaces and gently moves only the surrounding tissue (in a direction parallel to the scar). Questions regarding the appropriateness of initiating this massage should be discussed with the physician. If this intervention causes any increase in bleeding, exudate, or pain, the assistant should terminate the activity immediately and notify the supervising therapist. Scar massage is initiated once the incision is healed; at that point, the assistant can initiate gentle massage over the residual limb and the incision. If there are no adverse reactions, the assistant will progress to transverse friction massage over the incision to promote a mobile scar; the clinician can increase the intensity based on patient tolerance.

## Phantom Limb Pain and Sensation

**Phantom limb sensation** is the sensation that an amputated limb is still present. **Phantom limb pain (PLP)** is pain that feels as if it is coming from a body part that is no longer there. Approximately 79% of amputees reported lower extremity phantom limb sensation, and 72% reported PLP.[9] Pain that occurs in the early postoperative phase is often caused by the recent surgical trauma and is typically not directly related to PLP. The mechanism responsible for PLP is poorly understood. Peripheral causes (eg, neuroma formation) and spinal or brain changes (ie, plasticity related to the cortical representation of the residual limb or psychogenic mechanisms) are considered as potential causes of the pain. Each person's experience of the frequency, intensity, and quality of pain sensation is different.[9] Many pharmacologic and nonpharmacologic therapies are currently under investigation, but there is no one preferred treatment.[10-13]

### Considerations for the Physical Therapist Assistant

Ask the patient to describe the pain or sensation. Common descriptors of phantom limb sensations may include cold/warm, pulling, stuck, itchy, burning, stabbing, "electric shocks," pressure, aching, tired, squeezing, formication (bugs crawling), and "pins and needles."

Physical therapy interventions can provide a nonpharmacologic option to address PLP. Transcutaneous electric nerve stimulation may be useful; the clinician can apply electrodes to the intact limb in the area where the patient is describing pain on the amputated limb.[12] Treatment interventions that include muscle relaxation, mental imagery, and modified phantom limb exercise training are effective in reducing the intensity, rate, and bother of PLP and sensation; one such intervention program is the Santa Lucia Alleviation Intervention for Phantom in Amputees' Neurorehabilitation (the SAIPAN protocol).[11,13] Mirror therapy, residual limb wrapping, desensitization activities, and the containment/pressure that is incurred during prosthetic training have been investigated as potential interventions to decrease phantom pain. Common desensitization activities include tapping, rubbing the limb with fabrics of increasing texture, self-massage, motion with Theraband resistance, vibration, and weight bearing through the

**Table 17-4**

**General Skin Care Tips for a Residual Limb**

- Wash the residual limb daily with mild soap, rinse, and dry completely.
- Soaps should be nonscented and alcohol- and perfume-free.
- Avoid water temperature extremes when washing (ie, very hot or very cold water).
    - Do not use heating pads, hot packs, or cold packs on the residual limb.
- Do not soak the residual limb.
- Use lotion to maintain skin hydration (nonscented and alcohol and perfume free).
- Once the patient is a prosthetic candidate and may be using gel socks, review *any/all* lotion use with the prosthetist for safety.
- Avoid "home remedies" and any treatments touted to "toughen" the skin of the residual limb.

residual limb. Many persons with PLP will experience decreasing symptoms over time, but some patients will continue to experience pain.

Patients may experience pain from neuromas. A neuroma is an overgrowth of nerve tissue (it tends to be benign). A person with an amputation may also experience pain in the residual limb for any of the typical orthopedic reasons a therapist would screen for, including referred pain, joint pain, soft tissue pain, and pressure from the prosthesis. The therapist will determine the most appropriate treatment option based on the results of the physical therapy examination.

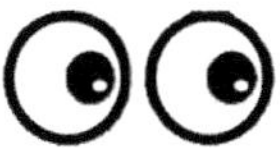

**Eye on the Research: Phantom Limb Pain**

Richardson and Kulkarni[10] reviewed current treatment options for PLP and concluded that there was not strong evidence for inclusion of any of the interventions. There was moderate support for pharmacologic management that included gabapentin, ketamine, or morphine. Mirror therapy, imagery, and virtual reality were associated with positive outcomes reported, but there were limitations (ie, small sample size) reported in these studies. Larger controlled studies are indicated.[10] Ferraro et al[11] published consensus recommendations that included the following: the use of morphine, gabapentin, or ketamine for a short-term analgesic effect. Nonpharmacologic treatments that could be considered include mirror therapy, mental imagery, phantom limb exercises, progressive muscle relaxation, and noninvasive brain stimulation.

## Exercises, Balance, and Gait Training

It is important to initiate ROM exercises for the residual limb (in all planes/directions) and strengthening of both lower extremities as soon as possible after surgery. Full hip extension and adduction ROM is important for normalizing gait for a person with a TFA; full hip and knee ROM (especially into extension) is important for normalizing gait for a person with a TTA.

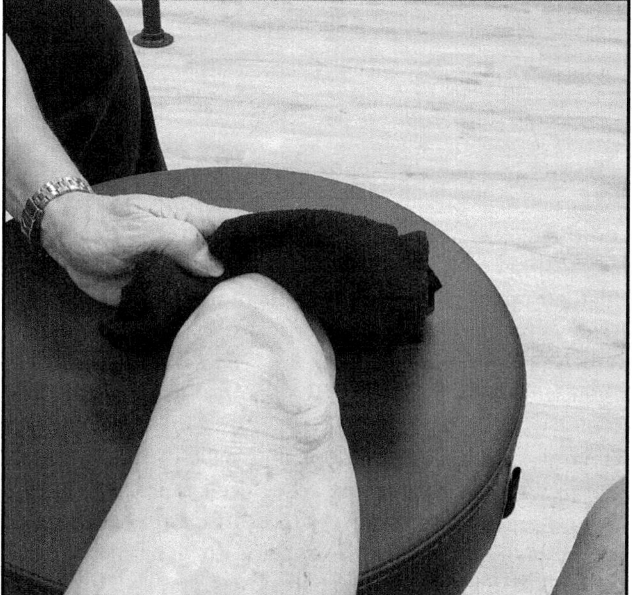

**Figure 17-8.** Desensitization of a residual limb with fabric.

Isometric exercises can begin day 1 postoperatively in medically stable patients. Residual limb hip extensor and abductor strengthening is progressed for eventual prosthetic training. People with TTAs will progressively strengthen the quadriceps and hamstrings in the residual limb to control the lower extremity (and prosthesis) during gait. Strengthening the residual limb lower extremity muscles (ie, modified bridging) is necessary for balance during the later phases of rehabilitation. Box 17-1 provides the list of priority exercises that should be included in an HEP early in the rehabilitation process for patients with TTAs or TFAs. Patients who are a higher level (more functional/independent) will benefit from the inclusion of

> **Box 17-1**
>
> **Minimum Exercises for Inclusion in Home Exercise Program**
>
> **Persons With a TTA**
>
> - Quadriceps sets and gluteal sets
> - Short-arc quadriceps
> - Long-arc quadriceps
> - Hip extension prone
> - Hip abduction
> - Prone lying
>
> **Persons With a TFA**
>
> - Gluteal sets
> - Hip extension prone
> - Hip abduction
> - Modified bridge
> - Prone lying

additional exercises. As each patient progresses in abilities and healing, additional exercises can be added to the HEP. Bilateral upper extremity strengthening, especially for the triceps brachii, is necessary for transfers and gait with an assistive device.

Patients with unilateral TTAs do not usually have difficulty with unsupported sitting. Patients with unilateral TFAs or bilateral amputations may have difficulty maintaining unsupported sitting. They need to learn to find a new center of mass because it has shifted after the loss of the limb(s). Progressing from static to dynamic balance training activities helps the patient to improve sitting balance and to weight shift and complete transfers.

During this phase, patients with lower extremity amputations who have impaired balance or endurance may use a walker for ambulation. Crutch training (using a 3-point gait pattern) is appropriate for patients with good balance, strength, endurance, and coordination. Ideally, patients will be ambulatory for short distances (ie, for toileting and walking from bed to chair) before being discharged from the acute care setting.

## Preprosthetic Training Phase

During the preprosthetic phase of rehabilitation, physical therapy interventions focus on increasing ROM, strength, and muscular and aerobic endurance and educating the patient about effective energy conservation techniques. Treatment goals include independence with residual limb care, avoiding contractures, performing self-care activities safely (either from the wheelchair or single-limb standing/walking without prosthesis), and increasing mobility to improve functional independence (ie, bed mobility and transfers). The patient typically continues with the exercises that were initiated in the preprosthetic training phase (Table 17-5) through the final phases of rehabilitation. The physical therapist assistant advances the therapy program based on patient presentation.

### *Standing Balance and Weight Bearing*

For many patients with a lower extremity amputation, a long-term goal is to ambulate with a prosthesis. The ability to walk safely and efficiently is dependent on both the patient's ability to bear weight into the residual limb and the patient's standing balance. Early training includes weight bearing through the residual limb and balance training tasks on the intact limb (in single-limb stance). Patients are taught to get up off the floor without the prosthesis. (There are a number of variations to the technique to get up from the floor; one option is depicted in Figure 17-9.) Functional activities that increase the patient's independence and confidence can be included in the treatment.

The initiation of weight bearing into the residual limb can be achieved in a sitting position and then gradually progressed into more challenging postures as the patient's tolerance for weight-bearing increases. When seated with the residual limb in the dependent position, the patient can wrap a towel so that the middle portion of the towel is under the residual limb (the patient holds both ends of the towel). The patient can gently push down into the towel; the clinician will guard as needed. Kneeling on a pillow positioned on the mat table and then weight shifting into the residual limb is a way to increase weight bearing into the lower extremity. Progress by placing a chair in the parallel bars with a pillow on it; the patient can stand next to the chair with the residual limb kneeling/supported on the pillow. As weight bearing onto the residual limb is progressed, the clinician monitors the patient's response and the integrity of the residual limb before, during, and after the intervention.

The patient's perception of their balance ability has a direct impact on their fear of falling and balance performance.[14] The clinician includes standing balance exercises on the intact limb early in this phase. The patient can begin with standing in the parallel bars with bilateral upper extremity support and progress to single-arm support and then standing on the intact limb unsupported (Figure 17-10A). Once the patient is stable and able to maintain standing on the intact limb for at least 30 seconds, progressions can include single-leg standing adding horizontal and vertical head movements and/or adding upper extremity motions (ie, AROM or throwing a ball) and/or standing on a foam mat (compliant surface) to improve the patient's balance performance and confidence (Figures 17-10B and 17-10C).

**Table 17-5**

**List of Recommended Therapeutic Exercises in the Preprosthetic Phase**

Begin with AROM; progress from gravity minimized to against gravity to progressive resistive exercises as tolerated (monitor patient and limb response).

See Chapter 13 for descriptions and photos of the varied exercises.

| Transtibial Amputation | Transfemoral Amputation |
|---|---|
| Hip flexor stretch: Start lying prone and then progress to prone on elbows and possibly prone press-up with straight elbows as tolerated/appropriate[a] | Hip flexor stretch: Start lying prone and then progress to prone on elbows and possibly prone press-up with straight elbows as tolerated/appropriate[a] |
| Passive stretch into knee extension[a] | Modified bridging[a] |
| Quadriceps sets[a] | Hip abduction[a] |
| Hamstring sets | Hip extensiona (start in side-lying position and progress to prone as tolerated) |
| Short-arc quadriceps[a] | Hip flexion |
| Long-arc quadriceps[a] | Hip adduction |
| Modified bridging[a] | Modified Thomas test stretch[a] |
| Straight leg raise[a] | Upper extremity strengthening[b] |
| Hip abduction[a] | Seated balance exercise[b] |
| Hip extension[a] (start in side-lying position and progress to prone as tolerated) | Standing tolerance and standing balance exercise[b] |
| Thomas test stretch | |
| Hip flexion | |
| Knee flexion | |
| Hip adduction | |
| Upper extremity strengthening[b] | |
| Seated balance exercise[b] | |
| Standing tolerance and standing balance exercise[b] | |

[a]Indicates priority exercise for this diagnosis.
[b]Include if indicated based on patient current status, goals, and presence of comorbidities

## Prosthetic Training Phase

The strongest predictors of return to effective functional mobility and ambulation with a prosthesis include amputation level, age, physical fitness, and the presence of fewer comorbidities. For patients who are prosthetic device candidates, patient education on prosthesis fit (and management) and prosthetic training are important parts of the rehabilitation process. The time from amputation to prosthesis fitting and prosthesis use (household vs community-level ambulation) will vary depending on the patient's overall health and whether the reason for the amputation was dysvascular or due to trauma. The time from amputation to prosthesis fitting is dependent on limb healing, which tends to be longer for persons with dysvascular causes for the amputation. If a patient is not a good candidate or cannot tolerate the increased energy demands of ambulating with a prosthesis, therapy goals will focus on maximizing the patient's independence at a wheelchair level of function.

A normal gait pattern will minimize deviations, reduce the risk of secondary impairments, conserve energy, and improve overall function. Gait deviations are common during prosthetic ambulation, and they can be due to inadequate gait training, poor habits, improper prosthesis fit or alignment, pain, and/or compensation for an impairment (ie, decreased strength or decreased ROM). Gait deviations that result from weakness or decreased ROM can be addressed by strengthening the weak muscles or stretching the muscles causing the restriction. Gait deviations can result from issues with the prosthesis. An in-depth review of prosthetic causes for gait deviations is outside the scope of this text; the reader is referred to the Suggested Resources provided at the end of the chapter.

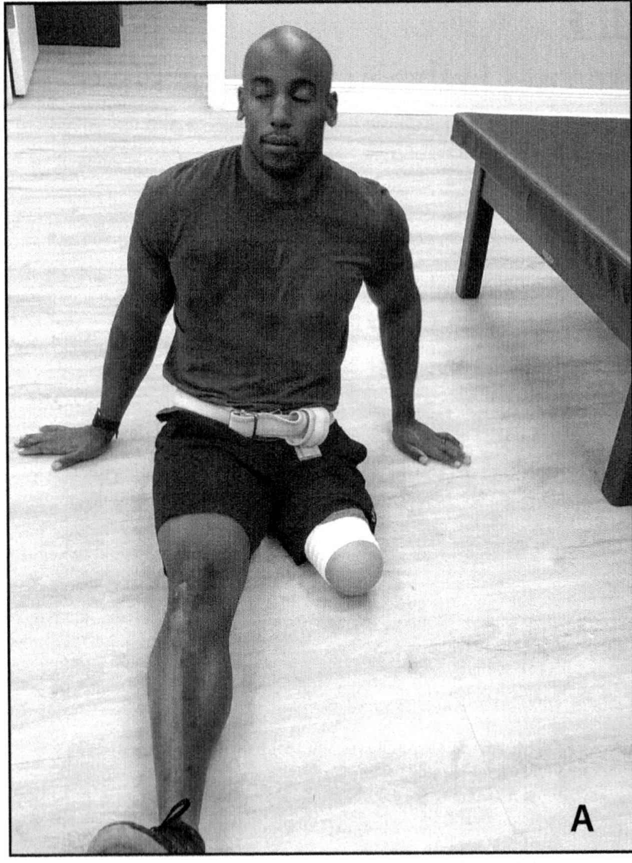


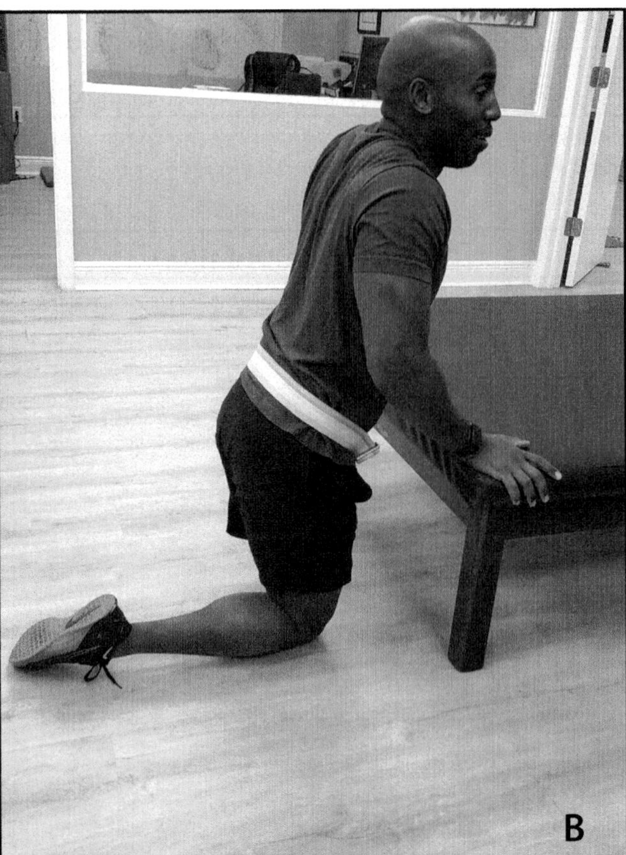


**Figure 17-9.** Floor-to-stand transfer without a prosthesis. (A) Beginning position: The patient is sitting on the floor and has "scooted" close to a sturdy mat (or chair). (B) The patient faces the mat, and transitions into a kneeling position. (C) The patient initiates a push-up from the mat, allowing him to shift the right foot underneath him, and he proceeds to standing.

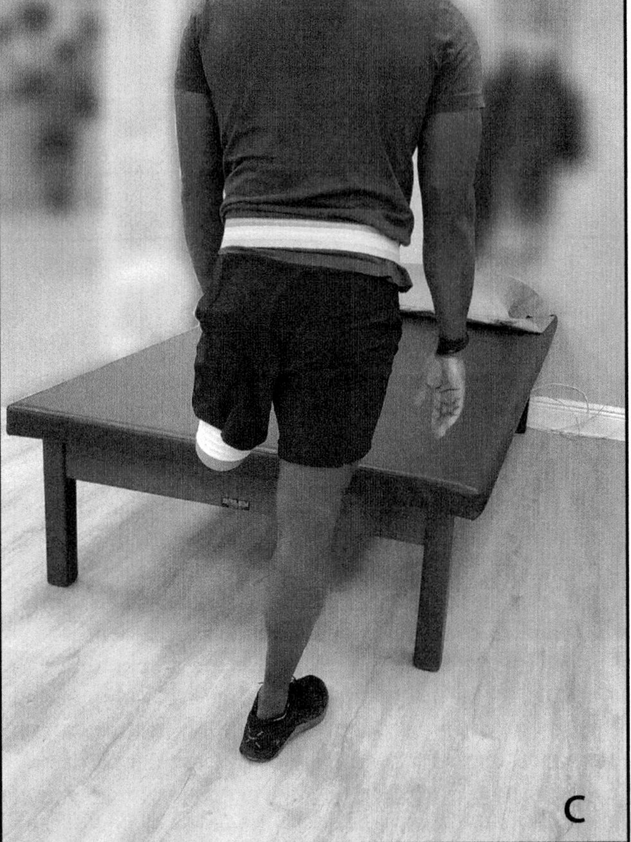

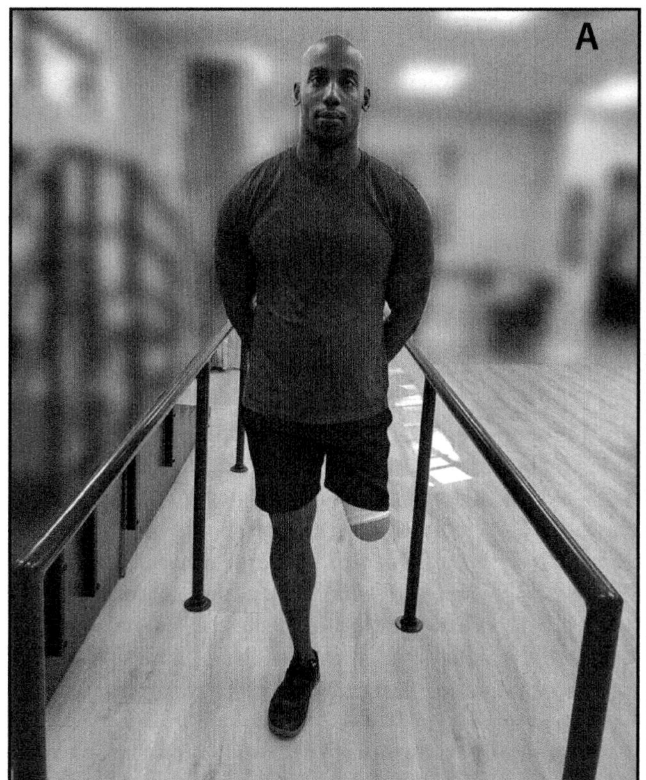


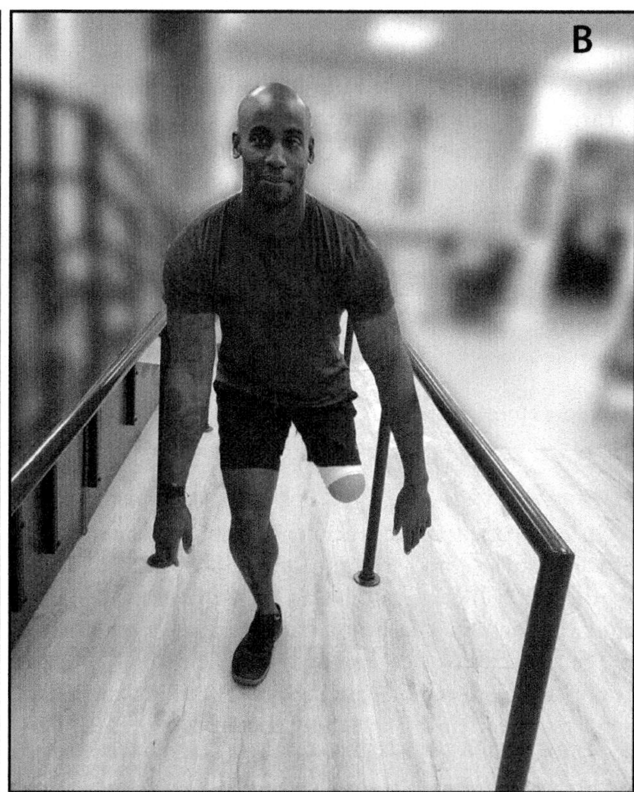


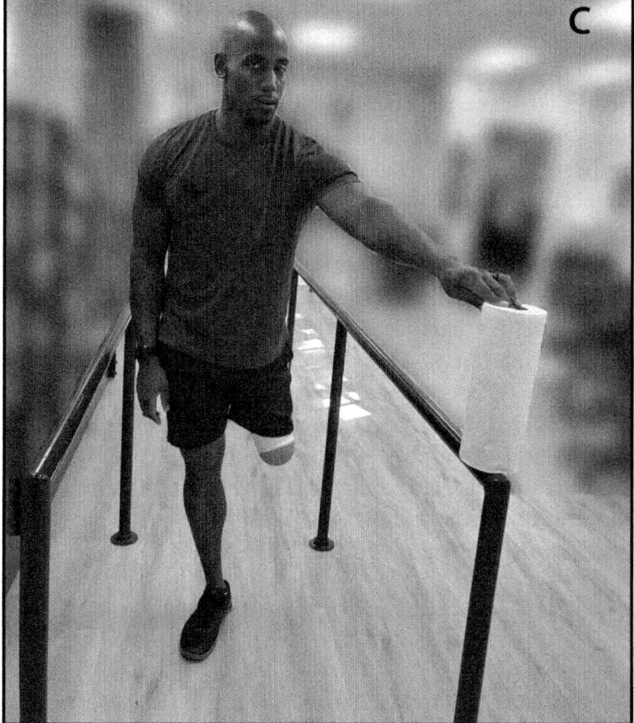


**Figure 17-10.** (A) Single-limb stance without a prosthesis. (B) Single-limb stance without a prosthesis, dynamic balance (mini-squat). (C) Single-limb stance without a prosthesis, dynamic balance (reaching).

Gait deviations increase the risk of future pain and pathology due to altered biomechanics. Focusing on early balance and proprioception training with the prosthesis, controlling the center of mass during weight shifting in all directions (Figure 17-11), and focused muscle strengthening can prevent or minimize future gait deviations. Table 17-6 and Figures 17-12 and 17-13 include interventions that can be used for balance and prosthetic gait training. The clinician uses appropriate guarding, and the patient uses upper extremity support as necessary (Figure 17-14). Consider starting in the parallel bars and then decrease both guarding and the patient's use of the upper extremities for balance as the patient improves. Not all patients will be able to complete all progressions. Interventions and progressions are selected based on the therapy goals and the patient's functional status.

The assistant should include interventions that specifically address the patient's impairments. Gait with a prosthesis may result in limited trunk rotation, pelvic rotation, and arm swing. To normalize the patient's gait using a prosthesis, the clinician may need to facilitate these motions by using rhythmic initiation and the resisted progression techniques illustrated in Figures 17-15 and 17-16.

### Clinical Tip

Providing cues that direct the patient's attention to proprioceptive feedback of the residual limb in the prosthesis improves functional outcomes.

Once a patient is independent with ambulation, the clinician can use higher-level training activities to facilitate the most efficient gait pattern. The use of a facilitated arm swing activity can help a patient improve arm swing and gait efficiency (see Figure 17-13). Clinicians include progressively more challenging interventions. Step-tap exercises for each lower extremity (Figure 17-17), unilateral weight bearing through the prosthetic limb (Figure 17-18), and high-level balance training tasks (Figure 17-19) can be initiated if indicated by the patient's status and the treatment goals. Floor transfer training should be included for most patients; 2 variations of floor-to-stand transfers are shown in Figures 17-20 and 17-21.

### Clinical Tip

Safety first! All prosthesis training interventions must be paired with a gradually progressed wearing schedule, skin inspection, and monitoring. Advanced training and exercising at increased intensity will affect prosthesis fit. Regular follow-up with the prosthetist is indicated during training.

## Functional Assessment Tools

Regular assessment of patient function allows the physical therapist assistant to quantify current functional level, measure improvement over time, provide the documentation/support for therapy services, and supply justification for prosthesis use. The Berg Balance Scale is a valid and reliable clinical instrument for assessing balance in individuals with a lower limb amputation, although it may not be useful as a predictor of fall risk with this population.[15] The L Test is a 20-meter test of basic mobility skills that includes 2 transfers and 4 turns used to assess a patient's fall risk. It has demonstrated good reliability and validity for this population.[16] The Timed Up and Go Test is a useful assessment tool for persons with amputations. In persons with a TTA, Timed Up and Go scores of 19 seconds or more are associated with an increased risk of having multiple falls with sensitivity of 85% and specificity of 74%.[17] The 6-Minute Walk Test has been shown to correlate well with other postamputation outcome tools. The 2-Minute Walk Test was highly predictive of the 6-Minute Walk Test distance, indicating that this tool may be appropriate to use with this population as well.[18]

The **amputee mobility predictor** is an outcome measure that assesses mobility and functional capability for people with unilateral lower limb amputations. It is a reliable and valid tool to assess functional mobility for amputees with or without a prosthesis. The amputee mobility predictor scores correlate to prosthetic K-levels.[19] K-levels are a rating system used to classify an amputee's activity level and indicate a person's rehabilitation potential.[20] The K-level is determined using the Medicare Functional Classification Level, and it is a primary factor in the decision on what prosthetic device is appropriate as well as the likelihood of insurance to pay for a specific prosthetic device.[20]

A patient's balance confidence can also provide useful information to the clinician. The Activities-Specific Balance Confidence Scale has been shown to be reliable and valid for use for persons with amputations.[21] Balance confidence, the ability to retrieve objects from the floor, turning to look behind, and placing an alternate foot on a stool were the most indicative skills for using a prosthesis successfully during mobility.[14]

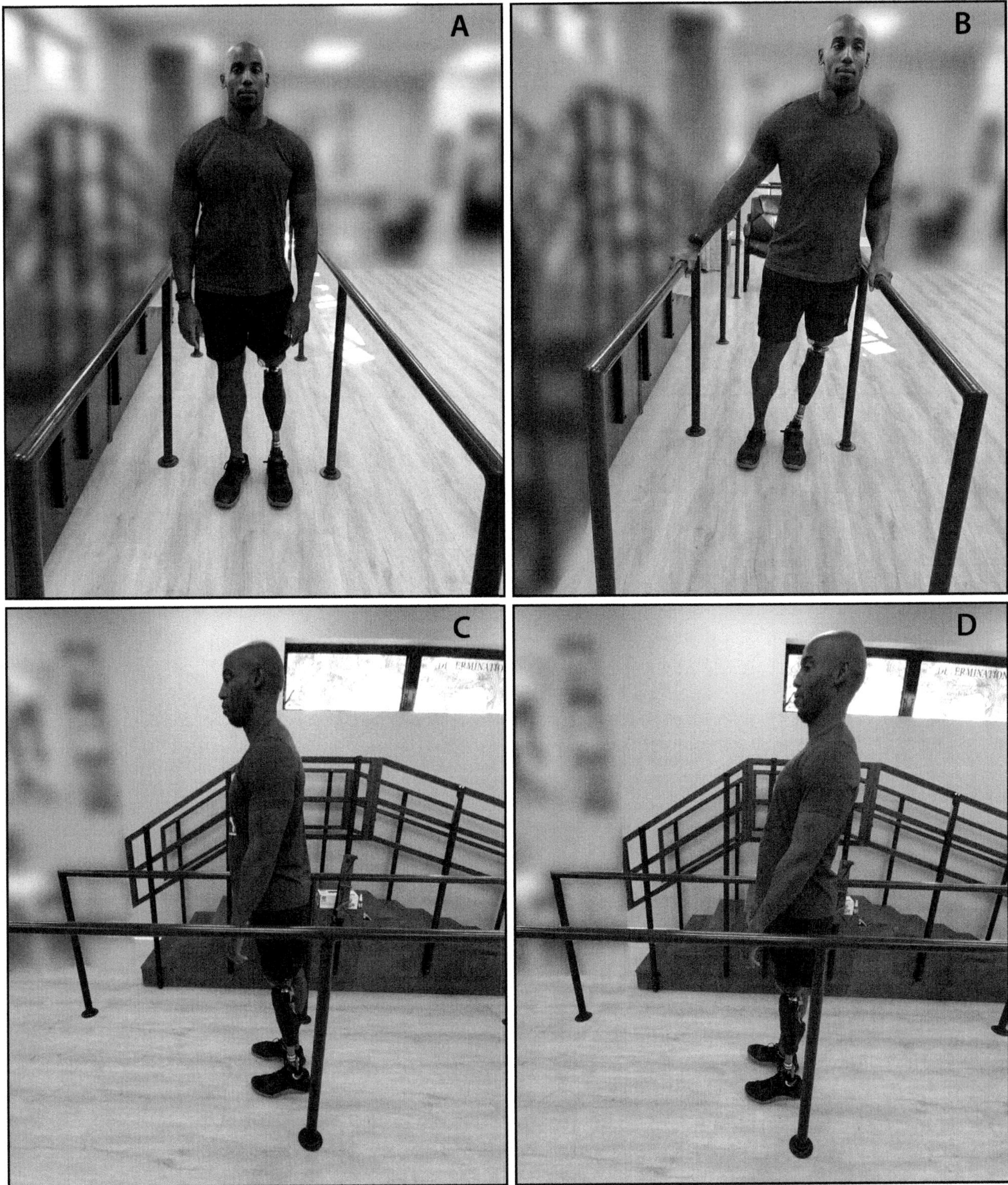

**Figure 17-11.** (A) Static stance with a prosthesis, unsupported. (B) Weight shift onto the prosthetic limb. (C) Anterior weight shift in stance with the prosthetic limb. (D) Posterior weight shift in stance with the prosthetic limb.

**Table 17-6**

**Balance and Gait Training Interventions With a Lower Extremity Prosthesis**

| Training Area of Focus | Intervention Suggestions |
|---|---|
| Improve proprioception in residual limb | • Using a reflex hammer, gently tap on the heel, then the big toe, and then the fifth toe on the unaffected limb. Have the patient verbalize location of the sensation on intact limb.<br>• Repeat on the prosthetic foot. Using a reflex hammer, gently tap on the heel, then the big toe, and then the fifth toe on the prosthetic foot. Have the patient push firmly into the socket and feel the area of vibration with each area that the clinician taps on. When tapping on the prosthesis, provide verbal cues to focus the patient's attention on the feedback/vibrations that the residual limb is feeling within the prosthetic socket. |
| Improve ability to balance over prosthetic limb | • Standing weight shifts in all directions (focus on weight shift over the prosthetic limb). Have the patient verbalize where they feel pressure/sensation in the prosthesis as they move in each direction.<br>*Consider using a mirror to increase feedback to patient.* |
| Improve single-limb stance and weight bearing through prosthesis | • Step taps with the intact limb. Start with a small step height, and ask the patient to gently tap the intact limb onto the step (weight bearing on the prosthetic limb). Increase the height of the step as the patient improves.<br>• Complete ball rolling with the sound limb. While weight bearing on the prosthetic limb, place a small ball under the intact limb and have the patient gently roll the ball under the foot. Start with a very small ball; increase to larger balls and then a basketball as the patient improves.<br>• Complete standing hip exercises with the unaffected limb while standing on the prosthetic limb. Complete "hip 4-ways" (hip flexion, extension, abduction, and adduction with the knee extended) with the intact limb. Progress to using resistance bands on the intact limb. *Emphasize hip abduction and extension.*<br>• Single-limb stance on the residual limb. Progress from bilateral to unilateral upper extremity support, to 2 fingers, to unsupported. *Time single-leg stance results weekly; this can serve as an indicator of compliance with HEP and patient progress.*<br>• Single-leg stance while completing upper extremity proprioceptive neuromuscular facilitation chop and lift patterns. Progress by using resistance bands. (Note: This is an advanced skill and not appropriate for all patients.)<br>*Watch for compensated (trunk lean) or uncompensated (pelvic drop) Trendelenburg during these activities.* |
| Restore pelvic motion during gait | • Stand with the prosthetic limb posterior and weight shift forward and back. Use rhythmic initiation at the pelvis (see Figure 17-12; progress active assisted ROM to AROM) and then resist the anterior/posterior motion as the patient steps forward and then back with that limb.<br>• Progress to resisted motion at the pelvis during gait. |
| Improve swing phase with the prosthesis during gait | • Step forward and back with the prosthetic limb (allow the knee to bend). *Use verbal/tactile cues to prevent hip hiking or circumduction.*<br>• Resisted walking at sternum facilitates hip extensors during terminal stance and helps to normalize swing phase.<br>*(continued)* |

**Table 17-6 (continued)**

**Balance and Gait Training Interventions With a Lower Extremity Prosthesis**

| Training Area of Focus | Intervention Suggestions |
|---|---|
| Improve trunk rotation and arm swing during ambulation | • Standing: Apply rhythmic stabilization (at the shoulders).<br>• Rhythmic initiation increases trunk rotation and facilitates arm swing in standing.<br>• Active trunk rotation standing to facilitate relaxed arm swings. Progress to walking.<br>• Standing in parallel bars, upper extremity proprioceptive neuromuscular facilitation chops/lifts. Progress by using resistance bands.<br>• Patient can use a cane or walking stick in each hand to promote arm swing. Advanced activity: Therapist ambulates holding onto canes behind the patient (see Figure 17-13). |
| Maximize participation in functional activities with the prosthesis | • Standing trunk flexion, extension, and lateral bending.<br>• Partial squats and lifting.<br>• Functional reach exercises at various angles.<br>• Ball toss (with one foot on step or standing on foam).<br>• Standing upper bike ergometer.<br>• Pick items up off floor.<br>• Side stepping, backward walking.<br>• Step-ups (lateral and forward).<br>• Gait training on stairs.<br>• Stepping over objects.<br>• Braiding.<br>• Getting up off of the floor.<br>• Ambulating on uneven surfaces. |

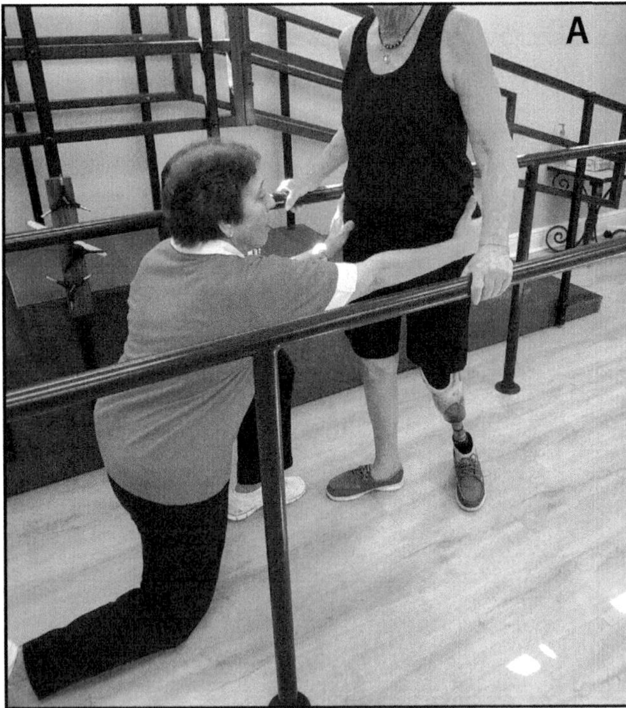


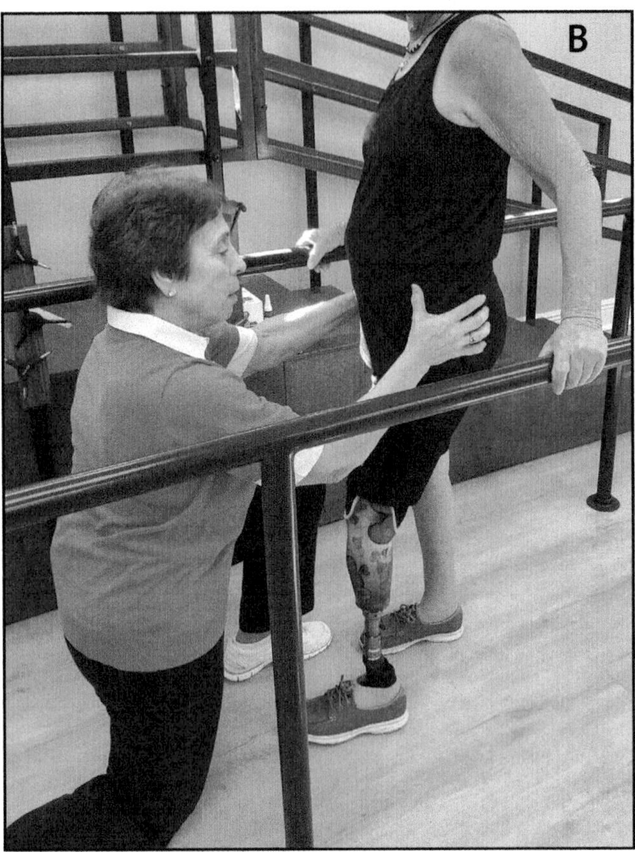


**Figure 17-12.** (A) Rhythmic initiation to facilitate pelvic rotation. Starting position. (B) Rhythmic initiation to facilitate pelvic rotation. The clinician facilitates anterior rotation of the pelvis as the patient steps forward with the prosthetic leg.

**Figure 17-13.** More advanced activity to facilitate arm swing during gait.

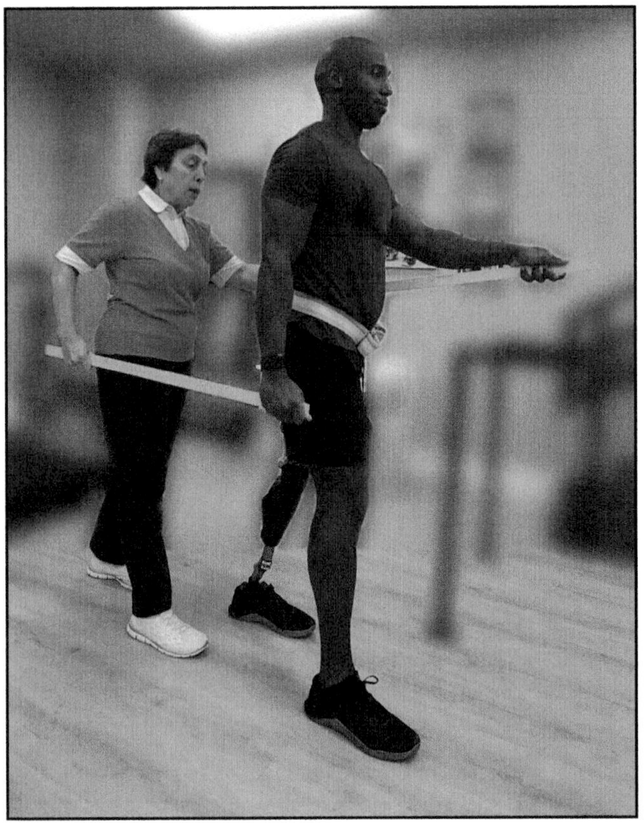

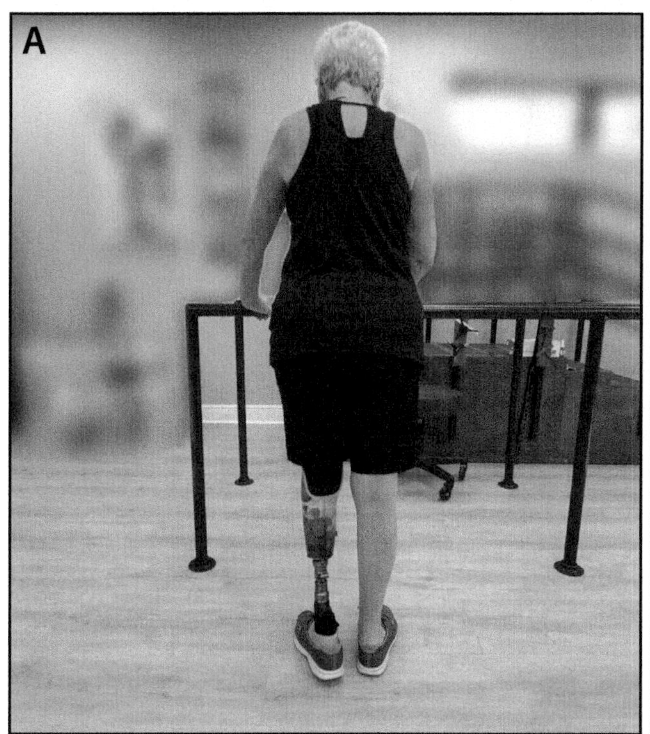


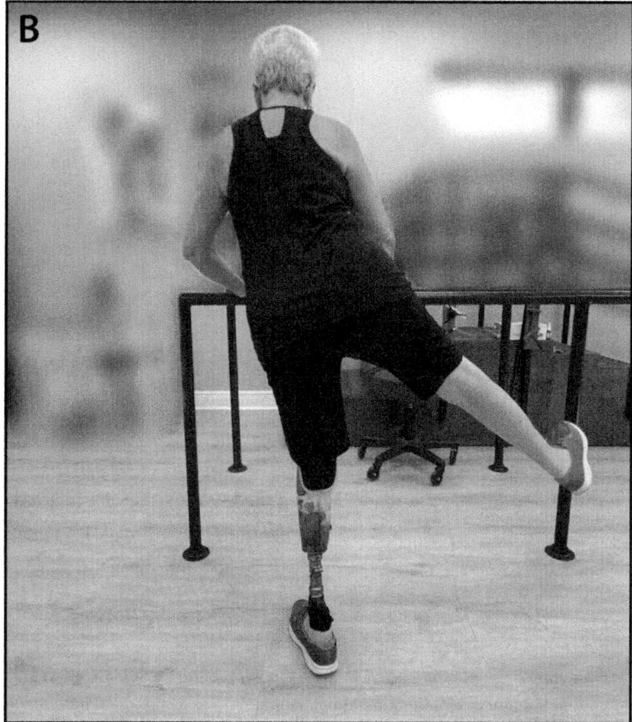


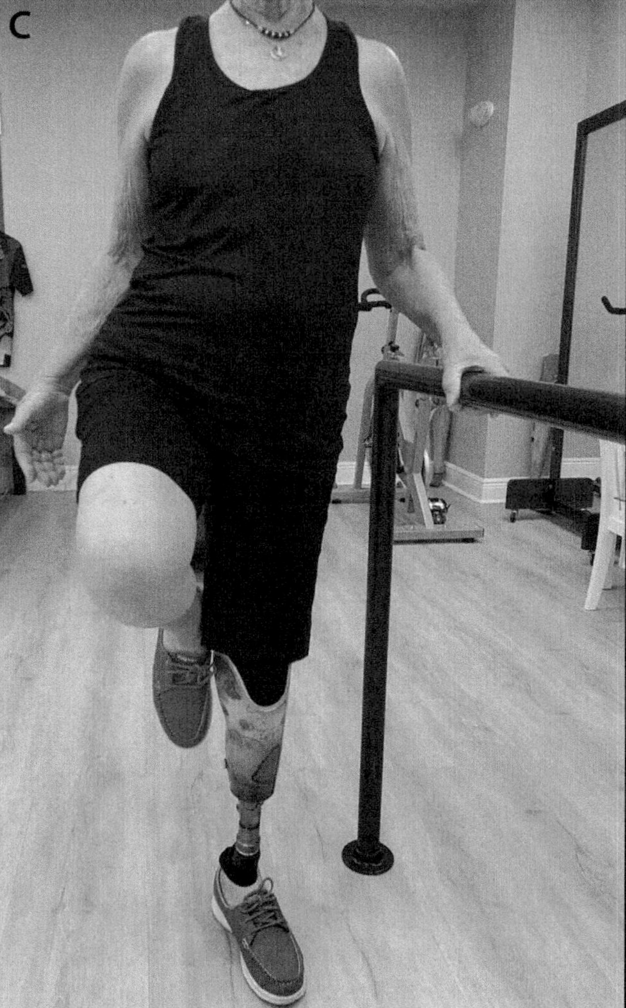


**Figure 17-14.** (A) Double-limb stance supported with the bilateral upper extremities. (B) Single-leg stance supported with the bilateral upper extremities. (C) Progress patient to single-leg stance supported with one upper extremity.

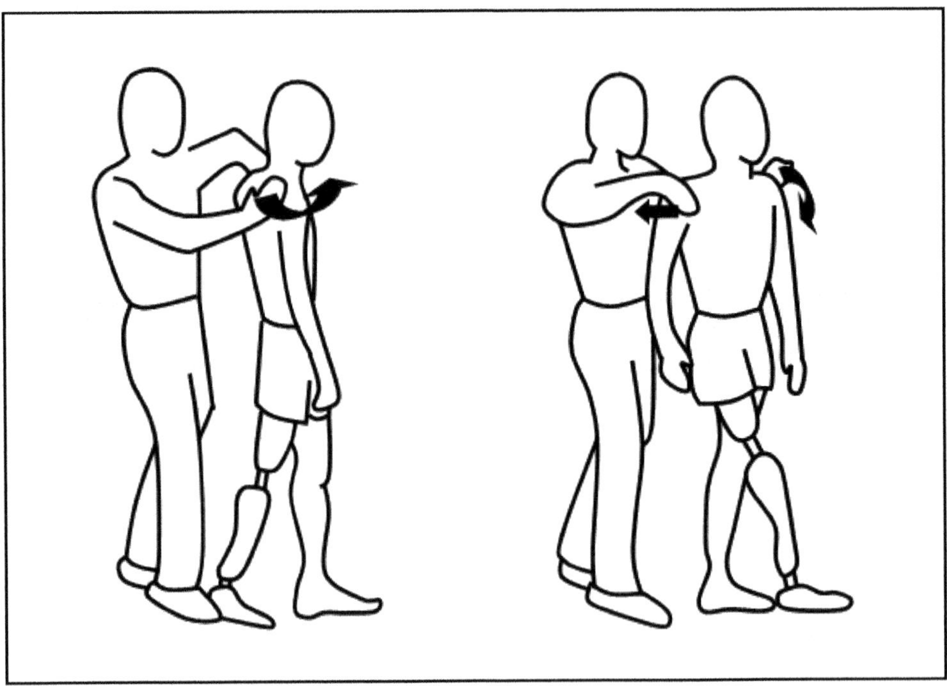

**Figure 17-15.** Rhythmic initiation at the shoulders will promote trunk rotation and arm swing. (Graphic created by John and Jimmy Kopack.)

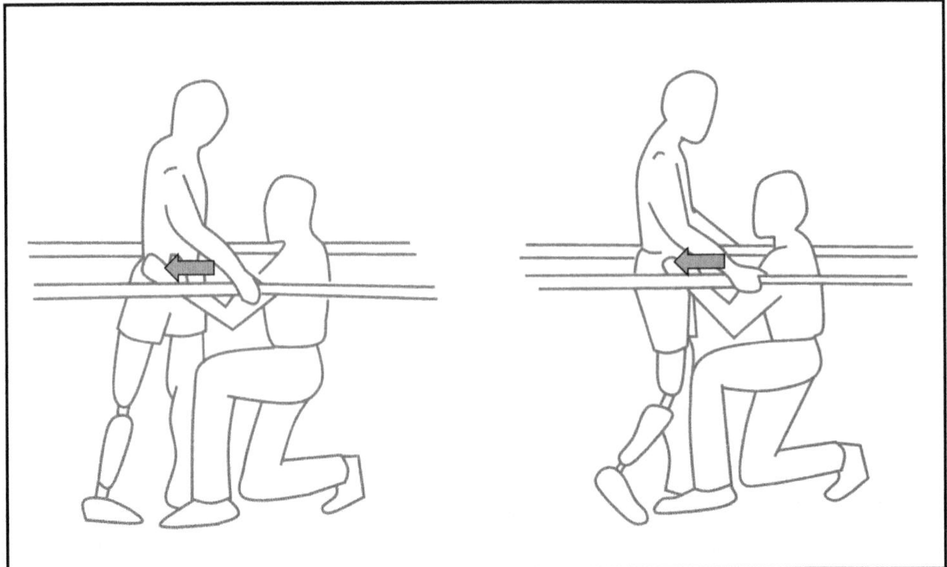

**Figure 17-16.** Resisted pelvic rotation with gait. (Graphic created by John and Jimmy Kopack.)

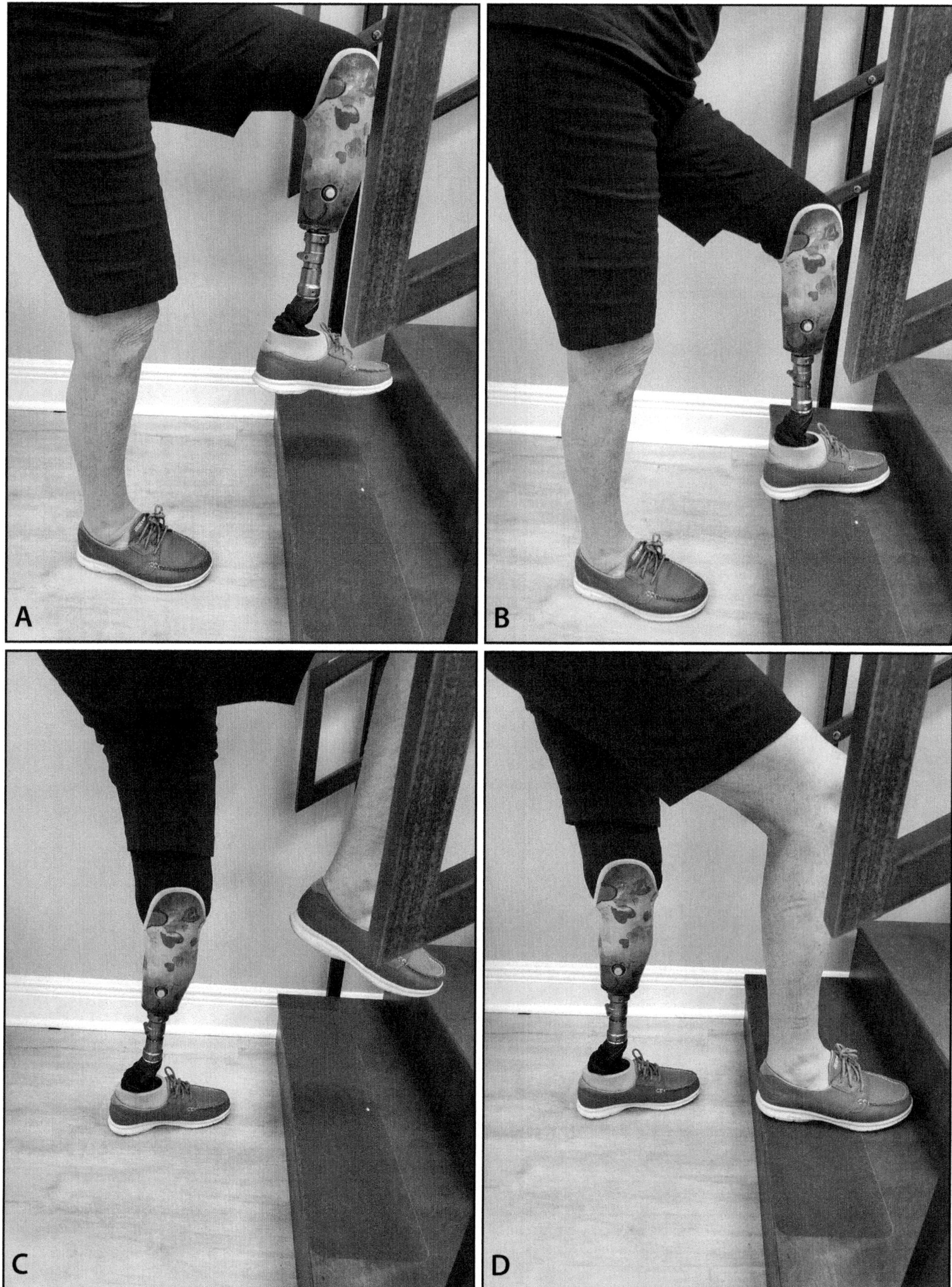


**Figure 17-17.** (A) Step tap, standing on the unaffected limb, initiation. (B) Step tap, standing on the unaffected limb, end position. (C) Step tap, standing on the prosthetic limb, initiation. (D) Step tap, standing on the prosthetic limb, end position.

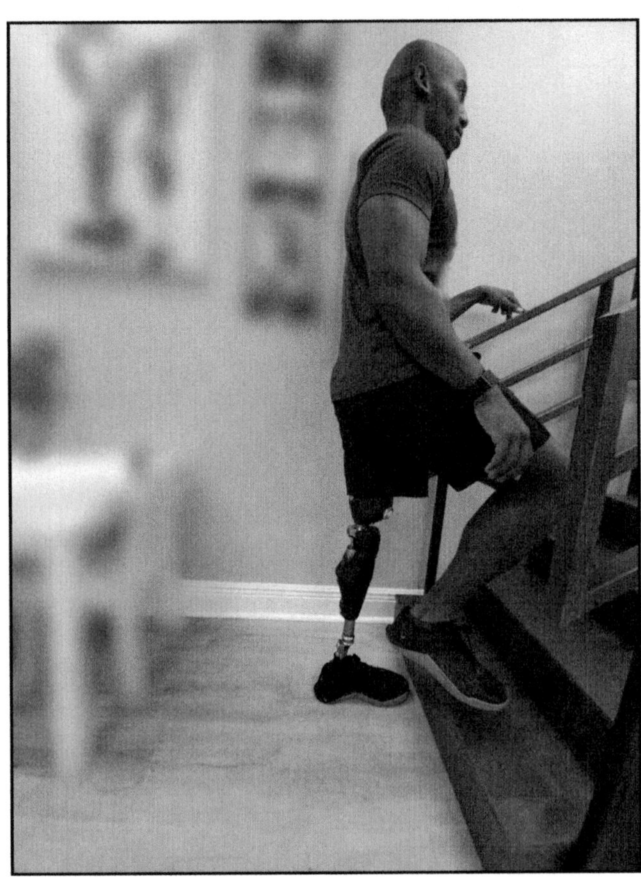

**Figure 17-18.** Unilateral weight bearing on the prosthetic limb.

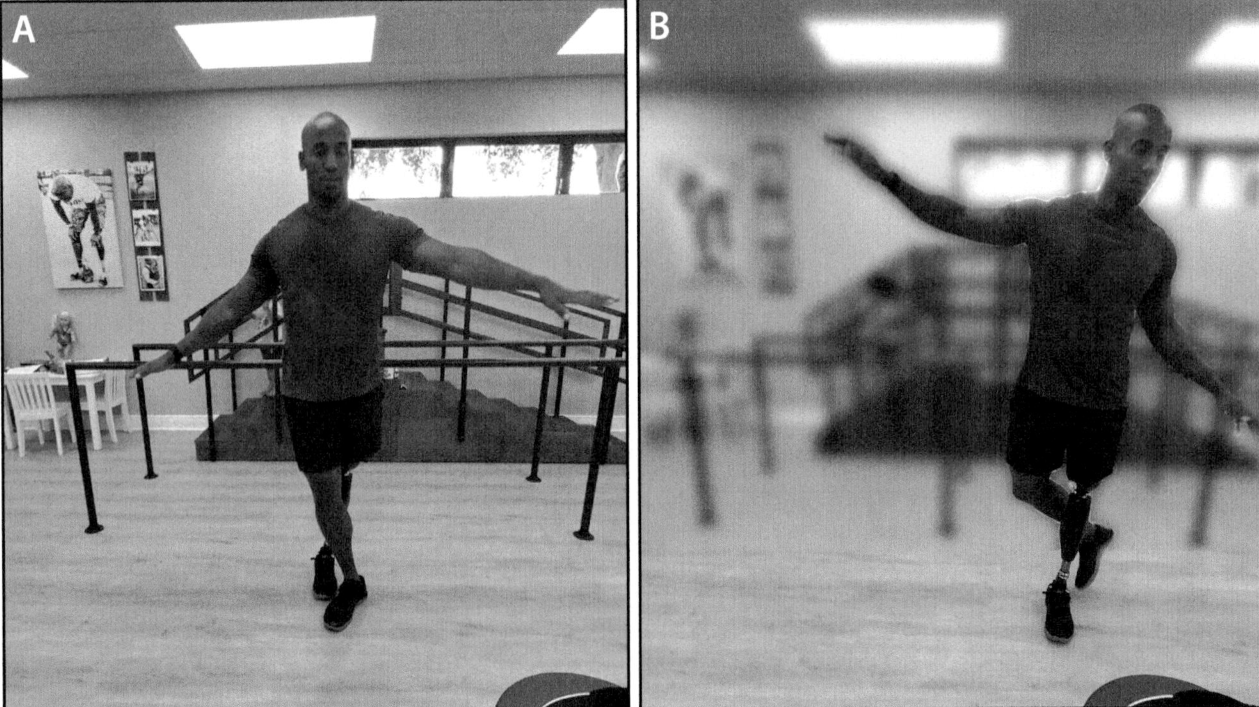

**Figure 17-19.** (A) High-level dynamic balance exercise. Lower extremity braiding exercise, start position. (B) High-level dynamic balance exercise. Lower extremity braiding exercise, transition 1. *(continued)*

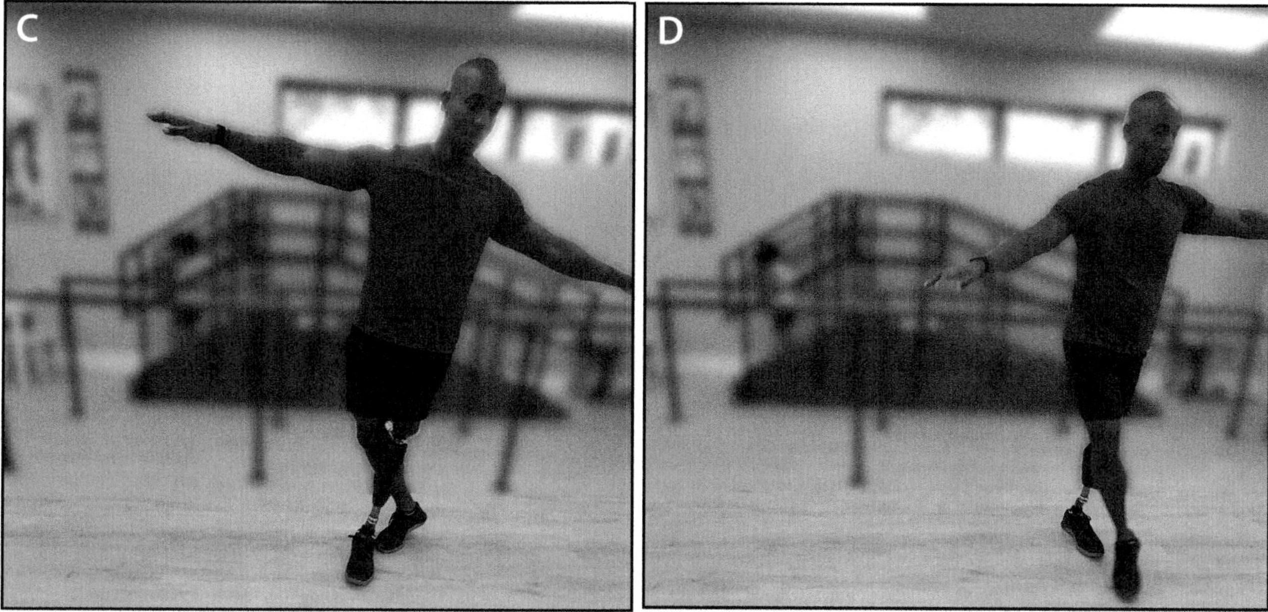

**Figure 17-19 (continued).** (C) High-level dynamic balance exercise. Lower extremity braiding exercise, transition 2. (D) High-level dynamic balance exercise. Lower extremity braiding exercise, end position.

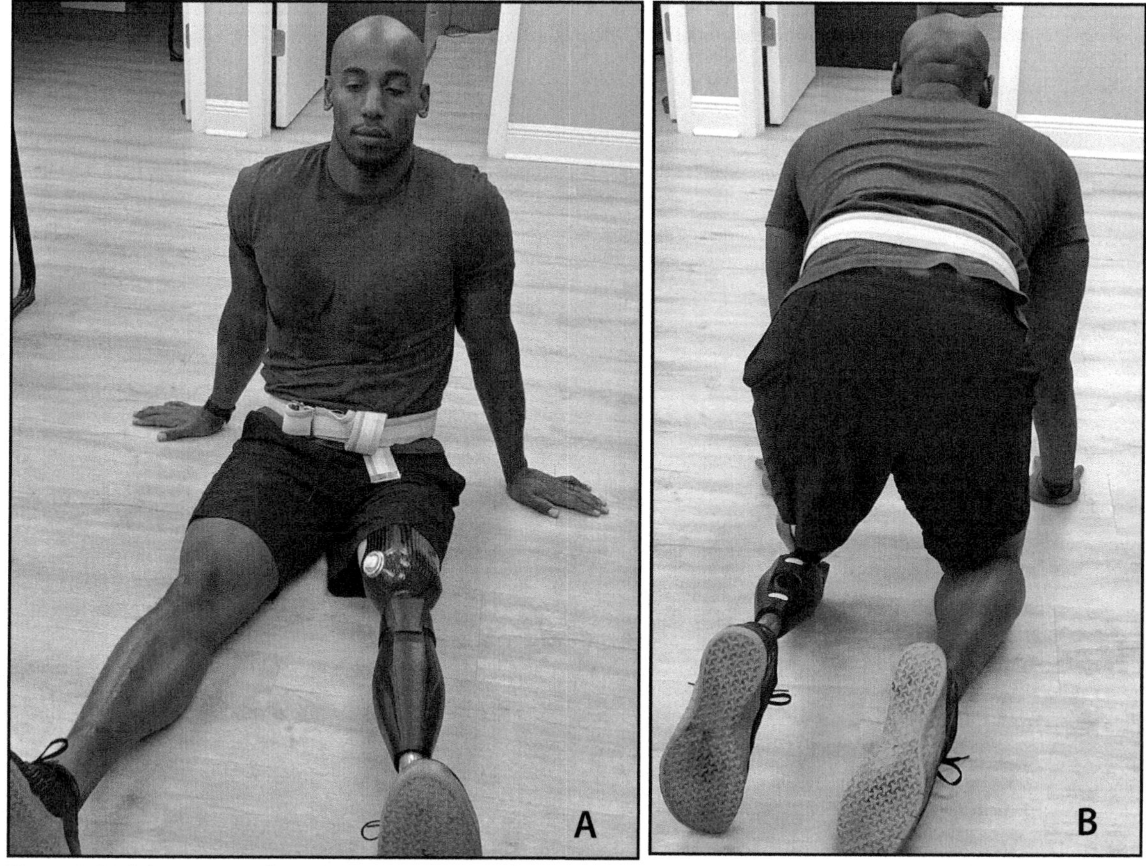

**Figure 17-20.** (A) A patient with a TFA prepares to get up off of the floor. (B) The patient moves to the quadruped position. *(continued)*

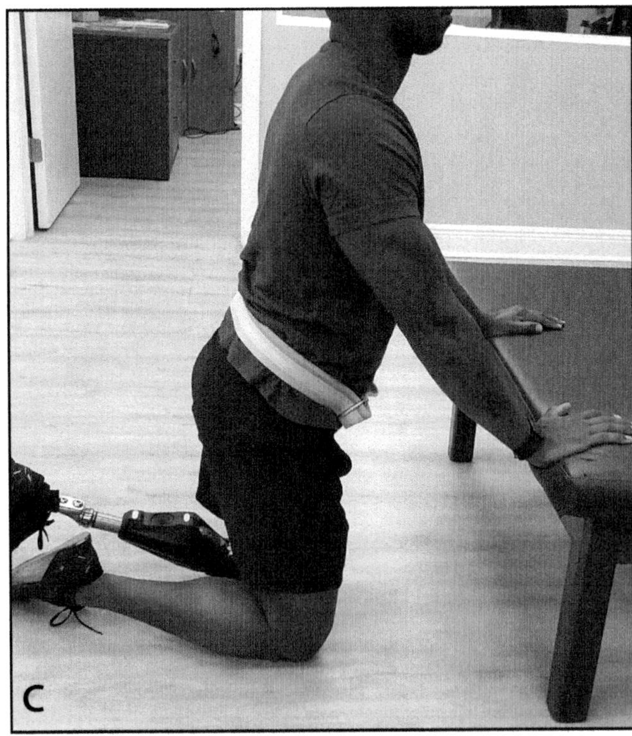


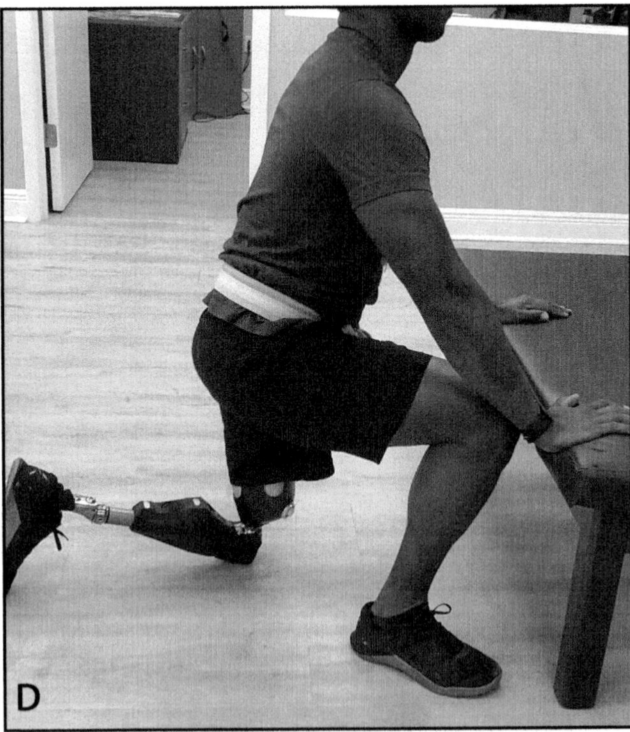


**Figure 17-20 (continued).** (C) The patient supports a positional shift with upper extremities. (D) The patient uses the sound leg to propel him to initiate standing. (E) The patient transitions to stand and maintains balance.

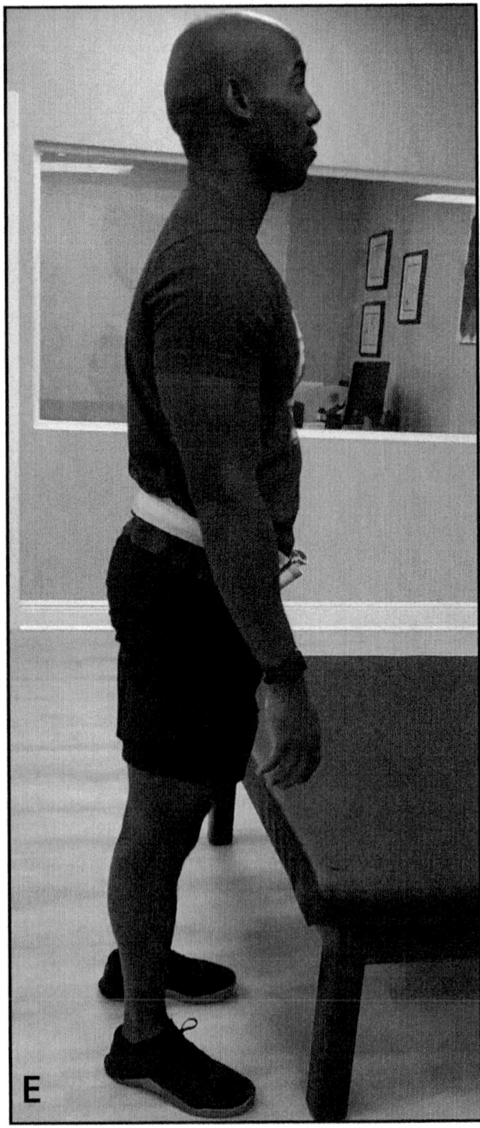

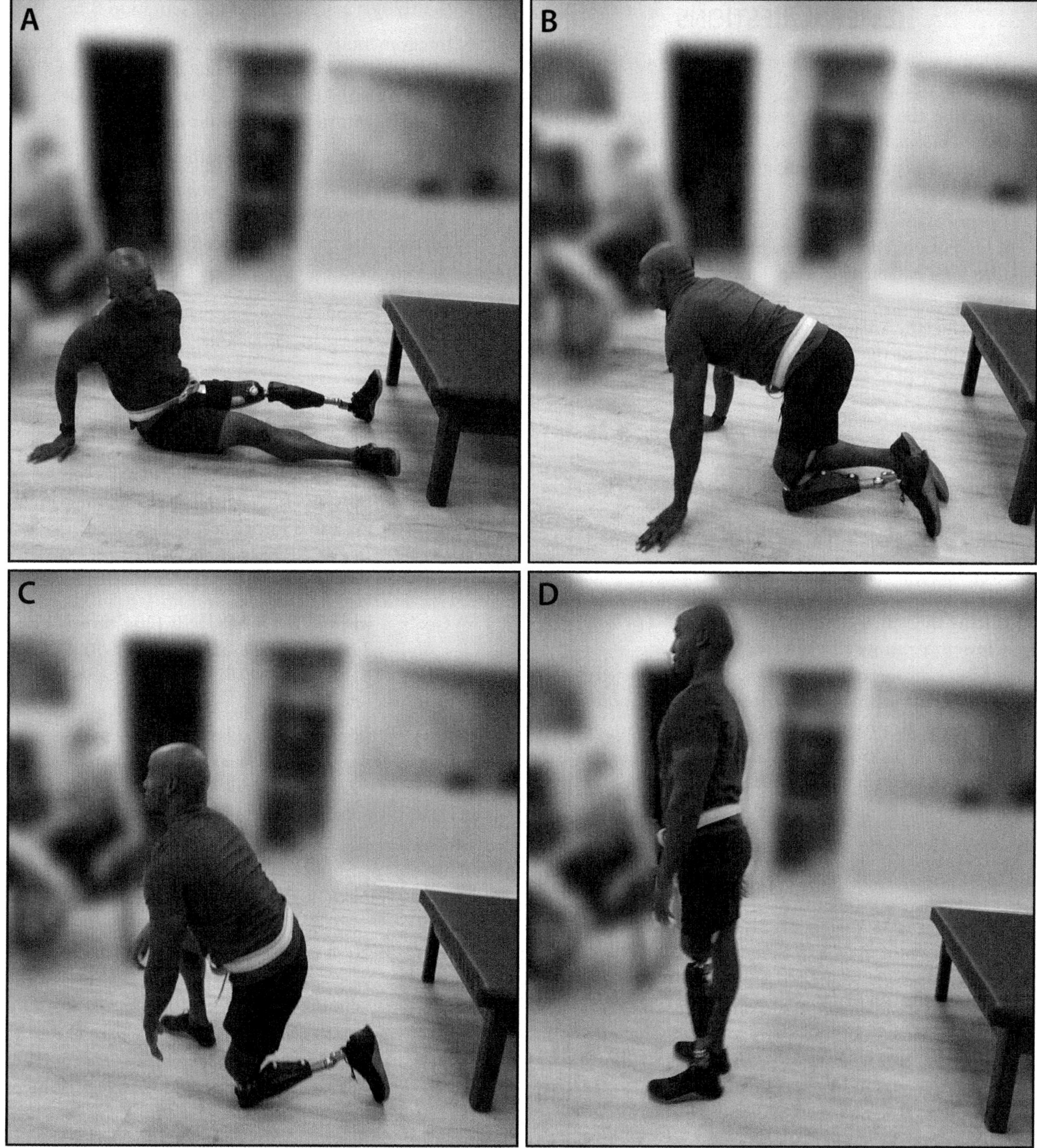


**Figure 17-21.** (A) Floor-to-stand transfer: Starting position. (B) Transition to quadruped. (C) Transition to half kneeling. (D) Transition to stand.

## Conclusion

Physical therapy is an important component of rehabilitation to maximize a patient's functional abilities after lower extremity amputation. The assistant will apply knowledge of the optimal exercises, residual limb care, and patient positioning when creating an individualized program to assist the patient in returning to the highest possible level of function. The assistant will guide the patient through a preprosthetic phase of treatment that prepares the patient and the limb for prosthetic wearing. The assistant will implement a training program that progressively challenges the patient to improve mobility once the patient is fitted with the prosthesis.

## Review Questions

1. What are contraindications to exercise after a lower extremity amputation?
2. Describe the treatment goals and priority treatment interventions that would be included in the rehabilitation for a person after amputation in the postsurgical phase.
3. Describe the treatment goals and priority treatment interventions that would be included in the rehabilitation for a person after amputation in the preprosthetic phase.
4. Describe the treatment goals and priority treatment interventions that would be included in the rehabilitation for a person after amputation in the prosthetic phase.
5. Which exercises are most appropriate for a person after a TFA?
6. Which exercises are most appropriate for a person after a TTA?
7. What patient education should be provided, specific to limb positioning, after a lower extremity amputation?
8. What should the physical therapist assistant monitor during therapy treatment when treating a person with a lower extremity amputation?
9. Outline an appropriate balance exercise progression for a person with a lower extremity amputation in the preprosthetic phase of rehabilitation.
10. Outline an appropriate balance exercise progression for a person with a lower extremity amputation in the prosthetic phase of rehabilitation.

## Case Study

The patient is 48-year-old 2 days status post right TTA as a result of a motor vehicle accident.

- SH: Lives with spouse and 2 children (13 and 15). Bedroom and bathroom are on the second floor, half bath on first floor. No steps to enter. The patient is employed as a computer programmer. Before onset, the patient was independent with all ADLs and instrumental ADLs, was a softball coach, and worked out regularly.
- O: Height: 5 ft 10 inches; weight: 165 pounds
    - Heart rate: 88 beats/minute
    - Blood pressure: 132/75 mm Hg
    - Respiratory rate: 14 breaths/minute
    - Neurologic assessment: Intact sensation B LE
    - Integumentary: Suture line/incision right LE clean with minimal clear exudate. Dressing and limb wrap intact. Left LE ABI 1.0 B UE AROM and strength within functional limits (WFL)
    - Left LE AROM WFL, strength 5/5 throughout
    - Right LE hip AROM WFL, strength 4/5. Right knee AROM 10 to 95 degrees, passive ROM 5 to 100 degrees, strength not assessed due to pain
    - Bed Mob Mod A due to pain
    - Transfers mod A
    - Balance: Sitting balance: Normal. Standing balance: S: G, D: P
    - Ambulation with B axillary crutches 150' with min A
    - Up/down 4 steps with mod A and B rails
    - WC propulsion I; I with brake management, requires VC and S for leg rest management.
- A: Decreased functional mobility and independence s/p TTA. Excellent rehab potential.
    - Goals: 1 week: R knee AROM 0-120 degrees, I Bed mobility, I transfers, I ambulation 250' with AD, up/down 12 steps with AD I; I with HEP, positioning and residual limb care
- P: Physical therapy twice a day to include patient education, therapy exercises, residual limb care, balance exercises, functional mobility training, modalities as needed, progress as appropriate, and initiate discharge planning

1. What are the implications of an ABI of 1.0?
2. Which exercises are the priority exercises for this patient?
3. Which education is most appropriate to provide to this patient?
4. What data should the physical therapist assistant collect?
5. Which functional assessment tool is most appropriate?
6. Create an appropriate 60-minute treatment plan for this patient.

## Suggested Resources

Gailey, RS, Clark CR. Physical therapy management of adult lower limb amputees (chapter 23). In: Bowker HK, Michael JW, eds. Atlas of Limb Prosthetics: Surgical, Prosthetic, and Rehabilitation Principles. American Academy of Orthopedic Surgeons; 1992. Accessed February 6, 2023. http://www.oandplibrary.org/alp/chap23-01.asp

International Committee for the Red Cross. *Exercises for Lower Limb Amputees.* September 2008. Accessed February 6, 2023. https://www.icrc.org/en/doc/assets/files/other/icrc_002_0936.pdf

## References


1. Ma VY, Chan L, Carruthers KJ. Incidence, prevalence, costs, and impact on disability of common conditions requiring rehabilitation in the United States: stroke, spinal cord injury, traumatic brain injury, multiple sclerosis, osteoarthritis, rheumatoid arthritis, limb loss, and back pain. *Arch Phys Med Rehabil.* 2014;95(5):986-995.
2. Ziegler-Graham K, MacKenzie EJ, Ephraim PL, et al. Estimating the prevalence of limb loss in the United States: 2005 to 2050. *Arch Phys Med Rehabil.* 2008;89(3):422-429.
3. Uustal H, Silevstri R, Callaghan S. Management of the lower extremity amputee. Paper presented at: Johnson Rehabilitation Institute; October 18, 2013; Edison, NJ.
4. Kahle JT, Highsmith MJ, Schaepper H, Johannesson A, Orendurff MS, Kaufman K. Predicting walking ability following lower limb amputation: an updated systematic literature review. *Technol Innov.* 2016;18(2-3):125-137. doi:10.21300/18.2-3.2016.125
5. Traugh GH, Corcoran PJ, Reyes RL. Energy expenditure of ambulation in patients with above-knee amputations. *Arch Phys Med Rehabil.* 1975;56(2):67-71.
6. Huang CT, Jackson JR, Moore NB, et al. Amputation: energy cost of ambulation. *Arch Phys Med Rehabil.* 1979;60(1):18-24.
7. Starholm IM, Mirtaheri P, Kapetanovic N, et al. Energy expenditure of transfemoral amputees during floor and treadmill walking with different speeds. *Prosthet Orthot Int.* 2016;40(3):336-342. doi:10.1177/0309364615588344
8. Mayo Clinic. Test ID: HBA1C hemoglobin A1c, blood. Accessed February 6, 2023. https://www.mayomedicallaboratories.com/test-catalog/Clinical+and+Interpretive/82080
9. Ehde DM, Czerniecki JM, Smith DG, et al. Chronic phantom sensations, phantom pain, residual limb pain, and other regional pain after lower limb amputation. *Arch Phys Med Rehabil.* 2000;81:1039-1044.
10. Richardson C, Kulkarni J. A review of the management of phantom limb pain: challenges and solutions. *J Pain Res.* 2017;10:1861-1870. doi:10.2147/JPR.S124664
11. Ferraro F, Jacopetti M, Spallone V, et al. Diagnosis and treatment of pain in plexopathy, radiculopathy, peripheral neuropathy and phantom limb pain. Evidence and recommendations from the Italian Consensus Conference on Pain on Neurorehabilitation (ICCPN). *Eur J Phys Rehabil Med.* 2016;52:855-866.
12. Mulvey MR, Fawkner HJ, Radford HE, Johnson MI. Perceptual embodiment of prosthetic limbs by transcutaneous electrical nerve stimulation. *Neuromodulation.* 2012;15(1):42-46; discussion 47. doi:10.1111/j.1525-1403.2011.00408.x
13. Brunelli S, Morone G, Iosa M, et al. Efficacy of progressive muscle relaxation, mental imagery, and phantom exercise training on phantom limb: a randomized controlled trial. *Arch Phys Med Rehabil.* 2015;96(2):181-187.
14. Wong CK, Chen CC, Benoy SA, Rahal RT, Blackwell WM. Role of balance ability and confidence in prosthetic use for mobility of people with lower-limb loss. *J Rehabil Res Dev.* 2014;51(9):1353-1364. doi:10.1682/JRRD.2013.11.0235
15. Major MJ, Fatone S, Roth EJ. Validity and reliability of the Berg balance scale for community-dwelling persons with lower-limb amputation. *Arch Phys Med Rehabil.* 2013;94(11):2194-2202. doi:10.1016/j.apmr.2013.07.002
16. Deathe AB, Miller WC. The L test of functional mobility: measurement properties of a modified version of the timed "up & go" test designed for people with lower-limb amputations. *Phys Ther.* 2005;85(7):626-635.
17. Dite W, Connor HJ, Curtis HC. Clinical identification of multiple fall risk early after unilateral transtibial amputation. *Arch Phys Med Rehabil.* 2007;88(1):109-114.
18. Reid L, Thomson P, Besemann M, Dudek N. Going places: does the two-minute walk test predict the six-minute walk test in lower extremity amputees? *J Rehabil Med.* 2015;47(3):256-261. doi:10.2340/16501977-1916
19. Gailey RS, Roach KE, Applegate EB, et al. The amputee mobility predictor: an instrument to assess determinants of the lower-limb amputee's ability to ambulate. *Arch Phys Med Rehabil.* 2002;83(5):613-627.
20. Balk EM, Gazula A, Markozannes G, et al. *Lower Limb Prostheses: Measurement Instruments, Comparison of Component Effects by Subgroups, and Long-Term Outcomes.* Agency for Healthcare Research and Quality; 2018. https://www.ncbi.nlm.nih.gov/books/NBK531517/table/ch2.tab1/
21. Miller WC, Deathe AB, Speechley M. Psychometric properties of the activities-specific balance confidence scale among individuals with a lower-limb amputation. *Arch Phys Med Rehabil.* 2003;84(5):656-661.

Chapter 18

# Pulmonary Conditions and Treatment Interventions

*Jacki Klaczak Kopack, PT, DPT*

**KEY TERMS** Active cycle of breathing | Adventitious breath sounds | Chest physical therapy | Diaphragmatic breathing | Positive expiratory pressure | Pursed lip breathing | Segmental breathing | Stacked breathing | Ventilatory or respiratory muscle training

## Chapter Objectives

1. Describe normal respiratory function and breath sounds.
2. Describe typical and atypical breathing patterns.
3. List the exercise considerations for persons with pulmonary disease.
4. Describe appropriate monitoring and activity/exercise progressions for a patient with pulmonary dysfunction.
5. Describe the commonly used breathing exercises and airway clearance techniques.
6. List the indications, precautions, and contraindications for respiratory muscle training.
7. Describe the impact medications can have on physiological responses to exercise and how to ensure safe and appropriate patient monitoring.
8. Given a physical therapy diagnosis and plan of care, design and progress a basic exercise and intervention program for a person with impaired respiratory function.

Respiratory system impairment can affect a patient's ability to participate in therapy as well as in functional activities and activities of daily living (ADLs) and will warrant additional monitoring on the part of the physical therapist and the physical therapist assistant. The more complex the patient's medical history or pulmonary dysfunction, the more likely that the rehabilitation team members will interact with the physician, respiratory therapist, occupational therapist, and nursing staff to provide coordinated multidisciplinary care. Respiratory treatment interventions are included not only for patients with pulmonary pathology but also for many of the other patient populations treated with physical therapy.

## Respiratory System Anatomy Review

The primary function of the respiratory system is to move air in and out of the body (ventilation) and to allow the exchange of oxygen and carbon dioxide within the lungs (respiration). The thoracic cage serves as protection for the lungs and as an attachment site for the muscles



Kopack JK, Cascardi KA.
*Principles of Therapeutic Exercise for the Physical Therapist Assistant* (pp 623-643).

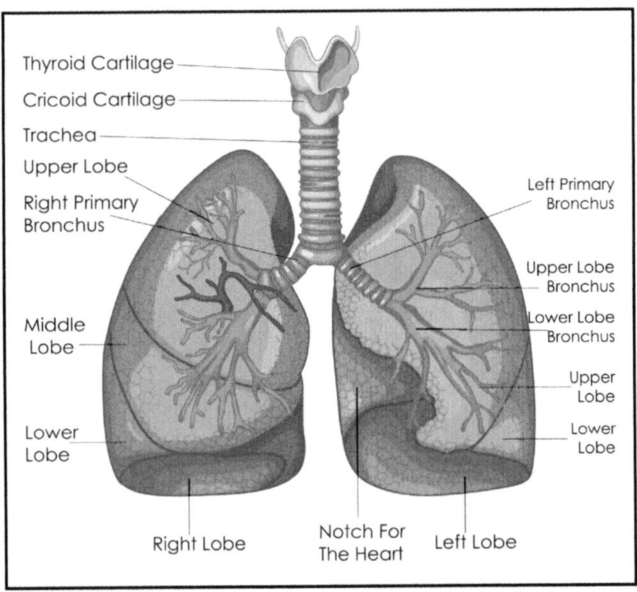


**Figure 18-1.** The respiratory tract anatomy (Vecton/Shutterstock.com).

**Table 18-1**

**Muscles of Respiration**

| Phases of Respiration | Muscles |
|---|---|
| Quiet inspiration (tidal breathing) | Diaphragm and external intercostals (pull upward on the rib cage) |
| Deep inspiration | Sternocleidomastoids, scalenes, levatores costarum, serratus posterior superior, and pectoralis major |
| Quiet expiration | Gravity and relaxation of external intercostals |
| Forced expiration | Abdominals (rectus abdominis, internal and external obliques, and transverse abdominis) contract forcing the diaphragm upward; internal intercostals contract pulling the ribs downward |

that assist with ventilation. Pulmonary function (alveolar ventilation) can adjust to meet the demands of activities in healthy individuals. Exercise/activity limitations in a healthy population are most often the result of muscle fatigue vs breathlessness, whereas breathlessness is a leading cause of activity limitation in persons with pulmonary disease.[1]

Air enters the body during inspiration through the nose or mouth and moves past the larynx and into the trachea (Figure 18-1). The trachea divides into the right and left bronchi. The bronchi divide into smaller bronchioles that lead to the alveolar sacs where actual gas exchange occurs. There are 3 types (level of effort) of inspiration (quiet, deep, and forced) and 2 types of expiration (quiet and forced). Muscle contraction drives the process of ventilation, and the number of muscles that are activated is dependent on the effort of breathing. The muscles of respiration are listed in Table 18-1. **Diaphragmatic breathing** is the most efficient method. The diaphragm is the primary muscle of inspiration, and it is innervated by the phrenic nerve (memory tip: C3, C4, C5 keep the diaphragm alive). When the diaphragm contracts, it lowers within the thorax, generating a negative pressure in the pleural space and pulling air into the lungs. The external intercostals also contract, raising the rib cage, increasing the diameter within the thoracic cage, and further opening the pleural space. Deep inspiration requires contraction of the accessory muscles and occurs during periods of increased activity when oxygen demand increases. Accessory muscle use increases the effort and the metabolic demand of breathing. When the upper extremities are stabilized, they create a closed kinetic chain, which allows the accessory muscles of respiration to assist with breathing via a reversal of muscle action (Figure 18-2). With forced inspiration, additional accessory muscles activate. The presence of pulmonary pathology typically necessitates accessory muscle contraction to maintain adequate ventilation.

Quiet expiration is a passive process that occurs as the diaphragm relaxes. The abdominals and internal intercostals actively contract during forced expiration. The internal intercostals pull the ribs down (decreasing the anterior/posterior diameter of the thoracic cage), and the abdominal muscles compress the abdominal contents (pushing them up), which pushes the diaphragm up and forces air from the lungs.

Breath sounds are heard during normal breathing by auscultating the front and back of the trunk. Breath sounds are described as either normal or abnormal (Table 18-2). Normal breath sounds vary based on the area being auscultated, and they are the sounds a clinician should hear in the absence of any disease/pathology. *Bronchial sounds* are heard over the large airways on the anterior chest near the second and third intercostal spaces. Sounds heard over the back of the trunk, between the scapulae, and on the center part of the anterior chest are called *bronchovesicular sounds*; sounds heard over lung tissue areas are called *vesicular sounds*.

**Adventitious breath sounds** are abnormal sounds, and they indicate pulmonary pathology. These sounds vary because of the presence of secretions or obstructions in different areas of the bronchi or lungs. Wheezes occur because of airway narrowing, whereas rhonchi result from secretions in the bronchial airways. These sounds are commonly found in patients with asthma or chronic obstructive pulmonary disease (COPD). Crackles are heard in patients who have bronchitis, pneumonia, or pulmonary edema.[2,3]

## Monitoring and Observing Patients With Pulmonary Disease

Common signs and symptoms of pulmonary disease include cough, dyspnea (shortness of breath), abnormal sputum production, hemoptysis, chest pain, cyanosis, digital clubbing, and altered breathing patterns.[4] The physical therapist screens for their presence during the initial evaluation and may perform lung auscultation as part of the patient examination. Auscultation is a systematic listening (using a stethoscope) over the patient's chest wall during a full inhalation/exhalation. The patient is instructed to sit upright and breathe fully in and out slowly through an open mouth. Beginning on the anterior thorax, the clinician listens during a full inspiration and expiration and then moves the stethoscope to each location shown in Figure 18-3A. The technique is repeated on the posterior thorax using the pattern shown in Figure 18-3B. Lung auscultation is completed to determine if there are areas of congestion. It is also completed after treatment to determine the effectiveness of airway clearance techniques.[2]

The physical therapist assistant should check for existing or new signs and symptoms before initiating treatment to determine the patient's overall physiological status and to verify that it is appropriate to proceed with treatment. The assistant should review the patient's vital sign trends (heart rate [HR], blood pressure, respiratory rate [RR], and oxygen saturation levels) and obtain these measurements before, during, and after treatment. Vital sign changes, changes in appearance, effort of breathing, perception of exertion, and breathing pattern provide information regarding the patient's endurance and activity tolerance. Knowledge of the expected changes associated with exercise allows the clinician to determine if a patient's response is atypical and if there is a need for assessment by the medical team.

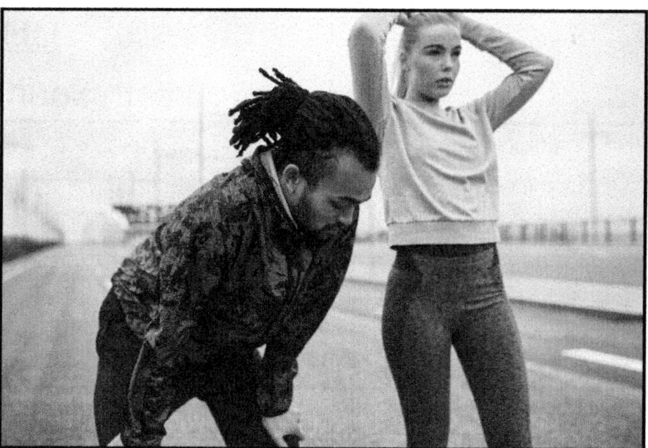

**Figure 18-2.** The accessory muscles during deep and forced inspiration: The reversal of muscle action with the upper extremities fixed (in a closed kinetic chain; Ground Picture/Shutterstock.com).

### Monitoring the General Appearance of Patients With Pulmonary Dysfunction

It is important to monitor the general appearance of patients with pulmonary conditions during treatment and over time. The assistant should observe body type, posture, skin tone, facial expressions, and preferred breathing techniques (ie, accessory muscle use and pursed lip or open mouth breathing). Patients who have increased abdominal adipose tissue may have difficulty breathing because of the physical restriction created by the abdomen pushing up on the diaphragm. Patients with end-stage emphysema are often thin and frail with general muscle wasting, and they may struggle to breathe, even at rest.

Postural deficits can affect pulmonary status. Significant kyphosis or scoliosis creates physical restrictions on lung expansion. Self-selected postures can also indicate the presence of pulmonary dysfunction. Patients in acute chronic heart failure (CHF) often have difficulty breathing when lying supine (orthopnea); they sit or elevate the head of the bed to improve respiration. Patients who sit leaning forward with the arms supported facilitate the activation of accessory muscles during inspiration, which increases the amount of air moving in and out of the lungs (tidal volume).[5] Patients with long-standing COPD tend to be barrel chested. The anterior-posterior diameter is larger in these patients (compared with patients without pulmonary pathology).

Skin tone may indicate general levels of oxygenation. The presence of a bluish tint to the lips/fingernail beds (observed in White people) or a grayish tint (observed in people with darker skin tones) is called *cyanosis*. Cyanosis is usually a sign of decreased oxygenation, although Raynaud's disease or other vascular issues can result in

**Table 18-2**

**Breath Sound Descriptions**

| | |
|---|---|
| Normal sounds | Depending on the area of auscultation:<br>Bronchial: Loud, high-pitched tubular sounds; expiratory sounds last longer than inspiratory sounds with a short pause between inspiration and expiration.<br>Bronchovesicular: Softer than bronchial sounds but a tubular sound; heard equally during inspiration and expiration.<br>Vesicular: Low soft, blowing, or rustling sounds; heard throughout inspiration and continue without pause partially through expiration. |
| Adventitious or abnormal sounds | Crackles or rales: Fine, discontinuous sounds, such as a bubbling, clicking, or crackling sound. Commonly heard during inspiration.<br>Wheezes: Continuous high-pitched sounds more common during exhalation.<br>Rhonchi: A rattling quality that is low pitched similar to snoring during inhalation.<br>Absent: No sound; indicates partial or total airway obstruction. |

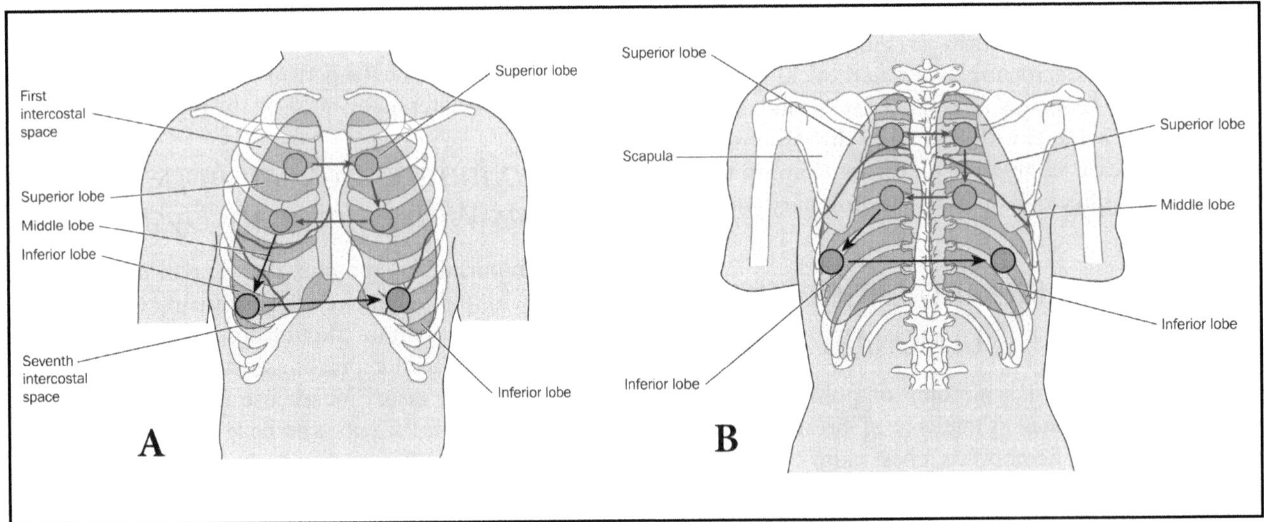


**Figure 18-3.** Lung auscultation. (A) The anterior view. (B) The posterior view (Blamb/Shutterstock.com).

cyanosis. Clubbing (bulbous distal joints and a downward angle of the nail bed) of the distal fingers/toes often indicates chronic hypoxia (Figure 18-4). The clinician observes facial expression for signs of distress, the position of the mouth/lips during exhalation, and neck musculature. **Pursed lip breathing** during exhalation is often used by patients with COPD to improve gas exchange. The presence of hypertrophied neck musculature, especially the sternocleidomastoid and scalene muscles, indicates a reliance on the accessory muscles for breathing (common in patients with chronic COPD).

## *Respiratory Rate and Breathing Pattern Monitoring*

The normal RR for adults is 12 to 20 breaths/minute. It should be assessed by inconspicuously observing the rise and fall of the patient's thorax for a full minute. If the patient is aware that the clinician is assessing their RR, they may subconsciously alter the rate. Observe the time spent during inhalation vs exhalation. The typical ratio is 1:2, but in patients with COPD, asthma, or chronic respiratory pathology, the ratio may increase to 1:4.[2]

The clinician documents breathing patterns and the effectiveness of cough. Patients who present with altered breathing patterns at rest may have difficulty meeting the increased metabolic demands of activity, requiring increased monitoring and gradual activity progression. Table 18-3 describes normal and atypical breathing patterns.[2,4] To assess cough, the clinician asks the patient to cough and assesses the strength and depth of the cough. Coughing is described as effective, weak, or absent. If the patient presents with a productive cough, the secretions/sputum should be described (ie, the amount, color, smell, and consistency).

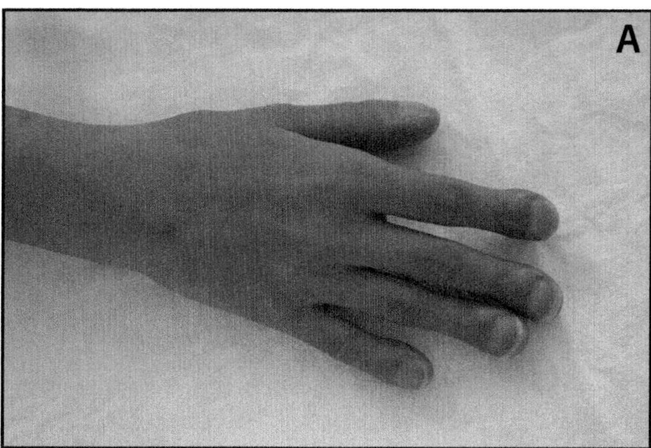


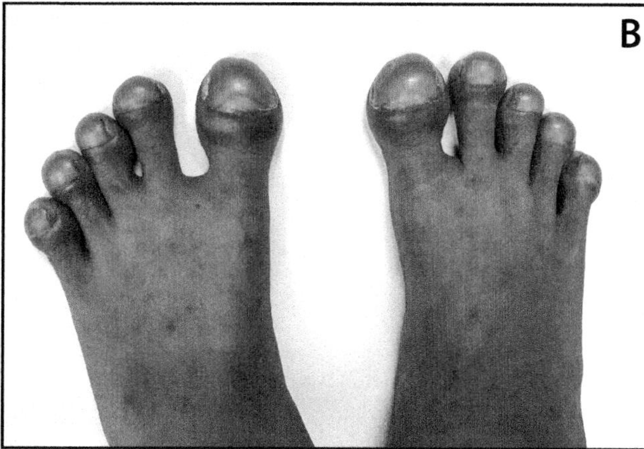


**Figure 18-4.** Clubbing of (A) fingers (kris4to/Shutterstock.com) and (B) toes (Chalie Chulapornsiri/Shutterstock.com).

**Table 18-3**

Breathing Patterns[2,4]

| Patterns | Description |
|---|---|
| Apnea | Absence of ventilation |
| Apneustic | Gasping (slow, deep) inspiration, short expiration followed by apnea |
| Biot | Slow, shallow respirations interspersed with fast deep breaths and periods of apnea |
| Bradypnea | Slow rate, normal rhythm |
| Cheyne-Stokes | Repeated cycle of deep breaths followed by shallow breaths or apnea |
| Dyspnea | Distressed, labored breathing; rapid rate, shallow depth, regular rhythm; associated with increased accessory muscle use |
| Eupnea | Normal rate, depth and rhythm |
| Hyperventilation | Fast rate, increased depth and regular rhythm |
| Orthopnea | Difficulty breathing in the supine position |
| Tachypnea | Fast rate, shallow depth, regular rhythm |

## *Monitoring Supplemental Oxygen Use and Rate of Perceived Dyspnea*

Patients with lung disease or pulmonary dysfunction may require supplemental oxygen to maintain adequate oxygen levels in their body (necessary for normal tissue and organ function). Supplemental oxygen is delivered via a nasal cannula (Figure 18-5) or mask (Figure 18-6; when higher concentrations of oxygen are needed). The assistant should ensure that the patient is wearing the cannula or mask correctly. The assistant monitors the patient's subjective reports (ie, the rate of perceived exertion or dyspnea), appearance (ie, skin color and breathing pattern), and hemoglobin saturation levels using a pulse oximeter. The most reliable way to monitor blood oxygen and carbon dioxide levels is by measuring arterial blood gas (arterial blood gas test), but this is an invasive technique. A pulse oximeter is a noninvasive way to measure oxygen saturation levels (Figure 18-7), and it is used to monitor the patient's response to activity.

**Considerations for the Physical Therapist Assistant**

A patient who has removed their nasal cannula may present with low oxygen saturation levels and/or confusion. Reapplication of the nasal cannula should reverse the deterioration.

Generally, the goal is to maintain oxygen saturation rates greater than 92% throughout treatment. Patients with significant respiratory disease/compromise may exhibit larger oxygen drops (desaturation) with activity. If the level drops below 92%, activity should be stopped until saturation levels rise to greater than 92%, and then activity can be resumed (assuming all other vital signs and patient presentation are appropriate). The assistant may cue the patient to complete pursed lip breathing during episodes of desaturation. The patient's response to activity should be regularly communicated to the medical team.

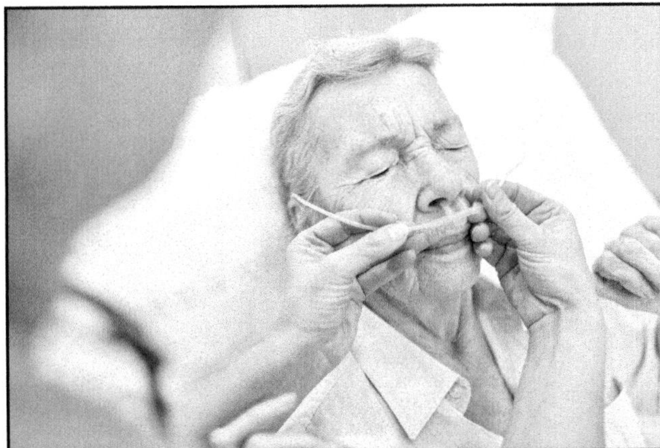

**Figure 18-5.** Adjusting a nasal cannula for the effective administration of lower levels of oxygen (True Touch Lifestyle/Shutterstock.com).

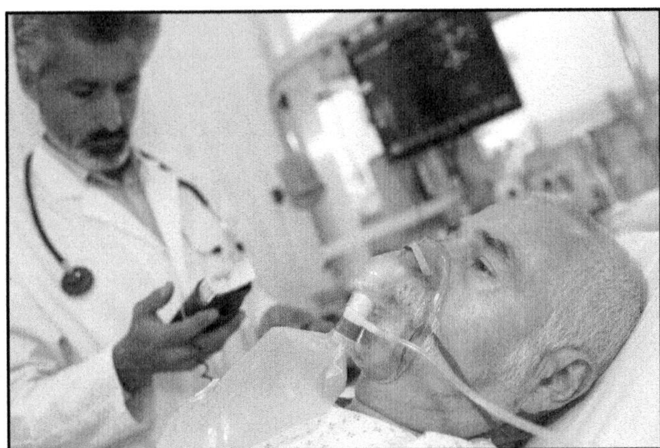

**Figure 18-6.** An oronasal/face mask for oxygen being delivered at a higher concentration (ALPA PROD/Shutterstock.com).

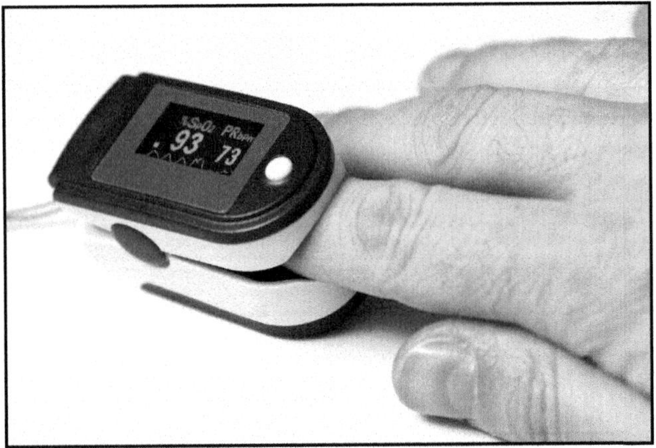


**Figure 18-7.** A pulse oximeter to measure oxygen saturation levels and HR (Juan R. Velasco/Shutterstock.com).

### Considerations for the Physical Therapist Assistant

For some people with severe pulmonary dysfunction, the oxygen saturation levels at rest and with activity may routinely drop lower than 90%. In these cases, the therapy team should discuss the situation with the physician. The physician will specify vital sign parameters for activity that are individualized for the patient.

The clinician should review the physician's order regarding supplemental oxygen and ensure that the oxygen is delivered as per the orders. For example, if the orders state 2 L $O_2$ increase to 4 L $O_2$ as needed to maintain oxygen saturation levels greater than 90%, the physical therapist assistant will use pulse oximetry to monitor the patient during the session. In this case, the assistant can increase the oxygen flow up to 4 L during activity if needed to maintain oxygen saturation levels above 90%.

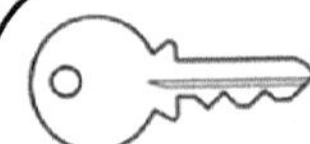

### Key Safety Considerations

The clinician should not increase oxygen concentrations without written orders from the physician. Some patients with COPD retain carbon dioxide, and titrating oxygen levels up may result in decreased respiratory drive.[2,4]

The clinician should monitor the patient's perceived level of dyspnea (shortness of breath) at rest and when performing a variety of activities. The rating of perceived dyspnea (RPD), which is included in Table 18-4, is an effective way to track a patient's dyspnea.[6-8] The clinician asks the patient to rate their difficulty breathing from 0 (no difficulty) to 10 (maximum difficulty/shortness of breath). RPD can be assessed in conjunction with vital signs (ie, HR, RR, and oxygen saturation) and functional performance.

## Pulmonary Testing and Functional Assessments

Pulmonary testing is performed to assess pulmonary function, to determine if pulmonary disease is present (and, if so, determine the severity), and to assess the impact of treatment on pulmonary function. Pulmonary testing measures lung capacities and lung volumes. These test results can be compared with age, weight, and sex-related norms. Volumes and capacities in patients with obstructive disease are atypical compared with healthy individuals. Lung volume measurements include the following: tidal volume, inspiratory reserve volume, expiratory reserve volume, and residual volume. Lung capacities include total lung capacity, forced vital capacity (FVC), inspiratory capacity, and functional residual capacity (Table 18-5).[3,9] These tests are

**Table 18-4**

**Rating of Perceived Dyspnea[7-9,53]**

| | |
|---|---|
| 0 | Nothing at all |
| 0.5 | Very, very slight |
| 1 | Very slight |
| 2 | Slight |
| 3 | Moderate |
| 4 | Somewhat severe |
| 5 | Severe |
| 6 | |
| 7 | Very severe |
| 8 | |
| 9 | Very, very severe |
| 10 | Maximal |

**Table 18-5**

**Lung Volumes and Capacities Descriptions**

| Lung Volumes |
|---|
| Tidal volume (TV) is the amount of air that is inhaled and exhaled during normal breathing. |
| Inspiratory reserve volume (IRV) is the additional (forcible) air that can be inhaled after a normal TV. Used for deep breathing. |
| Expiratory reserve volume (ERV) is the amount of air that can be forcibly exhaled after a normal TV exhalation. |
| Residual volume (RV) is the remaining air in the lungs after a full (or maximal) exhalation. |
| **Lung Capacities** |
| Total tung capacity (TLC) is the maximal amount of air that the lungs can handle. It is the sum of all volumes: TLC = TV + IRV + ERV + RV |
| FVC is the maximal amount of air that can be forcibly exhaled after maximal inhalation: FVC = TV + IRV + ERV |
| Inspiratory capacity (IC) is the maximal amount of air that can be inhaled: IC = TV + IRV |

used to determine if a patient has restrictive or obstructive lung disease or a combination of the 2. Spirometry testing (Figure 18-8) measures FVC and forced expiratory volume in 1 second ($FEV_1$). FVC is the volume of air that is exhaled after a deep inspiration, and it measures lung size (in liters). $FEV_1$ describes the amount of air exhaled in 1 second after a deep inspiration. Generally, test results that reveal a lower-than-expected FVC, $FEV_1$, and $FEV_1$/FVC ratio indicate obstructive lung disease (eg, COPD, cystic fibrosis, asthma). Test results that reveal a reduced FVC but a normal $FEV_1$/FVC ratio indicate the presence of restrictive lung disease (eg, scoliosis, pulmonary fibrosis, quadriplegia). Table 18-6 lists the lung volumes and lung capacity changes associated with obstructive and restrictive lung diseases.

**Study Tip**

Patients with **o**bstructive lung disease cannot get air **out**; patients with restr**i**cti**v**e lung disease have difficulty getting air **in**.

The Baseline Dyspnea Index (BDI)[10] and quality of life (QOL) assessments, such as the Chronic Respiratory Questionnaire[11] and the COPD Assessment Test (CAT), provide the clinician with useful data.[12] The BDI grades breathlessness as it relates to ADLs, and it assesses functional impairments, the magnitude of the task, and the magnitude of effort that provokes breathlessness.[10] The Chronic Respiratory Questionnaire is a 20-item questionnaire that

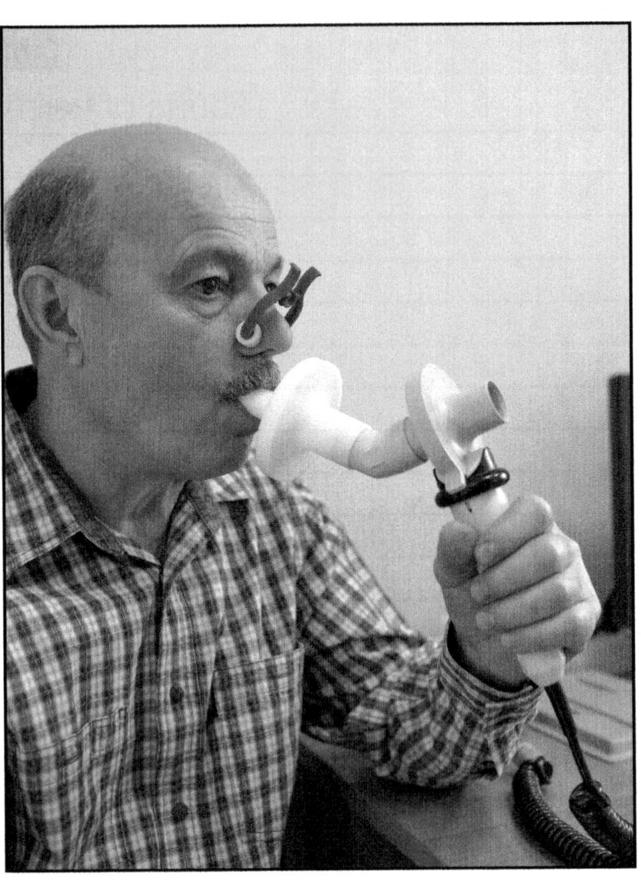

**Figure 18-8.** A pulmonary function test using a spirometer and lung volumes (Koldunov/Shutterstock.com).

**Table 18-6**

**Obstructive and Restrictive Lung Volumes and Capacities Compared With Normal Lung Values**

| Obstructive Disease | | Restrictive Disease | |
|---|---|---|---|
| Increased TV | ↑ | TV | ↓ All decreased |
| Increased RV | ↑ | IRV | ↓ All decreased |
| Increased TLC | ↑ | ERV | ↓ All decreased |
| Increased FRC | ↑ | RV | ↓ All decreased |
| Decreased IRV | ↓ | TLC | ↓ All decreased |
| Decreased ERV | ↓ | IC | ↓ All decreased |
| Decreased IC | ↓ | FVC | ↓ All decreased |
| Decreased FVC | ↓ | FRC | ↓ All decreased |

FRC = functional residual capacity.

measures physical function (quantifying dyspnea based on 5 self-selected ADLs) and emotional function (anxiety, depression, frustration, and fear of dyspnea).[11] The CAT is a quick and easy tool that determines how COPD impacts the patient's health status and ADL.[12] Links to the BDI and CAT are included in the Suggested Resources section at the end of this chapter.

The 6-Minute Walk Test (6MWT) and the Incremental (10-m) Shuttle Walk Test (ISWT) are useful tools to measure progress in patients with pulmonary disease. The 6MWT is commonly used because it is easy to administer and requires minimal equipment. A distance increase of approximately 35 meters for patients with moderate to severe COPD is considered clinically significant.[13] The

ISWT uses audio signals to determine an incremental increase in walking speed. This test is considered clinically significant with a change of 0.05 meter per second.[14] Links to 6MWT and ISWT instructions are included in the Suggested Resources section.

Other tests that may be appropriate include the bicycle ergometer test, treadmill test, and 6- or 12-Minute Walk Test. Exercise testing results are used to guide the physical therapist in prescribing safe levels of exercise. Testing allows objective tracking of changes in oxygenation during activities; it is completed with or without supplemental oxygen (based on the individual patient's presentation). Graded exercise testing should include continuous monitoring of vital signs and oxygen saturation levels for all pulmonary and cardiac patients.

Patients with pulmonary disease may exhibit decreased strength due to deconditioning and long-term steroid use. Decreased strength can have a negative long-term impact on patients with COPD. There is a correlation between upper limb muscle strength and exercise capacity.[15,16] Determining the patient's strength is important, but manual muscle testing may not be the best method because it can increase intrathoracic pressure if patients hold their breath (ie, the Valsalva maneuver) during maximal effort with resistance.[9]

### *Reasons to Terminate Testing*

In addition to the reasons an assistant would terminate exercise for any patient (eg, new-onset cardiac signs/symptoms, a significant change in patient status), the following are also reasons to terminate exercise testing and to check the patient's vital signs: the patient reports being too breathless to continue; the patient reaches 85% of their predicted maximum HR (maximum HR = 210 − 0.65 × age); or the patient exhibits or reports increasing mental confusion, lack of coordination or light-headedness, leg cramps or extreme leg muscle fatigue, or persistent oxygen saturation less than 85%.[17]

## Rehabilitation Goals and Treatment Interventions

General goals for pulmonary rehabilitation include independence with airway clearance and breathing techniques, increased cardiovascular endurance and muscle strength (ie, inspiratory and upper and lower extremity muscles) to reduce dyspnea and improve ADL and instrumental ADL abilities, and improved QOL. Interventions are selected to prevent airway obstruction and the accumulation of secretions, to improve cough effectiveness, and/or to improve ventilation. Treatment focuses on patient education (ie, disease self-management and realistic goals), energy conservation techniques, breathing and coughing exercises, and postural and **respiratory muscle training (RMT)**. Postural exercises can improve chest mobility as well as correct postural deformities to help support patient goals. Improvement in respiratory function can result in increased endurance and general activity tolerance via increasing the strength and power of the respiratory muscles.

### *Breathing Exercises and Techniques*

Breathing exercises can improve ventilation, prevent postoperative complications, improve the performance of respiratory musculature, correct inefficient breathing patterns, assist a patient during periods of dyspnea, and improve overall functional capacity.[3] Breathing exercise techniques include diaphragmatic breathing, pursed lip breathing, segmental breathing (includes lateral costal expansion), stacked breathing, and deep breathing (using an incentive spirometer). General instructions for these exercises are included in Table 18-7.

Diaphragmatic breathing decreases the energy cost associated with respiration and increases intrathoracic lung volumes (ie, tidal volume and inspiratory reserve volume). Diaphragmatic breathing requires less effort/energy compared with breathing using accessory muscles.[2,3] Diaphragmatic breathing is the most efficient breathing pattern, but it may not be appropriate for use with patients with COPD because it does not improve breathing mechanics.[18-21] Patients with COPD who demonstrate paradoxical breathing patterns or asynchronous thoracoabdominal motion experience increased dyspnea on exertion with diaphragmatic breathing.[20,21] Current research indicates that pursed lip breathing provides better universal outcomes for patients with COPD.[9,18-20,22]

**Pursed lip breathing** is helpful in decreasing a patient's sense of dyspnea or anxiety. It is especially useful in patients with COPD because these patients present with airway collapse during exhalation (which leads to hyperinflation of the alveoli). Pursing the lips creates resistance during exhalation and that resistance keeps the airways open, allowing better ventilation and preventing hyperinflation of the alveoli.[2,3,9,18] During exertion, using a pursed lip breathing strategy can reduce RR and aid in recovery in patients with COPD.[18]

**Segmental breathing** is used to encourage the expansion of segments/areas of the lungs. It is useful in addressing hypoventilation that occurs after surgery because of pain/guarding, atelectasis (a partial or total collapsed lung), and pneumonia.[2,3]

**Stacked breathing** is used with patients with atelectasis, hypoventilation, and an ineffective cough. It can improve thorax mobility, increase the depth of breaths, promote effective coughing, and help keep the lungs clear. The technique can be used with or without the assistance of a bag valve mask (Ambu bag [Ambu]).[23] Patient instructions for using this technique with an Ambu bag are included in the Suggested Resources section.

| **Table 18-7** |
|---|
| **Specific Instructions for Various Breathing Techniques** |
| Safety considerations: Obtain medical clearance before initiating breathing techniques. Discourage forcible exhalations.<br>Progressions: Start in a comfortable position (ie, hook lying or semi-Fowler's), progress to sitting, progress to standing, and progress to proper technique during activity. |
| Diaphragmatic breathing: The patient places one hand on their upper chest and one on their abdomen. Inhale slowly through the nose, looking for the hand on the abdomen to rise while the hand on the chest should stay as still as possible. Exhale slowly (cue patient to purse their lips).<br>Clinical tip: The therapist may provide tactile cues by placing the hand on the abdomen, moving a hand (immediately after exhalation) gently up and under the anterior thorax, and the cuing patient to "breathe/push into my hand." |
| Pursed lip breathing: Start to breathe in slowly through the nose (with the mouth closed) for a count of 3 to 4, and then open the mouth (into a whistling or puckering position) and exhale slowly for a count of 4 to 6. |
| Segmental breathing: The therapist places their hands on the patient's lateral lower ribs. As the patient exhales, provide a gentle squeezing pressure. Immediately before inhalation, provide a quick, gentle stretch down and in (to facilitate contraction of the intercostals). Provide light pressure during inhalation for increased sensory feedback. |
| Stacked breathing: The patient takes a deep breath in followed by a brief hold, then takes a second breath followed by a brief hold, and then a third breath (so they are stacked one on top of the other). Hold all of the inhaled air in for about 2 to 3 seconds. Then, the patient should exhale all of the air through the mouth in a controlled expiratory fashion. |
| Deep breathing with an incentive spirometer: The patient places the mouthpiece in their mouth and takes a deep breath in as forcefully as possible and holds up to 5 seconds followed by a normal exhalation. In the acute care setting, it is commonly recommended that the patient complete 10 repetitions per hour. |

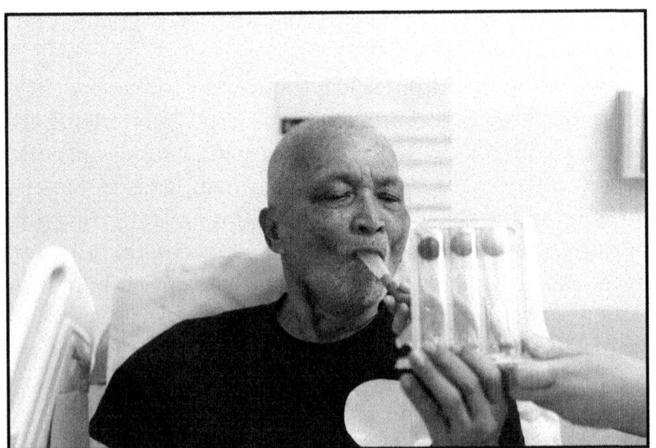

**Figure 18-9.** A patient using an incentive spirometer (PongMoji/Shutterstock.com).

Deep breathing using an incentive spirometer is useful to prevent or treat atelectasis and to stimulate an effective cough.[2,3] Incentive spirometer use is common after surgery or with pulmonary disorders (ie, pneumonia). Figure 18-9 shows a patient using an incentive spirometer.

Before initiating breathing exercises, the clinician should verify that the patient is cleared of any medical, orthopedic, or postsurgical precautions/contraindications and should observe the patient's resting RR. When performing any of these exercises, start in the hook-lying or the semi-Fowler position (allowing gravity to assist the diaphragm). Demonstrate the selected technique, and then provide manual and verbal cues as needed. Once the patient is able to correctly complete the exercise technique in the initial position, progressions include performing the exercise in sitting, then standing, and finally during activity. Instruct the patient to exhale normally; avoid forced exhalation because this may lead to bronchospasms or extremely prolonged exhalation (causing an irregular breathing pattern for subsequent breaths).

The clinician can also instruct patients on activity pacing strategies. Patients are instructed to listen to their body and only perform activities within their breathing capabilities. An activity can be broken down into stages or performed at a slower pace so that it does not exacerbate dyspnea. For example, a patient reports significant shortness of breath going up one flight of 10 steps. In this situation, the patient can ascend 5 or 6 steps, take 1 or 2 deep breaths, and then go up the remainder of the steps. With continued practice using pacing, the patient should progress to climbing all 10 steps as their endurance improves. Activity pacing is an effective strategy for patients with COPD and other pulmonary conditions.[9,24]

**Table 18-8**

**Respiratory Muscle Training Progressions[30]**

| Training Progression | Warm-Up | Intervention | Frequency |
|---|---|---|---|
| Foundational training | 2 sets of 30 breaths at 40% of the maximal inspiratory pressure | 30 breaths at 50% to 60% of the maximal inspiratory pressure | Twice a day daily for approximately 6 weeks |
| Functional training:<br>RMT (IMT used here as an example) | 2 sets of 30 breaths at 40% of the maximal inspiratory pressure | 30 breaths at up to 70% of the maximal inspiratory pressure | Twice a day 3 times a week (on opposing days, compete foundational sequence) |
| Maintenance | 2 sets of 30 breaths at 40% of the maximal inspiratory pressure | 30 breaths at up to 70% of the maximal inspiratory pressure | Minimum of once a day 3 times a week |

Note that examples are provided using IMT progressions; programs can isolate expiratory muscle training (EMT) as well or include a combination of the 2.
IMT = inspiratory muscle training.

## *Ventilatory or Respiratory Muscle Training*

**Ventilatory training or RMT** techniques are interventions to improve the function of respiratory muscles using specific exercises (Table 18-8). RMT includes breathing exercises and support exercises to increase the strength and endurance of the respiratory muscles, thereby improving respiration. RMT has been shown to be effective for patients after a cerebrovascular accident or spinal cord injury (SCI), patients with pulmonary disease (COPD or asthma), and athletes.[25-29] The use of RMT can increase a person's endurance by reducing exercise-limiting dyspnea and delaying the onset of fatigue during aerobic exercise.[29] Inspiratory muscle training (IMT) is an effective method of training for patients with COPD, resulting in decreased dyspnea during ADLs.[22,28] Although patient outcomes/improvements have been noted in the research, RMT has not been shown to increase maximum oxygen consumption.[30]

Respiratory muscles respond to training stimuli in a similar manner as skeletal muscles, achieving adaptations to their structure that are specific to the training stimulus. The training effects of RMT include a decreased effort of breathing (ie, less reliance on accessory muscles) and a decrease in respiratory muscle fatigue. RMT includes IMT, EMT, or a combination of both. Training using an RMT program can result in increased lung capacity.[30] Overload and reversibility are considerations when developing an effective RMT program. Exercise intensity, frequency, and duration are individualized to achieve a training effect.

It is easiest to initiate breathing exercises/RMT in a quiet environment after a thorough explanation and demonstration of the exercises.[2] Correct breathing technique (appropriate diaphragmatic breathing) is a critical factor for effective breathing exercises and RMT. The concurrent use of relaxation techniques may also be beneficial. Supine and semirecumbent postures impair respiratory muscle function; inspiratory muscle function is optimal in the upright position.[2] Training in seated and standing is most functional as long as the patient can tolerate activity in these postures.[2] Early modifications may include the use of semi-Fowler or supported sitting.[2] The breathing pattern should include the maximal range of motion of the rib cage and should maximize the recruitment of all inspiratory muscles (ie, the diaphragm and intercostals). Selection of an optimal training device and monitoring patient performance/technique are important. Performing IMT is likely to loosen pulmonary secretions. Patients should be trained in airway clearance techniques before initiating RMT.[30] The clinician will monitor vital signs, oxygen saturation, and general patient presentation throughout the training.

## *Developing a Respiratory Muscle Training Program*

The information in this section serves as an introduction to RMT exercises and monitoring. The reader is referred to *Respiratory Muscle Training: Theory and Practice*[30] for more detailed explanations and information.[1]

Program recommendations and monitoring were developed with the healthy population in mind. When using these techniques with patients with pulmonary pathology, increased patient monitoring is indicated. During the initial evaluation, the physical therapist will determine if the techniques are appropriate and safe for delegation based on the patient's presentation and acuity. Ensure the patient does not have contraindications to RMT. Precautions for RMT include recent cold or sinusitis and acute infection. Contraindications for RMT include a history of a spontaneous pneumothorax or recent pneumothorax, burst tympanic membrane (eardrum), other conditions of the middle

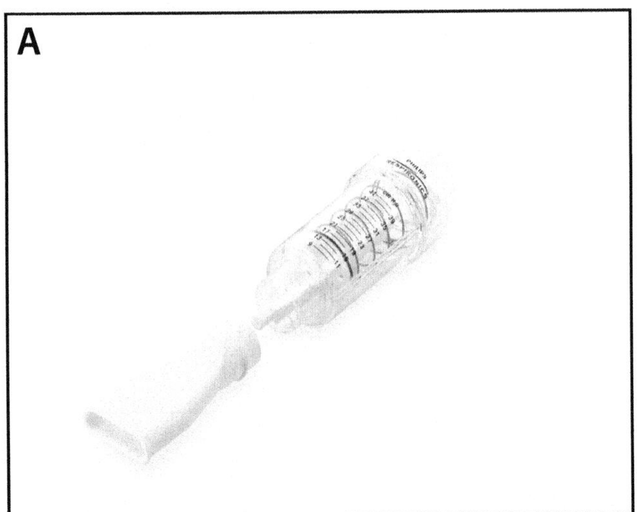

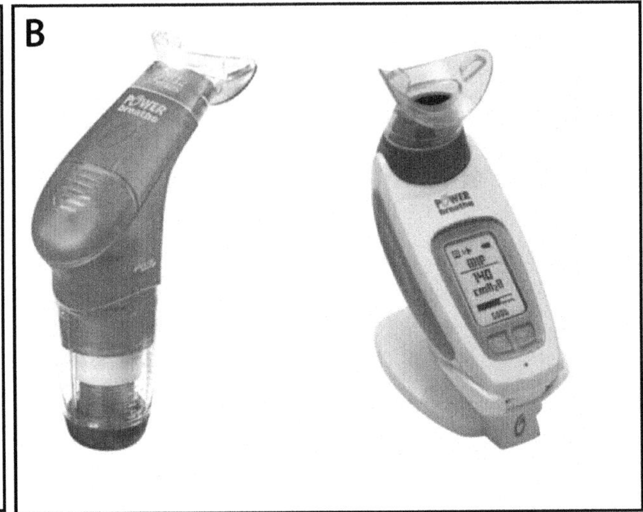

**Figure 18-10.** RMT devices. (A) Threshold IMT. (Courtesy of Philips. All rights reserved.) (B) Powerbreathe. (Reproduced with permission from POWERbreathe International Ltd.)

ear (infections or inflammation; ie, otitis media), and severe asthma with significant perception of dyspnea.[30]

There are various RMT training techniques, but the pressure threshold loading method is most commonly used and is well supported by research.[22,29,30] A small, handheld device (Figure 18-10) is used to provide calibrated resistance during inhalation; it is set specifically for the patient. The device has a pressure-loaded inspiratory valve (or spring) and an unloaded expiratory flap valve.

## Foundational Training

RMT can occur before or in conjunction with physical therapy interventions. The first phase of an RMT program incorporates foundational training exercises/activities, including general stretching and warm-ups, followed by submaximal IMT exercises. IMT warm-up includes 2 sets of 30 breaths at 40% of the maximal inspiratory pressure with a 1-minute rest between sets. Warm-up is followed by foundational training that includes 30 breaths at 50% to 60% of the maximal inspiratory pressure. The repetition maximum for inspiratory muscles is the repetition when the person is unable to achieve a satisfactory breath. A set of 25 to 35 training breaths is performed using an inspiratory training device. The patient is instructed to inhale using full effort as fast as possible and to breathe in and out as much/far as possible with each breath (ie, inhale and then exhale as fully as possible). The use of an appropriate breathing pattern is important. The exercises are completed twice a day, and the training load is increased at least once a week. The patient should keep an exercise log, noting any trends on days where the exercises might result in fatigue more quickly (ie, the time of day, ambient temperature or humidity, and mealtime). The recommended length of this phase is 4 to 6 weeks.

## Functional Training

Once the patient has completed the foundational program, a resistance training or endurance training (or a combination) program is implemented, and the patient is progressed to the functional phase. Respiratory muscle strength increases when exposed to high-load stresses over short periods of time, and an increase in endurance will occur when exposed to low-load stresses over prolonged periods. Stronger muscles use a lower percentage of their maximum capacity than weaker muscles do at a given workload and are able to sustain activity for longer periods of time. Because resistance training is less time consuming and it results in both strength and endurance improvements, it may be a preferred training method. IMT resistance training is achieved using a device (ie, Pflex resistive trainer device [Respironics Healthscan Inc] or Powerbreathe [Powerbreathe InternationalLtd]) to provide resistance to inspiration. EMT is completed using a device (ie, EMST-150 [Aspire Respiratory Products]) that resists exhalation; this training is indicated to improve cough or speech/swallow function. Resistance exercises are typically added after the patient is able to complete the foundational exercises, and they occur in conjunction with ongoing completion of the functional exercises.[30]

Many of the respiratory muscles perform ventilation and also play an important role in postural control and core stabilization. This may be why many patients complain of breathlessness with walking compared with riding a stationary bike. During walking, the demand on the respiratory muscles increases, and the postural muscles are challenged to maintain balance. For this reason, the functional training phase should include postural exercises, stretches to improve chest wall expansion, and strengthening and endurance exercises for the postural musculature.

Patients should perform IMT in challenging positions to facilitate and integrate the core/abdominal muscles and diaphragm. The clinician should monitor for correct breathing technique. This training can reduce the severity of dyspnea when the patient performs functional activities.[30] Progress is assessed by measuring inspiratory muscle function (maximal inspiratory pressure or peak inspiratory flow rate) and through the use of functional assessment tools (eg, the 6MWT).

### Maintenance Phase

Once the desired outcomes are achieved, the patient continues on a maintenance program. Respiratory muscles respond similarly to other muscles when training ends, so RMT should continue a minimum of once a day at least 3 times a week to maintain gains.[30]

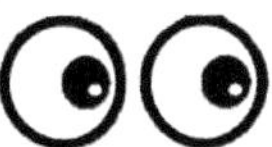

**Eye on the Research**

IMT can produce beneficial effects in patients with COPD, and IMT plus EMT can improve respiratory muscle strength.[31] IMT and EMT can be included within pulmonary rehabilitation with patients with severe to very severe COPD.[31]

## *Airway Clearance Techniques*

Airway clearance techniques are an important component of a pulmonary hygiene program. There are numerous pathologies that increase mucus production (eg, bronchitis, cystic fibrosis, pneumonia), decrease the abilities of the airways to remove secretions (eg, COPD, asthma), or decrease the patient's ability to cough and remove secretions (eg, high-level SCI, pain/chest wall injury). Adequate airway clearance is necessary to prevent the formation of mucus plugs, infection, pneumonia, and atelectasis. For patients with thick secretions, it may be beneficial to complete airway clearance techniques after a respiratory treatment (humidification or inhaled nebulizer treatments). Airway clearance is improved with the incorporation of coughing exercises, manually assisted cough, suctioning, active cycle of breathing exercises, **positive expiratory pressure (PEP)**, high-frequency chest wall oscillation, chest physical therapy, and postural drainage techniques.[2,3] The effectiveness of each of these techniques (with some variation based on pathology) and the selection of technique are dependent on the patient's preference and the individual patient's response to treatment.[32-38] Some of the evidence for using these techniques is not strong for hospitalized patients,[39] so the therapist should review the available research and discuss treatment options with the medical team to determine the optimal plan.[3]

### Coughing and Huffing

An effective cough is key to keeping the lungs clear of secretions. Coughing can be reflexive or voluntary. The therapist educates the patient about the importance of an effective cough and instructs and assists the patient in coughing. A normal cough requires a deep inspiration followed by closure of the glottis and contraction of the abdominals. For patients who cannot achieve this (ie, after SCI, thoracic surgery/pain, or rib fracture/pain), the therapist can instruct in components of the cough (ie, "K" cough and huffing). To assist the patient in learning how to control and close the glottis, ask the patient to make the "K" sound. The patient can then put their hands on the abdominals and make the "huff" sound to feel the contraction of the abdominals. The patient is instructed to complete either a series of 2 deep/forced expirations or a series of a few huffing (forced exhalation technique) coughs. The patient can be instructed to try to increase the force of contraction with each contraction.[2]

Coughing is typically easiest to perform in the seated position. The patient should be positioned either sitting upright or side lying when performing coughs. The clinician monitors the patient to ensure they do not gasp for breaths after coughing. Huffing (not forceful coughing) may be more appropriate for patients with a history of uncontrolled hypertension, cerebrovascular accident, and/or aneurysms.[2,3] For patients with chest wall pain caused by a recent surgery or trauma, the clinician should instruct the patient in splinted coughing. The clinician instructs the patient to press their hands or a pillow over the painful area to support it with each cough.[3] Splinted coughing is often used with patients after abdominal or open heart (median sternotomy) surgery.[3] The assistant will review the physician's orders and postoperative protocol before initiating any respiratory interventions with postoperative patients.

Patients with abdominal or respiratory muscle weakness may need assistance to perform an effective cough. The patient can be positioned supine or in a supported seated position; if the patient is seated in a wheelchair, the brakes should be engaged and the chair stabilized before starting the intervention. To start the intervention, instruct the patient to inhale deeply and to briefly hold the inhalation. The patient is instructed to attempt a cough, and the clinician can assist. There are a number of hand placements/techniques that can be used to manually assist a cough. The clinician can use the "butterfly" technique in which the clinician places both hands on the patient's stomach with the thumb of each hand together and the fingers spread apart (creating the shape of a butterfly; Figure 18-11A). The patient takes a couple of deep breaths, and then, as the patient exhales, the clinician instructs the patient to cough while the clinician assists by pushing up and in using a firm steady pressure in one smooth motion. The patient can be taught to self-assist a cough by placing their hands in the same position, applying an upward and inward pressure while leaning forward, and attempting a cough. Alternately, the hands can be placed around the

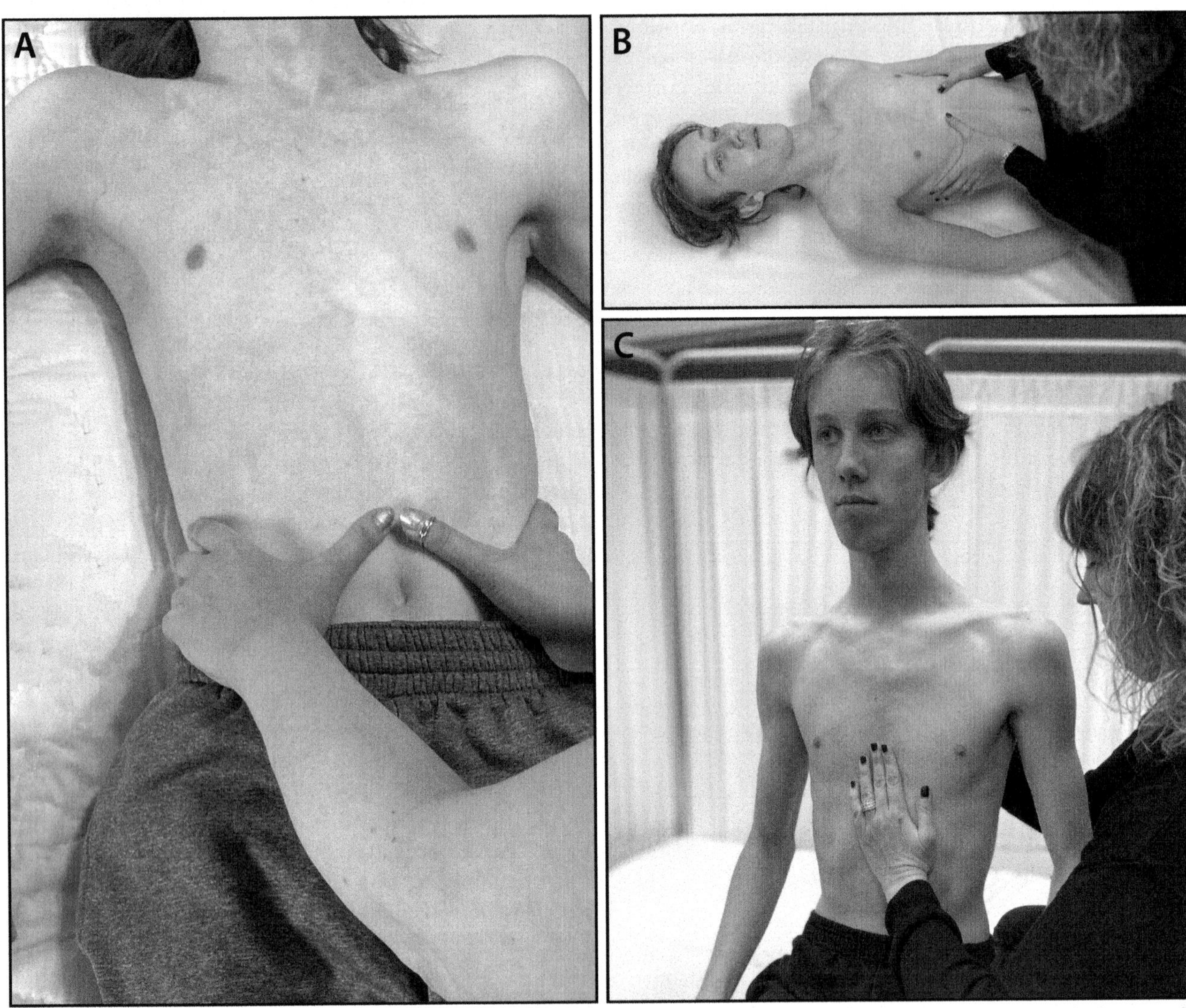


**Figure 18-11.** Manually assisted coughing. (A) The butterfly technique. (B) A manually assisted cough with rib compression. (C) The manually assisted cough abdominal thrust technique. (Note: The patient would typically be supported in a chair or in the supine position. The patient is unsupported to allow better visualization of hand placement.)

lower aspect of the ribs with the fingers wrapped laterally around the patient's sides, the fingers pointed posteriorly, and the thumbs pointing inward toward the center of the chest. The patient is asked to take a deep breath, and as the patient exhales, the clinician instructs the patient to cough; the clinician assists by gently compressing the ribs up and in using a firm steady pressure (Figure 18-11B).[3] Using an alternative hand position, the clinician can place their hand in the epigastric area, distal to the xiphoid process, as shown in Figure 18-11C. The patient is instructed to cough as the clinician simultaneously compresses the abdomen inward and upward (ie, the abdominal thrust method). The clinician should not apply direct pressure over the xiphoid.[3] This technique is less comfortable for the patient.

### Clinical Tips

Instruct the patient to turn their head away from the clinician when completing the cough. Use appropriate infection control precautions.

## Active Cycle of Breathing, Positive Expiratory Pressure, and Oscillation to Facilitate Cough

The **active cycle of breathing** technique is a directed cough technique that includes relaxed diaphragmatic breathing repetitions (breathing control phase) followed by deep breathing (thoracic expansion exercises) and a forced exhalation technique (huffing) to remove secretions. The breathing control phase includes at least 1 minute of relaxed breathing. The thoracic expansion includes 3 to 4 deep inhalations with a 3-second hold followed by another period of relaxed breathing. The patient assesses if there are secretions ready for removal; if so, the patient completes a couple of repetitions of huffing. If there are not secretions, the patient repeats the first 2 steps until readiness to huff is determined. The cycle continues until the secretions are removed.[2,9]

PEP uses exhalation against a fixed resistance to create an increase in airway pressure. The Acapella (Smiths Medical) and flutter valves are examples of PEP devices; they create PEPs and vibration to keep the airways open and to loosen sections (Figure 18-12). PEP is an effective way to remove airway secretions.[9]

High-frequency chest wall oscillation or high-frequency chest compression devices are effective at increasing pulmonary airflow and improving mucus expectoration. These devices include vests with air channels and a compressor that inflates and deflates the vest with air. The patient dons the vest, and vest inflation creates external pressure; the amount of "squeeze" (perception of pressure) and the vibration frequency can be modulated. This intervention can be used concurrently with aerosol respiratory treatments. The patient can complete this intervention without caregiver assistance.[9] A commonly prescribed vest is the SmartVest (Electromed, Inc).

### *Contraindications for Coughing Interventions*

Relative contraindications to the inclusion of directed cough interventions include infection with pathogens transmittable by droplet nuclei (ie, tuberculosis); elevated intracranial pressure; intracranial aneurysm; acute myocardial infarction; and acute unstable head, neck, or spine injury. Manually assisted directed coughing with pressure to the epigastrium may be contraindicated in the presence of potential for regurgitation/aspiration, acute abdominal pathology, abdominal aortic aneurysm, hiatal hernia, or pregnancy and an untreated pneumothorax. Manually assisted directed coughing with pressure to the thoracic cage is contraindicated in the presence of osteoporosis, rib fracture, and flail chest.[40]

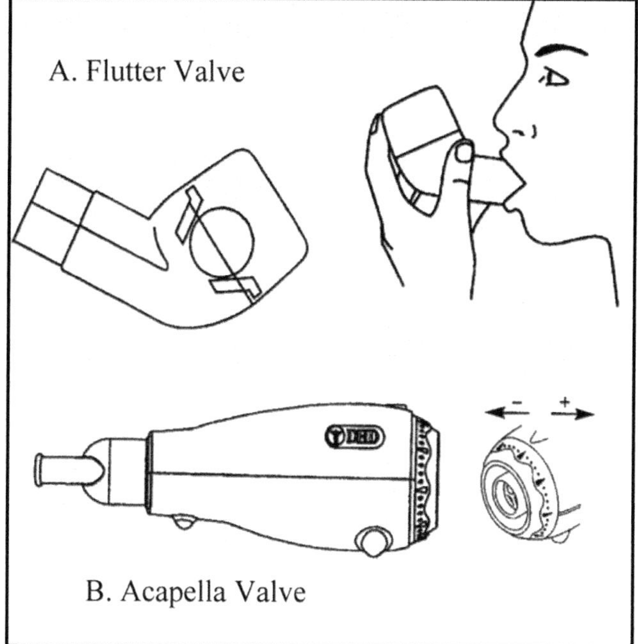


**Figure 18-12.** PEP devices. (A) A flutter valve. (B) The Acapella device. (Reproduced with permission from Volsko TA, Di Fiore JM, Chatburn RL. Performance comparison of two oscillating positive expiratory pressure devices: Acapella versus Flutter. *Respir Care.* 2003;48[2]:124-130.)

## Postural Drainage and Chest Physical Therapy

Postural drainage facilitates secretion mobilization out of a lung segment and into the central airway so it can be cleared by coughing. The patient is moved through a series of positions that target the drainage of each respective lung segment (Figure 18-13). Patient positions can be modified if needed based on the patient's presentation and/or medical pathologies/condition.

**Chest physical therapy** uses cupping/percussion and vibration manual techniques together with postural drainage positioning to mobilize secretions, improve ventilation, and prevent atelectasis. Percussion or cupping is performed by cupping the hands and striking the patient's chest wall over the affected lobe in a rhythmic manner. Appropriate hand position results in a hollow sound (vs a slapping sound) when contact is made with the patient's thorax. Percussion can be completed using plastic percussor cups or a mechanical percussor. Vibration or shaking is applied only during the expiratory phase of breathing over the affected area of the lung after postural drainage positioning and percussion. With both hands flat over the area of the thorax, the therapist uses quick, jerky, small upper extremity isometric contractions to create the vibration over the segment with pressure in the direction of the thorax movement that occurs during the respiratory cycle. The therapist initiates this treatment while the patient is in the postural drainage position for the most affected lobe first. After the vibrations, the patient is instructed to huff and/or cough to clear secretions. The patient moves into the next position. The patient's ability to tolerate positional changes and the length of treatment vary. Continuous monitoring of the patient's response is indicated.[2,3,9]

### *Contraindications and Precautions for Postural Drainage and Percussion*

Contraindications for the use of postural drainage include intracranial pressure greater than 20 mm Hg, rib fractures/osteoporosis, active untreated pneumothorax, unstable head/neck injuries, active hemorrhage, empyema, pulmonary emboli, surgical wounds, pulmonary edema/CHF, and the presence of a bronchopleural fistula. Precautions (especially in the Trendelenburg/head-down position) include increased intracranial pressure, acute CHF, hiatal hernia, uncontrolled hypertension, distended abdomen, aspiration, recent food consumption, and postoperative craniotomy.[2,3,9,41]

Contraindications/precautions for the use of percussion/vibration include osteoporosis, osteomyelitis, rib fractures/flail chest, tuberculosis, chest wall wounds/grafts, coagulopathy, frank hemoptysis, and long-term steroid use.[2,3,9,41]

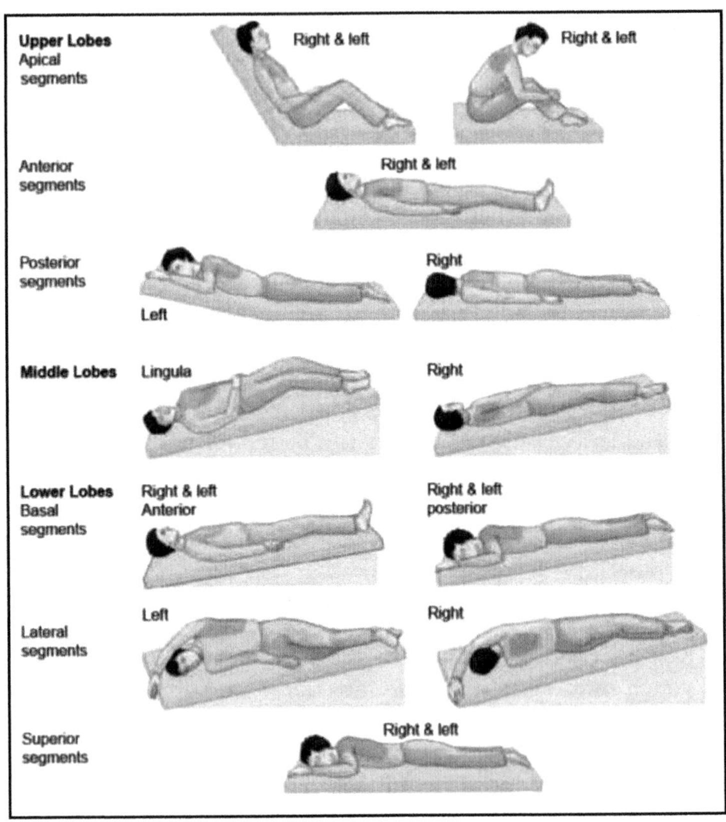


**Figure 18-13.** Postural drainage positions. (Reproduced with permission from Craven RF, Hirnle C, Henshaw C. *Fundamentals of Nursing: Concepts and Competencies for Practice*. 9th ed. Wolters Kluwer; 2020.)

## Implementing Aerobic and Strengthening Exercises

The aerobic training portion of a pulmonary rehabilitation session includes the following typical aerobic exercise components: warm-up, aerobic exercise, and cooldown. A graded exercise test with electrocardiographic monitoring provides parameters for exercise intensity. The therapist ensures that the patient has a rescue inhaler present (if indicated) and access to supplemental oxygen as appropriate. The most common modes of exercise include a treadmill, stationary bike, and arm ergometer. The duration and intensity of the exercise need to be carefully initiated, monitored, and progressed for patients with pulmonary compromise. Patients may have difficulty tolerating exercise sessions and often require frequent rest periods. Exercise progression focuses on increasing the duration of exercise and decreasing the rest periods. Once the patient can tolerate 20 minutes of exercise, then the therapist can increase the intensity or duration, but they should only adjust one variable at a time. Exercise intensity can be increased after the patient describes the current intensity as "too easy" or when the patient's exercise HR has dropped (compared with earlier sessions), indicating that the patient has adapted to the current workload. Patient monitoring during exercise should include HR, RR, oxygen saturation, RPD, and rate of perceived exertion.[9]

Performing upper and lower extremity strengthening exercises, either alone or in conjunction with endurance exercise, is beneficial for pulmonary patients. Increased strength can improve the ability to complete functional tasks and ADLs. Participation in a regular strengthening program is associated with greater survival rates for patients with COPD.[42,43]

## Monitoring and Intervention Considerations for Various Pulmonary Pathologies

The clinician should complete routine monitoring of HR, RR, blood pressure, RPD, and oxygen saturation before and after treatment.

### *Monitoring Related to Commonly Prescribed Medications*

Patients with respiratory diagnoses often take medication to assist with managing the disease. Each type of medication is typically prescribed to either prevent or ease a patient's symptoms or to maximize a patient's breathing ability or overall health. Some of the medications are taken daily, and some (eg, a rescue inhaler) are taken when the patient experiences an abrupt onset of difficulty breathing.

The patient (or caregiver) should have a clear understanding of when and how each medicine should be taken; questions regarding the medication timing or administration should be directed to the physician. Specific respiratory medications are described later; additional medications are listed in Appendix E.

Individuals with pulmonary pathology are often prescribed medications, including bronchodilators (to relieve shortness of breath), combination medications (bronchodilators/anti-inflammatories to relieve shortness of breath and to prevent flare-ups), and antibiotics (to treat infections).[44] Regular vaccinations (flu and pneumococcal) are recommended. Many medications used to manage respiratory disease are administered using an inhaler or a nebulizer. There are 2 main types of medications used to create bronchodilation (opening the airways for the patient): beta2-agonists and anticholinergics. Beta2-agonists are commonly used to relieve breathlessness. Short-acting beta2-agonists are used as a way to open airways quickly. The patient may call this a "rescue" inhaler. Long-acting beta2-agonists are prescribed to be taken regularly; they minimize symptoms for longer periods of time (to prevent/minimize episodes of shortness of breath). Anticholinergics relieve breathlessness, but they work in the body in a different way than beta2-agonists. They are inhaled medicines; there are short-acting and long-acting anticholinergics.[44] As the patient's disease worsens, they may take a number of these medications in combination.

Regular use of corticosteroids may increase the patient's risk of osteoporosis. The assistant should consider the benefits of weight-bearing exercises and be aware of contraindications and precautions for osteoporosis. Exercise should be terminated if oxygen saturation levels fall below 90% (unless other levels are documented in the physician's orders). The assistant should monitor the patient for side effects of bronchodilator medications (ie, palpitations, increased HR, nervousness, and cough) and observe for any new arrhythmia or signs and symptoms that may indicate toxicity (nervousness, confusion, and tremors).[44]

## Asthma

Patients with asthma should exercise in a trigger-free environment (ie, avoid cold, pollution, and smoke). Low-intensity exercise may minimize the occurrence of bronchospasms. If an inhaler is prescribed for pre-exercise use, ensure the patient uses it as prescribed. Patients can use a peak flow meter to monitor their expiratory capability. The device measures how fast air leaves the lungs during a forcible exhalation (Figure 18-14). Decreases in peak flow readings indicate a decline in pulmonary function; the assistant should discuss any changes with the physical therapist before proceeding with treatment.

A general goal is 20 to 30 minutes of aerobic activity 3 to 5 times a week at 50% of peak oxygen uptake or as tolerated by symptoms. A longer warm-up may help to minimize symptoms. Swimming is usually well tolerated by persons with exercise-induced asthma because the warm, moist air reduces the risk of triggering an asthma attack. If a patient experiences an asthma attack, assist the patient to a seated position and have the patient administer their fast-acting (rescue) inhaler. Encourage relaxed breathing and pursed lip exhalation. Immediate medical care should be obtained if a patient becomes cyanotic, peak flow is less than 250 (L/min), or the patient is still short of breath after 3 doses of the inhaler.[2,4,45]

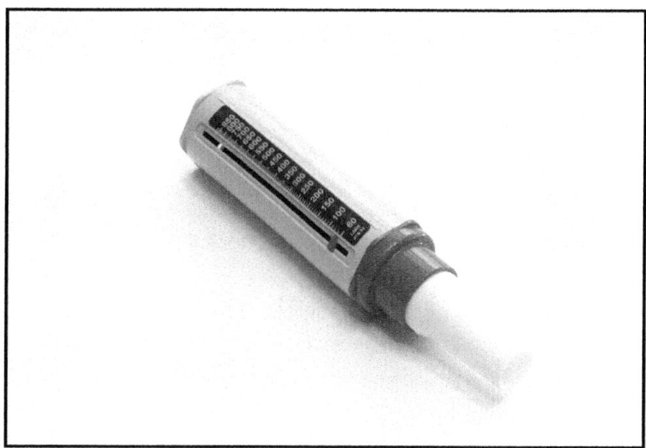

**Figure 18-14.** Peak flow meter measures expired air from the lungs (Blue Planet Earth/Shutterstock.com).

## Atelectasis

Atelectasis is a common breathing problem after surgery due to general anesthesia use. Early ambulation can reduce postoperative complications and promote airway clearance.[39] Deep breathing and coughing techniques help to prevent atelectasis. The incentive spirometer, segmental breathing techniques, and manual cues can facilitate expansion of the lower lobes.

## Chronic Obstructive Pulmonary Disease

Forced coughing should be avoided because it increases intrathoracic pressure and the closure of small airways in patients with COPD. Huffing allows a forced expiration while maintaining a stable open airway, making secretion removal more effective.[9] Upper and lower extremity resistance training/strengthening exercises using the FITT (frequency, intensity, time, type) parameters may lead to improved functional outcomes for patients with COPD.[42,43,46,47]

Light- and moderate-intensity aerobic exercise are associated with improved QOL, symptoms, and ADL abilities. The therapist should gradually increase the patient's program when appropriate to include aerobic exercise 3 to 5 days a week. Intensity can be light to vigorous based on the patient's tolerance.[46]

### Documentation Tip

When working with a patient with COPD who is using supplemental oxygen, document all aspects of patient presentation that are affected by exercise. For example, if a patient ambulates 50 feet (ft) during the therapy session, the assistant will document the patient's status throughout the activity. The documentation could look like the following:

Vital signs (VS) at rest: 118/78 mm Hg, 72 beats/minute, 16 RR, $O_2$ saturation of 95% on 2 L $O_2$ via nasal cannula (NC)

The patient ambulates 50 ft with rolling walker (RW) with one standing rest period. The patient requires verbal cues (VC) for pursed lip breathing as ambulation distance increases. VS postambulation: 138/78 mm Hg, 92 beats/minute, 24 RR, $O_2$ saturation 91% on 2 L $O_2$ via NC. VS recovery to resting rates after 2 minutes in seated with VC for pursed lip breathing. Patient reports distance is limited by fatigue.

## *Pulmonary Embolus*

A pulmonary embolus is an urgent condition requiring immediate medical attention. A pulmonary embolus results from a clot occluding a pulmonary artery, and if not treated emergently, it can lead to lung infarction and possible death. Signs or symptoms consistent with a pulmonary embolus include severe shortness of breath, fast RR, hemoptysis, rapid HR, pleuritic pain, and sudden anxiety/apprehension. These patients require immediate activation of the emergency medical system (call 911 or the inpatient emergency medical team).

## *Spinal Cord Injury*

Some patients with tetraplegia may have respiratory insufficiency because of the spinal level injury. Pneumonia is one of the most common complications and causes of death in patients with cervical SCI.[48] Oftentimes the respiratory muscles are weak, reducing lung volumes and the patient's ability to produce an effective cough. Manually assisted coughing techniques (see Figure 18-11) may be paired with the use of an abdominal binder to improve coughing.[3] RMT can improve expiratory muscle strength, vital capacity, and residual volume in patients with SCIs.[48]

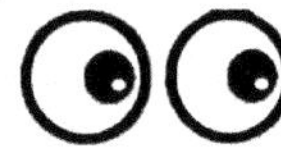

### Eye on the Research

The joint American College of Chest Physicians/American Association of Cardiovascular and Pulmonary Rehabilitation guidelines report that pulmonary rehabilitation and lower and upper extremity exercise training can improve dyspnea and health-related QOL.[49] Longer-term rehabilitation, maintenance strategies after rehabilitation, and the incorporation of education and strength training in pulmonary rehabilitation are beneficial. The guidelines note that pulmonary rehabilitation may be beneficial for patients with chronic lung diseases other than COPD.[49]

McCarthy et al[50] reported clinically significant improvements in dyspnea and fatigue, improved emotional function, and an increased sense of control after pulmonary rehabilitation. They reported improvement in health-related QOL and exercise capacity. Camillo et al[51] reported a correlation between patient improvement in functional performance after pulmonary rehabilitation programs and 5-year survival rates. Puhan et al[52] summarized that pulmonary rehabilitation results in improved QOL and exercise capacity. Australia and New Zealand recommend pulmonary rehabilitation and regular exercise for all patients with symptomatic COPD in their guidelines for the diagnosis and management of COPD.[53]

# Conclusion

Pulmonary rehabilitation programs include a supervised exercise program and a combination of any of the following activities: breathing exercises, RMT, strength training, aerobic exercise, patient education, and psychosocial support. Rehabilitation interventions are beneficial for patients with pulmonary pathologies. Patient outcomes are typically assessed subjectively using health QOL tools; strength, endurance, and functional mobility improvements are assessed using objective measures. The physical therapist assistant applies knowledge of the varied diagnoses and comorbidities to select the appropriate training techniques based on the patient's status and pulmonary conditions.

## Review Questions

1. Compare and contrast normal and abnormal breath sounds.
2. What should the physical therapist assistant monitor when treating a patient with a pulmonary diagnosis?
3. List and describe 2 breathing exercises.
4. Compare and contrast coughing and huffing. Which intervention might be more beneficial for a patient with COPD? Why?
5. List the contraindications for completing percussion on a patient as part of a pulmonary hygiene program.
6. With which diagnoses is the incorporation of postural drainage using the reverse Trendelenburg position contraindicated?
7. What is the most appropriate sequence of actions to complete in the following situation? A patient with COPD presents with an oxygen saturation of 97% before treatment. The physical therapist assistant is planning to have the patient perform seated exercises and then walk with a rolling walker. After the exercises are completed, the patient's oxygen saturation level is 88%.
8. Which pulmonary function test values are typically decreased for a patient with a restrictive lung disease?
9. List the indications and contraindications for completing respiratory muscle training.
10. Application for the athlete: Why does a person squat and brace hands on the thighs after completing a distance run when they are out of breath?

## Case Study

A 66-year-old with emphysema presents in the subacute setting with deconditioning after pneumonia (after 5 days of hospitalization). The patient is receiving nebulizer breathing treatments twice a day and continues on intravenous antibiotics. Before onset, the patient was independent community level, ambulating without an assistive device, using oxygen at 2 L continuously, driving, and completing all instrumental ADLs (with increased time and rest periods). Upper extremity and lower extremity strength are 4/5 throughout. The patient currently requires minimal assistance with all mobility and is ambulating 24 ft before needing to rest due to dyspnea on exertion. The patient is motivated but fatigues quickly, and tasks are limited by dyspnea on exertion. The physical therapy plan of care includes patient education, energy conservation training, progressive gait training, resistance exercise, balance exercises, and vital sign monitoring, with progression as tolerated.

1. What monitoring should the physical therapist assistant complete? When should the monitoring occur?
2. Which functional assessment tool is appropriate to complete with this patient?
3. Which breathing exercises are most appropriate?
4. List at least 3 exercises that are indicated given the patient's presentation.
5. Which functional training activities are most appropriate?

This same patient has made significant progress, and 6 weeks later has progressed from a skilled nursing facility and home care into an outpatient physical therapy setting. The patient can ambulate 150 ft with a rolling walker before needing to rest. The patient reports ongoing difficulty with ascending and descending stairs (requiring 2 rest periods to ascend/descend 12 steps). The patient's goal is to be able to "do stairs" without a rest, return to tai chi classes 3 times a week, and return to ambulation without an assistive device (patient reports ambulating community-level distances without a device before onset).

6. What monitoring should the physical therapist assistant complete? When should the monitoring occur?
7. Which functional assessment tool is appropriate to complete with this patient?
8. Which breathing exercises are most appropriate?
9. List at least 3 exercises that are indicated given the patient's presentation.
10. Which functional training activities are most appropriate?

## Suggested Resources

Baseline Dyspnea/Transition Index: https://www.ser.es/wp-content/uploads/2016/09/BDI-TDI-pdf.pdf

Breath stacking guidelines and handout for patients: https://www.physio-pedia.com/Breath_Stacking

COPD Assessment Test: https://www.catestonline.org/content/dam/global/catestonline/questionnaires/English_CAT_combined.pdf

Heart Online. Heart Education Assessment Rehabilitation Toolkit. Rating of perceived exertion: Borg scales. November 2014. https://www.heartonline.org.au/media/DRL/Rating_of_perceived_exertion_-_Borg_scale.pdf

Respiratory muscles exercise video: https://www.youtube.com/watch?v=Kp8WK4hFsTs

### *Assessment Tools for the Pulmonary Patient*

6MWT: Shirley Ryan Ability Lab. Six-minute walk test. April 3, 2013. Accessed February 7, 2023. https://www.sralab.org/rehabilitation-measures/6-minute-walk-test

ISWT: Lung Foundation Australia. Pulmonary rehabilitation toolkit: incremental 10-meter shuttle walk test. 2016. Accessed February 7, 2023. https://pulmonaryrehab.com.au/patient-assessment/assessing-exercise-capacity/incremental-shuttle-walking-test/

# References


1. Jolley C. Frontiers in sport and exercise science and medicine seminar on inspiratory muscle training. Centre for Sports Medicine and Human Performance, Brunel University; April 2013.
2. Hillegass E. *Essentials of Cardiopulmonary Physical Therapy.* 3rd ed. Elsevier; 2011.
3. Kisner C. Management of pulmonary conditions. In: Kisner C, Colby LA, eds. *Therapeutic Exercise Foundations and Techniques.* 5th ed. FA Davis; 2005:851-876.
4. Packel L. The respiratory system. In: Goodman CC, Fuller KS, eds. *Pathology: Implications for the Physical Therapist.* 4th ed. Elsevier; 2015:772-836.
5. Kim KS, Byun MK, Lee WH, Cynn HS, Kwon OY, Yi CH. Effects of breathing maneuver and sitting posture on muscle activity in inspiratory accessory muscles in patients with chronic obstructive pulmonary disease. *Multidiscip Respir Med.* 2012;7(1):9. doi:10.1186/2049-6958-7-9
6. Crisafulli E, Clini EM. Measures of dyspnea in pulmonary rehabilitation. *Multidiscip Respir Med.* 2010;5(3):202-210. doi:10.1186/2049-6958-5-3-202
7. Pianosi PT, Zhang Z, Hernandez P, Huebner M. Measuring dyspnea and perceived exertion in healthy adults and with respiratory disease: new pictorial scales. *Sports Med Open.* 2016;2:17.
8. Hareendran A, Leidy NK, Monz BU, Winnette R, Becker K, Mahler DA. Proposing a standardized method for evaluating patient report of the intensity of dyspnea during exercise testing in COPD. *Int J Chron Obstruct Pulmon Dis.* 2012;7:345-55. doi:10.2147/COPD.S29571
9. Starr JA. Chronic pulmonary dysfunction. In: O'Sullivan SB, Schmitz TJ, Fulk GD, eds: *Physical Rehabilitation.* 7th ed. FA Davis; 2014:434-464.
10. Mahler DA, Wells CK. Evaluation of clinical methods for rating dyspnea. *Chest.* 1988;93(3):580-586.
11. Wijkstra PJ, TenVergert EM, Van Altena R, et al. Reliability and validity of the chronic respiratory questionnaire (CRQ). *Thorax.* 1994;49(5):465-467.
12. Lanza FC, Castro RAS, de Camargo AA, et al. COPD assessment test (CAT) is a valid and simple tool to measure the impact of bronchiectasis on affected patients. *COPD.* 2018;15(5):512-519. doi:10.1080/15412555.2018.1540034
13. Puhan MA, Mador MJ, Held U, Goldstein R, Guyatt GH, Schünemann HJ. Interpretation of treatment changes in 6-minute walk distance in patients with COPD. *Eur Respir J.* 2008;32(3):637-643. doi:10.1183/09031936.00140507
14. Singh SJ, Puhan MA, Andrianopoulos V, et al. An official systematic review of the European Respiratory Society/American Thoracic Society: measurement properties of field walking tests in chronic respiratory disease. *Eur Respir J.* 2014;44(6):1447-1478. doi:10.1183/09031936.00150414
15. Kaymaz D, Candemir İÇ, Ergün P, Demir N, Taşdemir F, Demir P. Relation between upper-limb muscle strength with exercise capacity, quality of life and dyspnea in patients with severe chronic obstructive pulmonary disease. *Clin Respir J.* 2018;12(3):1257-1263. doi:10.1111/crj.12659
16. Dourado VZ, Antunes LC, Tanni SE, de Paiva SA, Padovani CR, Godoy I. Relationship of upper-limb and thoracic muscle strength to 6-min walk distance in COPD patients. *Chest.* 2006;129(3):551-557.
17. Lung Foundation Australia. Safety issues relating to exercise assessment. 2016. Accessed February 7, 2023. https://pulmonaryrehab.com.au/patient-assessment/assessing-exercise-capacity/safety-issues-relating-to-exercise-assessment-and/
18. Bott J, Blumenthal S, Buxton M, et al. BTS/ACPRC guidelines for the physiotherapy management of the adult, medical, spontaneously breathing patient. *Thorax.* 2009;64(suppl I):i1-i51. doi:10.1136/thx.2008.110726
19. Dechman G, Wilson CR. Evidence underlying breathing retraining in people with stable chronic obstructive pulmonary disease. *Phys Ther.* 2004;84(12):1189-1197.
20. Cahalin LP, Braga M, Matsuo Y, Hernandez ED. Efficacy of diaphragmatic breathing in persons with chronic obstructive pulmonary disease: a review of the literature. *J Cardiopulm Rehabil.* 2002;22(1):7-21.
21. Fernandes M, Cukier A, Feltrim MI. Efficacy of diaphragmatic breathing in patients with chronic obstructive pulmonary disease. *Chron Respir Dis.* 2011;8(4):237-244. doi:10.1177/1479972311424296
22. Crisafulli E, Costi S, Fabbri LM, Clini EM. Respiratory muscles training in COPD patients. *Intl J Chron Obstruct Pulmon Dis.* 2007:2(1):19-25.
23. Sarmento A, Dornelas de Andrade AF, Lima IN, Aliverti A, Augusto de Freitas Fregonezi G, Resqueti VR. Air stacking: a detailed look into physiological acute effects on cough peak flow and chest wall volumes of healthy subjects. *Respir Care.* 2017;6(4):432-433.
24. Hanania NA, O'Donnell DE. Activity-related dyspnea in chronic obstructive pulmonary disease: physical and psychological consequences, unmet needs, and future directions. *Int J Chron Obstruct Pulmon Dis.* 2019;14:1127-1138.
25. Geddes EL, O'Brien K, Reid WD, Brooks D, Crowe J. Inspiratory muscle training in adults with chronic obstructive pulmonary disease: an update of a systematic review. *Respir Med.* 2008;102(12):1715-1729. doi:10.1016/j.rmed.2008.07.005
26. Gomes-Neto M, Saquetto MB, Silva CM, Carvalho VO, Ribeiro N, Conceição CS. Effects of respiratory muscle training on respiratory function, respiratory muscle strength, and exercise tolerance in patients poststroke: a systematic review with meta-analysis. *Arch Phys Med Rehabil.* 2016;97(11):1994-2001. doi:10.1016/j.apmr.2016.04.018
27. Berlowitz DJ, Tamplin J. Respiratory muscle training for cervical spinal cord injury. *Cochrane Database Syst Rev.* 2013;7:CD008507. doi:10.1002/14651858.CD008507.pub2
28. O'Brien K, Geddes EL, Reid WD, Brooks D, Crowe J. Inspiratory muscle training compared with other rehabilitation interventions in chronic obstructive pulmonary disease: a systematic review update. *J Cardiopulm Rehabil Prev.* 2008;28(2):128-41. doi:10.1097/01.HCR.0000314208.40170.00
29. Sales AT, Fregonezi GA de F, Ramsook AH, Guenette JA, Lima INDF, Reid WD. Respiratory muscle endurance after training in athletes and non-athletes: a systematic review and meta-analysis. *Phys Ther Sport.* 2016;17:76-86.
30. McConnell A. Implementing respiratory muscle training. In: *Respiratory Muscle Training: Theory and Practice.* Elsevier; 2013.

31. Neves LF, Reis MH, Plentz RD, Matte DL, Coronel CC, Sbruzzi G. Expiratory and expiratory plus inspiratory muscle training improves respiratory muscle strength in subjects with COPD: systematic review. *Respir Care.* 2014;59(9):1381-1388. doi:10.4187/respcare.02793
32. Myers TR. Positive expiratory pressure and oscillatory positive expiratory pressure therapies. *Respir Care.* 2007;52(10):1308-1326; discussion 1327.
33. Fink JB. Forced expiratory technique, directed cough, and autogenic drainage. *Respir Care.* 2007;52(9):1210-1221; discussion 1221-1223.
34. van der Schans CP. Conventional chest physical therapy for obstructive lung disease. *Respir Care.* 2007;52(9):1198-1206; discussion 1206-1209.
35. Lee AL, Williamson HC, Lorensini S, Spencer LM. The effects of oscillating positive expiratory pressure therapy in adults with stable non-cystic fibrosis bronchiectasis: a systematic review. *Chron Respir Dis.* 2015;12(1):36-46. doi:10.1177/1479972314562407
36. McIlwaine M, Button B, Dwan K. Positive expiratory pressure physiotherapy for airway clearance in people with cystic fibrosis. *Cochrane Database Syst Rev.* 2015;6:CD003147. doi:10.1002/14651858.CD003147.pub4
37. Mckoy NA, Wilson LM, Saldanha IJ, Odelola OA, Robinson KA. Active cycle of breathing technique for cystic fibrosis. *Cochrane Database Syst Rev.* 2016;7:CD007862. doi:10.1002/14651858.CD007862.pub4
38. Morrison L, Innes S. Oscillating devices for airway clearance in people with cystic fibrosis. *Cochrane Database Syst Rev.* 2017;5:CD006842. doi:10.1002/14651858.CD006842.pub4
39. Strickland SL, Rubin BK, Drescher GS, et al. AARC clinical practice guideline: effectiveness of nonpharmacologic airway clearance therapies in hospitalized patients. *Respir Care.* 2013;58(12):2187-2193. doi:10.4187/respcare.02925
40. AARC clinical practice guideline. Directed cough. American Association for Respiratory Care. *Respir Care.* 1993;38(5):495-499.
41. Coglianese D. *Clinical Exercise Pathophysiology for Physical Therapy: Examination, Testing, and Exercise Prescription for Movement-Related Disorders.* SLACK Incorporated; 2015.
42. Liao WH, Chen JW, Chen X, et al. Impact of resistance training in subjects with COPD: a systematic review and meta-analysis. *Respir Care.* 2015;60(8):1130-1145. doi:10.4187/respcare.03598
43. Loprinzi PD, Sng E, Walker JF. Muscle strengthening activity associates with reduced all-cause mortality in COPD. *Chronic Illn.* 2017;13(2):140-147. doi:10.1177/1742395316657399
44. Ciccone C. *Pharmacology in Rehabilitation.* 4th ed. FA Davis; 2007.
45. Asthma. In: Goodman C, Helgeson K, eds. *Exercise Prescription for Medical Conditions: Handbook for Physical Therapists.* FA Davis; 2011.
46. Pescatello L, ed. *ACSM's Guidelines for Exercise Testing and Prescription.* 9th ed. Wolters Kluwer/Lippincott Williams & Wilkins, ACSM; 2014.
47. Iepsen UW, Jørgensen KJ, Ringbæk T, Hansen H, Skrubbeltrang C, Lange P. A combination of resistance and endurance training increases leg muscle strength in COPD: an evidence-based recommendation based on systematic review with meta-analyses. *Chron Respir Dis.* 2015;12(2):132-145. doi:10.1177/1479972315575318
48. Van Houtte S, Vanlandewijck Y, Gosselink R. Respiratory muscle training in persons with spinal cord injury: a systematic review. *Respir Med.* 2006;100(11):1886-1895.
49. Ries AL, Bauldoff GS, Carlin BW, et al. Pulmonary rehabilitation: joint ACCP/AACVPR evidence-based clinical practice guidelines. *Chest.* 2007;131(suppl):4S-42S.
50. McCarthy B, Casey D, Devane D, Murphy K, Murphy E, Lacasse Y. Pulmonary rehabilitation for chronic obstructive pulmonary disease. *Cochrane Database Syst Rev.* 2015;2:CD003793. doi:10.1002/14651858.CD003793.pub3
51. Camillo CA, Langer D, Osadnik CR, et al. Survival after pulmonary rehabilitation in patients with COPD: impact of functional exercise capacity and its changes. *Int J Chron Obstruct Pulmon Dis.* 2016:11:2671-2679.
52. Puhan MA, Gimeno-Santos E, Cates CJ, Troosters T. Pulmonary rehabilitation following exacerbations of chronic obstructive pulmonary disease. *Cochrane Database Syst Rev.* 2016;12:CD005305. doi:10.1002/14651858.CD005305.pub4
53. Yang IA, Brown JL, George J, et al. COPD-X Australian and New Zealand guidelines for the diagnosis and management of chronic obstructive pulmonary disease: 2017 update. *Med J Aust.* 2017:207(10):436-442. doi:10.5694/mja17.00686

Chapter 19

# Physical Therapy Interventions for Persons With an Oncologic and/or Lymphedema Diagnosis

*Kevin Kunkel, PT, MSPT, PhD*

**KEY TERMS** Axillary web syndrome | Complete decongestive therapy | Manual lymphatic drainage | Primary lymphedema | Radiation fibrosis | Secondary lymphedema

## Chapter Objectives

1. List the major types and stages of cancers and the resultant impairments that may indicate a need for physical therapy intervention.
2. Describe the impairments and functional limitations associated with cancer treatments.
3. Describe the stages of lymphedema.
4. Discuss the underlying premorbid postural deficits that could affect post–cancer treatment impairments.
5. Describe the contraindications and precautions for the treatment of a patient with lymphedema.
6. Discuss the signs and symptoms of cellulitis and erysipelas.
7. Describe the components of complete decongestive therapy (CDT).
8. Recognize the appropriate time to use a yoga-based breathing and upper extremity therapeutic exercise regimen for patient's with cancer and cancer survivors.

"Cancer is caused by the alterations in normal genes, especially those regulating cell growth and differentiation processes."[1] The American Cancer Association estimated 836,150 new cases in men, with the top 3 types being prostate, lung and bronchus, and colon and rectum. Other types of cancer noted in men include urinary/bladder, melanoma of the skin, kidney and renal pelvis, non-Hodgkin lymphoma, leukemia, oral cavity and pharynx, and liver and intrahepatic bile duct, which identify the top 10. New cases in women were estimated at 852,630 cases, with the top 3 being breast, lung and bronchus, and colon and rectum. Other types observed in women include uterine corpus, thyroid, melanoma of the skin, non-Hodgkin lymphoma, leukemia, pancreas and kidney, and renal pelvis.[2] Cancer survivorship has dramatically improved over the past several decades because of improvements in detection and treatment. The prevalence of cancer in our society is increasing as the population ages. More than 15.5 million Americans with a history of cancer were still alive as of January 2016, and it is estimated that by January 2026 more than 20 million Americans will be a survivor.[3]



Kopack JK, Cascardi KA.
*Principles of Therapeutic Exercise for the Physical Therapist Assistant* (pp 645-665).

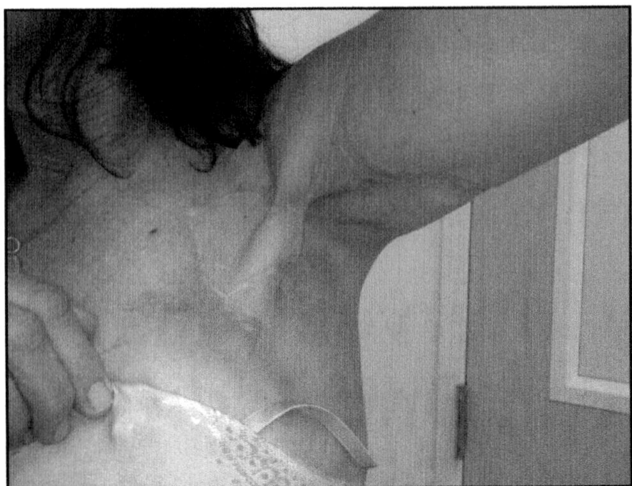

**Figure 19-1.** AWS.

Many health care practitioners are involved with the care of a person with cancer. Caregivers may include (but are not limited to) an internal medicine physician and/or nurse practitioner, oncologist, radiation oncologist, nurses, physical therapists, technicians, and aides. Which practitioner is responsible for creating a referral for physical therapy? Once the primary care professional has referred the patient to an oncologist, it may be months or 1 year before the patient returns to their care. If the oncologist refers the patient to a radiation oncologist and both physicians are treating the patient, either could make a referral. Recently, a subspecialty within physical medicine and rehabilitation physicians or physiatry has emerged, with physiatrists now specializing in cancer rehabilitation. However, when 97 physiatrists were surveyed, most of the physiatrists "considered themselves ill equipped to provide appropriate rehabilitation services."[4]

Once a referral for physical therapy is obtained, the patient must find a physical therapist who has the experience and knowledge to treat them. Practitioners trained and certified in treating lymphedema often treat patients with cancer. Unfortunately, only a small percentage of therapists and assistants obtain lymphedema certification, which creates a void in many communities in search for qualified therapists. The purpose of this chapter is to identify the impairments typically associated with cancer treatment and those impairments commonly observed in patients with lymphedema/edema. The information will serve as a guide to creating specific interventions and addressing the impairments that often accompany treatments for cancer or those associated with lymphedema.

The treatments for cancer are diverse and can include any of the following: surgery, chemotherapy, and radiation. Surgical procedures often are the first method of attempted eradication of the disease by physically removing the tumor. The use of chemotherapy and/or radiation therapy before, during, or after surgery are complementary courses of treatment. Individually or in combination, the interventions to treat cancer have the potential of resulting in physical impairments. These physical impairments may lead to functional limitations that affect a patient's ability to participate in activities of daily living (ADLs). Multiple systemic deficits can occur such as generalized weakness, cachexia, fatigue, and agility (the ability to move quickly and easily). Localized impairments such as trismus (lockjaw), **axillary web syndrome (AWS)**, and pelvic floor dysfunction can also occur. Trismus is a complication affecting the mastication muscles and is associated with head and neck cancer. AWS is a condition that develops in the axilla in which the soft tissue in the area becomes cord- or rope-like; this can cause pain and limit shoulder mobility (Figure 19-1). It usually occurs 1 to 2 months after breast cancer surgery. This condition and treatment are discussed in more depth later in this chapter.

The ability for the physical therapist to effectively evaluate and create a plan of care is important. The ability of the therapist or physical therapist assistant to deliver effective treatments and to perform appropriate therapeutic exercise is essential to the patient's recovery. Clinicians certified in lymphedema are specially trained in treating patients with cancer and/or lymphedema. Physical therapist assistants interested in working with this population will benefit from pursuing continuing education/certification.

## General Exercise Precautions

There are several considerations when developing an exercise program for patients who have undergone cancer treatment. For example, patients who have undergone surgery with specific nodal dissections are at risk of developing lymphedema. Lymphedema can result from damage to the lymphatic system, resulting in the inability of the body to remove interstitial fluid and return it to the blood circulatory system. When initiating an exercise program, the intensity should be at a low to moderate level to determine the effect and response on the body. If the patient's arm begins to feel heavy, it may be an indication of the onset of lymphedema. Wearing a prophylactic compression garment is suggested for patients who are at risk for developing lymphedema. Clinicians should avoid using thermal modalities to warm up tissues before exercise because this may increase the volume of edema or induce an episode of lymphedema.

Resistive exercises have traditionally been avoided because of the perceived risk of causing or exacerbating lymphedema in an at-risk extremity. However, one study found that there was no change in lymphedema status in 25 women who did not wear compression garments during a one-time resistance exercise session.[5] Another study indicated that there was a minimal risk of the development or exacerbation of lymphedema when resistive exercises were performed on patients with breast cancer–related lymphedema.[6] As stated earlier, patients who have or may potentially develop lymphedema often wear a compression garment or bandaging during exercise.

Blood pressure is usually taken as part of an initial evaluation and during exercise. Advisory warnings to avoid blood pressure readings, trauma, and/or injections to an extremity susceptible to developing or exacerbating lymphedema have been based on anecdotal information. The results of one study in which 3041 blood pressure readings were taken over a 9-year period suggested that there was no increase in the involved limb volume/weight when blood pressure readings, blood draws, or injections were performed on that limb.[7] However, an analysis of many peer-reviewed articles determined that limited evidence is available to change the guidelines, and further studies are recommended. For that reason, avoiding blood pressure readings, trauma, skin punctures, extreme temperatures, and infections on an ipsilateral extremity should be continued. It is also recommended that patients with lymphedema should wear their compression garments, especially when they fly.[8]

**Considerations for the Physical Therapist Assistant: Exercise Considerations/Precautions**

- Use low- to moderate-intensity exercise and monitor the patient's response to the exercise. Limb heaviness is usually indicative of/associated with lymphedema.
- Patients with lymphedema should wear their compression garments when exercising.
- Avoid using thermal modalities on patients who may be predisposed to developing or have lymphedema.
- Avoid application of cuff weights to an at-risk limb.
- Avoid taking blood pressure on a patient's extremity that may be susceptible to lymphedema.

# Types of Cancer and Associated Treatments

There are typically a number of treatment options after a person is diagnosed with cancer. Selected cancers have unique treatment plans. The treatment options are based on the specific diagnosis; cancer stage; and the oncologist's, radiation oncologist's, and surgeon's treatment plan. Staging is based on the size of the tumor and whether or not it has spread to the lymph nodes or other parts of the body. Treatments can include surgery, radiation, chemotherapy, endocrine therapy, biological therapy, or combinations of these interventions.[9]

## *Breast Cancer*

Breast cancer is the most common type of cancer. Surgical treatment for breast cancer can vary based on the diagnosis and extent of tumor growth. It has evolved over years toward a less destructive surgical approach in which the tumor is resected while preserving as much of the surrounding tissue as possible.[10] A lumpectomy or partial mastectomy involves the removal of the tumor from the breast tissue. To determine if the cancer has spread to the lymphatic system, a sentinel node biopsy may be performed. This procedure consists of an injection of a blue dye into the area of the tumor, which then migrates to the lymphatic system and specifically to the lymph nodes in the axilla. An axillary node dissection is performed to remove the first lymph node filled with the blue dye. The node is biopsied to determine if the cancer has spread. If it is determined that the cancer has spread, then additional lymph nodes are removed. This biopsy allows the surgeon to remove the lowest number of lymph nodes possible. This is important because lymph node removal impacts the development of lymphedema.

A radical mastectomy is performed when indicated due to progression of the cancer or other characteristics, such as multiple tumors, aggressiveness of the tumors, when postsurgical radiation treatment is contraindicated, and/or if patient preference includes the full removal of all tissue. A radical mastectomy includes surgical removal of all breast tissue with or without lymph node dissection. Some patients choose to undergo a prophylactic contralateral mastectomy as well.[10] Many patients choose to undergo surgical reconstruction of the breast, which can be performed during the mastectomy operation or delayed until a later time. Three approaches for breast reconstruction typically include (1) implants and skin expanders, (2) vascularized flaps (typically from abdominal tissue or latissimus dorsi tissue), and (3) fatty tissue use (transplanted from other areas of the body).[11]

Radiation therapy involves using high-energy radiation from either an external or an internal source to destroy cancer cells. Based on the types of the cancer, the radiation oncologist will determine the optimal treatment. Whole-breast radiation targets the majority of the breast tissue, creating a uniform distribution of the dose to the tissue and decreasing the risk of toxicity to the normal tissue. Another option is chest wall radiation; this is typically applied after a mastectomy (in which there was no lymph node involvement), and the radiation is focused on the chest wall, the surgical scar, and the locations where any drains exited the body postsurgery. Regional nodal radiation is targeted for the paraclavicular and axillary nodes.[9]

Chemotherapy is another adjuvant treatment that can be used before or after surgery. This treatment is designed to either kill the cancer cells or stop them from dividing. In the early years of cancer treatment, surgical procedures were typically aggressive (ie, radical mastectomies) with the thought to remove all possible areas of local cancer and prevent metastases. However, it was found that distant recurrence of the cancer continued to be a major clinical problem even with removal of all local tissue. As a result, there has been an increase in other types of adjuvant therapies including chemotherapy, endocrine therapy, and anti-HER2 therapy to reduce the spread of the cancer and a decrease in aggressive surgeries.[12]

## Colon and Rectum Cancer

Cancers of the colon and rectum that are staged at level I or II typically undergo a partial or total colectomy, and they may receive additional treatment (chemotherapy and/or radiation). A colectomy is a partial or total removal of the colon. In these cases, a colostomy is performed; this is a diversion of the colon to an opening in the abdominal wall to bypass the removed or damaged colon. An external pouch or bag collects the waste. In some patients who had a section of the colon removed, this procedure can be reversed to allow for normal function. Patients diagnosed with stage II or III colorectal cancer often are treated with chemotherapy plus radiation. Chemotherapy is the main treatment for patients with stage IV rectal cancers.

## Lung and Bronchus Cancer

Lung cancer has 2 classifications: small cell and non–small cell. Most patients with small-cell lung cancer undergo chemotherapy; however, the majority of patients with non–small-cell cancers will undergo surgery, with about 25% also receiving radiation and/or chemotherapy.[3] The extent of the surgery depends on the extent of the cancer. It can be as minimal as a wedge removed from a lobe of a lung or part of the lobe to the removal of a lobe or the entire lung.[13]

## Prostate, Urinary Bladder, and Uterine Cancer

Based on the location of these anatomical structures, they are grouped together because of the similarity of impairments that occur because of the treatment for the cancers. Prostate cancer treatment is dependent on the extent of the disease, the risk of recurrence, and other patient characteristics. For patients under 65 years old, 92% undergo a radical prostatectomy. Transurethral resection of the prostate involves inserting a surgical instrument into the urethra and then removing the prostate. Treatment can also include chemotherapy and/or radiation for more advanced disease. Radiation to the prostate bed directly affects the urethra.[3]

Nonmuscle urinary bladder cancers can undergo a procedure similar to transurethral resection of the prostate; this is called *transurethral resection of the bladder tumor*, which may be followed by chemotherapy within the bladder. However, if the tumor has invaded the muscle surrounding the bladder, about half will undergo transurethral resection of the bladder tumor, and about 40% will undergo a cystectomy with or without radiation. The radiation field will involve the lower abdomen and often the genital area.[3]

The uterus is divided into an upper section (uterine corpus) and a lower portion (cervix). Cancer of the uterine corpus is the second most prevalent type of cancer for women. The surgical option of a hysterectomy occurs in about 70% of patients at stage I and II, and 28% of these patients additionally receive radiation. The field of radiation usually covers similar areas of the urinary bladder and prostate. Approximately two-thirds of patients diagnosed with stage III or IV cancer will have surgical resection and radiation with or without chemotherapy.[3]

# Common Cancer Impairments and the Effects of Rehabilitation Interventions

Cachexia is a complex medical syndrome associated with cancer and other illnesses resulting in extreme involuntary weight loss, weakness, and muscle mass and/or fatty mass wasting.[14] Combatting the loss of weight and muscle strength requires a multidisciplinary team involving physicians, nutritionists, and therapists. After 6 months of diagnosis, 30% to 80% of patients with cancer will lose 5% of their weight. In addition, the heart's metabolism is affected by the inflammation associated with the cancerous tumor. As a result, both muscular strength and cardiopulmonary endurance are affected as a result of the tumor.[15]

There is also a phenomenon called *cancer-related fatigue (CRF)*, which is directly related to the cancer and/or treatment for it.[16] Multimodal exercise interventions that are able to counter the effects of either cachexia or CRF include stretching, endurance, and resistance training.[17] A consensus statement from the American College of Sports Medicine indicated that exercise was safe for patients with breast cancer who were concurrently receiving chemotherapy or radiation. The statement indicated exercise is associated with significant improvements in aerobic endurance, muscular strength, and lean mass with sporadic fatigue.[18] The inclusion of exercise is safe after chemotherapy and/or radiation and is associated with improvements in aerobic capacity, flexibility, fatigue, or energy levels and some improvement in body size and body composition.[18]

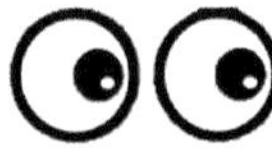

**Eye on the Research**

One study examined the use of an exercise rehabilitation program for patients with cancer, which involved 12 exercise sessions including 30 to 40 minutes of aerobic exercises and 20 to 30 minutes of resisted (dumbbell) exercises. The subjects were tested with a 6-Minute Walk Test, 30-second sit to stand, and handgrip assessment. The results identified improvements in aerobic capacity, muscular strength, and endurance and overall quality of life (QOL).[19]

Radiation treatment is part of the treatment regimen for cancer, and it can result in **radiation fibrosis.** The "underlying hallmark of cancer is their genomic instability."[20]

**Table 19-1**

**Recommendations for Exercise Duration, Frequency, and Intensity for Persons With Cancer[27]**

| |
|---|
| 150 minutes of moderate-intensity aerobic exercise over a 3- to 5-day period per week. |
| Resistance training should be at least 2 days per week. |
| Resistance training sessions should involve 8 to 10 major muscle groups 2 to 3 d/wk and 2 sets of 8 to 10 repetitions. |
| All sessions should include a 5- to 10-minute warm-up before and cooldown after any workout. |
| Refer to Chapter 9 for heart rate calculations and rate of perceived exertion. |

Radiation treatments are designed to damage the DNA of the rapidly replicating cells. However, there is significant "collateral damage to normal tissue and unwanted side effects" associated with radiation treatment.[20]

The impact of radiation fibrosis is illustrated in the example of patients with breast cancer who have undergone a mastectomy. The patients who also received radiation treatments have been shown to demonstrate joint impairments in 19% to 34% of the cases.[21] The addition of radiation treatment damages soft tissue in the radiation treatment field; this results in reduced elasticity in the affected tissues. When one considers the multiple areas of potential radiation treatment and the resultant potential loss of tissue mobility, one can imagine the losses in tissue range of motion (ROM) and the potential impact on joint ROM. Significant losses in joint ROM can impact and reduce function. Physical therapy interventions including manual therapy and therapeutic exercise can improve tissue extensibility and joint ROM and have positive effects in the recovery from cancer treatment.

A significant short- and long-term complication of breast cancer treatment after tumor resection and/or lymph node dissection is "cording" or AWS. Cording is defined as "an unusual form of superficial sclerosing thrombophlebitis."[22] The syndrome occurs after surgery and can present with cords of tissue that can originate at the site of the surgery. These cords traverse the axilla into the anterior medial upper arm and often continue to the wrist and thumb.[23] The cords cross joints, and their inelastic properties directly affect shoulder motions and at times the elbow and wrist. The anchor of the cords is usually at the chest wall region of the axilla; positions that put the cords on tension produce the highest tensile strength (see Figure 19-1). The loss of ROM mostly affects shoulder horizontal abduction, external rotation, and abduction. The loss of ROM is most apparent when attempting to complete these combined shoulder motions with elbow, wrist, and finger extension. Manual therapy and therapeutic exercise can improve patient mobility and agility of the upper extremity. One study found that patients who underwent a sentinel node biopsy were 45% more prone to develop cording. If patients underwent axillary clearance of further lymph nodes, the percentage who developed cording increased to 86%.[24]

Toxicity from chemotherapy varies and can be affected by the patient's age. One study reported that more than half of the patients receiving this treatment experienced toxicity requiring hospitalization.[25] Toxicity could result in the development of peripheral neuropathy. Peripheral neuropathy is characterized by a loss of sensory input from peripheral nerves that have been damaged by chemotherapy. The loss of motor fiber function affects the input of vibration sense, strength, movement, and proprioception from the affected area to the brain. The affected sensory fibers result in decreased information regarding pain and temperature being sent from the affected region to the brain.[26]

The diminished motor and sensory inputs (especially in the lower extremities) affect the ability of the nervous system to detect sway during static standing (refer to Chapter 8). As one shifts the center of gravity forward and backward, the proprioceptive sensors are stimulated, sending sensory input to the central nervous system, and the basal ganglia organizes the information to determine the appropriate motor output in response to the sensory input. In the case of a patient with peripheral neuropathy, there is diminished or total loss of sensory input, which alters the body's response to environmental changes and/or perturbations. During static posture on a firm surface, this loss of proprioceptive input may not be evident, but when standing on a compliant surface (eg, foam, grass, sand), the ability to appropriately respond to these conditions may result in a loss of balance and/or falls.

## Exercise Recommendations for Patients With Cancer

Exercise is beneficial for patients who have been diagnosed with cancer. QOL during and after treatment improves when cardiovascular and muscular exercise programs are implemented; programs are developed using the FITT-VP (frequency, intensity, time, type, volume, progression) parameters (refer to Chapter 5). Guidelines for aerobic exercises (refer to Chapter 9) and resistance exercises (refer to Chapter 6) can vary for different patient populations; recommendations for persons with cancer are included in Table 19-1.[27]

Patients with cancer were found to have lower functional performance compared with healthy individuals of the same age.[28] For this reason, these patients often need a multimodal rehabilitation approach because they may become deconditioned during their medical treatments. Physical therapist assistants should recognize that patients with cancer not only experience physiological changes but also may also experience psychosocial changes that can affect their QOL.[27] These patients may not only present with muscle weakness and reduced aerobic capacity but also display postural and balance deficits as a result of their cancer treatments. For example, patients who have developed peripheral neuropathy are prone to demonstrating balance and/or vestibular deficits. Patients who have gone through a mastectomy may present with thoracic kyphosis, rounded shoulders due to tight anterior (ie, pectoralis major) muscles, and forward head posture (refer to Chapter 7). Exercise performance and progression should focus on improving posture and balance and increasing the patient's exercise tolerance.

Physical therapist assistants should use objective measures to systematically alter and advance a patient's program. Patients with a diagnosis of cancer (during or after medical treatment) may require additional time to achieve their functional/fitness goals because of their common impairments (eg, reduced functional level, muscle weakness/flexibility, balance deficits). The clinician can vary the frequency, duration, and the mode of exercise based on patient presentation. For example, if a patient has a decrease in standing tolerance and the goal is to increase their tolerance, the patient can perform various upper and/or extremity exercises (eg, shoulder and elbow strengthening exercises) in standing and/or perform calf stretches (eg, anterior/posterior sway exercises). Each of these exercises addresses different impairments, but, collectively and simultaneously, they also address standing tolerance. Clinicians document the number of minutes the patient was able to continually stand without requiring a rest during the combined activities. This provides an objective time measurement so the standing tolerance goal can be documented and progressed. Educating the patient of their progression can motivate them.

## Treating Patients With Cancer and Balance Deficits

Agility decreases and fall risk increases with increased age due to a multitude of factors. These risks in older adults increase with the addition of a diagnosis of cancer and subsequent treatments. The side effects of chemotherapy, including fatigue, peripheral neuropathy, dehydration, and generalized weakness, can add to an increased risk of falls.[29]

The exercises used with patients with peripheral neuropathy work to enhance the visual and vestibular system because these patients have decreased proprioception. Exercises are designed to improve proprioceptive feedback by stimulating those receptors and increasing signal strength and frequency over a deficient or damaged system. However, because static balance is only a small portion of human performance, a dynamic group of exercises is also necessary to improve balance deficits. Balance improves by using progressively more difficult tasks to challenge patients while stimulating the sensory input to improve motor output.[30]

As discussed in Chapter 8, functional balance reactions rely on both the sensory and motor systems. The sensory system, which includes the visual, vestibular, and somatosensory systems, provides the input to the central nervous system that is organized in the basal ganglia, which then provides motor output in response.[31] To improve balance, these systems must be progressively stimulated and challenged. To improve balance, there should be a progressive reduction of the size of the patient's base of support, an increase in dynamic movement to disrupt the patient's center of gravity, and a reduction of sensory inputs (ie, eyes closed or on a compliant surface), which challenges the patient's postural responses and muscle responses.[32] Examples of progressions for static/dynamic balance and vestibular exercises are found in Tables 8-8 and 8-9 in Chapter 8.

When challenging and progressing patients with balance and/or vestibular problems, the physical therapist assistant should use a gait belt for safety. The purpose of challenging the patient's balance is to facilitate their ability to recover from a loss of balance and use the appropriate strategy sequence (ie, ankle, hip, and then stepping) to avoid falls.

## Cardiovascular and Endurance Issues Associated With Cancer

Many patients with breast cancer who are or have undergone treatment experience a decrease in aerobic capacity. The combined effect of the treatment itself and the decrease in activity cause this effect.[33] Using peak oxygen uptake ($VO_{2peak}$ [the tool used to identify cardiopulmonary function]), it was found that the average $VO_{2peak}$ was 27% (± 17%) lower than that of age-matched healthy sedentary women.[34] One-third of patients with breast cancer have a $VO_{2peak}$ less than the $VO_{2peak}$ considered necessary for functional independence. $VO_{2peak}$ was lowest in women with metastatic disease.[34] A leading cause of death in women who have nonmetastatic breast cancer is cardiovascular disease. Subjects who performed 3 to 5 sessions a week of moderate to vigorous exercise showed a reduction in mortality due to cardiovascular disease.[35]

Cachexia was previously identified as a systemic loss of muscle mass, but the heart (myocardium) can also experience cachexia because of chemotherapy and/or radiation treatments. It is important to introduce a controlled physical exercise program to improve cardiac function.[15] Cachexia in patients with cancer is present in 80% of severe cancer cases, and it is responsible for 30% of deaths.[36]

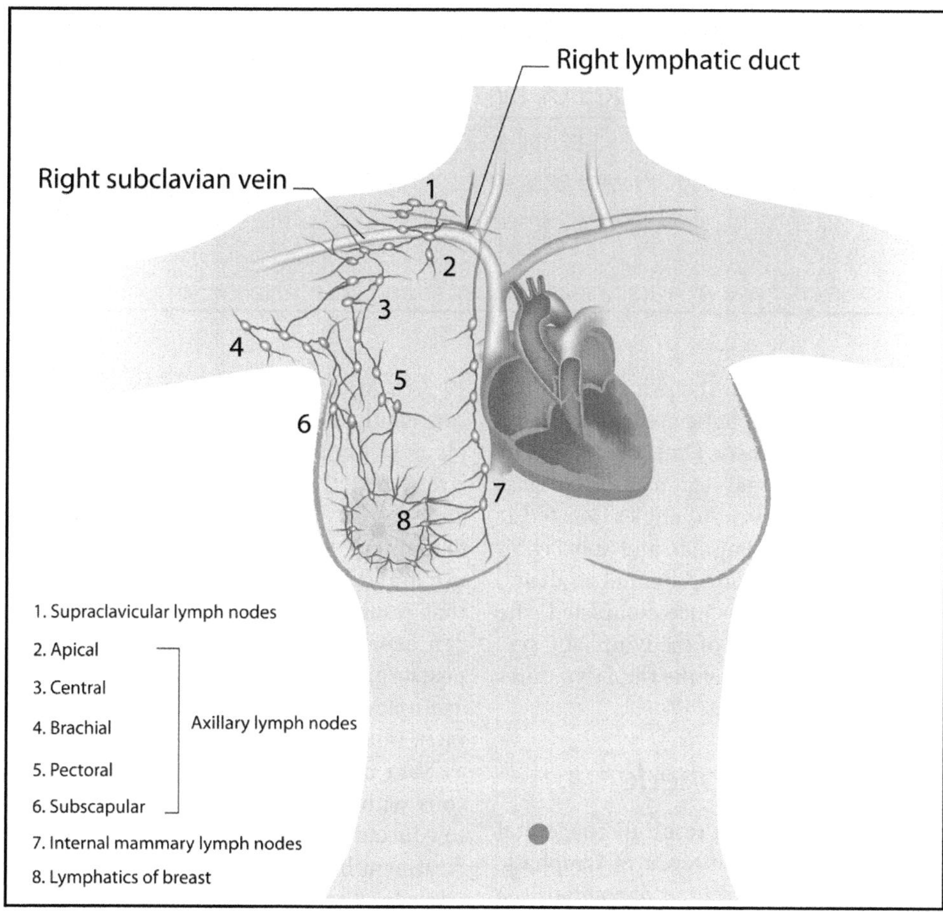


**Figure 19-2.** The lymphatic system (Alila Medical Media/Shutterstock.com).

Cancer cachexia results in earlier death when there is a faster progression of cachexia of the heart muscle. Aerobic exercise training has been shown to be an important adjunct therapy for these patients.[37]

## The Lymphatic System and Lymphedema

Lymphedema is the accumulation of excessive interstitial fluid due to the destruction of the lymphatic vessel system. The lymphatic system is a one-way vascular system that begins in the interstitial tissue area and migrates to the lymph nodes. The lymph nodes are pervasive throughout the body but are highly concentrated in areas including the cervical and abdominal regions with axillary and inguinal clusters to drain the limbs. The nodes also serve an immune function by destroying bacteria and viruses. The basic functions of the lymphatic system are to return filtered fluid, which has left the blood circulatory system, back into circulation through the subclavian veins leading into the heart and to transport white blood cells to the lymph nodes where immune responses are triggered.[38]

The body is divided into watershed regions, and each area of the body constitutes a different watershed. Watersheds divide the body into left and right as well as at the clavicular level and the abdominal level. Each region (watershed) drains to a particular region of lymph nodes. The lymph fluid passes through these nodes, and then it enters the larger lymphatic trunks deep within the body. After traveling through the lymphatic trunks, lymph fluid empties into the subclavian vein at the base of the neck.

The right cervical and neck region drains to the right supraclavicular region (Figure 19-2), and the left cervical region drains to the left supraclavicular region. The right upper limb and chest wall drains to the right axilla. The bilateral lower extremities drain to the corresponding inguinal node region and join at the cisterna chyli (a catchment area in the abdominal region). The thoracic duct continues to the cardiovascular system. Both lower extremities and the left upper extremity drain into the left supraclavicular region and eventually to the cardiovascular system.

The working unit of the lymphatic system is the lymphangion. The lymphatic vessels and the lymphangia can be imagined like a string of pearls in which the lymphangion (the pearl) contracts regularly, moving the lymph fluid through the vessels (the string) in waves. The lymphatic system has an automotoricity with a beat rate of 3 to 5 per minute. It is a one-way vessel system moving fluid from the interstitial spaces back to the blood circulatory system at the venous angle of the heart. The lymphangion can be stimulated by mechanical means to increase the beat rate to 15 to 20 per minute.[39]

**Table 19-2**

**Stages of Lymphedema[41]**

| Stages of Lymphedema |
|---|
| Stage 0: The lymphatic system is impaired, but physical signs are not yet evident. |
| Stage 1: Swelling is evident and is reduced with elevation. Pitting (indentation with finger pressure) may occur. |
| Stage 2: Swelling is consistent and rarely reduces when the limb is elevated. Pitting is prevalent with the development of fibrosis. |
| Stage 3: Significant tissue changes with an increase in fibrosis and skin character including thickness occur. |

The treatment pattern is based on the principles of the watersheds. In order to treat a lymphatic area of the body, it must first be prepared to be drained. Thus, the treatment begins with stimulating the proximal region at the cervical and supraclavicular regions at the venous angles (located at the junction between the internal jugular and subclavian veins). Then, preparation moves from proximal to distal, continuing to stimulate the system. Once completed, the process is reversed. Normal function of the lymphatic system is critical to maintaining balance of the fluid dynamics in the body.

## *Types and Stages of Lymphedema*

**Primary lymphedema** occurs as a result of congenital causes, such as a malformation or absence of lymphatic vessels. **Secondary lymphedema** is due to damage to the system caused by trauma, infection, malignancy, surgery, or radiation.[40] There are 4 stages of lymphedema (0 to 3) defined by the International Society of Lymphology Consensus Document; they are described in Table 19-2.[41]

## *Treating Lymphedema: Complete Decongestive Therapy and Diaphragmatic Breathing*

Lymphedema can be treated using a variety of methods. Oftentimes, 2 or more techniques are used either concurrently or sequentially. The course of treatment primarily includes an interventional technique called **CDT,** which is performed by certified therapists. CDT is considered the gold standard for the treatment of lymphedema, and it consists of 4 components: **manual lymphatic drainage (MLD),** skin care, compression therapy, and exercise.[42]

MLD is a manual technique that stimulates the lymphatic system to transport lymph fluid more effectively. This intervention should only be completed by a certified clinician. As stated earlier, the system has an automotoricity, which self-propels the fluid. MLD stimulates the system to work at a faster rate of contractility and is the first component of CDT. MLD involves a light tactile stretch of the skin in 3 dimensions, and the pressure is more superficial than an effleurage massage technique. The very light pressure of the clinician's hand is positioned and moved in a parallel plane to the body part, and the skin is stretched only to the point at which it can no longer stretch (Figure 19-3A). At that point, a rotational maneuver of the hands can gently stretch the skin in a relatively perpendicular plane (Figure 19-3B), again until the skin can no longer stretch. At this point, contact with the skin is released, and it snaps back into position. The certified clinician determines which strokes, sequences, and techniques to use in order to maximize treatment results. Any diagnosis that results in swelling or stagnation of interstitial fluid can benefit from MLD treatments. Venous insufficiency, postsurgical swelling, traumatic injury, and/or wounds are examples of conditions that may benefit from this treatment intervention.

Skin care is an important component of care for persons with lymphedema. It is the clinician's responsibility to educate patients regarding proper skin care during each treatment intervention. Skin care with moisturizing lotion precedes the application of compression wrapping. The compression wraps used for lymphedema are short-stretch bandages that only stretch about 40% to 50% greater than their resting length. These short-stretch bandages do not function like ACE (3M) elastic wraps. The long-stretch wraps (ie, ACE wraps) are capable of extending about 150% to 250% greater than their resting length. These long-stretch bandages are not appropriate for use with patients with lymphedema. A washable nonslip padding (Figure 19-4A) is first applied to help provide even pressure distribution; the pressure is applied using the short-stretch bandages, which are applied over the padding (Figure 19-4B). The short stretch permits low resting pressure because of the decreased recoil of the bandage. The bandages effectively maintain compression during movement, which is important, especially during the essential exercise component of CDT. Performing exercise while bandaged promotes an increase in lymphangiomotoricity, similar to the effects of MLD.

Proper breathing techniques supplement the treatment interventions for lymphedema. Diaphragmatic breathing exercises help stimulate the lymphatic system. During inhalation, negative pressure occurs within the lungs due to chest wall expansion. The negative pressure also creates a drawing or sucking effect on the lymphatic system. This effect facilitates the return of lymph to the blood circulatory system. To assist a patient in expanding the chest wall, understanding the mechanics of breathing is essential. To create negative pressure within the lungs, 4 processes occur. The diaphragm contracts and descends inferiorly to

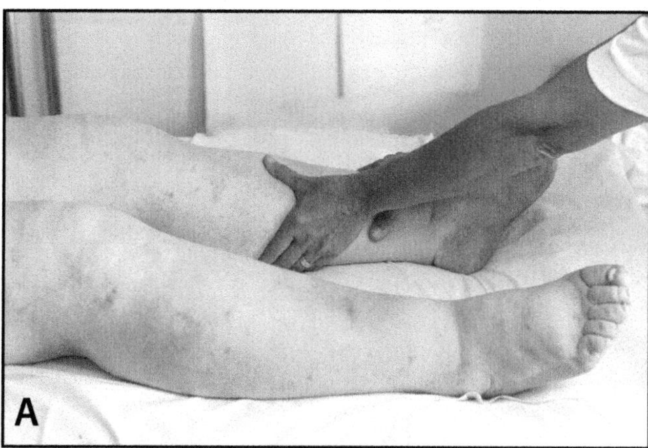


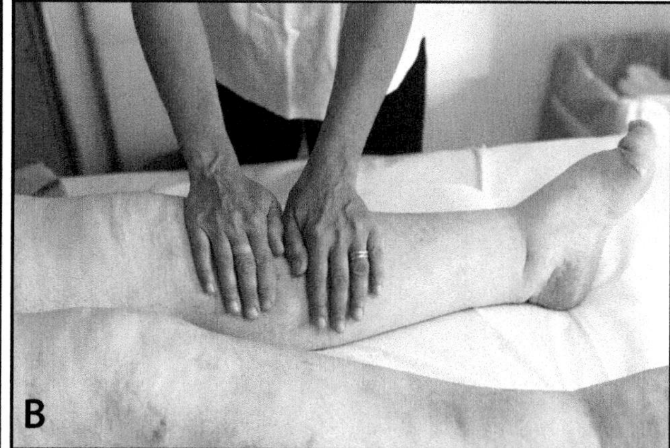


**Figure 19-3.** MLD being performed on a patient with lymphedema. (A) Parallel and (B) perpendicular strokes using light touch to stretch and release the skin (Valerio Pardi/Shutterstock.com).

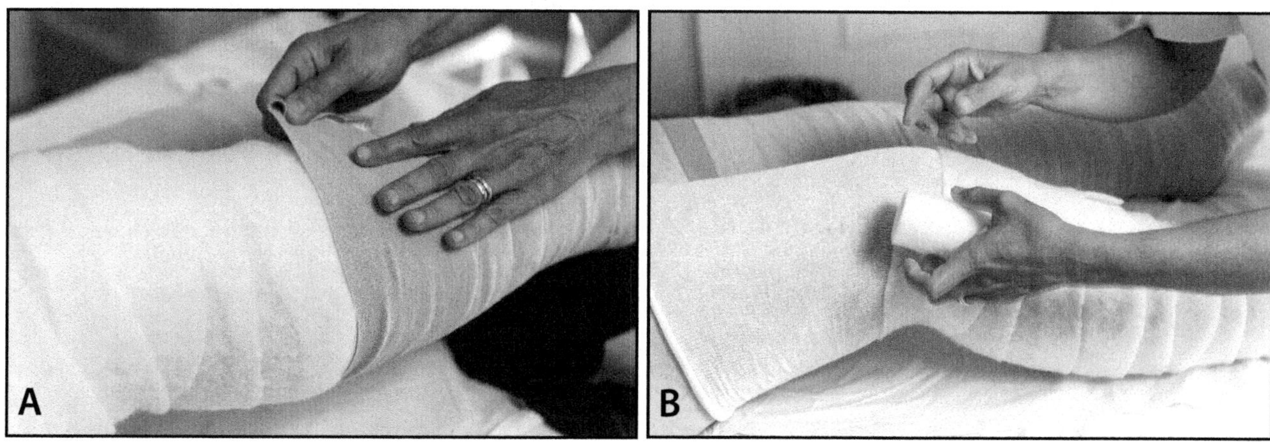


**Figure 19-4.** Compression therapy using various bandages to control the lymphedema. (A) Padding is first applied followed by (B) the short-stretch bandages (Valerio Pardi/Shutterstock.com).

increase the proximal to distal space. Then, the ribs translate laterally like the handle on a bucket, thus the term *bucket handle*. The next move occurs at the sternum, which expands in the anterior/posterior plane like the handle on a water pump, thus the term *pump handle*. These motions can be facilitated by the clinician as shown in Figures 19-5A and 19-5B. Patients should be able to perform diaphragmatic breathing independently after proper instruction. The clinician instructs the patient to place one hand on the sternum and the other on the abdomen (Figure 19-5C). The patient is instructed to inhale and feel the abdomen push outward with the lower hand first followed by movement felt in the upper hand as the patient continues to inhale and the anterior chest begins to expand. The sequence is reversed during exhalation.

Finally, the use of the accessory muscles of the cervical region elevates the rib cage in the opposite motion of the diaphragm (Figure 19-5D). This final motion occurs during heavy cardiovascular exertion when there is the need for a significantly increased intake of air.[43,44]

## Therapeutic Exercise for Patients With Lymphedema

There had been concerns that exercise could be counterproductive and possibly increase lymphedema. However, evidence has shown that exercise is safe for the majority of this patient population.[6] Exercise types will vary, but all therapeutic exercises should be performed while bandaged or wearing a compression garment. The intent of exercise is to stimulate the motoricity of the lymphatic system while compression continues to address the reduction of the swelling. The exercises are actively performed without resistance based on the location of the lymphedema.[6,45]

Each type of exercise (flexibility, strengthening, and aerobics) has a specific importance for the patient with lymphedema. The overall goal is to improve the patient's agility. Agility is the ability to move quickly and easily (not just joints but also the entire body). To be agile, one must have adequate ROM, strength, coordination, and speed. In patients with cancer, treatment often involves surgery and/

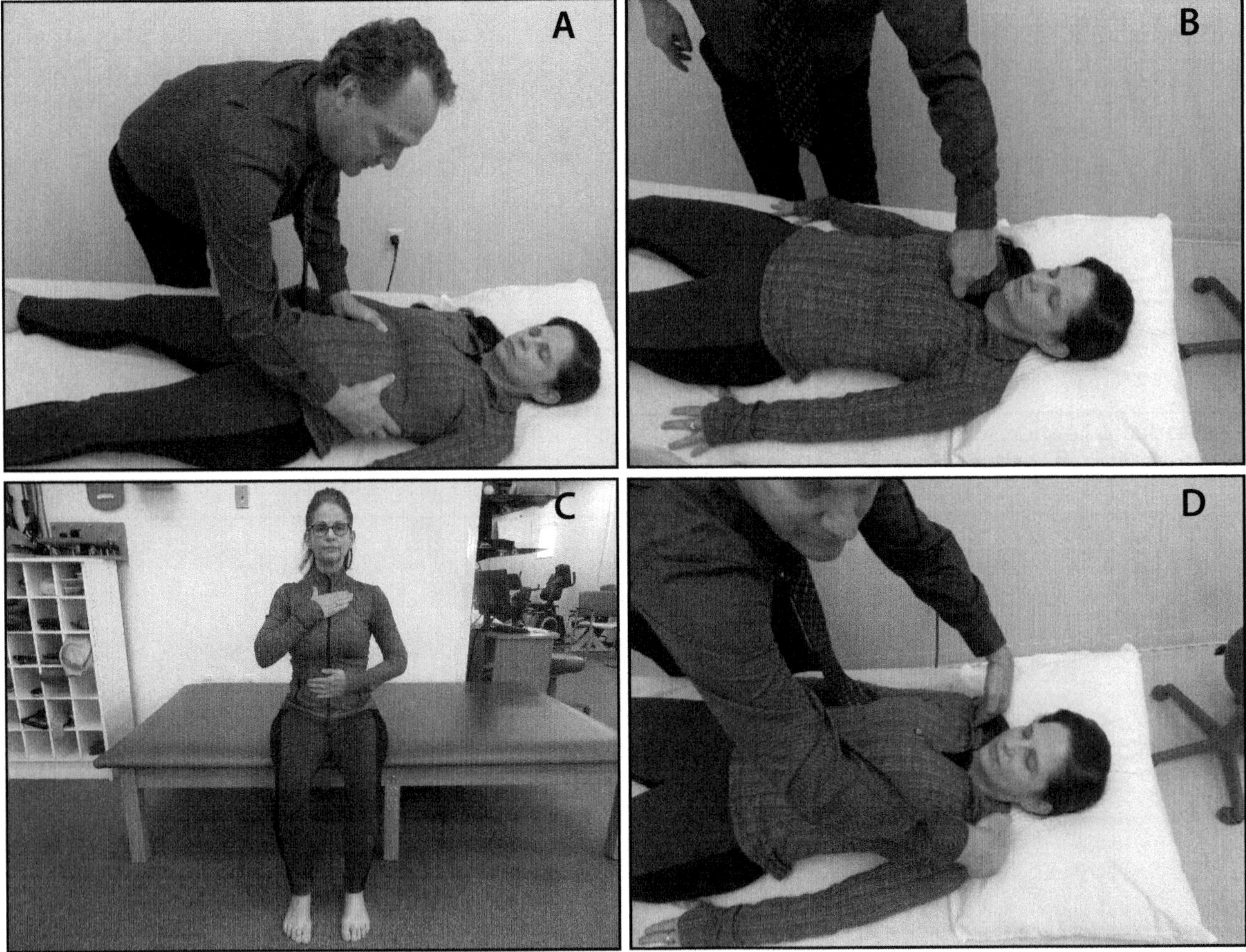


**Figure 19-5.** (A) Lateral rib excursion (bucket handle). Instruct the patient to expand the ribs into the clinician's hands during inspiration. (B) Instruct the patient to inhale into the clinician's hand placed on the sternum (pump handle). (C) Seated diaphragmatic breathing, first feeling it in the abdomen and then through the sternum during inhalation. (D) Facilitation of the accessory muscles during respiration. The clinician's hands are placed superior to the shoulders. Instruct the patient to elevate the shoulders while inhaling.

or radiation, which damages the lymphatic system. The development of scarring (or radiation fibrosis) may limit lymphatic flow, so maintaining or improving mobility and ROM in the involved and adjacent joints is essential. Lymphedema may not just limit joint mobility but can also restrict muscle function.

Strengthening can be initiated once flexibility has improved and ROM has increased. Resistive training has been shown to be beneficial for breast cancer survivors[46] and thus can be extrapolated to other cancer survivors. Coordination exercises such as proprioceptive neuromuscular facilitation have been shown to benefit patients with upper limb lymphedema.[47,48] Speed (the final component) can be added to the regimen of exercises through cues from the clinician to adjust the timing of a task or addressed in a reactive/responsive manner (ie, adding in task-specific activities, such as sport-related tasks/behaviors).

Many types of exercise can increase flexibility, muscle strength, and endurance, including yoga,[49] Pilates,[50] qigong,[51] and tai chi.[52] Aquatic therapy has also been shown to be beneficial for patients with lymphedema, but this is performed without compression wraps or a sleeve.[53] The water's hydrostatic pressure helps control lymphedema.

When considering the impairment of AWS and its association with lymphedema, one study combined MLD with a physical exercise program for 400 women. The exercise program defines specific criteria (one of the few found in the literature) associated with AWS (Table 19-3).[54] The protocol emphasizes mobility of the involved extremity and identifies taiji or tai chi as a useful intervention for patients with AWS. Tai chi is a "mind body exercise associated with reductions in chronic disease factors."[55] The practice focuses on specific fluid movements of the body, such as balancing and weight shifting.[55]

An alternative approach involves the philosophies based in yoga. The effects of yoga-based exercises result in a reduction in the volume of the affected extremity, a significant increase in bilateral shoulder flexion and external rotation ROM, and increased strength of shoulder abduction in women at risk for breast cancer–related lymphedema.[56] Samples of some yoga-based breathing exercises combined with upper extremity and trunk motions are

**Table 19-3**

**Exercise Criteria for Axillary Web Syndrome Associated With Lymphedema[54]**

| Stages | Duration | Training Focus |
|---|---|---|
| First stage | Surgical date until removal of the drainage tube (≤7 days) | • Passive shoulder ROM exercises.<br>• With limb relaxed, abduct and lift limb; move fingers, wrist, and elbow joints gently.<br>• Avoid using the affected limb for support. |
| Second stage | Date from removal of drainage tube to removal of the surgical sutures (7 to 30 days) | • Progress shoulder ROM from active assisted to active; use gentle progressions. Use fingers to touch ear and initiate wall climb exercises.<br>• Follow surgeon protocol to initiate soft tissue mobilization at shoulder and axilla areas. |
| Third stage | Date from removal day of the sutures to 3 months after surgery | • Patients are cleared to use the affected limb as they are able to (to comb hair, brush teeth, wash face, bathe, and other ADLs); restore range so patient can perform personal hygiene tasks and ADLs.<br>• Increase shoulder joint ROM. Abduct, lift, and spin the shoulder joint after softly massaging the shoulder and axilla.<br>• Initiate strengthening as per oncologist's protocol. |
| Fourth stage | 3 months postoperative to 6 months | • Initiate aerobic activity that is appropriate for the patient.<br>• Avoid vigorous activities; protect the affected limb.<br>• Strictly avoid using the limb for blood pressure measurements, collecting blood samples, or intravenous infusion or using cuff weights.<br>• Avoid heavy lifting, swinging arm, etc. |

found in Figures 19-6 and 19-7, and yoga-based exercise sequences in prone, supine, and standing are found in Figures 19-8 through 19-11. Other passive, active-assisted, and active exercises to improve shoulder range are beneficial for patients who are recovering from breast cancer surgery (refer to Chapter 12). Physical therapist assistants should follow the plan of care outlined by the evaluating physical therapist.

## Various Conditions Associated With Lymphedema and Exercise

Physical therapist assistants must be able to recognize various conditions, know when to implement exercises, and understand how to adjust the level of intensity when creating an appropriate treatment for patients with a cancer diagnosis.

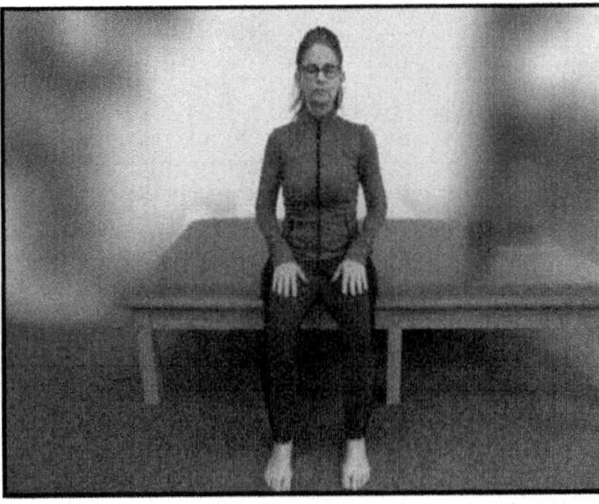

A. Centering of the posture

- Sitting with lower extremities parallel and hands placed on thighs with shoulders relaxed
- Have the patient move from posterior to an anterior pelvic tilt until pressure is felt on the ischial tuberosities
- Engage core muscles
- Shoulders should be depressed and retracted to neutral and cervical spine retracted to neutral

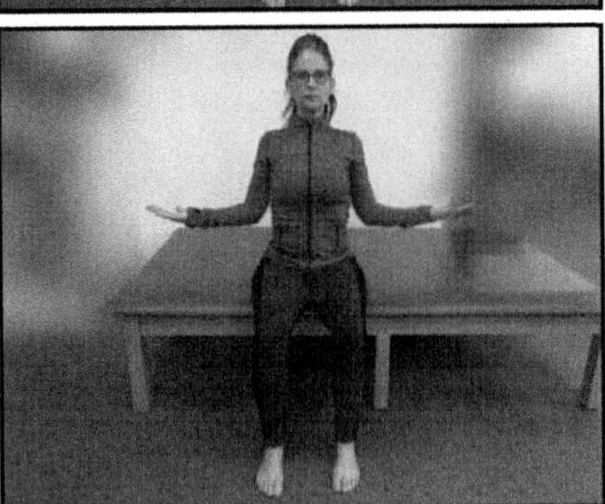

B. Opening of the chest

- Maintaining sitting posture
- While inhaling, move hands from thighs to the position shown in the photograph
- Shoulders are externally rotated and abducted while retracting the scapulae
- The forearms are supinated and wrists and fingers extended (palms face up)
- Slightly extend the cervical region while gazing upward
- Maintain this position while performing 5 expansive breathing cycles

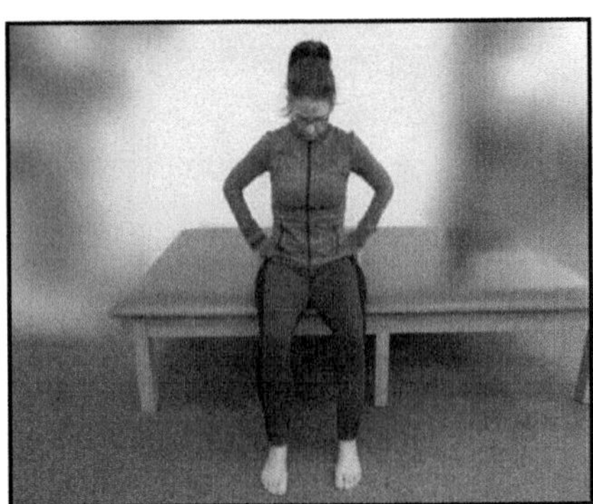

C. Posture reversal

- Maintain the sitting posture in Figure 19-6B
- While exhaling, move hands from the open chest position to the position shown in the photograph
- Internally rotate and adduct the shoulders while maintaining scapula retraction
- Make a fist by flexing the fingers and placing them on the lateral aspects of the pelvis
- Flex the cervical spine and gaze downward
- Maintain this position while performing 5 expansive cycles of breathing

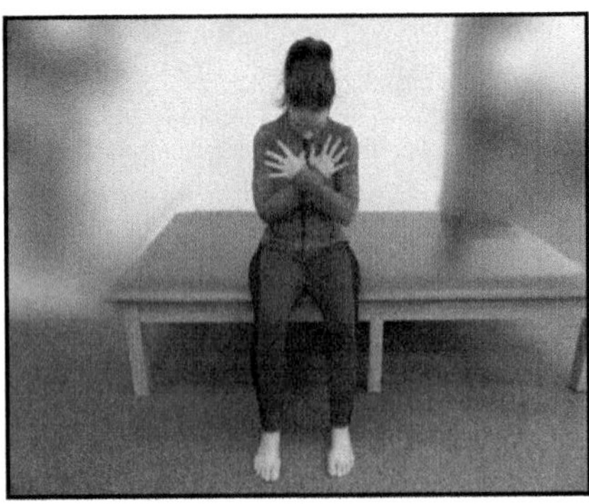

D. Closing of the chest

- Maintain the sitting posture in Figure 19-6C
- While exhaling, move the hands across the chest to opposite upper chest regions as shown in the photograph
- Protract the scapulae with fingers extended and separated
- Flex the cervical spine and gaze downward
- Slowly perform a posterior tilt and flex the spine during exhalation
- Maintain the position while performing 5 expansive cycles of breathing

Note: The pelvis and spine will move slightly into an anterior tilt and extension during inhalation. The pelvis and spine should move back into a posterior tilt and flexion during exhalation.

**Figure 19-6.** Yoga-based breathing exercises with bilateral upper extremity movements. (A) Centering of the posture. (B) Opening of the chest. (C) Posture reversal. (D) Closing of the chest.

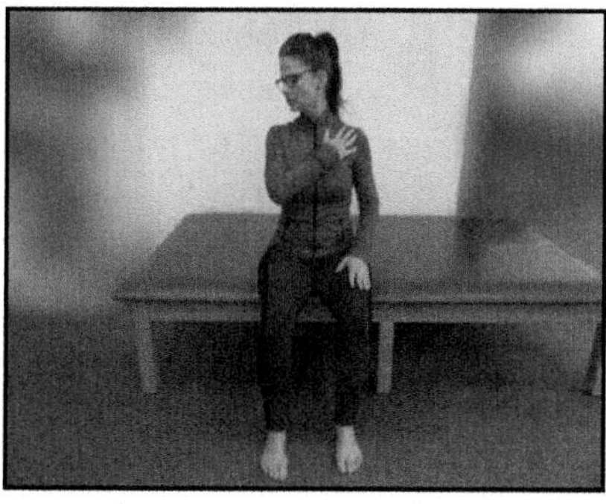

A. Unilateral closure shoulder girdle

- Start with the centering of posture shown in Figure 19-6A
- While exhaling, move one hand from the thigh to opposite upper chest position as shown in this photograph
- The shoulder is internally rotated and abducted while protracting the scapula
- Rotate the cervical region to the ipsilateral side as the active upper extremity
- Maintain the position while performing 5 expansive cycles of breathing
- Exercise can be repeated on the other side

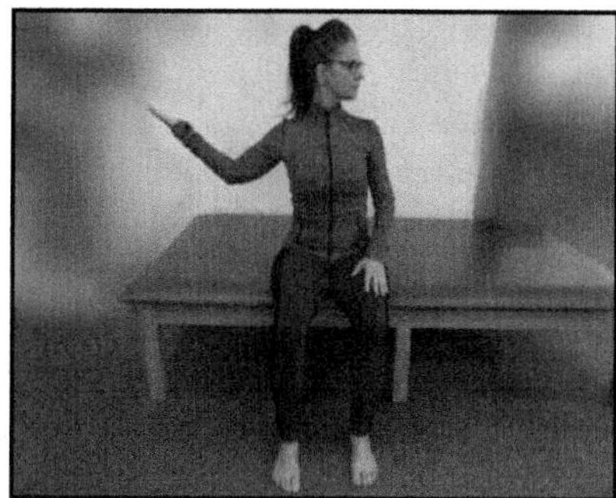

B. Unilateral opening shoulder girdle

- Start with the centering of posture shown in Figure 19-6A
- While exhaling, move one hand from the thigh out away from the body as shown in this photograph
- The shoulder is externally rotated and abducted to about 45 degrees while retracting the scapula
- Rotate the cervical region to the contralateral side of the active upper extremity
- Maintain the position while performing 5 expansive cycles of breathing
- Exercise can be repeated on the other side

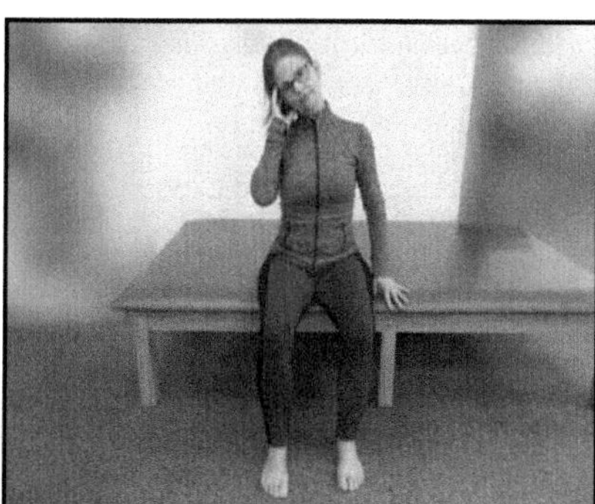

C. Unilateral cervical accessory muscle activation

- Start with the centering posture
- Maintain sitting posture
- While inhaling, move one hand from thigh to ipsilateral lateral facial region
- Side bend cervical region into the ipsilateral hand with finger placement on or posterior to the ear to avoid rotation
- Maintain position while performing 5 expansive cycles of breathing
- Repeat bilaterally

**Figure 19-7.** Yoga-based breathing exercises with unilateral upper extremity movements and cervical rotation. (A) Unilateral closure of the shoulder girdle. (B) Unilateral opening of the shoulder girdle. (C) Unilateral cervical accessory muscle activation.

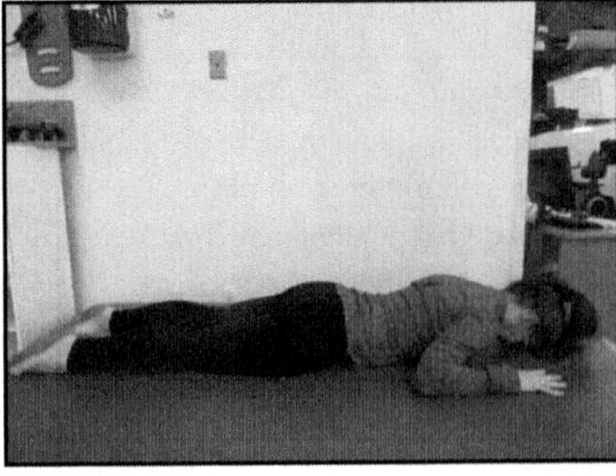

A. Prone starting position

- Start with prone
- Cervical in neutral
- Position with pillow under pelvis and/or chest region if structure of patient limits neutral prone position
- Scapulae are retracted
- Shoulders are extended slightly abducted and externally rotated
- Elbows are flexed with pronated forearms parallel to the torso
- Wrists in neutral and fingers extended

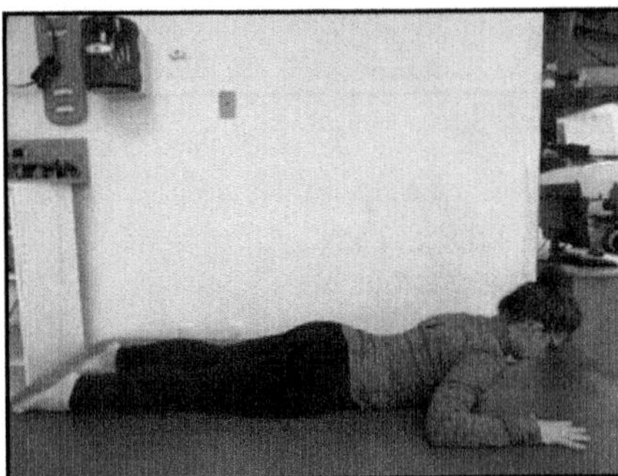

B. Prone thoracic extension

- Start in prone starting position
- Protraction of shoulder elevating chest
- Horizontal isometric adduction of bilateral shoulders
- Maintain cervical neutral position
- Passive extension of thoracic and lumbar spine

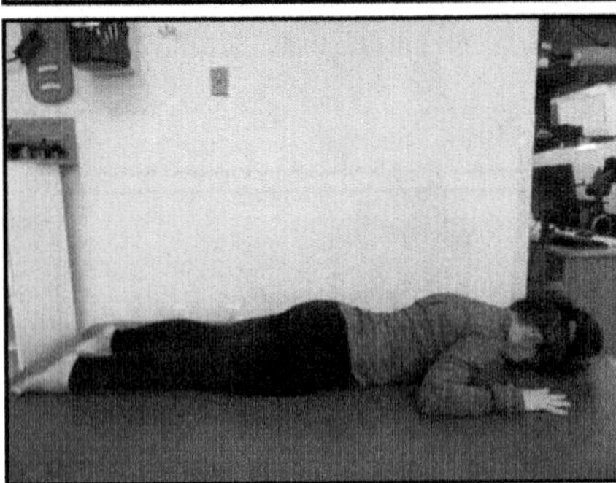

C. Prone starting position

- Start with prone
- Cervical in neutral
- Position with pillow under pelvis and/or chest region if structure of patient limits neutral prone position
- Scapulae are retracted
- Shoulders are extended slightly abducted and externally rotated
- Elbows are flexed with pronated forearms parallel to the torso
- Wrists in neutral and fingers extended

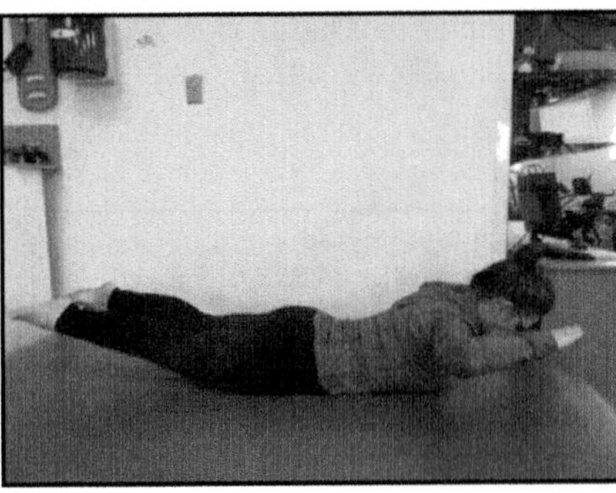

D. Symmetric elevations

- Start in prone thoracic extension
- Maintain position
- Externally rotate bilateral shoulders with hand moving toward forehead
- Simultaneously extend the bilateral hips while the knees are in neutral and ankles plantar flexed
- Hold position during breaths for up to 5 count or until position failure occurs and return to neutral

**Figure 19-8.** Yoga-based exercise sequence prone. (A) The prone starting position. (B) Prone thoracic extension. (C) Prone starting position. (D) Symmetric elevations.

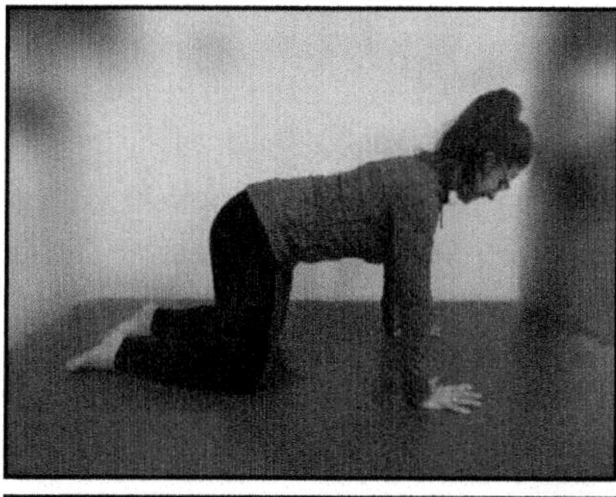

A. Quadruped transition position

- Start in prone starting position
- Flex hips and transition center of gravity inferior toward lower extremities
- Extend elbows and elevate torso
- Rotate pelvis posterior to position lumbar spine in neutral
- Hold position during breaths for up to 5 count or until position failure occurs and return to neutral

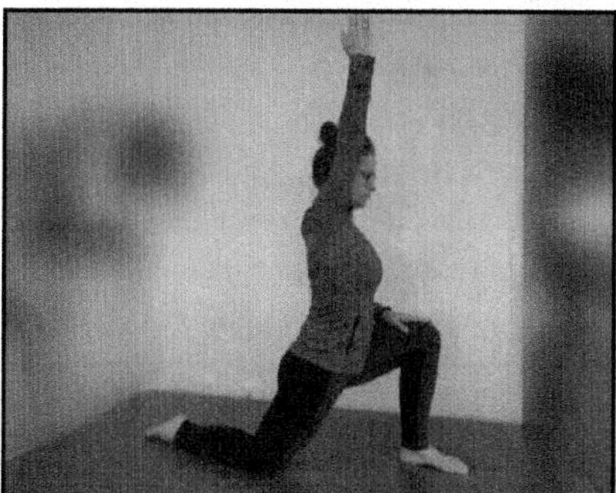

B. Half-kneeling position

- Start in quadruped transition position
- Extend trunk
- Simultaneously translate lower extremity into flexion and foot flat
- Elevate contralateral upper extremity into flexion while inhaling
- Hold position during breaths for up to 5 count or until position failure occurs and return to neutral

**Figure 19-9.** Yoga-based transition quadruped to half knee. (A) The quadruped transition position. (B) The half-kneeling position.

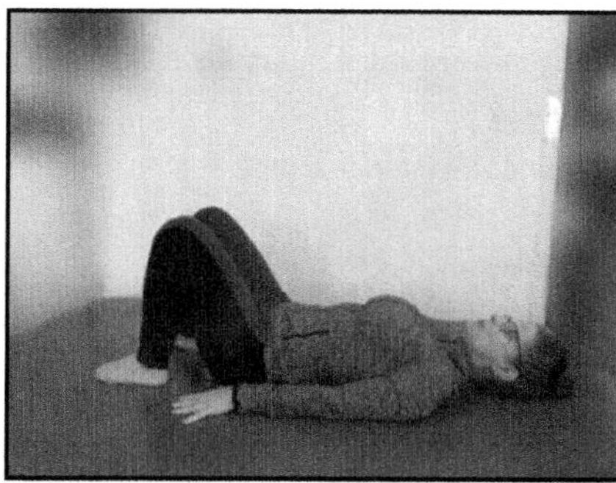

A. Supine starting position

- Start in supine
- Flex hips and knees such that both feet are flat and symmetric
- Bilateral and shoulder positioned in internal rotation
- Forearms pronated
- Wrist and fingers in neutral
- Hold position during breaths for up to 5 count

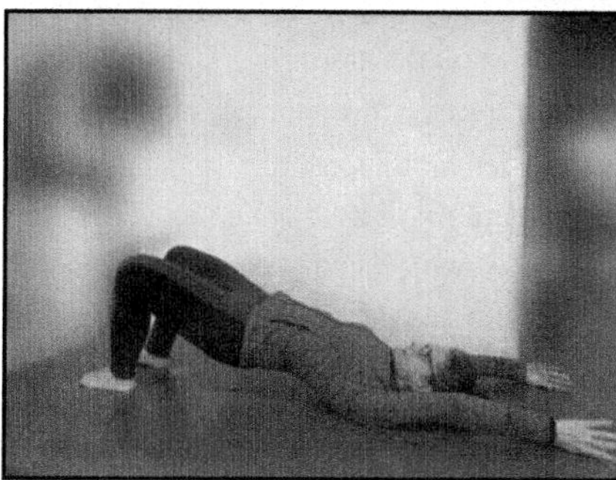

B. Bridge with shoulder flexion

- Start in supine starting position
- Extend the hip toward neutral
- Flex bilateral shoulders with external rotation
- Inhale during activity in previous bullet
- Hold position during breaths for up to 5 count

**Figure 19-10.** Yoga-based supine transitions. (A) The supine starting position. (B) Bridge with shoulder flexion. *(continued)*

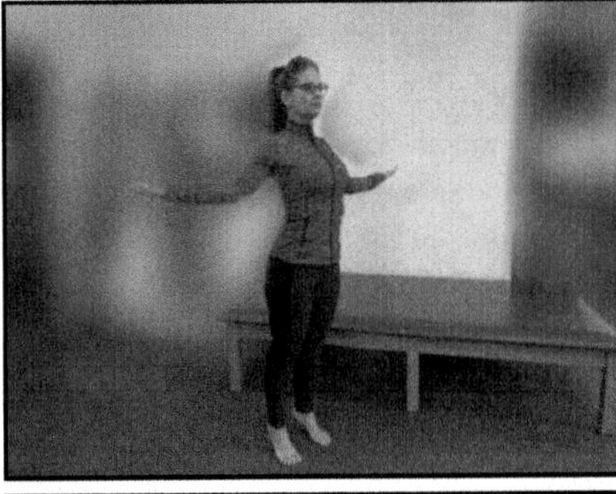

C. Standing elongation with shoulder external rotation and scapular retraction

- Begin in standing starting position
- Plantar flex bilateral ankle to maintain balance on toes
- Simultaneously, retract scapula, horizontally abduct and externally rotate shoulders with flexed elbows with supination of the forearm
- Inhalation occurs throughout the motions
- Return to starting point

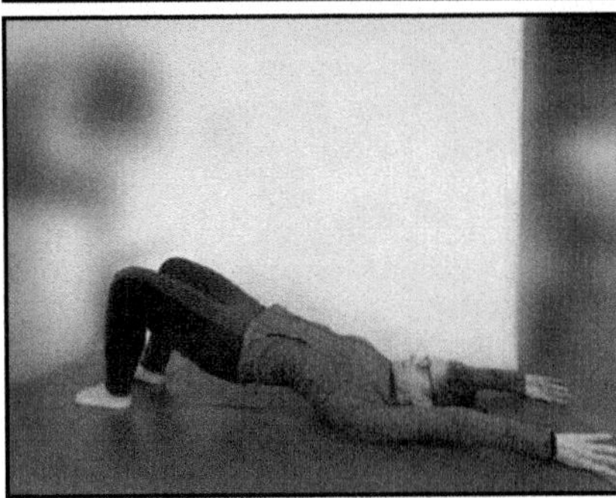

D. Bridge with shoulder flexion

- Start in supine starting position
- Extend hip toward neutral
- Flex bilateral shoulders with external rotation
- Inhale during activity in previous bullet
- Hold position during breaths for up to 5 count

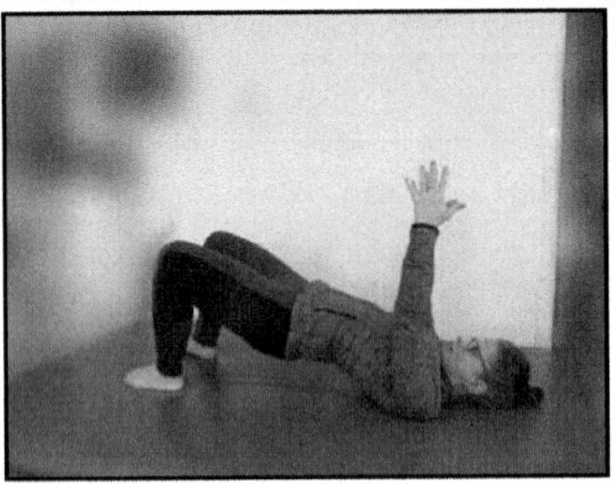

E. Bridge end point from shoulder abduction

- Continue from end point of bridge return from shoulder abduction
- Horizontally adduct bilateral shoulders
- Elbows extended
- Maintain neutral wrist and fingers
- Contact both hands at approximately 80 degrees flexion but perpendicular to the ground
- Hold position during breaths for up to 5 count

**Figure 19-10 (continued).** (C) Standing elongation with shoulder external rotation and scapular retraction. (D) Bridge with shoulder flexion. (E) Bridge end point from shoulder abduction.

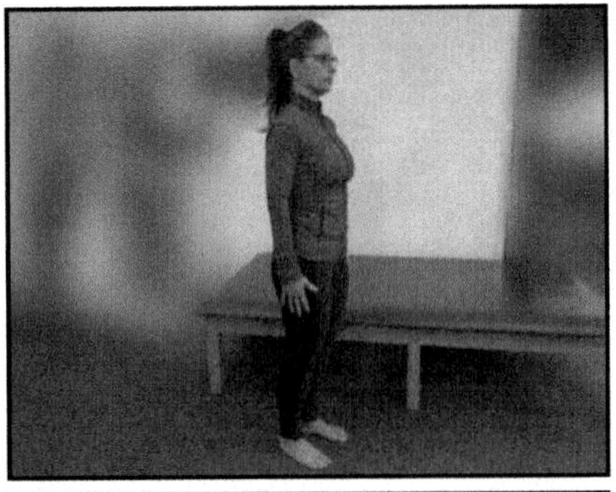

A. Standing starting position

- Position body in alignment
- Feet shoulder width apart
- Knees extended
- Neutral pelvis with minimal posterior rotation
- Shoulder retraction, depressed and internally rotated
- Chest expanded anteriorly and axial extension to neutral with chin tuck

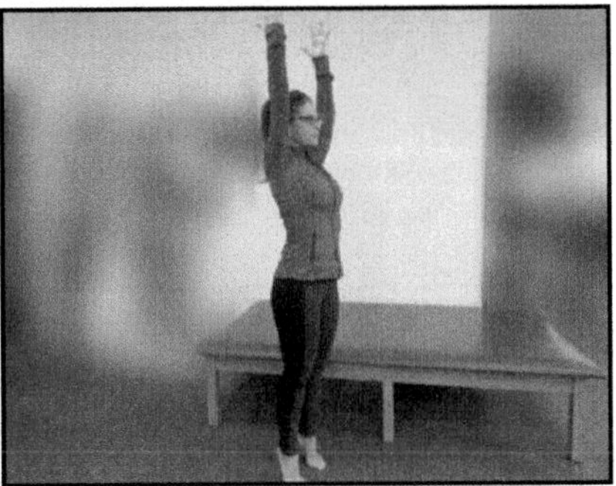

B. Standing elongation with shoulder flexion

- Begin in standing starting position
- Plantar flex bilateral ankle to maintain balance on toes
- Simultaneously flex shoulders with extended elbows and internally rotated shoulders
- Inhalation occurs throughout the motions
- Return to starting point

**Figure 19-11.** Yoga-based standing exercises. (A) The standing starting position. (B) Standing elongation with shoulder flexion. *(continued)*

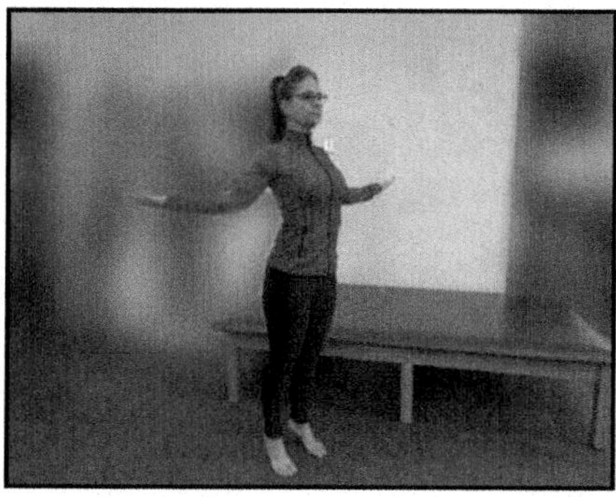

C. Standing elongation with shoulder external rotation and scapular retraction

- Begin in standing starting position
- Plantar flex bilateral ankle to maintain balance on toes
- Simultaneously, retract scapula, horizontally abduct and externally rotate shoulders with flexed elbows with supination of the forearm
- Inhalation occurs throughout the motions
- Return to starting point

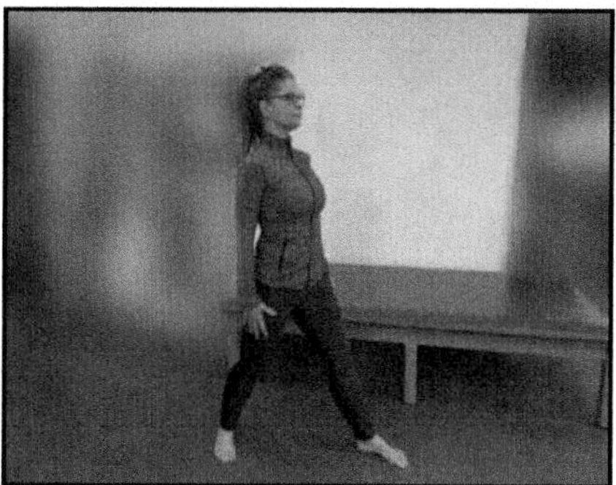

D. Asymmetrical stabilization

- Begin at standing starting position
- Advance one lower extremity similar to a stride in gait
- Maintain position avoiding loss of balance with rear foot in slight external rotation
- Advanced control can have rear foot internally rotate to parallel with the contralateral lower extremity

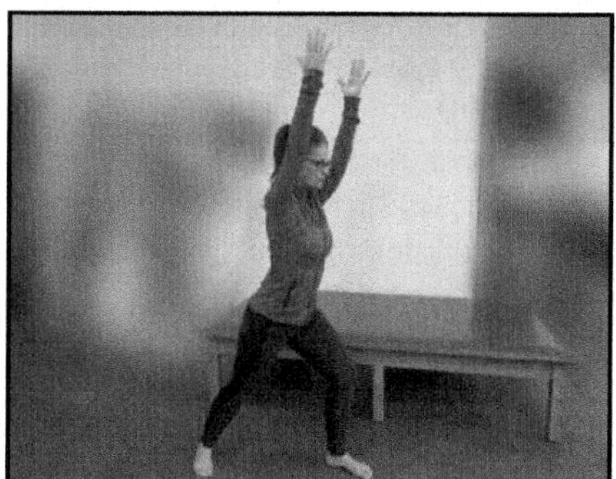

E. Transitional dynamic stability with should flexion

- Begin at asymmetrical stabilization position
- As bilateral shoulders flex, translate weight to forward limb
- Inhalation during the activity
- Hold and continue for a breath count of up to 5

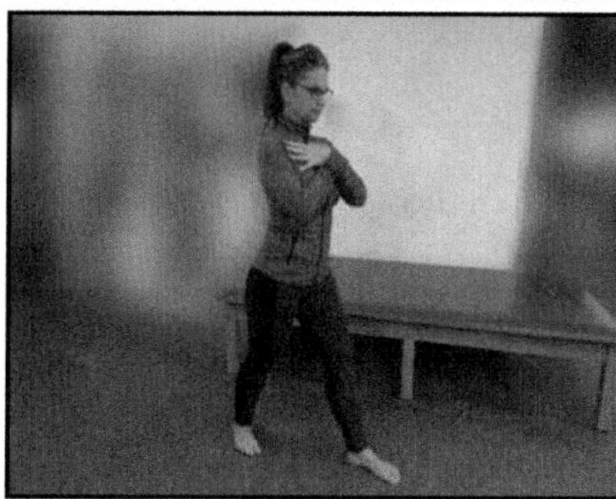

F. Translational dynamic stability with shoulder internal rotation

- Begin at translational dynamic stability with shoulder flexion
- As bilateral shoulders extend, translate weight to back limb
- Exhalation during the activity
- Hold and continue for a breath count of up to 5

**Figure 19-11 (continued).** (C) Standing elongation with shoulder external rotation and scapular retraction. (D) Asymmetrical stabilization. (E) Translational dynamic stability with shoulder flexion. (F) Translational dynamic stability with shoulder internal rotation.

A person with lymphedema or one at risk for developing lymphedema must be aware of the potential for cellulitis and erysipelas.[57,58] Cellulitis is a bacterial infection that can affect the dermis and subcutaneous tissues. Signs of cellulitis include inflammation, warmth, and pain with possible systemic fever.[58] Erysipelas is a type of cellulitis causing an inflammation to the superficial layer of the skin or upper dermis. It appears as a raised, red rash that is tender. These infections are more commonly seen on the involved limb after surgical cancer-related procedures. The infection can occur when damage to the skin allows bacteria to enter and proliferate. A regimen of antibiotics is the most common course of treatment.[57,58]

Clinicians must educate patients to avoid injury during exercise. Patients should be educated on preventing cellulitis by avoiding injury to the area, keeping their skin clean and moisturized, and keeping fingernails and toenails manicured.

Erysipelas or cellulitis can occur abruptly. Cellulitis is characterized by a change in the patient's skin appearance that includes an acute poorly demarcated erythema (rubor) that may also present with heat (calor). The other classic signs of inflammation that can occur are dolor (pain) and swelling. The onset of cellulitis can occur for the following reasons:

- A puncture to the skin in the edematous extremity that allows bacteria to infiltrate and then proliferate
- Trauma to the extremity that can initiate the inflammatory response
- Superficial fungal infections[56]

It is important for the physical therapist assistant to recognize and address potential cellulitis by immediately reporting the findings to the physical therapist and/or the referring physician. If the patient is being treated through direct access, an immediate referral to the emergency room is warranted. When treating patients with cancer, the assistant must be aware of and follow the contraindications and precautions discussed throughout this chapter.

### Considerations for the Physical Therapist Assistant: Pain and Exercise

- When initiating an exercise, the assistant should select a level that is the least physically stressful to determine the impact and the patient's response.
- If there is any report or indication of pain or inflammation, the exercise must be stopped immediately. Even the lowest levels of discomfort can be an indication of a potential situation that may increase swelling and should be reported to the physical therapist.

There are additional factors that must be considered when developing a treatment and exercise plan for patients with cancer. As stated earlier, thermal modalities should be avoided because of the potential for increase in lymphedema. Blood pressure should not be taken on an extremity that has or may be at risk for lymphedema. Constriction of the involved extremity may exacerbate or initiate an onset of lymphedema, so consider using dumbbells vs cuff weights. Physical therapist assistants should avoid applying any equipment to a limb that could rub or compress the affected area. Make adjustments to an exercise program gradually, avoiding large changes in intensity, duration, or frequency. The patient should be encouraged to wear their compression garment or wraps during exercise. Changes in a specific exercise are best when they occur in one parameter at a time to monitor the effects of the change on the patient. Ensure adequate rest periods occur to avoid overexertion as well.

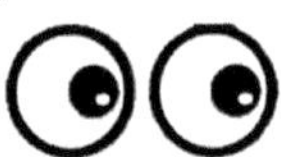

### Eye on the Research

A systematic meta-analysis reported that aerobic exercise showed better improvement in reducing CRF than aerobic and resistance exercise combined. High adherence to the exercise program had a greater effect on CRF than moderate to low adherence. Low-intensity exercise was more beneficial than high-intensity programs. Researchers noted that a high volume of exercise could have adverse effects on CRF, resulting in low adherence. Strenuous exercise is not needed to get positive results; low-intensity exercise may be adequate to reduce the effects of CRF.[59]

Additionally, researchers summarized that exercise programs have a positive impact on CRF because they reduced deconditioning and increased strength and physical fitness. However, physical therapist assistants need to monitor patients with cancer and survivors for any report or indication of pain, insomnia, depression, and anxiety because these can have a negative impact on CRF.[59]

### Certification Programs

Physical therapist assistants can become certified in CDT. The certification process varies among educators. Physical therapist assistants should review their state practice act to determine any specific practice considerations. It is advised that clinicians treating these patients be certified. The following institutions offer CDT training: the Norton School of Lymphatic Therapy (https://www.nortonschool.com), the Academy of Lymphatic Studies (https://www.acols.com), and the Dr. Vodder School (https://www.vodderschool.com).

## Conclusion

The physical therapist assistant participates as a member of the health care team in the treatment of persons diagnosed with cancer both during and after medical treatment concludes. The physical therapy team plays an important role in maximizing a person's recovery and function, providing patient education, and developing and progressing exercise interventions. Physical therapy team members who are lymphedema certified participate in lymphedema treatment and management. Effective treatment and appropriate therapeutic exercise is essential to the patient's recovery. The physical therapy team provides graded therapeutic interventions that consider the patient's comprehensive presentation. The physical therapist assistant incorporates knowledge of precautions, monitoring, and cancer-related risk factors to create individualized intervention programs that focus on maximizing the patient's quality of life and functional outcomes.

## Review Questions

1. Describe the stages of lymphedema.
2. What is the difference between primary and secondary lymphedema?
3. Discuss which physical therapy treatment interventions are indicated and which are contraindicated for a client with secondary right upper extremity lymphedema with a right shoulder passive ROM restriction?
4. What cancer-related treatment is most likely to lead to the development of fibrosis?
5. Define and list the signs and symptoms of cellulitis and erysipelas.
6. Describe the contraindications and precautions that need to be considered when treating patients with cancer.
7. List and describe the 4 components of CDT.
8. Discuss the potential indications for incorporating yoga within a treatment program for a person with cancer.

## Case Study

A 66-year-old woman was referred to physical therapy in October 2010 after desmoid tumor surgical excision with subsequent lymphedema to the left upper extremity (onset approximately 1 month prior). The patient reported pain and swelling that made it difficult for her to lift her arm and perform specific functional activities, including washing her hair, lifting any objects, or dressing using that arm.

Patient's cancer history: Initially diagnosed with breast cancer in December 2006.

- The patient underwent 16 rounds of chemotherapy in February 2007 before undergoing a bilateral mastectomy with removal of all left upper extremity lymph nodes in July 2007. During chemotherapy and radiation therapy, she noticed increased numbness and tingling in both feet. It decreased but still occurred in her toes. The symptoms were so severe that she was unaware of her spatial orientation, resulting in difficulty with walking, transfers, and ADLs.
- In January 2008, the patient underwent resection of the mastectomy due to heavy pulling and scar tissue. After 2 weeks of successful physical therapy treatment for lymphedema, the patient's function began to decline; she was referred to an oncologist and was diagnosed with a desmoid tumor in the left axillary region in August 2009. The patient then underwent intensive chemotherapy that reduced the size of the tumor enough to surgically excise it without damaging tissues surrounding the brachial plexus. The pectoral major muscle (75%) and the left lateral rib cage at the levels of ribs 2 to 4 were removed.

Patient's other previous medical history: Left anterior cruciate ligament repair and left patellar fracture from a fall, appendectomy, and a possible thyroid problem.

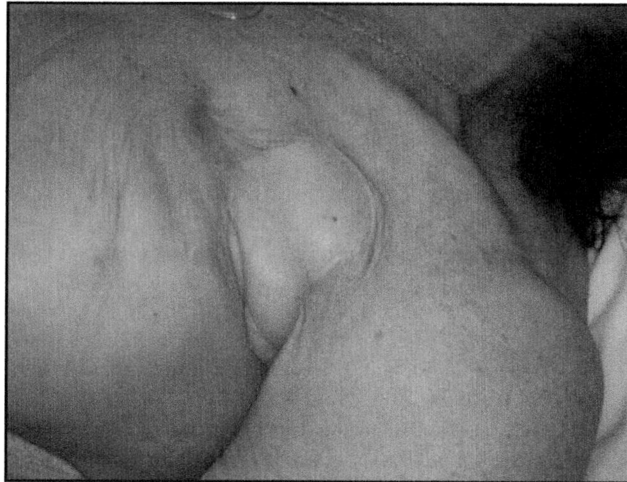

**Figure 19-12.** Left shoulder after mastectomy and skin graft following excision of desmoid tumor, pectoral muscle, and ribs 2 through 4.

Medications: Lexapro (escitalopram) for depression and anxiety, Arimidex (anastrozole) for the treatment of early breast cancer postmenopause, and vitamins for general health benefits. She demonstrated no signs or symptoms of acute distress at the initial evaluation and system pathology review. The patient reported a fair energy level, good response to emotional stress, good communication skills, good eating habits, fair sleeping patterns, and fair knowledge of exercise and fitness with no history of behavioral health risks.

Patient's prior functional status: Independent without pain or limitation in ambulation, instrumental ADLs, work, or recreation.

Goals of therapy: Reduce left upper extremity edema, increase left upper extremity strength and passive ROM, and decrease pain. Improve work performance, instrumental ADLs, recreational performance, and related activities to the patient's prior level of function (Figure 19-12).

1. What type of lymphedema does this patient have?
2. At what stage of lymphedema is this patient?
3. What intervention technique will facilitate the movement of the stagnant interstitial fluid?
4. Considering the removal of the desmoid tumor and resection of the rib cage, which therapeutic exercises are most appropriate to use initially?
5. Anticipating a postsurgical postural deficit, which muscle group would need lengthening and which muscle group would need strengthening?

## Acknowledgments

A special thank you to Cecilia D. Lester, PTA, LMT, ERYT 200, RYT 500, for her yoga-based therapeutic exercises and demonstration.

# References


1. Pierotti MA. The molecular understanding of cancer: from the unspeakable illness to a curable disease. *Ecancermedicalscience.* 2017;11:747. doi:10.3332/ecancer.2017.747
2. Siegel RL, Miller KD, Jemal A. Cancer Statistics, 2017. *CA Cancer J Clin.* 2017;67(1):7-30. doi:10.3322/caac.21387
3. Miller K, Siegel R, Lin C, et al. Cancer treatment and survivorship statistics, 2016. *CA Cancer J Clin.* 2016;66(4):271-289. doi:10.3322/caac.21349
4. Yang E, Chung S, Jeon J, et al. Current practice and barriers in cancer rehabilitation: perspectives of Korean physiatrists. *Cancer Res Treat.* 2015;47(3):370.
5. Singh B, Newton R, Cormie P, et al. Effects of compression on lymphoedema during resistance exercise in women with breast cancer-related lymphoedema: a randomised, crossover trial. *Lymphology.* 2015;48(2):80-92.
6. Kwan M, Cohn J, Armer J, et al. Exercise in patients with lymphedema: a systematic review of the contemporary literature. *J Cancer Surviv.* 2011;5(4):320-336.
7. Ferguson C, Swaroop M, Horick N, et al. Impact of ipsilateral blood draws, injections, blood pressure measurements, and air travel on the risk of lymphedema for patients treated for breast cancer. *J Clin Oncol.* 2016;34(7):691.
8. Asdourian MS, Skolny MN, Brunelle C, Seward CE, Salama L, Taghian AG. Precautions for breast cancer-related lymphoedema: risk from air travel, ipsilateral arm blood pressure measurements, skin puncture, extreme temperatures, and cellulitis. *Lancet Oncol.* 2016;17(9):392-405. doi:10.1016/s1470-2045(16)30204-2
9. Gradishar W, Anderson B, Balassanian R, et al. Breast Cancer Version 2.2015. *J Natl Compr Canc Netw.* 2015;13(4):448-475.
10. Piper M, Peled AW, Sbitany H. Oncoplastic breast surgery: current strategies. *Gland Surg.* 2015;4(2):154-163. doi:10.3978/j.issn.2227-684X.2015.03.01
11. Schmauss D, Machens HG, Harder Y. Breast reconstruction after mastectomy. *Front Surg.* 2016;2:71. doi:10.3389/fsurg.2015.00071
12. Anampa J, Makower D, Sparano JA. Progress in adjuvant chemotherapy for breast cancer: an overview. *BMC Med.* 2015;13(1):195. doi:10.1186/s12916-015-0439-8
13. Fernandez F, Kosinski A, Burfeind W, et al. STS lung cancer resection risk model: higher quality data and superior outcomes. *Ann Thorac Surg.* 2016;102(2):370-377. doi:10.1016/j.athoracsur.2016.02.098
14. Aoyagi T, Terracina KP, Raza A, Matsubara H, Takabe K. Cancer cachexia, mechanism and treatment. *World J Gastrointest Oncol.* 2015;7(4):17. doi:10.4251/wjgo.v7.i4.17
15. Belloum Y, Rannou-Bekono F, Favier FB. Cancer-induced cardiac cachexia: pathogenesis and impact of physical activity. *Oncol Rep.* 2017;37(5):2543-2552. doi:10.3892/or.2017.5542
16. Pfaff AK. Exercise and cancer related fatigue: an evidence-based analysis. 2017. Accessed February 7, 2023. https://www.semanticscholar.org/paper/Exercise-and-Cancer-Related-Fatigue%3A-An-Analysis-Pfaff/1d80af50eae4c957dc747e16939e02aad0c87575
17. Meneses-Echávez JF, González-Jiménez E, Ramírez-Vélez R. Effects of supervised multimodal exercise interventions on cancer-related fatigue: systematic review and meta-analysis of randomized controlled trials. *Biomed Res Int.* 2015;2015:328636. doi:10.1155/2015/328636
18. Schmitz K, Courneya K, Matthews C, et al. American College of Sports Medicine roundtable on exercise guidelines for cancer survivors. *Med Sci Sports Exerc.* 2010;42(7):1409-1426.
19. Smith T, Broomhall C, Crecelius A. Physical and psychological effects of a 12-session cancer rehabilitation exercise program. *Clin J Oncology Nurs.* 2016;20(6):653-659. doi:10.1188/16.cjon.653-659
20. O'Connor M. Targeting the DNA damage response in cancer. *Mol Cell.* 2015;60(4):547-560.
21. Ryttov N, Blichert-Toft M, Madsen E, et al. Influence of adjuvant irradiation on shoulder joint function after mastectomy for breast carcinoma. *Acta Radiol Oncol.* 1983;22(1):29-33.
22. Craythorne E, Benton E, Macfarlane S. Axillary web syndrome or cording, a variant of mondor disease, following axillary surgery. *Arch Dermatol.* 2009;145(10):1199-2000. doi:10.1001/archdermatol.2009.239
23. Leduc O, Fumiere E, Banse S, et al. Identification and description of the axillary web syndrome (AWS) by clinical signs, MRI and US imaging. *Lymphology.* 2014;47(04):164-176.
24. Leidenius M, Leppänen E, Krogerus L, et al. Motion restriction and axillary web syndrome after sentinel node biopsy and axillary clearance in breast cancer. *Am J Surg.* 2003;185(2):127-130.
25. Hurria A, Mohile S, Gajra A, et al. Validation of a prediction tool for chemotherapy toxicity in older adults with cancer. *J Clin Oncol.* 2016;34(20):2366-2371. doi:10.1200/jco.2015.65.4327
26. Marrs J, Newton S. Updating your peripheral neuropathy "know-how." *Clin J Oncol Nurs.* 2003;7(3):299-306. doi:10.1188/03.CJON.299-303
27. Segal R, Zwaal C, Green E, et al. Exercise for people with cancer: a clinical practice guideline. *Curr Oncol.* 2017;24(1):40.
28. Niederer D, Schmidt K, Vogt L, et al. Functional capacity and fear of falling in cancer patients undergoing chemotherapy. *Gait Posture.* 2014;39(3):865-869.
29. Naeim A, Reuben D. Geriatric syndromes and assessment in older cancer patients. *Oncology (Williston Park).* 2001;15(12):1567-1577.
30. Orr RM. Optimized conditioning practices for load carriage tasks. *TSAC Report.* 2012;2012(25):25.7-25.10.
31. Panek I, Bui T, Wright A, et al. Cutaneous afferent regulation of motor function. *Acta Neurobiol Exp (Wars).* 2014;74:158-171.
32. Borreani S, Calatayud J, Martin J, Colado JC, Tella V, Behm D. Exercise intensity progression for exercises performed on unstable and stable platforms based on ankle muscle activation. *Gait Posture.* 2014;39(1):404-409. doi:10.1016/j.gaitpost.2013.08.006
33. Neil-Sztramko S, Kirkham A, Hung S, et al. Aerobic capacity and upper limb strength are reduced in women diagnosed with breast cancer: a systematic review. *J Physiother.* 2014;60(4):189-200.
34. Jones L, Courneya K, Mackey J, et al. Cardiopulmonary function and age-related decline across the breast cancer survivorship continuum. *J Clin Oncol.* 2012;30(20):2530-2537. doi:10.1200/jco.2011.39.9014
35. Jones L, Habel L, Weltzien E, et al. Exercise and risk of cardiovascular events in women with nonmetastatic breast cancer. *J Clin Oncol.* 2016;34(23):2743-2749.
36. Tisdale M. Mechanisms of cancer cachexia. *Physiol Rev.* 2009;89(2):381-410.

37. Alves CRR, Cunha TFD, Paixão NAD, Brum PC. Aerobic exercise training as therapy for cardiac and cancer cachexia. *Life Sci.* 2015;125:9-14. doi:10.1016/j.lfs.2014.11.029
38. Moore JE Jr, Bertram CD. Lymphatic system flows. *Annu Rev Fluid Mech.* 2018;50:459-482. doi:10.1146/annurev-fluid-122316-045259
39. Chikly B. Lymph drainage therapy (LDT) manual lymphatic mapping and its clinical applications to lymphedema. *National Lymphatic Network.* 2000;12(3):1-7.
40. Stolldorf D, Dietrich M, Ridner S. A comparison of the quality of life in patients with primary and secondary lower limb lymphedema: a mixed-methods study. *West J Nurs Res.* 2016;38(10):1313-1334.
41. International Society of Lymphology Executive Committee. The diagnosis and treatment of peripheral lymphedema: 2016 consensus document of the International Society of Lymphology. *Lymphology.* 2016:49(4):170-184.
42. Pereira de Godoy LM, Pereira de Godoy Capeletto P, de Fátima Guerreiro Godoy M, Pereira de Godoy JM. Lymphatic drainage of legs reduces edema of the arms in children with lymphedema. *Case Rep Pediatr.* 2018;2018(4):1-3. doi:10.1155/2018/6038907
43. Park H, Kim Y, Kim T. The role of visual feedback in respiratory muscle activation and pulmonary function. *J Phys Ther Sci.* 2015;27(9):2883-2886.
44. Trevisan M, Boufleur J, Soares J, et al. Diaphragmatic amplitude and accessory inspiratory muscle activity in nasal and mouth-breathing adults: a cross-sectional study. *J Electromyogr Kinesiol.* 2015;25(3):463-468.
45. Boris M, Weindorf S, Lasinski B. Persistence of lymphedema reduction after noninvasive complex lymphedema therapy. *Oncology (Williston Park).* 1997;11:110-114.
46. Lite R, Mejia S. Resistance training for breast cancer survivors. *Strength Cond J.* 2010;32(5):60-62.
47. Hwang O, Ha K, Choi S. The effects of PNF techniques on lymphoma in the upper limbs. *J Phys Ther Sci.* 2013;25(7):839-841.
48. Hwang W, Chung S, Chung M, et al. Effect of proprioceptive neuromuscular facilitation D2 flexion and breathing exercises on lymphedema without a short stretch compression bandage. *J Phys Ther Sci.* 2015;27(10):3341-3343.
49. Narahari SR, Aggithaya MG, Thernoe L, Bose KS, Ryan TJ. Yoga protocol for treatment of breast cancer-related lymphedema. *Int J Yoga.* 2016;9(2):145-155. doi:10.4103/0973-6131.183713
50. Şener H, Malkoç M, Ergin G, et al. Effects of clinical pilates exercises on patients developing lymphedema after breast cancer treatment: a randomized clinical trial. *J Breast Health.* 2017;13(1):16-22.
51. Fong S, Ng S, Luk W, et al. Effects of qigong exercise on upper limb lymphedema and blood flow in survivors of breast cancer: a pilot study. *Integr Cancer Ther.* 2014;13(1):54-61.
52. Galantino M. Tai chi for well-being of breast cancer survivors with aromatase inhibitor-associated arthralgias: a feasibility study. *Altern Ther Health Med.* 2013;19(6):38-44.
53. Ambroza C, Geigle PR. Aquatic exercise as a management tool for breast cancer–related lymphedema. *Top Geriatr Rehabil.* 2010;26(2):120-127. doi:10.1097/tgr.0b013e3181dfd91f
54. Xin M, Zhang H, Zhong Q, et al. Combining manual lymph drainage with physical exercise after modified radical mastectomy effectively prevents axillary web syndrome. *J Phlebol Lymphol.* 2017;10(1):15-18.
55. Campo RA, Light KC, O'Connor K, et al. Blood pressure, salivary cortisol, and inflammatory cytokine outcomes in senior female cancer survivors enrolled in a tai chi chih randomized controlled trial. *J Cancer Surviv.* 2014;9(1):115-125. doi:10.1007/s11764-014-0395-x
56. Mazor M, Lee J, Peled A, et al. The effect of yoga on arm volume, strength, and range of motion in women at risk for breast cancer-related lymphedema. *J Altern Complement Med.* 2018;24(2):154-160.
57. de Godoy J, da Silva S. Prevalence of cellulitis and erysipelas in post-mastectomy patients after breast cancer. *Arch Med Sci.* 2007;3(3):249-251.
58. Morris AD. Cellulitis and erysipelas. *BMJ Clin Evid.* 2008;2008:1708.
59. Kessels E, Husson O, van der Feltz-Cornelis CM. The effect of exercise on cancer-related fatigue in cancer survivors: a systematic review and meta-analysis. *Neuropsychiatr Dis Treat.* 2018;14:479-494. doi:10.2147/NDT.S150464

Chapter 20

# Exercise for the Medically Complex Patient

*Jacki Klaczak Kopack, PT, DPT*

**KEY TERMS** Anemia | Arthritic diseases | Chronic kidney disease | Chronic liver disease | Critical illness myopathy | Diabetes mellitus | Osteoporosis

## Chapter Objectives

1. List the factors associated with a medical diagnosis that could affect a patient's participation in physical therapy.
2. Describe the appropriate monitoring and exercise progressions for a patient with a complex medical presentation.
3. Describe the intervention/treatment modifications that are indicated when a patient presents with selected medical conditions.
4. Describe the impact medications can have on physiological responses to exercise, and list ways to ensure safe patient monitoring.

The presence of medical conditions (comorbidities) can lead to a decrease in physical activity and deconditioning, which can result in decreased exercise capacity and an impaired response to exercise. This can result in a loss of function, an increased burden on caregivers, increased costs to assist/maintain independent living, and decreased quality of life (QOL). The importance of regular exercise is recognized by leading health organizations including the World Health Organization, the American Heart Association, the American College of Sports Medicine (ACSM), and the US Department of Health and Human Services.[1-4]

Most patients can safely participate in exercise. Physical therapists and physical therapist assistants are educated and knowledgeable about varied pathologies. Physical therapy team members are uniquely qualified to apply that knowledge while promoting a patient's increased activity and independence. Physical therapist assistants work in a variety of treatment settings, and they will assist in developing, monitoring, and progressing exercise programs for persons with multiple medical conditions.

The US Department of Health and Human Services, the American Heart Association, the World Health Organization, and the ACSM recommend regular physical activity, at least 150 minutes per week of moderate physical activity (or 75 minutes per week of vigorous activity) and muscle strengthening activities (for all major muscle groups) for 2 or more days a week.[1-4] The ACSM in its guidelines for exercise for older adults recommends that the activities reflect their current level of fitness and patient



Kopack JK, Cascardi KA.
*Principles of Therapeutic Exercise for the Physical Therapist Assistant* (pp 667-682).

response.[5] The ACSM has published exercise guidelines for persons with chronic disease/disability. These guidelines provide general guidance and activity recommendations, reflecting that many diseases require similar monitoring, that exercise is almost universally beneficial, and that the presence of chronic conditions can increase the likelihood of decline in function and independence.[1] It is beneficial to maintain strength, range of motion (ROM), and endurance because these affect a person's ability to maintain independence in functional mobility, activities of daily living (ADLs), and instrumental ADLs. The ACSM guidelines for persons with chronic disease are summarized in Table 20-1. Each person with a chronic condition should be physically active and should participate in regular exercise. Persons at an increased risk for falls should participate in an individualized program to address the factors that increase their fall risk.[1]

The guidelines provide a low-intensity starting point for exercise, and exercise should be modified based on patient presentation. The more acutely ill a patient is, the larger the number of comorbidities, or the greater the extent of deconditioning, the more monitoring and care the physical therapy team must use when increasing physical activity for a patient. Medications, medical procedures, and surgical interventions affect patient presentation. Certain medications can alter a patient's response to activity. Orthopedic or postsurgical precautions may alter a patient's ability to participate or significantly increase the energy expenditure of participation (ie, increased energy required for ambulation after a lower extremity amputation).

The primary physical therapy priority is to maintain patient safety. This is achieved using appropriate guarding, the use of a gait belt and safety equipment (ie, body weight–supported treadmill or LiteGait treadmill), and appropriate safety precautions (ie, proper footwear, a slow increase of activity parameters, ongoing monitoring of vital signs, and monitoring of the rate of perceived exertion [RPE]). The risk of adverse effects because of the medical pathology can be reduced by completing pre-exercise stress testing and using ongoing monitoring while gradually adjusting exercise intensity. There are few evidence-based guidelines for exercise parameters if an exercise test was not completed. The development and progression of an exercise program are often based on a therapist's clinical experience paired with careful observation of the patient's physiological responses to activity. The ACSM exercise recommendations for persons with chronic disease without exercise test results are listed in Table 20-2.

Slow, gradual progression and ongoing monitoring of the patient's response are indicated when implementing an exercise program with a medically complex patient. A patient may only tolerate a few minutes of activity at the initiation of the program; the patient may be limited quickly by fatigue. Many patients will begin to see increased exercise tolerance and decreased fatigue after only a few sessions. The risk of an adverse event occurring with exercise increases with high-intensity aerobic work, high-resistance exercise/heavy weights, and end-range/aggressive stretching. The physical therapist assistant should discuss any concerns about a patient's response to exercise with the supervising physical therapist. An adverse response to exercise that jeopardizes patient safety warrants activation of the emergency medical system.

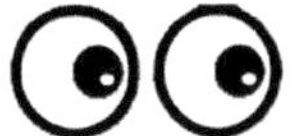

### Eye on the Research: Is There a Role for High-Intensity Interval Training for Patients With a Chronic Disease?

There is a newer body of evidence that considers the use of high-intensity interval training (HIIT) for patients with chronic diseases. Low-volume HIIT may have an advantage over moderate, continuous training because it has been shown to produce fewer negative training symptoms (ie, fewer complaints of dyspnea and leg discomfort). HIIT may be considered for patients with a chronic disease if the patient tolerates and prefers this training method because this may result in increased compliance. For the chronically ill patient, early integration of low-volume HIIT may include interspersing brief periods of faster walking followed by a recovery period. The physical therapist assistant should review current research before making a decision to try HIIT with a patient; much of the currently available research concludes that there is a need for further research with larger populations. A review of the current literature appears to indicate that HIIT presents little risk for stable patients when prescribed exercise protocols are followed and careful monitoring is in place.[1,6-10]

## Integrating Data From the Physical Therapist Examination

The physical therapist integrates data about the patient's comorbidities with the current medical status and functional performance to create a treatment plan and goals. Key information that the physical therapist assistant should review includes the patient's current level of assistance, balance, and activity tolerance. Exertional symptoms (eg, "I can walk one block before my legs cramp up," "I can stand at the sink for 4 minutes before I'm too tired to continue") and recovery time (how long the symptoms last after the patient has stopped the activity) are also important. This information assists the clinician in creating an appropriate baseline level of activity. For most pathologies, the physical therapist assistant will not ask the patient to work to the point of the onset of symptoms.

**Table 20-1**

American College of Sports Medicine Exercise Guidelines for Persons With Chronic Disease[1]

| Type | Frequency | Duration | Intensity | Progression |
|---|---|---|---|---|
| Aerobic | 4 to 5 days per week | Target goal of 40 minutes per session, but start at patient tolerance | Self-selected gait speed or alternate aerobic activity. Use RPE to monitor. | To RPE of 3 to 5/10, gradually increasing time to 40 minutes over 4 weeks |
| Resistive exercise | 2 to 3 days per week | 1 set of 8 to 12 repetitions to fatigue or functional activities (sit to stands, reach, step-ups, and biceps curls) | 50% to 70% of 1RM or functional activities: Goal is a minimum of 8 sit to stands, 10 step-ups (each foot), and 8 repetitions of arm curls | Increase repetitions as tolerated<br>Target goal of 2 sets of 10 repetitions; advance to this as tolerated |
| Flexibility | 3 days per week | 20 seconds per stretch | No pain | |
| Warm-up/cooldown | Every session | 10 to 15 minutes | RPE <3 | |

1RM = one-repetition maximum.

**Table 20-2**

American College of Sports Medicine Exercise Recommendations for Persons With Chronic Disease When No Exercise Test Results Are Available[1]

| Type of Exercise | Recommended Intensity/Parameters |
|---|---|
| Aerobic exercise | Activity at 2 to 4 metabolic equivalent level<br>Exercise HR = resting HR + 20 beats/minute<br>RPE not to exceed 11 to 14 (on the 6 to 20 Borg RPE Scale)<br>Ongoing physiological monitoring |
| Strengthening exercise | 2 sets of 30 seconds of sit to stands<br>2 sets of 8 biceps curls with 4 kg<br>2 sets of 10 step-ups<br>2 sets of seated chair reaches (30 seconds each to each side) |

HR = heart rate.

**Clinical Tip**

Knowledge of pathologies is important to keep the patient safe. The physical therapist assistant will typically avoid activities that reproduce symptoms. This is important for patient safety as well as for maximizing patient compliance. For example, a patient with a disk herniation will not be asked to complete exercises that cause radicular symptoms, numbness, or weakness. A patient with myopathy will not be asked to work those muscles to the point of fatigue or cramping. However, for certain pathologies, such as intermittent claudication, the therapist will ask the patient to exercise just to the point of discomfort (but never to the point of inducing pain or cramps). Patient education that emphasizes the goals and benefits of each exercise can encourage patient compliance.

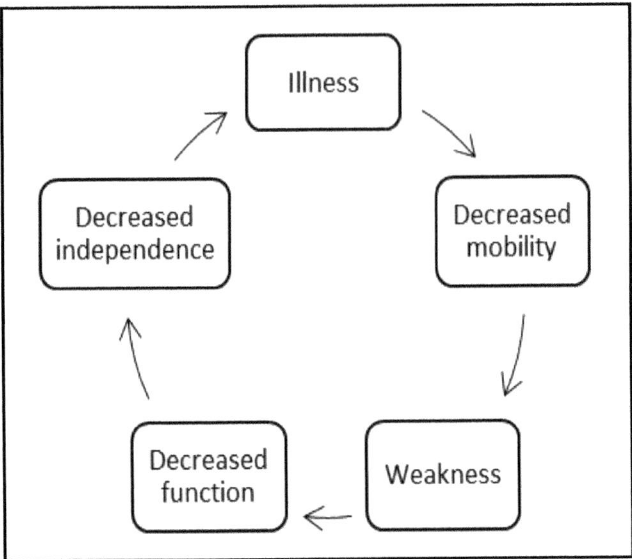


**Figure 20-1.** The downward spiral of illness.

## Preparing Mind and Body

A patient's willingness to participate and their desire to increase fitness levels can greatly affect the potential for improvement/success. The clinician can assess a patient's readiness to participate by considering the following: Does the patient see a benefit to exercising? Is the patient ready to try to exercise? and Is the patient motivated to build a habit of exercise? It is often easier to educate a patient who is self-motivated to improve. Patients with chronic illness or multiple comorbidities may be apprehensive and unable to see that exercise could lead to improvement. Inactivity and a lack of exercise can contribute to a loss of strength and endurance. The physical therapy team will treat patients who experience the downward spiral that often occurs after a significant or prolonged illness. Illness or pain can limit the patient's desire to move, which can lead to decreased strength and function, often resulting in a patient becoming more dependent on others (Figure 20-1).

A therapist who is able to inspire a patient can act as a coach for a patient who is initially reluctant or apprehensive or who demonstrates less internal motivation. Referring the patient to support groups, obtaining counseling, and having the medical team reinforce the benefits of increasing activity may increase the patient's willingness and motivation to exercise. Patients who acknowledge the need for exercise have already taken the first step to improving function! The physical therapy team can guide the patient and provide direction regarding optimal exercise interventions. Additionally, the assistant can encourage the patient when it is time to progress the exercise program.

The relationship with the patient begins during the initial evaluation when the physical therapist asks the patient their goals. This is especially important when working with patients with a complex medical presentation for whom motivation may be hampered by fear and initial mobility gains and progress may be slow. The therapist investigates areas in which increased activity and function can benefit the patient. The therapist gathers information regarding the patient's "big picture goals" (eg, "Walking on the beach with my grandkids," "Being able to climb 6 steps so that I can attend my child's sports game"). The therapist breaks the patient's big goal into manageable "chunks" or short-term goals. These short-term goals are linked to the functional long-term goals; yet, they are smaller and easier to attain. This can help the patient see progress and remain motivated. It is important for the therapist to provide feedback ("You walked 100 feet [ft] further this week; that gets you closer to the boardwalk ramp from the street") to keep the patient motivated and focused on their goals.

The clinician should monitor the patient before, during, and after exercise. Pre-exercise vital signs (HR, blood pressure [BP], respiratory rate, oxygen saturation, and pain) are assessed at each treatment. For patients with brittle control of diabetes, blood glucose should be assessed pretreatment as well. During exercise, vital signs are monitored (including RPE), and the therapist carefully observes the patient's response to the increased activity. Postexercise monitoring is indicated as well as a final assessment after cooldown is completed. As the patient becomes more familiar with the exercise program, the focus will shift to training the patient to self-monitor their vital signs (RPE and HR), promoting a shift to patient responsibility for the exercise program. The most effective physical therapy interventions result in discharging a patient at a higher level of function.

A common concern of patients with multiple medical comorbidities or significant deconditioning is the fear of increasing activity. Educating the patient about what is normal to experience during and after exercise as well as the signs/symptoms that warrant stopping exercise is helpful to minimize apprehension (Table 20-3).

## Commonly Used Assessment Tests

Validated assessment measurements create an objective baseline measurement to track the patient's progress. Many of these tests have normative reference values; this allows the clinician to categorize a patient's performance

**Table 20-3**

The Exercise Experience[1,5,11,12]

| What Exercises Can Do |
|---|
| • Result in feelings of increased energy<br>• Gradually improve fitness and activity tolerance<br>• For patients who are very ill, maintain function |
| **When Not to Exercise** |
| • With a fever (> 100 °F)<br>• With a new illness that has not been diagnosed<br>• If ambient temperature/humidity is excessive<br>• If the patient describes feeling ill |
| **Signs to Reduce Exercise Intensity** |
| • Borg RPE rating > 17/20 (very hard or very, very hard)<br>• Breathing too hard to talk<br>• Muscle soreness that lasts > 24 hours and prevents exercise the next day<br>• Excessive fatigue after exercise<br>• Does not feel recovered after an hour after exercise stopped |
| **When to Stop Exercise and Ask for Help*** |
| • New-onset chest pain<br>• Significant shortness of breath<br>• Dizziness<br>• Blurred vision<br>• Excessive fatigue<br>• Leg cramping that does not dissipate after exercise is terminated |
| *Red flags/safety note |

in comparison to a healthy population.[13,14] Data have been published that allow the clinician to compare the patient's performance to others with the same pathology.[15] Tests that may be useful for a patient who is medically complex or one who is deconditioned include the 2-Minute Walk Test, self-selected walking speed (or self-paced gait speed), the 30-Second Sit-to-Stand Test, the 5 Times Sit-to-Stand Test, and the Timed Up and Go Test. The Short Physical Performance Battery is a reliable, valid tool that has been used to predict disability (it assesses 4-meter gait speed, 5 repetitions of sit to stand, and balance).[16]

## *Considerations and Monitoring for Common Pathologies*

For patients with multiple medical issues, the general goal is to increase activity levels gradually and to reduce barriers to increasing activity. The clinician should consider how much of the patient's time is committed to disease management; this can affect motivation to exercise. Depending on the severity of the disease, improved function may not be a realistic goal, and the therapist may be focused on maintaining current abilities. The patient may also present with depression, which can impact motivation and performance.

Current research describing optimal exercise prescription for persons with chronic diseases is limited.[17] This chapter synthesizes the basic tenets of exercise, the available research, and medical management to provide an overview of appropriate modifications and necessary monitoring that are warranted to maximize patient safety. It is outside the scope of this text to provide a comprehensive review of the pathophysiology of each of these diseases. The reader should refer to pathophysiology textbooks to obtain comprehensive information about the varied conditions.

Some patients may have a medical pathology that has not yet been diagnosed. A comprehensive physical therapy examination will typically note any areas of concern that warrant a medical referral. Sometimes a systemic cause may not be fully evident during evaluation. In this situation, the physical therapist assistant may begin to note signs/symptoms that are inconsistent with the musculoskeletal diagnosis that is being treated. In this case, it is imperative that the physical therapist assistant carefully observe and document all new or changed findings and follow up with the supervising physical therapist. Physical therapy can effectively treat musculoskeletal pathologies. Musculoskeletal diagnoses have consistent symptom characteristics and presentations that can be reproduced with appropriate testing and assessment techniques. If the clinician cannot reproduce symptoms during the examination/testing, this may indicate a medical or systemic reason for the symptoms. Medical diagnoses and systemic issues require follow-up by the physician for medical management. It is important to remember that if we cannot reproduce it, we cannot treat it.

## Diabetes Mellitus

**Diabetes mellitus (DM)** is a metabolic disorder characterized by elevated blood glucose levels. DM occurs in people due to a decrease in the production of insulin, as a result of increased insulin resistance of the cells, or both. Type 1 diabetes (insulin-dependent DM) is characterized by an absolute inability to produce insulin; this patient must take insulin for survival. People with type 2 diabetes (non–insulin-dependent DM) typically have decreased production of insulin and cellular insulin resistance. Non–insulin-dependent DM is treated with diet, exercise, and oral medication. There is an increased risk of developing type 2 diabetes for individuals who are less active. Exercise training, especially when combined with dietary changes, has beneficial effects in improving glycemic control, cardiovascular risk profile, body composition, and cardiorespiratory fitness.[5,11] Recent research indicates that patients with type 2 diabetes may benefit from vigorous-intensity training (interval training) 5 to 7 days a week and regular strength training (at least twice a week).[5,18,19]

Normal fasting blood glucose levels are less than 100 mg/dL, and the normal nonfasting level is less than 140 mg/dL. Hypoglycemia is defined as blood glucose less than 70 mg/dL. Hypoglycemia can be a relative response as well; patients whose blood glucose level has been routinely elevated may experience signs/symptoms of hypoglycemia if there has been a rapid and significant drop from the prior elevated level. Hypoglycemic episodes tend to have rapid onset and present with the following signs/symptoms: weakness, shakiness, nervousness, tingling around mouth, pallor, sweating, and confusion. They can occur up to 12 hours after exercise.[11] Hyperglycemia is defined as blood glucose levels greater than 250 mg/dL, and patients experiencing hyperglycemia present with a flushed face, increased thirst, acetone/fruity breath scent, abdominal pain, and confusion.[11] Hyperglycemic episodes tend to have a more gradual onset.[11]

Generally, exercise should be avoided if blood glucose is less than 70 mg/dL or greater than 250 mg/dL (especially if there are ketones in the urine). If blood glucose is less than 100 mg/dL, administer a small carbohydrate snack before exercise (eg, handful of crackers, fruit). If a patient experiences hypoglycemia, stop the exercise and administer glucose (fruit juice or honey). Whenever possible, patients should exercise early in the day and at a consistent time. Supervised exercise is recommended in the event of a hypoglycemic episode. If the exercise period is longer than 30 minutes, snacks should be available.[11]

People with type 1 or type 2 DM with poor or inconsistent glucose control should test their blood glucose 15 minutes before exercise. The clinician should be aware of the patient's medical management of the disease, including whether the patient is injecting insulin or using an insulin pump. Exercise should be coordinated with mealtimes and the insulin dose to minimize the risk of hypoglycemia. Exercise should not coincide with peak insulin uptake times, and it should not target muscles where insulin was recently injected (because the insulin is then absorbed much more quickly). The patient may need to increase food or reduce insulin when new exercise is added or when exercise intensity is increased (dependent on the individual's glucose level response to activity). Strenuous or prolonged exercise increases the risk of severe hypoglycemia (the highest risk is 6 to 14 hours after exercise); therefore, adjusting food and insulin is important to avoid nocturnal hypoglycemia.[11,20] Patients often experience polyuria, so adequate hydration is important. Aquatic exercise (especially in a warm pool) can increase insulin absorption; patients' vital signs and blood glucose levels should be carefully monitored with aquatic exercise.[20] Patients with diabetes (especially type 1) are at increased risk of autonomic neuropathy. Autonomic neuropathy can affect BP, temperature control, digestion, and bladder function; it occurs when the nerves that control involuntary bodily functions are damaged (as occurs with poorly managed DM). Autonomic neuropathy can result in exercise intolerance if the patient's HR does not increase appropriately with increases in activity level. It creates an increased risk of myocardial infarction, which can occur without the warning signs of angina. Monitoring HR and BP responses to exercise is important; an atypical vital sign response should be reported to the supervising physical therapist.

Patients with DM have an increased risk of developing peripheral neuropathy and are at risk for impaired wound healing (increasing their risk for amputation). Educate the patient about proper foot and skin care (including routine skin checks of the feet) and the importance of wearing well-fitted supportive shoes. Peripheral neuropathy can result in impaired ankle strategies and decreased balance reactions; balance training may be beneficial.

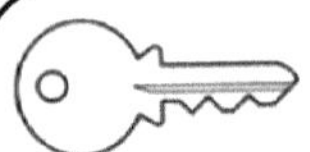

### Key Safety Considerations: Diabetes and Exercise

- Monitor blood glucose levels.
- Know the signs/symptoms of hypoglycemia and hyperglycemia.
- Have fruit juice or honey readily available.

## Cancer

Cancer treatments often result in decreased levels of physical activity and function. Exercise can improve health-related QOL, fatigue, and the overall level of fitness and independence during medical treatment and remission and after the cancer is cured.[21,22] Higher cardiorespiratory fitness and physical activity levels are associated with lower mortality rates in survivors.[23] Cancer survivors can follow the same exercise parameters as the general population, although the progression of intensity may be more gradual.[5] Modification to exercise will need to be made for survivors with metastatic bone disease and cardiac conditions.[5,11] The ability to maintain long-term outcomes is more likely when survivors participate in group exercise or supervised exercise programs with exercises performed at a moderate intensity (3 to 6 times the baseline resting state) on an ongoing basis.[22]

Cancer treatment protocols and treatment durations vary significantly depending on the type of cancer (see Chapter 19). The body's physiological response to different cancer treatments (eg, chemotherapy, radiation) can affect a patient's compliance with a fitness program and activity tolerance. Treatment (especially chemotherapy) can result in an increased risk of cardiac dysfunction; thorough screening is indicated before starting a new exercise program. The medical team will assess for the presence of peripheral neuropathies, musculoskeletal morbidities, cardiac issues, and signs/symptoms of metastasis.[22]

The physical therapist assistant will monitor vital signs before, during, and after each exercise session and check laboratory values before each session (especially during ongoing cancer treatments). The assistant should monitor HR, BP, respiratory rate, RPE, and oxygen saturation monitoring as well as observe for any signs indicating cardiorespiratory complications of treatment (eg, excessive fatigue, pallor, sweating, significant shortness of breath).

Precautions to participating in aerobic exercise include anemia, a low platelet count, and a low white blood cell count (see Chapter 2).[11] Patients with severe fatigue can try to complete gentle flexibility exercises daily and can include brief periods of activity. (Even 5 minutes is better than nothing, and the amount of time can be increased as the patient's tolerance improves.) Patients with significant neuropathy or gait or balance dysfunction may benefit from supported exercise options (eg, a recumbent bike, NuStep machine [NuStep, Inc]).[24] Patients with colon cancer who undergo an ostomy (colostomy or ileostomy) should begin resistance exercise with low resistance. Exercise intensity should be gradually progressed to limit the risk of herniation, and providing education to avoid the Valsalva maneuver is important. When exercising with patients postmastectomy, progress resistance training gradually, and begin with low resistance. Monitor for any signs or symptoms of lymphedema, and stop exercise if new symptoms arise (see Chapter 19). For patients with bony metastasis, exercise intensity and volume may need to be reduced, and moderate- or high-impact activities should be avoided. The aquatic environment should be avoided for survivors who are immunocompromised or receiving radiation and for those with indwelling lines (catheters, central lines, percutaneous endoscopic gastrostomy tubes, and ostomies).[5]

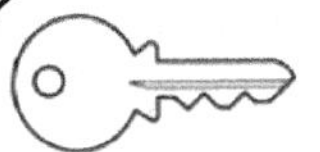

**Key Safety Considerations: Cancer and Exercise**

- Monitor vital signs and RPE.
- Follow up with the supervising physical therapist, and consider holding exercise/activity when hemoglobin is less than 10 g/dL, platelets are less than 50,000/mL, or the white blood cell count is less than 3,000/mL (or 10,000/mL with a fever).

Although research supports the benefits of physical activity for people with cancer, there is not widespread adherence to programs focused on increasing physical activity.[25] Barriers to exercise include physical capability, symptoms, comorbidities, previous sedentary lifestyle, psychological influences, and a lack of perceived relevance. Environmental factors (eg, access to services, resources, and time constraints) can lower compliance with exercise. Research has determined that the best "enablers" of promoting increased activity include knowledge of the anticipated benefits, frequent opportunity, and encouragement from clinicians. The clinician should prioritize educating the patient on the benefits of exercise. Proactively addressing barriers may help promote compliance.[26] Patients should be encouraged to continue with daily activity and exercise during treatment unless exercise worsens the patients' symptoms or specific complications develop that preclude exercise.

## Critical Illness Myopathy

Acutely and critically ill patients can benefit from a monitored, carefully progressed exercise and mobility program. The clinician must review all aspects of the patient's history, current medical status, and current physiological presentation. Early mobilization is beneficial.[27,28] The physical therapist evaluates the risk of mobility vs the risk of immobility, and the physical therapist assistant who participates in the care of these patients needs additional training beyond entry-level education. The clinician reviews the plan of care (POC) before initiating an episode of care, reviews the patient's current status with the nurse, checks the chart for any new orders, and reviews laboratory values and tests before entering the patient's room. Treatment begins with a review of vital signs and the patient's status to ensure that it is appropriate to initiate treatment. Treatment interventions are focused on increasing mobility and improving cardiorespiratory status, endurance, and muscle strength; interventions to address these goals are created based on the individual's current abilities.[11] Common interventions include progressive ROM exercises, submaximal resistance exercises, low-intensity endurance exercises, and function-based mobility training.

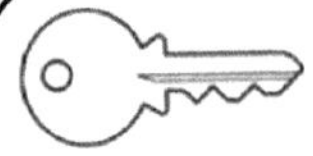

**Key Safety Considerations: Critical Illness Myopathy and Exercise**

- Monitor vital signs and RPE before, during, and after treatment.
- Check all laboratory values pretreatment.

## Chronic Kidney or Liver Disease

Patients with kidney and liver disease are often deconditioned and fatigue quickly. Exercise (as long as it is monitored and progressed gradually) is generally safe. These patients often will not tolerate formal exercise testing, but functional exercise testing and a gradual progressive program can be beneficial.[1]

**Chronic kidney disease** is a progressive deterioration of kidney function; the kidneys become less effective at filtering out toxins and maintaining fluid and electrolyte balance. Common causes of kidney dysfunction include diabetes, uncontrolled hypertension, congenital conditions, and autoimmune dysfunction. Chronic kidney disease can progress to end-stage renal disease (ESRD). Patients with ESRD often present with anemia, osteopenia, fatigue, myopathy, disorientation, shortness of breath, and an increased risk of cardiovascular disease.[11] Compliance with infection control protocols and handwashing is important because of the increased risk of infection. Patient compliance with the prescribed dietary and fluid restrictions is important.

The assistant will monitor laboratory values presession and assess vital signs and RPE each session. The therapist may assist in the patient's clinical care by recording the patient's weight and intake/output (depending on the treatment setting and what activities were completed during the treatment session). For patients with ESRD, the resting BP and HR may be elevated if a dialysis session was missed. For patients receiving dialysis, the therapist will need to coordinate therapy sessions around the scheduled dialysis treatments. Exercise can be completed before, during, or after dialysis (based on the patient's tolerance and preference). Note that completing exercises after dialysis may increase the risk of a hypotensive episode. The patient with ESRD with an arteriovenous shunt can exercise that limb (unless there are specific physician orders not to), but there should be no weight or pressure placed over the shunt, and the clinician should avoid taking BP in that limb.[11] Patients who receive continuous ambulatory peritoneal dialysis may be more comfortable if they drain any excess fluid before exercise.

The ACSM recommends initiating exercise at a low intensity using gradual progressions of intensity with a goal of aerobic exercise 3 to 5 days per week for 20 to 60 minutes and resistance exercise 2 to 3 days per week. The patient can start with intermittent bouts of aerobic activity (3 to 5 minutes if tolerated with a 1:1 rest period as needed; ie, 3 minutes of walking and 3 minutes of rest) with a goal of increasing activity time to 30 minutes as tolerated. Resistance exercise of at least one set of 10 repetitions at 70% of 1RM twice a week is recommended.[5]

**Chronic liver disease** is a progressive deterioration of liver function often caused by chronic inflammation (hepatitis) or alcohol abuse. These patients often present with weight loss, jaundice, coagulopathies, and weakness.[11] Frequent rest periods may be indicated to reduce the metabolic demand on the liver.[11] These patients will benefit from a slowly progressed, low-intensity exercise program. The goal may be to maintain current functional status; therapy interventions may not result in actual functional gains (depending on the severity of the disease).[1]

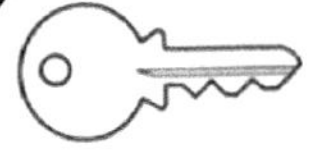

**Key Safety Considerations: Chronic Kidney or Liver Disease and Exercise**

- Check laboratory values pretreatment, and hold exercise if indicated.
- Monitor vital signs and RPE.
- For patients with ESRD with an arteriovenous shunt or fistula, no BP in the extremity that has the arteriovenous shunt and no pressure over the dialysis shunt with activity.
- No exercise if BP is greater than 200/100 mm Hg.
- Modify exercise and activity based on the individual's presentation every session.

## Anemia

Anemia occurs because of diseases or pathology that cause a decrease in the quantity or quality of red blood cells. A reduction in red blood cells causes a decrease in hemoglobin and a reduced ability to transport oxygen to the cells of the body. **Anemia** is defined as hemoglobin less than 14 g/dL for men and less than 12 g/dL for women. The symptoms include fatigue, weakness, and dyspnea.[11,20] Hemoglobin levels less than 8 g/dL are generally considered a reason to "hold" (postpone) therapy.[11] The clinician should review facility-specific protocols; some facility protocols may differ.

As hemoglobin levels decrease, activity tolerance decreases; therefore, activity expectations and treatment interventions must be modified. With lower hemoglobin levels, there is less oxygen circulating to the body's tissues and organs. As activity increases, organs and muscles require more oxygen, and these structures that were adequately oxygenated at rest become deprived during activity because of a decrease in oxygen availability. To meet the increased demand for oxygen, the HR and respiratory rate will increase at a faster rate than expected, even with low levels of activity. This increased workload increases the oxygen needed by the heart muscle. This is one of the reasons why a person with anemia may experience chest pain with exercise as well as fatigue and weakness. Tachycardia often occurs with light activity, so vital sign monitoring is indicated. Initial exercise interventions should be short with frequent rest periods as indicated by symptoms. Gradual increases in activity duration and intensity are appropriate.

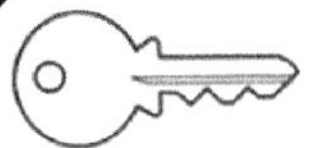

**Key Safety Considerations: Anemia and Exercise**

- Monitor vital signs and RPE.
- Check laboratory values pretreatment.
- Encourage a gradual increase in exercise intensity.

# HIV and AIDS

Infection with HIV affects the function of the body's immune system. Infection and disease progression is variable from person to person and is impacted by the medical treatments a person receives. The HIV infection progression moves through specific, defined stages that include seroconversion (postinfection, often presenting with flu-like symptoms), asymptomatic or stage 1 (can last many years), and symptomatic or stage 2 (symptoms and opportunistic diseases present). AIDS (stage 3) is defined by a CD4+ T-cell count less than 200 cells/µL and is characterized by severe weight and muscle loss and recurrent opportunistic infections.[29]

Advances in medical treatment and the broad use of antiretroviral medicines have resulted in significantly improved life expectancy for persons with HIV. The medical interventions (and their side effects) result in varied comorbidities, including an increased risk of dyslipidemia, insulin resistance, muscle atrophy, and peripheral neuropathy.[5,11] Patients living with HIV can have a widely varied presentation, from relatively healthy to extremely ill, based on the stage of disease. Regular exercise can contribute to maintaining muscle strength, decreasing body fat, and maintaining cardiorespiratory function, all of which may work to offset the increased risk of cardiometabolic disease.[30-33] Current evidence does not clearly indicate that exercise decreases viral load, but the positive psychological benefit of exercise paired with the physical advantages reinforce the importance of regular exercise for persons with HIV. There is preliminary research that appears to indicate that regular aerobic exercise may positively affect CD4+ counts in persons living with HIV, but further research is warranted.[34]

Transmission risk to a physical therapist or physical therapist assistant is typically low because transmission requires exposure to blood or infected body fluids (ie, amniotic fluid; cerebrospinal fluid; synovial, peritoneal, pleural, or pericardial fluid; semen; or vaginal secretions). The use of proper infection control procedures typically mitigates the risk to the clinician. Compliance with infection control is important regardless of the treatment setting; the Centers for Disease Control and Prevention estimates that approximately 20% of people who are HIV positive are unaware of their diagnosis.[29]

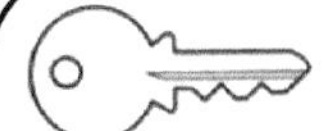

**Key Safety Considerations**

- Maintain compliance with infection control in all therapy settings and use protective barriers (eg, gloves, gowns, eye shields) when handling blood or bodily fluids.
- Do not treat patients if you have open/unhealed/uncovered wounds.
- Use caution to avoid needlesticks or scalpel sticks.
- If occupational exposure occurs, immediately follow up to obtain postexposure prophylaxis (follow facility-specific protocols).

Exercise is considered safe and beneficial for persons who are HIV positive. Patient education that reinforces the benefit of exercise and that encourages the creation of exercise as a habit promotes compliance. The physical therapist assistant will review the patient's physical therapy evaluation, paying attention to muscle strength, cardiac status/endurance, and any indication of peripheral neuropathy (which may indicate an increased fall risk or potential for gait disturbances). The assistant should verify that the patient's nutritional intake is adequate to support adding exercise. (Any concerns should be directed to the physical therapist and a dietician or nutritionist.) The clinician will check laboratory values before initiating an exercise program and will check vital signs after each intervention.

Exercise interventions are individualized based on the patient's disease stage and presentation. Generally, exercise recommendations for a person with asymptomatic HIV follow ACSM guidelines and include aerobic exercise training 3 to 4 times a week at 70% to 80% of the patient's maximal HR at an RPE of 14 or less. Intensity is adjusted based on the patient's presentation. Resistance training progressing to 2 to 3 times a week at 8 to 10 repetitions at 60% repetition maximum will be beneficial to maximizing/

maintaining strength.[1,5] As the disease progresses, the patient's tolerance for activity often decreases, and the program will be modified as needed. Interventions should reflect the patient's goals while still including a modified aerobic and strengthening program. Patients should not exercise to the point of fatigue, and additional rest/recovery time may be indicated.[11]

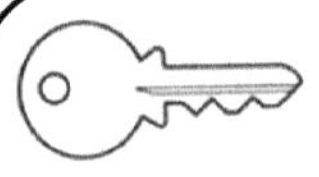

**Key Safety Considerations: HIV and AIDS and Exercise**

- Monitor vital signs and RPE.
- Check laboratory values pretreatment.
- Do not exercise to the point of fatigue.
- Hold exercise if acute myopathy or myositis is present.
- Institute fall precautions if gait disturbance or peripheral neuropathy is present.
- Refer to a nutritionist or dietician if there are concerns regarding nutritional intake.

## Obesity

Being overweight or obese is defined by having a body mass index greater than 25 or greater than 30, respectively.[35] Being overweight increases the risk of developing many other diseases (including, but not limited to, cardiac disease, diabetes, and musculoskeletal pain/disease), and the rates of obesity are increasing worldwide.[35] Being overweight creates barriers to exercise, but exercise is beneficial in improving health, assisting with weight loss, and maintaining weight loss. Being overweight can result in joint pain (especially foot, ankle, knee, hip, and low back) that can interfere with the ability to exercise.[1] The clinician should consider the impact that increased body weight has on exercise intensity. For example, walking may be a moderate-intensity activity for a person who is obese (vs mild intensity for a person with a much lower body mass index).

The therapy team can play a role in primary prevention by providing education regarding regular exercise and activity to the community, especially those at risk of being overweight.[1,5] The therapy team prescribes exercise for the person who is overweight and provides interventions to address the complications of obesity (eg, lymphedema, skin ulcers).

To maximize safety with exercise for patients who are overweight, the clinician monitors vital signs, educates the patient about cardiac signs/symptoms (reasons to terminate exercise), has the patient exercise in a climate-controlled environment, and monitors for overheating. The clinician selects activities to maximize patient enjoyment and minimize injury risk. The aquatic environment addresses a number of these issues, but not all patients are comfortable with initiating an aquatic exercise program (because of concerns about appearance or concerns about safety with entering/exiting the pool).

Exercise recommendations include moderate to vigorous aerobic exercise 30 minutes per day (increasing to up to 60 minutes per day) at least 5 days per week at a predetermined target HR.[1,5] Activity intensity and duration may be low initially. The addition of carefully progressed resistance training can assist with weight loss and maintenance. For best results, if weight loss is a goal, the overall medical plan should include behavioral modification and a personalized nutrition/eating plan.

There are varied surgical procedures that are available to treat obesity and promote bariatric weight loss. The patient's status post–bariatric surgery will often include abdominal surgery precautions, specific recommendations for activity, and exercise progression recommendations that are related to healing times and postoperative nutritional intake. The clinician should communicate closely with the medical team when developing exercise programs for these patients.

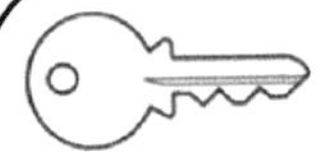

**Key Safety Considerations: Obesity and Exercise**

- Monitor vital signs and RPE.
- Use appropriate-size BP cuff.
- Avoid overheating.
- Select activities that minimize joint loading (consider an ergometer or bike).
- Alter activity if skin chafing occurs.

## Arthritis

Osteoarthritis (OA) or degenerative joint disease is a slowly progressive joint disease; the cartilage covering the joint surface wears down, and damage progresses to the underlying bone. OA is often associated with overuse and occurs more often in the weight-bearing joints (hips and knees) but may also be seen in the distal interphalangeal and proximal interphalangeal joints of the hand (most commonly in postmenopausal women). OA causes bony joint enlargement, decreases in ROM, pain, crepitus, and eventually joint deformity and loss of function.[11,12] Pain tends to increase with activity and decrease with rest, and patients often report stiffness after inactivity. The severity of symptoms does not correlate well with the presence of damage on radiography.[11]

Rheumatoid arthritis (RA) is a chronic, systemic, autoimmune, inflammatory disease that presents with articular and extra-articular symptoms. RA is a chronic multijoint arthritis that commonly affects joints bilaterally, with frequent involvement of the wrists, knees, hands, and feet. RA causes fatigue, diffuse pain, joint deformity, decreases in ROM, and loss of function. RA can also involve the cardiovascular, pulmonary, and gastrointestinal systems. There is a risk for atlantoaxial subluxation if there is cervical spine involvement. (Any new neurochanges or changes in bowel/bladder function should be reported to the physician emergently.) It is a disease of exacerbations and remissions. Pain tends to be the worst in the morning and after rest.[11]

For OA and RA, the focus of treatment interventions includes patient education, joint protection, proprioception exercises, and strengthening exercise. Joint protection includes recommendations for proper posture and minimizing joint compression.[11,12] Exercise in an aquatics environment or selecting biking vs running can provide joint protection. The clinician may recommend the use of an assistive device to off-load compressive forces or the use of a shoe orthotic to promote better alignment of the lower extremity. Lateral heel wedges or insoles are sometimes prescribed to reduce knee varus torque and decrease pain for patients with knee OA, but evidence does not consistently support this intervention.[36] Regular exercise, maintaining a healthy weight, and maximizing muscle strength around the affected joints can help lower the risk of disability associated with arthritis.[11,12] The supervising physical therapist will screen the joints above and below the affected joints and assess for impaired posture or biomechanics that may be contributing to the patient's symptoms.

Pain is a primary factor affecting compliance with exercise, so it is important to select exercises that are the least painful for the patient. Cycling is often preferred over treadmill walking. An extended warm-up may improve participation and decrease pain and swelling. The therapist should monitor the patient's symptoms throughout treatment. Aerobic training is generally recommended with a goal of greater than 150 minutes per week, although a patient may start with bouts of 5 to 10 minutes as indicated by their tolerance. Resistance training exercises are generally low to moderate resistance (10 to 15 repetitions at 40% to 60% 1RM). The inclusion of eccentric and weight-bearing exercises can be beneficial for strengthening as well as increasing proprioceptive feedback through the lower extremity joints as long as these exercises do not increase the symptoms.[5,12] A patient may experience an increase in discomfort after exercise, but any increase in pain that is significantly greater than pre-exercise values or lasts greater than 2 hours after exercise may indicate that the intensity was too high, necessitating program modification.[12]

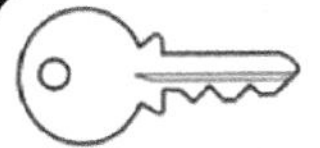

### Key Safety Considerations: Osteoarthritis and Rheumatoid Arthritis and Exercise[5,11,12]

- Monitor vital signs and pain.
- Report any new or concerning medication side effects to the physician.
- Consider aquatics (ideal temperature 83 °F to 88 °F).[37]
- Wear appropriate footwear (with good shock-absorbing soles).
- If mild swelling, ice before exercise. If moderate swelling, hold exercise, and consider use of ice and electrical stimulation to address swelling. Gentle ROM can be completed.
- Stretching is contraindicated over any areas of swelling.
- If patient cannot tolerate longer duration activity, consider shorter bouts throughout the day.
- Avoid high-impact activities (running and step machine).

**Additional Safety Considerations With Rheumatoid Arthritis**

- No stretching or resistance exercises to the involved joints during acute flare-up.
- Encourage compliance with splints (if needed).
- Any new onset of lower extremity weakness, balance changes, altered deep tendon reflex (DTR), or incontinence warrant immediate medical referral.

Resistance and aerobic exercise are beneficial to improve function and QOL for patients with RA.[38,39] Additional factors to address when treating a person with RA include ADL modification, energy conservation training, and education to minimize joint damage during flare-ups. During flare-ups, resistance, flexibility, and stretching activities should be discontinued around the inflamed joints and replaced with gentle ROM exercises.[11,12] RA can result in joint instability, so any new complaints or observations should be brought to the attention of the physical therapist and may require splinting for protection (especially during a flare-up). A person with RA (especially in the later stages) can be at increased risk of cervical instability, creating a risk for atlantoaxial subluxation or dislocation, which can be life-threatening.[11,20,40] The physical therapist should screen the neck before delegating any cervical exercises or interventions to the assistant. The assistant should immediately report any new symptoms that may indicate cervical cord compression (eg, new-onset lower extremity weakness, incontinence, gait disturbances, or changes in DTRs).[11,20,40]

## Thyroid Disease

The thyroid gland produces hormones that assist in regulating the metabolic rate of the body and the regulation of body functions. Thyroid disease can present as hyperthyroidism or hypothyroidism. Both of these diseases, if untreated or poorly managed, can result in cardiac failure. Thyroid disease should be stable (adequately controlled medically) before initiating exercise.[11] Hyperthyroidism is caused by oversecretion of thyroid hormones and often presents with signs/symptoms that include tremors, restlessness, tachycardia/palpitations, weakness, fatigue, heat intolerance, exophthalmos (protruding eyes), increased DTRs, and hypermetabolism (often presenting as weight loss without dieting). A patient can present with thyroid disease without any visible changes to the neck appearance.[11] Hypothyroidism occurs when there is a deficiency of thyroid hormone, and the patient often presents with fatigue, headache, report of slowed mental function (feeling "foggy" or forgetful), weakness, myalgia, bradycardia, intolerance to cold, paresthesia, coarse/thinning hair, weight gain (often reported without changes in diet/exercise), and constipation.[11]

The assistant should report any new onset of systemic signs/symptoms to the therapist. If a patient with well-controlled disease presents with new systemic signs/symptoms or a patient reports noncompliance with treatment/medications, this must also be brought to the supervising therapist's and physician's attention. Thyroid disease should be medically stable before adding exercise for the patient.[11,20] Once the disease is managed, exercise interventions can be gradually increased to match the parameters for the healthy individual. A gradual increase in intensity with careful monitoring of vital signs is important, especially for persons with newly treated hypothyroidism; it is possible that these patients will have decreased activity tolerance due to the hypometabolic rate.[11]

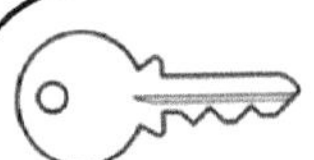

**Key Safety Considerations: Thyroid Disease and Exercise**

- Monitor vital signs and RPE.
- Report any new or changing systemic signs/symptoms.
- Gradually increase activity while ensuring compliance with medications and appropriate vital sign response to activity.

## Osteoporosis

**Osteoporosis** is a progressive skeletal disease that causes decreases in bone mass, bone mineral density, and bone quality, resulting in a decrease in bone strength and an increased risk of fractures.[1,11] The ACSM recommends weight-bearing exercise 3 to 5 days per week and resistance exercise 2 to 3 times a week.[5] Exercise should not cause pain. Patients with osteoporosis may present with postural changes (thoracic kyphosis is common), which may increase fall risk or create difficulty when attempting some exercises. A regular program of weight-bearing aerobic exercise may not have a significant impact on increasing bone strength, but it can improve functional mobility, endurance, and muscle endurance, thereby reducing fall risk. It is necessary to avoid maximal strengthening exercise as well as end-range joint mobilization assessment tests. Patients' status postfracture may exhibit prolonged healing times (resulting in the prolonged use of weight-bearing restrictions). People with postural changes or at risk for thoracic kyphosis should include exercises that address trunk extension. Trunk flexion exercises should be avoided, although posterior pelvic tilts and mini-crunches appear to be safe to include.[11,41]

## Burns

A patient who presents with burns is at increased risk of fluid and electrolyte imbalance, so laboratory values should be compared with the patient's prior values/normal ranges before treatment (see Chapter 2). Physical therapy treatment goals often include maintaining/increasing ROM; promoting wound healing; assisting with edema control; and increasing strength, functional mobility, and independence.[11] Patients with large or significant burns often report chronic joint pain/stiffness, difficulty walking or running, fatigue, weakness, and limited motion.[42] Therapy interventions are often uncomfortable and painful for a patient with significant burns, so timing therapy to coincide with peak pain medication performance is beneficial. Patients who are receiving modalities for wound care should be carefully screened for any contraindications associated with the modality. Strict adherence to infection control procedures should be maintained with all interventions. Maintaining ROM is an extremely important goal after a burn. A regular ROM program should occur at least 2 to 3 times per day because areas with wounds/burns are prone to contracture development. However, ROM exercises are contraindicated in the area of a recent skin graft. Typically, the ROM program will focus on moving the patient out of the comfort position of the joint. Careful attention to positioning is required for patients with burns as well as the consideration of ways to minimize pressure on any areas of at-risk or injured skin. Appropriate positioning can be attained with the use of pillows, towel rolls, splints, and multipodus boots and by alternating the use of supine, seated, side-lying, and prone positions. Position selection is based on patient presentation, burn location, medical status, and the ability to tolerate the position.[11,43] Optimal positions are described in Table 20-4. Functional mobility can be progressed per patient tolerance.

**Table 20-4**

Optimal Positioning for Various Burn Areas[11,43]

| Burn Area | Optimal Positioning |
|---|---|
| Neck | Extension if the anterior neck is burned, neutral if the posterior neck is burned |
| Axillary area | Arm abduction 90 to 110 degrees |
| Elbow | Arm extension, splint in minimal (< 10 degrees) flexion |
| Hand | Splint in the functional position of the hand (wrist extension, metacarpophalangeal flexion to 90 degrees, proximal interphalangeal/distal interphalangeal extension), using web spacers as needed |
| Hip | Hip extension, neutral for rotation |
| Knee | Knee extension (be sure to provide pressure relief for the heels) |
| Ankle | Neutral (including subtalar joint) |

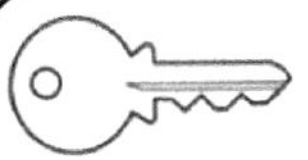

**Key Safety Considerations: Burns and Exercise**

- Monitor vital signs and oxygen saturation throughout treatment.
- Review laboratory values pretreatment (sodium, potassium, chloride, magnesium, serum albumin/prealbumin, hemoglobin, and white blood cells).
- Maintain compliance with infection control.
- Provide regular ROM (unless contraindicated because of a recent grafting procedure).
- Position the patient to maintain optimal function in the affected joint.
- Maintain all positioning precautions/restrictions per physician's orders (to protect healing graft tissue).

## The Impact of Medications on Patient Performance and Status

The medications that a patient takes can have an impact on a patient's performance in physical therapy. Although an in-depth presentation of medications is outside the scope of this text, a number of the more commonly prescribed medication classes are briefly described in Appendix E. Understanding how medications can affect the patient's response to exercise is an important component of providing holistic and safe patient care. Physical therapist assistants spend the majority of their time in direct patient contact; they are in the optimal position to observe and recognize side effects and adverse or toxic effects and to notify the physical therapist and physician. Adverse drug reactions describe unwanted or potentially harmful effects of a drug, and they can be mild, moderate, severe, or lethal. Medication side effects are predictable effects that are often unavoidable with appropriate dosing. The assistant will update the physical therapist and/or physician with any significant changes in patient status or if any new adverse effects are observed. The physical therapist assistant should be comfortable with looking up medication actions and side effects. Familiarity with medications and monitoring the patient appropriately help to keep the patient safe.

## Special Considerations in the Home Care Environment

A physical therapist assistant will encounter patients with many of these medical diagnoses when working in home care. Students often ask the following question: "Is home care a good treatment environment for a new graduate of a physical therapist assistant program?" In a number of states, new graduates are unable to work in home care (because there is not direct supervision from the physical therapist). It is the opinion of the authors that any new physical therapist assistant graduate (or new clinician in general) benefits from hands-on direction and mentoring from experienced clinicians. The home care environment is especially challenging because the clinician may be the only treating clinician "on the case." All clinicians in the home care setting act as the eyes and ears for the entire medical team. A novice clinician typically does not have the experience to recognize subtle changes in a patient's medical status that may lead to true emergencies. The physical therapist/physical therapist assistant treating patients in the home is often responsible for the following tasks in addition to the therapy interventions:

- Regular monitoring of vital signs (understanding baselines and assessing changes that may be early indicators of infection or change in status)
- Medication reconciliation (checking a patient's medication list, determining patient compliance, and reporting any changes in medications to the nurse/case manager)
- Education of the patient and caregiver

- Home modification recommendations
- Careful monitoring of patient presentation/medical status and providing regular updates to both the supervising physical therapist and the medical team manager

Effective and safe completion of these tasks is most appropriate for a clinician who has experience working with patients with multiple medical issues.

## Conclusion

Physical therapist assistants will treat patients of all ages in diverse clinical settings. Knowledge of medical diagnoses is needed for the provision of safe, effective care because the patient's medical conditions (comorbidities) and their medications can affect the patient's ability to participate in physical activities and exercise. A physical therapist assistant who is able to integrate information about a patient's primary treatment diagnosis, comorbidities, medications, and current presentation is better prepared to create safe and effective treatment plans.

## Review Questions

1. A patient with cancer who is undergoing chemotherapy is being treated in the hospital, and the physical therapy POC includes ambulation and light-resistance exercise. Which laboratory value results should the assistant review before treatment?
2. List 3 appropriate treatment interventions to include when treating a patient with critical illness myopathy.
3. What modifications to a treatment program are indicated for a patient with ESRD who has a right forearm arteriovenous fistula?
4. List the recommended exercise parameters for a patient with medically managed HIV.
5. Describe exercise modifications to increase compliance for a patient with RA.
6. Describe exercise parameters for a patient with moderate osteoporosis. What exercises are most appropriate? Which exercises are contraindicated?
7. Describe recommended positioning for a patient with moderate burns to the left axillary region.
8. List 3 objective assessment tools that are appropriate for use with a patient with multiple medical comorbidities.
9. What adverse side effects of corticosteroid use are likely to impact a physical therapy exercise program? What additional monitoring should the assistant plan to complete?
10. What is the medication Lopressor (metoprolol) indicated to treat? What monitoring is most appropriate for the assistant to complete when working with a patient who is taking Lopressor?

## Case Study

The patient is a 54-year-old presenting with the chief complaint of pain and difficulty completing job-related duties (which require walking the length of a 1000-ft warehouse).

- Past medical history: Type 2 DM, hypothyroidism
- Medical referral diagnosis: Right knee pain related to OA
- Medications: Metformin, Novolin N (insolin isophane; daily), NovoLog (insulin aspart; before meals based on blood sugar reading), Synthroid (levothyroxine), and Naprosyn (naproxen)
- Physical therapist evaluation notes: Pain at rest (right knee) 2 of 10, with gait 7 of 10
- Strength: 4+/5 bilateral lower extremity, except right knee 3+/5 with pain with resisted testing
- Crepitus present with ROM
- Active ROM within normal limits, except right knee 5 to 125 degrees, with passive ROM within normal limits
- Mild varus deformity right knee
- Mobility: Independent with transfers, gait 200 ft with single-point cane (limited by pain) and up down 12 steps (using step-to-gait pattern)
- Gait: Antalgic, with decreased stance time right and decreased step length left
- Physical therapy POC includes modalities for pain, resistance exercise, patient education, and aerobic exercise.
- Physical therapy short-term goals: Increase ambulation to 1000 ft without rest to promote ability to complete job duties, increase right knee strength to 4/5 to improve protection for joint and quality of gait, decrease pain with ambulation to 4 of 10 to promote increased ambulation distance, and patient independent with verbalizing and implementing joint protection strategies

1. List specific monitoring the physical therapist assistant should complete during each session given the medical diagnoses listed.
2. Which functional assessment tool is most appropriate?
3. The patient arrives at his 11:30 AM therapy appointment. The physical therapist assistant initiates treatment. The patient suddenly becomes pale and describes dizziness and feeling "shaky," What should the physical therapist assistant do first?

4. The patient has been coming to therapy for 3 weeks and has been making progress toward goals and describing decreased pain. During today's session, the patient states that since feeling better, the patient is thinking of stopping all medications. What should the physical therapist assistant do?
5. Create an exercise program (be specific) to address the patient's short-term goal.

## References


1. American College of Sports Medicine; Durstine JL, Moore G, Painter P, Roberts S. *ACSM's Exercise Management for Persons With Chronic Diseases and Disabilities.* 4th ed. Human Kinetics; 2016.
2. World Health Organization. Global recommendations on physical activity for health. 2010. Accessed February 7, 2023. https://www.who.int/dietphysicalactivity/publications/9789241599979/en/
3. United States Department of Health and Human Services. President's Council on Sports, Fitness & Nutrition. Importance of physical activity. Accessed February 7, 2023. https://www.hhs.gov/fitness/be-active/importance-of-physical-activity/index.html
4. American Heart Association. American Heart Association recommendations for physical activity in adults and kids. Reviewed April 18, 2018. Accessed February 7, 2023. https://www.heart.org/en/healthy-living/fitness/fitness-basics/aha-recs-for-physical-activity-in-adults
5. American College of Sports Medicine. *ACSM's Guidelines for Exercise Testing and Prescription.* 9th ed. Wolters Kluwer/Lippincott Williams & Wilkins; 2014.
6. Durstine JL, Gordon B, Wang Z, et al. Chronic disease and the link to physical activity. *J Sport Health Sci.* 2013;2(1):3-11.
7. Carl DL, Boyne P, Rockwell B, et al. Preliminary safety analysis of high-intensity interval training (HIIT) in persons with chronic stroke. *Appl Physiol Nutr Metab.* 2017;42(3):311-318. doi:10.1139/apnm-2016-0369
8. Toohey K, Pumpa KL, Arnolda L, et al. A pilot study examining the effects of low-volume high-intensity interval training and continuous low to moderate intensity training on quality of life, functional capacity and cardiovascular risk factors in cancer survivors. *PeerJ.* 2016;4:e2613.
9. Boyne P, Dunning K, Carl D, et al. High-intensity interval training and moderate-intensity continuous training in ambulatory chronic stroke: feasibility study. *Phys Ther.* 2016;96(10):1533-1544.
10. Ross L, Porter R, Durstine JL. High-intensity interval training (HIIT) for patients with chronic diseases. *J Sport Health Sci.* 2016;5(2):139-144. doi:10.1016/j.jshs.2016.04.005
11. Goodman C, Fuller K. *Pathology Implications for the Physical Therapist.* 4th ed. Elsevier; 2015.
12. Kisner C, Colby L. *Therapeutic Exercise Foundations and Techniques.* 6th ed. FA Davis; 2012.
13. Bohannon RW, Wang YC, Gershon RC. Two-minute walk test performance by adults 18 to 85 years: normative values, reliability, and responsiveness. *Arch Phys Med Rehabil.* 2015;96(3):472-477. doi:10.1016/j.apmr.2014.10.006
14. Bohannon RW, Wang YC, Bubela D, et al. Normative two-minute walk test distances for boys and girls 3 to 17 years of age. *Phys Occup Ther Pediatr.* 2018;38(1):39-45. doi:10.1080/01942638.2016.1261981
15. Bernabeu-Mora R, Medina-Mirapeix F, Llamazares-Herrán E, et al. The short physical performance battery is a discriminative tool for identifying patients with COPD at risk of disability [erratum in: Int J Chron Obstruct Pulmon Dis. 2016;11:623]. *Int J Chron Obstruct Pulmon Dis.* 2015;10:2619-2626. doi:10.2147/COPD.S94377
16. Treacy D, Hassett L. The short physical performance battery. *J Physiother.* 2018;64(1):61. doi:10.1016/j.jphys.2017.04.002
17. Pasanen T, Tolvanen S, Heinonen A, et al. Exercise therapy for functional capacity in chronic diseases: an overview of meta-analyses of randomised controlled trials. *Br J Sports Med.* 2017;51:1459-1465.
18. Hordern MD, Dunstan DW, Prins JB, et al. Exercise prescription for patients with type 2 diabetes and pre-diabetes: a position statement from Exercise and Sport Science Australia. *J Sci Med Sport.* 2012;15(1):25-31. doi:10.1016/j.jsams.2011.04.005
19. Buresh R, Berg K. Exercise for the management of type 2 diabetes mellitus. Factors to consider with current guidelines. *J Sports Med Phys Fitness.* 2018;58(4):510-524. doi:10.23736/S0022-4707.17.06969-9
20. Goodman C, Helgeson K. *Exercise Prescription for Medical Conditions: Handbook for Physical Therapists.* FA Davis; 2011.
21. American Cancer Society. Physical activity and the person with cancer. Revised March 16, 2022. Accessed February 7, 2023. https://www.cancer.org/treatment/survivorship-during-and-after-treatment/staying-active/physical-activity-and-the-cancer-patient.html
22. Segal R, Zwaal C, Green E, et al. Exercise for people with cancer: a clinical practice guideline. *Curr Oncol.* 2017;24(1):40-46. doi:10.3747/co.24.3376
23. Vainshelboim B, Müller J, Lima RM, et al. Cardiorespiratory fitness, physical activity and cancer mortality in men. *Prev Med.* 2017;100:89-94. doi:10.1016/j.ypmed.2017.04.014
24. Rock CL, Doyle C, Demark-Wahnefried W, et al. Nutrition and physical activity guidelines for cancer survivors [erratum in: CA Cancer J Clin. 2013;63(3):215]. *CA Cancer J Clin.* 2012;62(4):243-274. doi:10.3322/caac.21142
25. Tsai E, Robertson MC, Lyons EJ, et al. Physical activity and exercise self-regulation in cancer survivors: a qualitative study. *Psychooncology.* 2017;27(2):563-568. doi:10.1002/pon.4519
26. Granger CL, Connolly B, Denehy L, et al. Understanding factors influencing physical activity and exercise in lung cancer: a systematic review. *Support Care Cancer.* 2017;25(3):983-999. doi:10.1007/s00520-016-3484-8
27. Shepherd S, Batra A, Lerner DP. Review of critical illness myopathy and neuropathy. *Neurohospitalist.* 2017;7(1):41-48. doi:10.1177/1941874416663279
28. Schweickert WD, Pohlman MC, Pohlman AS, et al. Early physical and occupational therapy in mechanically ventilated, critically ill patients: a randomised controlled trial. *Lancet.* 2009;373(9678):1874-1882. doi:10.1016/S0140-6736(09)60658-9

29. Centers for Disease Control and Prevention. About HIV. Reviewed June 30, 2022. Accessed February 7, 2023. https://www.cdc.gov/hiv/basics/whatishiv.html
30. Leach LL, Bassett SH, Smithdorf G, et al. A systematic review of the effects of exercise interventions on body composition in HIV+ adults. *Open AIDS J.* 2015;9:66-79. doi:10.2174/1874613601509010066
31. O'Brien KK, Tynan AM, Nixon SA, et al. Effectiveness of progressive resistive exercise (PRE) in the context of HIV: systematic review and meta-analysis using the Cochrane Collaboration protocol. *BMC Infect Dis.* 2017;17(1):268. doi:10.1186/s12879-017-2342-8
32. O'Brien KK, Tynan AM, Nixon SA, et al. Effectiveness of aerobic exercise for adults living with HIV: systematic review and meta-analysis using the Cochrane Collaboration protocol. *BMC Infect Dis.* 2016;16:182. doi:10.1186/s12879-016-1478-2
33. Shephard RJ. Physical impairment in HIV infections and AIDS: responses to resistance and aerobic training. *J Sports Med Phys Fitness.* 2015;55(9):1013-1028.
34. Kamitani E, Sipe TA, Higa DH, et al. CDC HIV/AIDS Prevention Research Synthesis (PRS) Project. Evaluating the effectiveness of physical exercise interventions in persons living with HIV: overview of systematic reviews. *AIDS Educ Prev.* 2017;29(4):347-363. doi:10.1521/aeap.2017.29.4.347
35. Centers for Disease Control and Prevention. Defining adult overweight & obesity. Reviewed June 3, 2022. Accessed February 7, 2023. https://www.cdc.gov/obesity/adult/defining.html
36. Xing F, Lu B, Kuang MJ, et al. A systematic review and meta-analysis into the effect of lateral wedge arch support insoles for reducing knee joint load in patients with medial knee osteoarthritis. *Medicine (Baltimore).* 2017;96(24):e7168. doi:10.1097/MD.0000000000007168
37. Bukowski EL, Nolan TP. Hydrotherapy: the use of water as a therapeutic agent. In: Bellew JW, Michlovitz SL, Nolan TP Jr, eds. *Modalities for Therapeutic Intervention.* 5th ed. FA Davis; 2012:109.
38. Baillet A, Vaillant M, Guinot M, et al. Efficacy of resistance exercises in rheumatoid arthritis: meta-analysis of randomized controlled trials. *Rheumatology (Oxford).* 2012;51(3):519-527. doi:10.1093/rheumatology/ker330
39. Baillet A, Zeboulon N, Gossec L, et al. Efficacy of cardiorespiratory aerobic exercise in rheumatoid arthritis: meta-analysis of randomized controlled trials. *Arthritis Care Res (Hoboken).* 2010;62(7):984-992. doi:10.1002/acr.20146
40. Briggs AM, Fary RE, Slater H, et al. Physiotherapy co-management of rheumatoid arthritis: identification of red flags, significance to clinical practice and management pathways. *Man Ther.* 2013;18(6):583-587. doi:10.1016/j.math.2013.01.006
41. Broy SB. The vertebral fracture cascade: etiology and clinical implications. *J Clin Densitom.* 2016;19(1):29-34. doi:10.1016/j.jocd.2015.08.007
42. Holavanahalli RK, Helm PA, Kowalske KJ. Long-term outcomes in patients surviving large burns: the musculoskeletal system. *J Burn Care Res.* 2016;37(4):243-254.
43. Serghiou MA, Niszczak J, Parry I, et al. Clinical practice recommendations for positioning of the burn patient. *Burns.* 2016;42(2):267-275. doi:10.1016/j.burns.2015.10.007

Chapter 21

# Pelvic Floor and Women's Health Exercises

*Jacki Klaczak Kopack, PT, DPT*

**KEY TERMS** Continence | Diastasis recti | Functional incontinence | Micturition | Stress incontinence | Urge incontinence

## Chapter Objectives

1. Identify the basic anatomical structures of the pelvic floor.
2. Describe the common causes and clinical presentations of pelvic floor dysfunction and diastasis recti.
3. Identify the red flags and reasons for medical referral related to pelvic floor function.
4. Discuss the common treatment interventions used to address pelvic floor dysfunction.
5. Describe the changes that occur during pregnancy.
6. List the indications, contraindications, and safe progressions for exercise during pregnancy.
7. Given a patient diagnosis and a plan of care (POC), design and progress a basic exercise and intervention program to rehabilitate pelvic floor muscle weakness.

*Pelvic floor* is a general term referring to all structures of the lower pelvis (ie, the pelvic bone, pelvic organs, fascia, ligaments, and pelvic floor muscles). The pelvic floor muscles collectively include the layers of muscles that span from the pubic bone to the coccyx, and they serve to support the pelvic organs (ie, the bowel and bladder and the uterus in women). Normal function (strength, length, and neuromuscular control) of the pelvic floor muscles is critical to maintaining control of the bowel and bladder (the pelvic muscles control sphincter closure of the urethra, anus, and vagina), sexual function, and support of the abdominal structures. Pelvic floor muscles work together with other body structures, especially the pelvic girdle and lumbar and abdominal ("core") muscles to assist in postural stability and normal functional movement patterns. Pelvic floor muscles provide proprioceptive and sensory feedback, and these sensations contribute to sexual appreciation and function (in men, these muscles assist in achieving erections). The pelvic floor structures play an additional role for women during pregnancy and the birthing process. Weakness in pelvic floor musculature can result in impairments in any of these functions.



Kopack JK, Cascardi KA.
*Principles of Therapeutic Exercise for the Physical Therapist Assistant* (pp 683-704).

**Table 21-1**

Possible Indicators of Sexual Abuse[1]

| Children | Adolescents | Adults |
|---|---|---|
| • Nightmares or sleep problems without an explanation<br>• Distracted or distant at odd times<br>• Sudden change in eating habits<br>• Exhibits sudden mood swings<br>• Says things that seem likely to provoke a discussion about sexual issues<br>• New or unusual fear of certain people or places<br>• Refuses to talk about a secret shared with an adult or older child<br>• Writes, draws, plays, or dreams of sexual or frightening images<br>• Talks about a new older friend<br>• Suddenly has money, toys, or other gifts without reason<br>• Describes self or body as repulsive, dirty, or bad<br>• Shows adult-like sexual behaviors, language, and knowledge | • Self-injury behaviors (cutting and burning)<br>• Demonstrates sexual promiscuity<br>• Runs away from home<br>• Depression and anxiety<br>• Suicide attempts<br>• Fear of intimacy or closeness<br>• Compulsive eating or dieting<br>• Inadequate personal hygiene<br>• Drug and/or alcohol abuse | • Reminders of the assault generate fear<br>• Pervasive sense of anxiety and unsure of ever feeling safe again<br>• Assault flashbacks<br>• Difficulty concentrating<br>• Guilty feelings<br>• Negative self-image, feeling "dirty" inside or out<br>• Anger<br>• Depression<br>• Disruptions in close relationships<br>• Loss of interest in sex |

A thorough evaluation by an experienced physical therapist should guide the POC for persons with pelvic floor dysfunction. Given the functions of pelvic floor structures and the many potential origins of a patient's symptoms, the therapist's examination will include screening to rule out systemic, infectious, inflammatory, and visceral causes of pain because these would be reasons for a physician referral. The clinician gathers information regarding urogenital function, pregnancy/birth histories, and possibly sexual practices and history depending on the patient's presentation. Screening for a history of assault/intimate partner violence may also be indicated. Possible indications of sexual abuse for children, adolescents, and adults are found in Table 21-1.[1]

Physical therapist assistants should be aware of state/practice act requirements for reporting suspicion of abuse. Being sensitive to a history of abuse is especially important when treating the genitalia region. Many pelvic floor patients are initially uncomfortable, embarrassed, fearful, and/or anxious about pursuing treatment; these feelings may be exacerbated in patients with a history of abuse. Practitioners should demonstrate competent, evidence-based, and empathetic care at all times. Facility protocols and good judgment should be used during treatment interventions to prevent any suspicion of impropriety during treatment sessions. Recognizing the sensitive nature of providing treatment to an area of the body that is typically viewed as "private" (or to a patient with a history of abuse) requires clinicians to focus on the basic tenants of professionalism and to pair that focus with empathy and sensitivity. In all treatment situations, clinicians must create effective interactions by establishing trust and rapport; this is achieved by communicating clearly, watching body language carefully (yours and the patient's), and obtaining consent for each aspect of the treatment. If an intervention is not working or if the patient is uncomfortable, the clinician must consider alternatives (ie, another intervention or a different clinician). When possible, offer the patient a choice as to the preferred sex of the treating therapist. Recognize that a patient's comfort level may change from

**Table 21-2**

Common Misconceptions About Pelvic Floor Therapy[4]

| Misconception | Actual Facts |
|---|---|
| Only women are treated. | Men can and do receive pelvic floor retraining. |
| Only postpartum women need treatment. | Women can develop pain and incontinence after childbirth that requires treatment; other clinical indications for pelvic floor physical therapy include pelvic pain, coccyx pain, bowel incontinence, stress incontinence, and difficulty urinating. Initiating pelvic floor exercises during pregnancy can help prevent additional issues postpartum. |
| Pelvic floor retraining is only Kegel exercises. | Kegel exercises can be a beneficial component of a pelvic floor training program, but the exact exercise selection will be determined after a full physical therapy evaluation/assessment. Interventions may include modalities, biofeedback, core exercises, hip exercises, postural retraining, and pelvic floor exercises. |
| If a woman has a "medical diagnosis" or is "getting old," then physical therapy will not help. | As with other areas in the body, a medical diagnosis leading to pain/changes in posture can effectively be addressed by a therapist. This can occur in support of ongoing medical treatments. |

session to session so be prepared to modify interventions accordingly. It is important to provide ongoing education and communication regarding treatment interventions, pain, and anatomy with constant solicitation of regular feedback from the patient. If a patient is struggling with an aspect of treatment (eg, disrobing, positioning during treatment, privacy), seek alternatives to increase patient comfort. Offer information for other supportive services as indicated.[2]

Entry-level physical therapist assistants should know pelvic floor anatomy, the indications for treatment, and basic exercises and interventions. It is generally accepted that advanced training in anatomy, evaluation (including internal muscle palpation/evaluation and surface electromyographic testing), and assessment and treatment is indicated for therapists who intend to specialize in the treatment of pelvic floor dysfunction. The American Physical Therapy Association Academy of Pelvic Health Physical Therapy issued a position statement recognizing the use of the physical therapist assistant in treating women's health diagnoses. The Academy of Pelvic Health Physical Therapy recognizes and supports "beyond-entry level" training for all women's health practitioners and supports the specially trained assistant in participating as a team member. The physical therapist can delegate tasks to a qualified assistant, including assisting with biofeedback intervention, electrical stimulation interventions for the pelvic floor, internal pelvic floor muscle techniques that do not require ongoing assessment/evaluation, external pelvic floor muscle exercise, education in a pelvic floor muscle home exercise program, interventions using vaginal weights or dilators, behavioral interventions for the bowel and bladder, and internal pelvic floor tests and measures.[3]

There are misconceptions about pelvic floor dysfunction and treatment protocols (Table 21-2).[4] Clinicians can provide patients with information that better represents what pelvic floor physical therapy includes.

## Typical Pelvic Floor Anatomy

The bony support for pelvic structures is the pelvis. The pelvic bone includes the ilium, ischium, and pubic bones. The right and left pelvic bones are connected anteriorly by the pubic symphysis joint, and posteriorly these bones articulate with the sacrum (forming 2 sacroiliac [SI] joints). The bones serve as insertion points for the various ligaments that help provide support for the pelvic organs and SI joint stability.[5,6]

The primary ligaments supporting the anterior SI joint include the anterior longitudinal ligament, the sacrospinous ligament, and the anterior SI ligament. Together, these ligaments provide SI joint stability by resisting superior sacral motion and lateral motion of the ilium. The posterior SI ligaments include the short and long dorsal SI ligaments and the supraspinous, iliolumbar, and sacrotuberous ligaments. These posterior ligaments resist inferior and superior sacral motion and medial motion of the ilium.[5,6] Figure 21-1 depicts the primary ligaments of the pelvis and sacrum.

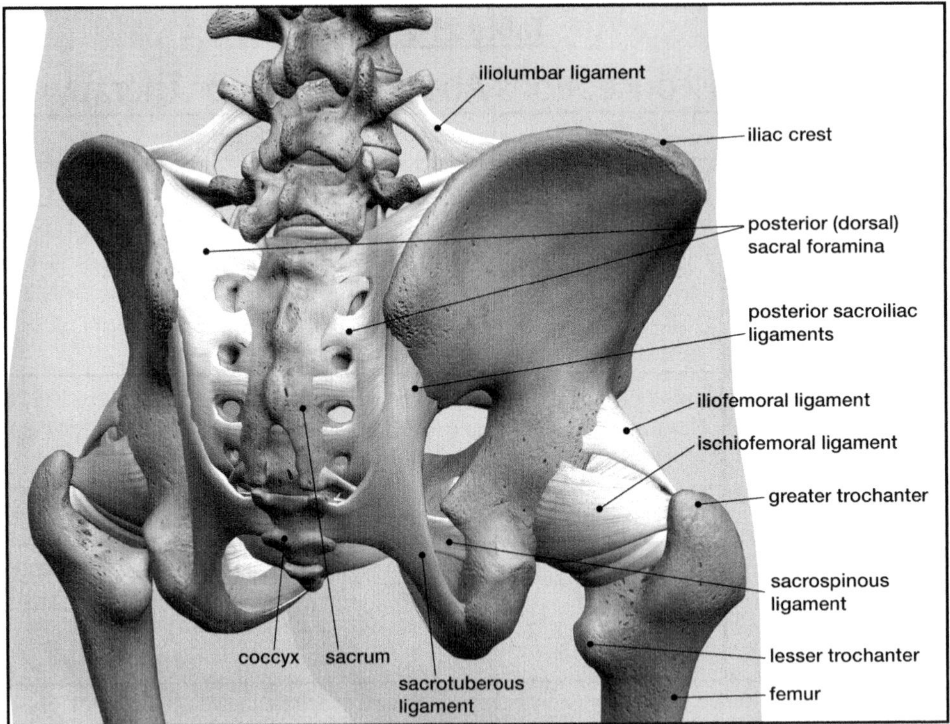


**Figure 21-1.** The primary ligaments of the pelvis and sacrum (Hank Grebe/Shutterstock.com).

The muscles of the pelvic floor are divided into superficial and deep muscles (Table 21-3).[7] The most superficial structure is the anal sphincter, which is innervated by S4 and functions to provide fecal continence. The anal sphincter is composed of both smooth and skeletal muscle.[6] The superficial genital muscles (Figure 21-2) include the bulbospongiosus, the ischiocavernosus, and the superficial and deep transverse perineal muscles. These muscles aid in sexual function. The deep pelvic floor muscles (Figure 21-3) aid in sexual function, maintaining continence, supporting pelvic organs, and assisting in postural stabilization. These muscles include the levator ani muscles (the puborectalis, pubococcygeus, and iliococcygeus) and the coccygeus muscle.

Pelvic floor muscles and the surrounding fascia support the pelvic organs. The ability to control bladder and bowel emptying (**continence**) occurs due to normal pelvic floor muscle function. Normal function includes a coordinated pattern of relaxation and contraction of these muscles, which allows controlled emptying of the bowel and bladder. **Micturition** is the physiological process of urination (Figure 21-4), including all reflexive activity. For urination to occur, the bladder detrusor muscle contracts, and the urethral sphincter relaxes (involuntary/autonomic nervous system control). The voluntary relaxation of the pelvic floor muscles (especially the levator ani muscle and the pubococcygeus) allows urination to occur in a controlled manner (so patients select an appropriate time and place to urinate, maintaining continence).[8]

Fecal continence requires a coordinated relaxation of the anal sphincter and puborectalis muscles (reflexive/autonomic nervous system control). Voluntary relaxation of the pelvic floor muscles and contraction of the abdominal muscles increase abdominal pressure (the Valsalva maneuver), allowing defecation to occur. The voluntary relaxation allows defecation in a controlled manner so patients can select an appropriate time and place to have a bowel movement.[5]

## Causes of Dysfunction

Pelvic floor muscles that are overactive or underactive (tight or weak) can result in impairments. Underactive pelvic muscles are also called *noncontracting pelvic muscles.* Common causes of underactive/weak or stretched pelvic floor muscles include vaginal birth, pregnancy, obesity, chronic/prolonged cough (pulmonary disease), menopause, chronic constipation, repeated straining (Valsalva with lifting/exercise), hysterectomy, pelvic muscle disuse atrophy, medical pathologies (eg, diabetes mellitus, thyroid disease), and increased age. Underactive pelvic floor muscles are often associated with weakness or increased muscle length, increased/stretched connective tissue length, muscle atrophy, impaired muscle endurance, or abdominal muscle weakness. Common medical diagnoses associated with underactive muscles include incontinence and pelvic organ prolapse.[1,5]

**Table 21-3**

Superficial and Deep Pelvic Floor Muscles[7]

| Superficial | |
|---|---|
| Bulbospongiosus | • Origin: Central tendon<br>• Insertion: Pubic arch (female), urogenital diaphragm (male)<br>• Innervation: Pudendal n.<br>• Action: Women—constricts vagina; men— assist in urethra emptying |
| Ischiocavernosus | • Origin: Ischial tuberosity<br>• Insertion: Pubic arch<br>• Innervation: Pudendal n.<br>• Action: Assists bulbospongiosis |
| Superficial and deep transverse perineal muscles | • Origin: Ischial tuberosity and rami<br>• Insertion: Central tendon, urogenital diaphragm<br>• Innervation: Pudendal n.<br>• Action: Supports pelvic viscera, stabilizes central tendon |
| **Deep** | |
| Puborectalis (levator ani) | • Origin: Pubis<br>• Insertion: Sacrum, coccyx<br>• Innervation: Pudendal n.<br>• Action: Controls defecation |
| Pubococcygeus (levator ani) | • Origin: Pubis<br>• Insertion: Coccyx<br>• Innervation: Pudendal n.<br>• Action: Supports pelvic floor, elevates/retracts anus |
| Iliococcygeus (levator ani) | • Origin: Ischial spine, pubis<br>• Insertion: Coccyx<br>• Innervation: Pudendal n.<br>• Action: Supports pelvic floor, elevates/retracts anus |
| Coccygeus | • Origin: Ischial spine<br>• Insertion: Lateral, inferior borders sacrum, coccyx<br>• Innervation: Inferior sacral n.<br>• Action: Supports pelvic floor |

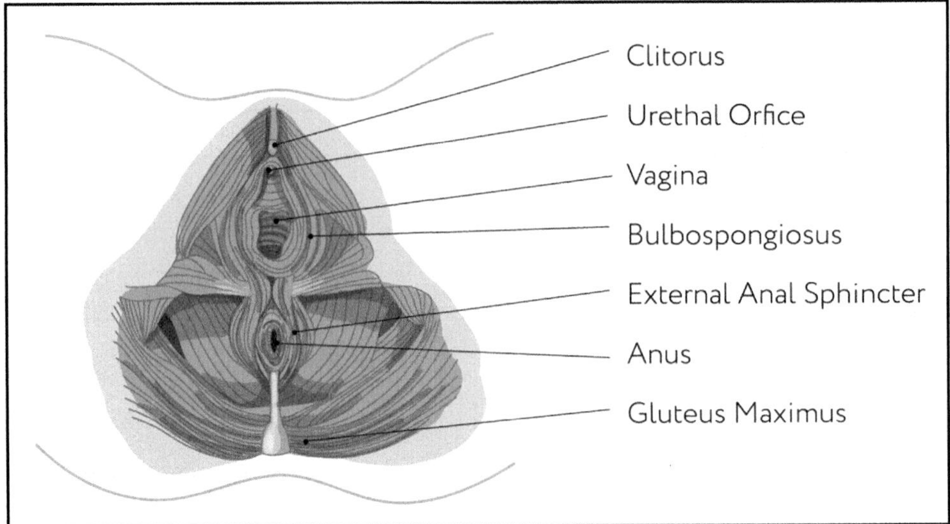


**Figure 21-2.** Superficial genital structures (molotoka/Shutterstock.com).

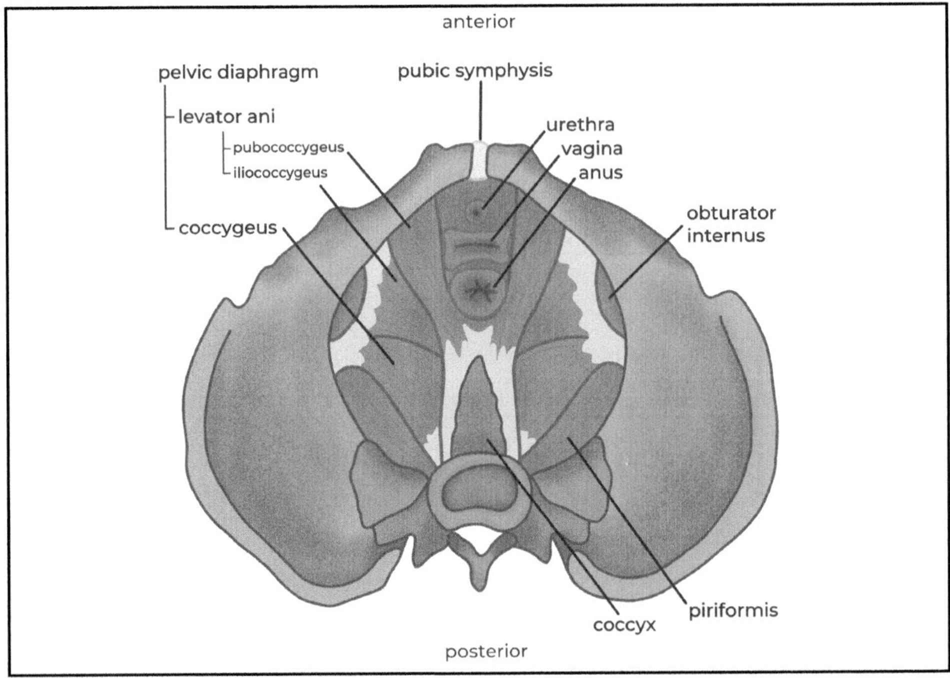


**Figure 21-3.** Deep pelvic floor muscles (superior view of the pelvis; Jinnicha/Shutterstock.com).

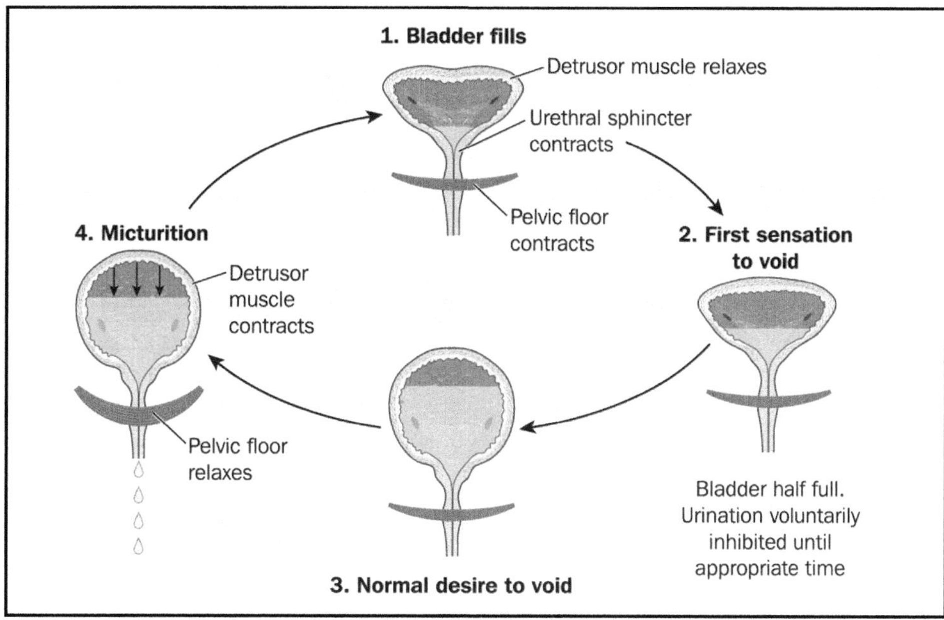


**Figure 21-4.** The process of urination (Blamb/Shutterstock.com).

Overactive muscles are also called *nonrelaxing pelvic floor muscles*. Some common causes of overactive pelvic floor muscles include back or pelvic pain or muscle imbalances, abdominal or pelvic scarring/adhesions, episiotomy or tearing during vaginal birth, pelvic surgery, endometriosis/interstitial cystitis, a history of sexually transmitted diseases, or recurrent perineal infections. Overactive pelvic floor muscles are often associated with the following diagnoses: levator ani syndrome, vulvodynia, vaginismus, and chronic pelvic pain.[1,5] Table 21-4 defines the clinical terms associated with pelvic floor dysfunction.[6,9,10]

## The Role of Physical Therapy

Common reasons patients seek out physical therapy treatment include incontinence and pelvic pain, both of which can affect women and men. Incontinence is not a disease but rather a symptom of an underlying medical diagnosis or physical problem or impairment. A thorough medical workup is typically indicated before the initiation of physical therapy services. The physical therapist reviews the medical findings and completes an examination to differentiate the type of incontinence, which guides the rest of the examination. An internal examination by the therapist or patient self-assessment examines resting tone, pelvic floor muscle strength and endurance, voluntary muscle relaxation, coordination, and the presence of trigger points and/or scar tissue; ultrasound imaging may be included.[1] The therapist creates a POC that targets the underlying impairments. The current clinical guidelines recommend the use of pelvic floor muscle training as a first line of treatment for stress urinary incontinence and pelvic floor muscle training and bladder training for persons with mixed incontinence.[11]

Pelvic pain can be caused by musculoskeletal disorders, and pelvic/abdominal organs can refer pain to the pelvic area (Appendix G).[12] There is a close anatomical relationship between pelvic floor muscles and the piriformis and the obturator internus; imbalances in the strength and length of these muscles can impact pelvic floor muscle function. The psoas major/minor, iliacus, and quadratum lumborum can cause low back or pelvic pain and should be ruled out as potential causes of pelvic floor dysfunction. Pelvic floor muscles that insert on the sacrum can create rotation and SI dysfunction/pain, especially if there are differences in the resting tone between the right and left musculature. Trigger points in the lumbopelvic muscles can also refer pain into the pelvic area.[13,14]

Because of the close functional relationship between the pelvic floor and low back, pelvic, and hip musculature, the physical therapist needs to carefully screen all of these areas before creating a problem list and treatment plan.[12] Evidence that indicates any underlying visceral or medical causes should be referred to the appropriate medical specialist.

### Clinical Tips: Finding and Treating the Causes of Symptoms Improves Outcomes

If patients are experiencing referred pain to the pelvic area (ie, tight/shortened hip adductor muscles with palpable trigger points), the treatment should target the cause of the pain (ie, decreasing trigger point irritability and stretching the hip adductors). In this case, normalizing muscle tone should decrease pelvic pain.

**Table 21-4**

**Clinical Terminology Associated With Pelvic Floor Dysfunction[6,9]**

| Term | Definition |
|---|---|
| Incontinence | Involuntary leakage of urine, feces, or gas |
| Stress incontinence | Urine leakage that occurs with exertion/pressure on the bladder (coughing, sneezing, laughing, exercising, and heavy lifting) |
| Urge incontinence | Sudden, intense urge to urinate followed by an involuntary loss of moderate to large amounts of urine |
| Mixed incontinence | Patients describe characteristics of more than one type of urinary incontinence |
| Overflow or retention incontinence | Frequent or constant dribbling of urine; straining to initiate urination, sensation of incomplete emptying |
| Functional incontinence | A physical or mental impairment prevents patient from making it to the toilet in time |
| Vulvodynia | Severe, often idiopathic pain in the external genitalia and perineal region |
| Vaginismus | Increased muscle tension in the muscle around the vagina and/or superficial or deep pelvic floor muscle layers, often causing dyspareunia |
| Coccygodynia | Pain located at the coccyx bone, often secondary to a fall on the buttocks or trigger points in pelvic floor muscles, gluteus maximus, piriformis, or obturator internus |
| Levator ani syndrome/ pelvic floor tension myalgia | Umbrella term that describes patients who present with vaginal or rectal pain |
| Anismus | Increased anal sphincter tone (called nonrelaxing puborectalis syndrome), resulting in severe pain with defecation and secondary constipation |
| Dyspareunia | Painful vaginal penetration/intercourse |
| Pudendal neuralgia | Intense pain in and around the pudendal nerve area (urethra, anus, rectum, perineum, and genitalia) is often caused by entrapment/compression of the pudendal nerve |
| Pelvic organ prolapse | Collapse or downward displacement of visceral structures (ie, uterus, bladder, or rectum) |
| Uterine prolapse | Collapse/downward displacement of the uterus (first, second, or third degree) |
| Cystocele | Protrusion of the urinary bladder against the vagina |
| Rectocele | Protrusion of the rectum against the vagina |
| Pessary | A device inserted into the vaginal area to assist with nonsurgical treatment of stress urinary incontinence or pelvic organ prolapse. The device is typically considered temporary and often paired with pelvic floor muscle re-education. A recent systematic review recommends pessary use as a first line of treatment for patients with stress urinary incontinence.[10] |

If the cause of a patient's musculoskeletal symptoms is correctly determined, physical therapy interventions can treat the dysfunction:

- If it is weak, strengthen it.
- If it is tight, stretch it.
- If there is pain, determine the cause and use appropriate interventions, modalities, and patient education to alleviate/control the pain. Education is critical, and it is the clinician's responsibility to educate patients! This is especially true when discussing misconceptions about incontinence.

Physical therapist assistants collect patient information each session to help the physical therapist determine if a more in-depth evaluation is warranted. The assistant will share the patient's responses to the following questions: Do you ever leak urine or bowel movements? Do you ever wear a pad because of urine leakage? and Do you experience pain during intercourse?[6] The presence of any of the red flag signs/symptoms (Table 21-5) may indicate the presence of a systemic, visceral, inflammatory, or infectious cause of pain.[15] New onsets of these symptoms, changes in continence, or new pelvic symptoms should be reported to the supervising therapist before treatment.

**Table 21-5**

Red Flag Items for the Pelvic Region[15]

- New onset of fever (in older adults, increased confusion may present in lieu of fever), generalized malaise, nausea, and vomiting
- Pain relieved by passing gas or having a bowel movement
- New onset of gastrointestinal, urologic, or gynecologic signs/symptoms (any abdominal pain at the same level as back pain); any change in symptoms associated with eating patterns; persistent but vague gastrointestinal symptoms; early satiety
- Any change in bowel or bladder habits, including changes in continence
- Blood present in urine or stool
- Pelvic pain increases with prolonged standing
- Positive McBurney's sign or pinch-an-inch test (rule out appendicitis)
- Positive iliopsoas/obturator test (rule out appendicitis and peritonitis)
- Pelvic pain aggravated by the Valsalva maneuver/increased abdominal pressure (coughing, sneezing, standing, and sexual intercourse)
- Missed menses with new-onset cramping and/or shoulder pain and/or low back pain (rule out ectopic pregnancy)
- New/atypical vaginal or penis discharge
- New reports of a "lump" or pressure in the vaginal or perineal area, especially if presents with new report of constipation and feeling of incomplete rectal emptying (rule out prolapse, cystocele, and rectocele)
- Pain that is constant/does not change with treatment or movement testing
- Pain that increases at night and is constant
- New (unplanned) weight loss/extreme fatigue

Pelvic pain and difficulty controlling muscle contractions or relaxation can result in incontinence or pelvic pain that can disrupt everyday activities and/or sexual function. Pelvic floor dysfunction and the sequelae can have a negative impact on a patient psychologically and socially. In a large systematic review, it was determined that many women with incontinence are reluctant to seek medical treatment for incontinence.[16] Incontinence is often viewed as shameful and has a negative impact on activities of daily living (ADLs), socialization, and intimacy/sexual satisfaction.[16,17] Men and women living with incontinence report increased incidences of depression and anxiety and decreased health-related quality of life.[18] The clinician's ability to address a patient's concerns in an empathetic manner can help the patient in feeling more comfortable with pursuing treatment and, ultimately, improving function and quality of life.

## Physical Therapy Interventions

Pelvic floor treatment refers to a comprehensive intervention program supervised by an experienced clinician that includes exercise, behavioral, and conservative treatments; lifestyle changes (ie, bladder training with urge suppression); internal and external palpation of the pelvic floor muscles; manual stretching of the pelvic floor muscles; manual soft tissue work; trigger point massage and scar massage (often internal techniques); use of dilators; vaginal cones; biofeedback; and electrical stimulation.[19] Unfortunately, often when a layperson hears "pelvic floor treatment," they think only of pelvic floor muscles/Kegel exercises. Comprehensive treatment extends beyond entry-level practice expectations. Physical therapist assistants who want to include all available interventions into pelvic floor treatments should complete additional training/certification after graduation. Physical therapists may complete portions of the treatment and then delegate pelvic floor exercises, postural muscle training/exercises, and patient education to the assistant. Studies indicate that patients who participate in pelvic floor training programs overseen by a pelvic floor specialist have better outcomes than patients who attempt the exercises unsupervised.[20] Researchers found that despite evidence-based research indicating the efficacy and cost-effectiveness in the treatment of urinary incontinence, comprehensive programs are not commonly used as a first-line treatment in clinical practice in the United States.[19,21]

Intervention selection is based on the patient's type of incontinence. The types of incontinence and common treatments are described in Table 21-6. Although incontinence is often considered a women's health issue, incontinence can impact men as well. Men can benefit from targeted treatment programs to address incontinence and pelvic floor

**Table 21-6**

**Common Pelvic Floor Interventions Based on Type of Incontinence[6]**

| Type of Incontinence | Typical Presentation | Treatment Interventions |
|---|---|---|
| Urge | Sudden, strong urge to urinate<br>Loss of control over when urination occurs<br>Frequent urination day and night | Acupuncture<br>Percutaneous tibial nerve stimulation<br>Pelvic floor muscle strengthening<br>Timed voiding program |
| Stress | Leak urine | Kegel exercises<br>Pelvic floor muscle strengthening<br>Biofeedback<br>Electrical stimulation<br>Vaginal pessaries |
| Functional | Incontinence due to inability to access toilet in timely manner | Transfer training<br>Gait training<br>Use of assistive devices/ compensatory techniques<br>ADL retraining<br>Strength/balance training |
| Mixed | Patients present with signs of more than one type | Patients are prescribed interventions from each category as indicated in the POC |

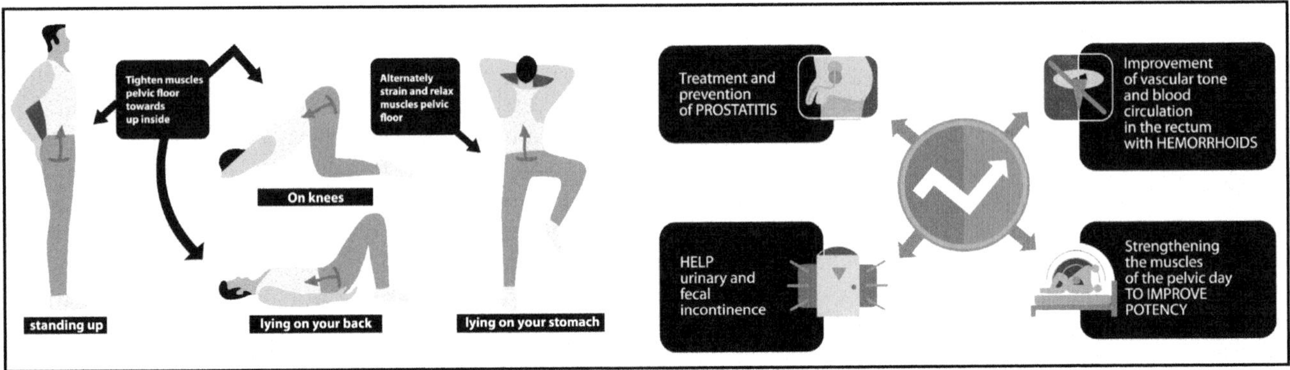


**Figure 21-5.** The benefit of pelvic floor exercises for men (sergfear/Shutterstock.com).

diagnoses (Figure 21-5). To maximize patient performance and compliance, clinicians should educate them regarding pelvic anatomy and provide visual information so that the patient can begin to understand where the muscles are and how they work. The duration of the contraction and the number of repetitions/sets are individualized and should reflect the patient's performance on the evaluation. Pelvic floor muscle training exercises and progression (Box 21-1) are often prescribed during pregnancy, and there are safety considerations and monitoring considerations (see the Obstetric Patient section).

## *Pelvic Floor Exercises*

Typical exercises for pelvic floor dysfunction include a combination of exercises (quick and long contraction holds and relaxation) that target strength, endurance, and relaxation of the pelvic floor muscles.[22] Short/quick contraction exercises include quickly contracting and relaxing the pelvic floor muscles. Each contraction is typically 1 to 2 seconds while cuing the patient to breathe normally (no breath holding). The patient should count how many contractions can be completed in one set.[23] When performing long/endurance contraction exercises, patients are instructed to tighten and hold the pelvic floor muscles for as long as possible (8 to 10 seconds per repetition). If the patient can hold a contraction for 4 seconds, they should be instructed to relax the muscles fully (a 10-second rest), and then repeat the long hold contraction. In the early stages of training, the rest period may need to be longer, but as the muscle strength and endurance improve, rest periods can be decreased as long as full muscle relaxation between repetitions occurs.[22] After each long/endurance contraction and/or between sets of short/quick contractions, the patient is instructed to fully relax. Deep breathing helps patients achieve complete relaxation of the pelvic floor muscles. Patients should complete both types of contractions several times during the day, achieving the ultimate goal of completing up to 60 pelvic floor muscle contractions per day.[22] As the patient becomes more skilled, these contractions can be completed during daily activities as well (especially during tasks/activities that may be a trigger for urine leakage). Quality is more important than quantity; performing exercises correctly results in improvements, but performing the exercises incorrectly does not!

The physical therapist assistant can incorporate the following cues and guidelines when educating patients[9,22]:

- Contract the correct muscles. If patients try to stop urination midstream, the pelvic floor muscles are contracting. Although this cue may help guide patients in identifying the correct muscles, patients should be educated NOT to practice stopping their urine stream because this can lead to incomplete bladder emptying/infection. Instead, cuing patients to place an index finger on the perineum (the skin between the vagina or penis and rectum) while contracting the pelvic floor muscles is advised. The patient should feel the tissues move away from the finger but should not feel the anus or the perineal tissue move closer to the finger. Initially, patients should practice these contractions lying down. If the patient feels "bulging" under the finger, the technique should be reviewed with the clinician.
- Practice! Tighten the pelvic floor muscles and hold the contraction for ___ seconds, and then relax for 5 seconds. Complete ___ in a row. Repeat ___ times a day. Clinicians should fill in the blanks based on the patient's hold time and repetitions from the evaluation/current session.
- Patients should keep a daily log. Have the patient record how long the contraction is held (up to 8 to 10 seconds), how many repetitions were completed with the hold (long contractions), and how many short/quick contractions can be completed.
- Maintain focus. For best results, instruct the patient to focus on tightening only the pelvic floor muscles and focusing on breathing easily during the exercises.
- Once the patient is independent with exercises and correct form has been verified, patients should be instructed to use Kegel exercises as part of their daily routine (eg, sitting at a traffic light or work desk, during ADLs).

## Box 21-1

### Pelvic Floor Muscle Training Progressions

Positioning progressions: Supine (gravity neutral) ⇨ seated ⇨ standing ⇨ with activity

Muscle contraction progressions: Facilitation by local muscles (contract abdominals, adductors, and gluteal muscles with pelvic floor muscles) ⇨ isolated contraction

At no point should the patient complete an abdominal contraction with bearing down.

Feedback progressions: With feedback (vaginal palpation, biofeedback, or visual feedback) ⇨ self-assessment

Exercise parameters: The initial dosage should be based on the patient's ability during examination. Repetitions, sets, and rest periods should be matched to the patient's current ability while promoting strength and compliance.

- Remind patients that a realistic outcome is not a "quick fix"; it may take 3 to 6 months to see the full benefit of a pelvic floor strengthening program.
- Check the patient's form (maximize their ability to isolate and contract the pelvic floor muscles) as follows:
  - Educate/instruct proper sitting posture, including appropriate lumbar lordosis
  - Avoid the Valsalva maneuver
  - Educate the patient to gently contract abdominal muscles before contracting the pelvic floor muscles (ensure the abdomen is not "pushed out" and the patient is not trying to bear down during a pelvic floor muscle contraction).

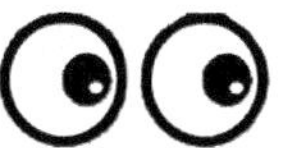

### Eye on the Research: First-Line Treatment

To attain the best results for patients with incontinence, first-line treatment should include a pelvic floor muscle training program overseen by a physical therapist or nurse specially trained in incontinence. A daily minimum of 24 pelvic floor muscle contractions (8 repetitions 3 times a day) should be completed for a 3-month trial. Successful treatment transitions into a maintenance program.[20]

Dumoulin et al[21] summarized that the inclusion of pelvic floor muscle training for women with incontinence generally improved patient outcomes (improved or cured incontinence and/or improved sexual outcomes) without risk of adverse effects. They recommended that pelvic floor muscle training be included as a first-line treatment for conservative management of incontinence. Participants who completed a 12-week program of customized behavioral urinary incontinence treatments that included 150 minutes of weekly walking and twice weekly strength training classes reported a statistically significant improvement in continence (compared with the control group).[24]

## *Exercise Progression*

Clinicians should verify that the patient performs exercises correctly. The clinician reviews the patient's exercise log, and then adjusts the number of repetitions/sets/hold and rest time as strength/endurance improves. The clinician questions if the episodes of incontinence and/or pain (if referred pain was present) are decreasing. Once the patient is independent with the exercises and is incorporating Kegel exercises as part of their daily routine, the clinician can educate/instruct the patient to contract the pelvic floor muscles before coughing, sneezing, laughing, or lifting/straining to prevent urine leakage.[20,25]

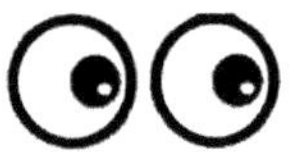

### Eye on the Research: Positioning—Does Footwear Matter?

A systematic review summarized that when treating women with urinary incontinence, pelvic floor muscle training should be performed while standing with the ankles in a neutral position or dorsiflexion to facilitate a more effective pelvic floor muscle contraction. Researchers reported that decreased resting activity of the pelvic floor muscle in plantar flexion indicates that high heel wearers with urinary incontinence may potentially experience more leakage during exertion in a standing position. They recommended that women with stress incontinence be advised to wear flat shoes.[26]

# Special Population Considerations

## *The Older Adult Patient*

Adequate functional mobility and strength are critical for maintaining one's independence. Consider the following: Can a patient walk to the bathroom safely (adequate balance and lower extremity strength) in the appropriate amount of time (speed) and distance required (endurance), and, once in the bathroom, can the patient maintain their balance while managing clothing and hygiene (before voiding)? Between 22.5% and 46.7% of older adults have mobility limitations.[27] Mobility issues can be an early indicator of health decline, and they affect a person's ability to safely access the bathroom and maintain continence.[27] This decline in mobility paired with pelvic floor muscle weakness can result in **functional incontinence**. The physical therapy team can provide compensatory strategies to improve function and reduce the underlying impairments that result in functional incontinence.

### Implications for the Physical Therapist Assistant

The following are ideas for interventions based on treatment goals. If the goal is to restore function, consider including the following treatment options: lower extremity strengthening and endurance exercises, shoulder depression and elbow extension strengthening exercises, aerobic/gait training (walking) at increased speed, balance exercises, and task-specific training (sit to stand). Compensatory techniques that can be helpful include elevating the seat (or toilet) height, using chairs with arms, using a portable commode (at a closer distance than where the bathroom is located/shortening the distance to walk), installing grab bars next to/around the toilet, using an assistive device during ambulation, finding an easier way to manage clothing (sweatpants/elastic waist vs zipper/buttons), and/or using incontinence pads (absorbent pads/disposable pull-ups).

## *The Obstetric Patient*

Pregnancy results in numerous physiological changes to support the growth of a fetus. Physical therapist assistants must be aware of the changes associated with pregnancy to safely implement an exercise program for the patient.[28,29] The common physiological changes that are associated with pregnancy are outlined in Table 21-7. These specific changes can affect a woman's tolerance and willingness to exercise and can increase the risk of injury/harm during exercise. Gastrointestinal changes and discomfort associated with pregnancy may result in lower motivation to exercise and/or a need to avoid certain positions (eg, supine). A person with anemia may experience decreased exercise and activity tolerance and an increased heart rate response at lower levels of activity. Changes in posture and increased lordosis may increase the likelihood of low back pain/SI pain and changes in balance. These symptoms may be exacerbated during weight-bearing exercise, so non–weight-bearing or aquatic exercise may be more appropriate. Motionless exercise postures/positions (certain yoga positions and prolonged static standing) and lying in a supine position may result in decreased venous return and hypotension, all of which should be avoided.

Activities requiring high-level balance responses or rapid changes in movements (aerobic dance programs, yoga, and bike riding) may be difficult to complete as pregnancy progresses and may need to be modified or replaced with other modes of exercise. The American College of Obstetricians and Gynecologists (ACOG) notes that decreases in respiratory reserve may result in a decreased ability to complete exercise and that the ability to meet the demand of strenuous aerobic exercise and strenuous

**Table 21-7**

## Physiological Changes Associated With Pregnancy[6,29,30]

| | |
|---|---|
| Cardiovascular | • Cardiac output increases by 30% to 50%, peaking between 24 and 30 weeks of gestation, and vascular resistance decreases. Heart rate and stroke volume increase. Resting heart rate tends to increase 8 to 20 beats/minute. Blood pressure may drop in the second trimester.<br>• After week 30, cardiac output will vary based on body position; recumbent positioning places pressure on the vena cava, with a resultant drop in cardiac output.<br>• Increase in blood flow to the kidneys to improve the removal of metabolic waste products (increased urine production) occurs.<br>• Increased blood flow to the skin (temperature regulation) occurs.<br>• Premature atrial and ventricular beats are common. |
| Hematologic | • The total blood volume increases proportionally with cardiac output (plasma volume increases more than red blood cell mass, resulting in a relative lowering of hemoglobin).<br>• A slight increase in white blood cells during pregnancy and significant leukocytosis (≥20,000/μL) during labor and for the first few days postpartum.<br>• Iron requirements increase (typically supplements are required to prevent further decrease in hemoglobin). |
| Urinary | • Kidney filtration rate increases 30% to 50%.<br>• Postural changes affect renal function more during pregnancy (supine increases renal function, and upright positions decrease renal function). Positional changes result in a greater need to urinate when trying to sleep. |
| Respiratory | • Carbon dioxide ($CO_2$) levels decrease; tidal volume, minute volume, and respiratory rate increase, causing an increase in plasma pH.<br>• Oxygen consumption increases 20% (due to increased metabolic needs of the fetus, placenta, and maternal organs).<br>• Decrease in inspiratory and expiratory reserve, residual volume and capacity, and plasma partial pressure of carbon dioxide. No change in vital capacity or partial pressure of oxygen.<br>• Thoracic circumference increases.<br>• Mild dyspnea during exertion is typical; deep respirations are more frequent. |
| Gastrointestinal and hepatobiliary | • Pressure from the enlarging uterus (on rectum and lower colon) may cause constipation.<br>• Gastrointestinal motility decreases (elevated progesterone levels relax smooth muscle).<br>• Heartburn is common (delayed gastric emptying/gastroesophageal reflux due to relaxation of the lower esophageal sphincter).<br>• There is a possible increase in incidence of gallbladder disorders. |
| Endocrine | • Pregnancy alters the function of most endocrine glands.<br>• Increased levels of relaxin, estrogen, and progesterone cause fluid retention, ligament laxity, and reduced smooth muscle tone occur.<br>• Levels of estrogen and progesterone increase.<br>• Placenta produces hormones resulting in thyroid stimulation (increased thyroid activity) and increased levels of adrenal hormones, especially aldosterone and cortisol (causing increased edema and insulin resistance).<br>  ○ Possible complication: development of gestational diabetes.<br>• Pituitary gland enlarges by about 135% during pregnancy (plasma prolactin increases to ensure lactation).<br><br>*(continued)* |

**Table 21-7 (continued)**

Physiological Changes Associated With Pregnancy[6,29,30]

| | |
|---|---|
| Basal metabolic rate | • Increases 15% to 30%, requiring about 300 kcal more per day to meet increased metabolic demand<br>• Heat production/sweating increase |
| Musculoskeletal system | • Weight gain (significant variance observed; recommendations for weight gain are based on prepregnancy weight/body mass index).<br>• Center of gravity shifts upward and anterior, resulting in compensatory increased lumbar lordosis and sometimes increased thoracic kyphosis and forward head posture.<br>• Increased mechanical stress on the abdominal and pelvic floor muscles occurs.<br>• Joint laxity and hypermobility; may cause low back pain/SI pain and increased foot pronation (changes in lower extremity biomechanics).<br>• Weight gain and redistribution cause a wider base of support and increased hip external rotation with ambulation. |
| Changes with exercise | • With exercise, cardiac output, heart rate, oxygen consumption, and respiratory volume per minute increase more during pregnancy. |

work may lag; this impact is more significant for women who are overweight. For this reason, aerobic exercise at a lower intensity may be indicated; using the Borg Rating of Perceived Exertion (RPE) Scale to monitor the perceived workload is helpful. Because of changes in temperature regulation and increased metabolic demands, women should be well hydrated and avoid high heat and humidity; exercising in an air-conditioned setting is preferred. To meet the increased metabolic demand, women who exercise regularly may need an additional 300 to 500 kcal per day during pregnancy and the breastfeeding period (depending on exercise intensity/duration).

## Common Pathologies Associated With Pregnancy and Indicated Treatment Interventions

The changes associated with pregnancy (ante- or postpartum) can result in pain, dysfunction, or pathology for some women. Changes in ligamentous laxity and posture can increase the development of low back and SI pain.[6,30] Low back pain can be effectively treated with postural exercises, low back strengthening exercises (with positioning modifications for pregnancy), and body mechanics training. Modality use (deep heat, traction, and electrical stimulation) and stretching exercises should be avoided during pregnancy. The treatment of SI pain can include activity modification education, stabilization exercises, and the use of SI belts to provide external stabilization and support to the joint. Activity modification to reduce asymmetrical forces on the pelvis includes avoiding single-limb weight-bearing standing/exercises, crossing the legs when seated, excessive hip abduction, and end-range hip flexion or hyperextension (ie, climbing steps 2 or 3 at a time). Additionally, the patient should be instructed to use logrolling for bed mobility, to use a pillow between the knees in the side-lying position, and to enter/exit a car by sitting and then moving both legs into/out of the car simultaneously. The patient should be instructed to activate the transverse abdominis (drawing/bracing maneuvers) and pelvic floor muscles during transitional movements and lifting.

Increases in blood volume and increased pressure on the vena cava from the growing uterus can lead to the development or worsening of varicose veins.[6,30] The patient should be instructed to wear lower extremity compression stockings, minimize lower extremity–dependent positioning, and elevate the legs as much as possible.

Stresses on the abdominal muscles from the expanding uterus can cause **diastasis recti,** which is the separation of the rectus abdominis at the linea alba (Figure 21-6).[6,30] Additional information and management tips for diastasis recti are discussed later in the chapter.

Nerve compression can occur as a result of hormonal shifts, increased edema, circulatory compromise, or postural changes. Nerve compression syndromes more commonly associated with pregnancy include carpal tunnel syndrome and thoracic outlet syndrome. Carpal tunnel syndrome that begins during pregnancy typically resolves after delivery. Patients are often issued night splints to promote alignment and decrease symptoms (refer to Chapter 12).[6,30]

Gestational diabetes is glucose intolerance that develops during pregnancy, and it occurs in about 14% of pregnancies in the United States. Regular exercise can assist in maintaining better glucose control and may delay or prevent the need for insulin therapy.[6,30] A patient with gestational diabetes should participate in exercise with

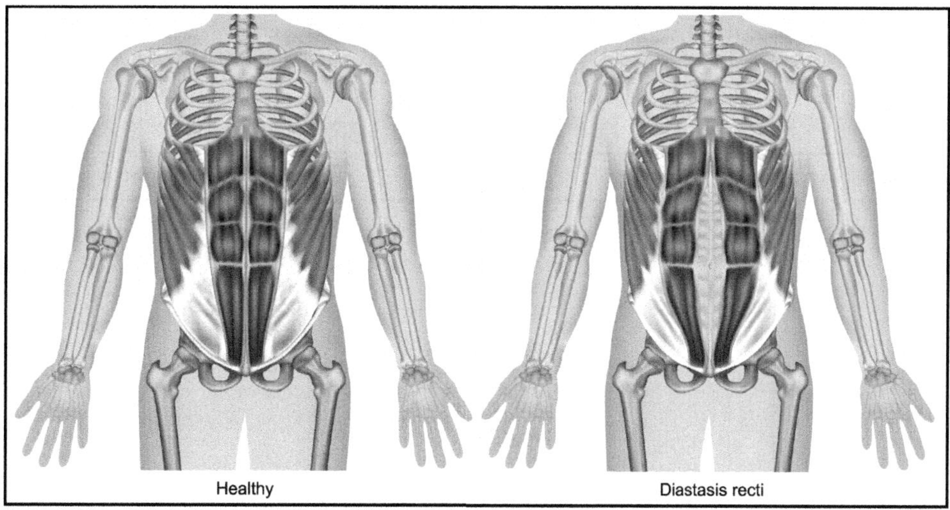


**Figure 21-6.** Diastasis recti (medicalstocks/Shutterstock.com).

medical supervision; the physical therapist will create an individualized exercise program. Monitoring during exercise is indicated, and it is recommended that the patient follow up with a dietician to pair exercise with appropriate dietary choices and meal timing.

Mechanical pressure, stretching, and tearing (or episiotomy) during labor and delivery can result in pelvic floor dysfunction. Pelvic floor muscle strengthening should be initiated during pregnancy and continued postpartum. Pelvic floor management may be added as indicated based on the individual's presentation in the postpartum period.[6,30]

## Benefits of Exercise During Pregnancy

Regular aerobic exercise during pregnancy can maintain physical fitness levels (or in some cases improve it). There is no evidence of harm as long as contraindications and appropriate monitoring are observed. The benefits of exercise include decreased incidence or improved management of gestational diabetes, decreased incidence of cesarean delivery, and decreased postpartum recovery time. Exercise may help prevent preeclampsia and is associated with very modest decreases in overall antepartum weight gain. Additionally, exercise can prevent or manage low back pain, diastasis recti, and pelvic floor dysfunction while improving muscle tone, increasing stabilization, and preventing injury caused by connective tissue laxity.[28] Regular exercise has been shown to decrease deep vein thrombosis risk and venous stasis as well as elevate mood and decrease the risk for postpartum depression.[31] The ACOG summarized that 30 minutes of strenuous exercise is well tolerated by women and fetuses in active as well as inactive women.[28]

## Exercise Prescription for the Patient Who Is Pregnant: Uncomplicated Pregnancy

Exercise prescription for patients who are pregnant can be initiated after a comprehensive physical therapist examination. In the absence of medical complications or concerns, the exercise principles discussed in Section I of this textbook should be followed with some modifications to accommodate for pregnancy. The program can include up to moderate-intensity exercise for 20 to 30 minutes per day (based on the individual's fitness level and medical presentation) during the ante- and postpartum periods. Vital sign monitoring is indicated, and the Borg RPE Scale should be used. (The goal with moderate exercise is a level of exertion of 13 to 14 on the Borg 6 to 20 Scale.) Education regarding warning signs to stop exercise, proper hydration, and avoiding overexertion is important and should be provided before starting any exercise program.[28]

Women who were sedentary and did not exercise regularly before pregnancy should begin exercising at a low intensity and frequency, and physical therapist assistants should gradually increase activity as indicated by the patient's response to the exercise. Women who are obese should begin with low-intensity and short-duration exercise paired with education about a healthy lifestyle and diet. Activity should also be gradually progressed based on the patient's response. Women who exercised regularly before pregnancy should be able to tolerate moderate- to high-intensity exercise (matched to prepregnancy activity levels) with no adverse effects. Competitive athletes may require closer monitoring due to adhering to a more rigorous training schedule and returning to high-intensity, full training activities earlier postpartum. High-intensity or prolonged exercise may lead to hypoglycemia and hyperthermia. The clinician should guide the patient in planning to increase calorie intake, maintaining hydration, and monitoring exercise intensity to minimize these risks.[28] Physical therapy clinicians must educate their pregnant patients about the absolute and relative contraindications related to aerobic exercise during pregnancy according to the ACOG guidelines (Table 21-8).

Selecting appropriate exercise interventions should be based on individual presentation and the physical

**Table 21-8**

**Absolute and Relative Contraindications During Aerobic Exercise When Pregnant[28]**

| Absolute Contraindications | Relative Contraindications |
|---|---|
| • Hemodynamically significant heart disease<br>• Restrictive lung disease<br>• Incompetent cervix or cerclage<br>• Multiple gestation at risk of premature labor<br>• Persistent second or third trimester bleeding<br>• Placenta previa after 26 weeks of gestation<br>• Premature labor during current pregnancy<br>• Ruptured membranes<br>• Preeclampsia or pregnancy induced hypertension<br>• Severe anemia | • Anemia<br>• Unevaluated maternal cardiac arrhythmia<br>• Chronic bronchitis<br>• Poorly controlled type 1 diabetes<br>• Extreme morbid obesity<br>• Extreme underweight (body mass index < 12)<br>• History of extreme sedentary lifestyle<br>• Intrauterine growth restriction on current pregnancy<br>• Poorly controlled hypertension<br>• Orthopedic limitations<br>• Poorly controlled seizure disorder<br>• Poorly controlled hyperthyroidism<br>• Heavy smoker |

therapy POC. Safe activities and high-risk activities/exercises that should be avoided are listed in Table 21-9. Goals and indications for exercise include improving/maintaining aerobic capacity/endurance, decreasing lumbopelvic pain, improving posture, increasing/maintaining strength, preventing diastasis recti, and addressing urine leakage/incontinence. Interventions that can address these goals during pregnancy include the following[6,30]:

- Abdominal strengthening exercises (if performed in supine, frequent position changes are indicated) including pelvic tilts, quadruped posterior pelvic tilts, supine heel slides, and hip abduction in the hook-lying position (maintain posterior pelvic tilt)
- Pelvic floor strengthening exercises
- Postural correction exercises (the typical focus includes chin tucks, scapular retraction, and the drawing-in maneuver [bringing the pelvis to neutral])
- Aerobic exercise: Walking and swimming are great options; monitor vital signs and RPE with activity

Although exercise is generally deemed safe (low risk) and beneficial when performed during an uncomplicated pregnancy, appropriate monitoring is still indicated. Most injuries sustained during pregnancy are musculoskeletal, so clinicians must be aware of signs/symptoms that are associated with an inappropriate reaction to exercise.[28] However, if a woman presents with any of the signs or symptoms listed in Table 21-10, exercise should be terminated immediately, vital signs should be reassessed, and the physical therapist assistant should complete the appropriate follow-up (notify the physical therapist, contact the physician, and/or initiate emergency medical services).

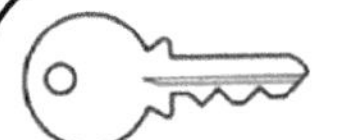

**Key Safety Considerations: The Healthy Obstetric Patient**

- Maintain appropriate vital sign response to activity.
- No exercise if absolute contraindications are present (see Table 21-8).
- Monitor for signs/symptoms to terminate exercise (see Table 21-10).
- Verify patients use the appropriate form with all exercises.
- Verify patients use the drawing-in maneuver and pelvic floor muscle contraction with movement transitions.
- Avoid unsafe positions (quadruped, unilateral weight bearing, and full supine after second trimester).

## Safety Considerations for High-Risk Pregnancy

Pregnancies are deemed high risk if there are maternal or fetal factors that jeopardize the potential for a healthy full-term birth (ie, preeclampsia, placenta previa, breech presentation, or placenta abruption).[6] Treatment for serious complications often includes bed rest or a cesarean section. Preeclampsia is diagnosed when a patient who is pregnant presents with high blood pressure; protein in their urine; and swelling in their legs, feet, and hands. This usually occurs late in pregnancy, and the presentation can range from mild to severe. Preeclampsia can progress to eclampsia, which can be fatal; the only cure for preeclampsia is to give birth. Placenta previa occurs when the placenta covers

**Table 21-9**

**Safe and High-Risk Activities/Exercises During Pregnancy**

| Activities/Exercises That Are Safe to Continue During Uncomplicated Pregnancy (With Obstetrician Clearance)[28] | Activities to Avoid* |
|---|---|
| • Walking<br>• Swimming<br>• Stationary cycling<br>• Low-impact aerobics<br>• Modified Pilates/yoga (caution with positions that can cause hypotension)<br>• Safe to continue only if the following activities were completed before: Jogging/running, racket sports (intact balance), and strength training | • Bilateral straight-leg raise/lowering<br>• Supine position (avoid > 5 minutes after first trimester)<br>• Single-limb weight bearing<br>• Ballistic stretching<br>• End-range stretching/overstretching<br>• Quadruped fire hydrant exercise<br>• Quadruped hip hyperextension<br>• Avoid the Valsalva maneuver<br>• Contact sports (hockey, boxing, and soccer)<br>• Activities with a high fall risk (skiing, surfing, water skiing, gymnastics, and horseback riding)<br>• Scuba diving<br>• Skydiving<br>• Hot yoga or hot Pilates |

*Note: If a pregnant person participated in these before pregnancy, clear continuing antepartum with obstetric MD.[2,6,30]

**Table 21-10**

**Reasons to Terminate Exercise During Pregnancy[28]**

- Vaginal bleeding
- Regular painful contractions
- Amniotic fluid leakage
- Dizziness
- Headache
- Dyspnea before exertion
- Chest pain
- Muscle weakness affecting balance
- Calf pain or swelling

all or part of the cervix. Breech presentation occurs when a baby is positioned feetfirst toward the cervix in the final trimester; typically, the baby is positioned head down in the mother's uterus. Placental abruption is a serious pregnancy complication in which the placenta detaches from the uterus before delivery, which can deprive the baby of oxygen and nutrients.

Although it is the ACOG position that "bed rest should not be routinely recommended," bed rest may be prescribed in situations in which the mother or baby is at risk because of pregnancy-related or medical complications. Patients on bed rest or with restricted physical activity have an increased risk of venous thromboembolism, bone demineralization, and deconditioning.[28] These patients may be referred to physical therapy to try to minimize the impact of bed rest. The goals of a therapeutic exercise program should include minimizing the risk of complications, improving circulation, minimizing deconditioning, decreasing pain, and promoting proper positioning.[6,28] Contraindications to activity/exercise include vaginal bleeding, increased contractions, increased blood pressure or leakage of amniotic fluid, and unstable conditions.[6,28]

If physical therapy is deemed appropriate, the determination as to which clinician will treat the patient is based on the clinical judgment of the supervising physical therapist. If there are ongoing medical changes or significant acuity requiring ongoing assessment of status, the therapist should treat the patient. The following exercises may be appropriate to include: ankle pumps; side-lying knee flexion/extension and knee to chest; supine cervical active range of motion (AROM) and chin tucks; scapular retraction; unilateral heel slides; shoulder, elbow, and wrist AROM; and side-lying upper extremity AROM (with light resistance if appropriate). The clinician should monitor vital signs, RPE, and symptoms during the completion of all exercises. Patient education regarding proper exercises, activity safety, and appropriate exercise progression should be emphasized. This education includes the need to limit lower extremity motion against gravity (because it may increase bleeding/contractions), avoid lower extremity resistance exercise, progress activities slowly, avoid fatigue, avoid the Valsalva maneuver, avoid abdominal muscle contractions, and stop exercise immediately if symptoms increase and contact the physician.

### Postpartum Exercises and Exercises After a Cesarean Section

A cesarean section is a surgical procedure for delivering a baby through the abdominal and vaginal wall. Cesarean sections may be indicated in situations in which the maternal or fetal health may be compromised with a vaginal delivery (ie, placenta previa, breech presentation, fetal distress, or failure of labor to progress).[6,30] Because these patients are abdominal postoperative surgical patients, the typical postoperative precautions/protocols implemented include early mobilization (getting the patient up, out of bed, and walking as soon as medically appropriate), abdominal splinting with mobility, deep breathing exercises (eg, huffing and splinted coughing), using an incentive spirometer, ankle pumps, and lower extremity compression stockings/pumps. The patient is instructed in pelvic floor exercises and bed mobility training including supine to side lying to sit to minimize stresses on the incision, and postural exercises may be indicated. Once the sutures are removed and the incision is healed, scar massage can be initiated. All other considerations for postpartum exercise (as noted previously) should also be followed for the patient after a cesarean section.

Generally, after an uncomplicated cesarean delivery, exercise can be restarted once the patient is cleared by the physician and feels able to restart exercise. Typical goals/indications for exercise include improving or maintaining aerobic capacity/endurance, increasing/maintaining strength, improving diastasis recti, and addressing urine leakage/incontinence. Interventions that can address these goals include the following[6,30]:

- Pelvic floor strengthening exercises
- Diastasis recti correction
- Aerobic exercise: Begin with low intensity and increase as tolerated. Ensure adequate warm-up/cooldown.
- Strength training: Begin with low intensity and increase as tolerated. Exercises to be avoided during the postpartum period include any exercise in which the hips and/or pelvis are positioned higher than the patient's chest (eg, bridging, knee to chest, inverted postures/positions) because there is a small risk of a potentially fatal air emboli.[6] Exercises should be terminated if there is an increase in vaginal bleeding. During breastfeeding, attention to dietary intake to ensure adequate calories is important.[6,30]

## *Diastasis Recti Abdominis and Treatment Interventions*

As defined earlier, diastasis recti abdominis (DRA) is a painless separation of the rectus abdominis muscle centrally and longitudinally at the linea alba (see Figure 21-6). The linea alba is the tendinous seam between the left and right rectus abdominis muscles running from the sternum to the pubic symphysis. Diastasis recti can occur in newborns (typically with spontaneous reduction), men, and/or women, although it is most prevalent and associated with pregnancy.[32] During pregnancy, the growing fetus creates a mechanical tension/stress on the linea alba. The increased tension together with the increased anterior pelvic tilt and hormonal changes associated with pregnancy can create DRA in some women. A separation greater than 2 to 2.7 cm[33] is considered to be a diastasis recti. Many DRAs will reduce spontaneously during the postpartum period.

Diastasis recti is measured by 1 of 3 techniques: fingertip measurement, calipers, or ultrasound imaging. Oftentimes clinicians will use the fingertip measurement to assess for the presence of DRA, although the reliability of this technique is not high.[34] To measure for diastasis recti, the patient is positioned in the supine hook-lying position with their arms at their sides. The clinician instructs the patient to chin tuck and then complete a partial crunch (scapula clearing the mat). The therapist places their fingers approximately 2 inches (in; 5.08 cm) below, 2 inches above, and at the level of the umbilicus (central in the linea alba). Each finger that can fit in the space is equivalent to 1 cm/0.39 in.

There are mixed reports in the research regarding pain, low back pain, pelvic floor dysfunction, postural deficits, and ADL limitations associated with DRA, with some research showing evidence of these deficits and other research indicating women with diastasis recti are not at higher risk for these impairments. There is mixed evidence on the effectiveness of physical therapy and exercise training in the treatment of DRA as well. Regular exercise before and throughout pregnancy may decrease the development of DRA, and women who are physically fit before pregnancy appear to have a lower incidence of DRA. Common physical therapy interventions include DRA correction, exercises increasing/progressing core stability and strengthening exercises, taping/bracing, and postural education/body mechanics training.[35] An overview of the more commonly used exercises is included later; the reader should review the latest evidence when creating/carrying out treatment plans for persons with DRA.

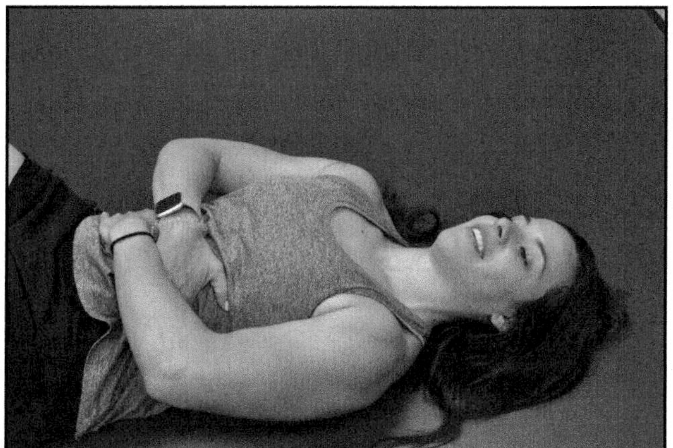

**Figure 21-7.** Manual correction of diastasis recti.

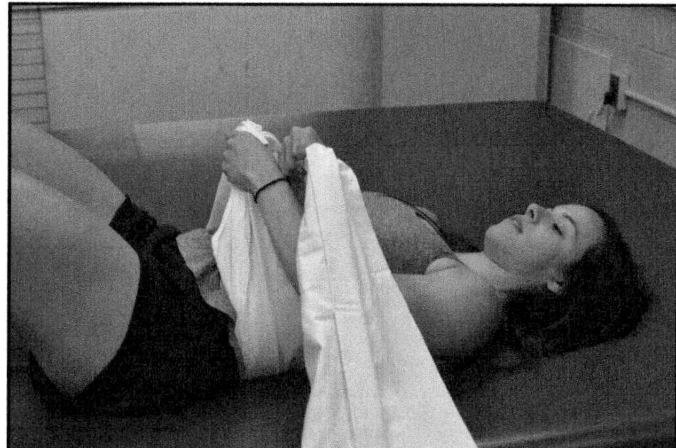

**Figure 21-8.** The correction of diastasis recti facilitated with a sheet.

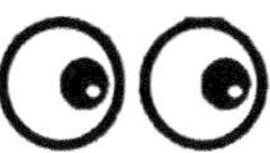

## Eye on the Research: Diastasis Recti Abdominis

Exercise during pregnancy can reduce the likelihood of developing DRA, but a recent systematic review was unable to conclusively state that postpartum exercise was effective in resolving DRA.[33] Mommers et al[36] noted that physical therapy can achieve a limited reduction in DRA during muscle contractions. A study examined 175 post-partum women and concluded that supervised abdominal exercise was no more effective at decreasing DRA than no treatment, but it did not include specific exercises to address the correction of DRA (ie, Noble's exercise or the Tupler technique) nor did it target the transverse abdominis muscle before the addition of core strengthening.[37] Tuttle et al[38] concluded that a transverse abdominis exercise protocol for postpartum women with DRA (with or without taping) was significantly better than taping alone or no intervention at reducing the intrarectus distance. Further research is indicated to determine if exercise that includes manual correction of DRA with core strengthening is beneficial to improve DRA.

An intervention commonly recommended for correcting DRA occurs with the patient in a supine hook-lying position with the arms crisscrossed over the abdomen while manually approximating the rectus abdominis (Figure 21-7). The patient slowly exhales while performing a posterior pelvic tilt and lifts the head/neck and scapulae from the mat. This is referred to as *Noble's exercise*.[39] An alternate option is to facilitate the closure by placing a sheet around the patient's torso and having the patient pull the sheet across the body for additional support (Figure 21-8).

The drawing-in maneuver, which targets and strengthens the transverse abdominis, is beneficial. To complete this maneuver, a patient is instructed to place their hands on the lower stomach area, take a deep breath in, and on the exhalation draw the abdomen in ("pull the belly button toward the spine"). The patient is then instructed to try to hold the contraction while avoiding the Valsalva maneuver. If the patient is able to hold the contraction without breath holding, the exercise can be progressed by asking the patient to hold the belly in that position and take small breaths while keeping the belly flat. On exhalation, the patient should try to pull the belly in closer toward the spine. The patient can work up to holding this position for a full minute. Once the patient is able to complete this activity, practice is progressed to completing it in seated, quadruped, and finally standing. If the patient can complete the exercise in these positions, they should practice it during functional tasks. There should be no increase in bulging of the DRA during exercise. Early use of crunches/sit-ups should be avoided because they can increase the DRA. Once the patient is able to correct the DRA with drawing in, the clinician can assess to see if the patient can maintain the reduction with postural and core strengthening exercises. As the patient progresses, the clinician should monitor performance to ensure there is no increase in the DRA.

Clinicians will continually address modifications to mobility tasks to minimize DRA with functional activities. Early use of supine to side lying to sit with abdominal bracing is more appropriate than supine to sit. Using abdominal splinting, binders, or Kinesiotape may provide additional feedback to the patient and serve as a reminder to complete the drawing-in maneuver. The patient should complete this drawing-in/abdominal bracing maneuver when lifting objects (including lifting the baby), and they should be educated in the tenants of proper body mechanics. Caution with carrying and lifting heavy loads and limiting the use of front body baby slings may be appropriate, but clinicians should observe these activities and determine the impact on the DRA when making individualized recommendations to the patient.

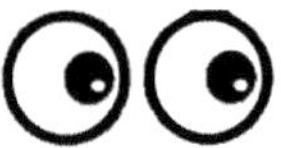

### Eye on the Research: Antepartum Pain Clinical Practice Guidelines

The Women's Health and Orthopedic Sections of the American Physical Therapy Association have created clinical practice guidelines for treating pelvic girdle pain (PGP)[40]; these recommendations include that evaluating therapists should differentiate PGP from serious disease/psychological factors. Self-reported outcomes questionnaires should be used in combination with clinical examination results to create a clinical diagnosis. The guidelines suggest that postural changes should not be considered indicative of the development of PGP (moderate evidence). The use of support belts and exercise can be considered, but there is conflicting evidence to support this premise. There is weak evidence to support the use of manual therapy in treating PGP.[40]

## Conclusion

Physical therapy can play an important role in the treatment and care of pelvic floor dysfunction, pelvic floor–related pain, incontinence, and pregnancy-related musculoskeletal issues. Knowledge of pelvic floor anatomy and the causes of pelvic floor dysfunction guides the clinician in creating appropriate treatment interventions. Knowledge, empathy, and the ability to effectively educate the patient are requirements for any clinician treating patients with pelvic floor or women's health diagnoses. The physical therapist assistant who is interested in providing all of the interventions that could be included in the treatment of pelvic floor diagnoses will pursue additional training.

## Review Questions

1. Describe the function of the pelvic floor muscles.
2. List common causes of pelvic floor dysfunction and pain.
3. Describe appropriate exercises and interventions that can be included in the treatment of a patient with pelvic floor dysfunction.
4. Compare and contrast the types of incontinence.
5. What are red flags indicating a patient receiving physical therapy for a pelvic floor diagnosis might need a medical referral?
6. How do treatment interventions differ for a person with stress incontinence vs functional incontinence?
7. What are typical changes that occur in the body during pregnancy?
8. What modifications should be made when implementing an exercise program for an obstetric patient? What additional considerations are there if the pregnancy is considered to be high risk?
9. List contraindications to exercise and reasons to terminate exercise for a person who is pregnant.
10. What is DRA? How can physical therapy help to address DRA?

## Case Study 1

The patient is a 28-year-old woman 3 months after the birth of her first child. She reports a "bulge above my belly button" and reports needing to get out of bed using a supine-to-side-to-sit maneuver because supine to sit via a sit-up "feels weird." The physical therapist evaluation notes diastasis recti, and the POC includes DRA correction exercises.

1. Determine the appropriate exercises to address this, and practice patient education.
2. What clinical signs indicate that it is appropriate to advance the exercise interventions to abdominal strengthening?

## Case Study 2

A 45-year-old patient presents with a report of incontinence that developed after the birth of her third child. The patient states she "has been dealing with it" but wants to begin running again and states she is "leaking" urine when she runs. The physical therapy examination records a diagnosis of stress incontinence, and the POC includes pelvic floor muscle training and patient education.

1. Determine the appropriate exercises to address this, and practice performing patient education.
2. List the key information the physical therapist assistant should gather from the patient during the follow-up visits.
3. What information will the physical therapist assistant use to determine when it is appropriate to advance the exercise interventions?
4. Describe an appropriate treatment progression.

## Case Study 3

An 83-year-old woman presents with a diagnosis of incontinence. The physical therapy evaluation includes a Timed Up and Go score of 20 seconds and a 30-second chair rise score of 20 repetitions. The patient ambulates independently without an assistive device with a wide base of support and an occasional loss of balance. Standing dynamic balance is fair. The patient states "I just can't make it to the bathroom in time once I feel the need to go." The physical therapy examination includes a diagnosis of functional incontinence and urge incontinence, and the POC includes pelvic floor muscle training, functional mobility training, and patient education.

1. Determine the appropriate exercises to include.
2. List the key information the assistant should gather from the patient during the follow-up visits.

3. What information will the assistant use to determine when it is appropriate to advance the exercise interventions?
4. Describe an appropriate treatment progression.

# References


1. IUGA ICS joint report on terminology female pelvic floor dysfunction. August 20, 2009. Accessed June 16, 2018. http://wiki.ics.org/file/view/IUGA_ICS_Joint_Report_On_Terminology_Female_Pelvic_Floor_Dysfunction_17.pdf
2. Schachter C, Stalker C, Teram E. Toward sensitive practice: issues for physical therapists working with survivors of childhood sexual abuse. *Phys Ther.* 1999;79(3):248-261. doi:10.1093/ptj/79.3.248
3. APTA. Physical therapist assistant (PTA) education statement: section on women's health. Updated April 2016. Accessed June 10, 2018. https://aptapelvichealth.org/wp-content/uploads/2021/01/Physical-Therapist-Assistant-PTA-Education-Statement-01-11-2021-1.pdf
4. Pelvic Guru. 10 common misconceptions about pelvic physical therapy. Accessed May 31, 2018. https://pelvicguru.com/10-common-misconceptions-about-pelvic-physical-therapy/
5. Eickmeyer SM. Anatomy and physiology of the pelvic floor. *Phys Med Rehabil Clin N Am.* 2017;28(3):455-460. doi:10.1016/j.pmr.2017.03.003
6. Brody L, Hall C. *Therapeutic Exercise: Moving Towards Function.* 4th ed. Wolters/Kluwer Health; 2018.
7. Moini J. *Anatomy and Physiology for Health Professionals.* 2nd ed. Jones and Bartlett; 2016.
8. Chermansky CJ, Moalli PA. Role of pelvic floor in lower urinary tract function. *Auton Neurosci.* 2016;10(200):43-48. doi:10.1016/j.autneu.2015.06.003
9. Mayo Clinic. Urinary incontinence. Accessed February 7, 2023. https://www.mayoclinic.org/diseases-conditions/urinary-incontinence/symptoms-causes/syc-20352808
10. Al-Shaikh G, Syed S, Osman S, Bogis A, Al-Badr A. Pessary use in stress urinary incontinence: a review of advantages, complications, patient satisfaction, and quality of life. *Int J Womens Health.* 2018;10(4):195-201. doi:10.2147/IJWH.S152616
11. Culbertson S, Davis AM. Nonsurgical management of urinary incontinence in women. *JAMA.* 2017;317(1):79-80. doi:10.1001/jama.2016.18433
12. Prather H, Camacho-Soto A. Musculoskeletal etiologies of pelvic pain. *Obstet Gynecol Clin North Am.* 2014;41(3):433-442. doi:10.1016/j.ogc.2014.04.004
13. MyoRehab. The trigger point and referred pain guide. Accessed June 13, 2018. http://triggerpoints.net/all-muscles
14. Travell J, Simons D, Simons L. *Myofascial Pain and Dysfunction: The Trigger Point Manual.* 2nd ed. Lippincott, Williams & Wilkins; 1999.
15. Goodman C, Snyder T. *Differential Diagnosis for Physical Therapists.* 5th ed. Elsevier Saunders; 2013.
16. Mendes A, Hoga L, Gonçalves B, Silva P, Pereira P. Adult women's experiences of urinary incontinence: a systematic review of qualitative evidence. *JBI Database System Rev Implement Rep.* 2017;15(5):1350-1408. doi:10.11124/JBISRIR-2017-003389
17. Wyman JF. The psychiatric and emotional impact of female pelvic floor dysfunction. *Curr Opin Obstet Gynecol.* 1994;6(4):336-339.
18. Coyne KS, Kvasz M, Ireland AM, Milsom I, Kopp ZS, Chapple CR. Urinary incontinence and its relationship to mental health and health-related quality of life in men and women in Sweden, the United Kingdom, and the United States. *Eur Urol.* 2012;61(1):88-95. doi:10.1016/j.eururo.2011.07.049
19. Lamin E, Parrillo LM, Newman DK, Smith AL. Pelvic floor muscle training: underutilization in the USA. *Curr Urol Rep.* 2016;17(2):10. doi:10.1007/s11934-015-0572-0
20. Price N, Dawood R, Jackson SR. Pelvic floor exercise for urinary incontinence: a systematic literature review. *Maturitas.* 2010;67(4):309-315. doi:10.1016/j.maturitas.2010.08.004
21. Dumoulin C, Hay-Smith EJ, Mac Habée-Séguin G. Pelvic floor muscle training versus no treatment, or inactive control treatments, for urinary incontinence in women. *Cochrane Database Syst Rev.* 2014;5:CD005654. doi:10.1002/14651858.CD005654.pub3
22. National Association for Continence. What are Kegel exercises? 2017. Accessed February 7, 2023. https://www.nafc.org/kegel
23. UCSF Health. Bladder retraining. Accessed February 7, 2023. https://www.ucsfhealth.org/education/bladder_training
24. Talley KM, Wyman JF, Bronas U, Olson-Kellogg BJ, McCarthy TC. Defeating urinary incontinence with exercise training: results of a pilot study in frail older women. *J Am Geriatr Soc.* 2017;65(6):1321-1327. doi:10.1111/jgs.14798
25. McLean L, Varette K, Gentilcore-Saulnier E, Harvey MA, Baker K, Sauerbrei E. Pelvic floor muscle training in women with stress urinary incontinence causes hypertrophy of the urethral sphincters and reduces bladder neck mobility during coughing. *Neurourol Urodyn.* 2013;32(8):1096-1102. doi:10.1002/nau.22343
26. Kannan P, Winser S, Goonetilleke R, Cheing G. Ankle positions potentially facilitating greater maximal contraction of pelvic floor muscles: a systematic review and meta-analysis. *Disabil Rehabil.* 2019;41(2):2483-2491. doi:10.1080/09638288.2018.1468934
27. Musich S, Wang SS, Ruiz J, Hawkins K, Wicker E. The impact of mobility limitations on health outcomes among older adults. *Geriatr Nurs.* 2018;39(2):162-169. doi:10.1016/j.gerinurse.2017.08.002
28. American College of Obstetricians and Gynecologists. Committee Opinion No. 650. Physical activity and exercise during pregnancy and the postpartum period. *Obstet Gynecol.* 2015;126:e135-e142.
29. Mittelmark RA. Physiology of pregnancy. October 2016. Accessed June 24, 2018. https://www.merckmanuals.com/professional/gynecology-and-obstetrics/approach-to-the-pregnant-woman-and-prenatal-care/physiology-of-pregnancy
30. Kisner C, Colby L. *Therapeutic Exercise Foundations and Techniques.* 7th ed. FA Davis; 2018.
31. Poyatos-León R, García-Hermoso A, Sanabria-Martínez G, Álvarez-Bueno C, Cavero-Redondo I, Martínez-Vizcaíno V. Effects of exercise-based interventions on postpartum depression: a meta-analysis of randomized controlled trials. *Birth.* 2017;44(3):200-208. doi:10.1111/birt.12294

32. Michalska A, Rokita W, Wolder D, Pogorzelska J, Kaczmarczyk K. Diastasis recti abdominis - a review of treatment methods. *Ginekol Pol.* 2018;89(2):97-101. doi:10.5603/GP.a2018.0016
33. Benjamin DR, van de Water AT, Peris CL. Effects of exercise on diastasis of the rectus abdominis muscle in the antenatal and postnatal periods: a systematic review. *Physiotherapy.* 2014;100(1):1-8.
34. Bursch SG. Interrater reliability of diastasis recti abdominis measurement. *Phys Ther.* 1987;67(7):1077-1079.
35. APTA. Move forward guide. The physical therapist guide to diastasis rectus abdominus. Accessed June 23, 2018. https://www.choosept.com/guide/physical-therapy-guide-diastasis-rectus-abdominis
36. Mommers EH, Ponten JE, Al Omar AK, de Vries Reilingh TS, Bouvy ND, Nienhuijs SW. The general surgeon's perspective of rectus diastasis. A systematic review of treatment options. *Surg Endosc.* 2017;31(12):4934-4949. doi:10.1007/s00464-017-5607-9
37. Gluppe SL, Hilde G, Tennfjord MK, Engh ME, Bø K. Effect of a postpartum training program on the prevalence of diastasis recti abdominis in postpartum primiparous women: a randomized controlled trial. *Phys Ther.* 2018;98(4):260-268. doi:10.1093/ptj/pzy008
38. Tuttle L, Fasching J, Keller A, et al. Noninvasive treatment of postpartum diastasis recti abdominis: a pilot study. *J Womens Health Phys Ther.* 2018;42(2):65-75.
39. Noble E. *Essential Exercise for the Childbearing Year.* 4th ed. New Life Images; 2003.
40. Clinton S, Newell A, Downey PA, Ferreira K. Pelvic girdle pain in the antepartum population: physical therapy clinical practice guidelines linked to the International Classification of Functioning, Disability, and Health from the Section on Women's Health and the Orthopaedic Section of the American Physical Therapy Association. *J Womens Health Phys Ther.* 2017;41(2):102-125.

Chapter 22

# Workplace Rehabilitation, Ergonomics, and Safety

*Jacki Klaczak Kopack, PT, DPT*

**KEY TERMS** Ergonomics | Functional capacity evaluation | Work conditioning | Work hardening | Work rehabilitation program

## Chapter Objectives

1. Identify and describe the common causes of workplace injuries.
2. Identify the red flags and reasons to obtain medical referral related to common workplace injuries.
3. Identify the components of proper body mechanic techniques during patient transfers.
4. Discuss patient education instructions for safe lifting, reaching, and moving tasks.
5. Define ergonomics and list the basic principles of an ergonomic training program.
6. Discuss the benefits of a workplace ergonomic assessment, corrective modifications, and exercises that can reduce the risk of work-related injury.
7. Compare and contrast outpatient physical therapy, work conditioning, work hardening, and transitional programs.
8. Define and describe the goals of a functional capacity evaluation (FCE).
9. List the treatment interventions commonly incorporated in a work hardening program.
10. Describe task modifications that can reduce the risk of work-related injury.
11. Design and progress a basic exercise and intervention program for a patient after a work-related back injury based on their job description.

## Introduction to Work-Related Injuries

Physical therapists and physical therapist assistants can work with employers and employees to decrease the likelihood of workplace-related injury. They can work with injured workers to promote a safe return to the workplace. The US Bureau of Labor Statistics reported that there were approximately 2.8 million nonfatal workplace injuries and illnesses in 2018 (2.8 cases per 100 full-time equivalent workers), resulting in approximately 900,400 lost workdays. Common nonfatal injuries included sprains/strains/dislocations (about 345,000), back injuries (about 142,200), and injuries from falls (about 240,160).[1,2] It is estimated that overexertion injuries (work-related lifting, pushing,



Kopack JK, Cascardi KA.
*Principles of Therapeutic Exercise for the Physical Therapist Assistant* (pp 705-717).

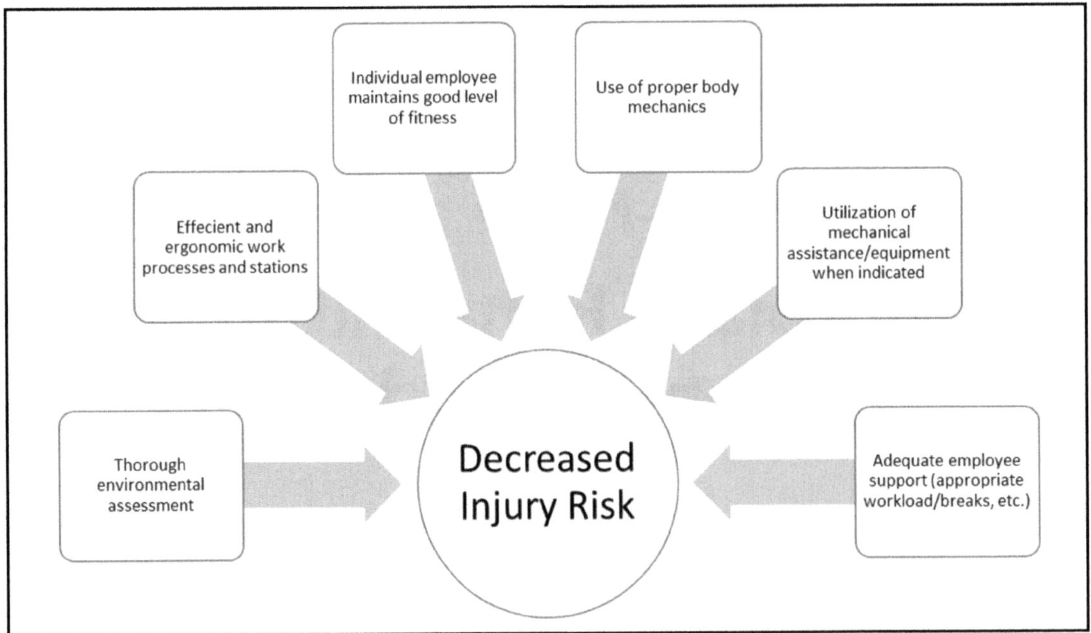


**Figure 22-1.** Factors that decrease work-related injury risk.

pulling, holding, carrying, and throwing), repetitive use of tools and/or equipment, and falls were the top 3 most common causes of nonfatal injuries. Health care and social assistance workers accounted for 544,800 nonfatal injuries during 2017 to 2018.[3] Serious, nonfatal workplace injuries result in billions of dollars in direct US workers' compensation costs.[4] Overexertion injuries accounted for 23.4%, and falls accounted for 19.2% of work-related injuries, costing businesses over $13 billion and $11 billion, respectively.[4] Each work environment and profession has individual risk factors for injury. Environmental assessment, maximizing workflow (for efficiency and ergonomics), and promoting the fitness and health of each employee can mitigate some of these risks for injury. The physical therapy team is uniquely qualified to address each of these factors (Figure 22-1).

Common workplace injuries include sprains/strains/dislocations, low back injuries, and almost 80,000 fractures in a year.[2] Musculoskeletal injuries can occur as a result of repetitive tasks; falls; or from tasks that incorporate lifting, reaching, pushing, or pulling. Excessive repetition, awkward postures, and heavy lifting are the most common factors associated with work-related musculoskeletal disorders (MSDs).[5] Some specific job duties (ie, data entry/computer work, painting, or playing an instrument) increase the risk of overuse injuries such as carpal tunnel syndrome, and high-volume overhead work increases the risk of rotator cuff injuries. Construction workers who use a jackhammer or pneumatic drill are at risk for vibration-related injuries to the low back and upper extremities. These patients can benefit from physical therapy, and the goal is to return the individual back to work safely and to make recommendations to reduce the risk of reinjury.

## *Physical Therapy Work-Related Musculoskeletal Injuries and Body Mechanics*

Job duties of physical therapists and physical therapist assistants create an increased risk of injury for these clinicians. The highest annual prevalence of work-related injuries for physical therapists was in the low back (45%) followed by the wrists and hands (29.6%); upper back (28.7%); neck (24.7%); and shoulders, elbows, hips and thighs, knees, and ankles and feet (each less than 20%).[6] The lifetime prevalence of injury is reported to be 55% to 91%.[7] The lower back area is the most frequently affected (lifetime prevalence ranging from 26% to 79.6%) followed by injuries to the neck, upper back, and shoulders.[7,8] The major risk factors for work-related low back pain include lifting, transferring, repetitive movements, awkward and static postures, increased physical load, treating a large number of patients in a single day, working while injured, and/or years of experience on the job.[7,8] Many physical therapists and assistants alter their method of treatment or change the type of patients (ie, inpatient vs outpatient) to reduce their pain or discomfort due to injury. Investigators determined that physical therapy clinicians tend to self-treat their injuries.[8] There is an increased incidence of low back pain in women, younger therapists, and therapists working in rehabilitation settings. Although therapists are trained in proper body mechanics and lifting techniques, these skills do not appear to prevent work-related injuries.[7] Consistent with general findings and recommendations by the National Institute for Occupational Safety and Health (NIOSH), the use of mechanical aids and equipment for patient lifting and for manual therapy techniques should be used more consistently.[7,9]

**Table 22-1**

**Body Mechanics and Instructions for Physical Therapist Assistants During Patient Transfers**

- Plan the move.
  - Assess the environment (position of intravenous lines/equipment and/or wheelchair; ensure a clear path).
  - Be familiar with the level of assistance the patient requires and the patient's ability to follow directions.
- Communicate with the patient.
- Place the gait belt snugly around the patient.
- Lower the bed and then scoot patient to the edge of the bed until the patient's feet are on the floor (if weight bearing is permitted).
- Get close; the clinician's center of gravity should be close to the object/patient's center of gravity.
- Stand with a wide BOS (staggered foot placement).
- Maintain proper spinal position (maintain a slight lumbar lordosis) and engage the core.
- Bend your knees and use your legs, not your back.
- Prepare the patient for the move.
  - Use short commands: "We'll stand (or go) on 3."
  - Gently rock the patient to a count of 3 (to prepare the patient for the move) and then stand or transfer the patient on 3.
- Exhale during the exertion/lifting phase of the motion.
- Wait and check the patient's status before moving.
- Turn by moving the feet to step around to position the patient before sitting. Do not flex or rotate your back.

Note: Ask for assistance if the patient is too heavy or use mechanical equipment!

How a person positions and moves during a task is referred to as *body mechanics*. There are 4 elements that need to be addressed when assessing proper body mechanics during task performance: posture/body position, center of mass/base of support (BOS), the use of large muscle groups, and task execution. The elements of body mechanics are typically addressed throughout the educational curriculum for physical therapist assistants; this section provides a brief summary of the key components related to clinician and patient safety. The reader is referred to physical therapy foundational textbooks for additional information.

The physical therapist assistant should use proper body mechanics during all tasks; this is especially important during transfers for the safety of both the clinician and the patient (Table 22-1). During every patient interaction that involves physically assisting in moving a patient, the 2 individuals need to create one coordinated mechanical motion to complete the task (Figure 22-2). The assistant must be able to recognize their physical abilities and limitations when moving patients. There is mechanical equipment available to aid clinicians when transferring overweight or dependent patients (Figure 22-3). Clinicians should incorporate this equipment to lower injury risk.

Physical therapist assistants instruct patients how to use proper body mechanics in different situations (ie, pushing, pulling, and reaching overhead/below the waist) and in the selection of appropriate lifting techniques (ie, traditional, power, and stoop lifts). The goal of proper body mechanics is to use safe, efficient, and coordinated movements while maintaining a stable and balanced BOS and conserving energy. The assistant should modify body mechanics instructions based on a patient's physiological abilities and limitations. Table 22-2 provides body mechanics instructions for patients.

**Clinical Tips**

Work smarter, not harder! Include safe patient handling techniques in all patient care interventions. Physical therapist assistants should maintain or increase their personal physical fitness through regular strength training and cardiovascular exercise.

**Figure 22-2.** When assisting with sit-to-stand transfers, the clinician will apply a gait belt to the patient before initiating the transfer. Note the clinician's body mechanics (ie, knees bent and slight lumbar lordosis). The clinician is positioned close to the patient.

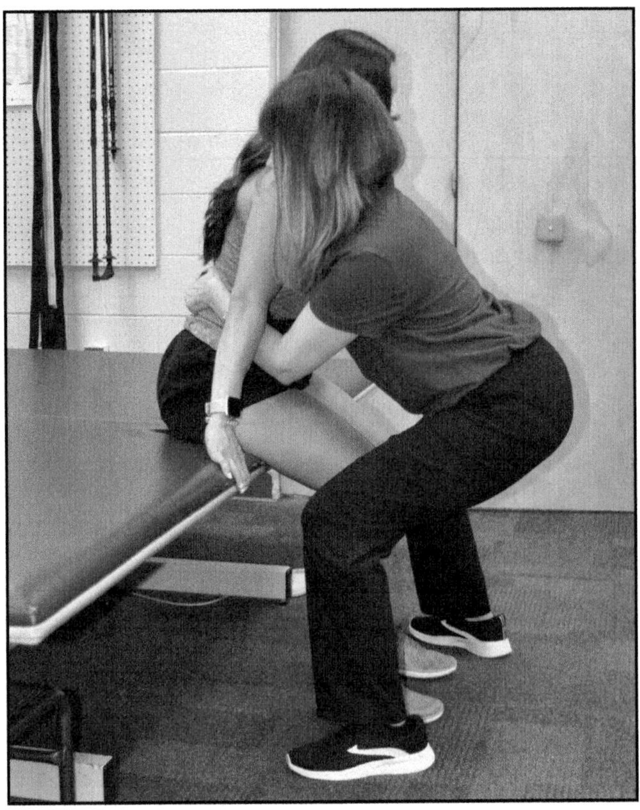

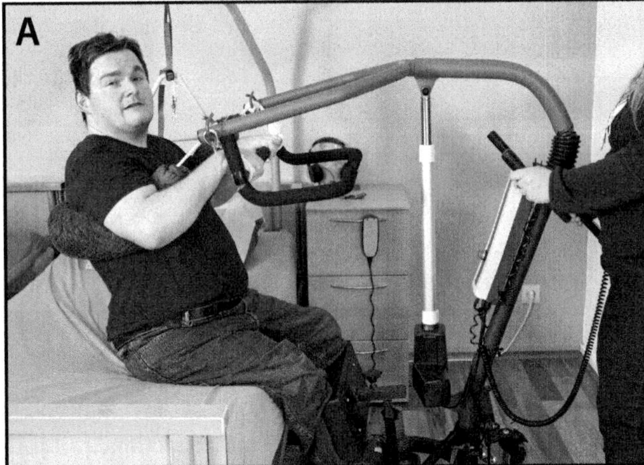


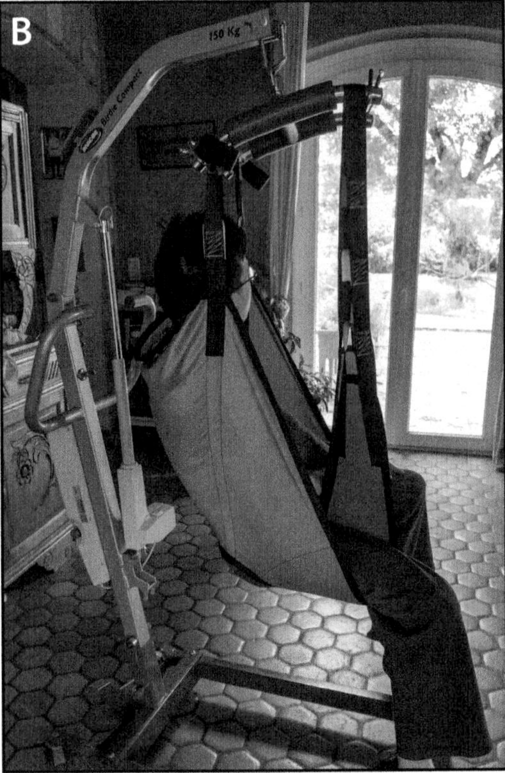


**Figure 22-3.** Equipment to assist clinicians or caregivers to transfer patients. (A) Lift to assist sit to standing (Belushi/Shutterstock.com). (B) Lift that can transfer patients from a supine or seated position and move patients from bed to chair/wheelchair (Spech/Shutterstock.com).

**Table 22-2**

**Proper Body Mechanics Instructions for Patients for Lifting, Reaching, and Moving Objects**

Lifting instructions:

- Plan the move ahead of time.
- Stand close to the object/load and place feet shoulder-width apart or stagger your stance.
- Tighten abdominal (core) muscles, but don't hold your breath!
- Maintain a slight arch in the low back.
- Bend the knees to squat down to the object/load.
- Get a good grasp on the load with both hands and bring the load close to the center of your body (pelvis).
- Use your legs (not your back) to stand; keep your spine vertical when lifting the load.
- Take small steps with your feet when turning to move the object. Do not twist your spine!
- Bend your knees and lower the object slowly to its new location.

Other important tips for lifting, reaching, or moving objects:

- Avoid bending and rotating the trunk simultaneously.
- Use a foot stool or stable ladder (preferably with a hand support) to reach for objects overhead.
- Know your lifting limits! (Do you have the strength and muscle control to move the object?)
- Get assistance or use equipment when lifting or moving heavy or awkwardly shaped objects.
- Roll, push, or slide objects instead of lifting. Push objects vs pulling whenever possible.

## Ergonomic Assessments and Work-Related Treatment Intervention Programs

According to the Occupational Safety and Health Administration (OSHA), most work-related musculoskeletal injuries can be prevented. It is the responsibility of the employer to provide a safe and healthy workplace for employees. OSHA has developed ergonomic program guidelines that can be implemented by employers for different work environments (eg, poultry and meatpacking plants, grocery store, shipyards, nursing homes) to prevent MSDs.[10] The guidelines are based on work-related injury prevention research and recommendations provided to OSHA by NIOSH. The physical therapy team can review the research and guidelines to assist patients and employers in reducing injuries in the workplace. Resources that are individualized to varied workplace settings/jobs are found in the Suggested Resources section at the end of the chapter. Implementing these guidelines can increase safety and efficiency and reduce company costs (ie, workers' compensation).

**Ergonomics** is "an applied science concerned with designing and arranging things people use so that the people and things interact most efficiently and safely."[11] Ergonomic programs address 4 basic principles: neutral posture or joint positions, grip types (for workers who use hand tools), muscle fatigue and back/neck pain, and proper lifting.[12] These principles are used to teach workers the best ways to avoid awkward positions, repetitive activities, and poor lifting mechanics. This instruction can improve job efficiency, lessen muscle fatigue, and reduce the number and severity of injuries. The Health and Human Services, Centers for Disease Control and Prevention, and NIOSH have developed a guide for clinicians who provide ergonomic assessments and training. These resources highlight MSD risk factors and ways to reduce them (see Suggested Resources).

### Clinical Tips

The neutral position for most joints is within the midrange of the available joint motion. Muscles tend to be at their normal resting length in this position and can generate maximal muscle force. When joints are positioned awkwardly (fully flexed or extended), muscles are unable to generate maximal force, and they fatigue faster, creating stress on joints and muscle and increasing the risk for injury.[12] Consider the following: What is the most efficient way to use a screwdriver? How are the elbow and wrist positioned? Which screwdriver handle diameter is optimal for use (ie, small, medium, or large)? Record and explain your response before reading on.

Consider that keeping the shoulder in neutral (next to the trunk) and the elbow at waist height is the most efficient way to use a screwdriver. Positions: elbow at 90 degrees and wrist in neutral. The grip size of the screwdriver depends on the size of the person's hand, but it should allow for the comfortable use of a power grip.

**Table 22-3**

**Elements of an Ergonomic Training Program**

- Identifying risk factors: Assess for the presence of risk factors based on the 4 basic principles of ergonomics. Use an ergonomic assessment checklist (see Suggested Resources section).
- Train management and workers: Training should be targeted to the audience's job and type of work environment. Use easy-to-understand terms. Workers should be instructed on how to recognize risk factors and signs/symptoms and how to report MSD. Workers should also understand how to address and remediate the risk factors and hazards. If they cannot remediate the risk factors, they should be instructed to report them appropriately.
- Collect evidence (medical/health): Data collection determines the scope of the problems. How many workers have experienced the same or similar MSD? Perform a job analysis to assess tools/equipment being used, workstation layout, environment (eg, lighting, temperature), and job demands.
- Fix the problem by employing remediation techniques: This improves overall safety for the workers. For example, replace equipment that is problematic or use best practice interventions to reduce injury.
- Assess the effectiveness: Determine the impact of the actions taken.
- Promote a healthy workplace: Perform workplace assessment to better understand job requirements. If possible, employers should accommodate workers when they return to work (eg, modified jobs, restricted duties, transfer to a temporary position).
- Maintain open communication between a committed management and involved workers: Management must be committed to reducing MSD and should encourage workers to report real or potential job hazards and find ways to reduce the hazards.

Companies may contract with a local therapy company to provide ergonomic assessments, training, and education. Engaging workers is an important component of an effective work site assessment. Identification, modification, and/or correction of ergonomic problems is part of the training provided; the education is individualized to the work site and job requirements of the workers. Successful programs encourage workers to report issues and injuries early and use a regular process for evaluating progress and program outcomes.[10] Implementation of the processes recommended by NIOSH helps to ensure an effective ergonomic training program (Table 22-3).[13]

## Ergonomic Training Programs

Effective education includes language that is appropriate for the audience (layperson's terms), demonstrations, and skill practice. The trainer should be mindful of the primary language of the workers who are attending the session. A common ergonomic training activity that a physical therapy department in a hospital coordinates is the facility's annual body mechanics/back school education program. The target audience is typically facility/hospital workers, and the content varies from session to session depending on the specific group attending (based on the jobs/duties of those attending). For example, ergonomic education provided to medical billing staff may focus on proper computer or workstation positioning. The focus for nursing assistants includes the use of proper body mechanics specific to lifting/transferring patients. Training frontline health care workers typically includes basic education on spinal anatomy; a description of risky work-related activities; an overview, demonstration, and practice of proper sitting and standing postures; instruction, demonstration, and practice of proper lifting/transfer techniques; and instruction in the use of gait belts and supplemental mechanical assistance equipment. The clinician explains the role of the physical therapy team in ergonomic assessments, rehabilitation, and the importance of general physical conditioning/fitness for all workers. The clinician provides participants a list of injury-reducing ergonomic tips (Table 22-4), including how to modify task sequences to maximize efficiency and strategies to reduce repetitive motion, avoid prolonged postures, and eliminate awkward postures.

## Ergonomic Assessments

Clinicians can assess an employee's workstation or job/task requirements using a detailed checklist (see Suggested Resources) and then make recommendations to increase efficiency and safety. Employees can complete a self-assessment of their work space (see Suggested Resources). Self-assessment helps to determine other issues that may be present. The clinician recommends work space modifications based on the clinician's data collection, the individual employee's assessment of their work space and job/task requirements, and the clinical ergonomic assessment (Table 22-5). The clinician considers proper alignment and joint angles when assessing a worker positioned at a

**Table 22-4**

**General Ergonomic Tips to Reduce Risk of Injury**

- Avoid or interrupt prolonged static positions and/or repetitive motions.
- Maintain a neutral spine position when sitting (a lumbar support may be suggested).
- If prolonged standing is required, alternate placing one foot on a low stool and/or standing on a padded mat (eg, GelPro) to reduce low back stress.
- Make a plan before moving objects.
- Minimize joint and muscle forces when performing a task; push rather than pull and use mechanical lifting equipment whenever possible.
- Minimize pressure on bony contact points: Add pressure relief padding to sitting/standing surfaces; modify hand tools (ie, add padding) to reduce pressure or vibratory forces.
- Rearrange work spaces to reduce overhead or lateral reaching.
- Arrange sitting or standing workstation heights to allow for proper posture.
- Minimize muscle fatigue: Modify activities, vary task sequences, and add modifications to minimize joint stress (ie, built-up grips or adaptive equipment).
- Change positions often and move throughout the day: Every 30 to 45 minutes take 30 seconds to 1 minute to stretch between prolonged positioning or repetitive work tasks.
  - If sitting, stand and extend the trunk; if standing, flex forward as long as it does not cause pain.
  - Take brief walks around the office.
  - If doing computer work or other repetitive wrist/hand/finger tasks, stretch those muscles often.
- "Sedentary is the new smoking."[14] Keep physically active and avoid sedentary lifestyles.

computer workstation regardless of the desk height (Figure 22-4). Common modifications include the use of standing desks, keyboard modifications, workstation adjustments or seating alterations, modification of task sequencing, instruction in safe patient handling equipment and practices, or the use of vibration dampeners.

**Clinical Tips**

"Sitting is the new smoking"[14] has led to an increase in the use of standing desks. Standing desks are not for everyone because prolonged standing may result in fatigue or leg or back pain for some people. A healthy work environment allows frequent position changes, minimizes high-risk activities, and offers opportunities for motion interspersed throughout the day.[14]

## *Work Rehabilitation: Work Conditioning, Work Hardening, and Transitional Programs*

There are opportunities for physical therapist assistants to treat persons with work-related injuries and to facilitate return to work; physical therapist assistants can also participate in the work environment assessment. Assistants will complete on-the-job training and continuing education coursework to become competent and proficient in this specialty area. There are several continuing education courses with certifications that are available for physical therapist assistants to pursue in the field of ergonomics, such as office and industrial ergonomic evaluator certification, work hardening/work conditioning/return-to-work training, and **FCE** certification courses. A physical therapist assistant can also become a certified industrial rehabilitation specialist.

Physical therapy helps assist workers with their transition back to work as safely and as soon as possible after injury. This is referred to as *work rehabilitation*.[15,16] **Work rehabilitation programs** include work conditioning, work hardening, and transitional programs.[16] Treatment interventions and patient education are geared toward having the employee return to work. A worker whose job has high physical demands (eg, firefighter, construction worker) requires more extensive training to meet the needs of their job requirements. **Work conditioning** and **work hardening** programs are treatment interventions that can meet those needs and bridge the gap between traditional therapy and returning to work. According to the American Physical Therapy Association (APTA) guidelines, a work conditioning program is an intensive, work-related, and goal-oriented treatment program specifically designed to restore an individual's systemic, neurologic, musculoskeletal, and cardiopulmonary functions. The overarching program goals are to restore the patient's physical capacity and function, prevent the recurrence of the same injury, and decrease their fear of returning to work. Typically, work conditioning programs are held in outpatient physical therapy settings. Treatment sessions are usually for 2 to 4 hours 5 days a week for 4 to 8 weeks.[15]

**Table 22-5**

Workplace Assessment Checklist

| Employee Name: ______ Job Title: ______<br>Date: ______ Assessment Completed by: ______ | | | |
|---|---|---|---|
| | Yes | No | Recommendations |
| ***Does the Seated Workspace Meet Ergonomic Design Principles?*** | | | |
| Screen at eye level? | | | |
| Seat height allows feet to fully contact floor? | | | |
| Chair allows lumbar lordosis and fully upright posture? | | | |
| Keyboard height allows elbows to remain at side, wrist neutral? | | | |
| Knees relaxed and at or just below hip height (about 90 degrees)? | | | |
| Hips at 90 degrees? | | | |
| Approximate time seated without position changes: ______ | | | |
| ***Does the Standing Workspace Meet Ergonomic Design Principles?*** | | | |
| Computer monitor height allows neutral neck position? | | | |
| Screen at eye level? | | | |
| Keyboard height allows elbows to remain at side, wrist neutral? | | | |
| Standing pad/cushion available? | | | |
| Approximate time standing without position changes: ______ | | | |
| ***Does the Employee Perform Repetitive Tasks? If Yes, Estimate Time/Task*** | | | |
| Describe task: ______ Time/task: ______ | | | |
| Describe task: ______ Time/task: ______ | | | |
| Describe task: ______ Time/task: ______ | | | |
| Describe task: ______ Time/task: ______ | | | |
| ***Task assessment. Does the Employee: If yes, Estimate Time/Task*** | ***Time*** | | |
| Perform tasks that require repeated lifting of object > 20 pounds? | | | |
| Perform tasks that require occasional lifting of object > 50 pounds? | | | |
| Perform tasks that require repeated lifting of object > 50 pounds? | | | |
| Perform tasks with neck positioned in flexion, lateral bending, rotation, or extension? | | | |
| Perform tasks with back positioned in flexion, lateral bending, rotation, or extension? | | | |
| Perform tasks with awkward elbow position for prolonged time/with high force? | | | |
| Perform tasks with a prolonged wrist flexion position or with high-force application? | | | |
| Perform tasks with a prolonged hip flexion position or with high-force application? | | | |
| Perform tasks with prolonged or repeated reaching overhead or with high force? | | | |
| Perform tasks with prolonged extreme reaching or with high force application? | | | |
| Are high-impact tools used routinely? If yes, list: | | | |
| Are high-vibration producing tools used routinely? If yes, list: | | | |

*(continued)*

**Table 22-5 (continued)**

| Workplace Assessment Checklist | | |
|---|---|---|
| Observation of Employee Task Completion | | |
| *Task Observed* | *Quality of Motion/Task Completion* | *Recommendations for Physical Therapy Interventions* |
| | | |
| | | |
| | | |
| | | |

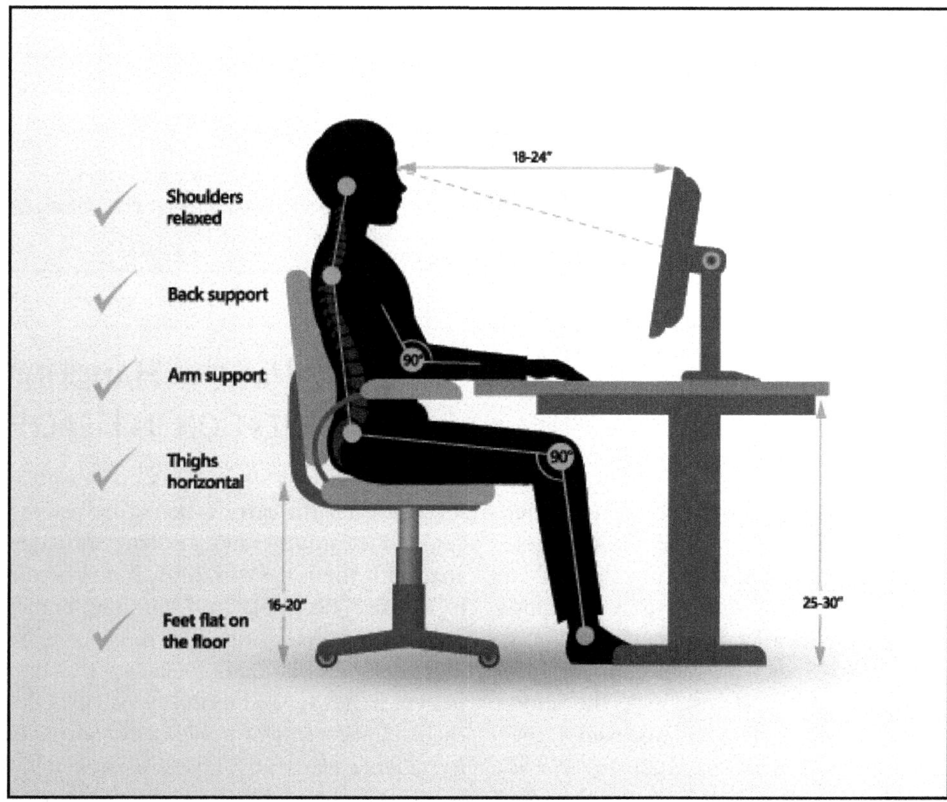


**Figure 22-4.** Proper seated positioning (3DBear/Shutterstock.com).

A work hardening program is a highly structured and individualized program using work-simulated or real work activities; it is multidisciplinary in nature. These sessions are usually progressive multihour programs (up to 8 hours a day) 5 days a week for 4 to 8 weeks. Work simulation training often includes the use of additional equipment or special work areas. Some examples of work-related equipment include multisized boxes, weight sleds, weight boxes, stools, lifting stations with various shelf heights, push/pull weighted carts, and assembly simulation stations based on job duties. Some specialty clinics have ladders, stairs, and/or construction area simulation areas (eg, sand pile with shovels, woodworking areas). The goal of the program is to restore physical, behavioral, and vocational functions. In addition to physical/occupational therapy interventions, the multidisciplinary team may also provide psychological counseling and job coaching and perform an individualized ergonomic evaluation. Patients in work hardening programs have strict requirements (ie, consistent attendance and must make objective progress) that must be followed in order to participate in the program. Patients are discharged if these requirements are not met, if the patient experiences medical/psychosocial complications, or if the patient has met all outlined goals. "Transitional work programs focus on the specific work tasks and work environment, with recommendations by the treatment team for task and environmental modifications to enhance work performance at the job site."[16]

Delays in entering into a work rehabilitation program may have serious negative effects on patients' ability to return to work; early intervention is critical when treating patients with a work-related injury.[16] The physical therapist assistant monitors for any changes in a patient's presentation (ie, any new or changing signs/symptoms above or below the injury site) and any red or yellow flags and promptly relays this information to the physical therapist (refer to Chapter 11 [Table 11-2]).

## Functional Capacity Evaluations

The therapist completes a comprehensive functional evaluation. A physical therapist completes a typical physical therapy examination (vital signs, posture, ambulation ability/distance, transfers, bed mobility, balance, range of motion, and strength). Then, the physical therapist evaluates the injury, reviews the patient's function in relation to their job, and completes an FCE to identify specific physical limitations and functional deficits that prevent the patient from returning to full-duty work.[15,16] The APTA defines the FCE as "a comprehensive battery of performance-based tests that are commonly used to determine ability for work, activities of daily living, or leisure activities."[15] FCEs are modified to reflect individual job duties, and they use standardized and objective repeatable testing measures. The FCE measures strength, endurance, and the ability to tolerate positional demands and physical demands of a job. Additionally, the therapist collects information specific to the amount/load a patient can push, pull, lift (from varied heights), and carry as well as sitting and standing tolerance. The purpose of an initial or baseline FCE is to determine the patient's current level of physical activity (sedentary, light, medium, or high), aerobic capacity (poor, fair, average, good, or excellent), grip strength, and mobility and strength (core and/or joint specific) in relation to their injury. A full FCE usually takes several hours to complete, and because of the extensive amount of testing, data collection may be split over 2 days. Commonly used FCEs include the Physical Work Performance Evaluation (ErgoScience, Inc), the Isernhagen Work Systems Functional Capactity Evaluation (Isernhagen Work Systems, Inc), the short-form FCE, the Blankenship System (Blankenship, Inc), Ergos Work Simulator (Work Recovery, Inc), the WEST-EPIC 5 (Work Evaluation Systems Technology), Key Method Functional Capacity Assessment (Key Functional Assessments, Inc). Specific hand strength and endurance assessment tools include the ARCON Grip (Applied Rehabilitation Concepts, Inc) and the Hanoun Medical Pinch (Hanoun Medical, Inc).[17] Each facility (or corporation) typically selects 1 or 2 FCE tools to use. The consistent use of 1 or 2 tools can improve the clinician's competence/reliability in the use of that tool.

The therapist uses the results of the FCE to create an individualized program designed to increase the patient's current physical abilities. This often includes medium- to high-intensity cardiovascular and strengthening exercises as well as stretching and additional conditioning activities specifically tailored to the tasks required to perform the patient's job. The FCE data are also used to determine the patient's potential ability to return to preinjury job duties, patient progress, and the need for potential accommodations, as well as to make recommendations for ongoing training/interventions.

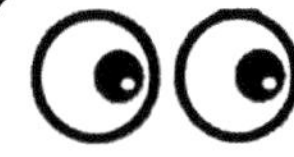

### Eye on the Research: Functional Capacity Evaluation Protocols

De Baets et al[18] examined 9 different FCEs and summarized that although many of the well-known FCE methods have been rigorously studied, some of the research indicates areas of weakness in reliability and validity. The 2 tools noted to have high predictive validity were the Physical Work Performance Evaluation and the short-form FCE. The Isernhagen Work System FCE was found to have moderate to high test-retest, intra-, and inter-rater reliability. The clinician should research the reliability and validity of the selected tool and implement strategies to maximize reliability (eg, ensure adequate training with a given tool/assessment and inter-rater reliability).[18]

## Safe Patient Handling and Mobilization in Health Care

Manual lifting of patients creates an increased risk of injury for health care workers; the use of mechanical lifts can reduce injury rates and the subsequent costs associated with them.[19-25] In 2005, Texas became the first state to require hospitals and nursing homes to implement safe patient handling and movement programs, which increased the national focus on the importance of safe patient handling and mobility (SPHM). Texas law required the establishment of policies to control the risk of injury to patients and staff that were associated with lifting and moving patients. It created limitations for the use of manual lifting techniques and mandated that each patient scenario be assessed to determine if mechanical equipment was indicated.[19] Since then, 11 more states have signed similar legislation.[22]

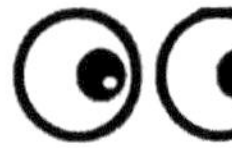

### Eye on the Research

The implementation of an SPHM program can result in substantial injury reduction. Researchers reviewed data from 27 studies and summarized that extended follow-up and education were associated with greater injury prevention; the greatest reduction in injuries occurred in the intensive care setting. Researchers recommended further study to determine the most effective interventions for different patient care levels/settings.[26]

Many professional organizations have created statements and actions to support SPHM.[21-24] Research indicates that when SPHM programs are implemented, the quality of patient care improves and the costs to hospital organizations are reduced. The Alliance between OSHA and the Association of Occupational Health Professionals published a resource guide for SPHM in the acute care setting (see Suggested Resources). OSHA published a brochure that provides information regarding the cost benefits of implementing a safe patient handling program, highlighting examples that included reduced costs related to fewer patient injuries (eg, falls, pressure ulcers), fewer staff sick days related to injury/illness, and a reduction in nursing staff attrition. The cost to recruit, hire, orient, and train one new nurse to replace one who has left the profession can range from $27,000 to $103,000.[25] One hospital reduced their overall nurse turnover rate to 5%, resulting in $170,000 savings (in 1 year) as well as a 92% reduction in workers' compensation costs associated with patient handling injuries after implementing the SPHM program.[25] The APTA states that physical therapists and physical therapist assistants should be leaders in the development, implementation, refinement, and maintenance of SPHM programs. The APTA promotes leadership by example, stating that the physical therapy team should always use SPHM and should provide leadership in multidisciplinary SPHM training programs. The APTA recommends that therapists and assistants should have appropriate access to a variety of safe patient handling equipment and that therapy departments should have appropriate policies and training in safe patient handling procedures.[23]

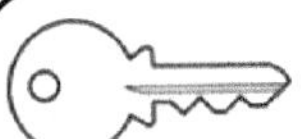

**Key Safety Considerations**

- Always practice proper body mechanics.
- Maintain personal fitness levels.
- Use mechanical equipment or get additional assistance when appropriate.
- Practice SPHM. In situations in which there is a perceived gap in the available support, speak up. Offer your expertise as a movement specialist; provide suggestions to improve staff and/or patient safety.

## Conclusion

The physical therapy team plays an important role in workplace safety, the prevention of workplace-related injuries, and facilitating return to function and work after injury. Physical therapist assistants participate in work conditioning and work hardening programs as well as in workplace training and ergonomic training programs. Knowledge of ergonomics, proper body mechanics, and the elements of an ergonomic training program supports the rehabilitation of persons with work-related injuries. Physical therapy interventions can minimize workplace-related injuries, and physical therapist assistants can assist in implementing programs to maximize the health of the workforce.

## Review Questions

1. List 3 possible factors that could contribute to workplace injury.
2. List the principles of proper body mechanics.
3. Is personal fitness an important consideration in work-related injury prevention? Why/why not?
4. Define ergonomics and list the components of an ergonomics training program.
5. A patient asks for some tips for setting up a work space to lower risk for injury. What information should you share?
6. What are the goals and purposes of an FCE?
7. List at least 3 advantages of implementing SPHM.
8. Which tasks increase the risk of injury for a physical therapist assistant? What are the best ways to reduce these risks?
9. What is the difference between work conditioning and work hardening? When are these programs most appropriate to implement?
10. What red flags indicate the need to follow up with the physical therapist/physician when working with a patient who presents with a work-related injury?

## Case Study 1

The student physical therapist assistant has been asked by their clinical supervisor to present a mock "back school" education in preparation for educating a patient with a recent lumbosacral strain. The patient's job duties include sitting (50%), standing/walking (25%), and lifting floor to waist with a load of 10 to 15 pounds (25%). Outline the appropriate education to include, and practice presenting this information to a peer.

## Case Study 2

The physical therapist assistant is preparing to see a patient with Guillain-Barré syndrome who has just been transferred to acute care from the intensive care unit. The patient has upper extremity return but no lower extremity return yet, and rehabilitation placement is pending. The patient is stable and cleared for physical therapy with goals of increasing upper extremity active range of motion, increasing bed mobility from maximum assistance to moderate assistance, supine to sit from maximum assistance of 2 to maximum assistance of 1, improving sitting balance, and increasing tolerance out of bed in chair. What is the optimal positioning of the bed when assisting the patient with exercises and bed mobility? Consider the treatment environment, and outline the factors that the assistant should consider specific to ergonomics and workplace safety. Is the use of a mechanical lift appropriate?

## Suggested Resources

### *Ergonomic Assessment Forms and Checklists for Various Work Environments*

OSHA various workplace ergonomic assessment forms: https://www.osha.gov/dte/grant_materials/fy14/sh-26336-sh4/Ergonomic-Assessment-Checklist.pdf

### *Ergonomic Program Guidelines and Principles*

Department of Health and Human Services, Centers for Disease Control and Prevention, NIOSH. Practical demonstrations of ergonomic principles. https://stacks.cdc.gov/view/cdc/57870/cdc_57870_DS1.pdf?

OSHA. Ergonomic assessment checklist: https://www.osha.gov/sites/default/files/2018-12/fy14_sh-26336-sh4_Ergonomic-Assessment-Checklist.pdf

OSHA ergonomic program guidelines for various work environments and NIOSH research for prevention of work-related injuries: https://www.osha.gov/SLTC/ergonomics/

### *Computer Workstation Self-Assessment Checklist*

National Institute of Health. Computer workstation ergonomics: self-assessment checklist. https://ors.od.nih.gov/sr/dohs/Documents/checklist-ergonomics-computer-workstation-self-assessment.pdf

### *Safe Patient Handling and Mobility Program Resource Guides*

Association of Occupational Health Professionals in Healthcare, Kabuto A, Gruden MA, Pionk C, Smir S. *Beyond Getting Started. A Resource Guide: Implementing a Safe Patient Handling and Mobility Program in the Acute Care Setting.* 4th ed. 2020. Accessed February 7, 2023. https://aohp.org/aohp/Portals/0/Documents/ToolsForYourWork/BGSpublication/20-06%20BGS%20Safe%20Patient%20Handling.pdf

## References


1. US Bureau of Labor Statistics. Injuries, illness, fatalities. Accessed February 7, 2023. www.bls.gov/IIF
2. US Bureau of Labor Statistics. Injuries, illness, fatalities. Table R13, Accessed February 7, 2023. https://www.bls.gov/iif/oshwc/osh/case/cd_r13_2018.htm
3. Work Injury Source. Workplace injury statistics–2019 year-end data for workplace accidents, injuries, and deaths. February 12, 2020. Accessed February 7, 2023. https://workinjurysource.com/workplace-injury-statistics-2019/
4. Liberty Mutual Insurance. Liberty mutual workplace safety index. February 2018. Accessed February 7, 2023. https://business.libertymutualgroup.com/business-insurance/Documents/Services/Workplace%20Safety%20Index.pdf
5. da Costa RB, Vieira ER. Risk factors for work-related musculoskeletal disorders: a systematic review of current longitudinal studies. *Am J Ind Med.* 2010;53:285-323.
6. Bork BE, Cook TM, Rosecrance JC, et al. Work-related musculoskeletal disorders among physical therapists. *Phys Ther.* 1996;76(8):827-835.
7. Milhem M, Kalichman L, Ezra D, Alperovitch-Najenson D. Work-related musculoskeletal disorders among physical therapists: a comprehensive narrative review. *Int J Occup Med Environ Health.* 2016;29(5):735-747. doi:10.13075/ijomeh.1896.00620
8. Sharan D, Ajeesh PS. Injury prevention in physiotherapists--a scientific review. *Work.* 2012;41(suppl 1):1855-1859. doi:10.3233/WOR-2012-0397-1855
9. Centers for Disease Control and Prevention. The National Institute for Occupational Safety and Health (NIOSH). Safe patient handling and mobility. Reviewed August 2, 2013. Accessed February 7, 2023. https://www.cdc.gov/niosh/topics/safepatient/
10. United States Department of Labor, Occupational Safety and Health Administration. Ergonomics: prevention of musculoskeletal disorders in the workplace. Accessed February 7, 2023. https://www.osha.gov/SLTC/ergonomics/
11. Merriam-Webster. Ergonomics. Accessed February 7, 2023. https://www.merriam-webster.com/dictionary/ergonomics

12. Moore SM, Torma-Krajewski J, Steiner LJ; Health and Human Services, Center for Disease Control, The National Institute for Occupational Safety and Health. Practical demonstrations of ergonomic principles. July 2011. Accessed February 7, 2023. https://stacks.cdc.gov/view/cdc/57870/cdc_57870_DS1.pdf
13. Center for Disease Control, The National Institute for Occupational Safety and Health. Elements of ergonomics programs. Accessed July 23, 2020. https://www.cdc.gov/niosh/topics/ergonomics/ergoprimer/default.html
14. Mula A. Ergonomics and the standing desk. *Work.* 2018;60(2):171-174. doi:10.3233/WOR-182736
15. American Physical Therapy Association. Guideline occupational health physical therapy: advanced work rehabilitation guidelines. Rescinded May 2011. Accessed February 7, 2023. https://www.orthopt.org/uploads/content_files/OHSIG_Guidelines/OHSIG_guidelines_2/Work_Rehab_Guideline_Final_Draft_4_1_11.pdf
16. Voss MR, Homa JK, Singh M, Seidl JA, Griffitt WE. Outcomes of an interdisciplinary work rehabilitation program. *Work.* 2019;64(3):507-514. doi:10.3233/WOR-193012
17. Chen JJ. Functional capacity evaluation & disability. *Iowa Orthop J.* 2007;27:121-127.
18. De Baets S, Calders P, Schalley N, et al. Updating the evidence on functional capacity evaluation methods: a systematic review. *J Occup Rehabil.* 2018;28(3):418-428. doi:10.1007/s10926-017-9734-x
19. Hudson MA. Texas passes first law for safe patient handling in America: landmark legislation protects health-care workers and patients from injury related to manual patient lifting. *J Long Term Eff Med Implants.* 2005;15(5):559-566.
20. Association of Occupational Health Professionals in Healthcare, Carbuto A, Gruden MA, Pionk C, Smir S. *Beyond Getting Started. A Resource Guide: Implementing a Safe Patient Handling and Mobility Program in the Acute Care Setting.* 4th ed. 2020. Accessed February 7, 2023. https://aohp.org/aohp/Portals/0/Documents/ToolsForYourWork/BGSpublication/20-06%20BGS%20Safe%20Patient%20Handling.pdf
21. Wood, D. AMN Healthcare. The new national standards in safe patient handling and mobility. June 28, 2013. Accessed February 7, 2023. https://www.amnhealthcare.com/latest-healthcare-news/new-national-standards-safe-patient-handling-mobility/
22. Powell-Cope G, Rugs D. What elements of the 2013 American Nurses Association safe patient handling and mobility standards are reflected in state legislation? *Am J Safe Patient Handl Mov.* 2015;5(1):13-18.
23. American Physical Therapy Association. The role of physical therapy in safe patient handling HOD P06-12-21-20 [position]. Updated August 22, 2012. Accessed July 27, 2018. https://www.apta.org/siteassets/pdfs/policies/pt-and-pta-safe-patient-handling.pdf
24. Association of Rehabilitation Nurses. Safe patient handling toolkit for the interdisciplinary team. Accessed February 7, 2023. https://rehabnurse.org/resources/sph-toolkit
25. Occupational Safety and Health Act. Safe patient handling: effectiveness and cost savings. Accessed February 7, 2023. https://www.osha.gov/Publications/OSHA3279.pdf
26. Teeple E, Collins JE, Shrestha S, Dennerlein JT, Losina E, Katz JN. Outcomes of safe patient handling and mobilization programs: a meta-analysis. *Work.* 2017;58(2):173-184. doi:10.3233/WOR-172608

# Chapter 23
# Considerations for Athletes

*Karen A. Cascardi, PhD, MS, ATC, PTA*

**KEY TERMS** Exertional heat stroke | Exertional rhabdomyolysis | Preparticipation physical screens | Sports prehabilitation | Sports specialization

## Chapter Objectives

1. Discuss how flexibility, strength training, and performance training regimens affect injury risk.
2. Describe the components of a prehabilitation program.
3. Explain the role of preparticipation physical screening.
4. Summarize the American Academy of Pediatrics recommendations to reduce adolescent sports injuries.
5. Identify the indications for movement/mobility screening.
6. Define the basic components of an injury prevention program.
7. List the sports-related concussion recovery steps.
8. Identify the signs of heat acclimatization and the key components of a heat acclimatization protocol.
9. Identify the signs, symptoms, risk factors, treatments, and suggested return-to-play guidelines for exertional heat stroke (EHS).
10. Identify the signs, symptoms, risk factors, treatments, and return-to-play guidelines for exertional rhabdomyolysis.

Physical therapist assistants work with physical therapists to develop training programs that optimize sports performance, maximize athlete safety, and reduce the risk of injury. Incorporating evidence-based exercises and protocols in training can improve a patient's ability to participate in sports. The therapy team uses functional movement screens (FMSs) to identify weaknesses or asymmetries and applies that information when creating individualized prehabilitation programs. The therapy team is attentive to sports-specific risk factors, including concussions, heat-related illness, and **exertional rhabdomyolysis**. The physical therapist team modifies interventions based on the patient's response to treatment, the stage of tissue healing, and evolving evidence.

## The Effects of Stretching on Sports Performance

Varied stretching techniques are used before and after competitive events, practices, or training programs as well as in rehabilitation. The effect of flexibility on muscle performance has been vigorously debated. Some studies found



Kopack JK, Cascardi KA.
*Principles of Therapeutic Exercise for the Physical Therapist Assistant* (pp 719-734).

that flexibility training improved performance, whereas others reported it had no effect or a negative effect on performance.[1-3] Many training programs include stretching exercises to prevent injuries, but there is not substantial evidence to support this.[1,4]

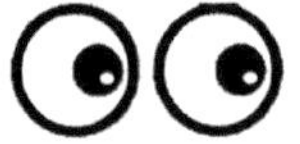

### Eye on the Research: Inconclusive Effects of Stretching on Performance

Research results regarding the effect of stretching on athletic performance are inconclusive. Tsolakis et al[1] studied the effect of static or ballistic stretching on the flexibility and power of fencers and determined that neither static nor ballistic stretching affected the fencers' flexibility, jumping ability, or lower extremity performance tests. Prior studies had concluded that static stretching before athletic performance had a negative effect on a variety of performance variables, such as sprinting, agility, and vertical jumping.[1] Beedle et al[2] reported that stretching performed after a workout did not improve flexibility more than stretching before a workout.

An active aerobic warm-up may increase hamstring flexibility, and static stretching after warm-up may result in additional increases in flexibility. However, aerobic warm-up followed by dynamic stretching can result in a decrease in flexibility.[3] The impact of the type of stretching may be dependent on the actual sport or type of sport.[4,5] Peck et al[5] reported that incorporating dynamic stretches during warm-up was beneficial for speed- and agility-dominant sports/activities.

The consensus appears to indicate that dynamic stretching is beneficial before athletic activity, and static and/or proprioceptive neuromuscular facilitation stretching is useful after athletic participation.[5] Because of the variability in the existing recommendations, the assistant will benefit from ongoing review of research in this area.

## Injury Prevention: Prehabilitation, Preparticipation, and Functional Movement Screens

Prehabilitation prepares a patient for surgery (refer to Chapter 3), but it is also used to improve sports performance and prevent injury. **Sports prehabilitation** programs rely on the clinician having knowledge of the common injuries associated with each sport. The clinician will select interventions that are specific to the sport that are targeted to reduce injury through consideration of the common mechanisms of injury. An effective program includes targeted strengthening and stretching and progresses to include challenging movement patterns/plyometrics to improve the patient's mobility and motor control in activities that replicate the sport.[6]

**Preparticipation physical screens**, pre/postseason training, and return-to-sports (after injury) training programs are important in preventing or reducing sports-related injuries or reinjuries. The physician typically performs preparticipation screens; the physical therapy team can also identify existing impairments that may predispose the patient to an increased risk for injury or reinjury. Athletes participate in training programs for several weeks, and the clinician's role is to (1) observe and provide feedback on joint mechanics/positions during athletic performance of technical skills (eg, jumping, hopping, lateral movements) and (2) train the patient-athlete in safe and effective ways to react to unexpected events (eg, sudden changes of direction, starts/stops).

### *Prehabilitation Programs and Preparticipation Screens*

Prehabilitation is an exercise program that is focused on preventing injuries before they occur; it can also be an exercise program that is performed preoperatively to enhance recovery. Patients who complete a structured exercise program before surgical interventions have lower postoperative complications and a shorter functional limitation period with activities of daily living (ADLs) performance compared with those not involved in prehabilitation.[6,7]

Avoiding anterior cruciate ligament (ACL) injuries is a common focus for screenings and prehabilitation programs. Joint kinematics and biomechanical and neuromuscular characteristics each have a role in reducing injuries to the ACL.[6-10] Participation in pre- and post-training programs is effective in reducing injuries for male amateur soccer players.[11] Programs that include stretching, plyometrics, strengthening to improve the quadriceps/hamstring ratio, balance training (ie, neuromuscular and proprioceptive activities and single-leg dynamic balance), and agility drills have been shown to reduce the risk of ACL injuries.[6,8-10,12-14] These activities should be performed in multiplanes and during unexpected decision-making situations.[9] Providing technical feedback related to joint mechanics (specifically as it pertains to ways to decrease valgus stresses) during these activities is an essential component for ACL injury prevention.[8]

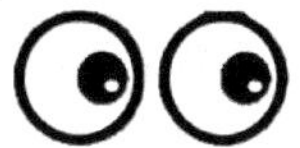

## Eye on the Research: Reducing the Risk of Female Athlete Anterior Cruciate Ligament Injuries

There are unique biomechanical, anatomical, and hormonal factors that predispose female athletes to specific injuries, including ACL injuries. Research is focused on clarifying these specific risk factors so exercise prevention and treatment programs can be developed more effectively.

A large systematic review of ACL primary prevention programs for girls in various sports concluded that in-season training was more effective than preseason training for ACL injury prevention and that a combination of strength training, plyometrics, balance training, and technique monitoring with feedback produced the most favorable results.[12] Sugimoto et al[13] determined that the dosage of neuromuscular training, exercise variations within neuromuscular training, and the use of verbal feedback optimize the preventative effects of neuromuscular training in reducing ACL injury reduction in female athletes. An effective component to reduce the risk of ACL injuries is the inclusion of neuromuscular training techniques with younger clients (middle and high school athletes). Neuromuscular training is most appropriate when supervised by trained personnel who use functional lower extremity strengthening exercises (ie, lunges, calf raises, closed chain eccentric hamstring curls, or Nordic curls) and who include a focus on correct performance of controlled and stable landings after jumps and hops.[14]

Before beginning a prehabilitation program, each athlete should understand the risks associated with the sport (eg, football, soccer, volleyball, swimming, tennis). The repetitive nature of sport-specific skills can predispose the athlete to muscle imbalances (eg, throwing athletes tend to develop tight rotator cuff muscles, excessive anterior shoulder range of motion [ROM], and weakness in the scapular stabilizers). The physical therapist will evaluate the athlete's posture, joint alignment, strength, flexibility, and the various movement patterns associated with the particular sport and the athlete's position (eg, lineman, running back/wide receiver, kicker in football). Knowledge of the physical demands and typical sports movement patterns helps the clinician to individualize the patient's program.

The FMS is a tool that can identify areas of weaknesses or asymmetries that can increase the risk of an athlete sustaining an injury.[15] The individual performing the screen must know how to score each of the items correctly. The test has 7 items that are scored from 0 to 3 with a maximum possible score of 21 (Table 23-1). A score of less than 14 indicates the need for additional assessment by a physical therapist, sports medicine physician, or athletic trainer.[15] This screen can be used before sport-specific conditioning programs.[16,17] Any physiological issues or concerns can be addressed within an individualized prehabilitation program; physical therapy is indicated if pain, significant weakness, or muscle imbalances are present. The Suggested Resources section at the end of the chapter includes links to the full screening form, the scoring grid used with the FMS, and the FMS website (for continuing education and certification courses).

A prehabilitation program can facilitate improvements in static and/or dynamic posture, and it can promote increased core stability, muscle strength, flexibility, endurance, power, proprioception, and motor control as well as address faulty movement patterns. Addressing impairments in these areas will reduce injury risk and improve sport-specific movement patterns. An effective prehabilitation program targets the athlete's individual physical presentation while taking into consideration the required skills, level of competition (ie, novice, intramural, high school, collegiate, or professional) and demands of the specific sport.

There is evidence that implementing the Fédération Internationale de Football Association *The 11: Prevention Program* is an effective way to reduce injuries.[11] This program has 3 separate parts; the program should be performed in a sequential order at the start of each preseason session. The program focuses on using good body control and proper positioning/alignment, and it prioritizes the provision of feedback for correcting faulty mechanics. Part 1 includes 6 various slow running activities. Part 2 includes 6 exercises that focus on progressively increasing strength (legs and core), single-leg balance, and plyometric (jumping) exercises. The last part of the program includes higher-intensity running activities and incorporates abrupt speed changes, skipping for height, and abrupt stops with cutting movements. A link for the *11* manual is provided in the Suggested Resources section.

Other factors that can increase injury risk include the athlete's age; length of uninterrupted playing time; the amount of rest periods within and between games; the individual's available ROM, muscle strength, and endurance; and the particular demands of the given sport. The therapy team should consider all of these variables when creating an intervention program that is individualized to the particular patient's presentation and training needs.

**Table 23-1**

## Overview of the Functional Movement Screen[16,17]

Each motion listed below is graded using these scoring criteria:
0: The movement is painful and requires physical therapist or physician referral
1: Inability to perform or complete the movement pattern
2: Able to perform the movement pattern but evidence of compensation
3: Performs the movement pattern without hesitation or compensation

| Task | Purpose |
|---|---|
| Deep squat | Screens hips, knees, ankles, spine, and shoulders |
| Hurdle step | Screens hips, knees, and ankles |
| In-line lunge | Screens hip, knee, and ankle strength and stability |
| Shoulder mobility | Screens shoulder internal and external rotation |
| Active straight leg raise | Screens hamstring and gastrocnemius flexibility and pelvic stability |
| Push-up | Screens core and trunk strength/stability and triceps strength |
| Ipsilateral arm and leg lifts | Screens pelvic, core, and trunk stability |

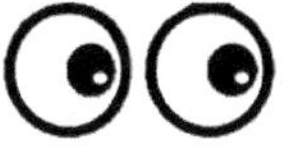

### Eye on the Research: Is Early Specialization in One Sport Indicated?

Specialization is the participation and training for only one sport, oftentimes year round. Youth **sports specialization** at earlier ages continues to be prevalent despite reported consequences (eg, increased injury rates and burnout). Swindell et al[18] concluded that young athletes, coaches, and parents continue to have misconceptions about the necessity of early sports specialization, resulting in inappropriate encouragement to focus on a single sport at a young age. Interestingly, early sports specialization is uncommon among National Collegiate Athletic Association Division I athletes for most team sports, a fact that is contrary to the perceived need to specialize early.[18]

Bell et al[19] determined that specialization in one sport is associated with an increased risk of overuse musculoskeletal injuries. Athletes who specialized in one sport had an increased risk of sustaining an overuse injury compared with athletes with low or moderate levels of specialization. Athletes with moderate specialization were at a higher risk of injury compared with those with low specialization.[19] Jayanthi et al[20] reported higher rates of injury, increased psychological stress, and increased likelihood of quitting sports at a young age with early specialization. Summary recommendations published in the *American Journal of Sports Medicine* corroborate that high levels of specialization are associated with a history of injuries and that athletes who exceeded volume recommendations were more likely to have a history of overuse injuries.[21]

Guidelines published by the American Academy of Pediatrics summarized that programs that address the long-term needs of children include diverse and varied play and sports activities.[22] Participation in diverse sports and activities lowers dropout rates, helps to foster positive peer interactions, and creates intrinsic motivation to maintain participation because the activities are perceived as enjoyable. The American Academy of Pediatrics noted that although early specialization in certain sports (eg, figure skating, gymnastics, diving) may be required because peak performance occurs before full physical maturation, it is not known whether the training required for such sports poses a risk for athletes' long-term health and well-being. The general recommendations proposed by the American Academy of Pediatrics include an early, diversified training program that includes flexibility, balance, and motor skill development. Regular rest and recovery periods should be built in, as should participation in a variety of sports. Specialization in a specific sport is not recommended until late adolescence.[22]

## Preparticipation Cardiac Screenings: Key Safety Considerations

Cardiac screening preparticipation guidelines exist to help keep young athletes safe while participating in sports. There are rare cardiac complications that can occur during vigorous competitive athletics; many of these occur because of undiagnosed diseases associated with heart muscle problems, coronary artery abnormalities, or electrical problems with the heart. Cardiac screening guidelines aim to identify individuals with cardiovascular abnormalities who may be at risk for sudden cardiac death and to initiate an appropriate treatment to mitigate the risk. A cardiac screening program typically includes the assessment of 3 areas: personal medical history, family medical history, and a physical examination.[23] The personal history indicates if there are any key signs or symptoms that indicate potential cardiac risk, including fainting episodes, unexplained extreme exhaustion (with minimal physical activity), chest pain brought on by exercise, and/or palpitations associated with exercise. Family history is reviewed to determine if there are any family members with serious cardiac conditions or sudden cardiac death or any family members who died suddenly at a young age without explanation. The physical examination focuses on assessing cardiac sounds (the presence of a heart murmur or other abnormal cardiac sounds that may raise concern), blood pressure (especially if elevated), an unexplained fast heart rate (tachycardia), an irregular heart rhythm, abnormal lung sounds, and/or abnormal peripheral pulses. An atypical or concerning finding in any of these screening areas often results in a cardiology referral for further testing, which may include a comprehensive cardiac examination, an electrocardiogram, an echocardiogram, Holter or event monitoring, exercise testing, and/or cardiac magnetic resonance imaging.[23]

The American Medical Society for Sports Medicine (AMSSM) guidelines acknowledge that early detection of cardiovascular conditions associated with sudden cardiac arrest and death in athletes is important, but the absence of outcomes-based research precludes AMSSM from endorsing a single or universal cardiovascular screening strategy for all athletes. AMSSM currently recommends/supports individual physician autonomy to implement the most appropriate cardiovascular screening strategy (unique to their athlete population and community resources). The inclusion of routine electrocardiographic testing remains controversial; physicians incorporating electrocardiography in the screening process should optimize strategies to ensure accurate electrocardiographic interpretation. Screening does not provide absolute protection against sudden cardiac arrest/death; AMSSM recommends a comprehensive emergency action plan and access to an automated external defibrillator to improve outcomes from sudden cardiac arrest in athletes.[23]

The American Academy of Family Physicians and the American College of Physicians recommend cardiac and musculoskeletal screening (as noted previously) before sports training, but they do not recommend annual electrocardiography or any other annual cardiac screening for asymptomatic, low-risk patients. The American Heart Association recommends additional medical screening for patients who present with any of the key symptoms (listed earlier) during the interview of personal and family history.[24]

## Contraindications for Sports Participation

The American Academy of Family Physicians includes the following contraindications to participation in sports: active myocarditis or pericarditis, acute spleen or liver enlargement, presence of an eating disorder (paired with noncompliance with therapy), recent concussion with post-concussion symptoms, long QT syndrome, hypertrophic cardiomyopathy, severe uncontrolled hypertension, sickle cell disease, poorly controlled seizures, recurrent episodes of upper extremity pain or weakness, episodic quadriplegia (until spinal stability is ascertained), and suspected coronary artery disease until fully evaluated. Patients with impaired resting left ventricular systolic function less than 50%, exercise-induced ventricular dysrhythmias, or exercise-induced ischemia on exercise stress testing are at the greatest risk of sudden death, and these individuals should not participate in sports.[24]

# Concussions and Return to Play

Hundreds of articles have been written on sport-related concussions (SRCs), but as new knowledge emerges, modifications to care recommendations must be made.[25,26] The primary focus in this section is to provide physical therapist assistants a basic strategy for a gradual return-to-sport participation following a concussion; however, concussion evaluation, testing, and rehabilitation discussions are beyond the scope of this textbook. The assistant should report all patient subjective data and objective findings regarding patient presentation during the recovery stage to the physical therapist.

Emerging research indicates that prolonged inactivity may have adverse effects on postconcussion recovery. Once the athlete is asymptomatic at rest, it is important to assess responses to exercise exertion with the initiation of light aerobic exercise. Approaches that include specific activities with gradually increasing intensity have been shown to be more beneficial for athletes emotionally, cognitively, and physically.[25,27,28] Researchers determined that children and adolescents who began exercise 7 days postconcussion (to tolerance) had reduced persistent symptoms 28 days postconcussion compared with those who did not participate in any physical activity.[29] Physical activity is associated with a lowered risk for the physical and mental deconditioning that can occur with prolonged rest. However, researchers acknowledge that additional randomized trials need to be conducted.[29]

If an athlete has increased complaints of dizziness or blurred vision when running during an exertion test, the clinician should consider selecting a different type of aerobic activity (eg, upper body ergometer or stationary bike) for aerobic conditioning. Dizziness or blurred vision (due to vestibulo-ocular reflex deficits) can also be addressed using vestibular rehabilitation interventions (refer to Chapter 8). The assistant should monitor vital signs and the patient's grading of their symptoms at rest and during activity. Aerobic activity intensity can be increased as the patient reports a reduction in their symptoms. Once the patient is tolerating aerobic exercise, gradual reintroduction of sport-specific skills is initiated. Consider sport-specific demands; if the athlete needs to return to running and performing the ball-handling skills associated with soccer, the clinician should assess those sport-specific tasks that provoke symptoms, and as symptoms decrease, sport-related activity can be increased. The goal is for the athlete to remain asymptomatic during high-intensity demands of the specific sport during practice before returning to competition.

Table 23-2 provides a guide for return to play after concussions; progressions are dependent on the athlete's age, concussion history, sport, and level of participation. When an athlete is preparing to return to play, investigators have suggested a 6-step[25,26] and a 7-step (for pediatrics)[30] guide. Table 23-2 provides a 5-step guideline. It does not include the "no activity" or "limited ADL activity" steps that are included within the 6- and-7-step guidelines; these steps preclude the initiation of the return-to-activity sequence described in Table 23-2. The return-to-play sequence is initiated after physician clearance.

After a mild concussion, a physical and cognitive initial rest period of 24 to 48 hours is typically recommended. Once the athlete is asymptomatic at rest, ADLs that do not exacerbate symptoms can be initiated. The athlete should avoid physical and cognitive activities that provoke symptoms. Light aerobic activity such as walking, swimming, or stationary cycling can be initiated only when ADLs are performed asymptomatically for 24 hours. Resistance training should be avoided during the first 2 steps of the program because it can result in increased intracranial pressure that may increase symptoms. Once symptoms are stable, assessment of resistance training tolerance is important to allow the athlete to proceed to the next phase of rehabilitation.[25,30] The athlete can progress to the next level if they remain asymptomatic for 24 hours. If the athlete remains asymptomatic at each level, it would take a minimum of 1 week to complete the protocol. If the athlete experiences symptoms (during or 24 hours after exercise) at the current level of exercise, the athlete needs to revert to the previous level where they were asymptomatic. They can attempt the next level again as long as no symptoms recur for 24 hours at the lower level.[25] If the athlete is not able to progress to the next level after 3 attempts because of complaints of symptoms, the assistant should notify the therapist, and the physician should be contacted.[30]

The recovery period for children (ages 5 to 12 years) and adolescents (ages 13 to 18 years) is longer than that for college athletes. A more conservative approach for these younger athletes should be considered when deciding when to allow them to return to play.[26] No athlete should be allowed to return to play on the same day of injury occurrence. The athlete should be referred to a physician if symptoms persist for more than 1 month in children or more than 10 days to 2 weeks for adults.[25,26]

**Table 23-2**

Postconcussion Return-to-Play Guidelines

| Level | Exercise/Skills | Objective |
|---|---|---|
| 1<br>Light aerobic exercise[a] | Walking, stationary bike, upper bike ergometer, and swimming at a normal or medium pace about 10 to 20 minutes; no resistance training | To increase heart rate; light to moderate rate of perceived exertion |
| 2<br>Sport-specific skills/ exercise | Jogging about 20 to 30 minutes; running play routines or simulated drills in football or soccer, base running in baseball/softball, and ice hockey skating drills. No activities that provide impact to the head (eg, avoid heading the ball in soccer). Depending on presentation, it may be possible to initiate light resistance training (eg, light elastic bands or 1 to 2 pounds). | Increasing movement patterns and speed of movements staying below symptom threshold |
| 3<br>Noncontact training drills | Increase level of difficulty and speed of sport-specific drills. Quick cutting, start/stop, and direction changing drills on command; initiate ball handling and passing in soccer, football, ice hockey, baseball/ softball, and lacrosse with helmet. Vertical jumping drills. Initiate progressive resistive exercises and weight training. | Working on coordination (ie, eye/hand, eye/foot), power, and agility; put athlete in noncontact decision-making situations<br>Full aerobic conditioning program |
| 4<br>Full-contact practice (after physician clearance) | Contact drills with pads and helmet in football, hockey, and lacrosse; ball heading in soccer. Return to full training and practice activities. | Increase confidence by resuming normal participation. Increase comfort level of skills performance. Monitoring for symptoms every 30 minutes by athletic trainer. |
| 5<br>Return to sport competition | Participate in all sport-related competition | Resume normal competitive sport activities. Continue to monitor for symptoms. |

These steps are initiated after physician clearance.

[a]Physical and cognitive rest is recommended for the first 24 to 48 hours before introducing non–symptom-provoking ADLs. The athlete must be asymptomatic for 24 hours with ADLs before beginning any exercise. School- or work-related activities should be introduced gradually. Increase or return of symptoms indicates the need to return to lower-level activities.

Adapted from Halstead ME, Walter KD, Moffatt K; Council on Sports Medicine and Fitness. Sport-related concussion in children and adolescents. *Pediatrics.* 2018;142(6):e20183074. doi:10.1542/peds.2018-3074 and May KH, Marshall DL, Burns TG, Popoli DM, Polikandriotis JA. Pediatric sports specific return to play guidelines following concussion. *Int J Sports Phys Ther.* 2014;9(2):242-255.

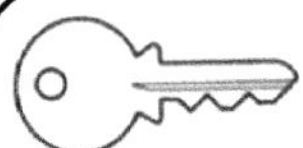

**Key Safety Considerations: Postconcussion**

- Avoid physical and cognitive activities that provoke symptoms.
- If the athlete experiences symptoms (during or 24 hours after exercise) at the current level of exercise, revert to the previous level where they were asymptomatic.
- Persistent symptoms warrant referral back to the physician.

## *Prevention of Sport-Related Concussions: Physical Therapy Implications*

Many patients with SRCs present with cervical strains and sprains due to the common whiplash actions that can occur during injury.[26] The physical therapy team assesses cervical and scapula ROM and muscle strength and treats areas of impairment. Cervical muscle strength has been shown to be a predictor of SRCs; a study of high school athletes indicated that for every 1-pound increase in cervical muscle strength, the odds of sustaining a concussion was reduced by 5%.[27] Exercises that target the cervical musculature should be considered as part of the training or prehabilitation program for athletes of all ages.

## Heat Acclimatization Guidelines

Athletes participating in any activity in which preseason practice or play occurs outdoors during warmer seasons need to acclimate to warm and hot environments. This is especially important for sports that have an endurance component like long-distance running or cycling, soccer, football, field hockey, and tennis, but heat acclimatization is relevant for any participants in prolonged outdoor activities (eg, golf, marching band). Athletes should complete a preparticipation medical screening before sport participation to rule out any health concerns or risks that may predispose the athlete to exertional heat illnesses. There are 7 key recommendations summarized in Table 23-3 that are supported by the National Athletic Trainers' Association and other organizations to significantly reduce the risk of heat-related illnesses among high school athletes.[31]

To achieve heat acclimatization, there must be a gradual yet repetitive exposure to heat; the exposures must increase core and skin temperature in order to produce profuse sweating during exercise. This acclimatization process reduces the risk of heat illness and improves performance. This usually occurs during the warmer months of preseason, and the process takes approximately 1 to 14 days.[31,32] The most effective way to acclimate to the heat is through exposure to the warm-hot weather daily for a minimum of 90 minutes or a maximum of 2 hours that is broken down into two 60-minute sessions. Once the athlete can exercise for 100 minutes comfortably, the intensity is gradually increased each day for the 14-day acclimatization period. Indicators that heat acclimatization is occurring include a lower heart rate, lower core and skin temperature, and earlier onset and higher sweat rate during exercise in the heat (compared with preacclimation values). The sweat rate improves the body's ability to cool down through evaporation. There is a difference between desert and tropical heat; athletes need to acclimate to the type of climate where the competition is to be held. Staying hydrated is also important. (Athletes tend to underhydrate as they become more acclimated to the heat.) Prehydration (ie, drinking an adequate amount prepractice) is an important part of the process. Encourage hydration with liquids with electrolytes during the acclimatization period; this is important because electrolytes are sweated out at higher rates before the athlete acclimating to the heat. The body becomes more efficient at regulating electrolytes after acclimatization.[32]

Clinicians must recognize the signs and symptoms of each level of heat illnesses. It is beyond the scope of this chapter to discuss specific emergency treatment procedures when treating heat illnesses, but therapists should be aware of basic first aid procedures. Physical therapist assistants working with this population must familiarize themselves with facility/team protocols used to address medical emergencies. Table 23-4 provides a general overview of the required interventions. Athletic trainers and emergency medical technician staff are trained to follow specific procedures when treating heat-related illness. Refer to the exertional heat illness booklet published by the National Athletic Trainers' Association (see Suggested Resources) to review these procedures. **EHS** is a medical emergency.

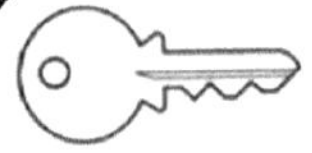

**Key Safety Considerations: Heat-Related Illness**

- Athletes should complete a preparticipation medical screening before any sport participation.
- Maintain careful compliance with heat acclimatization protocols.
- Monitoring for symptoms every session.
- Reinforce the need for adequate hydration.
- Know the signs and symptoms of heat-related illness.
- Immediately terminate practice and initiate first aid and medical interventions if athletes present with heat-related illness signs/symptoms.

**Table 23-3**

**Recommendations for Heat Acclimatization Before Full Athletic Participation/Practice for High School Athletes (14 Days)[31]**

| Days 1 Through 5 |
|---|
| • Maintain adequate prehydration as well as adequate activity and postactivity hydration levels.<br>• Athletes are permitted to participate in only 1 practice per day.<br>• Total practice time should not exceed 3 hours (even if practice is interrupted by inclement weather or excessive heat conditions).<br>• Walk-throughs for a 1-hour maximum are permitted during these initial days, but a period of 3 hours for recovery between practice and walk-through should occur. A walk-through means the athlete can only wear shoes and helmets (if required) and use the ball during play reviews.<br>• Days 1 and 2: Helmets (if required) are the only protective equipment to be worn for these days.<br>• Days 3 to 5: Only helmets and shoulder pads (if required) can be worn during this period.<br>• Days 3 to 5 football (only): Contact drills using blocking sleds and tackling dummies can be initiated. |
| **Days 6 Through 14** |
| • Beginning on this day, all protective equipment can be worn, and full-contact drills can be initiated. This is the earliest day when full-contact live drills should begin and will be continued through day 14.<br>• Walk-throughs are permitted on single practice days. A 3-hour rest period must occur between single-day practices and walk-throughs.<br>• A double-practice day must be followed by a single-practice day (or a full day of rest). |
| **Double-Practice Days** |
| • Neither of these practice sessions should be longer than 3 hours, and the total practice time must be <5 hours over the course of both sessions. Note: Warm-up, stretching, conditioning and weight training, walk-throughs, and cooldowns are all included in the total practice time.<br>• Double practices should be separated by a minimum of 3 continuous hours of rest in a cool environment.<br>• If a double-practice day is followed by a full rest day, then another double-practice day is permitted on the following day.<br>Note: Because of the high risk of heat-related illnesses during the acclimatization period, it is strongly recommended that a board-certified, licensed athletic trainer be present during and after all practices to assist in monitoring the athletes. |
| All practice recommendations are guidelines *only* and must be adjusted to reflect the individual athlete's presentation and abilities. Practice escalations should be carefully monitored and individualized for each athlete. Progressions should include adequate hydration and rest schedules and careful monitoring for any signs/symptoms of heat-related illness. Any signs or symptoms of heat-related illness should result in immediate termination of activity, transition to a cool/shaded area, rehydration, and monitoring. Any increased or continued symptoms warrant follow-up with the medical team or emergency medical services based on the severity of the symptoms (see Table 23-4). |

## *Exertional Heat Stroke and Exertional Rhabdomyolysis*

EHS and exertional rhabdomyolysis are complex systemic medical conditions that can cause organ damage and death if not appropriately treated. There is an increased risk of recurrence for athletes who return to play too early and have not fully recovered. There is limited evidence to guide return-to-play protocols and assist medical professionals when making decisions regarding if and when athletes with one of these conditions should return to play.[33]

EHS is one of the leading causes of preventable death among high school athletes.[31] It is defined as a having an elevated core temperature greater than 104 °F (or 40 °C). It is a multisystem condition associated with central nervous system changes, signs of tissue damage and organ failure from strenuous exercise, and excessive heat exposure resulting in severe hyperthermia.[33-35] Prevention, including careful acclimatization, hydration, and monitoring, is the best intervention. EHS is a life-threatening condition and medical emergency that must be addressed immediately. Heat stroke occurs when the body is overwhelmed

**Table 23-4**

Heat-Related Illnesses

<table>
<tr><th>What to Look For</th><th>What to Do</th></tr>
<tr><td colspan="2">Heat Stroke</td></tr>
<tr><td>• High body temperature (103 °F or higher)<br>• Hot, red, dry, or damp skin<br>• Fast, strong pulse<br>• Headache<br>• Dizziness<br>• Nausea<br>• Confusion<br>• Losing consciousness (passing out)</td><td>• Call 911 right away—heat stroke is a medical emergency<br>• Move the person to a cooler place<br>• Help lower the person's temperature with cool cloths or a cool bath<br>• Do not give the person anything to drink</td></tr>
<tr><td colspan="2">Heat Exhaustion</td></tr>
<tr><td>• Heavy sweating<br>• Cold, pale, and clammy skin<br>• Fast, weak pulse<br>• Nausea or vomiting<br>• Muscle cramps<br>• Tiredness or weakness<br>• Dizziness<br>• Headache<br>• Fainting (passing out)</td><td>• Move to a cool place<br>• Loosen your clothes<br>• Put cool, wet cloths on your body or take a cool bath<br>• Sip water<br>Get medical help right away if:<br>• You are throwing up<br>• Your symptoms get worse<br>• Your symptoms last longer than 1 hour</td></tr>
<tr><td colspan="2">Heat Cramps</td></tr>
<tr><td>• Heavy sweating during intense exercise<br>• Muscle pain or spasms</td><td>• Stop physical activity and move to a cool place<br>• Drink water or a sports drink<br>• Wait for cramps to go away before you do any more physical activity<br>Get medical help right away if:<br>• Cramps last longer than 1 hour<br>• You're on a low sodium diet<br>• You have heart problems</td></tr>
<tr><td colspan="2">Sunburn</td></tr>
<tr><td>• Painful, red, and warm skin<br>• Muscle pain or spasms</td><td>• Stay out of the sun until your sunburn heals<br>• Put cool cloths on sunburned areas or take a cool bath<br>• Put moisturizing lotion on sunburned areas<br>• Do not break blisters</td></tr>
<tr><td colspan="2">Heat Rash</td></tr>
<tr><td>• Red clusters of small blisters that look like pimples on the skin (usually on the neck, chest, groin, or in elbow creases)</td><td>• Stay in a cool, dry place<br>• Keep the rash dry<br>• Use powder (like baby powder) to soothe the rash</td></tr>
<tr><td colspan="2">Reproduced with permission from Centers for Disease Control and Prevention. Warning signs and symptoms of heat-related illness. Reviewed September 1, 2017. Accessed February 8, 2023. https://www.cdc.gov/disasters/extremeheat/warning.html</td></tr>
</table>

**Table 23-5**

## American College of Sports Medicine Return-to-Play Guidelines After Exertional Heat Stroke[33,36]

- No exercise for a minimum of 7 days after release from medical care.
- Seven days after the incident, the athlete must be asymptomatic; laboratory values and diagnostic organ imaging must be normalized, and physician clearance must be obtained before athletic participation.
- Begin exercise in a cool climate-controlled environment with a gradual increase of intensity, duration, and exposure to heat over a 2-week period to initiate acclimatization and heat tolerance. (Refer to Table 23-2 for acclimatization program). Progress activities as follows (allot at least 3 days at each stage as tolerated). The athlete must be asymptomatic throughout the stage to advance to the next stage.
  - Light to moderate activities in a cool environment
  - Vigorous or strenuous activities in a cool environment
  - Light to moderate activities in the heat
  - Vigorous or strenuous activities in the heat
  - Moderate practice activities with helmet progress to vigorous (if applicable) in the heat
  - Moderate practice activities with full pads/equipment progress to full practice or training in the heat
- If the athlete cannot tolerate vigorous activity over a 4-week period because of recurrent symptoms, they should be referred for an exercise heat tolerance test and be re-evaluated.
- Once the athlete can participate fully in conditioning/training in the heat for 2 to 4 weeks, full competition can be resumed as long as the athlete is still asymptomatic.

and is no longer able to regulate heat production, resulting in thermoregulatory system failure. The central nervous system (the hypothalamus senses core temperature), the cardiovascular system, and the skin all interact to play a role in thermoregulation. The body's response to an increase in core temperature is tachycardia, tachypnea, and cutaneous vasodilation.

There are both intrinsic and extrinsic factors that contribute to an increased risk of EHS. Some intrinsic factors include a previous history of exertional heat illnesses, lack of or a poor acclimatization preparation program, low fitness level, being overweight or obese, recent infection or fever, poor hydration, sleep deprivation, alcohol use, and certain medications (eg, diuretics, antihistamines, weight loss supplements). Extrinsic factors include high air temperature, humidity and/or sun exposure for days in a row, intense and/or long exposure to hot environments with inadequate breaks, rest or fluid intake during practice, use of equipment during practice, double practices before heat acclimatization, lack of athlete and parent education on heat illnesses, and/or inability to recognize early signs and symptoms of heat illnesses.[31]

EHS is determined by using a rectal thermometer, and the best plan to reduce the athlete's core temperature as quickly as possible is to submerge the athlete in a total body ice bath that is on site before transferring the athlete emergently to a hospital. The core temperature should be constantly monitored because it is imperative to reduce the temperature below 104 °F (or 40 °C) quickly. The risk of morbidity and mortality increases the longer the core temperature stays at or above this critical level. Longer periods of core temperature elevation above 104 °F are associated with prolonged recovery times as well. According to the current literature, most athletes recover from EHS within a few weeks as long as proper immediate care was implemented.[33,34]

Return-to-play guidelines for athletes after EHS are not standardized, but they typically reflect a gradual progression back to activity. A gradual re-entry to practice is only appropriate once symptoms resolve and significant laboratory values have returned to normal. Close attention should be paid to the athlete's response to the reintroduction of training regimens; the athlete needs to be reacclimatized at a slower rate than preinjury protocols outline. The risk of recurrence is a major concern with these athletes, and the athletic training staff, coaches, and all available medical staff should monitor all progressions. The increased risk of recurrence results in a decrease in heat tolerance for the athlete for up to 1 year postoccurrence. The return-to-play guidelines are described in Table 23-5.[33,36] The primary goal is to prevent heat illnesses, especially as athletes begin training in late summer, by implementing safe training regimens and acclimatization programs. Early recognition and immediate care of heat cramps and heat exhaustion will reduce the chances of athletes experiencing EHS. Prevention and early detection are keys to maintaining athletes' safety.

Rhabdomyolysis is not common, but it can have long-term debilitating results and can be fatal if not diagnosed and treated quickly; it is a medical emergency. Some causes of rhabdomyolysis include hyperthermia (prolonged high fever), crush injuries, high doses of statins (the medication class commonly used to treat high cholesterol), prolonged tourniquet application, compartment syndrome, and vigorous exercise (especially in combination with dehydration or excessive heat). These causes have only one commonality—experiencing a direct or indirect muscle injury. Because the purpose of this chapter is focusing on return to play and injury prevention for athletes, only exertional rhabdomyolysis is discussed. Exertional rhabdomyolysis is defined as a breakdown of striated muscle tissue due to insult or injury most commonly caused by intense, repetitive, and/or prolonged exercise. Eccentric exercises and total muscle fatigue are also associated with exertional rhabdomyolysis.[33,37] This condition can occur under any environmental condition, but there is a higher risk for exertional rhabdomyolysis during hot and humid weather. Exertional rhabdomyolysis has been reported to occur in military personnel during basic training, recreational athletes, weekend warriors (ie, those who participate in bouts of excessive weight training and CrossFit or similar high-intensity training protocols), and elite athletes. Exertional rhabdomyolysis has also been reported in a variety of sports including football, swimming, bodybuilding, and running.[37-39]

The breakdown and necrosis of muscle tissue release creatine kinase, myoglobin, potassium, and organic acids into the body. Elevated creatine kinase levels (5 to 10 times higher than the normal range of 10 to 205 units/L) are characteristic of exertional rhabdomyolysis. The clinical presentation of exertional rhabdomyolysis includes severe muscle pain during active and passive movements, delayed-onset muscle soreness, weakness, pain, and swelling within 24 to 72 hours after strenuous prolonged activities.[33,37-39] Elevated myoglobin released into systemic circulation may lead to cola- or tea-colored urine, and this causes acute kidney problems. This very dark urine is a primary indicator of rhabdomyolysis. Muscle damage results in elevated potassium levels (hyperkalemia), which can increase the athlete's risk for cardiac dysrhythmias. Elevated organic acids can result in metabolic acidosis. Reduced electrolyte levels due to extreme sweating in endurance athletics is a major concern, especially in warmer humid temperatures. Dehydration and warm/hot temperatures not only increase the risk of exertional rhabdomyolysis but also increase the risk of heat-related illnesses.[31,37] In addition to heat illness and dehydration, other factors that contribute to the increased risk of exertional rhabdomyolysis include sickle cell trait (most commonly noted in Black athletes), sudden and drastic increases in training programs, strenuous exercise while unfit, and poor conditioning or acclimatization programs.

The severity of exertional rhabdomyolysis is directly proportionate to the amount of muscle degradation. Exertional rhabdomyolysis often goes undiagnosed in mild cases, which resolve with rest and hydration. These athletes have elevated creatine kinase and minimal muscle pain but no other significant clinical findings. In severe cases of exertional rhabdomyolysis, the muscle pain is significant, and swelling or weakness is evident. These patients have significant clinical findings and require hospitalization for intravenous hydration and dialysis. Rest, monitoring for renal failure and electrolyte abnormalities, an electrocardiogram (due to hyperkalemia), and cardiac monitoring are necessary in severe cases.[33]

There are no specific evidence-based guidelines regarding return to play after recovery from exertional rhabdomyolysis. There are 3 considerations before having an athlete return to play: a follow-up evaluation to determine the risk for recurrence, a timeline for the athlete to safely return to sport participation and competition, and what restrictions (if any) need to be put in place to promote a safe return to the prior level of sport participation.[33,38] Before returning to sports, athletes need to be categorized as either a high or low risk for exertional rhabdomyolysis recurrence (Table 23-6). The Consortium for Health and Military Performance and the Heller Institute of the Israeli Defense Force composed a list of conservative return-to-play guidelines for those at low risk of exertional rhabdomyolysis recurrence.[33,38,39] If an athlete is at a high risk for recurrence, the athlete should be continually monitored by the appropriate medical specialist and should not return to play. Once the athlete is no longer considered high risk, they can follow the return-to-play guidelines (Table 23-7) once they are cleared by a medical specialist. These guidelines are conservative, but they reduce the chance of missing athletes who are at risk for recurring exertional rhabdomyolysis, and they maximize the safety of all affected patients.[38]

Physical therapists, physical therapist assistants, and health care professionals need to remember that the largest risk and most common cause for exertional rhabdomyolysis is the performance of excessive exercise (ie, exercise performed at too high of an intensity for too long of a time or with too rapid of a progression).[37] Careful monitoring, graded acclimatization, and careful progression of exercise intensity and duration can help prevent the occurrence of exertional rhabdomyolysis.

**Table 23-6**

Athletes at High and Low Recurrence Risk for Exertional Rhabdomyolysis[38]

| Low Risk[a] | High Risk |
|---|---|
| • Creatine kinase normalized and rapid clinical recovery after exercise restrictions<br>• Well-conditioned or elite athletes who experienced exertional rhabdomyolysis after a vigorous/high-intensity period of exercise<br>• No personal or familial history of rhabdomyolysis<br>• No history of exercise-induced muscle pain or cramping that was severe or debilitating<br>• No personal history of familial hyperthermia<br>• Other reported incidents of exertional rhabdomyolysis by a group or team while performing the same exercise sessions<br>• Reported or documented concomitant infectious diseases or viral/bacterial infections<br>• Taking drugs (eg, statins, erythromycin, amphetamines), illegal drugs (eg, lysergic acid diethylamide, ecstasy, cocaine), or dietary supplements that contributed to the exertional rhabdomyolysis event | • Delayed recovery > 1 week after exercise restrictions<br>• After > 2 weeks of rest, creatine kinase levels are persistently elevated and > 5 times the upper limits of normal values.<br>• Any degree of acute renal injury due to exertional rhabdomyolysis<br>• Personal or familial history of exertional rhabdomyolysis<br>• Personal or familial history of sport-, exercise-, or ADLs-induced severe muscle pain or recurrent debilitating cramping<br>• Personal or familial history of sickle cell trait or disease<br>• Personal history of heat stroke<br>• Experienced muscle injury after low to moderate exercise/physical work |

[a]To be categorized as low risk, the athlete must exhibit at least one of the conditions in this column and none of the conditions in the high-risk column.

**Table 23-7**

**Return-to-Play Guidelines for Low-Risk Athletes After Exertional Rhabdomyolysis[38]**

| Phase 1 (Initial 72 Hours) | 72-Hour Follow-Up | Phase 2 | Phase 3 |
|---|---|---|---|
| • Rest for 72 hours and stress the importance of hydration by mouth.<br>• Encourage the athlete to have 8 hours of uninterrupted sleep for several nights.<br>• If exertional rhabdomyolysis was heat related, the athlete should stay in an environment that is thermally controlled. | • Repeat creatine kinase and urinalysis.<br>• If creatine kinase is <5 times the normal upper limit and urinalysis is normal, progress to phase 2.<br>• If creatine kinase is abnormal, follow up every 72 hours until creatine kinase is within the safe range and urinalysis is normal.<br>• At 2 weeks, if creatine kinase and urinalysis are still abnormal, follow up with medical specialist. | • Initiate light activities and avoid strenuous exercise.<br>◦ Activities should be self-paced and tolerable distance.<br>• At end of 1 week, follow up with physician/health care provider.<br>• If athlete is clinically asymptomatic and laboratory tests are normalized, progress to phase 3.<br>◦ If symptomatic, stay in phase 2, and continue with 1-week follow-up until normal.<br>◦ Athlete can progress to phase 3 if no complaints of muscle pain, soreness, or weakness. | • Gradually return to sport-specific activities and training.<br>• Follow up with physician/health care provider as needed. |

## Conclusion

The physical therapist assistant participates as a member of the health care team in the medical management of athletes and sports participants. The physical therapy team plays a role in injury prevention, patient education, and postinjury rehabilitation. Prehabilitation programs, patient/family education, and implementation of necessary preseason training protocols (eg, screening, heat acclimatization) are beneficial in preventing and reducing injury risk for athletes. The physical therapy team can effectively implement prehabilitation programs for athletes participating in any sport; targeted prehabilitation programs can lower injury risks for participants. The physical therapy team will participate in managing and progressing patients who have experienced SRCs and heat-related illnesses. The implementation and compliance with existing return-to-sport protocols and ongoing monitoring are critical to safe return to sport. The health care professional team is focused on maintaining safety and ensuring safe return to play for athletes of all ages and level of participation.

## Review Questions

1. Briefly describe the benefits and indications for flexibility and strength training programs for an athletic population.
2. When should a clinician use the FMS?
3. What is prehabilitation? List 3 scenarios when prehabilitation could be beneficial.
4. What are the indications for and the purpose of a preparticipation physical screening?
5. List 3 ways to reduce the incidence of pediatric sports-related injuries.
6. What is the 11+ warm-up program? Describe how a physical therapist assistant could incorporate parts of this program into a prehabilitation or rehabilitation program for a patient.
7. What are the signs and symptoms of concussion? Briefly describe the protocol that determines readiness to return to sport after a concussion.

8. What are the signs and symptoms of heat-related illness? What are the signs and symptoms of exertional rhabdomyolysis?
9. Describe the components of an effective heat acclimatization program.
10. What are the benefits and pitfalls of pediatric sports specialization?

## Case Study

The patient is a 15-year-old boy referred by his pediatrician for a prehabilitation program. The patient discontinued long-distance track after 1 season 9 months ago because of symptoms related to Achilles tendinopathy. He has played team soccer for the prior 8 years and is planning to restart with his team in 8 weeks. His parents have requested a conditioning program because of an overall decrease in exercise/activity after the diagnosis. The patient had and used heel orthotics during track only and reports that he has been symptom free since he quit track.

- Posture: Within normal limits (WNL)
- Upper extremity screen: WNL
- Bilateral lower extremity active ROM: WNL, except bilateral hamstring length 60 degrees
- Bilateral lower extremity strength: 5/5
- The physical therapy plan of care includes therapeutic exercises, aerobic conditioning, and patient education.

1. Outline an appropriate training program for this patient for the first week after the evaluation.
2. List the criteria the assistant should use to progress or modify the exercise program.
3. What education should be provided to the patient?

## Suggested Resources

FMS overview of the screen with photographs of each item: https://www.functionalmovement.com/files/Articles/572a_FMS_Article_NoBleed_Digital.pdf

FMS scoring grid: https://www.functionalmovement.com/files/Articles/717a_650a_FMS_ScoreSheet_V4.pdf

FMS website listing courses and certifications: https://www.functionalmovement.com/

*The 11: The Prevention Program:* https://jacobstirtonmd.com/wp-content/uploads/2019/07/The-FIFA-11-Soccer-Injury-Prevention-Program.pdf

## References


1. Tsolakis C, Douvis A, Tsigganos G, Zacharogiannis E, Smirniotou A. Acute effects of stretching on flexibility, power and sport specific performance in fencers. *J Hum Kinet.* 2010;(26):105-114. doi:10.2478/v10078-010-0054-x
2. Beedle BB, Leydig SN, Carnucci JM. No difference in pre- and postexercise stretching on flexibility. *J Strength Cond Res.* 2007;21(3):780-783. doi:10.1519/R-20736.1
3. O'Sullivan K, Murray E, Sainsbury D. The effect of warm-up, static stretching and dynamic stretching on hamstring flexibility in previously injured subjects. *BMC Musculoskelet Disord.* 2009;10:37. doi:10.1186/1471-2474-10-37
4. Witvrouw E, Mahieu N, Danneels L, McNair P. Stretching and injury prevention: an obscure relationship. *Sports Med.* 2004;34(7):443-449. doi:10.2165/00007256-200434070-00003
5. Peck E, Chomko G, Gaz DV, Farrell AM. The effects of stretching on performance. *Curr Sports Med Rep.* 2014;13(3):179-185. doi:10.1249/JSR.0000000000000052
6. James LP, Beckman E, Kelly VG. The impact of prehabilitation on the development of strength and power in a block periodised training plan. *J Aust Strength Cond.* 2014;22(1):5-16.
7. Wynter-Blyth V, Moorthy K. Prehabilitation: preparing patients for surgery. *BMJ.* 2017;358:j3702. doi:10.1136/bmj.j3702
8. Monajati A, Larumbe-Zabala E, Gross-Sampson M, Nacierio F. The effectiveness of injury prevention programs to modify risk factors for non-contact anterior cruciate ligament and hamstring injuries in uninjured team sports athletes: a systematic review. *PLoS One.* 2016;11(5):e0155272. doi:10.1371/journal.pone.0155272
9. Sugimoto D, Alentorn-Geli E, Mendiguchía J, Samuelsson K, Karlsson J, Myer GD. Biomechanical and neuromuscular characteristics of male athletes: implications for the development of anterior cruciate ligament injury prevention programs. *Sports Med.* 2015;45(6):809-822. doi:10.1007/s40279-015-0311-1
10. Meir R, Diesel W, Archer E. Developing a prehabilitation program in a collision sport: a model developed within English premiership rugby union football. *Strength Cond J.* 2007;29(3):50-62.
11. Al Attar WSA, Soomro N, Pappas E, Sinclair PJ, Sanders RH. Adding a post-training FIFFA 11+ exercise program to the pre-training FIFFA 11+ injury prevention program reducing injury rates among male amateur soccer players: a cluster randomized trial. *J Physiother.* 2017;63:235-242.
12. Michaelidis M, Koumantakis GA. Effects of knee injury primary prevention programs on anterior cruciate ligament injury rates in female athletes in different sports: a systematic review. *Phys Ther Sport.* 2014;15(3):200-210. doi:10.1016/j.ptsp.2013.12.002
13. Sugimoto D, Myer GD, Barber Foss KD, Pepin MJ, Micheli LJ, Hewett TE. Critical components of neuromuscular training to reduce ACL injury risk in female athletes: meta-regression analysis. *Br J Sports Med.* 2016;50(20):1259-1266. doi:10.1136/bjsports-2015-095596
14. Petushek EJ, Sugimoto D, Stoolmiller M, Smith G, Myer GD. Evidence-based best-practice guidelines for preventing anterior cruciate ligament injuries in young female athletes: a systematic review and meta-analysis. *Am J Sports Med.* 2019;47(7):1744-1753. doi:10.1177/0363546518782460
15. Orser KS. Review of the literature: the effectiveness of the functional movement screen at predicting injuries in athletes aged 18-35 years old. *J Aust Strength Cond.* 2018;26(1):44-48.
16. Cook G, Burton L, Hoogenboom BJ, Voight M. Functional movement screening: the use of fundamental movements as an assessment of function-part 1. *Int J Sports Phys Ther.* 2014;9(3):396-409.

17. Cook G, Burton L, Hoogenboom BJ, Voight M. Functional movement screening: the use of fundamental movements as an assessment of function-part 2. *Int J Sports Phys Ther.* 2014;9(4):549-563.
18. Swindell HW, Marcille ML, Trofa DP, et al. An analysis of sports specialization in NCAA division I collegiate athletics. *Orthop J Sports Med.* 2019;7(1):2325967118821179. doi:10.1177/2325967118821179
19. Bell D, Post E, Biese K, Bay C, Valovich McLeod T. Sport specialization and risk of overuse injuries: a systematic review with meta-analysis. *Pediatrics.* 2018;142(3):e20180657. doi:10.1542/peds.2018-0657
20. Jayanthi N, Pinkham C, Dugas L, Patrick B, Labella C. Sports specialization in young athletes: evidence-based recommendations. *Sports Health.* 2013;5(3):251-257. doi:10.1177/1941738112464626
21. Post EG, Trigsted SM, Riekena JW, et al. The association of sport specialization and training volume with injury history in youth athletes. *Am J Sports Med.* 2017;45(6):1405-1412. doi:10.1177/0363546517690848
22. Brenner J; Council on Sports Medicine and Fitness. Sports specialization and intensive training in young athletes. *Pediatrics.* 2016;138(3):e20162148. doi:10.1542/peds.2016-2148
23. Drezner JA, O'Connor FG, Harmon KG, et al. AMSSM MSSM position statement on cardiovascular preparticipation screening in athletes: current evidence, knowledge gaps, recommendations and future. *Br J Sports Med.* 2017;51(3):153-167. doi:10.1136/bjsports-2016-096781
24. Mirabelli M, Singh J, Mendoza M. The preparticipation sports evaluation. *Am Fam Physician.* 2015;92(5):371-376.
25. McCrory P, Meeuwisse W, Dvorak J, et al. Consensus statement on concussion in sport-the 5th international conference on concussion in sport held in Berlin, October 2016. *Br J Sports Med.* 2017;51(11):838-847.
26. Halstead ME, Walter KD, Moffatt K; Council on Sports Medicine and Fitness. Sport-related concussion in children and adolescents. *Pediatrics.* 2018;142(6):e20183074. doi:10.1542/peds.2018-3074
27. Mucha A, Cara Troutman-Enseki C. Clinical summary on concussions. *PT Now.* February 8, 2023. Accessed November 26, 2018. https://www.ptnow.org/clinical-summaries-detail/concussion-3
28. NCAA Sport Science Institute Interassociation consensus: diagnosis and management of sport related concussion best practices. Accessed October 14, 2018. https://www.ncaa.org/sports/2016/7/20/concussion-safety-protocol-management.aspx
29. Grool AM, Aglipay M, Momoli F, et al. Association between early participation following acute concussion and persistent postconcussive symptoms in children and adolescents. *JAMA.* 2016;316(23):2504-2514. doi:10.1001/jama.2016.17396
30. May KH, Marshall DL, Burns TG, Popoli DM, Polikandriotis JA. Pediatric sports specific return to play guidelines following concussion. *Int J Sports Phys Ther.* 2014;9(2):242-255.
31. Casa DJ, Csillan D; Inter-Association Task Force for Preseason Secondary School Athletics Participants. Preseason heat-acclimatization guidelines for secondary school athletics. *J Athl Train.* 2009;44(3):332-333. doi:10.4085/1062-6050-44.3.332
32. Sawka MN, Périard JD, Racinais S. Heat acclimatization to improve athletic performance in warm-hot environments. *Sport Sci Exchange.* 2015;(28)153:1-6. Accessed February8, 2023. https://www.gssiweb.org/sports-science-exchange/article/sse-153-heat-acclimatization-to-improve-athletic-performance-in-warm-hot-environments
33. Asplund CA, O'Connor FG. Challenging return to play decisions: heat stroke, exertional rhabdomyolysis, and exertional collapse associated with sickle cell trait. *Sports Health.* 2015;8(2):117-125. doi:10.1177/19417381156174
34. O'Connor FG, Heled Y, Deuster PA. Exertional heat stroke, the return to play decision, and the role of heat tolerance testing: a clinician's dilemma. *Curr Sports Med Rep.* 2018;17(7):244-248. doi:10.1249/JSR.0000000000000502
35. Casa DJ, DeMartini JK, Bergeron MF, et al. National Athletic Trainers' Association Position Statement: Exertional Heat Illnesses [published correction appears in J Athl Train. 2017 Apr;52(4):401]. *J Athl Train.* 2015;50(9):986-1000. doi:10.4085/1062-6050-50.9.07
36. O'Connor FG, Casa DJ, Bergeron MF, et al. American College of Sports Medicine roundtable on exertional heat stroke—return to duty/return to play: Conference proceedings. *Curr Sports Med Rep.* 2010;9(5):314-321.
37. Furman J. When exercise causes exertional rhabdomyolysis. *JAAPA.* 2015;28(4):38-43. doi:1097/01.JAA.0000458861.78559.3b
38. O'Connor FG, Brennan FH Jr, Campbell W, Heled Y, Deuster P. Return to physical activity after exertional rhabdomyolysis. *Curr Sports Med Rep.* 2008;7(6):328-331. doi:10.1249/JSR.0b013e31818f0317
39. Tietze DC, Borchers J. Exertional rhabdomyolysis in the athlete: a clinical review. *Sports Health.* 2014;6(4):336-339. doi:10.1177/1941738114523544

# Glossary

## A

**Active cycle of breathing** is a combined breathing and cough technique used to remove secretions.

**Active insufficiency** occurs when a multijoint muscle is unable to continue developing tension when contracting across more than one joint simultaneously.

**Adhesive capsulitis** is characterized by a progressive loss of both active and passive shoulder mobility.

**Adventitious breath sounds** are abnormal breath sounds.

**Aerobic or cardiorespiratory endurance** is the ability of the circulatory and pulmonary systems to provide oxygen during sustained physical activity.

**Allograft** uses tissue taken from another donor (commonly a cadaver) to replace a damaged tissue in a patient.

**Amputee mobility predictor** is an outcome measure that assesses mobility and functional capability for people with unilateral lower-limb amputations.

**Anemia** is defined as a low number of red blood cells.

**Arthritic diseases** (including osteoarthritis and rheumatoid arthritis) cause joint pain and deformity.

**Arthrodesis** is the fusing of a joint to stabilize a joint that is lax or unstable.

**Arthroplasty** is a joint replacement that uses one or more implant (ie, partial/hemiarthroplasty replacing one joint surface or total arthroplasty replacing both joint surfaces).

**Autogenic inhibition** describes the protective relaxation of a muscle, which results from Golgi tendon organ activation in response to a high-tension contraction.

**Autograft** uses tissue taken from one part of a patient's body to replace damaged tissue elsewhere in the body.

**Axillary web syndrome** is a condition that develops in the axilla when the soft tissue in the area becomes cord or rope-like, resulting in pain and decreased shoulder mobility.

## B

**Balance** is the ability to maintain one's center of mass over a base of support.

**Ballistic stretching** is a quick (high intensity) repetitive bouncing movement that is completed in an attempt to increase flexibility.



Kopack JK, Cascardi KA.
*Principles of Therapeutic Exercise for the Physical Therapist Assistant* (pp 735-740).

**Bankart lesion** is an avulsion of the anterior-inferior glenoid labrum; it may include an inferior glenohumeral ligament tear and/or bony damage to the inferior aspect of the glenoid fossa.

**Benign paroxysmal positional vertigo** is the most common cause of vertigo, which gives a patient a false sensation of spinning or moving; pathologic nystagmus can be observed.

**Body functions** are the physiologic functions of the various body systems.

**Body structures** are anatomical parts such as organs, limbs and their components.

**Buoyancy** is the power of a fluid to exert an upward force on a body placed in it.

## C

**Capsular patterns** are joint-specific patterns of restriction associated with a loss of passive motion.

**Cardiac rehabilitation** is a formal, coordinated intervention focused on decreasing the morbidity and mortality associated with cardiac diseases/procedures.

**Carpal tunnel syndrome** is compression of the median nerve at the wrist, where it passes through a narrow space between the carpal bones and transverse ligament.

**Chest physical therapy** uses cupping/percussion, vibratory manual techniques, and postural drainage positioning to mobilize secretions and improve ventilation.

**Chondromalacia patella** is a softening and deterioration of the articular cartilage on the posterior surface of the patella, which may be associated with patellofemoral pain syndrome.

**Chronic kidney disease** is a progressive deterioration of kidney function, which decreases the body's ability to filter out toxins and maintain fluid and electrolyte balance.

**Chronic liver disease** is a progressive deterioration of liver function often caused by chronic inflammation (hepatitis) or alcohol abuse.

**Closed kinetic chain exercises** are exercises performed when the distal segment of a limb is fixed.

**Closed-pack position** is the position where joint surfaces are most congruent and the joint is most stable.

**Cluster tests** are a group of special tests that are used to rule in or rule out musculoskeletal diagnoses. Current research supports the use of a selected group of tests vs a single test to more reliably diagnosis a pathology.

**Compensatory training** includes task training that occurs in an effort to use substitution for loss of motor ability.

**Complete decongestive therapy** is the gold standard for treatment of lymphedema. It includes manual lymphatic drainage, skin care, compression therapy, and exercise.

**Concentric contraction** occurs when the muscle's origin and insertion move closer together as the muscle shortens.

**Continence** is the ability to control one's bladder and bowel function.

**Contractures** are an adaptive shortening of muscles and soft tissue at a joint resulting in a loss of motion.

**Counternutation** occurs when the base of the sacrum tilts in a posterior and superior direction, and the coccyx moves anteriorly as the ilium rotates anteriorly.

**Critical illness myopathy** is the most common cause of neuromuscular weakness in the intensive care setting.

## D

**Delayed-onset muscle soreness** occurs when exercise intensity is increased too aggressively; signs and symptoms include severe soreness, localized tenderness or pain and decreased range of motion (ROM).

**Density** determines whether an object will float or sink. Objects that are denser than water will sink, whereas lighter objects will float.

**Diabetes mellitus** is a metabolic disorder characterized by elevated blood glucose levels.

**Diaphragmatic breathing** is an energy efficient breathing pattern where air moves into the lungs as the diaphragm contracts.

**Diastasis recti** is the separation of the rectus abdominis at the linea alba, which may occur during pregnancy.

**Directional preference** is a motion in a specific direction that reduces radicular pain (or peripheralization) and centralizes symptoms.

**Dive reflex** is a decrease in cardiac workload resulting from the effect of buoyancy and the cooling effect of the water during immersion.

**Drag force** is the resistance to motion that occurs in water.

**Dynamic posture** is the ability to maintain appropriate alignment of the body while in motion.

## E

**Eccentric contraction** is a contraction that occurs during controlled lengthening of a muscle, when the origin and insertion move away from each other.

**Epley maneuver or canal repositioning techniques** are treatment interventions commonly used to treat benign paroxysmal positional vertigo for anterior and posterior canalithiasis.

**Ergonomics** is an applied science that involves designing and/or organizing areas in a workplace to improve worker efficiency and safety.

**Evidence-based practice** is the integration of best available research, clinical expertise, and patient information in the development of treatment plans.

**Exertional heat stroke** is associated with strenuous exercise and excessive heat exposure; it presents with an elevated core temperature greater than 104 °F (or 40 °C); it causes central nervous system changes, tissue damage and organ failure.

**Exertional rhabdomyolysis** is associated with a breakdown of striated muscle tissue due to insult or injury most commonly caused by intense, repetitive, and/or prolonged exercise.

**Extrinsic (augmented) feedback** is applied or given by an external source.

## F

**FITT (frequency, intensity, time, and type) principle** includes treatment parameters, elements or variables that include frequency, intensity, time, and type.

**Flexibility** is the ability of periarticular soft tissue and muscle lengthening to allow a joint (or series of joints) to move in an unrestricted, pain-free ROM.[3,4,5]

**FOOSH (falling on an outstretched hand)** means falling on an outstretched hand. This is a common mechanism of injury that can result in an upper extremity injury.

**Fracture** is defined as a disruption in bone continuity.

**Functional capacity evaluation** includes a battery of performance-based tests that are used to determine the patient's capacity to work.

**Functional incontinence** is incontinence due to the inability to access the toilet in timely manner.

**Function-induced recovery** occurs as a result of practicing a task, due to CNS adaptation following a brain insult.

## G

**Gait cycle** is the period from ipsilateral heel strike to ipsilateral heel strike.

**Global muscles** are larger, superficial muscles that cross many vertebral segments and generate movement (ie, erector spinae).

**Graded exercise tests** are used to assist with detecting heart disease, to predict patient response/risk and maximal exercise intensity, and to assist with monitoring a patient's response to an exercise program.

## H

**Herniated disk (protrusion)** occurs when the nucleus pulposus pushes outward (commonly posteriorly) but does not completely rupture the annulus.

**Hill-Sachs lesion** is a compression fracture type of defect (or indentation) of the posterolateral humeral head commonly caused by a humeral head dislocation.

**Human movement system** represents the integration of the various bodily systems (cardiovascular, pulmonary, endocrine, integumentary, nervous, and musculoskeletal) as they generate and maintain movement and function.

**Hydrostatic pressure** is the pressure exerted on a person's body by the water surrounding it.

## I

**Impairment** is a problem with a body structure or function.

***International Classification Functioning, Disability and Health* model** is a biopsychosocial model that reflects the biological, social and individual factors that impact a patient's ability to function in society.

**Intrinsic feedback** is feedback that occurs within the patient/learner.

**Isokinetic exercise** occurs when the speed or velocity is fixed, regardless of the amount of force applied to overcome the resistance. The amount of muscle force generated can vary depending on joint position and the patient's ability to meet the speed/velocity.

**Isometric contractions** produce tension in a muscle without joint motion occurring.

**Isotonic or dynamic contractions** include concentric and eccentric contractions; the tension generated by a muscle varies as the joint angle changes.

## J

**Joint position sense** is the ability of an individual to accurately return to a neutral head posture following the performance of specific active cervical motions.

## K

**Knowledge of performance** is feedback regarding the components of task performance.

**Knowledge of results** is feedback about the outcome of a motor task.

**Kyphosis** is an exaggerated flexed curvature of the thoracic spine.

## L

**Lateral epicondylalgia** also known as *tennis elbow*. Pain is present at the attachment of the common wrist extensor tendons.

**Limb advancement** is the phase of the gait cycle where the leg is advancing; it includes pre-swing, initial swing, mid-swing, and terminal swing.

**Limit of stability** is the maximal sway angle from a vertical position in any given direction that can be achieved without loss of balance or sudden change in base of support.

**Local muscles** are small deep/intrinsic muscles that attach directly or via a fascia attachment to the lumbar vertebrae, providing intervertebral segmental stability (ie, transverse abdominis, multifidus).

**Lordosis** is an exaggerated anterior curvature of the spine that is most commonly seen in the cervical or lumbar spine.

**Lumbar neutral spine position** is a position of the lumbar spine that is midway between extreme lordosis and a flat back posture.

**Lumbopelvic rhythm** is the coordinated activity or movement of the lumbar spine and pelvis in the sagittal plane in the open kinetic chain.

## M

**Manual lymphatic drainage** is a manual technique that stimulates the lymphatic system to transport lymph fluid more effectively.

**Mechanical Diagnosis and Therapy** is a classification-based musculoskeletal examination and intervention system that classifies patients into treatment categories based upon the patient's response to repeated end range and sustained movement testing.

**Mechanism of injury** is the description of how an injury occurs.

**Medial epicondylalgia** also known as *golfer's* or *Little League elbow.* Pain is present at the attachment of the common wrist flexor tendons.

**Metabolic equivalent task** standardizes the relative intensity of work/activity.

**Micturition** is the technical term referring the physiologic process of urination, including all reflexive activity.

**Motor learning** involves both skill acquisition and retention through repetitive practice. There are 3 stages of motor learning: cognitive, associative, and autonomous.

**Motor performance** is the patient's ability to perform a task or skill.

**Movement system–based approach** examines a patient's motor control, coordination, and movement quality, as well as considering the patient's strength, ROM, medical diagnosis, and special test results. These data are used to create an impairment-based diagnosis.

**Muscle endurance** is the ability of the muscle to repeatedly contract over a period of time.

## N

**Neuroplasticity** is the brain's ability to form and reorganize nerve cell connections in the remaining/undamaged areas of the brain.

**Nutation** occurs when the base of the sacrum moves/tilts in an anterior and inferior direction, and the coccyx moves posteriorly as the ilium rotates posteriorly.

## O

**Open kinetic chain exercises** are exercises performed when the distal segment of a limb is moving freely.

**Open-packed position** is the position where the joint structures are least congruent allowing the greatest amount of joint play.

**Osteoporosis** is a progressive skeletal disease that causes decreases in bone mass, bone mineral density and bone quality.

**Overload principle** states that for muscle strength to increase, a resistance or external force must be greater than the normal stresses placed on the muscle.

## P

**Pain neuroscience education** is used to decrease a patient's perception of pain by incorporating education about the neurophysiology of pain and pain processing by the nervous system.

**Passive insufficiency** occurs when a multijoint muscle is lengthened to its maximal extent across 2 or more joints.

**Patellofemoral pain syndrome** often occurs due to activity-related repetitive knee flexion/extension, resulting in anterior knee pain.

**Pathoanatomical approach** labels musculoskeletal conditions by identifying a specific tissue pathology that is presumed to be the cause of the client's pain or dysfunction.

**Phantom limb pain** is a noxious sensation (pain) that feels as if it is coming from a body part that is no longer there.

**Phantom limb sensation** is the sensation that an amputated limb is still present.

**Physical activity** is any movement that results in a substantial increase in energy expenditure.

**Physical fitness** encompasses the characteristics that provide a person the ability to perform physical activity.

**Plyometrics** are intense, ballistic, power-generating activities often completed during sports performance.

**Positive expiratory pressure** is a technique that uses exhalation against a fixed resistance to create an increase in airway pressure.

**Postural control** is the ability to maintain one's body in a stable manner under various conditions.

**Prehabilitation** includes interventions to prepare a patient/client for surgery (or an athlete for sports activities) with a goal of maximizing performance and to minimizing injury risk.

**Preparticipation physical screens** determine general health, fitness level of the participant and detect conditions that may increase injury risk.

**Primary lymphedema** occurs as a result of congenital cause, such as a malformation or absence of lymphatic vessels.

**Protrusion/retrusion** is the action of moving the mandible anteriorly/posteriorly.

**Psychologically informed care** acknowledges the contextual factors about a patient and their pain, in addition to considering the pain and the musculoskeletal diagnosis.

**Pursed lip breathing** is a technique used to decrease a patient's sense of dyspnea.

## R

**Radiation fibrosis** is the formation of fibrotic tissue subsequent to radiation treatments, resulting in reduced tissue extensibility and joint ROM.

**Radiculopathy** are symptoms that can occur along the distribution of a specific nerve due to compression, traction, or inflammation of a spinal nerve.

**Rate of perceived exertion** is a method of measuring a person's perception of how hard they are working while performing physical activity.

**Reciprocal inhibition** describes the reflexive relaxation of an antagonist muscle when the agonist muscle contracts.

**Red flags** are observations or events that indicate that a high risk or medically significant event is evolving.

**Reference of correctness** is an internal cognitive map/plan for how the task should look for the patient.

**Referred pain** is a generalized perceived pain pattern that is generated from one anatomical source and is felt in another location (or structure) but does *not* follow a dermatomal and/or myotomal pattern.

**Regional interdependence model** is an approach that focuses on the assessment of the affected area and the surrounding regions of the body because of the relationship that is purported to exist between regions of the body.

**Rehabilitation management approach** is one of the 3 treatment options in the initial triage of a patient within the treatment-based classification approach.

**Rocabado 6 × 6** are exercises to treat temporomandibular joint disorders, which consist of 6 exercises performed for 6 repetitions, 6 times per day.

## S

**Scoliosis** is a lateral curvature of the spine, commonly affecting the thoracic and/or lumbar spines.

**Screw-home mechanism** occurs at the end of knee extension when the tibia rotates to lock the knee in order to increase joint stability.

**Secondary lymphedema** results from damage to the lymphatic system caused by trauma, infection, malignancy, surgery, or radiation.

**Segmental breathing** is used to encourage the expansion of the lung segments and address hypoventilation.

**Selective stretching** is a technique that allows for stretching of selected joints and muscles while restricting motion at other joints.

**Single-limb stance** occurs during midstance and terminal stance phases of the gait cycle, and only one foot is in contact with the floor.

**SLAP (superior labrum anterior to posterior) lesion** is a tear of the superior glenoid labrum anterior to posterior; this injury can result in shoulder instability.

**SAID (Specific Adaptation to Imposed Demands) principle** states that the body will adapt to those demands placed on it.

**Spinal stenosis** is a narrowing of the spinal canal causing pressure on the cord or nerve roots.

**Spondylolisthesis** occurs when one vertebra slips forward on the vertebra below (most commonly occurs at L5-S1).

**Spondylolysis** is a fracture of the pars interarticularis.

**Spondylosis** is a degenerative process that affects the facet joints and vertebral disks.

**Sports prehabilitation** are exercise programs created using knowledge of common injuries associated with each sport to reduce injury risk.

**Sports specialization** is participation and training for only one sport, often times year round.

**Spasticity** is a condition characterized by muscle tightness due to increased involuntary muscle tone paired with a velocity-dependent resistance to ROM.

**Sprain** is an injury to ligaments.

**Stacked breathing** is used with patients with atelectasis, hypoventilation, or an ineffective cough to improve thorax mobility and increase depth of breaths.

**Static posture** is the ability to maintain the body and its segments at rest.

**Static stretching** occurs when a muscle is placed on a stretch and that position is held for a predetermined amount of time.

**Strain** is an injury to tendons and/or muscles.

**Strength, resistance, and weight training** is a physical conditioning program that uses isometric, isotonic, or isokinetic exercises to strengthen muscles.

**Stress incontinence** is characterized by leakage of urine; this often occurs with exercise or laughter.

**Stretch reflex** is a reflexive contraction in response to a quick stretch.

**Stretching** is the process of a muscle/muscle group elongation beyond the patient's available ROM.

**Subacromial impingement** refers to shoulder pain that arises from an impingement of the supraspinatus tendon, subacromial bursa, and/or long head of the biceps brachii tendon situated below the acromion process (subacromial space).

**Substitution patterns or compensation** are altered movement patterns or use of other muscles to assist those muscles that are normally responsible for creating a desired motion.

**Synergy pattern** is a primitive pattern of movement that interferes with normal coordinated motions.

## T

**Tendinopathy** is a broad term used to describe tendon-associated conditions.

**Therapeutic exercise** is the performance of specific physical motions to improve or prevent impairments, enhance functional ability, reduce risk of disease, or improve overall health, fitness, and well-being.

**Thoracic outlet syndrome** is an irritation or compression to the brachial plexus and/or vascular structures. The thoracic outlet area lies between the cervical spine and the upper chest region.

**Transfemoral amputation** is a limb amputation at the level of the femur.

**Transtibial amputation** is a limb amputation at the level of the tibia.

**Treatment-based classification** categorizes a patient based on their clinical presentation into a classification where the patient is most likely to respond favorably.

## U

**Unhappy/terrible triad** is an injury that occurs to the anterior cruciate ligament, medial meniscus, and medial collateral ligament.

**Urge incontinence** is bladder incontinence that is characterized by a sudden, strong urge to urinate and loss of control related to when urination occurs.

## V

**Ventilatory or respiratory muscle training** are interventions to improve the function of respiratory muscles by using specific exercises.

**Vertigo** typically presents with nystagmus and dizziness that is associated with positional changes of the head.

**Viscosity** is the resistance of a fluid to flow or motion.

**Volkmann ischemic contracture** is a vascular complication that can result from an elbow fracture, and presents with limb positioning in elbow flexion, forearm pronation, wrist flexion, and metacarpophalangeal joint extension. This is a red flag item.

## W

**Weight acceptance** occurs as body weight transfers onto a limb during initial contact (heel strike) and loading response (foot flat).

**Windlass mechanism** occurs during the pre-swing (heel off) phase of gait; the plantar fascia shortens the distance between the calcaneus and metatarsals and elevates the medial longitudinal arch.

**Work conditioning** is a work-related, goal-oriented treatment program designed to restore an individual's function.

**Work hardening** is a multidisciplinary, structured, and individualized program using work-simulated or real work activities to rehabilitate a patient.

**Work rehabilitation program** includes return-to-work strategies to assist workers with their transition back to work as early and safely as possible following injury.

## Y

**Yellow flags** are psychological, social, or environmental risk factors that (if present) may prolong disability, or result in pain becoming more chronic in nature.

Appendix A

# Therapeutic Exercise/ Orthopedic Progressions



Kopack JK, Cascardi KA.
*Principles of Therapeutic Exercise for the Physical Therapist Assistant* (pp 741-742).

Therapeutic exercise/orthopedic progressions Diagnosis:______________________________

Common structure(s) injured: ______________________________

Common structure(s) that are tight? ______________________________ *Consider stretching options.*

Common structure(s) that are stretched? ______________________________ *Consider strengthening options.*

Common structure(s) that are weak? ______________________________ *Consider strengthening options.*

Review PT evaluation (screening for reasons to modify your selection of exercise).

Are there other areas of weakness in the joints above/below that may be contributing to symptoms (sx)/presentation? ____________________

Are there other areas of tightness in the joints above/below that may be contributing to sx/presentation? ____________________

| Phase | |
|---|---|
| Acute Phase | • Exercise focus:<br>• Most appropriate exercises:<br>• Precautions/considerations: |
| Subacute Phase | • Exercise focus:<br>• Most appropriate exercises:<br>• Precautions/considerations: |
| Return-to-Function Phase | • Exercise focus:<br>• Most appropriate exercises:<br>• Precautions/considerations: |

Appendix B

# Treatment Plan Development Guide



Kopack JK, Cascardi KA.
*Principles of Therapeutic Exercise for the Physical Therapist Assistant* (pp 743-744).

Patient diagnosis: ____________ Treatment focus based on diagnosis: ____________

Pertinent comorbidities: ____________

Contraindication/precautions to review for: ____________

Problem list: ____________

| Problem | PT STG | Treatment Ideas | Rationale |
|---|---|---|---|
| | → | • <br>• <br>• | → <br>→ <br>→ |
| | → | • <br>• <br>• | → <br>→ <br>→ |
| | → | • <br>• <br>• | → <br>→ <br>→ |
| | → | • <br>• <br>• | → <br>→ <br>→ |
| | → | • <br>• <br>• | → <br>→ <br>→ |
| | → | • <br>• <br>• | → <br>→ <br>→ |

Verify:

- Are selected activities included in the physical therapist plan of care?
- Does final treatment plan address STG? Does it account for any contraindications/precautions?
- Are activities appropriate for patient's current functional level?
    - Do activities consider patient's balance? Level of assist? Ortho issues? Communication abilities? Cognitive status?
- Did you address positioning needs?
- Did you address education? (Patient, caregiver, or family [caregiver] instruction?)

# Appendix C
# Sample Exercise Prescription

The clinician can use an exercise prescription to increase the perceived importance of the recommendations for the patient.

This type of form is used as a master tracking form, allowing the physical therapist assistant to list categories and tasks in one place for the patient. This allows the patient and therapist to determine which exercise types are a priority and to consider how to schedule for best compliance. The therapist can supply the patient with diagrams to reference as they complete the recommended exercises in each category.



Kopack JK, Cascardi KA.
*Principles of Therapeutic Exercise for the Physical Therapist Assistant* (pp 745-746).

Rx

Name: ____________________

Date: ____________________

Prescribing Therapist: ____________ Phone: ____________

| | Monday | Tuesday | Wednesday | Thursday | Friday | Saturday | Sunday |
|---|---|---|---|---|---|---|---|
| Aerobic exercise<br>Type: ______<br>Frequency: ______<br>Intensity: ______<br>Time: ______ | | | | | | | |
| Strengthening<br>Refer to diagrams issued by physical therapist<br>Frequency: ______<br>Intensity/Resistance: ______<br>Flexibility<br>Refer to diagrams issued by physical therapist<br>Frequency: ______<br>Reps: ______<br>Hold Time: ______ | | | | | | | |
| Balance<br>Refer to diagrams issued by physical therapist<br>Frequency: ______<br>Time: ______ | | | | | | | |

If you have any questions regarding your exercise prescription, please ask your physical therapist.

If you have pain that occurs during exercise, stop exercise and contact your physical therapist.

If you experience chest pain, left arm or jaw pain, dizziness, or severe shortness of breath, please stop exercise and call 911.

## Appendix D

# Student Worksheet

## Home Exercise Program Prescription

Student learner study suggestion: use the following grid to practice recording recommended parameters for persons with a medical diagnosis (ie, a patient with Parkinson disease or multiple sclerosis).

Clinician tips:

- Create a reasonable program; do not overload the patient!
- Select exercises that *best* address the priority issues and that the patient is able to complete using proper form without cues.
- Provide clear instruction before issuing program, demonstrate, and request return demonstration of all exercises before issuing.
- Provide pictures or video links to specific exercises whenever possible.
- Follow up with the patient each session to review home exercise program performance and encourage compliance.
- Provide positive reinforcement.
- Initiate home exercise program early in the rehab process; the longer a patient completes this regularly, the more likely it is to become a habit.



Kopack JK, Cascardi KA.
*Principles of Therapeutic Exercise for the Physical Therapist Assistant* (pp 747-748).

# Personalized Exercise/Training Plan

Patient name: ______________________________

Date: ______________________________

| Type of Exercise | Frequency | Intensity | Type/Mode Specific Exercise/Joint | Time | Progress When ... |
|---|---|---|---|---|---|
| *Postural Exercise* | | | | | |
| *Range of Motion* | | | | | |
| *Stretching* | | | | | |
| *Strengthening* | | | | | |
| *Aerobic* | | | | | |
| *Balance* | | | | | |

Complete exercises as prescribed by your therapist. If you have any questions regarding the exercises, contact your therapist ____________________ at ____________________.

If you experience new onset of pain with any of the exercises, stop the activity and contact your therapist.

If you experience chest pain, nausea, dizziness, or left arm or jaw pain, stop the exercise immediately. If the pain does not go away, call 911.

# Appendix E

# Common Indications



Kopack JK, Cascardi KA.
*Principles of Therapeutic Exercise for the Physical Therapist Assistant* (pp 749-758).

## Common Medications: Indications for Use, Adverse Side Effects, and Appropriate Physical Therapist Assistant Monitoring/Action[1-5]

| Medication Class/ Examples* | Indication for Use | The Physical Therapist Assistant Monitors for Signs/Symptoms of Adverse Side Effects | Implications for the Physical Therapist Assistant | Action |
|---|---|---|---|---|
| Nonsteroidal anti-inflammatory drugs/ salicylates and nonsalicylates<br><br>COX-2 inhibitors<br>Aspirin<br>Diclofenac (Voltaren-XR, Zorvolex), ibuprofen (Motrin, Advil)<br>Indomethacin (Indocin)<br>Celecoxib (Celebrex) | Commonly used to treat muscle and joint pain, inflammation, and fever | Gastric irritation or peptic ulcer presenting with indigestion, nausea, vomiting, thoracic pain, and melena (black, tarry stools)<br>COX-2 inhibitors: Hypertension and arrhythmia | Monitor for adverse effects. Monitor vital signs. | Notify the physical therapist and physician. |
| Chondroitin | Over-the-counter supplement used to promote joint protection. Chemically similar to anticoagulant medications. | Unexplained back or shoulder pain, excessive bruising, and new episodes of bleeding | Monitor for adverse effects. | Notify the physical therapist and physician. |
| Insulin<br>Lispro (Humalog)<br>Aspart (Novolog)<br>Velosulin (for use in the insulin pump)<br>NPH (N)<br>Insulin glargine (Lantus) | Helps the cells in the body to absorb glucose and use energy | Hypoglycemia: Weakness, shakiness, nervousness, tingling around mouth, pallor, sweating, and confusion | Monitor for signs/symptoms of hypo- or hyperglycemia. Monitor blood sugar. Know when patient last injected insulin/type of insulin. | Administer glucose/sugar.<br>Notify physical therapist. |

(continued)

| Common Medications: Indications for Use, Adverse Side Effects, and Appropriate Physical Therapist Assistant Monitoring/Action[1-5] (continued) | | | | |
|---|---|---|---|---|
| Medication Class/ Examples* | Indication for Use | The Physical Therapist Assistant Monitors for Signs/Symptoms of Adverse Side Effects | Implications for the Physical Therapist Assistant | Action |
| Antiretroviral medications<br><br>Atazanavir/ATV (Reyataz)<br>Didanosine/ddl (Videx)<br>Rilpivirine/RPV (Edurant)<br>Ritonavir/RTV (Norvir)<br>Zidovudine/ZDV (Retrovir) | Stopping virus replication in the body; allow the immune system to repair itself and prevent further damage | New dyslipidemia, appetite loss, diarrhea, fatigue, high cholesterol, mood changes, nausea, and vomiting | Monitor for adverse effects. | Notify the physical therapist and physician. |
| Corticosteroids (glucocorticoids)<br><br>Hydrocortisone (A-Hydrocort, Cortef)<br>Cortisone (Cortone)<br>Prednisone (Deltasone, Rayos)<br>Dexamethasone (Decadron, DexPak, Ozurdex)<br>Prednisolone (Flo-Pred, Pediapred, Orapred, Omnipred)<br>Methylprednisolone (Medrol)<br>*Study hint: Common suffix: -sone or -olone* | Used to decrease inflammation for local or systemic conditions for immunosuppression (ie, organ transplants, CA, SLE, scleroderma, RA, and asthma)<br>*Affects carbohydrates and protein metabolism as well as immune system*<br>May be used to treat pain/swelling (associated with CA metastasis, cerebral edema, lymphedema, and nerve pain) | Increased risk of infection, new onset of proximal muscle weakness (may indicate steroid-induced myopathy), drug-induced Cushing syndrome, gastrointestinal ulcers, glaucoma, insomnia, development of osteoporosis (prolonged use), and fluid retention.<br>*Note that all steroid medications should be tapered down before discontinuation.* | Monitor for adverse effects.<br>Careful compliance with infection control procedures.<br>Monitor blood pressure.<br>If patient complains of pain (especially with long-term use), rule out fracture.<br>After steroid joint injection, limit joint weight bearing and vigorous activity × 1 to 2 days.<br>Encourage weight-bearing activities and closed chain strengthening exercises (to minimize effect of myopathy and osteoporosis).<br>Monitor vital signs and laboratory values. | Notify the physical therapist and physician if new weakness or signs/symptoms of infection. |

*(continued)*

## Common Medications: Indications for Use, Adverse Side Effects, and Appropriate Physical Therapist Assistant Monitoring/Action[1-5] (continued)

| Medication Class/ Examples* | Indication for Use | The Physical Therapist Assistant Monitors for Signs/Symptoms of Adverse Side Effects | Implications for the Physical Therapist Assistant | Action |
|---|---|---|---|---|
| Opioids/narcotic analgesics<br><br>Morphine (MS Contin)<br>Hydromorphone (Dilaudid)<br>Hydrocodone (Vicodin)<br>Methadone (Dolophine)<br>Oxycodone (OxyContin)<br>Percocet (includes acetaminophen)<br>Meperidine (Demerol) | Class of analgesics used to treat moderate to severe pain | Side effects include sedation, muscle weakness, impaired coordination, addictive, CNS depression, vertigo, HA, nervousness, euphoria, and cognitive disorders. | Schedule treatment 1 hour after medications. Treat when sedation is minimal. Implement fall precautions. | Notify the physical therapist/ physician if blunted respiratory response to exercises. |
| Skeletal muscle relaxants<br><br>Carisoprodol (Soma)<br>Cyclobenzaprine (Amrix, Flexeril)<br>Metaxalone (Skelaxin)<br>Methocarbamol (Robaxin)<br>Orphenadrine (Norgesic, Norflex, Banflex) | Commonly used to treat muscle spasm.<br>(Muscle spasms typically occur as a result of musculoskeletal injury or peripheral nerve injury [not CNS injury]). | Side effects include drowsiness, dizziness, may relax muscles in other regions of body, sedation, nausea/ vomiting, tolerance, and dependence. | May see reduced coordination. Monitor for orthostasis and falls. Maximize muscle relaxation with stretching, relaxation exercise, and modalities. | Notify the physical therapist regarding any significant change in patient symptoms or presentation. |
| Antispasticity medications<br><br>Baclofen (Lioresal)<br>Dantrolene (Dantrium)<br>Tizanidine (Zanaflex) | Commonly used to treat spasticity; increased tone due to upper motor neuron diagnoses (SCI, CVA, MS, or CP) | Side effects include drowsiness, confusion, HA, dizziness, generalized muscle weakness, ataxia, tolerance, and dependence. | If tone/spasticity is contributing to function (ie, ability to stand); may see a decline in function with the initiation of medication. Monitor for orthostasis and falls. | Notify the physical therapist/ physician regarding the patient's functional status, especially as medication amounts are adjusted. |

*(continued)*

| Common Medications: Indications for Use, Adverse Side Effects, and Appropriate Physical Therapist Assistant Monitoring/Action[1-5] (continued) | | | | |
|---|---|---|---|---|
| **Medication Class/ Examples*** | **Indication for Use** | **The Physical Therapist Assistant Monitors for Signs/Symptoms of Adverse Side Effects** | **Implications for the Physical Therapist Assistant** | **Action** |
| Diuretics<br><br>Chlorothiazide (Diuril)<br>Furosemide (Lasix)<br>Spironolactone (Aldactone) | Promote an increase in excretion of water and diminish volume in circulatory system.<br>Used to treat HTN, edema, and CHF. | Light-headedness, vertigo, weakness, restlessness, insomnia, fatigue, fluid depletion, and electrolyte imbalance | Increased urinary urgency; may increase risk of falls. Monitor vital signs. | Contact the physical therapist/physician if the patient reports dizziness, light-headedness, or arrhythmia/muscle cramps (may indicate hypokalemia). |
| Digitalis preparations<br><br>Digoxin, digitoxin (Lanoxin) | Increases force of heart contraction and slows the HR, resulting in increased ventricular filling and increased cardiac output. Used in the treatment of CHF.<br>*High toxicity (patient will have routine laboratory monitoring)* | Visual disturbances,[a] confusion, hallucinations,[a] nausea and vomiting, diarrhea, and cardiac disturbances[a] | Monitor vital signs; monitor for signs/symptoms of toxicity | Contact the physical therapist/physician immediately if cardiac disturbances or seizures. Contact the physician if HR < 60 or > 100 at rest. |
| Nitrates<br><br>Nitroglycerin (Isordil, Nitro patch, Nitrostat) | Dilate the coronary arteries. This increases the blood available to the heart muscle, decreasing oxygen demand and the workload of the heart.<br>*Medications may increase exercise and activity threshold by increasing the anginal threshold.* | HA, dizziness, and postural hypotension | Monitor vital signs, do not overtax patient, and insure that patient brings medication to every treatment session. | Contact the physical therapist/physician with any change in the patient's angina symptoms.<br><br>*(continued)* |

Common Medications: Indications for Use, Adverse Side Effects, and Appropriate Physical Therapist Assistant Monitoring/Action[1-5] (continued)

| Medication Class/ Examples* | Indication for Use | The Physical Therapist Assistant Monitors for Signs/Symptoms of Adverse Side Effects | Implications for the Physical Therapist Assistant | Action |
|---|---|---|---|---|
| Beta blockers<br>Propanolol (Inderal)<br>Atenolol (Tenormin)<br>Metoprolol (Lopressor)<br>Carteolol (Cartrol)<br>*Study hint: Common suffix: -olol (generic)* | Used to treat HTN, angina, and arrhythmia. Reduces the workload of the heart, which decreases oxygen demand of the heart.<br>Decreases HR and BP (resting and after exercise). | Fatigue, depression, excessive decrease in HR, light-headedness, and dizziness | These medications[b] inhibit (blunt) HR response to exercise/activity. HR after exercise is decreased at any exercise intensity. Use RPE with activity.<br>Do not overtax.<br>Monitor vital signs. | Contact the physical therapist/physician if the patient reports dizziness or asthmatic attacks. |
| Alpha adrenergic antagonist agents<br>Doxazosin (Cardura)<br>Prazosin (Minipress)<br>Terazosin<br>Clonidine (Catapres)<br>Methyldopa (Aldomet, Aldoril, Dopamet) | Used to treat HTN, benign prostatic and hyperplasia<br>Medications reduce peripheral vascular tone, causing vasodilation and a decrease in BP (resting and after exercise) | Orthostatic hypotension, dizziness, and palpitations | Fall risk; monitor for orthostatic hypotension. Monitor vital signs. Use RPE with activity. | Contact the physical therapist/physician with any new cardiac signs/symptoms. |
| Angiotensin-converting enzyme inhibitors<br>Enalapril (Vasotec)<br>Lisinopril (Prinivil)<br>Benazepril (Lotensin)<br>Captopril (Capoten)<br>*Study hint: Common suffix: -pril (generic)* | Used to treat HTN and CHF.<br>Medications work by decreasing peripheral vascular resistance. | Hypotension, hyperkalemia, cough, skin rash, weakness, palpitations, and fainting | Monitor vital signs; fall precautions | Contact the physician with dizziness or fainting. |

*(continued)*

| Common Medications: Indications for Use, Adverse Side Effects, and Appropriate Physical Therapist Assistant Monitoring/Action[1-5] (continued) | | | | |
|---|---|---|---|---|
| Medication Class/ Examples* | Indication for Use | The Physical Therapist Assistant Monitors for Signs/Symptoms of Adverse Side Effects | Implications for the Physical Therapist Assistant | Action |
| Calcium channel blocker<br><br>Diltiazem (Cardizem)<br>Nifedipine (Procardia)<br>Amlodipine (Norvasc)<br>Verapamil (Calan)<br>*Study hint: Common suffix: -ipine* | Used to treat HTN and angina<br>Prevents vasoconstriction and promotes vasodilation in coronary and peripheral arteries | HA, dizziness, flushing, peripheral edema, fatigue, and bradycardia | Monitor vital signs; fall precautions. Avoid modalities that produce widespread vasodilatation.<br>These drugs lower resting and exercise BP. Know reference values for the patient. Use RPE with exercise. | Contact the physical therapist/physician with new-onset dizziness. |
| Antiarrhythmics<br><br>Procainamide (Procan)<br>Propafenone (Rythmol)<br>Disopyramide (Norpace) | Used to treat abnormalities in heart rhythm | Dizziness, nausea, and visual disturbances | Monitor vital signs; fall precautions. Faintness/dizziness may be a sign of arrhythmia. | Alert the physician with new-onset dizziness or if HR rhythm changes. |
| Anticoagulants<br><br>Warfarin (Coumadin)<br>Heparin<br>Clopidogrel (Plavix)<br>Enoxaparin sodium (Lovenox) | Used to prevent blood clot formation<br>(Platelet inhibitors such as aspirin may also be used.) | Easy bruising, hemorrhage, joint/abdominal pain, difficulty breathing or swallowing, and nosebleeds | Monitor for joint/abdomen pain or difficulty breathing or swallowing and for blood in urine or stool. Be extremely cautious with wound care; fall precautions. Check PTT/INR with warfarin/heparin use. | Contact the physical therapist/physician if signs/symptoms of a bleed are present. Check laboratory values pretreatment. |

*(continued)*

**Common Medications: Indications for Use, Adverse Side Effects, and Appropriate Physical Therapist Assistant Monitoring/Action[1-5] (continued)**

| Medication Class/ Examples* | Indication for Use | The Physical Therapist Assistant Monitors for Signs/Symptoms of Adverse Side Effects | Implications for the Physical Therapist Assistant | Action |
|---|---|---|---|---|
| Benzodiazepines<br><br>Triazolam (Halcion)<br>Flurazepam (Dalmane)<br>Temazepam (Restoril)<br>Lorazepam (Ativan)<br>Oxazepam (Serax)<br>Diazepam (Valium)<br>Alprazolam (Xanax) | Used to reduce anxiety; function by sedating, relaxing muscles | Drowsiness, lethargy, confusion, and addiction may occur; may have a rebound effect when discontinued | Schedule treatment when sedation is minimal; fall precautions | Alert the physical therapist/ physician with any new onset of adverse effects. |
| Antidepressants<br><br>Amitriptyline (Elavil)<br>Nortriptyline (Pamelor)<br>Phenelzine (Nardil)<br>Sertraline (Zoloft)<br>Fluvoxamine (Luvox)<br>Paroxetine (Paxil)<br>Citalopram (Celexa)<br>Fluoxetine (Prozac)<br>Venlafaxine (Effexor) | Used to manage depression. Mechanism of action depends on the drug type (selective serotonin reuptake inhibitors [SSRIs]), serotonin-noradrenaline reuptake inhibitors, noradrenaline and specific serotonergic antidepressants, tricyclic antidepressants, and monoamine oxidase inhibitors | Tachycardia, arrhythmia, orthostatic hypotension, increased appetite, dry mouth, blurred vision, and insomnia | Monitor vital signs; fall precautions | Report to the physician any suicidal ideation or any new onset of adverse effects. |

(continued)

## Common Medications: Indications for Use, Adverse Side Effects, and Appropriate Physical Therapist Assistant Monitoring/Action[1-5] (continued)

| Medication Class/ Examples* | Indication for Use | The Physical Therapist Assistant Monitors for Signs/Symptoms of Adverse Side Effects | Implications for the Physical Therapist Assistant | Action |
|---|---|---|---|---|
| Antipsychotics<br><br>Haloperidol (Haldol)<br>Chlorpromazine (Thorazine)<br>Aripiprazole (Abilify)<br>Quetiapine (Seroquel)<br>Clozapine (Clozaril)<br>Risperidone (Risperdal)<br>Olanzapine (Zyprexa)<br>Carbamazepine (Tegretol) | Used in the treatment of psychoses, including schizophrenia | Side effects can be very serious, especially with long-term use, including dystonia, akathisia, pseudoparkinsonism, tardive dyskinesia | For patients with extrapyramidal effects, monitor for change in posture and balance; fall precautions | Notify the physician of new onset of side effects. |
| Basal ganglia dysfunction agents<br><br>Carbidopa/levodopa (Sinemet) | Used to treat Parkinson disease<br>Strict medication timing regimen required to maximize function | "On-off" phenomenon, tolerance, dystonia, choreiform movement, confusion, agitation, rigidity, behavioral changes, difficulty initiating movement, arrhythmia, and orthostatic hypotension | Fall precautions | Notify the physician of new onset of side effects. |

*List is *not* inclusive of all medications in drug class
[a]Possible toxicity
[b]Karvonen's formula not valid
BP = blood pressure; CA = cancer; CHF = congestive heart failure; CNS = central nervous system; COX-2 = cyclooxygenase-2; CP = cerebral palsy; CVA = cerebrovascular accident; HA = headache; HTN = hypertension; HR = heart rate; INR = international normalized ratio; MS = multiple sclerosis; NPH = neutral protamine hagedorn; PTT = partial thromboplastin time; RA = rheumatoid arthritis; RPE = rate of perceived exertion; SCI = spinal cord injury; SLE = systemic lupus erythematosus.

## Suggested Resource

Beers Criteria Medication List. Potentially inappropriate medication for the elderly according to the Revised Beers Criteria. https://dcri.org/beers-criteria-medication-list/

## References

1. Pescatello L, ed. *ACSM's Guidelines for Exercise Testing and Prescription*. 9th ed. Wolters Kluwer/Lippincott Williams & Wilkins; 2014.
2. Goodman C, Fuller K. *Pathology Implications for the Physical Therapist*. 4th ed. Elsevier; 2015.
3. Drugs.com. Find Drugs & Conditions. Accessed March 28, 2023. https://www.drugs.com/
4. Ciccone C. *Pharmacology in Rehabilitation*. 5th ed. FA Davis; 2015.
5. Ciccone C. *Davis's Drug Guide for Rehabilitation Professionals*. FA Davis; 2013.

Appendix F

# Dermatome Map

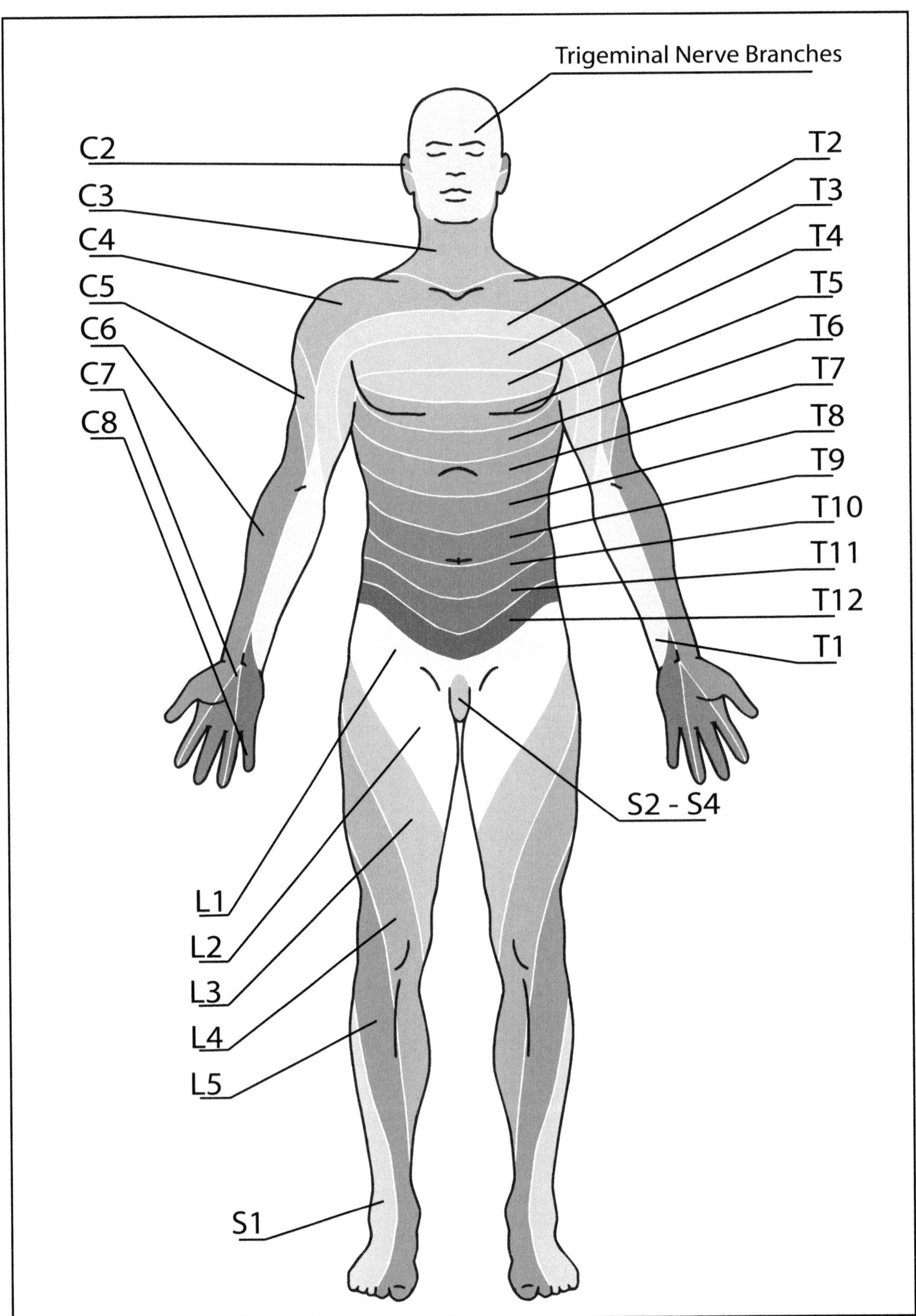


(Shutterstock.com/stihii)

# Appendix G

# Referred Pain Patterns of the Organs



Kopack JK, Cascardi KA.
*Principles of Therapeutic Exercise for the Physical Therapist Assistant* (pp 761-763).

Musculoskeletal pain is reproducible. Pain that cannot be reproduced or that does not match the patterns we expect (based on the type of tissue that was injured/is involved) may indicate that the symptoms are not musculoskeletal in nature. If in doubt, refer out. The first person the physical therapist assistant should report this information to is the supervising physical therapist.

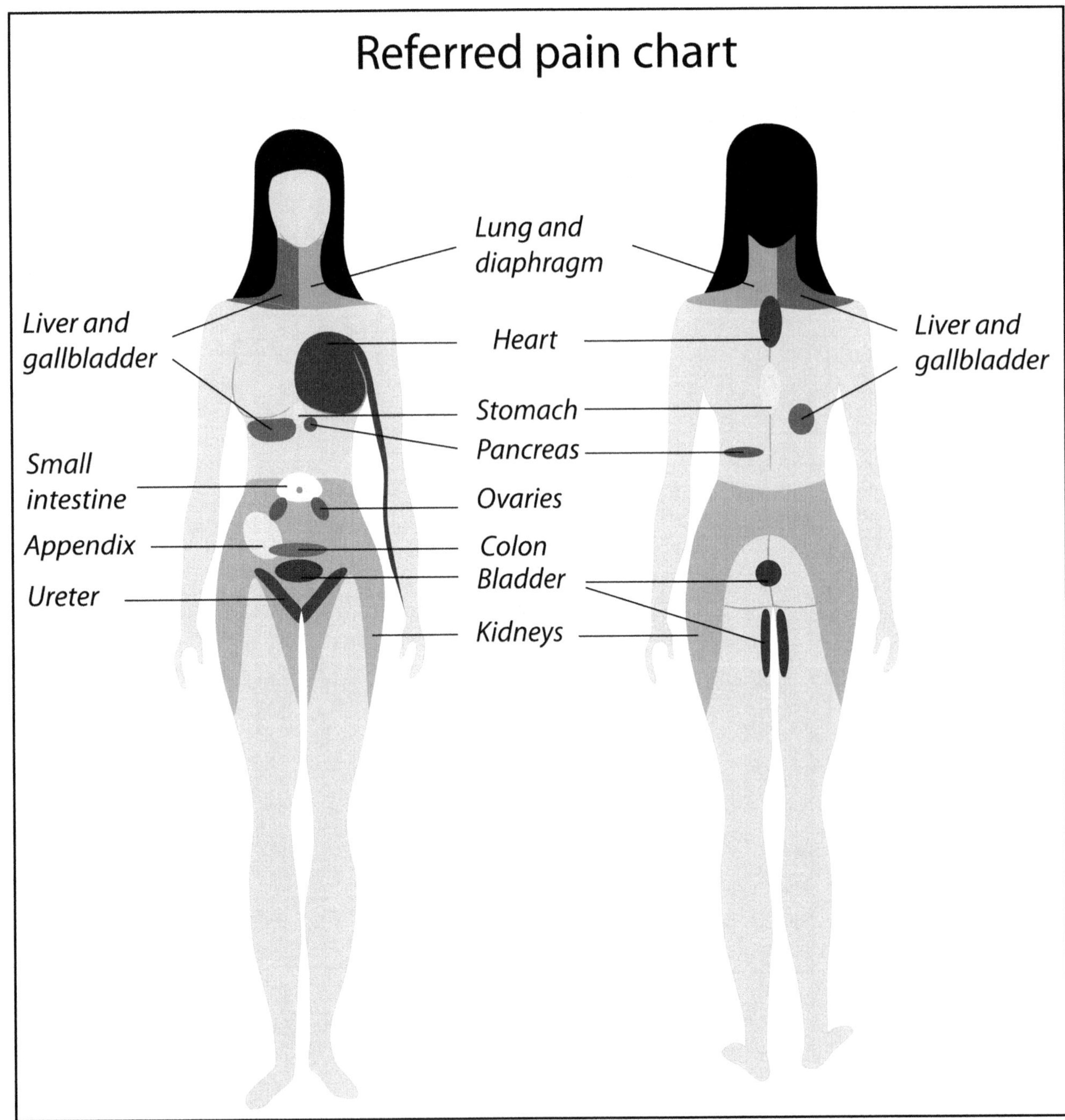


(Shutterstock.com/Alila Medical Media)

| Referred Pain Pattern/Location | Organ |
|---|---|
| Cervical spine, upper trapezius region | Diaphragm |
| Chest; left neck, jaw, or arm; midscapular region (more typical in women) | Heart |
| Thoracic spine | Lungs |
| Substernal region, upper abdominal region | Esophagus |
| Upper abdomen, thoracic spine | Stomach |
| Lower thoracic and upper lumbar spine, upper abdomen | Pancreas |
| Thoracic spine, upper abdomen | Bile duct |
| Right upper quadrant, right thoracic spine | Gallbladder |
| Right upper quadrant or right side, thoracic spine | Liver |
| Abdomen, thoracic spine | Intestines |
| Lower abdomen, sacral region | Ovaries/testicles |
| Flank, abdomen, lumbar spine | Kidney |
| Thoracic/lumbar junction, sacral region | Uterus/prostate |
| Suprapubic region, sacrum | Ureter |
| Data Source: Goodman C, Fuller K. *Pathology Implications for the Physical Therapist.* 4th ed. Elsevier; 2015 and Standring S, ed. *Gray's Anatomy.* 41st ed. Elsevier; 2015. | |

# Financial Disclosures

*Dr. Kenneth R. Amsler* reported no financial or proprietary interest in the materials presented herein.

*Dr. Karen A. Cascardi* reported no financial or proprietary interest in the materials presented herein.

*Dr. Patricia A. Crane* reported no financial or proprietary interest in the materials presented herein.

*Dr. Jacki Klaczak Kopack* reported no financial or proprietary interest in the materials presented herein.

*Dr. Kevin Kunkel* reported no financial or proprietary interest in the materials presented herein.

*John Morris* reported no financial or proprietary interest in the materials presented herein.

# Index